Sixth Edition

Motor Control

Translating Research into Clinical Practice

Sixth Edition

Motor Control

Translating Research into Clinical Practice

Anne Shumway-Cook
PT, PhD, FAPTA
Emeritus Professor
Division of Physical Therapy
Department of Rehabilitation Medicine
University of Washington
Seattle, Washington

Jaya Rachwani
PT, MS, PhD
Assistant Professor
Department of Physical Therapy
Hunter College
City University of New York
New York, New York

Marjorie H. Woollacott
MA, PhD
Emeritus Professor
Department of Human Physiology
Institute of Neuroscience
University of Oregon
Eugene, Oregon

Victor Santamaria
PT, MS, PhD, PCS
Associate Research Scientist
Robotics and Rehabilitation Lab
Mechanical Engineering Department
Columbia University
New York, New York
Lead Pediatric Physical Therapist
International Institute for the Brain
New York, New York

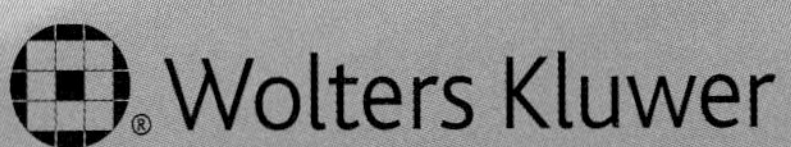

Philadelphia • Baltimore • New York • London
Buenos Aires • Hong Kong • Sydney • Tokyo

Acquisitions Editor: Matt Hauber
Development Editor: Greg Nicholl (freelance), Amy Millholen
Editorial Coordinator: Remington Fernando
Editorial Assistant: Parisa Saranj
Marketing Manager: Phyllis Hitner
Production Project Manager: Catherine Ott
Design Coordinator: Stephen Druding
Art Director: Jennifer Clements
Manufacturing Coordinator: Margie Orzech
Prepress Vendor: Lumina Datamatics

Sixth Edition, Revised Reprint

9 8 7 6 5 4 3 2 1

Printed in Singapore

Library of Congress Cataloging-in-Publication Data

978-1-9752-0956-8

Cataloging in Publication data available on request from publisher.

shop.lww.com

MKO1122

It is with great love and gratitude that we dedicate this book to the many people, including professional colleagues and patients, who have contributed to the development of the ideas presented here. We also gratefully acknowledge the divine source of our enthusiasm, wisdom, and joy. The sweet mix of inspiration and effort involved in the creation of this book was truly a delight.

Anne Shumway-Cook and Marjorie H. Woollacott

To our beloved children, Nathan and Natalie, and our parents for their unconditional love and support. To all our patients who were part of our professional journey and have been the inspirational source of much of the work included in the book.

Jaya Rachwani and Victor Santamaria

PREFACE

In recent years, there has been a growing emphasis on evidence-based clinical practice, which is characterized by the integration of the best available research with expert clinical judgment and patient preferences regarding assessment and treatment of motor control problems. However, the integration of research into clinical practice is easier said than done. The explosion of new research in the field of neuroscience and motor control has created an ever-widening gap between research and clinical practice. This book is dedicated to reducing this gap by reviewing current research in the area of motor control and exploring the translation of this research into best clinical practices.

AN OVERVIEW OF THE SIXTH EDITION

The overall framework of the sixth edition continues the legacy established from previous editions with four parts. Part I, the Theoretical Framework, reviews current theories of motor control, motor learning, and recovery of function after neurological insult. The clinical implications of various theories of motor control are discussed, as are the physiological basis of motor control and motor learning. This section also includes a suggested conceptual framework for clinical practice (Chapter 6) and a chapter on the pathophysiology of sensory, motor, and cognitive impairments affecting motor control. The first section is the foundation for the major thrust of the book, which addresses motor control issues as they relate to the control of posture and balance (Part II), mobility (Part III), and upper-extremity function (Part IV).

The chapters in each of these sections follow a standard format:

- The first chapter in each section discusses issues related to normal control processes.
- The second and third chapters describe development and age-related issues, respectively.
- The fourth chapter presents research on abnormal function.
- The final chapter in each section discusses clinical strategies related to assessment and treatment of problems in each of the three functional areas and reviews the underlying research that supports these strategies.

This book will be of use in several ways. First, we envision it as a textbook used in both undergraduate and graduate courses on normal motor control, motor development across the life span, and rehabilitation in the area of physical and occupational therapy, as well as kinesiology and exercise science. We also envision that the book will assist clinicians in staying connected to some of the research that serves as the foundation for evidence-based clinical practice. A strength of *Motor Control: Translating Research into Clinical Practice* is its summary of a broad range of research papers and the translation of this research into clinical practice. However, reading summaries cannot replace the insights that are gained by delving into the original research papers. A book by its very nature summarizes only research available before its publication; therefore, it is critical that clinicians and students alike continue to read emerging research.

Motor Control: Translating Research into Clinical Practice, sixth edition, seeks to provide a framework that will enable the clinician to incorporate current theory and research on motor control into clinical practice. More importantly, it is our hope that the book will serve as a springboard for developing new, more effective approaches to examining and treating patients with motor dyscontrol.

Changes to the Sixth Edition

As has been true for all previous editions, the sixth edition of *Motor Control* includes updated research and significant revisions to the four parts: theoretical framework, posture and balance, mobility, and upper-extremity function. The theoretical framework has been edited with the most up-to-date knowledge in Neuroscience and its clinical implications. Almost all chapters include new figures to highlight the main outcomes of critical research. In order to emphasize essential knowledge, the last chapter on upper-extremity function (Chapter 20) has been heavily revised and synthesized. We continue to have the honor of co-authoring Chapter 20 with Susan V. Duff, EdD, MPT, OT/L, CHT, associate professor at the Physical Therapy Department at Chapman University (Irvine, California).

Online Resources for Students and Faculty

Videos associated with the case studies are referred to throughout the text. The videos are included as part of the online resources and are intended to be used along with the book.

Teaching materials to accompany the sixth edition of *Motor Control* are available to faculty and include the following:

- An image bank
- PowerPoint slides
- A test bank

For more information, please see the inside front cover.

A Final Note

We are very happy to introduce Jaya Rachwani, PT, MS, PhD and Victor Santamaria PT, MS, PhD, PCS as co-authors of this sixth edition of *Motor Control: Translating Research into Clinical Practice*. Dr. Rachwani and Dr. Santamaria come to this endeavor with excellent credentials, having received their Physical Therapy degrees in Spain and having performed graduate work with Dr. Woollacott and Dr. Shumway-Cook during their PhD program at the University of Oregon in the Dept. of Human Physiology. More recently Dr. Rachwani was a postdoctoral fellow at NYU with Dr. Karen Adolph, before becoming a professor at Hunter College in Manhattan. Dr. Santamaria performed postdoctoral research with Dr. Andrew Gordon at Teachers College and is now an Associate Research Scientist at Columbia University and a Lead Pediatric Physical Therapist at the International Institute for the Brain. We have collaborated with them for many years and their research on development of postural and reaching skills in both typical children and children with cerebral palsy and in adult patients after stroke has been featured in the previous edition of this textbook. We are happy that they are now part of the writing team for our sixth edition of *Motor Control*. Welcome Dr. Rachwani and Dr. Santamaria!

Anne Shumway-Cook
Marjorie H. Woollacott

We would like to express our most sincere gratitude to Dr. Shumway-Cook and Dr. Woollacott for enlightening the clinical and research careers of many of us. Their dedication and efforts are truly admirable. Thank you for giving us the opportunity to be part of this seminal book.

Jaya Rachwani
Victor Santamaria

CONTENTS

PART I

Theoretical Framework

"*Movement is essential to our ability to walk, run, and play; to seek out and eat the food that nourishes us; to communicate with friends and family; and to earn our living—in essence to survive.*"

CHAPTER 1

Motor Control: Issues and Theories

Learning Objectives

Following completion of this chapter, the reader will be able to:

1. Define motor control and discuss its relevance to the clinical treatment of patients with movement pathology.
2. Discuss how factors related to the individual, the task, and the environment affect the organization and control of movement.
3. Define what is meant by a theory of motor control and describe the value of theory to clinical practice.
4. Compare and contrast the following theories of motor control: reflex, hierarchical, motor programming, systems, and ecological, including the individuals associated with each theory, critical elements used to explain the control of normal movement, limitations, and clinical applications.
5. Discuss the relationship between theories of motor control and the parallel development of clinical methods related to neurologic rehabilitation.
6. Compare and contrast the neurofacilitation approaches to the task-oriented approach with respect to assumptions underlying normal and abnormal movement control, recovery of function, and clinical practices related to assessment and treatment.

INTRODUCTION

What Is Motor Control?

Movement is a critical aspect of life. It is essential to our ability to walk, run, and play; to seek out and eat the food that nourishes us; to communicate with friends and family; and to earn our living—in essence to survive. The field of motor control is directed at studying the nature of movement and how movement is controlled. **Motor control** is defined as the ability to regulate or direct the mechanisms essential to movement. It addresses questions such as the following: How does the central nervous system (CNS) organize the many individual muscles and joints into coordinated functional movements? How is sensory information from the environment and the body used to select and control movement? How do our perceptions of ourselves, the tasks we perform, and the environment in which we are moving influence our movement behavior? What is the best way to study movement, and how can movement problems be quantified in patients with motor control problems?

Why Should Therapists Study Motor Control?

Physical and occupational therapists have been referred to as applied motor control physiologists (Brooks, 1986). This is because therapists spend a considerable amount of time retraining patients who have motor control problems producing functional movement disorders. Assessment and treatment of movement disorders depend on a number of factors, including knowledge of the neural basis for normal movement control and pathophysiology of impaired movement. Assessment and treatment strategies must be consistent with current knowledge regarding the neural basis for movement disorders. Therapeutic strategies are designed to improve the quality and quantity of postures and movements essential to function. Thus, understanding motor control and, specifically, the nature and control of both normal and abnormal movement is critical to clinical practice.

We will begin our study of motor control by discussing important issues related to the nature and control of movement. Next, we will explore different theories of motor control, examining their underlying assumptions and clinical implications. Finally, we will review how theories of motor control relate to past and present clinical practices.

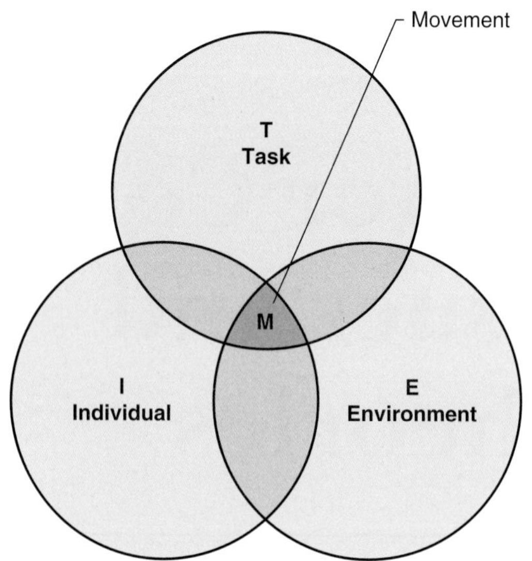

Figure 1.1 Movement ($\bar{M}$) emerges from interactions between the individual ($\bar{I}$), the task ($\bar{T}$), and the environment ($\bar{E}$).

UNDERSTANDING THE NATURE OF MOVEMENT

Movement emerges from the interaction of three factors: the individual, the task, and the environment. Movement is organized around both task and environmental demands. The individual generates movement to meet the demands of the task being performed within a specific environment. In this way, we say that the organization of movement is constrained by factors within the individual, the task, and the environment. The individual's capacity to meet interacting task and environmental demands determines that person's functional capability. Motor control research that focuses only on processes within the individual without taking into account the environment in which that individual moves or the task that they are performing will produce an incomplete picture. Thus, in this book, our discussion of motor control will focus on the interactions of the individual, the task, and the environment. Figure 1.1 illustrates this concept.

Individual Systems Underlying Motor Control

Within the individual, movement emerges through the cooperative effort of many brain structures and processes. The term "motor control" in itself is somewhat misleading, since movement arises from the interaction of multiple systems, including sensory/perceptual, cognitive, and motor/action.

Motor/Action Systems

Understanding motor control requires knowledge of how the motor systems, including both the neuromuscular and biomechanical systems, contribute to functional movement control. The body is characterized by a high number of muscles and joints, all of which must be controlled during the execution of coordinated, functional movement. There are also multiple ways a movement can be carried out (multiple equivalent solutions). This problem of choosing among equivalent solutions and then coordinating the many muscles and joints involved in a movement has been referred to as the "degrees of freedom problem" (Bernstein, 1967). It is considered a major issue being studied by motor control researchers and will be discussed in later chapters. So, the study of motor control includes the study of the motor systems that control *functional movement*.

Sensory/Perceptual Systems

Sensation and perception are essential to the control of functional movement. Perception is the integration of sensory impressions into psychologically meaningful information. Perception involves both peripheral sensory mechanisms and higher-level processing that adds interpretation and meaning to incoming afferent information. Sensory/perceptual systems provide information about the state of the body (e.g., the position of different body parts in space) and features within the environment critical to the regulation of movement. Sensory/perceptual information is clearly integral to the ability to act effectively within an environment (Rosenbaum, 1991). Thus, understanding movement requires the study of systems controlling sensation and perception and their role in functional movement control.

Cognitive Systems

Since movement is not usually performed in the absence of intent, cognitive processes are essential to motor control. In this book, we define cognitive processes broadly to include attention, planning, problem solving, motivation, and emotional aspects of motor control that underlie the establishment of intent or goals. Motor control includes perception and action systems that are organized to achieve specific goals or intents. Thus, the study of motor control must include the study of cognitive processes as they relate to perception and action.

As shown within Figure 1.2, within the individual (I), many systems interact in the production of functional movement. While each of these systems categorized as sensory/perceptual (S/P), cognitive (C), and motor/action (M/A) can be studied in isolation, we believe a true picture of the nature of motor control cannot be achieved without a synthesis of information from all three.

Task Constraints on Movement Control

In everyday life, we perform a tremendous variety of functional tasks requiring a multiplicity of movement strategies. The type of task being performed has a great impact on the neural organization of movement. For example, open movement tasks such as playing soccer or tennis require performers to adapt movement strategies to a constantly changing and often unpredictable environment. This requires a constant monitoring of sensory inputs, which are then used to update, modify, and regulate motor output. In contrast, closed movement tasks are performed in relatively fixed or predictable environments and are less dependent on the constant monitoring of sensory inputs related to environmental change. See Table 1.1 for a classification scheme for different types of movement tasks. Thus, understanding motor control requires an awareness of how tasks regulate neural mechanisms controlling movement. Figure 1.2 illustrates the three motor control tasks featured in this book.

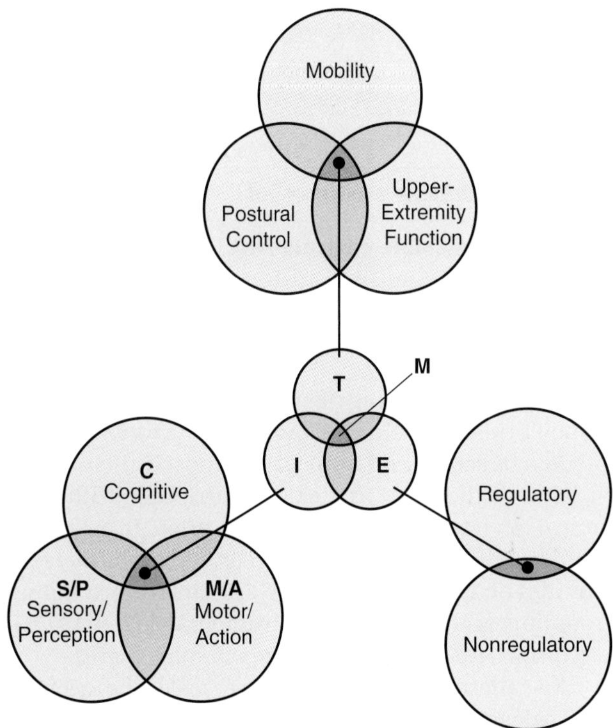

Figure 1.2 Individual ($\bar{I}$), task ($\bar{T}$), and environmental ($\bar{E}$) contributions to movement control. Within the individual, movement emerges from the interaction of sensory/perceptual ($\bar{S}/\bar{P}$), cognitive ($\bar{C}$), motor/action ($\bar{M}/\bar{A}$) systems. Environmental constraints ($\bar{E}$) on movement are divided into regulatory and nonregulatory factors. Finally, attributes of the task ($\bar{T}$) contribute to the organization of functional movement. This book focuses on the neural control of three tasks: Postural Control, Mobility, and Upper-Extremity Function.

The importance of practicing tasks in the rehabilitation of patients with movement disorders is well accepted by clinicians. However, what tasks should be practiced, in what order, and at what time, is less

TABLE 1.1 Classification Scheme for Different Types of Movement Tasks

Category of tasks	Distinguishing attribute
Discrete vs. Continuous	Discrete movement tasks, such as kicking a ball or moving from sitting to standing or lying down, have a recognizable beginning and end. In continuous movements such as walking or running, the end point of the task is not an inherent characteristic of the task but is decided arbitrarily by the performer (Schmidt, 1988b).
Closed vs. Open	Open movement tasks such as playing soccer or tennis require performers to adapt movement strategies to a constantly changing and often unpredictable environment. Closed movement tasks are performed in relatively fixed or predictable environments.
Stability vs. Mobility	Stability tasks such as sitting or standing are performed with a nonmoving base of support, while mobility tasks such as walking or running require moving the base of support.
Manipulation vs. Nonmanipulation tasks	Manipulation tasks involve movement of the upper extremities.

TABLE 1.2 A Taxonomy of Tasks Combining Stability–Mobility and Closed–Open Task Continua

	Stability (nonmoving BOS)	Mobility (moving BOS)
Closed, predictable environment	Sitting or standing on a nonmoving surface	Walking/nonmoving surface
Open, unpredictable environment	Sitting or standing on foam or a rocker board	Walking on an uneven or moving surface

BOS, Base of support.

clear. An understanding of task attributes can provide a framework for structuring tasks into a taxonomy. Tasks can then be sequenced from least to most difficult based on their relationship to a shared attribute. Within the clinical environment, tasks are most often grouped into broad functional categories, such as bed mobility tasks, activities of daily living (ADLs) (e.g., dressing, toileting, grooming, and feeding), or instrumental ADLs (IADLs) (e.g., work, housekeeping, money management).

An alternative to classifying tasks functionally is to categorize them according to a critical attribute. Table 1.2 summarizes and defines some categories of tasks. A taxonomy of tasks can provide a useful framework for assessment and treatment. It allows a therapist to identify the specific kinds of tasks that are difficult for the patient to accomplish. In addition, the set of tasks can serve as a progression for retraining functional movement in the patient with a neurologic disorder. An example of a taxonomy of tasks using two attributes—stability/mobility and environmental predictability—is shown in Table 1.2. Once the taxonomy is developed, the therapist must decide the order in which tasks will be practiced. For example, the easiest tasks to begin with are the stability tasks practiced in a closed environment. The most difficult are the mobility tasks practiced in an open environment. However, whether stability tasks in an open environment should be practiced prior to beginning to practice mobility tasks in a closed environment will depend on the patient. Lab Activity 1.1 offers you an opportunity to develop your own taxonomy of tasks and to consider the order in which you would expect to progress a patient through your taxonomy. The answers to this activity may be found at the end of this chapter.

LAB ACTIVITY 1.1

Objective: To develop your own taxonomy of movement tasks.

Procedure: Make a graph like the one illustrated in Table 1.2. Identify two categories of tasks you would like to combine. You can begin by using one or more of the categories described in Table 1.1, or alternatively you can create your own based on attributes of movement tasks we have not discussed. In our example, we combined the stability–mobility continuum with the open–closed continuum.

Assignment

1. Fill in the boxes with examples of tasks that reflect the demands of each of the continua.
2. Think about ways you could "progress" a patient through your taxonomy. What assumptions do you have about which tasks are easiest and which the hardest? Is there a "right" way to move through your taxonomy? How will you decide what tasks to use and in what order?

Environmental Constraints on Movement Control

Tasks are performed in a wide range of environments. Thus, in addition to attributes of the task, movement is also constrained by features within the environment. In order to be functional, the CNS must take into consideration attributes of the environment when planning task-specific movements. As shown in Figure 1.2, attributes of the environment that affect movement have been divided into regulatory and nonregulatory features (Gordon, 1987). Regulatory features specify aspects of the environment that shape the movement itself. Task-specific movements must conform to regulatory features of the environment in order to achieve the goal of the task. Examples of regulatory features of the environment include the size, shape, and weight of a cup to be picked up and the type of surface on which we walk (Gordon, 1997). Nonregulatory features of the environment may affect performance, but movement does not have to conform to these features. Examples of nonregulatory features of the environment include background noise and the presence of distractions.

Thus, understanding features within the environment that both regulate and affect the performance of movement tasks is essential to planning effective intervention. Preparing patients to perform in a wide variety of environments requires that we understand the features of the environment that will affect movement performance and that we adequately prepare our patients to meet the demands in different types of environments.

We have explored how the nature of movement is determined by the interaction of the individual, the task, and the environment. Thus, the movement we observe in patients is shaped not just by systems within the individual, such as sensory, motor, and cognitive impairments, but also by attributes of the task being performed and the environment in which the individual is moving. We now turn our attention to examining the control of movement from a number of different theoretical views.

THE CONTROL OF MOVEMENT: THEORIES OF MOTOR CONTROL

Theories of motor control describe viewpoints regarding how movement is controlled. A **theory of motor control** is a group of abstract ideas about the control of movement. A **theory** is a set of interconnected statements that describe unobservable structures or processes and relate them to each other and to observable events. Jules Henri Poincare (1905/2001, p. 141) said, "Science is built up of facts, as a house is built of stone; but an accumulation of facts is no more a science than a heap of stones is a house." A theory gives meaning to facts, just as a blueprint provides the structure that transforms stones into a house (Miller, 2002).

However, just as the same stones can be used to make different houses, the same facts are given different meaning and interpretation by different theories of motor control. Different theories of motor control reflect philosophically varied views about how the brain controls movement. These theories often reflect differences in opinion about the relative importance of various neural components of movement. For example, some theories stress peripheral influences; others may stress central influences, while still others may stress the role of information from the environment in controlling behavior. Thus, motor control theories are more than just an approach to explaining action. Often, they stress different aspects of the organization of the underlying neurophysiology and neuroanatomy of that action. Some theories of motor control look at the brain as a *black box* and simply study the rules by which this black box interacts with changing environments as a variety of tasks are performed. As you will see, there is no one theory of motor control that everyone accepts.

Value of Theory to Practice

Do theories really influence what therapists do with their patients? Yes! Rehabilitation practices reflect the theories, or basic ideas, we have about the cause and nature of function and dysfunction (Shepard, 1991). In general, then, the actions of therapists are based on assumptions that are derived from theories. The specific practices related to examination and intervention used with the patient who has motor dyscontrol are determined by underlying assumptions about the nature and cause of movement. Thus, motor control theory is part of the theoretical basis for clinical practice. This will be discussed in more detail in the last section of this chapter.

What are the advantages and disadvantages of using theories in clinical practice? Theories provide the following:

- A framework for interpreting behavior
- A guide for clinical action
- New ideas
- Working hypotheses for examination and intervention

Framework for Interpreting Behavior

Theory can help therapists to interpret the behavior or actions of patients with whom they work. Theory allows the therapist to go beyond the behavior of one patient and broaden the application to a much larger number of cases (Shepard, 1991).

Theories can be more or less helpful depending on their ability to predict or explain the behavior of an individual patient. When a theory and its associated assumptions do not provide an accurate interpretation of a patient's behavior, it loses its usefulness to the therapist. Thus, theories can potentially limit a therapist's ability to observe and interpret movement problems in patients.

Guide for Clinical Action

Theories provide therapists with a possible guide for action (Miller, 2002; Shepard, 1991). Clinical interventions designed to improve motor control in the patient with neurologic dysfunction are based on an understanding of the nature and cause of normal movement, as well as an understanding of the basis for abnormal movement. Therapeutic strategies aimed at retraining motor control reflect this basic understanding.

New Ideas: Dynamic and Evolving

Theories are dynamic, changing to reflect greater knowledge relating to the theory. How do these affect clinical practices related to retraining the patient with motor dyscontrol? Changing and expanding theories of motor control need not be a source of frustration to clinicians. Expanding theories can broaden and enrich the possibilities for clinical practice. New ideas related to examination and intervention will evolve to reflect new ideas about the nature and cause of movement.

Working Hypotheses for Examination and Intervention

A theory is not directly testable, since it is abstract. Rather, theories generate hypotheses, which are testable. Information gained through hypothesis testing is used to validate or invalidate a theory. This same approach is useful in clinical practice. So-called hypothesis-driven clinical practice transforms the therapist into an active problem solver (Rothstein & Echternach, 1986; Rothstein et al., 2003). Using this approach to retrain the patient with motor dyscontrol calls for the therapist to generate multiple hypotheses (explanations) for why patients move (or do not move) in ways to achieve functional independence. During the course of therapy, therapists will test various hypotheses, discard some, and generate new explanations that are more consistent with their results.

Each of the many theories that will be discussed in this chapter has made specific contributions to the field of motor control, and each has implications for clinicians retraining patients with motor dyscontrol. It is important to understand that all models are unified by the desire to understand the nature and control of movement. The difference is in the approach.

Reflex Theory

Sir Charles Sherrington, a neurophysiologist in the late 1800s and early 1900s, wrote *The Integrative Action of the Nervous System* in 1906. His research formed the experimental foundation for a classic reflex theory of motor control. The basic structure of a reflex is shown in Figure 1.3. For Sherrington, reflexes were the building blocks of complex behavior. He believed that complex behavior could be explained through the combined action of individual reflexes that were chained together (Sherrington, 1947). Sherrington's view of a reflexive basis for movement persisted unchallenged by many clinicians for 50 years, and it continues to influence thinking about motor control today.

Limitations

There are a number of limitations of a reflex theory of motor control (Rosenbaum, 1991). First, the reflex cannot be considered the basic unit of behavior if both spontaneous and voluntary movements are recognized as acceptable classes of behavior, because the reflex must be activated by an outside agent.

Second, the reflex theory of motor control does not adequately explain and predict movement that occurs in the absence of a sensory stimulus. It has been shown that animals can move in a relatively coordinated fashion in the absence of sensory input (Taub & Berman, 1968).

Third, the theory does not explain fast movements, that is, sequences of movements that occur too rapidly to allow for sensory feedback from the preceding movement to trigger the next. For example, an experienced and proficient typist moves from one key to the next so rapidly that there is no time for sensory information from one keystroke to activate the next.

Fourth, the concept that a chain of reflexes can create complex behaviors fails to explain the fact that a single stimulus can result in varying responses depending on context and descending commands. For example, there are times when we need to override reflexes to achieve a goal. Normally, touching something hot results in the reflexive withdrawal of the hand. However, if our child is in a fire, we may override the reflexive withdrawal in order to pull the child from the fire.

Finally, reflex chaining does not explain the ability to produce novel movements. Novel movements put together unique combinations of stimuli and responses according to rules previously learned. A violinist who has learned a piece on the violin and also knows the technique of playing the cello can play that piece on the cello without necessarily having practiced it on the cello. The violinist has learned the rules for playing the piece and has applied them to a novel situation.

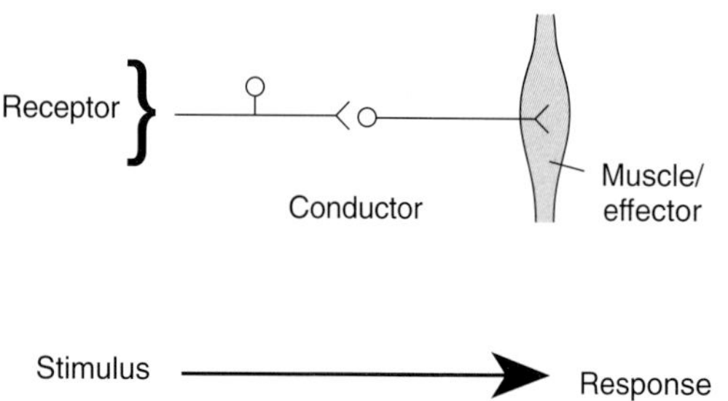

Figure 1.3 The basic structure of a reflex consists of a receptor, a conductor, and an effector.

Clinical Implications

How might a reflex theory of motor control be used to interpret a patient's behavior and serve as a guide for the therapist's actions? If chained or compounded reflexes are the basis for functional movement, clinical strategies designed to test reflexes should allow therapists to predict function. In addition, a patient's movement behaviors would be interpreted in terms of the presence or absence of controlling reflexes. Finally, retraining motor control for functional skills would focus on enhancing or reducing the effect of various reflexes during motor tasks.

Hierarchical Theory

Many researchers have contributed to the view that the nervous system is organized as a hierarchy. Among them, Hughlings Jackson, an English physician, argued that the brain has higher, middle, and lower levels of control, equated with higher association areas, the motor cortex, and spinal levels of motor function (Foerster, 1977).

Hierarchical control in general has been defined as organizational control that is top down. That is, each successively higher level exerts control over the level below it, as shown in Figure 1.4. In a strict vertical hierarchy, lines of control do not cross and there is never bottom–up control.

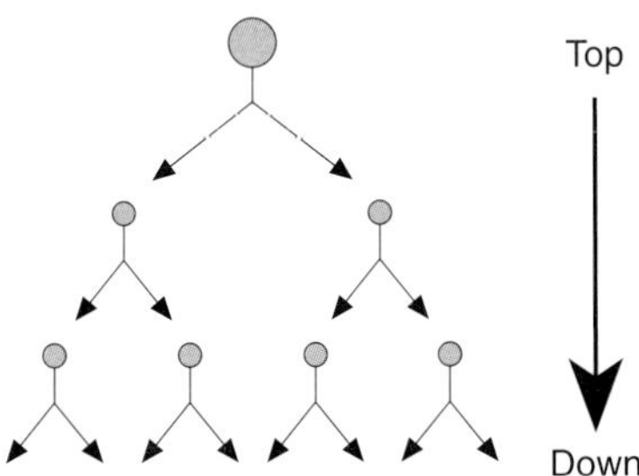

Figure 1.4 The hierarchical control model is characterized by a top-down structure, in which higher centers are always in charge of lower centers.

In the 1920s, Rudolf Magnus began to explore the function of different reflexes within different parts of the nervous system. He found that reflexes controlled by lower levels of the neural hierarchy are present only when cortical centers are damaged. These results were later interpreted to imply that reflexes are part of a hierarchy of motor control, in which higher centers normally inhibit these lower reflex centers (Magnus, 1925, 1926).

Later, Georg Schaltenbrand (1928) used Magnus's concepts to explain the development of mobility in children and adults. He described the development of human mobility in terms of the appearance and disappearance of a progression of hierarchically organized reflexes. He went on to say that pathology of the brain may result in the persistence of primitive lower-level reflexes. He suggested that a complete understanding of all the reflexes would allow the determination of the neural age of a child or of a patient with motor control dysfunction.

In the late 1930s, Stephan Weisz (1938) reported on hierarchically organized reflex reactions that he thought were the basis for equilibrium in humans. He described the ontogeny of equilibrium reflexes in the normally developing child and proposed a relationship between the maturation of these reflexes and the child's capacity to sit, stand, and walk.

The results of these experiments and observations were drawn together and are often referred to in the clinical literature as a reflex/hierarchical theory of motor control. This theory suggests that motor control emerges from reflexes that are nested within hierarchically organized levels of the CNS.

In the 1940s, Arnold Gesell (Gesell, 1954; Gesell & Armatruda, 1947) and Myrtle McGraw (McGraw, 1945), two well-known developmental researchers, offered detailed descriptions of the maturation of infants. These researchers applied the current scientific thinking about reflex hierarchies of motor control to explain the behaviors they saw in infants. Normal motor development was attributed to increasing corticalization of the CNS, resulting in the emergence of higher levels of control over lower-level reflexes. This has been referred to as a neuromaturational theory of development. An example of this model is illustrated in Figure 1.5. This theory assumes that CNS maturation is the primary agent for change in development. It minimizes the importance of other factors, such as musculoskeletal changes, during development.

Current Concepts Related to Hierarchical Control

Since Hughlings Jackson's original work, a new concept of hierarchical control has evolved. Modern neuroscientists have confirmed the importance of elements of hierarchical organization in motor control. The concept of a strict hierarchy, in which higher centers are always in control, has been modified. Current concepts describing hierarchical control within the nervous system recognize the fact that each level of the nervous system can act on other levels (higher and lower), depending on the task. In addition, the role of reflexes in movement has been modified. Reflexes are not considered the sole determinant of motor control, but only as one of many processes important to the generation and control of movement.

Limitations

One of the limitations of a reflex/hierarchical theory of motor control is that it cannot explain the dominance of

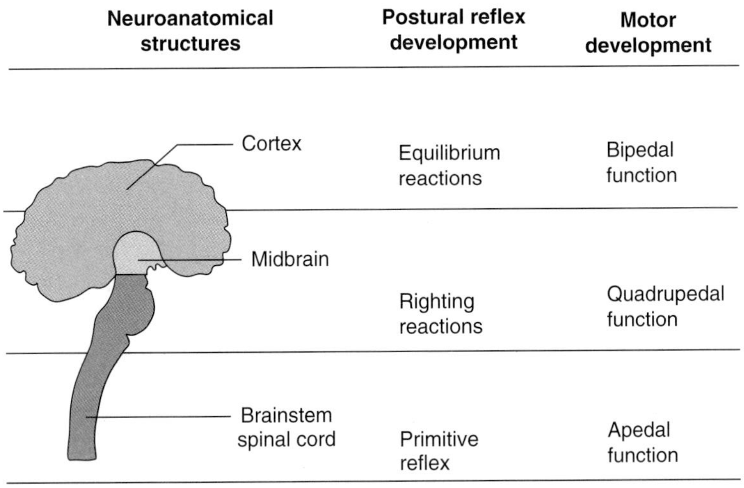

Neuroanatomical structures	Postural reflex development	Motor development
Cortex	Equilibrium reactions	Bipedal function
Midbrain	Righting reactions	Quadrupedal function
Brainstem spinal cord	Primitive reflex	Apedal function

Figure 1.5 The neuromaturational theory of motor development is based on the reflex/hierarchical theory of motor control and attributes motor development to the maturation of neural processes, including the progressive appearance and disappearance of reflexes.

reflex behavior in certain situations in normal adults. For example, stepping on a pin results in an immediate withdrawal of the leg. This is an example of a reflex within the lowest level of the hierarchy dominating motor function. It is an example of bottom–up control. Thus, one must be cautious about assumptions that all low-level behaviors are primitive, immature, and nonadaptive, while all higher-level (cortical) behaviors are mature, adaptive, and appropriate.

Clinical Implications

Many clinicians have used the concept of abnormalities of reflex organization to explain disordered motor control in patients with neurologic disorders. Signe Brunnstrom, a physical therapist who pioneered early stroke rehabilitation, used a reflex hierarchical theory to describe disordered movement following a motor cortex lesion. She stated, "When the influence of higher centers is temporarily or permanently interfered with, normal reflexes become exaggerated and so-called pathological reflexes appear" (Brunnstrom, 1970, p. 3).

Berta Bobath, an English physical therapist, in her discussions of abnormal postural reflex activity in children with cerebral palsy, interpreted that the release of motor responses integrated at lower levels from restraining influences of higher centers, especially that of the cortex, leads to abnormal postural reflex activity (Bobath, 1965; Mayston, 1992). The clinical applications of the reflex/hierarchical theory are discussed in more detail in the last section of this chapter.

Motor Programming Theories

More recent theories of motor control have expanded our understanding of the CNS. They have moved away from views of the CNS as a mostly reactive system and have begun to explore the physiology of actions rather than the physiology of reactions. Reflex theories have been useful in explaining certain stereotyped patterns of movement. However, an alternative way to view reflexes is to consider that one can remove the stimulus, or the afferent input, and still have a patterned motor response (VanSant, 1987). If we remove the motor response from its stimulus, we are left with the concept of a central motor pattern. This concept of a central motor pattern, or motor program, is more flexible than the concept of a reflex because it can be activated either by sensory stimuli or by central processes. Scientists who contributed to the development of this theory include individuals from clinical, psychological, and biological backgrounds (Bernstein, 1967; Keele, 1968; Wilson, 1961).

A motor program theory of motor control has considerable experimental support. For example, experiments in the early 1960s studied motor control in the grasshopper or locust and showed that the timing of the animal's wing beat in flight depended on a rhythmic pattern generator. Even when the sensory nerves were cut, the nervous system by itself could generate the output with no sensory input; however, the wing beat was slowed (Wilson, 1961). This suggested that movement is possible in the absence of reflexive action. Sensory input, while not essential in driving movement, has an important function in modulating action.

These conclusions were further supported by work examining locomotion in cats (Grillner, 1981). The results of these experiments showed that in the cat, spinal neural networks could produce a locomotor rhythm with neither sensory inputs nor descending patterns from the brain. By changing the intensity of stimulation to the spinal cord, the animal could be made to walk, trot, or gallop. Thus, it was again shown that reflexes do not drive action, but that central pattern generators (CPGs) (spinally mediated motor programs) by themselves can generate such complex movements as they walk, trot, and gallop. Further experiments showed the important modulatory effects of incoming sensory inputs on the CPG (Forssberg et al., 1975).

These experiments led to the motor program theory of motor control. This term has been used in a number of ways by different researchers, so care should be taken in determining how the term is being used. The term "motor program" may be used to identify a CPG, as described previously, that is, a specific neural circuit like that for generating walking in the cat. In this case, the term represents neural connections that are stereotyped and hardwired.

Schmidt (1975; Schmidt and Lee, 2011) believed that previousmotor program theories could not explain the control of movement in the absence feedback, as it is observed in quick or ballistic movements, or could not explain how motor programs could generate novel movements. He thus preferred to adopt the concept of generalized motor program, which is a broader concept than the earlier understanding of motor programs. In the generalized motor program view, there is an abstract representation that can be used to create a class of movements with certain invariant features such as the order of events, the relative timing of events, and the relative force with which the events are produced. The generalized motor program then specifies how a particular movement will be performed, using parameters such as overall movement duration, overall force of contractions, and the muscles involved. This modification in the conceptualization of motor programs provides for the possibility of many different movements performed by using the same motor program and also for the creation of novel movements through the specification of new parameters. (See Chapter 2 for more information on Schmidt's concepts on generalized motor programs.)

Thus, in this case the term "motor program" is used to describe higher-level motor programs that represent actions in more abstract terms. A significant amount of research in the field of psychology has supported the

LAB ACTIVITY 1.2

Objective: To apply the concept of motor program to functional movement.

Procedure: Write your signature as you normally would on a small piece of paper. Now write it larger, on a blackboard. Now try it with your other hand.

Assignment

1. Examine the three signatures carefully, looking for common elements found in all of them.
2. Write down the common elements you found. What do you think are the causes for both the common elements and the differences? How do your results support or contradict the theory of motor programs?

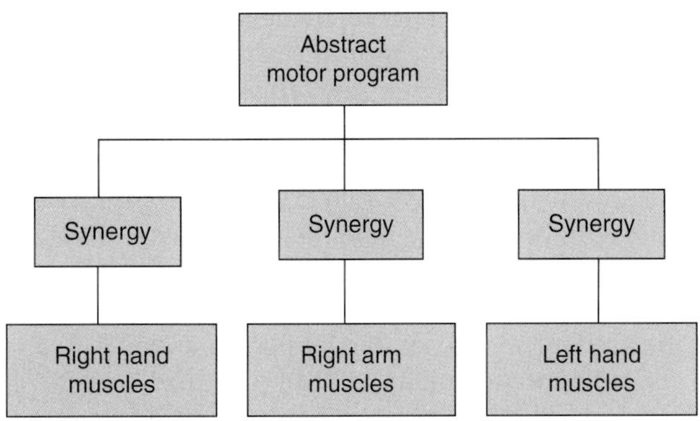

Figure 1.6 Levels of control for motor programs and their output systems. Rules for action are represented at the highest level, in abstract motor programs. Lower levels of the hierarchy contain specific information, including muscle response synergies, essential for effecting action.

existence of hierarchically organized motor programs that store a set of abstract rules that direct the execution ofmovements so that we can perform motor tasks with a variety of effector systems (Keele, 1968). You can see this for yourself in Lab Activity 1.2.

As shown in Figure 1.6, it has been hypothesized that the rules for writing a given word are stored as an abstract motor program at higher levels within the CNS. As a result, neural commands from these higher centers used to write your name could be sent to various parts of the body that act as the effector. Yet elements of the written signature remain constant regardless of the part of the body used to carry out the task (Bernstein, 1967).

Limitations

The concept of CPGs expanded our understanding of the role of the nervous system in the control of movement. However, we must be careful to realize that the CPG concept was never intended to replace the concept of the importance of sensory input in controlling movement. It simply expanded our understanding of the flexibility of the nervous system in creating movements to include its ability to create movements in isolation from feedback.

An important limitation of the motor program concept is that a central motor program cannot be considered to be the sole determinant of action (Bernstein, 1967). Two identical commands to the elbow flexors, for example, will produce different movements depending on whether your arm is resting at your side or you are holding your arm out in front of you. The forces of gravity will act differently on the limb in the two conditions and thus modify the movement. In addition, if your muscles are fatigued, similar nervous system commands will yield different results. Thus, the motor program concept does not take into account that the nervous system must deal with both musculoskeletal and environmental variables in achieving movement control.

Clinical Implications

Motor program theories of motor control have allowed clinicians to move beyond a reflex explanation for disordered motor control. Explanations for abnormal movement have been expanded to include problems resulting from abnormalities in CPGs or in higher-level motor programs. In patients whose higher levels of motor programming are affected, the motor program theory suggests the importance of helping patients relearn the correct rules for action. In addition, intervention should focus on retraining movements important to a functional task, not just on reeducating specific muscles in isolation.

Systems Theory

In the early and mid-1900s, Nicolai Bernstein (1896–1966), a Russian scientist, was looking at the nervous system and body in a whole new way. Previously, neurophysiologists had focused primarily on neural control aspects of movement. Bernstein, who also participated in the development of motor program theories, recognized that you cannot understand the neural control of movement without an understanding of the characteristics of the system you are moving and the external and internal forces acting on the body (Bernstein, 1967).

In describing the characteristics of the system being moved, Bernstein looked at the whole body as a mechanical system, with mass, and subject to both external forces such as gravity and internal forces such as both inertial and movement-dependent forces. He thus showed that the same central command could result in quite different movements because of the interplay between external forces and variations in the initial conditions. For the same reasons, different commands could result in the same movement. Bernstein also suggested that control of integrated movement was probably distributed throughout many interacting systems working cooperatively to achieve movement. This gave rise to the concept of a distributed model of motor control (Bernstein, 1967).

How does Bernstein's approach to motor control differ from the approaches presented previously? Bernstein asked questions about the organism in a continuously changing situation. He found answers about the nature and control of movement that were different from those of previous researchers because he asked different questions, such as "How does the body as a mechanical system influence the control process?" and "How do the initial conditions affect the properties of the movement?"

In describing the body as a mechanical system, Bernstein noted that we have many degrees of freedom that need to be controlled. For example, we have many joints, all of which flex or extend and many of which can be rotated as well. Furthermore, there exist many different muscles responsible for controlling the joint displacements in addition to the motor neurons in the CNS that control and coordinate these muscles. This situation complicates movement control incredibly. He said, "Coordination of movement is the process of mastering the redundant degrees of freedom of the moving organism" (Bernstein, 1967, p. 127). In other words, it involves converting the body into a controllable system. As a solution to the degrees of freedom problem, Bernstein hypothesized that hierarchical control exists to simplify the control of the body's multiple degrees of freedom. He framed his model in relation to the evolution of the nervous system and proposed that each level of the hierarchy solves a particular class of movement problem. This hierarchical neural model is built anatomically bottom–up with higher levels of the nervous system functionally activating lower levels in a top–down fashion to take advantage of the functional capabilities of the lower levels and then reduce the involvement of higher levels in movement control. Despite the hierarchical view to understand each level of movement control, as it is presented in his work on the "levels of construction of movements," Bernstein emphasized that the integrity of the whole system is required to control movements (Profeta & Turvey, 2018).

The hierarchical neural model contains four main levels (Fig. 1.7). The first level, level of tonus, is known as the "muscle language." It resides in the spinal cord and is never considered a leading level—its function is to prepare the motor apparatus to respond appropriately upon upper-level commands. The second level, the level of synergies, resides in the middle brain and is responsible for constraining the degrees of freedom of the motor apparatus. The third level, the level of space, leads to purposeful, goal-oriented, and dexterous movements within the environment. This third level receives a rich sensory influx in combination with previous experiences to objectively perceive the body and the external space and to operate accordingly. Finally, the last level, the level of action, resides in the frontal cortex. It controls and organizes movement sequences to attain the action's goal.

The different elements that comprise the sequence can be organized in many different ways to achieve the same motor goal. Therefore, the level of action is characterized by flexibility to find several potential motor solutions for the same movement problem—commonly known as *motor equivalence* (Profeta & Turvey, 2018). Any movement would require at least a *leading level*, an upper level that controls a goal-directed movement, and a *background level*, the level that provides support so that the movement can be executed. Background levels cannot anticipate or compensate for non-mechanical environmental perturbations.

Contemporary motor control scientists have revisited Bernstein's levels of construction of movements to represent the control of purposeful movements without burdening the "conscious," or cognitive aspect of the nervous system (Latash & Turvey, 1996; Profeta & Turvey, 2018; Turvey & Carello, 1996). The functional hierarchical scheme described by Bernstein proposes a solution to the degrees of freedom problem, in such a way that when the demands of a task increase, the control signal to the synergy increases; which leads to parallel increases in the activation of all muscles within a synergy.

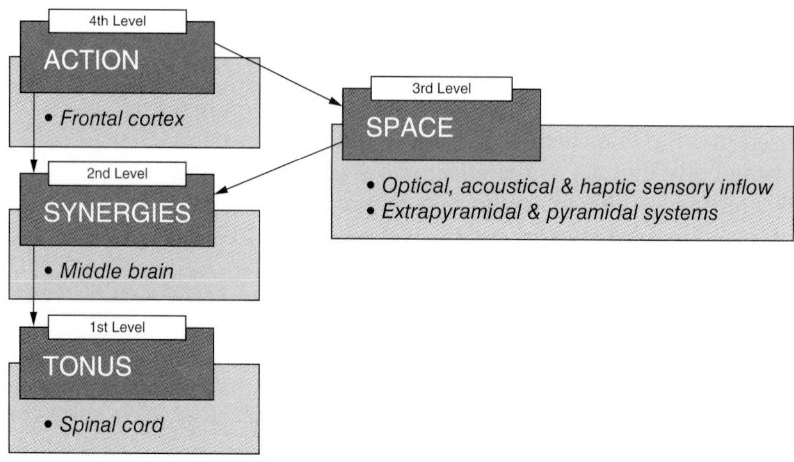

Figure 1.7 Schematic representation of Bernstein's levels of construction of movements and the interaction among them. Arrows indicate direction of dominance between levels, from leading to background levels. (Adapted from Profeta VLS, Turvey MT. Bernstein's levels of movement construction: A contemporary perspective. *Hum Mov Sci.* 2018;58:111–133.)

We can think of our movement repertoire to be like sentences made up of many words. The letters within the words are the muscles and the muscle tonus, the words themselves are the synergies, and the sentences are the actions themselves. Thus, Bernstein believed that synergies play an important role in solving the degrees of freedom problem by constraining certain muscles to work together as a unit. He hypothesized that although there are few synergies, they make possible almost the whole variety of movements we know. For example, he considered some simple synergies to be the locomotor, postural, and respiratory synergies.

Since Bernstein first proposed the concept of synergies, research has continued to examine this concept, and as a result, our understanding of the nature of synergies continues to evolve and change. For example, Latash and others (Latash & Anson, 2006; Latash et al., 2007) have proposed a new definition of the term "synergy." In this definition, synergies are not used by the nervous system to eliminate redundant degrees of freedom, but instead to ensure flexible and stable performance of motor tasks. They call this the "principle of abundance." They define synergy as a neural organization of a multielement system (e.g., muscles) that (a) organizes sharing of a task among a set of elemental variables (e.g., muscles) and (b) ensures covariation among elemental variables with the purpose of stabilizing performance variables (e.g., center of mass in posture control or the end point in a reaching task). Thus, synergies show both stability against perturbations and flexibility to solve concurrent tasks (Latash et al., 2007; Newell et al., 1984). Ting and colleagues (Torres-Oviedo & Ting, 2007) examined the organization and structure of muscle synergies used for balance control. In traditional views of synergies, a muscle belongs to only one synergy, and muscles within a synergy are activated equally as a unit. Newer views of synergies suggest that a muscle can belong to multiple synergies; in addition, an individual muscle has a unique contribution to each synergy. Finally, the total activation of a muscle is dependent on both the simultaneous activation of multiple synergies containing that muscle and the relative contribution of that muscle within each of these synergies. Thus, the concept of synergies has evolved from Bernstein's concept of fixed action patterns to a more recent understanding of the dynamic, flexible, and adaptive nature of synergies. The research examining the role of synergies in postural control is described in more detail in Chapter 7.

Since Bernstein first put forth the principles of systems theory, a number of researchers have expanded and built upon this approach. One of the most popular theories is the "dynamic systems theory" (Kamm et al., 1991; Kelso & Tuller, 1984; Kugler & Turvey, 1987; Perry, 1998; Thelen et al., 1987). In principle, the theories are very similar at their foundation; thus, either term may be used when people discuss this framework. The dynamic systems theory comes from the broader study of dynamics or synergetics within the physical world and asks the following questions: How do the patterns and organization we see in the world come into being from their orderless constituent parts? How do these systems change over time?

Self-organization is commonly found in nature. Patterns of cloud formations and the movement of water as it goes from ice to liquid to boiling to a gaseous state are examples of the principle of *self-organization*. This principle states that when a system of individual parts comes together, its elements behave collectively in an ordered way. There is no need for a "higher" center issuing instructions or commands in order to achieve coordinated action. This principle applied to motor control predicts that movement could emerge as a result of interacting elements, without the need for specific commands or motor programs within the nervous system. The dynamic systems perspective also tries to find mathematical descriptions of these self-organizing systems.

Another critical feature of dynamic systems is their nonlinear properties (Harbourne & Stergiou, 2009; Kugler & Turvey, 1987). What is nonlinear behavior? A nonlinear system is one whose output is not proportional to its input (Harbourne & Stergiou, 2009). A nonlinear behavior is one that transforms into a new configuration when a single parameter of that behavior is gradually altered and reaches a critical value. For example, as an animal walks faster and faster, there is a point at which, suddenly, it shifts into a trot. As the animal continues to move faster, there is a second point at which it shifts into a gallop. This is shown in Figure 1.8.

What causes this change from one behavioral pattern (e.g., a walk) to a new behavioral pattern (e.g., a trot)? Dynamic theory suggests that the new movement emerges because of a critical change in one of the systems, called a "control parameter." A control parameter is a variable that regulates change in the behavior of the entire system. In our example, the control parameter is velocity. When the animal's walking velocity, a control parameter, reaches a critical point, there is a shift in the animal's behavior, from a walk to a trot. Thus, the dynamic action

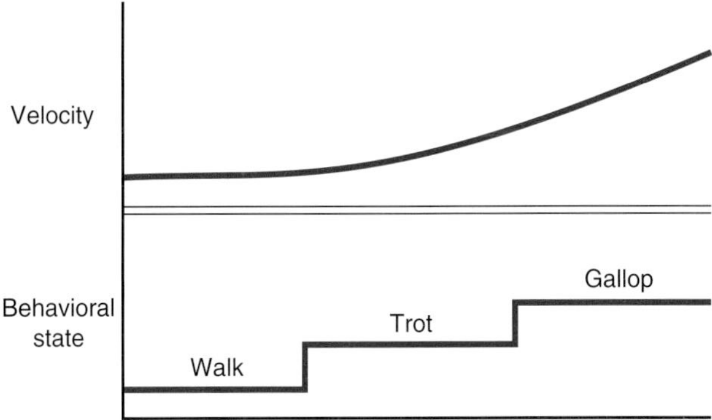

Figure 1.8 A systems model predicts discrete changes in behavior resulting from changes in the linear dynamics of a moving system. For example, as locomotion velocity increases linearly, a threshold is reached that results in a nonlinear change in the behavioral state of the moving animal from a walk to a trot to a gallop.

perspective has de-emphasized the notion of commands from the CNS in controlling movement and has sought physical explanations that may contribute to movement characteristics as well (Perry, 1998).

An important concept in describing movement from a dynamic systems theory perspective is the role of variability in the control of movement. In the dynamic systems theory, human movement, like behavior in other complex nonlinear systems, has inherent variability that is critical to optimal function (Harbourne & Stergiou, 2009). Movement variability includes variations that occur normally in motor performance across multiple repetitions of a task (Stergiou et al., 2006). However, the role of variability in motor control in dynamic systems theory is viewed differently from other theories of motor control. For example, in motor program theory, variability is considered to be the consequence of errors in motor performance, with the assumption that as performance improves during skill acquisition, error—and consequently variability—decreases. In contrast, in dynamic systems theory, variability is not considered to be the result of error, but rather as a necessary condition of optimal function. Optimal variability provides for flexible, adaptive strategies, allowing adjustment to environmental change and as such is a central feature of normal movement. Too little variability can lead to injury (as in repetitive strain problems), while too much variability leads to impaired movement performance, such as occurs in persons with ataxia.

In dynamic systems theory, a small amount of variability indicates a highly stable behavior. Highly stable behaviors are often viewed as an attractor state. Attractor states may be considered highly stable, preferred patterns of movement; many are used to accomplish common activities of daily life. Animals all habitually walk at a preferred pace that represents an attractor state for walking speed specific to the individual. Walking at other speeds is possible, but barring outside influences, individuals tend to walk at a preferred pace, which is energetically most efficient. The degree to which the flexibility exists to change a preferred pattern of movement is characterized as an attractor well. This concept is shown in Figure 1.9. The deeper the well, the harder it is to change the preferred pattern, suggesting a stable movement pattern. A shallow well suggests an unstable pattern.

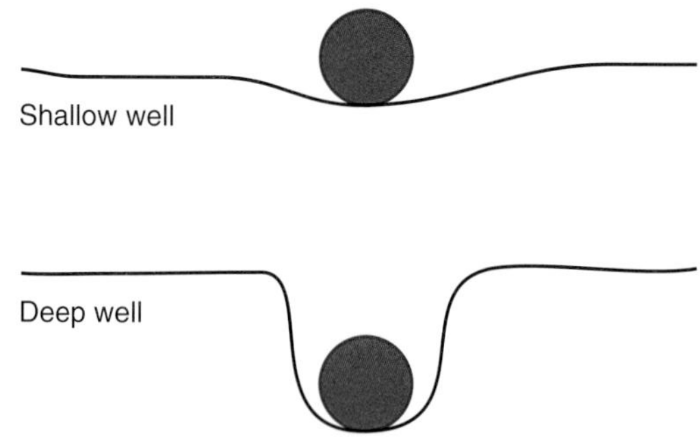

Figure 1.9 Attractor wells describe the variability in a preferred pattern of movement. Deep attractor wells represent a pattern of movement with low variability. Shallow attractor wells represent a pattern of movement with high variability.

Attractor wells may be viewed as riverbeds. When a riverbed is quite deep, the likelihood that the river will flow outside the established riverbed is slight. The river flows in the preferred direction established by the riverbed, which is a deep attractor well. Alternatively, if the riverbed is quite shallow, the river will be more likely to flow in areas not established by the riverbed. In this case, the shallow riverbed is a shallow attractor well. Similarly, movement patterns in patients could be characterized as stable or unstable based on the difficulty associated with changing them. It will be much easier to change an unstable movement pattern that has a shallow attractor well than to change a stable movement pattern that has a deep attractor well.

Kelso and Tuller (1984) have shown that stable movement patterns become more variable, or unstable, just prior to a transition to a new movement pattern. For example, if persons are asked to move their two index fingers of the right and left hand out of phase (i.e., one finger is flexing while the other is extending) while making the movements faster and faster, an abrupt phase transition occurs between the two fingers. The asymmetrical out-of-phase mode shifts suddenly to a symmetrical in-phase mode (both fingers flexing) involving a shift to activation of homologous muscle groups. Researchers have documented an increase in variability prior to the emergence of new, more stable patterns of behavior during the acquisition of new movement skills in both children and adults (Gordon, 1987; Harbourne & Stergiou, 2009; Harbourne et al., 2007; Woollacott & Shumway-Cook, 1990). Thus, it may be possible for therapists to view variability in movement behavior as an antecedent to change in some patients. In comparison to some of the other theories of motor control, the systems (dynamical systems) theory is quite complex with many important points. Table 1.3 summarizes the main concepts associated with this theory.

Limitations

What are some of the limitations of the systems theory of motor control? This is the broadest and most complex of the theories discussed so far. Because systems theory takes into account not only the contributions of the nervous system to action but also the contributions of the muscle and skeletal systems, as well as the forces of gravity and inertia, it predicts actual behavior much better than did previous theories. This theory reminds us that the nervous system in isolation will not allow the prediction of movement. However, a limitation of some variations of this model can be the presumption that the nervous system has a less important role in determining the animal's behavior, giving mathematical formulas and principles of body mechanics a more dominant role in describing motor control. Understanding the

TABLE 1.3 Critical Concepts Associated with the Systems and Dynamic Systems Theory of Motor Control

Concept	Definition
Degrees of freedom	Body as a mechanical system with many degrees of freedom. Systems theory stresses the importance of the whole body as a mechanical system with many degrees of freedom. Coordination of movement is the process of mastering the redundant degrees of freedom of the moving organism.
Synergies	Synergies proposed as a solution to the degrees of freedom problem; concept of synergies modified to reflect the flexible, adaptive nature of synergies rather than fixed stereotypical patterns of activity.
Self-organization	Principles of self-organization found in nature are applied to motor control. The degrees of freedom problem is solved through self-organization. Organization emerges from the interaction of elements and does not require central commands.
Nonlinear behavior	Self-organizing systems often have nonlinear properties. A nonlinear behavior is one that transforms into a new configuration when a single parameter of that behavior is gradually altered and reaches a critical value (e.g., walk, trot, and gallop emerging from a change in velocity).
Variability	Systems theory believes that variability of movement is not due to error, rather a necessary condition for optimal function. The concept of attractor wells is used to characterize the variability and flexibility of a movement pattern. The deeper the well, the less variable and flexible the movement. A shallow well suggests an unstable pattern. There is a significant increase in variability of a movement just prior to a change to a new movement pattern (a shift to a new attractor well). For example, walking patterns become more variable just prior to a shift from walk to trot.

application and relevance of this type of analysis to clinical practice can be very difficult.

Clinical Implications

The systems theory has a number of implications for therapists. First, it stresses the importance of understanding the body as a mechanical system. Movement is not determined solely by the output of the nervous system but is the output of the nervous system as filtered through a mechanical system, the body. When working with the patient who has a CNS deficit, the therapist must be careful to examine the contribution of impairments in the musculoskeletal system, as well as the neural system, to overall loss of motor control. The systems theory suggests that examination and intervention must focus not only on the impairments within individual systems contributing to motor control but also on the effect of interacting impairments among multiple systems.

In addition, one of the major implications of the systems theory is the view that movement is an emergent property—that is, it emerges from the interaction of multiple elements that self-organize based on certain dynamic properties of the elements themselves. This means that shifts or alterations in movement behavior can often be explained in terms of physical principles rather than necessarily in terms of neural structures. What are the implications of this for treating motor dyscontrol in patients? If, as clinicians, we understand more about the physical or dynamic properties of the human body, we can make use of these properties in helping patients to regain motor control. For example, velocity can be an important contributor to the dynamics of movement. Often, patients are asked to move slowly in an effort to move safely. Yet this approach to retraining fails to take into account the interaction between speed and physical properties of the body, which produce momentum, and therefore can help a weak patient move with greater ease.

Variability as a characteristic feature of normal movement has important clinical implications for therapists involved in retraining movement in patients with neural pathology. When variability is viewed as a consequence of error, therapists will use therapeutic strategies designed to reduce error, guiding patients toward an optimal and stable movement pattern. In contrast, when variability is viewed as a critical element of normal function, therapists will encourage patients to explore variable and flexible movement patterns that will lead to success in achieving performance goals (Harbourne & Stergiou, 2009).

Ecological Theory

In the 1960s, independent of the research in physiology, a psychologist named James Gibson was beginning to explore the way in which our motor systems allow us to interact most effectively with the environment in order to perform goal-oriented behavior (Gibson, 1966). His research focused on how we detect information in our environment that is relevant to our actions and how we use this information to control our movements. The ability to use perceptions to guide action emerges early in life. For example, by 15 weeks of age, infants do not automatically reach for every object that passes by, but instead they are able to use perceptions related to velocity to determine in advance whether or not they can catch a ball (von Hofsten & Lindhagen, 1979).

This view was expanded by students of Gibson (Lee & Young, 1986; Reed, 1982) and became known as the ecological approach to motor control. It suggests that motor control evolved so that animals could cope with the environment around them, moving in it effectively in order to find food, run away from predators, build shelter, and even play (Reed, 1982). What was new about this approach? It was really the first time that researchers began focusing on how actions are geared to the environment. Actions require perceptual information that is specific to a desired goal-directed action performed within a specific environment. The organization of action is specific to the task and the environment in which the task is being performed.

Whereas many previous researchers had seen the organism as a sensory/motor system, Gibson stressed that it was not sensation per se that was important to the animal, but perception. Specifically, what is needed is the perception of environmental factors important to the task. He stated that perception focuses on detecting information in the environment that will support the actions necessary to achieve the goal. From an ecological perspective, it is important to determine how an organism detects information in the environment that is relevant to action, what form this information takes, and how this information is used to modify and control movement (Lee & Young, 1986).

In summary, the ecological perspective has broadened our understanding of nervous system function from that of a sensory/motor system, reacting to environmental variables, to that of a perception/action system that actively explores the environment to satisfy its own goals.

Limitations

Although the ecological approach has expanded our knowledge significantly with regard to the interaction of the organism and the environment, it has tended to give less emphasis to the organization and function of the nervous system that led to this interaction. Thus, the research emphasis has shifted from the nervous system to the organism–environment interface.

Clinical Implications

A major contribution of this view is in describing the individual as an active explorer of the environment. The active exploration of the task and the environment in which the task is performed allows the individual to develop multiple ways to accomplish a task. Adaptability is important not only in the way we organize movements to accomplish a task but also in the way we use perception.

An important part of intervention is helping the patient explore the possibilities for achieving the goal of a functional task in multiple ways, given the constraints of different environments, since features in the environment impact the selection and execution of goal-directed movements. Effective motor control requires the patient learn to perceive the critical aspects of an environment (affordances) that impact how movement is organized. This suggests that an important aspect of the rehabilitation process is controlling and manipulating the environment so that patients can learn to perceive critical features and adapt movements accordingly.

Which Theory of Motor Control Is Best?

So which motor control theory best suits the current theoretical and practical needs of therapists? Which is the most complete theory of motor control, the one that really predicts the nature and cause of movement and is consistent with our current knowledge of brain anatomy and physiology?

As you no doubt can already see, there is no one theory that has it all. We believe the best theory of motor control is one that combines elements from all of the theories presented. A comprehensive or integrated theory recognizes the elements of motor control we do know about and leaves room for the things we do not. Any current theory of motor control is in a sense unfinished, since there must always be room to revise and incorporate new information.

Many people have been working to develop an integrated theory of motor control (Gordon, 1987; Horak & Shumway-Cook, 1990; Woollacott & Shumway-Cook, 1990). In some cases, as theories are modified, new names are applied. As a result, it becomes difficult to distinguish among evolving theories. For example, systems, dynamic, dynamic action, and dynamic systems theory are all terms that are often used interchangeably.

Previously, we (Woollacott & Shumway-Cook, 1990, 1997) have called the theory of motor control on which we base our research and clinical practice a systems approach. We have continued to use this name, although our concept of systems theory differs from Bernstein's systems theory and has evolved to incorporate many of the concepts proposed by other theories of motor control. In this book, we will continue to refer to our theory of motor control as a systems approach. This approach argues that it is critical to recognize that movement emerges from an interaction between the individual, the task, and the environment in which the task is being carried out. Thus, movement is not solely the result of muscle-specific motor programs or stereotyped reflexes but results from a dynamic interplay between perception, cognition, and action systems. This theoretical framework will be used throughout this textbook, and it is the basis for clinical methods related to examination and intervention in the patient with movement control problems. We have found the theory useful in helping us to generate research questions and hypotheses about the nature and cause of movement.

PARALLEL DEVELOPMENT OF CLINICAL PRACTICE AND SCIENTIFIC THEORY

Much has been written about the influence of changing scientific theories on the treatment of patients with movement disorders. Several excellent articles discuss in detail the parallel developments between scientific theory and clinical practice (Carr & Shepherd, 1992; Gordon, 1987; Horak, 1991).

Although neuroscience researchers identify the scientific basis for movement and movement disorders, it is up to the clinician to develop the applications of this research. Thus, scientific theory provides a framework that allows the integration of practical ideas into a coherent philosophy for intervention. A theory is not right or wrong in an absolute sense, but it is judged to be more or less useful in solving the problems presented by patients with movement dysfunction (Gordon, 1987; Horak, 1991).

Just as scientific assumptions about the important elements that control movement are changing, so too, is clinical practice. New assumptions regarding the nature and cause of movement are replacing old assumptions. Clinical practice evolves in parallel with scientific theory, as clinicians assimilate changes in scientific theory and apply them to practice. This concept is shown in Figure 1.10. Let us explore in more detail the evolution of clinical practice in light of changing theories of motor control.

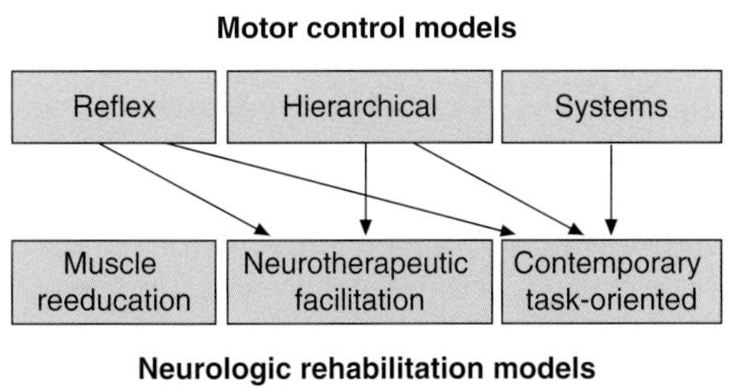

Figure 1.10 The parallel development of theories of motor control and clinical practices designed to examine and treat patients with motor dyscontrol. (Adapted from Horak F. Assumptions underlying motor control for neurologic rehabilitation. In: Contemporary management of motor control problems. Proceedings of the II Step Conference. Alexandria, VA: American Physical Therapy Association, 1992:11, with permission.)

Neurologic Rehabilitation: Reflex-Based Neurofacilitation Approaches

In the late 1950s and early 1960s, the so-called neurofacilitation approaches were developed, resulting in a dramatic change in clinical interventions directed at the patient with neurologic impairments (Gordon, 1987; Horak, 1991). For the most part, these approaches still dominate the way clinicians treat the patient with a neurologic deficit.

Neurofacilitation approaches include the Bobath approach, developed by Bobath and Bobath (1984), the Rood approach, developed by Margaret Rood (Stockmeyer, 1967), Brunnstrom's approach, developed by Signe Brunnstrom (1966), proprioceptive neuromuscular facilitation (PNF), developed by Kabat and Knott (1954) and expanded by Voss et al. (1985), and sensory integration therapy, developed by Jean Ayres (1972). These approaches were based largely on assumptions drawn from both the reflex and hierarchical theories of motor control.

Prior to the development of the neurofacilitation approaches, therapy for the patient with neurologic dysfunction was directed largely at changing function at the level of the muscle itself. This has been referred to as a muscle reeducation approach to intervention (Gordon, 1987; Horak, 1991). Although the muscle reeducation approach was effective in managing movement disorders resulting from polio, it had less impact on altering movement patterns in patients with upper motor neuron lesions. Thus, the neurofacilitation techniques were developed in response to clinicians' dissatisfaction with previous modes of intervention and a desire to develop approaches that were more effective in solving the movement problems of patients with neurologic dysfunction (Gordon, 1987).

Clinicians working with patients with upper motor neuron (motor cortex and pyramidal tract) lesions began to direct clinical efforts toward modifying the CNS itself. Neurofacilitation approaches focused on retraining motor control through techniques designed to facilitate and/or inhibit different movement patterns. *Facilitation* refers to intervention techniques that increase the patient's ability to move in ways judged to be appropriate by the clinician. Inhibitory techniques decrease the patient's use of movement patterns considered to be abnormal (Gordon, 1987). Further information on the underlying assumptions behind the neurofacilitation approach, including the clinical applications may be found in Extended Knowledge 1.1.

Task-Oriented Approach

One of the newer approaches to retraining is the task-oriented approach to clinical intervention, based on newer theories of motor control. In previous publications, we have referred to this approach as a systems approach (Woollacott & Shumway-Cook, 1990). Others

Extended Knowledge 1.1

Neurofacilitation: Underlying Assumptions and Clinical Applications

Underlying Assumptions

Neurofacilitation approaches are largely associated with both the reflex and hierarchical theories of motor control. Thus, clinical practices have been developed based on assumptions regarding the nature and cause of normal motor control, abnormal motor control, and the recovery of function.

This approach suggests that normal movement results from a chain of reflexes organized hierarchically within the CNS. Thus, control of movement is top down. Normal movement requires that the highest level of the CNS, the cortex, be in control of both intermediate (brainstem) and lower (spinal cord) levels of the CNS. This means that the process of normal development, sometimes called "corticalization," is characterized by the emergence of behaviors organized at sequentially higher and higher levels in the CNS. A great emphasis is placed on the understanding that incoming sensory information stimulates and, thus, drives a normal movement pattern.

Explanations regarding the physiological basis for abnormal motor control from a reflex and hierarchical perspective largely suggest that a disruption of normal reflex mechanisms underlies abnormal movement control. It is assumed that lesions at the highest cortical levels of the CNS cause release of abnormal reflexes organized at lower levels within the CNS. The release of these lower-level reflexes constrains the patient's ability to move normally.

Another prevalent assumption is that abnormal or atypical patterns of movement seen in patients with motor cortex lesions are the direct result of the lesion itself, as opposed to considering some behaviors as developing either secondary to the lesion or in response to the lesion (i.e., compensatory to the lesion). Thus, it is predicted that in the child with motor cortex lesions, the process of increasing corticalization is disrupted and, as a result motor control, is dominated by primitive patterns of movement organized at lower levels of the CNS. In addition, in the adult with acquired motor cortex lesions, damage to higher levels of the CNS probably results in a release of lower centers from higher-center control. Likewise, primitive and pathologic behaviors organized at these levels reemerge to dominate, preventing normal patterns of movement from occurring.

A central assumption concerning the *recovery of function* in the patient with a motor cortex lesion is that recovery of normal motor control cannot occur unless higher centers of the CNS regain control over lower centers. According to this approach, recovery of function, in a sense, recapitulates development, with higher centers gradually regaining their dominance over lower centers of the CNS.

Two key assumptions are that (a) functional skills will automatically return once abnormal movement patterns are inhibited and normal movement patterns facilitated, and (b) repetition of these normal movement patterns will automatically transfer to functional tasks.

Clinical Applications

What are some of the clinical applications of these assumptions? First, examination of motor control should focus on identifying the presence or absence of normal and abnormal reflexes controlling movement. Also, intervention should be directed at modifying the reflexes that control movement. The importance of sensory input for stimulating normal motor output suggests an intervention focus of modifying the CNS through sensory stimulation (Gordon, 1987; Horak, 1991).

A hierarchical theory suggests that one goal of therapy is to regain independent control of movement by higher centers of the CNS. Thus, intervention is geared toward helping the patient regain normal patterns of movement as a way of facilitating functional recovery.

The neurofacilitation approaches still dominate the way clinicians examine and intervene with patients who have CNS pathology. However, just as scientific theory about the nature and cause of movement has changed in the past 30 years, so too, have many of the neurofacilitation approaches changed their approach to practice. Currently within the neurofacilitation approaches, there is a greater emphasis on explicitly training function and less emphasis on inhibiting reflexes and retraining normal patterns of movement. In addition, there is more consideration of motor learning principles when developing intervention plans. The boundaries between approaches are less distinct, as each approach integrates new concepts related to motor control into its theoretical base.

---

have referred to these new clinical methods as a motor control or motor learning approach (Carr & Shepherd, 1992). Whatever the label is, these newer methods of clinical practice are based on concepts emerging from research in the fields of motor control, motor learning, and rehabilitation science. Clinical practice is dynamic, changing in response to emerging evidence. We will continue to refer to the clinical approach presented in this book as a "task-oriented" approach, although specific examination and treatment strategies will by necessity change as new research in the field emerges.

Underlying Assumptions

Assumptions underlying a task-oriented approach are quite different from those underlying the neurofacilitation techniques. In the task-oriented approach, it is assumed that normal movement emerges as an interaction among many different systems, each contributing different aspects of control. In addition, movement is organized around a behavioral goal and is constrained by the environment. Thus, the role of sensation in normal movement is not limited to a stimulus/response reflex mode but is essential to predictive and adaptive control of movement as well.

Assumptions regarding abnormal motor control suggest that movement problems result from impairments within one or more of the systems controlling movement. Movements observed in the patient with a motor cortex lesion represent behavior that emerges from the best mix of the systems remaining to participate. This means that what is observed is not just the result of the lesion itself but also of the efforts of the remaining systems to compensate for the loss and still be functional. However, the compensatory strategies developed by patients are not always optimal. Thus, a goal in intervention may be to improve the efficiency of compensatory strategies used to perform functional tasks.

Clinical Applications

These assumptions suggest that when retraining movement control, it is essential to work on identifiable functional tasks rather than on movement patterns for movement's sake alone. A task-oriented approach to intervention assumes that patients learn by actively attempting to solve the problems inherent in a functional task rather than by repetitively practicing normal patterns of movement, independent of a specific task goal. Adaptation to changes in the environmental context is a critical part of recovery of function. In this context, patients are helped to learn a variety of ways to solve the task goal rather than a single-muscle activation pattern.

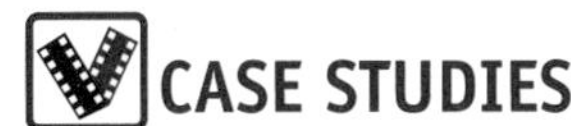

CASE STUDIES

The underlying intent of this book is to impact therapeutic interventions designed to improve the functional capacity and quality of life of patients with movement disorders. Research is a critical part of determining the therapeutic strategies used to modify motor control problems. Thus, this book is intended to discuss motor control research and show its application to the management of patients with movement disorders. To help the reader better understand motor control research and its clinical applications, we use a series of case studies to help explain and apply the material covered in this book. Table 1.4 introduces the patients we will be referring to throughout this textbook. Further information on each patient may be found on his or her video case study.

TABLE 1.4 Introduction to Case Studies

John 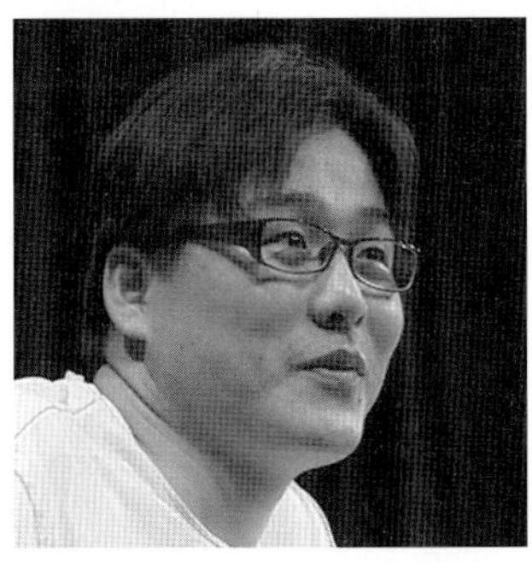	John is a 33-year-old man with spinocerebellar ataxia type 2, a genetic disorder causing degeneration of the cerebellum. He is single, living with his parents, and working part-time. His primary concerns are his balance and gait; he has had several falls.
Jean 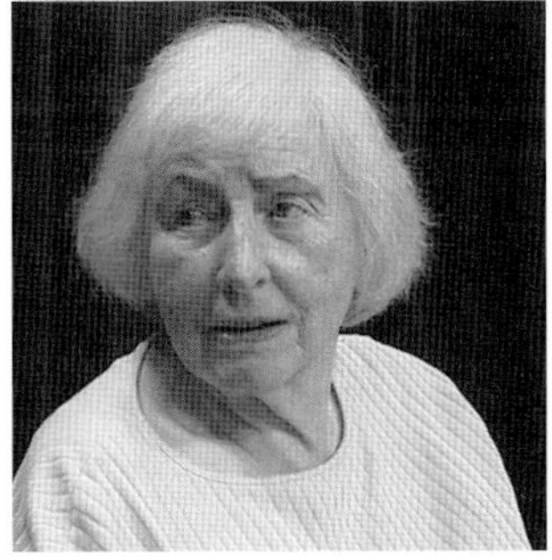	Jean is an 82-year-old woman who had a left cerebral vascular accident 6 years ago, leaving her with a residual right hemiparesis. She lives by herself in an apartment within an assisted living facility. Her primary concerns are her reduced ability to use her right arm and hand and her poor balance, which affects her walking. She falls once or twice a month, most often during walking and transfers.
Mike 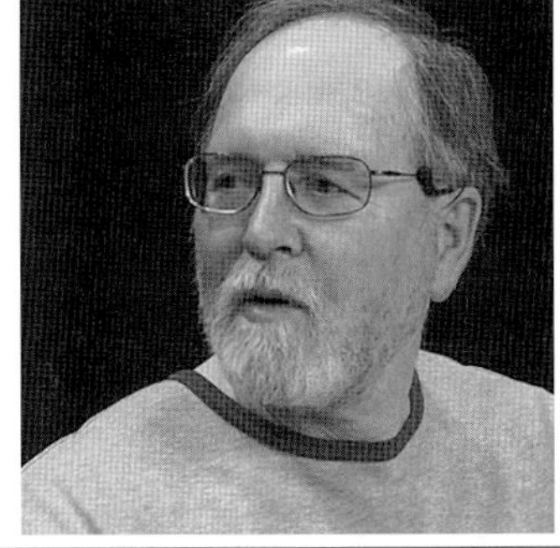	Mike is a 67-year-old man diagnosed with Parkinson's disease 11 years ago. He is married, living in his own home, and retired. He takes anti-Parkinson medications, but motor impairments fluctuate over his medication cycle. His concerns relate to balance and walking. He falls occasionally, particularly when his medication wears off.

(continued)

TABLE 1.4 Introduction to Case Studies (*continued*)

Bonnie 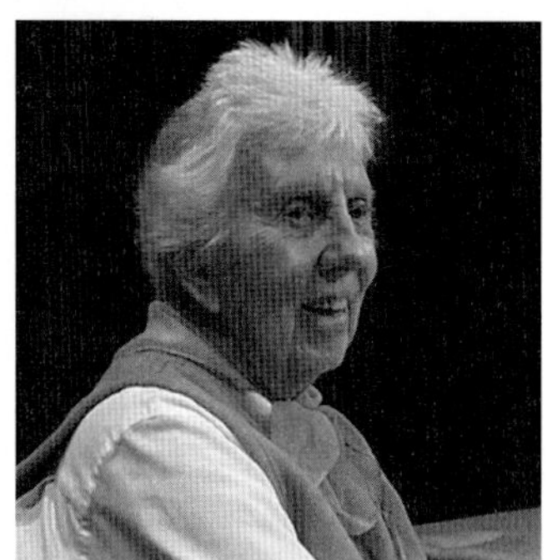	Bonnie is a 90-year-old woman with impaired balance resulting in multiple falls, two of which required hospitalization. She lives alone in an apartment and has a home health aide 3 days a week to assist her with shopping, cooking, and cleaning. Her main concerns relate to maintaining her physical and cognitive function so she can remain in her apartment and to reduce her falls.
Thomas 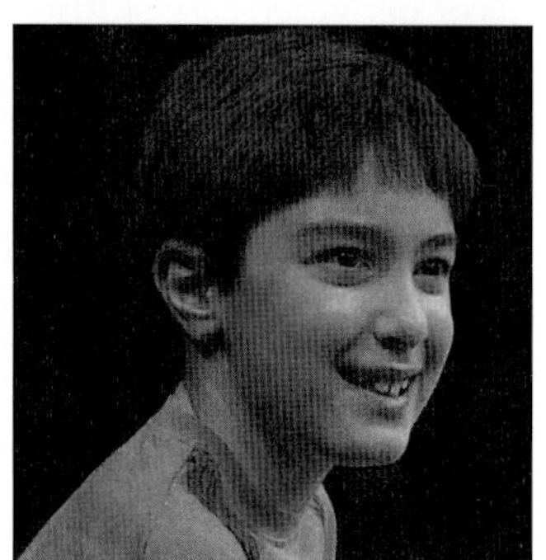	Thomas is a 7-year-old boy with spastic diplegia cerebral palsy. He is moderately involved and classified as a 3 on the Gross Motor Function Classification Scale. He lives with his parents and sister and likes to play piano and computer games. He receives therapy at school and twice a week at an outpatient clinic. Like his parents, his major concerns are his balance and walking since he falls several times a week.
Malachi 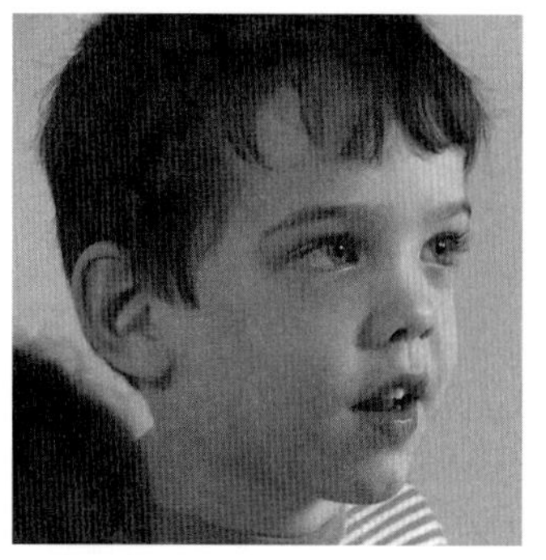	Malachi is a 4-year-old boy with mixed-type cerebral palsy (athetoid and spastic). He is severely involved and classified as a 4 on the Gross Motor Function Classification Scale. He lives with his parents and twin brother and likes to play with toys that have sound and light effects. His parents' major concerns relate to his oral motor function, which affects speech and feeding. In addition, they want to see Malachi gain his independence in functional motor skills, including sitting and upper-extremity function.
Genise 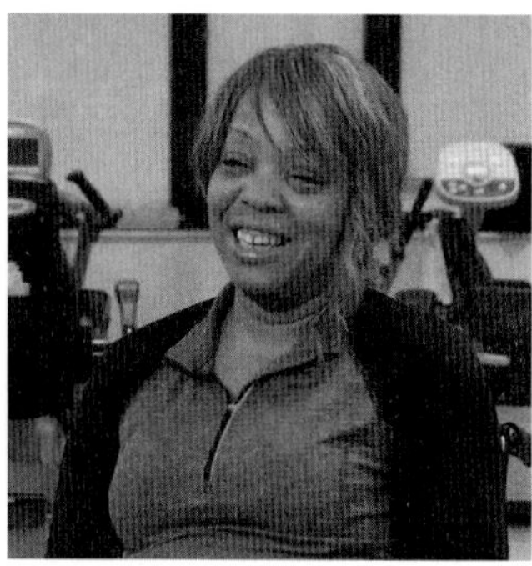	Genise is a 53-year-old woman who had a left cerebral vascular accident resulting in a right hemiparesis. Prior to her stroke, she was living independently with her husband. She was admitted to acute care for 4 days before being transferred to inpatient rehabilitation for 2 weeks. She was discharged home and continued to participate in outpatient therapy for 6 months. This video case study follows her recovery.

TABLE 1.4 Introduction to Case Studies (*continued*)

Sue 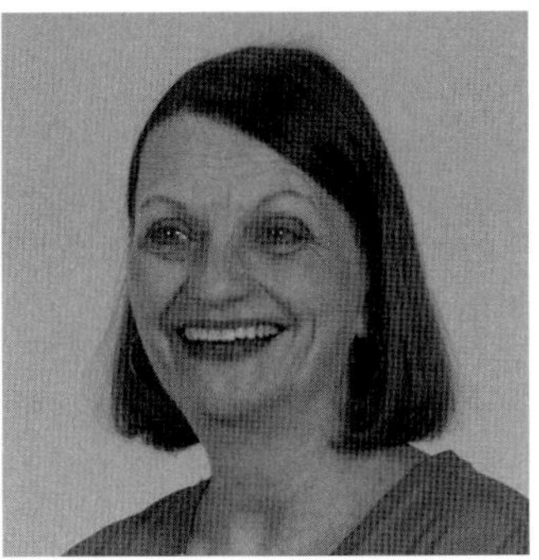	Sue is a 66-year-old woman who was diagnosed with relapsing–remitting multiple sclerosis 28 years ago. She lives with her husband and is retired. She is independent in personal ADLs but requires assistance with home care. Her concerns relate to impaired balance, weakness, and fatigue, all of which contribute to multiple falls.

ADLs, activities of daily living.

SUMMARY

1. Motor control is the ability to regulate the mechanisms essential to movement. Thus, the field of motor control is directed at studying the nature of movement and how that movement is controlled.
2. The specific practices used to examine and treat the patient with motor dyscontrol are determined by underlying assumptions about how movement is controlled, which come from specific theories of motor control.
3. A theory of motor control is a group of abstract ideas about the control of movement. Theories provide (a) a framework for interpreting behavior, (b) a guide for clinical action, (c) new ideas, and (d) working hypotheses for examination and intervention.
4. Rehabilitation practices reflect the theories or basic ideas we have about the nature of function and dysfunction.
5. This chapter reviews many motor control theories that influence our perspective regarding examination and intervention, including the reflex theory, hierarchical theory, motor programming theories, systems theory, and ecological theory.
6. In this textbook, we use a systems theory as the foundation for many clinical applications. According to systems theory, movement arises from the interaction of multiple processes, including (a) perceptual, cognitive, and motor processes within the individual and (b) interactions between the individual, the task, and the environment.
7. Clinical practices evolve in parallel with scientific theory, as clinicians assimilate changes in scientific theory and apply them to practice. Neurofacilitation approaches to intervention were developed in parallel with the reflex and hierarchical theories of motor control. New approaches to intervention, such as the task-oriented approach, are being developed in response to changing theories of motor control.

ANSWERS TO LAB ACTIVITY ASSIGNMENTS

Lab Activity 1.1

1. As you do this lab, you will find there are many ways to organize a taxonomy of tasks, since there are many attributes you could use to order tasks. You may also find that as therapists we often order tasks according to the stability demands associated with tasks.
2. You will find that it is easy to distinguish the easiest tasks (e.g., sitting with support) from the hardest tasks (e.g., walking on uneven surfaces while holding a cup of water), but it is not always easy to order intermediate tasks. This suggests that there is no "one" way to move through a progression of tasks, particularly the tasks that reflect an intermediate level of difficulty.

Lab Activity 1.2

1. You should see that regardless of the size or hand used to write your signature, there are common elements in each of the signatures.
2. These common elements may include the relationship of one letter to another, how certain letters are formed, and the tendency to stop and start certain letters in relatively the same place. These commonalities support the theory of motor programs.

CHAPTER 2

Motor Learning and Recovery of Function

Learning Objectives

Following completion of this chapter, the reader will be able to:

1. Define motor learning and discuss the similarities and differences between learning, performance, and recovery of function.
2. Understand the concept of attention and its relevance in the learning of new motor skills and during the retrieval of movement-related information.
3. Compare and contrast implicit and explicit forms of learning and give examples of each.
4. Discuss the basic concepts, clinical implications, and limitations of the following motor learning theories: Schmidt's schema theory and Newell's ecological theory.
5. Compare and contrast the following theories related to stages of motor learning: Fitts and Posner's three-stage theory, systems three-stage theory, and Gentile's two-stage theory.
6. Define intrinsic versus extrinsic feedback, give examples of each, and discuss their importance in teaching motor skills.
7. Discuss factors that have an impact on the structure of practice and describe their effect on performance versus learning.
8. Define recovery of function and describe the differences between recovery and compensation.
9. Discuss the effect of preinjury and postinjury factors on recovery of function following central nervous system injury.

INTRODUCTION TO MOTOR LEARNING

Before her stroke, Mrs. Genise T., a 53-year-old, was living independently in her own home with her husband and adult son. She enjoyed composing and performing songs, gardening, and socializing with her family and friends. She had an ischemic stroke affecting her left internal capsule resulting in a right hemiparesis. She spent 4 days in the hospital and then was transferred to an inpatient rehabilitation unit for 2 weeks of rehabilitation. She was discharged home and is continuing to receive outpatient therapy for residual problems related to her stroke. She is gradually regaining the ability to stand, walk, and perform personal activities of daily living (ADL), such as feeding, grooming, and dressing herself but has not regained her prestroke functional status. What are the factors that contribute to her recovery of motor function, and what are the factors that constrain it? How much of her initial recovery is due to "spontaneous recovery"? How much of her recovery may be attributed to therapeutic interventions? How much will she continue to improve? How many of the motor skills acquired in the rehabilitation facility will be retained and used when she returns home? These questions and issues reflect the importance of motor learning to clinicians involved in retraining the patient with motor control problems.

WHAT IS MOTOR LEARNING?

In Chapter 1, we defined the field of motor control as the study of the nature and control of movement. We define the field of motor learning as the study of the acquisition and/or modification of skilled actions. While motor control focuses on understanding the control of movement already acquired, motor learning focuses on understanding the acquisition and/or modification of skilled actions.

The field of motor learning has traditionally referred to the study of the acquisition or modification of movement in normal subjects. In contrast, recovery of function has referred to the reacquisition of movement skills lost through injury. While there is nothing inherent in the term "motor learning" to distinguish it from processes involved in the recovery of movement function, the two are often thought of as separate. This separation between recovery of function and motor learning may be misleading. Issues facing clinicians concerned with helping patients reacquire skills lost as a result of injury are similar to those faced by people engaged in motor learning research (Schmidt, 1991). Questions common to both include the following: How can I best structure practice (therapy) to ensure learning? How can I ensure that skills learned in one context transfer to others? Will simplifying a task (i.e., making it easier to perform) result in more efficient learning? What is the best way to promote neural plasticity and adaptation underlying the (re) acquisition of movement skills critical to the recovery of function? It is clear that learning underlies the recovery of function and the development of new skills in the face of neurologic and other disabling conditions (Fitts & Posner, 1967; Higgens & Spaeth, 1979; Winstein et al., 2014). Thus, motor learning research designed to answer these and other questions has important implications for therapists involved in helping patients to relearn skilled actions following acquired brain injury (Schmidt, 1991; Winstein et al., 2014).

In this chapter, we use the term "motor learning" to encompass both the acquisition and the reacquisition of movement. We will begin our study of motor learning by discussing important issues related to the nature of motor learning. Following this, we will explore different theories of motor learning, examining their underlying assumptions and clinical implications. We will discuss the practical applications of motor learning research. Finally, we will discuss issues related to recovery of function, including the many factors that affect a patient's ability to recover from brain injury.

NATURE OF MOTOR LEARNING

Early Definitions of Motor Learning

Learning has been described as the process of acquiring knowledge about the world; motor learning has been described as a set of processes associated with practice or experience leading to relatively permanent changes in the capability for producing skilled action. This definition of motor learning reflects four concepts: (a) learning is a process of acquiring the capability for skilled action; (b) learning results from experience or practice; (c) learning cannot be measured directly—instead, it is inferred from behavior; and (d) learning produces relatively permanent changes in behavior; thus, short-term alterations are not thought of as learning (Schmidt & Lee, 2011).

Broadening the Definition of Motor Learning

In this chapter, the definition of motor learning has been expanded to encompass many aspects not traditionally considered as part of motor learning. Motor learning involves more than motor processes; it involves learning new strategies for sensing as well as moving. Thus, motor learning, like motor control, emerges from a complex of perception, cognition, and action processes.

Previous views of motor learning have focused primarily on changes in the individual. But the process of motor learning can be described as the search for a task solution that emerges from an interaction of the individual with the task and the environment. Task solutions are strategies for perceiving and acting (Newell, 1991).

Similarly, the recovery of function involves the search for new solutions in relationship to specific tasks and environments given the new constraints imposed on the individual by neural pathology. Thus, one cannot study motor learning or recovery of function outside the context of how individuals solve functional tasks in specific environments.

Relating Performance and Learning

Traditionally, the study of motor learning has focused solely on motor outcomes. Earlier views of motor learning did not always distinguish it from performance (Schmidt & Lee, 2011). Changes in performance that resulted from practice were usually thought to reflect changes in learning. However, this view failed to consider that certain practice effects improved performance initially but were not necessarily retained, which is a condition of learning. This led to the notion that learning could not be evaluated during practice but rather during specific retention or transfer tests. Thus, learning, defined as a relatively permanent change, has been distinguished from a change in performance, defined as a temporary change in motor behavior seen during practice sessions (e.g., sensorimotor adaptation).

For example, Genise, our patient with an acute stroke, has shown an improved ability to sit and stand symmetrically (with weight evenly distributed to both legs) at the end of her daily therapy session, but when she returns to therapy the following day, she again stands with all her weight on her noninvolved leg. This suggests that while performance had improved in response to therapy, learning had not yet occurred. When on subsequent days Genise demonstrates a more symmetric weight-bearing stance even as she arrives for therapy, we may suggest that learning (a permanent change in behavior) is occurring.

Attention and Motor Learning

Learning new actions is a complex procedure in which a person needs to attend to a continuous influx of information from the action *per se* and the surrounding environment. However, the person might opt to focus on the environment, movement itself (internal focus), or movement outcomes (external focus) (Magill & Anderson, 2014). The cognitive process by which people can detect, select, sustain, or shift awareness among a myriad of relevant information and stimuli is known as attention.

Attention is limited, complex, and multidimensional (Song, 2019). Attention presents itself in a broad diversity of forms with distinct components. Attention may be selective when improvements in performance are observed for a particular task, an object, or a stimulus feature that is significant to the individual; in addition, attention may be nonselective, as when a certain level of effort (i.e., arousal) is required to maintain a high level of performance across different tasks (Luo & Maunsell, 2019). Attention can also be either externally driven (i.e., exogenous attention) or internally generated (i.e., endogenous attention). Exogenous attention requires bottom–up control, which is stimulus driven and automatically controlled by a salient stimulus, such as sounds or fast-moving and colorful objects. In contrast, endogenous attention uses top–down control and is goal oriented and internally driven (Knudsen, 2007; Miller & Buschman, 2013). The main constructs that comprise attention—focused, sustained, selective, alternating, and divided—are reviewed in Chapter 5.

Attention and working memory are highly interrelated. Attentional processing is used (a) to detect and select essential information from the environment, (b) during memory storage, and (c) when selecting the domain (e.g., verbal, mathematical, or visuospatial) that will be accessed by working memory—a process defined as competitive selection. In seconds, working memory can store a limited amount of critical information needed to plan and elaborate more complex behaviors (Knudsen, 2007). Thus, cognitive resources such as attention and memory are a cornerstone for both motor learning and motor performance. Studies show an interaction between attention and motor skill acquisition, between attention and motor memory (procedural memory), and between internally and externally driven attentional processing and motor performance (Song, 2019).

This interaction between cognitive and motor systems is particularly relevant in complex real-life situations, which require processing multiple sensory inputs (both expected and unexpected) in order to adapt actions to changing conditions, thus increasing the attentional processing demands. Let's examine how this complex interaction between cognitive and motor systems impacts gait retraining in Genise, our patient with an acute stroke. Genise's gait training program includes improving her ability to walk in the clinic as well as in her community. The clinic is often a controlled environment, characterized by little variability; thus, walking in this environment requires relatively low levels of sustained attention. However, walking in the community requires adapting gait to complex environmental demands such as negotiating a curb while crossing a road or avoiding collisions with people and objects. In this situation, Genise will need to recall and modify previously learned gait patterns to a complex environment, and this will increase the cognitive demands associated with walking. When walking in the community, she will need to use attentional resources to process relevant information such as surface features (e.g., uneven or slippery grounds), navigate curbs, monitor traffic lights for the "go" or "stop" signal, and identify objects or other people walking nearby that must be avoided, while simultaneously disregarding distracting stimuli (e.g., noise or car sounds). In addition, she will have to overcome difficulties (e.g., poor light and rough weather) that may interfere in the control of balance and gait, placing her at risk for a fall. Walking in a complex community environment requires Genise to use internally driven attentional resources to identify relevant environmental features that impact the planning and execution of an appropriate gait pattern. In addition, externally driven attentional processes will be required to detect unexpected environmental stimuli such as a changing traffic light or the sudden approach of a car so that she can adapt her gait pattern quickly to the new environmental demands.

Forms of Learning

The recovery of function following injury involves the reacquisition of complex tasks. However, it is difficult to understand the processes involved in learning using the study of complex tasks. Therefore, many researchers have begun by exploring simple to more complex forms of learning, with the understanding that these simple forms of learning are the basis for the acquisition of skilled behavior.

We begin by reviewing different forms of learning and discussing some of their clinical applications. We then consider theories of motor learning that have been developed to describe the acquisition of skilled behavior and suggest how each might be used to explain the acquisition of a skill such as reaching for a glass of water. At the outset, we provide an overview of the categories of memory and learning.

Basic Forms of Long-Term Memory: Nondeclarative (Implicit) and Declarative (Explicit)

Studies of patients with memory deficits due to bilateral medial temporal lobe lesions have shown that these patients show a profound loss of the ability to remember factual knowledge. This type of memory, usually called "declarative memory" or "explicit memory," involves the association of information related to people or things one has encountered, places one has been, and the meaning of these bits of information. On the other hand, the patients still possess other forms of long-term memory related to motor skills and simple learning tasks such as habituation, sensitization, and classical conditioning. Figure 2.1 shows two major categories of long-term memory that we will discuss next, nondeclarative (or implicit) and declarative (or explicit), and the different types of learning embedded within them. We will see that much of motor learning is nondeclarative or implicit.

Nondeclarative (Implicit) Forms of Learning

As you see in Figure 2.1, nondeclarative learning can be divided into a number of subtypes, each controlled by different parts of the brain. We will begin our discussion of nondeclarative learning with nonassociative forms of learning, which are the simplest forms of learning, involving reflex pathways.

Nonassociative Forms of Learning. Nonassociative learning occurs when animals are given a single stimulus repeatedly. As a result, the nervous system learns about the characteristics of that stimulus. Habituation and sensitization are two very simple forms of nonassociative learning. Habituation is a decrease in responsiveness that occurs as a result of repeated exposure to a nonpainful stimulus (Kandel et al., 2000b).

Habituation is used in many different ways in the clinical setting. For example, habituation exercises are used to treat dizziness in patients with certain types of vestibular dysfunction. Patients are asked to repeatedly move in ways that provoke their dizziness. This repetition results in habituation of the dizziness response. Habituation also forms the basis of therapy for children whose behavior is termed "tactile defensive," that is, children who show excessive responsiveness to cutaneous stimulation. Children are repeatedly exposed to gradually increasing levels of cutaneous inputs in an effort to decrease their sensitivity to this stimulus.

Sensitization is an increased responsiveness following a threatening or noxious stimulus (Kandel et al., 2000b). For example, if I receive a painful stimulus on the skin and then a light touch, I will react more strongly than I normally would to the light touch. After a person has habituated to one stimulus, a painful stimulus can dishabituate the response to the first. That is, sensitization counteracts the effects of habituation.

There are times when increasing a patient's sensitivity to a threatening stimulus is important. For example, increasing a patient's awareness of stimuli indicating likelihood for impending falls might be an important aspect of balance retraining.

Associative Forms of Learning. A second type of nondeclarative or implicit learning is associative learning. What is associative learning? It is through associative learning that a person learns to predict relationships, either relationships of one stimulus to another (classical conditioning) or the relationship of one's behavior to a consequence (operant conditioning). For example, when a patient recovering from a stroke, through repeated practice, begins to learn to redefine their stability limits so that they do not put so much weight on their involved limb that they fall, they are undergoing associative learning and, specifically, operant

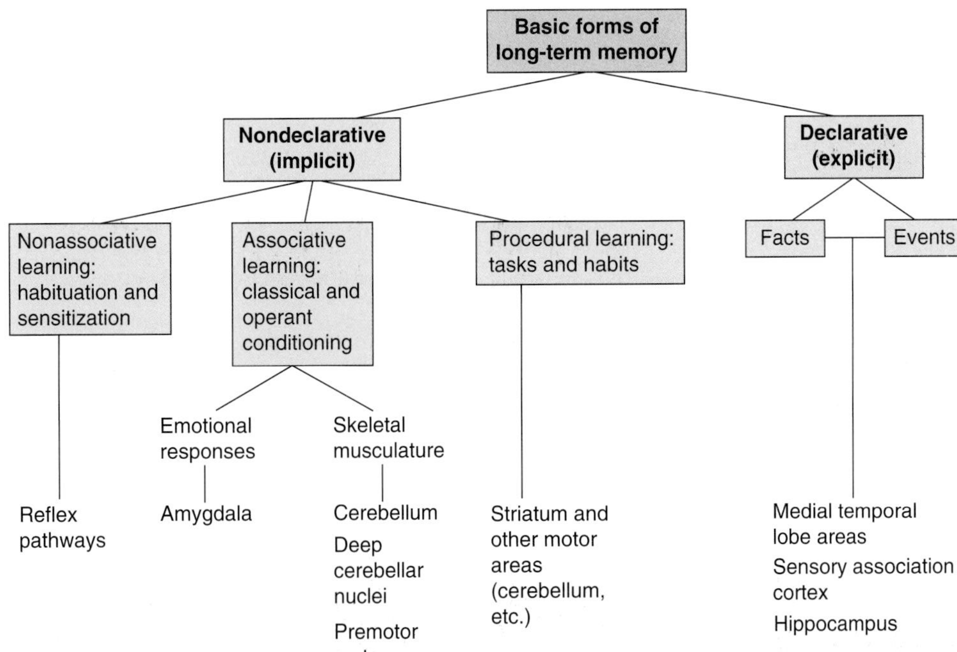

Figure 2.1 Basic forms of long-term memory.

conditioning. That is, they are learning that stability is associated with a new strategy of weight support.

It has been suggested that associative learning has evolved to help animals learn to detect causal relationships in the environment. Establishing lawful and therefore predictive relationships among events is part of the process of making sense and order of our world. Recognizing key relationships between events is an essential part of the ability to adapt behavior to novel situations (Kandel et al., 2000b).

Patients who have suffered an injury that has drastically altered their ability to sense and move in their world have the task of reexploring their body in relationship to their world in order to determine what new relationships exist between the two. Pavlov studied how humans and animals learn the association of two stimuli through the simple form of learning that is now called "classical conditioning."

Classical conditioning. Classical conditioning consists of learning to pair two stimuli. During classical conditioning, an initially weak stimulus (the conditioned stimulus [CS]) becomes highly effective in producing a response when it becomes associated with another, stronger, stimulus (the unconditioned stimulus [UCS]). The CS is usually something that initially produces no response (like a bell). In contrast, the UCS, which could be food, always produces a response. After repeated pairing of the CS and the UCS, one begins to see a conditioned response (CR) to the CS. Remember, it originally produced no response (Kandel et al., 2000b).

What the subject is doing in this type of learning is to predict relationships between two stimuli or events that have occurred and to respond accordingly. For example, in a therapy setting, if we repeatedly give patients a verbal cue in conjunction with physical assistance when making a movement, they may eventually begin to make the movement with only the verbal cue.

Thus, as patients gain skills, we see them move along the continuum of assistance, from hands-on assistance from the therapist to performing the task with verbal cues and eventually to performing the action unassisted.

It has been shown that we generally learn relationships that are relevant to our survival; it is more difficult to associate biologically meaningless events. These findings underscore an important learning principle: the brain is most likely to perceive and integrate aspects of the environment that are most pertinent. With regard to therapy, patients are most likely to learn tasks in environments that are relevant and meaningful to them.

Operant conditioning. Operant, or instrumental, conditioning is a second type of associative learning (Kandel et al., 2000b). It is basically trial-and-error learning. During operant conditioning, we learn to associate a certain response, from among many that we have made, with a consequence. The classic experiments in this area were done with animals that were given food rewards whenever they randomly pressed a lever inside their cages. They soon learned to associate the lever press with the presentation of food and the frequency of lever pressing became very high.

The principle of operant conditioning could be stated as follows: behaviors that are rewarded tend to be repeated at the cost of other behaviors. And likewise, behaviors followed by aversive stimuli are not usually repeated. This has been called the "law of effect" (Kandel et al., 2000b).

Operant conditioning plays a major role in determining the behaviors shown by patients referred for therapy. For example, the frail older adult who leaves her home to go shopping and experiences a fall is less likely to repeat that activity. A decrease in activity results in declining physical function, which in turn increases the likelihood that she will fall. This increased likelihood for falls will reinforce her desire to be inactive, and on it goes, showing the law of effect in action. Therapists may make use of a variety of interventions to assist this patient in regaining her activity level and in reducing her likelihood of falling. One intervention may be the use of desensitization to decrease her anxiety and fear of falling—for example, practicing walking in outdoor situations that have engendered fear in the past.

Operant conditioning can be an effective tool during clinical intervention. Verbal praise by a therapist for a job well done serves as a reinforcer for some (though not all) patients. Setting up a therapy session so that a particular movement is rewarded by the successful accomplishment of a task desired by the patient is a powerful example of operant conditioning.

Regions of the brain that contribute to these types of implicit memory include the cerebellum and the deep cerebellar nuclei for movement conditioning (e.g., for certain types of classical conditioning and to gain control of reflexes, such as the vestibuloocular reflex), the amygdala for adaptation involving the emotions (e.g., for conditioned fear, such as the fear of falling in an older adult, after an injurious fall), and the lateral dorsal premotor areas of the cortex (for associating a particular sensory event with a specific movement). As shown in Figure 2.1, regions of the brain that contribute to these types of implicit memory. (Kandel et al., 2000b; Krakauer & Ghez, 2000).

Procedural Learning. Another type of nondeclarative or implicit learning is procedural learning, which refers to learning tasks that can be performed automatically without attention or conscious thought, like a habit. Procedural learning develops slowly through repetition of an act over many trials, and it is expressed through improved performance of the task that was practiced. Like other forms of implicit learning, procedural learning does not require awareness, attention, or other higher cognitive processes. During motor skill acquisition, repeating a movement continuously under varying circumstances would typically lead to procedural learning. That is, one automatically learns the movement itself, or the rules for moving, called a "movement schema."

For example, when teaching a patient to transfer from chair to bed, we often have the patient practice the task repeatedly in order to learn a movement strategy that is effective in performing a transfer task. To better prepare patients to transfer effectively in a wide variety of situations and contexts, patients practice under different conditions in order to learn to move from chairs of differing heights and at different positions relative to the bed. They thus begin to form the rules associated with the task of transfer. The development of rules for transferring will allow them to safely transfer in unfamiliar circumstances. Practicing tasks repeatedly under varying contexts results in efficient procedural learning underlying the reacquisition of effective and safe transfers. As shown in Figure 2.1, the striatum of the basal ganglia is critical to procedural learning (Kandel et al., 2000b).

Declarative or Explicit Learning

While nondeclarative or implicit learning is more reflexive, automatic, or habitual in character and requires frequent repetition for its formation, declarative learning results in knowledge that can be consciously recalled and thus requires processes such as awareness, attention, and reflection (Kandel et al., 2000b). As noted previously, it involves the ability to remember factual knowledge (often related to objects, places, or events). Declarative learning can be expressed in declarative sentences: "first I button the top button, then the next one." Therapists often use declarative learning when helping patients reacquire functional skills. They may teach a specific sequence to a patient who is having difficulty moving from sitting to standing: first move to the edge of the chair, lean forward "nose over toes," and then stand up. Constant repetition can transform declarative into nondeclarative or procedural knowledge. In our example, when patients are first learning to stand, they may verbally describe the steps as they do them. However, with repetition, the movement of standing up becomes an automatic motor activity—that is, one that does not require conscious attention and monitoring.

The advantage of declarative learning is that it can be practiced in ways other than the one in which it was learned. For example, expert ski racers, when preparing to race down a slalom hill at 120 miles an hour, rehearse in their minds the race and how they will run it. Also, prior to getting on the ice, figure skaters preparing to perform will often mentally practice the sequences they will skate.

In therapy, when helping patients reacquire skills lost through injury, should the emphasis be on procedural (implicit) learning or declarative (explicit) learning? This is a complex issue and depends in part on the location and type of central nervous system (CNS) pathology. As discussed in more detail in Chapter 5, some types of neural pathology impair implicit learning, while others affect explicit learning. Since declarative learning requires the ability to verbally express the process to be performed, it cannot easily be used with patients who have cognitive and/or language deficits that impair their ability to recall and express knowledge. Teaching movement skills declaratively would, however, allow patients to rehearse their movements mentally, increasing the amount of practice available to them when physical conditions such as fatigue would normally limit it.

Neural circuitry underlying declarative learning includes input from the sensory association cortices that synthesize somatosensory, visual, and auditory sensations; medial temporal lobe areas (including parahippocampal and perirhinal cortices, the entorhinal cortex, and the dentate gyrus); the hippocampus; and the subiculum. The right hippocampus is especially important for spatial representation—that is, memory for space and context—and the left hippocampus is more important for memories of words and objects. A lesion to any one of these components would have a major impact on declarative learning and memory. However, long-term memory is stored in the association cortices, so damage to these areas does not affect early memories (Kandel et al., 2000b).

Declarative or explicit learning also involves four different types of processing: encoding, consolidation, storage, and retrieval. Encoding involves the circuitry just described and requires attention. The extent of the encoding is determined by the level of motivation, the extent of attention to the information, and the ability to associate it meaningfully with information that is already in memory. Consolidation includes the process of making the information stable for long-term memory storage and involves structural changes in neurons. Storage involves the long-term retention of memories and has a vast capacity compared to the limited capacity of short-term or working memory. Retrieval involves the recall of information from different long-term storage sites. It is subject to distortion, since an individual reconstructs the memories from a combination of different sites. Interestingly, it is most accurate when retrieved in the same context in which it was created (Kandel et al., 2000b).

One last type of memory that is critical for the encoding and recall of long-term memory is working, or short-term, memory. This memory system consists of an attentional control system, also known as the central executive (located in the prefrontal cortex), and two rehearsal systems, the articulatory loop for rehearsing language and the visuospatial sketch pad for vision and action (located in different parts of the posterior parietal or visual association cortex).

This information suggests that teaching movement skills can be optimized when the patient is highly motivated, attending fully to the task, and able to relate or integrate the new information to information they already know about the task. When retraining gait, it would thus be important to find a goal that is important to the patient, such as being able to walk to the mailbox for the newspaper, to work with them in an environment in which they can attend fully to the task instructions and their own performance outcome, and to relate instructions for improved gait characteristics to previous knowledge so that they can remember them after the therapy session is over.

THEORIES OF MOTOR LEARNING

Just as there are theories of motor control, there are theories of motor learning, that is, a group of abstract ideas about the nature and control of the acquisition or modification of skilled action. Theories of motor learning, like theories of motor control, must be based on current knowledge regarding the structure and function of the nervous system. The following sections review theories of motor learning; also included is a brief discussion of several theories related to recovery of function.

Schmidt's Schema Theory

In the 1970s, Richard Schmidt, a researcher from the field of physical education, proposed a new motor learning theory, which he called the "schema theory." It emphasized open-loop control processes and the generalized motor program concept (Schmidt, 1975). Although the concept of motor programs was considered essential to understanding motor control, no one had yet addressed the question of how motor programs can be learned. As had other researchers before him, Schmidt proposed that motor programs do not contain the specifics of movements but instead contain generalized rules for a specific class of movements. He predicted that when learning a new motor program, the individual learns a generalized set of rules that can be applied to a variety of contexts.

At the heart of this motor learning theory is the concept of schema, which has been important in psychology for many years. The term "schema" originally referred to an abstract representation stored in memory following multiple presentations of a class of objects. For example, after seeing many different types of dogs, it is proposed that we begin to store an abstract set of rules for general dog qualities in our brain, so that whenever we see a new dog, no matter what size, color, or shape, we can identify it as a dog. The schema theory of motor learning is equivalent to the motor programming theory of motor control. At the heart of both theories is the generalized motor program. The generalized motor program is considered to contain the rules for creating the spatial and temporal patterns of muscle activity needed to carry out a given movement (Schmidt & Lee, 2011).

Schmidt proposed that, after an individual makes a movement, four things are available for brief storage in short-term memory: (a) the initial movement conditions, such as the position of the body and the weight of the object manipulated; (b) the parameters used in the generalized motor program (overall duration, overall force, and muscle-selection); (c) the outcome of the movement, in terms of knowledge of results (KR); and (d) the sensory consequences of the movement—that is, how it felt, looked, and sounded. This information is stored in short-term memory only long enough to be abstracted into two schemas: the recall schema (motor) and a recognition schema (sensory).

The recall schema is used to select a specific response. Schmidt and Lee (2011) suggest that it may be created in the following way. Each time a person makes a movement with a particular goal in mind, they use a particular movement parameter, such as a given force, and then receive input about the movement's accuracy. After making repeated movements using different parameters causing different outcomes, the nervous system creates a relationship between the size of the parameter and the movement outcome. Each new movement adds a new data point to the internal system to refine the rule. After each movement, the sources of information are not retained in the recall schema but only the rule that was created.

When making a given movement, the initial conditions and desired goal of the movement are inputs to the recall schema. The initial conditions (e.g., lifting a heavy vs. a light object) may alter, for example, the slope of the line, representing the rule.

The recognition schema is used to evaluate the response. In this case, the sensory consequences and outcomes of previous similar movements are coupled with the current initial conditions to create a representation of the expected sensory consequences. This is then compared to the sensory information from the ongoing movement in order to evaluate the efficiency of the response. When a person makes a movement, they select the outcome wanted and choose the initial conditions. With the recognition schema rule, the person can determine the expected sensory consequences, which help with movement evaluation. When the movement is over, any error information is fed back into the schema and the schema is modified as a result of the sensory feedback and KR. Thus, according to this theory, learning consists of the ongoing process of updating the recognition and recall schemas with each movement that is made.

One of the predictions of schema theory is that variability of practice should improve motor learning. Schmidt hypothesized that learning was affected not only by the extent of practice but by the variability of practice. Thus, with increased variability of practice, the generalized motor program rules were made stronger. A second prediction is that a particular movement may be produced accurately, even if it has never been made before, if it is based on a rule that has previously been created as part of a similar movement that has been practiced earlier.

Clinical Implications

What are some of the clinical implications of schema theory? According to schema theory, when our patient Genise is learning a new movement task such as reaching for a glass of milk with her affected limb, optimal learning will occur if this task is practiced under many different conditions. This will allow her to develop a set of rules for reaching (recall schema), which then could be applied when reaching for a variety of glasses and cups. As she practices reaching and lifting, sensory information about the initial conditions and consequences of her reaches will be used to form a recognition schema, which will be used to evaluate the accuracy of future reaches. As rules for reaching improve, Genise will become more capable of generating appropriate reaching strategies for picking up an unfamiliar glass, with less likelihood of dropping the glass or spilling the drink. Practicing reaching under many different conditions is essential then to forming accurate recall and recognition schemas.

Limitations

Is schema theory supported by research? Yes and no. As mentioned previously, one of the predictions of schema theory is that when practicing a skill, variable forms of practice will produce the most effective schema or motor program. Research to test this prediction has used the following paradigms. Two groups of subjects are trained in a new task, one given constant practice conditions and the other given variable practice conditions. Both groups are then tested on a new but similar movement. According to schema theory, the second group should show higher-level performance than the first, because they have developed a broad set of rules about the task, which should allow them to apply the rules to a new situation. On the other hand, the first group should have developed a very narrow schema with limited rules that would not be easily applicable to new situations.

In studies on normal adults, the support is mixed. Many studies show large effects of variable practice, while some studies show very small effects or no effect at all. However, with regard to studies in children, there has been strong support. For example, 7- and 9-year-old children were trained to toss beanbags over variable distances or a fixed distance. When asked to throw at a new distance, the variable practice group produced significantly better scores than the fixed practice group (Kerr & Booth, 1977). Why might there be differences between children and adults in these experiments? It has been suggested that it may be difficult to find experimental tasks for which adults do not already have significant variable practice during normal activities, while children, with much less experience, are more naive subjects (Shapiro & Schmidt, 1982). Therefore, the experiments may be more valid in children.

Another limitation of the theory is that it lacks specificity. It does not predict how the generalized motor program or the other schemata are created—that is, how a person makes their first movement before any schema exists. In addition, because of its generalized nature, there are few recognizable mechanisms that can be tested. Thus, it is not clear how schema processing itself interacts with other systems during motor learning and how it aids in the control of that movement.

Ecological Theory

Karl Newell drew heavily from both systems and ecological motor control theories to create a theory of motor learning based on the concept of search strategies (Newell, 1991). In the previous learning theory proposed by Schmidt (1975), practice produced a cumulative continuous change in behavior due to a gradual buildup of the strength of motor programs. It was proposed that, with practice, a more appropriate representation of action is developed.

In contrast, Newell suggests that motor learning is a process that increases the coordination between perception and action in a way that is consistent with the task and environmental constraints. What does he mean by this? He proposes that during practice, there is a search for optimal strategies to solve the task. Part of the search for optimal strategies involves not merely finding the appropriate motor response for the task but finding the most appropriate perceptual cues as well. Thus, both perception and action systems are incorporated or mapped into an optimal task solution.

Critical to the search for optimal strategies is the exploration of the perceptual and motor workspaces. Exploring the perceptual workspace involves exploring all the possible perceptual cues in order to identify those that are most relevant to the performance of a specific task. Perceptual cues that are critical to the way in which a task is executed are also called "regulatory cues" (Gentile, 1972). Likewise, exploring the motor workspace involves exploring the range of movements possible in order to select the optimal or most efficient movements for the task. Optimal solutions then incorporate relevant perceptual cues and optimal movement strategies for a specific task. Newell believes that one useful outcome of his theory will be the impetus to identify critical perceptual variables essential to optimal task-relevant solutions. These critical variables will be useful in designing search strategies that produce efficient mapping of perceptual information and movement parameters.

According to the ecological theory, perceptual information has a number of roles in motor learning. In a prescriptive role, perceptual information relates to understanding the goal of the task and the movements to be learned. This information has typically been given to learners through demonstrations.

Another role of perceptual information is as feedback, both during the movement (concurrent feedback, sometimes called "knowledge of performance [KP]"), and on completion of the movement (KR). Finally, it is proposed that perceptual information can be used to structure the search for a perceptual or motor solution that is appropriate for the demands of the task. Thus, in this approach, motor learning is characterized by optimal task-relevant mapping of perception and action, not by a rule-based representation of action.

Newell discusses ways to augment skill learning. The first is to help the learner understand the nature of the perceptual or motor workspace. The second is to understand the natural search strategies used by performers in exploring space. The third is that of providing augmented information to facilitate the search. One central prediction of this theory is that the transfer of motor skills is dependent on the similarity between the two tasks, but more specifically on the similarity between the optimal perceptual/motor strategies. Transfer of motor skills in this theory is relatively independent of the muscles used or the objects manipulated in the task.

In summary, this new approach to motor learning emphasizes dynamic exploratory activity of the perceptual/motor workspace in order to create optimal strategies for performing a task.

Clinical Implications

What are the clinical implications of the ecological theory of motor learning? As in the schema theory, when our patient Genise is relearning a movement with her affected arm, such as reaching for a glass, repeated practice with reaching for a variety of glasses that contain a variety of substances within them results in learning to match the appropriate movement dynamics for the task of reaching. But in addition, the ecological theory suggests that Genise must also learn to distinguish the relevant perceptual cues important to organizing action. Relevant perceptual cues for reaching and lifting a glass of milk include the size of the glass, how slippery the surface is, and how full it is. Thus, in order to relearn to reach, Genise must not only develop effective motor strategies, she must also learn to recognize relevant perceptual cues and match them to optimal motor strategies. If a perceptual cue suggests a heavy glass, she will need to grasp with more force. If the glass is full, the speed and trajectory of the movement must be modified to accommodate the situation. If Genise is unable to recognize these essential perceptual cues, a motor strategy that is less than optimal will be generated. That is, she may spill the fluid outside the glass or the glass may slip.

Perceptual cues such as the color of the glass are nonregulatory cues, which are not essential to the development of optimal movement strategies for grasping. Thus, during recovery of motor skills, an important part of "motor learning" is learning to discriminate relevant from irrelevant perceptual cues.

Limitations

Though this theory takes into account more of the variables that need to be considered in motor learning (dealing with interactions between the individual, the task, and the environment), it is still a very new theory. One of its major limitations is that it has yet to be applied to specific examples of motor skill acquisition in any systematic way.

THEORIES RELATED TO STAGES OF LEARNING MOTOR SKILLS

Another set of theories focuses on motor learning from a temporal perspective and attempts to more carefully characterize the learning process. These theories begin by describing initial stages of skill acquisition and describe how learning occurs over time.

Fitts and Posner's Three-Stage Model

Fitts and Posner (1967), two researchers from the field of psychology, described a theory of motor learning related to the stages involved in learning a new skill. They suggest that there are three main phases involved in skill learning. In the first stage, the learner is concerned with understanding the nature of the task, developing strategies that could be used to carry out the task, and determining how the task should be evaluated. These efforts require a high degree of cognitive activity, such as attention. Accordingly, this stage is referred to as the "cognitive stage of learning."

In this stage, the person experiments with a variety of strategies, abandoning those that do not work while keeping those that do. Performance tends to be quite variable, perhaps because many strategies for performing the task are being sampled. However, improvements in performance are also quite large in this first stage, perhaps as a result of selecting the most effective strategy for the task.

Fitts and Posner call the second stage in skill acquisition "the associative stage." By this time, the person has selected the best strategy for the task and now begins to refine the skill. Thus, there is less variability in performance during this stage, and improvement also occurs more slowly. It is proposed that verbal/cognitive aspects of learning are not as important at this stage because the person focuses more on refining a particular pattern rather than on selecting among alternative strategies (Schmidt & Lee, 2011). This stage may last from days to weeks or months, depending on the performer and the intensity of practice.

The third stage of skill acquisition has been called the "autonomous stage." Fitts and Posner define this stage by the automaticity of the skill and the low degree of attention required for its performance, as shown in

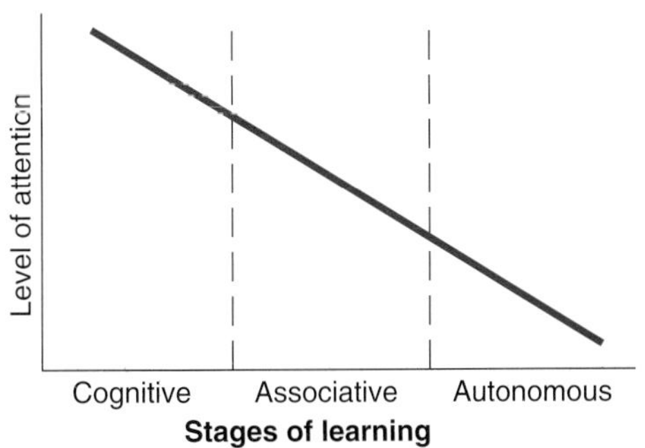

Figure 2.2 The changing attentional demands associated with the three stages of motor skill acquisition outlined by Fitts and Posner (1967).

Figure 2.2. Thus, the person can begin to devote their attention to other aspects of the skill in general, like scanning the environment for obstacles that might impede performance, or they may choose to focus on a secondary task (like talking to a friend while performing the task) or to save their energy, so as not to become fatigued.

Several research studies have supported the hypothesis that during later stages of motor learning, as a motor skill becomes more automated, it requires less attentional resources, and in fact paying too much attention to the elements of the task may reduce performance (Beilock et al., 2002; Wulf & Weigelt, 1997). For example, Perkins-Ceccato et al. (2003) have shown that when asked to focus attention on the motor elements of a task, such as focusing on the form of the golf swing and adjusting the force for the distance they were from the target (internal focus), novices, who were just learning the skill, became better as compared with using an external focus (hitting the ball as close to the target as possible). In contrast, experts in the skill actually showed the opposite effect, with performance decrements when using internal focus on the elements of the swing. In a study by Beilock et al. (2002), experienced golfers were more accurate at putting under dual-task conditions than when focusing attention on step-by-step putting performance. In addition, expert soccer players performed better at dribbling under dual-task conditions with their dominant right foot but performed better in the skill-focused condition when using their less-skilled left foot. Novices also performed better when skill focused, regardless of the foot they used. This suggests that performance of a well-learned task can actually be improved when practiced with a secondary task. Why would this happen? It is possible that focusing cognitive resources on a well-learned task that has become automated actually interferes with the automatic motor control processes.

Clinical Implications

How can the three-stage model help us to understand the acquisition of motor skills in patients? This theory suggests that Genise (our patient who has had stroke) would learn to reach for a glass in the following way. When first learning to reach for the glass, the task would require a great deal of attention and conscious thought. Genise would initially make a lot of errors and spill a lot of water, while she experimented with different movement strategies to accomplish the task. When moving into the second stage, however, her movements toward the glass would become refined as she developed an optimal strategy. At this point, the task would not require her full attention. In the third autonomous stage, Genise would be able to reach for the glass while carrying on a conversation or being engaged in other tasks.

Bernstein's Three-Stage Approach to Motor Learning: Mastering Degrees of Freedom

Another theory related to the stages of motor learning comes originally from work by Bernstein (1967) and was subsequently extended by researchers in the area of dynamical systems theory and motor development (Fentress, 1973; Newell & van Emmerik, 1989; Southard & Higgins, 1987). In this theory, the emphasis is on controlling degrees of freedom of the body segments involved in the movement as a central component of learning a new movement skill. In the first stage, there is a reduction of the number of degrees of freedom of the joints to be controlled to a minimum—a reduced joint range of motion with a high correlation between the movement of paired joints. This theory suggests that when a novice or an infant is first learning a new skill, the degrees of freedom of the body are constrained as they perform the task, in order to make the task easier to perform (i.e., freezing the degrees of freedom strategy). A recent review indicates that the CNS strategy of freezing the degrees of freedom to learn novel movements and sport skills has been investigated in a great diversity of scenarios such as handwriting with the non-preferred hand, dart throwing, skiing simulators, football kicking, volleyball serve, or walking on hands and feet (Guimarães et al., 2020). For example, a person first learning to use a hammer may co-contract agonist and antagonist muscles at the wrist joint to stiffen this joint and primarily control hammer movement at the elbow. The learner can perform the task reasonably accurately at this stage, but the movement is not energetically efficient, and the performer is not able to deal flexibly with environmental changes. As the task is gradually mastered, the learner begins to release the degrees of freedom at the wrist and learns to coordinate the movements at the two joints, which allows for more movement efficiency, freedom, and exploration and, thus, overall skill. It seems that the interaction between the skill class (i.e., discrete vs. continuous) and the objective of the skill (e.g., balance, velocity, or accuracy) could determine the level of freezing/freeing of degrees of freedom (Guimarães et al., 2020). This tendency to freeze degrees of freedom during the early stages of learning a task can be seen during the development of balance control. A newly standing infant may freeze the degrees of freedom of the legs and trunk and sway only about the ankle joints in response to threats to balance. Gradually, with experience and practice, infants may increase the degrees of freedom used, as they learn to control sway at the hip as well (Woollacott et al., 1998).

Vereijken et al. (1992) have taken this approach and used it to develop a model of the stages of motor learning. They suggest that the first stage of motor learning is the novice stage, in which the learner simplifies the movement in order to reduce the degrees of freedom. They suggest that this is accomplished by constraining or coupling multiple joints, so they move in unison, and by fixing the angles of many of the joints involved in the movement. These constraints are made at the cost of efficiency and flexibility in response to changing task or environmental demands.

In the second stage, called the advanced stage, the performer begins to release additional degrees of freedom, by allowing movements at more joints involved in the task. Now, the joints can be controlled independently as necessary for the task requirements. Simultaneous contraction of agonist and antagonist muscles at a joint would be reduced, and muscle synergies across a number of joints would be used to create a well-coordinated movement that is more adaptable to task and environmental demands. For example, in postural development, it might be hypothesized that this would allow the infant to begin to balance using hip, knee, and ankle joints equally, as more complex balance tasks are mastered (Bernstein, 1967; Newell & Vaillancourt, 2001).

In the third stage, called the "expert stage," the individual now has released all the degrees of freedom necessary to perform the task in the most efficient and coordinated way. Bernstein predicts that there is also an exploitation of reactive phenomena of forces of one segment that influence another segment. That is, the person uses passive forces increasingly in movement control, allowing less expenditure of active forces and more efficient use of energy, and consequently reducing fatigue. Thus, the individual has learned to take advantage of the mechanics of the musculoskeletal system and of the environment and to optimize the efficiency of the movement. They can exploit the mechanical and inertial properties of the limbs to increase movement characteristics such as speed and to reduce energy costs (Rose, 1997; Schmidt & Lee, 2011; Vereijken et al., 1992).

These general hypotheses regarding stages of motor skills have been supported by a number of studies. For example, in adult skill learning, Arutyunyan et al. (1969) have shown that pistol shooters first use control at the shoulder joint in their aiming movements, freezing the other joints of the arm in order to reduce the degrees of freedom. With increasing practice, the degrees of freedom of the arm are increased to include the distal joints. Broderick and Newell (1999) also found that the progression of skill in basketball bouncing started with movements of the shoulder and wrist and progressed to release of the previously constrained elbow joint with further training. This has also been supported in the development of leg kicking and early walking in infants, with progression from mainly proximal (hip) control with few adjustments to distal (knee and ankle) control, accompanied by increased adjustments and modulation (Hallemans et al., 2007; Jensen et al., 1995; Newell & Vaillancourt, 2001).

Interestingly, the final stage of Bernstein's motor learning model has also received supporting evidence from the motor control literature. Schneider and Zernicke (1989) found that after practicing an arm motion task pattern, subjects were able to use active muscle forces as complementary forces to the passive interactive components of the moving limb, thus exploiting reactive forces and reducing their own need to generate tension.

Clinical Implications

Bernstein's three-stage theory of motor learning has a number of clinical implications. First, it suggests a possible explanation for the presence of coactivation of muscles during the early stages of acquiring a motor skill and as an ongoing strategy in patients who are unable to learn to control a limb dynamically. One explanation is that coactivation serves to stiffen a joint and therefore constrain the degrees of freedom. This strategy may in fact be a reasonable solution to the underlying problem: inability to control the degrees of freedom of a limb segment.

This theory offers a new rationale for using developmental stages in rehabilitation. Traditionally, recapitulating developmental stages in the adult patient was based on a neuromaturational rationale. Alternatively, motor development could be viewed from a biomechanical perspective as a gradual release of degrees of freedom. For example, the progression from supporting oneself on all fours to upright kneeling to an independent stance can be viewed as a gradual increase in the number of degrees of freedom that must be controlled. Thus, having a patient practice maintaining an upright kneeling position before learning to control stance could be justified using this theory from a mechanical (i.e., controlling degrees of freedom) rather than a neural perspective.

Finally, this theory suggests the importance of providing external support during the early phases of learning a motor skill in patients with coordination problems. Providing external support constrains the degrees of freedom that the patient initially has to learn to control. As coordinative abilities improve, support can be systematically withdrawn as the patient learns to control more and more degrees of freedom.

You can see the effect of controlling degrees of freedom on function in the video case study of Malachi, who has severe cerebral palsy.

Malachi has significantly impaired trunk postural control that constrains his ability to use his arms. External support is provided by the therapist at different trunk segments in order to limit the degrees of freedom (i.e., trunk segments) that Malachi has to control. Once the level of trunk support provided by the therapist is optimal relative to Malachi's ability to control the unconstrained trunk segments, postural control as a constraint on upper-extremity function is lessened and Malachi is freer to explore his capability for upper-extremity movement.

This concept of systematically controlling the degrees of freedom in order to facilitate greater and greater control is the basis for targeted training, a method for training trunk postural control in children like Malachi. To see an example of how targeted training is used, refer to the video case study on assessment and treatment of segmental trunk control.

Limitations to the Three-Stage Model/Approach

It has been noted that little research has been focused on the autonomous or expert stage of learning, partly because it would take months or years to bring many subjects to this skill level on a laboratory task. Thus, the principles that govern motor learning processes to lead to this last stage of mastery are largely unknown (Schmidt, 1988a).

Gentile's Two-Stage Model

In contrast to the three-stage theories discussed previously, Gentile (1972, 1987) proposed a two-stage theory of motor skill acquisition that describes the goal of the learner in each stage. In the first stage, the goal of the learner is to develop an understanding of the task dynamics. At this stage, they are just getting the idea of the requirements of the movement (Gentile, 1972). This includes understanding the goal of the task, developing movement strategies appropriate to achieving the goal, and understanding the environmental features critical to the organization of the movement. An important feature of this stage of motor learning is learning to distinguish relevant, or regulatory, features of the environment from those that are nonregulatory.

In the second stage, called the "fixation/diversification stage," the goal of the learner is to refine the movement. Refining movement includes both developing the capability of adapting the movement to changing task and environmental demands and performing the task consistently and efficiently. The terms "fixation" and "diversification" refer to the distinct requirements of open versus closed skills. As discussed in Chapter 1, closed skills have minimal environmental variation and thus require a consistent movement pattern with minimal variation. The concept is illustrated in Figure 2.3A, which is a representation of the movement consistency that occurs with repeated practice under unchanging conditions. Movement variability decreases with practice. In contrast, open skills are characterized by changing environmental conditions and therefore require movement diversification. This concept of movement diversification is illustrated in Figure 2.3B (Higgins & Spaeth, 1979).

Stages of Motor Program Formation

Finally, researchers have hypothesized that hierarchical changes may occur in movement control as motor programs are assembled during the learning of a new task (MacKay, 1982; Schmidt & Lee, 2011). Motor programs for controlling a complex behavior might be created by combining programs that control smaller units of the behavior, until the whole behavior is controlled as a unit. The example given by MacKay

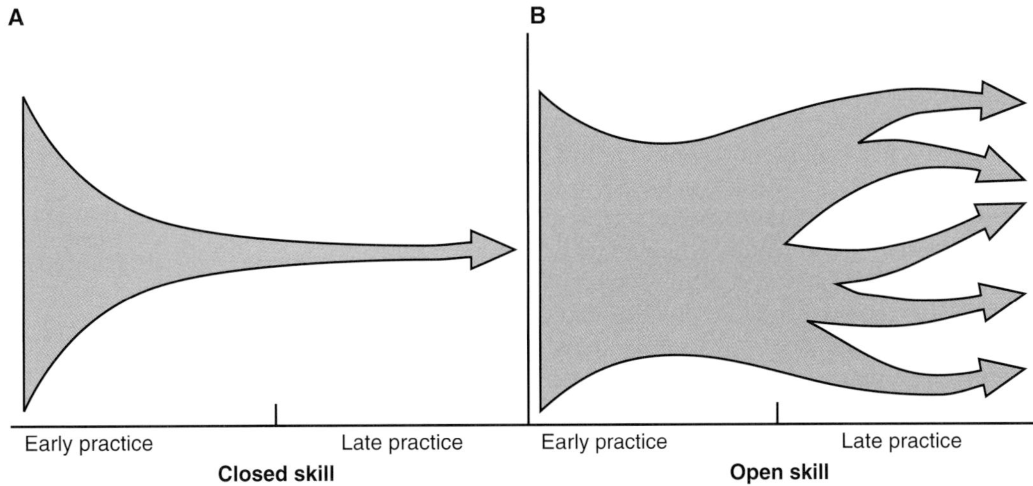

Figure 2.3 Schematic representation of movement patterns associated with closed **(A)** versus open **(B)** motor skills. Closed skills require refinement of a single or limited number of movement patterns (movement consistency); in contrast, open skills require a diversity of movement patterns (movement diversity). (Adapted with permission from Higgens JR, Spaeth RA. Relationship between consistency of movement and environmental condition. *Quest*. 1972;17:65.)

illustrates the process of learning to shift gears in a car with manual transmission. In this example, in the early stages of practice, each of the seven components of the skill (accelerator up, clutch down, shift lever forward, shift lever to right, shift lever forward, clutch up, accelerator down) is controlled by a separate motor program. As the learner improves their ability to shift, components of the behavior are grouped and controlled together, such as when we combine control of the clutch and accelerator. This is the middle practice stage. Finally, in late practice, all seven components of the gear-shifting process are controlled by a single motor program.

In our example of Genise learning to move from sitting to standing, initially during early practice, she may develop a motor program for each component of the movement—for example, sliding forward on the seat, shifting her feet back, leaning her trunk forward, putting her hands on the chair arms, and standing up. During middle practice, she may begin to combine units of the behavior—for example, sliding forward on the seat and repositioning her feet. Finally, in late practice, all parts of the movement are combined into one program for the movement of sitting to standing.

PRACTICAL APPLICATIONS OF MOTOR LEARNING RESEARCH

During Genise's rehabilitation, her therapist may have many questions regarding how best to organize her treatment sessions. The therapist may wonder, What is the best way to structure my therapy sessions in order to optimize learning? How often should Genise practice a particular task? Is the type of feedback that I am giving Genise concerning the quality of her movements really effective? Could I give a different form of feedback that might be better? Should I give feedback with every trial that Genise makes, or would it be better to withhold feedback occasionally and make Genise try to discern for herself whether her movement is accurate or efficient? What is the best timing for feedback? In this section, we discuss research in motor learning that has attempted to answer these questions. We review the research in relation to the different motor learning factors that are important to consider when retraining patients, like Genise, with motor control problems, including practice frequency, feedback, practice conditions, and variability of practice, and consider how this information could impact how Genise's therapist organizes her therapy sessions.

Practice Levels

The most important factor in retraining motor skills is the amount of practice. According to research by Fitts (1964), Newell and Rosenbloom (1981), and others, practice on many different tasks, using widely different performance measures, showed the same result: a logarithmic law of practice, described by Schmidt and Lee (2011) as the power law of practice. The logarithmic relationship shows that the rate of improvement during any part of practice is linearly related (on a log scale) to the amount left to improve. This means that early in practice of a new task, performance improves rapidly, while after much practice, it improves more slowly. It also shows that performance may improve for many years, although increments may be small. One application of this law has been as an explanation of the efficacy of constraint-induced therapy. It is possible that one reason for the substantial improvement in motor skills for patients undergoing this intensive training (about 6 hours a day for 2 weeks) is simply the massive numbers of practice trials they have performed (Schmidt & Lee, 2011). What are the implications of this research to Genise's therapy sessions? They reinforce the importance of practice—lots of practice. This includes not just the number of repetitions Genise does when practicing a task within a therapy session but the importance of extending practice beyond therapy sessions. Extending practice may include establishing an "in-room" program of exercises (when she is an inpatient), a home program of exercises (when she is an outpatient), and finally a discharge "forever" exercise program that she will continue after her final discharge.

Feedback

We have already discussed the importance of feedback in relation to motor learning. Clearly, some form of feedback is essential for learning to take place. In this section, we describe the types of feedback that are available to the performer and the contributions of these different types of feedback to motor learning.

The broadest definition of feedback includes all the sensory information that is available as the result of a movement that a person has produced. This is typically called response-produced feedback (also called "movement-produced feedback"). This feedback is usually further divided into two subclasses: intrinsic (or inherent) feedback and extrinsic (or augmented) feedback (Schmidt & Lee, 2011; Shea et al., 1993).

Intrinsic Feedback

Intrinsic (or inherent) feedback is feedback that comes to the individual simply through the various sensory systems as a result of the normal production of the movement. This includes such things as visual information concerning whether a movement was accurate as well as somatosensory information concerning the position of the limbs as one was moving (Schmidt & Lee, 2011).

Extrinsic Feedback

Extrinsic (or augmented) feedback is information that supplements intrinsic feedback. For example, when you tell a patient that they need to lift their foot higher to clear an object while walking, you are offering extrinsic feedback.

Extrinsic feedback can be given concurrently with the task and in addition at the end of the task, in which case it is called "terminal feedback." An example of concurrent feedback would be verbal or manual guidance to the hand of a patient learning to reach for objects. An example of terminal feedback would be telling a patient after a first unsuccessful attempt to rise from a chair, to push harder the next time, using the arms to create more force to stand up.

In her therapy sessions, Genise may have difficulty using intrinsic feedback due to her sensory impairments. In this case, the use of extrinsic feedback, to augment her limited intrinsic feedback, will be quite important. For example, Genise is having problems establishing a symmetrical base of support during standing in part due to impaired sensation in her paretic limb (limiting the available intrinsic feedback related to this task). Genise's therapist has her practice in front of a mirror so she can visually see her postural orientation (extrinsic feedback). Genise also practices symmetrical stance using two bathroom scales, another form of extrinsic feedback.

Knowledge of Results. KR is one important form of extrinsic feedback. It has been defined as terminal feedback about the outcome of the movement, in terms of the movement's goal (Schmidt & Lee, 2011; Shea et al., 1993). This is in contrast to KP, which is feedback relating to the movement pattern used to achieve the goal.

Research has been performed to determine the types of feedback that are the best to give a subject. Almost all of the research that has been performed involves examining the efficacy of different types of KR. Typically, research has shown that KR is an important learning variable; that is, it is important for learning motor tasks (Bilodeau et al., 1959). However, there are certain types of tasks for which intrinsic feedback (e.g., visual or kinesthetic) is sufficient to provide most error information, and KR has only minimal effects. For example, in learning tracking tasks, KR only minimally improves the performance and learning of a subject.

When should KR be given for optimal results? Should it be given right after a movement? What delay is best before the next movement is made, to ensure maximum learning efficiency? Should KR be given after every movement? These are important questions for the therapist who wants to optimize the learning or relearning of motor skills in patients with motor disorders.

Experiments attempting to determine the optimal KR delay interval have found very little effect of KR delay on motor learning efficacy. The same is true of the post-KR delay interval. There may be a slight reduction in learning if the KR delay is very short, but any effects are very small. However, it has been shown that it is good not to fill the KR delay interval with other movements, since these appear to interfere with the learning of the target movements. Research on the effects of filling the post-KR delay interval (the interval between KR and the next trial) with extraneous activities is less clear. Apparently, this interval is not as important as the KR delay interval for the integration of KR information. It has also been recommended that the intertrial interval should not be excessively short, but the literature in this area shows conflicting results (Salmoni et al., 1984) concerning the effects of different lengths of intertrial intervals on learning.

What happens to learning efficacy if KR is not given for every trial? For example, if you ask a patient to practice a reaching movement and give the patient feedback only on the accuracy of the movement every 5 or 10 trials, what do you think might happen? One might assume that decreasing the amount of KR given would have a detrimental effect on learning. However, experiments in this area have shown surprising results.

In one study, Winstein and Schmidt (1990) manipulated KR to produce what they called a "fading schedule," giving more KR early in practice (50% frequency) and gradually reducing it later in practice. They compared the performance of this group to one given a 100% frequency feedback condition (feedback on every trial). No difference in performance was found during acquisition, but the 50% fading frequency condition gave better scores on a delayed retention test. Why would this be the case? They propose that on no-KR trials, the subject needs to use other cognitive processes, such as those related to error detection. In addition, when KR is given in 100% of trials, this produces dependency on the KR (Shea et al., 1993; Winstein & Schmidt, 1990).

In another set of studies, Lavery (1962) compared the performance of (a) subjects who had KR feedback on every trial; (b) subjects who had summary KR, that is, KR for each of the trials only at the end of an entire block of 20 trials; and (c) subjects who had both types of feedback. It was found that at the end of the acquisition trials, performance was best if KR was given after every trial (groups 1 and 3 had far better performance than group 2). However, when performance was then compared for the groups on transfer tests, for which no KR was given at any time, the group that was originally the least accurate, the summary KR-only group (group 2), was now the most accurate (Lavery, 1962).

These results suggest that summary KR is the best feedback; but if this were so, group 3 should have been as good as group 2, and this was not the case. It has thus been concluded that immediate KR is detrimental to learning, because it provides too much information and allows the subject to rely on the information too strongly (Schmidt & Lee, 2011).

What is the best number of trials to complete before giving KR? This appears to vary depending on the task. For very simple movement timing tasks, in which KR was given after 1 trial, 5 trials, 10 trials, or 15 trials, the performance on acquisition trials was best for the most frequent feedback, but when a transfer test was given, the performance was best for the 15-trial summary group. In a more complex task, for which a pattern of moving lights had to be intercepted by an arm movement (like intercepting a ball with a bat), the most effective summary length for learning was 5 trials, and anything more or less was less efficient (Schmidt et al., 1989; Schmidt & Lee, 2011).

How precise must KR be in order to be most effective? The answer varies for adults versus children. For adults, quantitative KR appears to be best, with the more precise KR giving more accurate performance, up to a point, beyond which there is no further improvement. For adults, units of measure (e.g., inches, centimeters, feet, and miles) do not seem to be important, with even nonsense units being effective. However, in children, unfamiliar units or very precise KR can be confusing and reduce learning (Newell & Kennedy, 1978; Schmidt & Lee, 2011).

How might this research on KR influence Genise's therapy sessions? It suggests that KR is an important facilitator of motor learning and therefore needs to be incorporated in each therapy session. As Genise is practicing functional tasks, her therapist is careful to institute a fading schedule in her use of KR. For example, the therapist does not allow Genise to see the results from either the mirror or the scales on every trial, so that Genise does not become dependent on extrinsic feedback but increases the use of intrinsic feedback. In addition, her therapist is careful not to introduce distractions (including practice of other tasks) during the KR interval (e.g., between the practice and the KR). It is important to remember that if the therapist provided KR after every trial, Genise's performance might improve quickly, but her long-term learning will be reduced.

Practice Conditions

We have already discussed the importance of KR to learning. A second variable that is also very important is practice. Typically, the more practice you can give a patient, the more the patient learns, with other things being equal. Thus, in creating a therapy session, the number of practice attempts should be maximized. But what about fatigue? How should the therapist schedule practice periods versus rest periods? Research to answer these questions is summarized in the following sections.

Massed versus Distributed Practice

To answer the questions previously mentioned, researchers have performed experiments comparing two types of practice sessions: massed and distributed. Massed practice is defined as a session in which the amount of practice time in a trial is greater than the amount of rest between trials. This may lead to fatigue in some tasks. Distributed practice is defined as a session in which the amount of rest between trials is equal to or greater than the amount of time for a trial. For continuous tasks, massed practice has been proven to decrease performance markedly while it is present, but it affects learning only slightly when learning is measured on a transfer task in distributed conditions. In this case, fatigue may mask the original learning effects during massed practice, but the effects become apparent on the transfer tasks. For discrete tasks, the research results are not as clear, and they appear to depend considerably on the task (Schmidt & Lee, 2011).

How does this information impact Genise and her therapist? It is important to remember that massed practice leading to excessive fatigue may increase Genise's risk of injury and this may be somewhat dangerous for her when she practices tasks, which places her at risk for falls. In this case, a more distributed schedule of practice may be a better choice since it is less likely to overfatigue Genise, decreasing her risk for injury.

Constant versus Variable Practice

The ability to generalize learning to novel situations is considered a very important variable in motor learning. In general, research has shown that variable practice increases this ability to adapt and generalize learning. For example, in one experiment, one group of subjects practiced a timing task (they had to press a button when a moving pattern of lights arriving at a particular point) at variable speeds of 5, 7, 9, and 11 miles per hour, while a second group (constant practice) practiced at only one of those speeds. Then, all subjects performed a transfer test, in which they performed at a speed outside their previous range of experience. The absolute errors were smaller for the variable than for the constant practice group (Catalano & Kleiner, 1984; Schmidt & Lee, 2011). Thus, in this example, variable practice allowed a person to perform significantly better on novel variations of the task. Using variable practice may be most essential when learning tasks that are likely to be performed in variable conditions. Tasks that require minimal variation and will be performed in constant conditions may best be practiced in constant conditions (Rose, 1997).

This research suggests that variable practice is a better choice during Genise's therapy sessions, since it is more likely to result in better long-term learning and transfer. So when Genise is practicing transfer tasks, for example, sit to stand, her therapist will insure that she has the opportunity to practice from a variety of chairs with different characteristics. This will allow Genise to develop a schema for the sit-to-stand task, insuring her ability to carry out this task in novel and unfamiliar environments and conditions.

Random versus Blocked Practice: Contextual Interference

Surprisingly, it has also been found that factors that make performing a task more difficult initially very often make learning more effective in the long run. These types of factors have been called "context effects." For example, if you were to ask Genise to practice five different tasks in random order (e.g., sit to stand, supine to sit, sit to supine, sit to walk, and walk to sit) versus blocking the trials (i.e., practicing one task [such as sit to stand]) for a block of trials and then moving on to the next task (sit to walk), you might presume that Genise would learn to perform each task faster using the blocked design. However, this is not the case. Although performance is better during the acquisition phase (i.e., when Genise is first learning the tasks) when trials are in a blocked design, when tested on a transfer task, her performance will actually be better in the randomly ordered conditions. Thus, contextual interference occurs when multiple skills are practiced within a single session.

Is it always the case that random practice is better than blocked practice? It appears that a number of factors related to both the task and the learner must be considered when deciding whether to use random versus blocked practice (Magill & Hall, 1990). Random practice appears to be most effective when used with skills that use different patterns of coordination and thus different underlying motor programs (Magill & Hall, 1990). In addition, characteristics of the individual, such as level of experience and intellectual abilities, may also influence the effectiveness of random practice (Rose, 1997). Researchers have found that random practice may be inappropriate until learners understand the dynamics of the task being learned (Del Rey et al., 1983; Goode, 1986). In addition, research by Edwards et al. (1986) on motor learning in adolescents with Down syndrome suggests that random practice was not superior to blocked practice in this group of learners. To understand the clinical applications of contextual interference, complete Lab Activity 2.1.

You can repeat this lab activity exploring how the structure of a therapy session would vary if you were using constant versus variable practice, guided versus discovery learning, or KR versus KP.

LAB ACTIVITY 2.1

Objective: To understand the clinical applications of contextual interference.

Procedure: Your patient is John C., a 33-year-old with degenerative spinocerebellar ataxia. He requires assistance with most of his ADL because of dysmetria and discoordination. Today's therapy session is focusing on training transfers (bed to wheelchair and wheelchair to toilet) and bed mobility skills (supine to prone [rolling], supine to sitting on edge of bed, and sitting to standing).

Assignment

Your job is to plan a therapy session showing how your therapy strategies would vary depending on the motor learning strategies you are using. Consider the effects of these different strategies on John's recovery of function.

1. Outline a therapy session to teach these skills based on a random practice schedule.
2. How would your therapy session differ if you were focusing on training using a blocked practice schedule?
3. What will be the effects of each approach to practice on the initial acquisition of skills, and what effect will each approach have on long-term retention and transfer to novel conditions?

Whole versus Part Training

One approach to retraining function is to break the task down into interim steps, helping the patient to master each step prior to learning the entire task. This has been called "task analysis," and it is defined as the process of identifying the components of a skill or movement and then ordering them into a sequence. How are the components of a task defined? They are defined in relation to the goals of the task. So, for example, a task analysis approach to retraining locomotion would be to break the gait pattern into naturally occurring components such as step initiation, stability during stance, and push-off to achieve progression. During locomotor retraining, the patient would practice each of these components in isolation, before combining them into the whole gait pattern. But each of these components must be practiced within the overall context of gait. For example, having a patient practice hip extension while prone will not necessarily increase the patient's ability to achieve the goal of stance stability, even though both require hip extension. Thus, part-task training can be an effective way to retrain some tasks, if the task itself can be naturally divided into units that reflect the inherent goals of the task (Schmidt, 1991; Winstein, 1991).

The research on part versus whole practice suggests that within each therapy session, Genise should be encouraged to practice functional tasks under both part and whole conditions. As stated previously, Genise may practice parts of gait in isolation (part practice), but it is also essential that she practice the entire task of walking. This is also true for other types of functional tasks such as transfers that are often broken down into segments. This type of practice will facilitate the development of motor programs for controlling complex tasks, by combining smaller units of the behavior into larger and larger units, until the whole behavior is controlled automatically as a unit. In Genise's treatment case study video, you can see examples of part and whole practice being used in locomotor training.

Transfer

A critical issue in Genise's rehabilitation is how well her training transfers, either to a new task or to a new environment. For example, will learning a task in a clinical environment transfer to her home environment? Or does practice in standing balance transfer to a dynamic balance task such as walking around the house? What determines how well a task learned in one condition will transfer to another? Researchers have determined that the amount of transfer depends on the similarity between the two tasks or the two environments (Lee, 1988; Schmidt et al., 1989). A critical aspect in both appears to be whether the neural processing demands in the two situations are similar. For example, training Genise to maintain standing balance in a well-controlled environment, such as on a firm, flat surface in a well-lit clinic, will not necessarily enable her to balance in her home environment that contains thick carpets, uneven surfaces, and visual distractions. The more closely the processing demands in the practice environment resemble those in the actual environment, the better the transfer will be (Schmidt & Lee, 2011; Winstein, 1991). This means that in order to ensure that Genise's functional improvements transfer to her home environment when she is discharged, her therapist needs to make sure Genise practices functional tasks under a range of conditions that will mimic her home or community environment.

Mental Practice

It has been shown that mentally practicing a skill (the act of performing the skill in one's imagination, with no action involved) can produce large positive effects on the performance of the task. For example, Hird et al. (1991) taught subjects in different groups a pegboard task, putting pegs of different colors and shapes into holes in the pegboard, or a pursuit rotor task, in which the subject was asked to follow a target moving in a circular pattern. Groups were given seven sessions of training using different combinations of physical and mental practice, with a control group getting practice on a totally separate task (a stabilometer task). Results showed that the group given 100% mental practice was more effective at the task than the control group but not nearly as effective as the group given the same amount of physical practice (100%). The groups given different combinations of mental and physical practice showed learning that was proportional to the time spent in physical practice. These results suggest that physical practice is definitely the best type of practice, but mental practice is an effective way to enhance learning during times when physical practice is not possible.

Why is this the case? One hypothesis is that the neural circuits underlying the motor programs for the movements are actually triggered during mental practice, and the subject either does not activate the final muscle response at all or activates responses at very low levels that do not produce movement. In Chapter 3, we discuss experiments showing that one part of the brain, the supplementary motor cortex, is activated during mental practice.

This research has a lot of implications for Genise in her rehabilitation program. Because she fatigues easily, use of mental practice can facilitate her motor learning. In addition to physical practice, her therapist can assign her mental practice of functional tasks during her home (or in-room) program, another way of extending practice.

Guidance versus Discovery Learning

One technique often used in therapy is guidance; that is, the learner is physically guided through the task to be learned. Research has again explored the efficiency of this form of learning versus other forms of learning that involve trial-and-error discovery procedures. In one set of experiments (Schmidt & Lee, 2011), various forms of physical guidance were used in teaching a complex elbow movement task. When performance was measured on a no-guidance transfer test, physical guidance was no more effective than simply practicing the task under unguided conditions. In other experiments (Singer, 1980), practice under unguided conditions was found to be less effective for acquisition of the skill but was more effective for later retention and transfer. This is similar to the results just cited, which showed that the conditions that made the performance acquisition more difficult enhanced performance in transfer tests.

This does not mean that her therapist should never use guidance in teaching skills to Genise, but it does imply that if guidance is used, her therapist should limit it to when she is learning a new task (the acquisition stage), to acquaint Genise with the characteristics of the task to be learned. Then, guidance should gradually be replaced by discovery learning, so that Genise can explore the perceptual motor workspace associated with learning the task. In Genise's case, when initially learning to do a reach and grasp task with her paretic limb, she may initially be guided through the task (guided learning); however, for optimal learning, she needs to be exposed to a range of reaching tasks so that she can discover through trial and error the relevant perceptual cues and movement strategies appropriate to different reaching tasks.

In summary, using motor learning research, Genise's therapist has a good sense of how to structure her therapy sessions to enhance the acquisition of functional motor skills and ensure that those skills transfer to both new environments and other tasks. Genise's therapist understands that many of these motor learning strategies may initially slow the acquisition of tasks but ensure long-term learning, transfer, and generalization. Using a motor learning approach can be very challenging because of her insurance; Genise has limited access to rehabilitation services. Genise's therapist is under pressure to increase Genise's functional status as quickly as possible, increasing the temptation to use strategies that improve performance quickly, with less consideration of long-term retention and generalizability of skills.

As you can see, there are many factors that need to be considered when planning a therapy program, including characteristics of the learner (patient), the task being taught, and the learning environment, including conditions of practice. This can be challenging since we lack a comprehensive framework for organizing the learning environment taking into consideration the characteristics of the learner, the task being learned, and the conditions of practice (Winstein et al., 2014). The challenge point framework (CPF) has been proposed as a theoretical framework for organizing the learning environment, taking these factors into consideration (Guadagnoli & Lee, 2004). Information on the CPF may be found in Extended Knowledge 2.1.

Extended Knowledge 2.1

The Challenge Point Framework: A Framework for Optimizing Motor Learning

There are many factors that need to be considered when planning a therapy program, including characteristics of the learner (patient), the task being taught, and the learning environment, including conditions of practice. The CPF is a theoretical framework for organizing the learning environment by taking into consideration the characteristics of the learner, the task being learned, and the conditions of practice (Guadagnoli & Lee, 2004). According to CPF, learning is intimately related to the amount of information available to the person when learning a task. Information is viewed as a challenge to the performer. Optimal information leads to optimal learning; however, too little or too much information can slow the learning process. The optimal challenge point for learning is determined by the characteristics of the learner (e.g., skill level), the difficulty of the task, and the environment (defined by the conditions of practice and feedback) (Guadagnoli & Lee, 2004).

In CPF, task difficulty is conceptualized as both nominal (i.e., constant) and functional. Nominal task difficulty reflects factors such as some of the perceptual and motor processing requirements of the task that are constant. In contrast, functional task difficulty is variable, depending on the skill level of the performer and the conditions under which a task is being performed. Thus, while every task contains a specific nominal level of difficulty, the conditions under which the task is practiced and the skill level of the performer will change the functional level of difficulty (Guadagnoli & Lee, 2004). For example, in the task of walking, nominal difficulty is determined by the perceptual and motor requirements of walking and is an invariant and inherent characteristic of the task. In contrast, functional difficulty will vary according to the skill level of the performer and the conditions of practice. In our example, functional difficulty associated with walking on a level, unobstructed surface is low for a healthy young adult but high for a person in the acute stages of recovering from a stroke. As recovery progresses and the skill level of the patient increases, the functional level of difficulty associated with walking on level ground declines. The therapist can increase the functional difficulty of the learning environment by changing the conditions of practice, taking into consideration the skill level of the learner and the difficulty of the task being learned.

In our example, in the acute recovery stage, when the skill level of the patient is low, walking may be best learned under blocked conditions (repetitive practice of walking on level ground, followed by repetitive practice of walking over obstacles, followed by repetitive practice of walking with a load) with high-frequency KR (feedback after every repetition). As the patient's skill level increases, learning may be best when walking is practiced under random conditions (walking on level ground, obstacles, loads, and dual-task conditions) with low-frequency KR. Using CPF, the therapist can optimize the potential for learning in each therapy session by manipulating the conditions of practice, taking into consideration the skill level of the patient and the difficulty of the task.

Onla-or and Winstein (2008) tested the predictions of the CPF for motor learning in Parkinson's disease (PD) through the systematic manipulation of three factors: the learner's skill level (control vs. PD), conditions of practice (random vs. blocked practice order and frequency of KR), and nominal task difficulty (low vs. high). Twenty adults with PD and 20 controls (without disability) practiced a goal-directed arm movement under low (1,500 ms movement time) versus high (900 ms movement time) levels of nominal task difficulty and under low-demand (blocked practice order with 100% KR) and high-demand (random practice order with 60% KR) practice conditions. The difference between goal and participant-generated movement (root mean square error) was used to quantify learning 1 day after practice. The results from this study partially supported the predictions made by the CPF. Under low-demand practice conditions, individuals with moderately severe PD demonstrated learning comparable to that of controls when nominal task difficulty was low but demonstrated learning deficits when nominal task difficulty was high. Under high–nominal-demand practice conditions, individuals with PD demonstrated learning comparable to that of controls only when the context of the recall test was the same as that during practice (e.g., random retention test in the random practice conditions or blocked practice retention test in the blocked practice conditions). In other words, they could not generalize or transfer learning to a new context, unlike the controls, suggesting that further refinements are needed to this model.

While the CPF provides a potentially useful framework to help therapists make decisions regarding how to organize the practice environment, taking into consideration both the skill level of the patient (learner) and the difficulty of the tasks being learned, further research is needed to validate this approach in patients with neurologic pathology.

RECOVERY OF FUNCTION

Motor learning is the study of the acquisition or modification of movement in normal subjects. In contrast, recovery of function has referred to the reacquisition of movement skills lost through injury. However, as we noted at the beginning of this chapter, there is a strong relationship between motor learning and the process of rehabilitation designed to promote recovery of function.

Concepts Related to Recovery of Function

To understand the concepts related to recovery of function, it is necessary first to define terms such as "function" and "recovery."

Function

Function is defined here as the complex activity of the whole organism that is directed at performing a behavioral task (Craik, 1992). However, the term "function" does not in itself imply level of skillfulness. Rehabilitation that focuses simply on the recovery of "function" may downplay the importance of achievement of skilled movement in the service of functional tasks (Winstein et al., 2014). In this book, when we use the term "function," we are referring to the recovery of skilled action.

Recovery

The term "recovery" has a number of different meanings pertaining to regaining function that has been lost after an injury. A stringent definition of recovery requires achieving the functional goal in the same way it was performed before injury, that is, using the same processes used prior to the injury (Almli & Finger, 1988). Less-stringent definitions define recovery as the ability to achieve task goals using effective and efficient means but not necessarily those used before the injury (Slavin et al., 1988). Thus, the term "recovery" has been used to refer simultaneously to the restitution of damaged structures or functions and as a term to describe clinical improvements regardless of how these may have occurred (i.e., through restitution or adaptation) (Levin et al., 2009).

Recovery versus Compensation

Is recovery the same as or different from compensation? Remember, the strict definition of recovery is achieving function through original processes. Compensation is defined as behavioral substitution; that is, alternative behavioral strategies are adopted to complete a task. However, there is considerable confusion regarding the use of these terms (Levin et al., 2009). Levin et al. (2009) define recovery of motor performance as the reappearance of motor patterns present prior to CNS injury. In contrast, motor compensation is defined as the appearance of new motor patterns resulting from either (a) the adaptation of remaining motor elements or (b) substitution, meaning that functions are taken over, replaced, or substituted by different end effectors or body segments. Levin and colleagues have presented a framework for distinguishing between recovery and compensation based on the International Classification of Function (ICF) (see Chapter 6 for a detailed discussion of the ICF framework). Table 2.1 summarizes their classification scheme.

A question of concern to many therapists is, Should therapy be directed at recovery of function or compensation? The response to this question has changed over the years as our knowledge about the plasticity and malleability of the adult CNS has changed (Gordon, 1987). For many years, the adult mammalian CNS was characterized as both rigid and unalterable. On maturation, function was believed to be localized to various parts of the CNS. Research at the time suggested that regeneration and reorganization were not possible within the adult CNS. This view of the CNS naturally led to therapy directed at compensation, since recovery, in the strict sense of the word, was not possible. More recent research in the field of neuroscience has begun to show that the adult CNS has great plasticity and retains an incredible capacity for reorganization. Studies on neural mechanisms underlying recovery of function are covered in Chapter 4.

Sparing of Function

When a function is not lost, despite a brain injury, it is referred to as a spared function (Craik, 1992). For example, when language develops normally in children who have suffered brain damage early in life, retained language function is said to be spared.

Stages of Recovery

Several authors have described stages of recovery from neural injury. Stages of recovery are based on the assumption that the process of recovery can be broken down into discrete stages. Classically, recovery is divided into spontaneous recovery and forced recovery. Forced recovery is recovery obtained through specific interventions designed to have an impact on neural mechanisms (Bach-y-Rita & Balliet, 1987).

The presumption is that different neural mechanisms underlie these relatively discrete stages of recovery. Chapter 4 describes how research on neural mechanisms might contribute new methods to improving and speeding the various stages of recovery.

Factors Affecting Recovery of Function

A number of factors can affect the outcome of damage to the nervous system as well as the extent of subsequent recovery, including both endogenous (within the individual) and exogenous (external to the individual) factors (Chapman & McKinnon, 2000). In addition, both

TABLE 2.1 Definitions of Motor Recovery and Motor Compensation at Three Different Levels

Level	Recovery	Compensation
ICF: Health Condition: Neuronal	Restoring function in neural tissue that was initially lost after injury. May be seen as reactivation in brain areas previously inactivated by the circulatory event. Although this is not expected to occur in the area of the primary brain lesion, it may occur in areas surrounding the lesion (penumbra) and in the diaschisis.	Neural tissue acquires a function that it did not have prior to injury. May be seen as activation in alternative brain areas not normally observed in individuals without disability.
ICF: Body Structure and Function (performance)	Restoring the ability to perform a movement in the same manner as it was performed before injury. This may occur through the reappearance of premorbid movement patterns during task accomplishment (voluntary joint range of motion, temporal and spatial interjoint coordination, etc.).	Performing an old movement in a new manner. May be seen as the appearance of alternative movement patterns (i.e., recruitment of additional or different degrees of freedom, changes in muscle activation patterns such as increased agonist/antagonist coactivation, delays in timing between movements of adjacent joints, etc.) during the accomplishment of a task.
ICF: Activity (functional)	Successful task accomplishment using limbs or end effectors typically used by individuals without disability.	Successful task accomplishment using alternate limbs or end effectors, for example, opening a pack of chips using 1 hand and the mouth instead of 2 hands.

ICF, International Classification of Function.

Source: Reprinted with permission from Levin MF, Kleim JA, Wolf SF. What do motor "recovery" and "compensation" mean in patients following stroke? *Neurorehabil Neural Repair*. 2009;23:313–319. Table 1, page 316.

preinjury and postinjury factors influence the extent of injury and the recovery of function. Figure 2.4 illustrates some of the factors that have an impact on recovery of function after brain injury. The following section reviews the research examining some, but not all, of the effects of both preinjury and postinjury factors on recovery of function. At the end of this review, we consider the implications of this research on the recovery of function in Genise, our patient who has had a stroke.

Effect of Stage of Development (Age)

How does the stage of development or the age of the person at the time of CNS lesion affect recovery? Does outcome vary if brain damage occurs early versus later in life? Early views on age-related effects on recovery of brain function proposed that injury during infancy caused fewer deficits than damage in the adult years. For example, in the 1940s, Kennard (1940, 1942) performed experiments in which she removed the motor cortex of infant versus adult monkeys and found that infants were able to learn to feed, climb, walk, and grasp objects, while adults were not able to recover these functions. In humans, this effect has been noted in language function, in which damage to the dominant hemisphere shows little or no effect on speech in infants but causes different degrees of aphasia in adults. However, there is research to suggest that early injury can result in reduced brain plasticity and may interfere with later emerging functions. For example, young children with injuries to the frontal areas of the cortex may appear to function normally until they reach an age at which frontal skills are more apparent (Anderson et al., 1999). Thus, the age of the individual at the time of the lesion affects recovery of function, but it does so in a complex manner, depending on the location of the lesion and the function it subserves (Chapman & McKinnon, 2000; Held, 1987; Stein et al., 1995). If an area is mature, injury will typically cause similar damage in infants and adults. But if another area that is functionally related is not yet mature, it may assume the function of the injured area. In addition, if an immature area is damaged and no other area assumes its function, no problems may be seen in infancy, but in later years, deficits may become apparent. In summary, what the data on age-related effects on brain injury suggest is that "the brain reacts differently to injury at different stages of development" (Stein et al., 1995, p. 77).

With respect to our patient Genise, the age at which she had her stroke has an impact on her capacity to

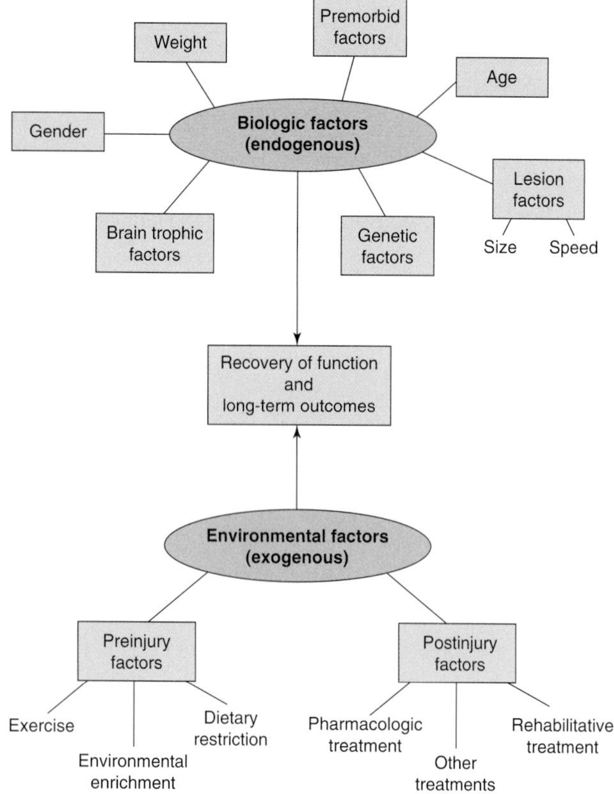

Figure 2.4 Factors that influence recovery of function and outcomes after CNS pathology are complex and include both endogenous (biologic factors within the individual) and exogenous (environmental factors, external to the individual) factors occurring prior to and following injury. (Adapted with permission from Chapman SB, McKinnon L. Discussion of developmental plasticity: factors affecting cognitive outcome after pediatric traumatic brain injury. *J Commun Disord.* 2000;33:335.)

recovery. Having a stroke at the age of 53, she has a better prognosis for recovery than Jean (our case study on chronic stroke), who had her stroke at the age of 76.

Characteristics of the Lesion

In addition to age, characteristics of the lesion also affect the extent of recovery from injury (Held, 1987). In general, researchers have shown a fairly strong relationship between injury severity and long-term functional outcomes; however, there is considerable variability in recovery even among individuals with severe brain injury. This suggests that the injury severity may be an indicator rather than a predictor of recovery (Chapman & McKinnon, 2000). Researchers have also found that patients with a small lesion have a greater chance of recovery, as long as a functional area has not been entirely removed. In addition, slowly developing lesions appear to cause less functional loss than lesions that happen quickly. This phenomenon has been explored experimentally by making serial lesions in animals, with the animal being allowed to recover between lesions (Craik, 1992). If a single large lesion is made in the motor cortex (Brodmann's areas 4 and 6), animals become immobilized; in contrast, function is spared if a similar lesion is produced serially over a period of time. If serial lesions are made, the animal recovers the ability to walk, feed, and right itself with no difficulty (Travis & Woolsey, 1956).

Other factors, such as the age of the animal, also influence the effect of serial lesions. In younger animals, function is spared even when serial lesions are performed close together. In contrast, older animals may not show any sparing of function, regardless of how much time has elapsed between lesions (Stein et al., 1995).

Preinjury Neuroprotective Factors

A number of preinjury factors have been shown to moderate the effect of pathology (degenerative and traumatic) on CNS function. Preinjury exercise, environmental enrichment, and dietary restriction are all examples of neuroprotective factors. Researchers have shown that preinjury exercise can protect against some of the damaging effects of aging, neurodegeneration, and brain injury. In animal studies, prestroke exercise was found to reduce infarct size, although the mechanisms underlying this finding are not clear. Neuroprotective aspects of exercise may be due to an increase in exercise-induced neuroplasticity and/or angiogenesis to support collateral blood flow. In addition, preinjury exercise may serve to decrease processes such as apoptosis, edema, and the inhibition of neurite growth–inhibiting molecules (Kleim et al., 2003). Genise was very active and had a history of exercise prior to her stroke, indicating many positive preinjury protective factors that will positively influence her recovery.

Experiments have shown that preinjury environmental enrichment protects animals against certain deficits after brain lesions. For example, two sets of rats received lesions of the cortex, one group with preoperative enrichment and a control group. After surgery, the enriched animals made fewer mistakes during maze learning and in fact performed better than control animals without brain damage (Held, 1998).

In a second study by Held et al. (1985), the effect of preoperative and postoperative enrichment was compared for a locomotor task following removal of sensorimotor cortex. They found that preoperatively enriched rats were no different from enriched controls with sham lesions on both behavioral and fine-grained movement analyses. The group that was only postoperatively enriched was mildly impaired in locomotor skills but recovered more quickly than the controls with lesions, although they never regained full locomotor function. Thus, postoperative enrichment is effective, but it does not allow the same extent of recovery as preoperative enrichment.

Held et al. suggest that enriched subjects may have functional neural circuitry that is more varied than that of restricted subjects, and this could provide them with a greater ability to reorganize the nervous system after a lesion or simply to use alternative pathways to perform a task. You can see that Genise, who was actively engaged in a rich and varied life prior to her stroke, had many positive preinjury factors that will potentially moderate the effect of her stroke.

Postinjury Factors

Effect of Pharmacology

Another factor that can affect recovery of function after brain injury is the use of pharmacological treatments that reduce the nervous system's reaction to injury and promote recovery of function. There are several excellent articles that review basic scientific and clinical studies on pharmacological strategies for behavioral restoration following brain damage (Feeney & Sutton, 1987; Goldstein, 1993, 2003). These studies suggest that certain drugs can have profound effects on the recovery process; however, while some drugs are beneficial to the recovery of function, others may be detrimental.

Scientists are studying the effects of a number of different types of drugs on recovery of function following brain injury, including the following:

1. Drugs that affect trophic factors, promoting regeneration and cell survival
2. Drugs that replace neurotransmitters lost because of cell death
3. Drugs that prevent the effects of toxic substances produced or released by dead or dying cells
4. Drugs that restore blood circulation
5. Antioxidants, such as vitamin E, that block the effects of free radicals that destroy cell membranes (Stein et al., 1995)

Overall, results from drug studies following brain injury are very promising and suggest that pharmacologic treatment can enhance recovery of function following brain injury (Feeney & Sutton, 1987; Goldstein, 2003; Stein et al., 1995). Further information on the effects of drugs on recovery of function may be found in Extended Knowledge 2.2.

Neurotrophic Factors

Research on the role of neurotrophic factors and their role in brain plasticity in animals and humans is still growing and is a complex subject. Although we offer an overview of the role of these molecules in neural plasticity, a complete discussion is beyond the scope of this book.

Extended Knowledge 2.2

The Effects of Pharmacology on Recovery of Function

Amphetamine is a well-studied drug that appears to facilitate recovery following brain injury. Amphetamine works by enhancing the effects of neurotransmitters such as adrenaline, noradrenaline, serotonin, and dopamine (Braun et al., 1986; Feeney et al., 1981, 1982; Goldstein, 2003; Hovda & Feeney, 1985; Stein et al., 1995). Several studies have shown that following stroke, treatment with amphetamines in conjunction with physical therapy produced a better outcome in motor performance on the Fugl–Meyer test than either intervention in isolation (Crisostomo et al., 1988; Walker-Batson et al., 1992).

The inhibitory neurotransmitter gamma-aminobutyric acid (GABA) also affects recovery of function—drugs that were GABA agonists impeded recovery from brain damage in the rat, while GABA antagonists were beneficial (Goldstein, 1993). Administration of cholinergic agents appears to facilitate recovery (van Woerkom et al., 1982). However, the administration of various drugs that block specific types of glutamate receptors has had mixed results (Goldstein, 1993, 2003).

There is considerable debate about the use of antioxidants such as vitamin E in both traumatic and neurodegenerative diseases such as PD. Considerable destruction of cell tissue that leads to the production of free radicals occurs during early stages of trauma. Free radicals are molecules of hydrogen, oxygen, and iron that have extra electrons, making them highly destructive to other living cells. Free radicals destroy the lipid membrane of a cell, allowing toxic substances to enter the cell and essential substances inside the cell to leave. Drugs such as vitamin E, which block the effects of free radicals, are called "antioxidants" (Stein et al., 1995). Stein and colleagues (1995) demonstrated that rats that were given vitamin E directly after frontal lobe damage were able to perform a spatial learning task as well as noninjured rats. A study by Fahn (1991) looked at the effect of vitamin E in patients in the early stages of PD and found that it appeared to slow the progression of the disease. Unfortunately, other studies have not been as successful in showing the beneficial effects of vitamin E on slowing the progression of PD.

Finally, drugs that are used to treat commonly occurring comorbidities in older patients can have a deleterious effect on recovery of function following stroke. For example, antihypertensive and sedative agents have been shown to slow recovery of motor and language functions following stroke (Goldstein, 1993; 2003; Goldstein & Davis, 1988).

In addition to drug-related factors, many factors within the individual influence the effect of drugs on brain recovery, including age, sex, health status at the time of injury, and type and extent of injury (stroke, trauma, or ischemia). For example, several researchers have shown that hormonal levels have a profound effect on both extent of damage following brain trauma and response to medication. Because of hormonal differences, the effect of a drug varies between male and female patients. Metabolic status can influence drug reactions as well. This is particularly important in light of the fact that systemic metabolism can change quickly following brain injury (Stein et al., 1995). For example, hypermetabolism can cause the breakdown of a drug too quickly, reducing its effectiveness.

According to the neurotrophic factor hypothesis, which was based on studies of Hamburger and Levi-Montalcini (1949; Jessell & Sanes, 2013), many biochemical properties of a neuron are determined by signals from surrounding cells. In fact, the very survival of a neuron depends on factors released from surrounding cells. For example, the size of their muscle target is critical for the survival of spinal motor neurons. Thus, the target cell appears to produce a limited amount of an essential trophic factor that is taken up by nerve terminals and transported to the neuronal cell bodies to promote their survival (Jessell & Sanes, 2013). There is a great diversity of neurotrophic factors. Neurotrophins are one type with specific relevance to rehabilitation, since therapeutic strategies used during rehabilitation can stimulate their local production to modulate multiple neurotransmitter systems and enhance sprouting of compensatory relay networks (Griffin & Bradke, 2020).

Some neurotrophins involved in neuronal survival and neural plastic changes are nerve growth factor (NGF) for nociceptive neurons; neurotrophin-3 (NT-3) for muscle spindle–related proprioceptive sensory neurons and the mechanoreceptive neurons that innervate Merkel cells; and glial cell line–derived neurotrophic factor (GDNF) for motor, sensory, and sympathetic neurons (Jessell & Sanes, 2013). Another well-studied neurotrophin is the brain-derived neurotrophic factor (BDNF). BDNF has been shown to have an impact on neural plasticity in animal models (Pham et al., 2002; Sherrard & Bower, 2001). In humans, BDNF expression is linked to activity-dependent practice and also acute aerobic exercise. BDNF has a wide variety of functions for neurite expression, neuronal communication efficacy, neuroprotection, axonal and dendritic growth and remodeling, synaptogenesis, and even metabotrophic effects—it reduces food intake, increases oxidation of glucose, lowers blood glucose levels, and increases insulin sensitivity (Knaepen et al., 2010).

Effect of Exercise and Training

Postinjury training is a different form of exposure to enriched environments in that the activities used are specific rather than generalized (Held, 1998). Ogden and Franz (1917) performed an interesting study in which they produced hemiplegia in monkeys by making lesions in the motor cortex. They then gave four types of postoperative training: (a) no treatment, (b) general massage of the involved arm, (c) restraint of the noninvolved limb, and (d) restraint of the noninvolved limb coupled with stimulation of the involved limb to move, along with forced active movement of the animal. The last condition was the only one to show recovery, and in this condition, it occurred within 3 weeks.

A study by Black et al. (1975) examined recovery from a motor cortex forelimb area lesion. They initiated training immediately after surgery or 4 months after surgery, with training lasting 6 months. They found that training of the involved hand alone, or training of the involved and normal hand together, was more effective than training of the normal hand alone. When training was delayed, recovery was worse than when it was initiated immediately following the lesion.

The effect of postinjury rehabilitation training on neural plasticity and recovery of function is complex and is affected by many factors, including the location and type of injury and the timing and intensity of intervention. It is not always the case that early and intense intervention is best. In animal models of recovery of function, researchers have found that early and intense motor enrichment may promote neural plasticity in the contralesional hemisphere, but it exaggerated the effects of injury in the perilesional area. Forced motor enrichment (simulating forced-use paradigms) in the first week after injury exaggerated the extent of the cortical injury (Humm et al., 1999; Risedal et al., 1999). In contrast, a more gradual and modest increase in motor therapy facilitated neural plasticity and recovery of function in perilesional areas (Schallert et al., 2003).

It appears that if postinjury stimulation is to have an effect on recovery of function, it must incorporate active participation of the patient in order for full recovery to occur (Stein et al., 1995). When rats with unilateral lesions of the visual cortex were exposed to visual shapes, only the rats that were allowed to move freely in the environment and to interact with the visual cues showed good recovery of visual function. The rats that were exposed to the visual cues within their environment but were restrained from moving were very impaired (Stein et al., 1995).

Research on animal models with spinal cord injury (SCI) have shown that, aside from the contextual benefit (i.e., enriched environment), the type of training seems to be critical to promote regeneration and plasticity and further prune and refine the underlying circuits relevant to the motor task under practice (Griffin & Bradke, 2020). A study investigated rats with incomplete SCI that underwent three different training modalities: quadrupedal treadmill training, swim training, and stand training. Quadrupedal treadmill training reduced allodynia—neuropathic pain that results from increased sensitivity to nonpainful stimulation—and restored sensation in rats; swim training only reduced allodynia, and stand training did not have any benefits. Therefore, the type of training should be task specific and intensive enough to promote changes within the nervous system (Griffin & Bradke, 2020; Hutchinson et al., 2004).

New research is investigating the synergistic effects of combinatory approaches that include genetic manipulation, pharmacological drugs, electro-chemical stimulation, and robotic assistive devices during simultaneous task-specific practice. For instance, a study in SCI rodents shows that the application of electrochemical neuromodulation to the injured lumbar segment enabled robotic gravity-assisted gait training. The training program reinforced and reorganized the reticulospinal tracts under the level of injury and rerouted corticospinal projections. The result was a motor cortex-dependent recovery of walking and also swimming in the absence of neuromodulation (Asboth et al., 2018). In humans, research done in children with cerebral palsy showed that a regimen of activity-based practice that includes motor learning principles (i.e., goal-oriented, intensity, age-appropriate, variability, task-progression, feedback, attention, and engagement) with upper and lower extremities promotes long-term motor, functional, and neuroplastic changes within the corticospinal tract (Bleyenheuft et al., 2020; Brandão et al., 2014; Friel et al., 2016).

Clinical Implications

By now, it should be clear that the field of rehabilitation has much in common with the field of motor learning. Therapists involved in the treatment of the adult patient with a neurologic injury are concerned with issues related to motor relearning, or the reacquisition of movement. The pediatric patient who is born with a CNS deficit or who experiences injury early in life faces the task of acquisition of movement in the face of unknown musculoskeletal and neural constraints. In either case, the therapist is concerned with structuring therapy in ways to maximize acquisition and/or recovery of function.

When considering Genise's recovery of function, we can see that it cannot be attributed to any one factor. Some of her functional return will be due to recovery, that is, regaining control of original mechanisms; some will be due to compensatory processes. In addition, both positive and negative preinjury factors will influence the degree of function regained.

Genise has been, and is, receiving excellent therapy as well! She is involved in carefully organized therapy sessions that are contributing to reacquisition of task-relevant skilled behaviors. Both associative and nonassociative forms of learning are playing a role in her recovery. Trial-and-error learning (operant conditioning) is used to help her discover optimal solutions to many functional tasks. Her therapist carefully structured her environment so that optimal strategies are reinforced.

Functionally relevant tasks are being practiced under wide-ranging conditions. Under optimal conditions, this will lead to procedural learning, ensuring that Genise will be able to transfer many of her newly gained skills to her home environment. Practicing tasks under varied conditions is aimed at the development of rule-governed actions or schemata. Recognizing the importance of developing optimal perceptual and motor strategies, her therapist structures her therapy sessions so that Genise has the opportunity to explore the perceptual environment. This is designed to facilitate the optimal mapping of perceptual and motor strategies for achieving functional goals. Finally, therapy is directed at helping Genise repeatedly solve the sensorimotor problems inherent in various functional tasks, rather than teaching her to repeat a single solution.

SUMMARY

1. Motor learning, like motor control, emerges from a complex set of processes, including perception, cognition, and action.
2. Motor learning results from an interaction of the individual with the task and environment.
3. Forms of learning include nondeclarative or implicit learning and declarative or explicit learning. Nondeclarative learning can be divided into nonassociative, associative, and procedural learning.
4. Nonassociative learning occurs when an organism is given a single stimulus repeatedly. As a result, the nervous system learns about the characteristics of that stimulus.
5. Habituation and sensitization are two very simple forms of nonassociative learning. Habituation is a decrease in responsiveness that occurs as a result of repeated exposure to a nonpainful stimulus. Sensitization is increased responsiveness following a threatening or noxious stimulus.
6. In associative learning, a person learns to predict relationships, either relationships of one stimulus to another (classical conditioning) or the relationship of one's behavior to a consequence (operant conditioning).
7. Classical conditioning consists of learning to pair two stimuli. During operant conditioning, we learn to associate a certain response, from among many that we have made, with a consequence.
8. Procedural learning refers to other nondeclarative learning tasks that can also be performed automatically without attention or conscious thought, like a habit.
9. Declarative or explicit learning results in knowledge that can be consciously recalled and thus requires processes such as awareness, attention, and reflection.
10. There are many different theories of motor learning including Schmidt's schema theory, the ecological theory of learning as exploration, and a number of theories on the stages of motor learning.
11. Classical recovery is divided into spontaneous recovery and forced recovery, that is, recovery obtained through specific interventions designed to have an impact on neural mechanisms.
12. Experiments show that several preinjury factors, including exercise, environmental enrichment, and nutrition, are neuroprotective; that is, they minimize the effects of neurodegenerative and acquired brain injury.

13. Postinjury factors such as exercise and training can have a positive effect on recovery of function, but the optimal timing, frequency, and intensity of training depend on the location of injury.

ANSWERS TO LAB ACTIVITY ASSIGNMENTS

Lab Activity 2.1

1. In a random practice schedule, John would practice each skill only once or twice before moving to the next skill. A random practice approach requires preplanning and a good physical setup.
2. In contrast, if you were organizing your therapy session on a blocked schedule of practice, you would practice each of the specific skills one at a time. That is, you would first have John practice wheelchair-to-bed transfers for a concentrated period of time; then switch to a different skill, wheelchair-to-toilet transfers; and practice that repeatedly before switching to the next task.
3. In the random practice schedule, if all the tasks to be practiced are not physically close to one another, too much time is wasted moving to site-specific areas for practice, which is not realistic in the amount of time available for therapy. Traditional methods for retraining motor skills, by having a patient practice one skill repeatedly, may initially result in the speedy acquisition of a skill, but long-term learning and the ability to transfer skills to novel conditions are limited. In contrast, encouraging the patient to practice a number of tasks in random order may slow down the initial acquisition of skills but will be better for long-term retention (Schmidt & Lee, 2011).

CHAPTER 3

Physiology of Motor Control

Learning Objectives

Following completion of this chapter, the reader will be able to:

1. Discuss the differences between parallel and hierarchical processing in motor control and give examples of each.
2. Describe the anatomical connections and functional contributions to movement control for each of the major components of the brain (spinal cord, brainstem, cerebellum, basal ganglia, and each cortical area).
3. Describe the electrical properties of an action potential and a resting potential and the process of synaptic transmission.
4. Describe the components of the somatosensory system, including sensory receptors, ascending pathways, and higher-level centers that process information from this system relative to other sensory inputs.
5. Discuss elements in the dorsal versus ventral stream pathways in the visual system and explain the role of each system in visual processing.
6. Discuss the contributions of basal ganglia, cerebellum, motor cortex, brainstem, and descending pathways to both internally generated and externally triggered movements.

INTRODUCTION AND OVERVIEW

Motor Control Theories and Physiology

As mentioned in Chapter 1, theories of motor control are not simply a collection of concepts regarding the nature and cause of movement. They must take into consideration current research findings about the structure and function of the nervous system. Movement arises from the interaction of perception and action systems, with cognition affecting both systems at many different levels. Within each of these systems are many levels of processing, which are illustrated in Figure 3.1. For example, perception can be thought of as progressing through various processing stages. Each stage reflects specific brain structures that process sensory information at different levels, from initial stages of sensory processing to increasingly abstract levels of interpretation and integration in higher levels of the brain.

Movement control is achieved through the cooperative effort of many brain structures that are organized both hierarchically and in parallel. This means that a signal may be processed in two ways. A signal may be processed hierarchically, within ascending levels of the central nervous system (CNS). In addition, the same signal may be processed simultaneously among many different brain structures, showing parallel distributed processing. Hierarchical processing, in conjunction with parallel distributed processing, occurs in the perception, action, and cognitive systems of movement control.

When we talk about hierarchical processing in this chapter, we are describing a system in which higher levels of the brain are concerned with issues of abstraction of information. For example, within the perceptual system, hierarchical processing means that higher brain centers integrate inputs from many senses and interpret incoming sensory information. On the action side of movement control, higher levels of brain function form motor plans and strategies for action. Thus, higher levels might select the specific response to accomplish a particular task. Lower levels of processing would then carry out the detailed monitoring and regulation of the response execution, making it appropriate for the context in which it is carried out. Cognitive systems overlap with perception and action systems, and involve high-level processing for both perception and action. In addition, many structures of the brain (e.g., the spinal

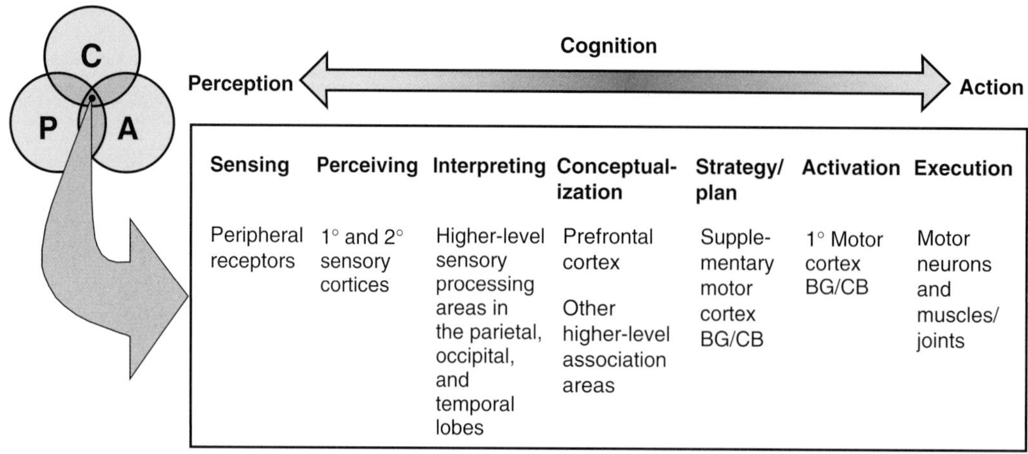

Figure 3.1 Model of the interaction between perceptual, action and cognitive processes involved in motor control. BG, basal ganglia; CB, cerebellum.

cord, brainstem, cerebellum, and association cortex) have both perception and action components.

In parallel distributed processing, the same signal is processed simultaneously among many different brain structures, although for different purposes. For example, the cerebellum and the basal ganglia process higher-level motor information simultaneously before sending it back to the motor cortex for action. Parallel processing can also be found within the same neural pathway in which neuronal groups convey computations simultaneously to increase the speed and reliability of the information processed by the CNS. A benefit of parallel processing is that damage of a specific brain area or pathway does not necessarily result in a total loss of neural function. Thus, the function or behavior is partially maintained or even recovered after the structural reorganization of related neural networks (Pearson & Gordon, 2013).

This chapter reviews the processes underlying the production of human movement. The first section of this chapter presents an overview of the major components of the CNS and the structure and function of a neuron, the basic unit of the CNS. The remaining sections of this chapter discuss in more detail the neural anatomy (the basic circuits) and the physiology (the function) of the systems involved in the production and control of movement. The chapter follows the neural anatomy and physiology of movement control from perception into cognition and action, recognizing that it is often difficult to distinguish where one ends and others begin.

Overview of Brain Function

Brain function underlying motor control is typically divided into multiple processing levels, including the spinal cord, the brainstem (the midbrain, or mesencephalon, medulla oblongata, and pons), the cerebellum (which is sometimes included with the brainstem areas of medulla and pons, as part of the hindbrain), and the forebrain, including the cerebral cortex, thalamus, hypothalamus, the basal ganglia, amygdala, and hippocampus (Amaral, 2000; Patton et al., 1989).

Spinal Cord

At the lowest level of the perception or the action hierarchy is the spinal cord. The circuitry of the spinal cord is involved in the initial reception and processing of somatosensory information (from the muscles, joints, ligaments, and skin) and the reflex and voluntary control of posture and movement through the motor neurons. At the level of spinal cord processing, we can expect to see a fairly simple relationship between the sensory input and the motor output. At the spinal cord level, we see the organization of reflexes, the most stereotyped responses to sensory stimuli, and the basic flexion and extension patterns of the muscles involved in leg movements, such as kicking and locomotion (Amaral, 2000; Kandel, 2000b).

Sherrington (1906) called the motor neurons of the spinal cord the "final common pathway," since they are the last processing level before muscle activation occurs. Figure 3.2A shows the anatomist's view of the nervous system with the spinal cord positioned caudally. Figure 3.2B shows an abstract model of the nervous system with the spinal cord (segmental spinal networks) positioned at the bottom of the hierarchy, with its many parallel pathways. In this view, the sensory receptors are represented by the box labeled "afferent input" and send information (represented by thin arrows) to the spinal cord (segmental spinal networks) and higher parts of the brain. After processing at many levels, including the segmental spinal networks, the output (represented by thick arrows) modulates the activity of the skeletal muscles.

Brainstem

The spinal cord extends rostrally to join the next neural processing level, the brainstem. The brainstem contains important nuclei involved in postural control and locomotion, including the vestibular nuclei, the red nucleus, and the reticular nuclei. It also contains ascending and descending pathways transmitting sensory and motor information to other parts of the CNS. The brainstem receives somatosensory inputs from the skin and muscles of the head, as well as sensory inputs from the vestibular and visual systems. In addition, nuclei in the brainstem control the motor output to the neck, face, and eyes and are critical to the functions of hearing and taste. In fact, all the descending motor pathways except the corticospinal tract originate in the brainstem. Finally, the reticular formation is a widespread distributed network of command excitatory and inhibitory neurons that extends from the caudal midbrain through the pons and medulla. The reticular formation regulates movement (muscle tone

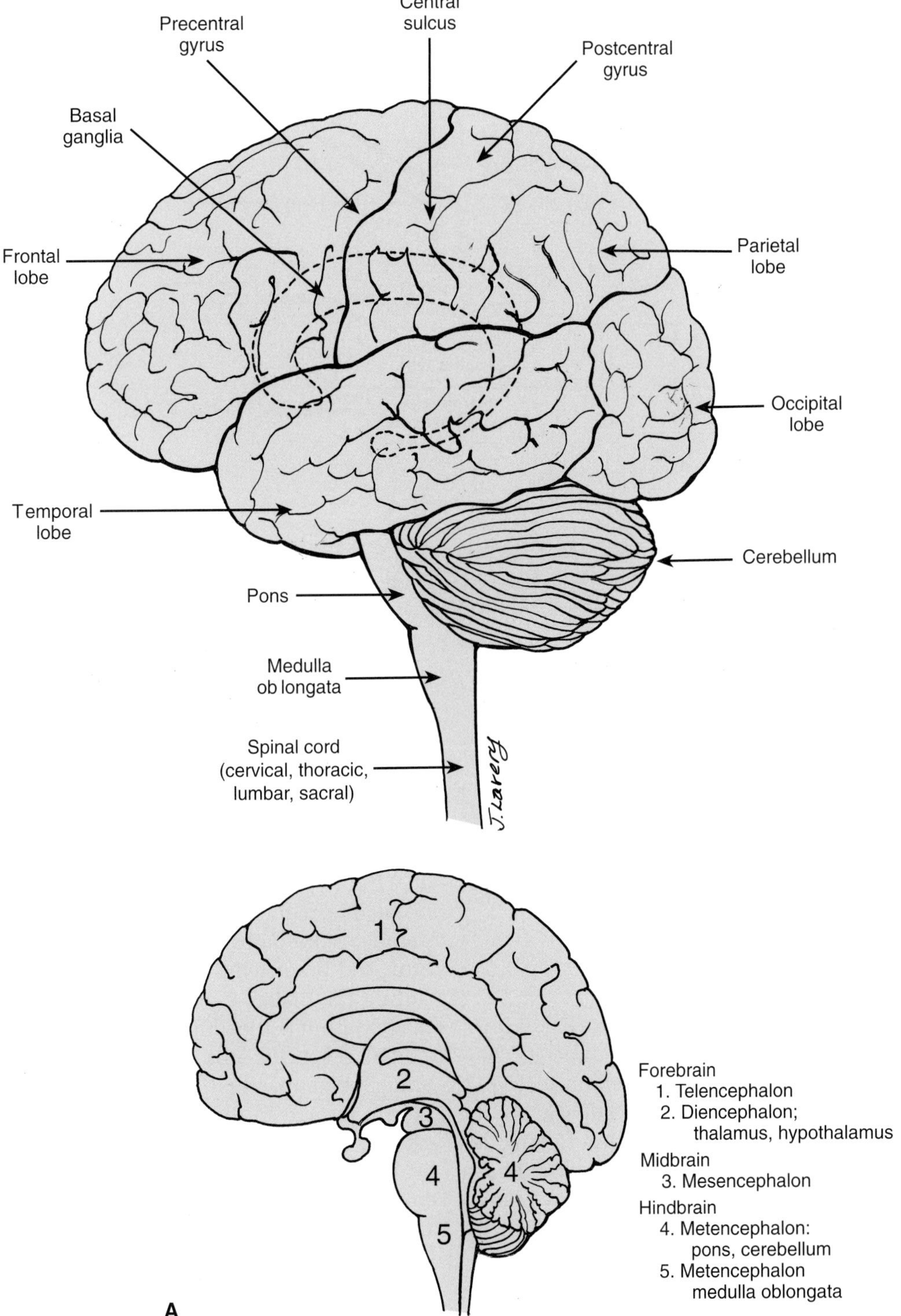

Figure 3.2 (A) The nervous system from an anatomist's point of view.

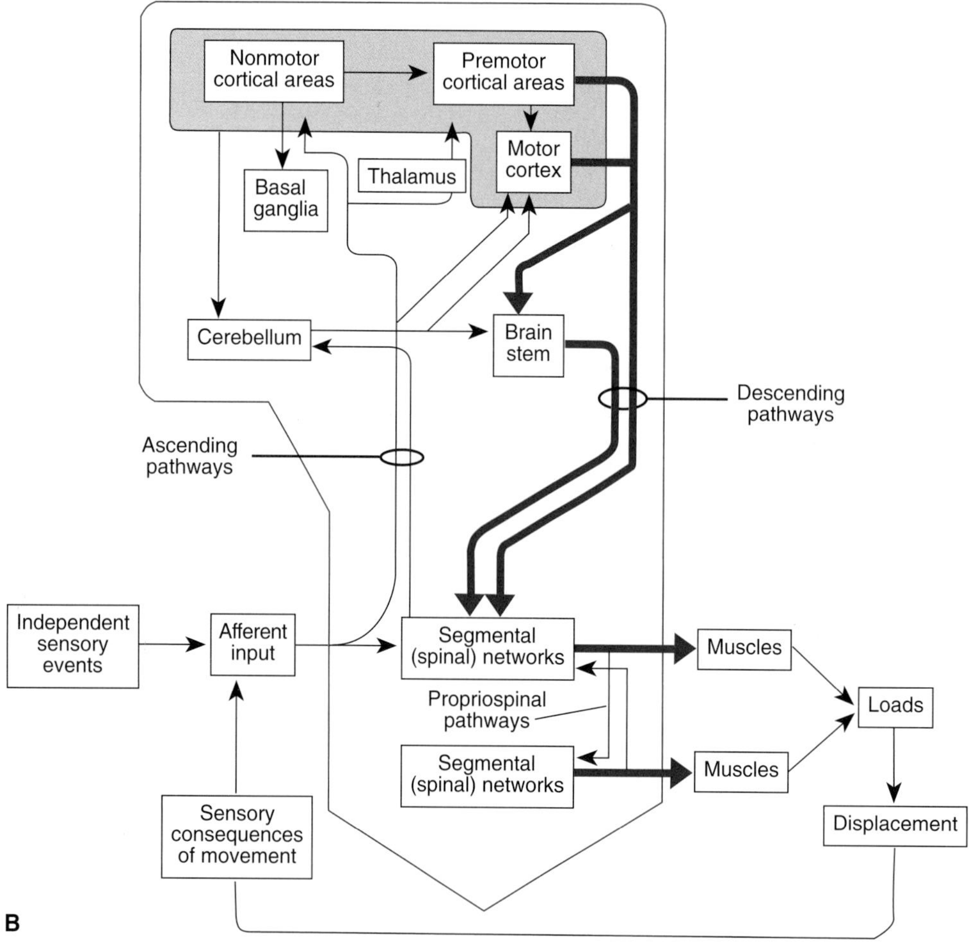

Figure 3.2 *(continued)* **(B)** An abstract model of the nervous system. (Adapted from Kandel ER, Schwartz JH, Jessell TM, eds. *Principles of Neuroscience*, 3rd ed. New York, NY: Elsevier, 1991:8; figure 1-2.)

and reciprocal flexion–extension and right–left movements) as well as the states of arousal and awareness (Amaral, 2000; Brownstone & Chopek, 2018).

The anatomist's view of the brainstem (Fig. 3.2A) shows divisions from caudal to rostral into the medulla, pons, and midbrain, while the abstract model (Fig. 3.2B) shows its input connections from the spinal cord and higher centers (the cerebellum and motor cortex) and its motor pathways back to the spinal cord.

Cerebellum

The cerebellum lies behind the brainstem (Fig. 3.2A) and is connected to it by tracts called "peduncles." As you can see from Figure 3.2B, the cerebellum receives inputs from the spinal cord (giving it feedback about movements) and from the cerebral cortex (giving it information on the planning of movements), and it has outputs to the brainstem. The cerebellum has many important functions in motor control. One is to adjust our motor responses by comparing the intended output with sensory signals, and then to update the movement commands if they deviate from the intended trajectory. The cerebellum also modulates the force and range of our movements and is involved in motor learning (from simple adaptation through more complex learning).

Diencephalon

As we move rostrally in the brain, we next find the diencephalon (Fig. 3.2A), which contains the thalamus and the hypothalamus. The thalamus processes most of the information coming to the cortex from the many parallel input pathways (from the spinal cord, cerebellum, and brainstem). These pathways stay segregated during the thalamic processing and during the subsequent output to the different parts of the cortex (Kandel, 2000b). A specific area of the thalamus, the motor thalamus, encompasses the thalamic nuclei that are primarily located in the ventral thalamic region and are glutamatergic. The motor thalamus is interconnected with cortical motor areas and receives afferents mainly from the basal ganglia (substantia nigra [SN] pars reticulata and internal segment of the globus pallidus [GP]), cerebellum (dentate and interposed nucleus), and reticular thalamic nuclei and from the superior colliculus, pedunculopontine nucleus, and somatosensory spinal cord. The motor thalamus function is hypothesized to be related to motor learning processes and postural and movement control (Bosch-Bouju et al., 2013).

Cerebral Hemispheres (Cerebral Cortex and Basal Ganglia)

As we move higher, we find the cerebral hemispheres, which include the cerebral cortex and basal ganglia. Lying at the base of the cerebral cortex, the basal ganglia (Fig. 3.2A) receive input from most areas of the cerebral cortex and send their output back to the motor cortex via the thalamus. Some of the functions of the basal ganglia involve higher-order cognitive aspects of motor control, such as the planning of motor strategies (Kandel et al., 1991).

The cerebral cortex (Fig. 3.2A) is often considered the highest level of the motor control hierarchy. The parietal and premotor areas, along with other parts of the nervous system, are involved in identifying targets in space, choosing a course of action, and programming movements. The premotor areas send outputs mainly to the motor cortex (Fig 3.2B), which sends its commands on to the brainstem via corticopontine and corticobulbar projections and to the spinal cord via the corticospinal system. The corticopontine fibers coming from the frontal lobes establish an indirect communication with the contralateral cerebellum—through the middle cerebellar peduncle—after relaying in the pontine nuclei to coordinate planned motor functions (Rea, 2015).

In light of these various subsystems involved in motor control, clearly, the nervous system is organized both hierarchically and "in parallel." Thus, the highest levels of control not only affect the next levels down but also can act independently on the spinal motor neurons. This combination of parallel and hierarchical control allows a certain overlap of functions, so that one system is able to take over from another when environmental or task conditions require it. This also allows a certain amount of recovery from neural injury, by the use of alternative pathways.

To better understand the function of the different levels of the nervous system, let us examine a specific action and walk through the pathways of the nervous system that contribute to its planning and execution. For example, perhaps you are thirsty and want to pour some milk from the carton in front of you into a glass. Sensory inputs come in from the periphery to tell you what is happening around you, where you are in space, and where your joints are relative to each other: they give you a map of your body in space. In addition, sensory information gives you critical information about the task you are to perform: how big the glass is and what size and how heavy the milk carton is. Higher centers in the cortex make a plan to act on this information in relation to the goal: reaching for the carton of milk.

From your sensory map, you make a movement plan (using, possibly, the parietal lobes and supplementary and premotor cortices). The plan includes reaching over the carton of milk in front of you. This plan is sent to the motor cortex, and muscle groups are specified. The plan is also sent to the cerebellum and basal ganglia, and they modify it to refine the movement. The cerebellum sends an update of the movement output plan to the motor cortex and brainstem. Descending pathways from the motor cortex and brainstem then activate spinal cord networks, spinal motor neurons activate the muscles, and you reach for the milk. If the milk carton is full, when you thought it was almost empty, spinal reflex pathways will compensate for the extra weight that you did not expect and activate more motor neurons. Then, the sensory consequences of your reach will be evaluated, and the cerebellum will update the movement—in this case, to accommodate a heavier milk carton.

Neuron: The Basic Unit of the CNS

The lowest level in the hierarchy is the single neuron in the spinal cord. How does it function? What is its structure? To explore more fully the ways neurons communicate between the levels of the hierarchy of the nervous system, we need to review some of the simple properties of the neuron, including the resting potential, the action potential, and synaptic transmission.

Remember that the neuron, when at rest, always has a negative electrical charge or potential on the inside of the cell, with respect to the outside. Thus, when physiologists record from a neuron intracellularly with an electrode, they discover that the inside of the cell has a resting potential of about −70 mV with respect to the outside (Fig. 3.3). This electrical potential is caused by an unequal concentration of chemical ions on the inside versus the outside of the cell. Thus, K^+ ions are high on the inside of the cell and Na^+ ions are high on the outside of the cell, and an electrical pump within the cell membrane keeps the ions in their appropriate concentrations. When the neuron is at rest, K^+ channels are open and keep the neuron at this negative potential (Kandel, 1976; Koester & Siegelbaum, 2000; Patton et al., 1989).

When a neuron is excited, one sees a series of dramatic jumps in voltage across the cell membrane. These are the action potentials, nerve impulses, or spikes. They do not go to zero voltage, but to +30 mV (as shown in Fig. 3.3). That is, the inside of the neuron becomes positive. Action potentials are also about 1 ms in duration, and the membrane is quickly repolarized. The height of the action potential is always about the same: −70 to +30 mV = ~100 mV.

How does the neuron communicate this information to the next cell in line? It does this through the process of synaptic transmission. A cleft, 200 Å wide, separates neurons. Each action potential in a neuron releases a small amount of transmitter substance. It diffuses across the cleft and attaches to receptors on the next cell, which open up channels in the membrane and depolarize the

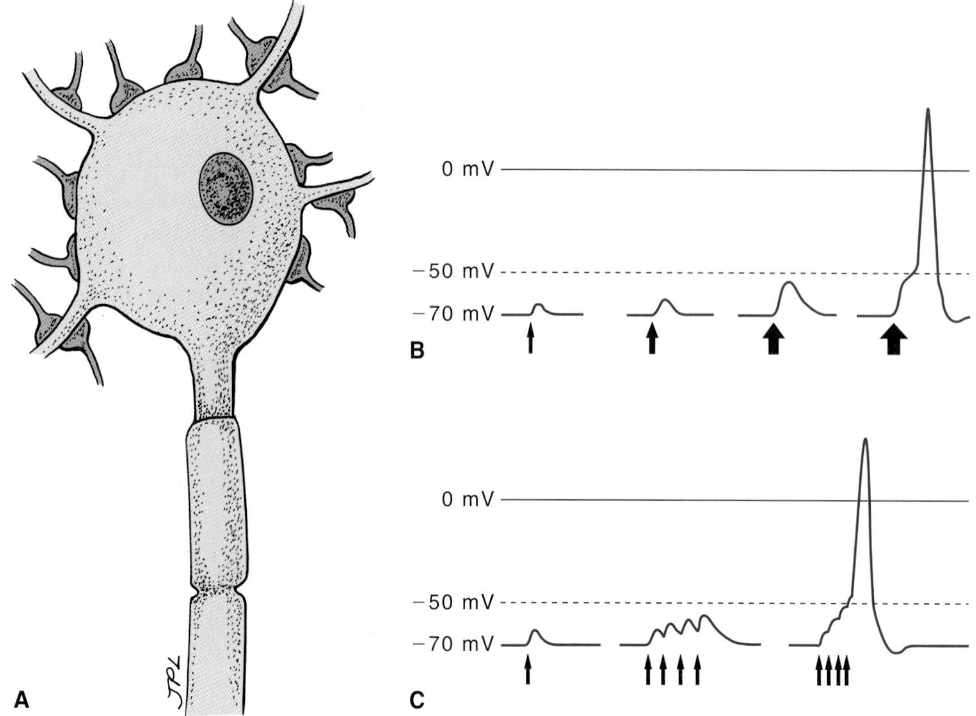

Figure 3.3 (A) A neuron with many synaptic connections on the cell body and dendrites. **(B)** Example of spatial summation, in which progressively larger numbers of presynaptic neurons are activated simultaneously (represented by progressively larger arrows) until sufficient transmitter is released to activate an action potential in the postsynaptic cell. **(C)** Example of temporal summation, in which a single presynaptic neuron is activated once, four times at a low frequency, or four times at a high frequency (*arrows* indicate timing of presynaptic potentials). Note that with a high-frequency stimulus the postsynaptic potential does not decay back to resting levels, but each successive potential sums toward threshold, to activate an action potential.

cell. One action potential makes only a small depolarization, called an excitatory postsynaptic potential (EPSP). The EPSP normally dies away after 3 to 4 ms, and as a result, the next cell is not activated (Patton et al., 1989).

But if the first cell fires enough action potentials, there is a series of EPSPs, and they continue to build up depolarization to the threshold voltage for the action potential in the next neuron. This is called summation. There are two kinds of summation, temporal and spatial, and these are illustrated in Figure 3.3B,C. Temporal summation results in depolarization because of synaptic potentials that occur close together in time (Fig. 3.3C). Spatial summation produces depolarization because of the action of multiple cells synapsing on the postsynaptic neuron (Fig. 3.3B). Spatial summation is really an example of parallel distributed processing, since multiple pathways are affecting the same neuron (Kandel & Siegelbaum, 2000).

The effectiveness of a given synapse changes with experience. For example, if a given neuron is activated over a short period of time, it may show synaptic facilitation, in which it releases more transmitter and therefore more easily depolarizes the next cell. Alternatively, a cell may also show defacilitation (or habituation). In this case, the cell is depleted of transmitter, and thus is less effective in influencing the next cell. Many mechanisms can cause synaptic facilitation or habituation in different parts of the nervous system. Increased use of a given pathway can result in synaptic facilitation. However, in a different pathway, increased use could result in defacilitation or habituation. Variations in the coding within the neuron's internal chemistry and the stimuli activating the neuron will determine whether it will respond to these signals in one mode or another. For more information, see Chapter 4, which describes the physiology of simple and complex forms of learning (Kandel, 2000b).

With this overview of the essential elements of the nervous system, we can now turn our attention to the heart of this chapter, an in-depth discussion of the sensory and motor processes underlying motor control.

SENSORY AND PERCEPTUAL SYSTEMS

What is the role of sensation in the production and control of movement? In Chapter 2, on motor control theories, there were divergent views about the importance of sensory input in motor control. Current neuroscience research suggests that sensory information plays many different roles in the control of movement.

Sensory inputs serve as the stimuli for reflexive movement organized at the spinal cord level of the nervous system. In addition, sensory information has a vital role in modulating the output of movement that results from the activity of pattern generators in the spinal cord (e.g., locomotor pattern generators). Likewise, at the spinal cord level, sensory information can modulate movement that results from commands originating in higher centers of the nervous system. One reason that sensation can modulate all these types of movement is that sensory receptors converge on both spinal interneurons and the motor neurons, which are considered the final common pathway. But another role of sensory information in movement control is accomplished via ascending pathways, which contribute to the control of movement in much more complex ways.

Somatosensory System

The somatosensory system, including neurons from the lowest to the highest level of the CNS hierarchy, and going from the reception of signals in the periphery to the integration and interpretation of those signals relative to other sensory systems in association cortex, is described in this section. Notice how both hierarchical and parallel distributed processing contributes to the analysis of somatosensory signals.

Peripheral Receptors

Muscle Spindle. Most muscle spindles are encapsulated spindle-shaped sensory receptors located in the muscle belly of skeletal muscles. They consist of (a) specialized very small muscle fibers, called intrafusal fibers (extrafusal fibers are the regular muscle fibers); (b) sensory neuron endings (group Ia and group II afferents) that wrap around the central regions of these small intrafusal muscle fibers; and (c) gamma motor neuron endings that activate the polar contractile regions of the intrafusal muscle fibers. Figure 3.4 shows a muscle spindle with its intrafusal muscle fibers (nuclear chain and nuclear bag fibers), the sensory neuron endings (Ia and II), and the motor neuron endings (gamma).

Muscle spindles detect both absolute muscle length and changes in muscle length, and along with the monosynaptic reflex, help to finely regulate muscle length during movement. In humans, the muscles with the highest spindle density (spindles per muscle) are the extraocular, hand, and neck muscles. It should not be surprising that neck muscles have such a high spindle density, because we use these muscles in eye and head coordination as we reach for objects and move about in the environment (Gordon & Ghez, 1991).

The different types of muscle fibers and sensory and motor neurons innervating the muscle spindle are designed to support two muscle spindle functions, the signaling of (a) static length of the whole muscle, and (b) dynamic changes in muscle length. In the following paragraphs, we will explain the way each part of the spindle supports this role.

Intrafusal muscle fibers. The two types of intrafusal muscle fibers are called "nuclear bag" (divided into both static and dynamic types) and "nuclear chain" (static type) fibers. The nuclear bag fiber has many spherical nuclei in its central noncontractile region (looking like an elastic bag of nuclei), which stretches quickly when lengthened because of its elasticity, while the nuclear chain fiber has a single row of nuclei, and, being less elastic, stretches slowly (Fig. 3.4A).

Groups Ia and II afferent neurons. These afferent neurons have cell bodies located in the dorsal-root ganglia of the spinal cord. Primary endings (type Ia) have larger diameter and faster conduction than secondary endings (type II). Each muscle spindle has only one Ia afferent ending and comprises numerous spirals that wrap around the equatorial region (which is very elastic) of both bag and chain intrafusal muscle fibers. The result is that Ia afferents respond quickly to stretching, sensing the rate of muscle length change. The group II endings wrap around the polar region (the area next to the equator), which is less elastic and thus less responsive to stretching. The Ia afferents go to both bag and chain fibers, while the group II afferents go mainly to the chain fibers (Fig. 3.4A). Thus, the group Ia afferent neurons are most sensitive to the rate of change or dynamic muscle length, and the group II afferent neurons are most responsive to steady-state or static muscle length. The groups Ia afferents (but not the group II afferents) respond well to slight tendon taps, sinusoidal stretches, and even vibration of the muscle tendon, since these stimuli cause fast changes in muscle length. However, in contrast to low velocity muscle contractions or muscle contractions against a load, Ia afferent activity may be silenced during rapid volitional muscle fiber contractions due to insufficient fusimotor drive—activity from gamma motor neurons 20 to 50 ms after the muscle fiber contraction—which typically functions to overcome the unloading response of intrafusal fibers and maintain the intrinsic muscle spindle discharge to the rapid muscle shortening (Macefield & Knellwolf, 2018; Pearson & Gordon, 2000).

Gamma motor neurons. Both the bag and chain muscle fibers are activated by axons of the gamma motor neurons. The cell bodies of the gamma motor neurons are inside the ventral horn of the spinal cord, intermingled with the alpha motor neurons, innervating the extrafusal (regular skeletal muscle) fibers. The gamma motor neuron axons (fusimotor fibers) terminate at the polar, striated region of the bag and the chain muscle fibers, as shown in Figure 3.4A. There are two types of gamma motor neurons: (a) the gamma dynamic, activating only dynamic bag muscle fibers, and (b) the gamma static, innervating both static bag and chain muscle fibers. Gamma dynamic motor neurons influence Ia afferent output under certain conditions, but have little effect on the activity of type II fibers. For example, though dynamic gamma motor neurons do not have a significant effect on Ia afferent activity

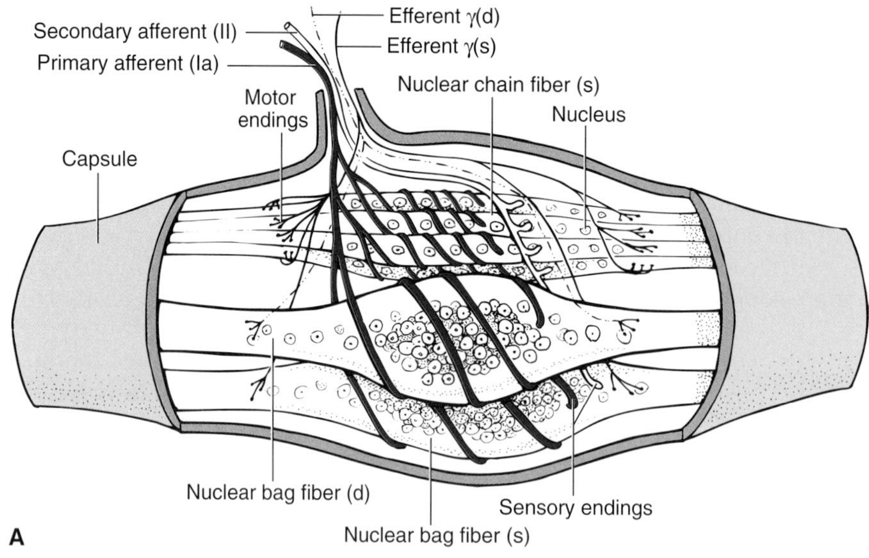

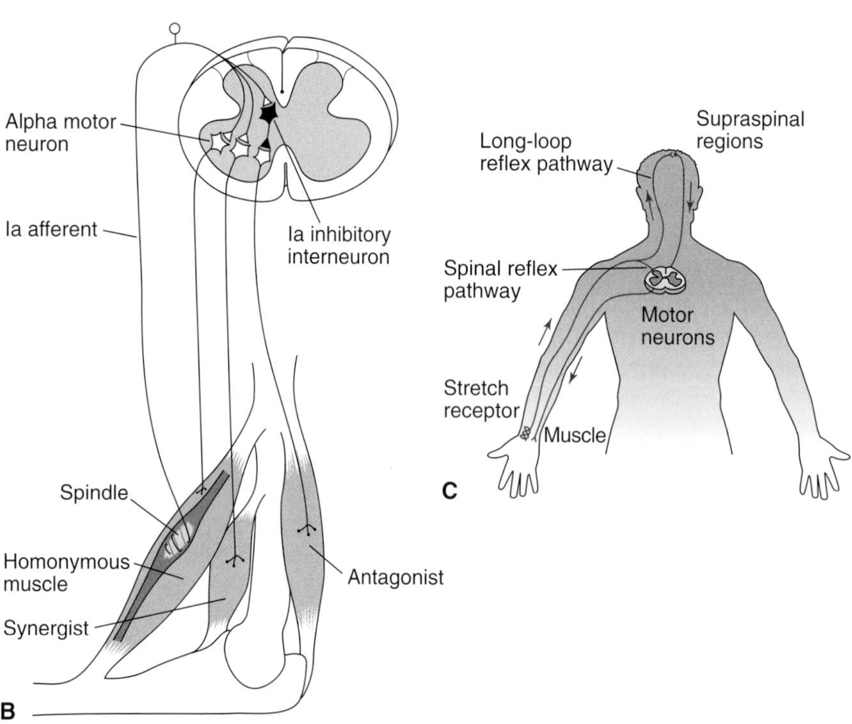

Figure 3.4 Anatomy of the muscle spindle. **(A)** Drawing of a muscle spindle showing: (1) dynamic and static nuclear bag fibers and static nuclear chain muscle fibers; (2) the group Ia and II afferent neurons that wrap around their central regions, sensing muscle length and change in length; and (3) the gamma efferent motor neurons that cause their polar regions to contract in order to keep the central regions from going slack during contractions of the whole muscle in which the muscle spindle is embedded. **(B)** Neural circuitry of the monosynaptic stretch reflex, showing the muscle spindle in the biceps muscle, the Ia afferent pathway to the spinal cord, with monosynaptic connections to the alpha motor neuron of the biceps and its synergist, and its connection to the Ia inhibitory interneuron that inhibits the motor neuron to the antagonist triceps muscle. **(C)** Muscle spindle information contributes to both a spinal reflex pathway and a long loop reflex pathway. *S*, static; *D*, dynamic. (Parts **B** & **C**, adapted from Kandel ER, Schwartz JH, Jessell TM, eds. *Principles of neural science*, 4th ed. New York, NY: Elsevier, 2000.)

when the length of muscle fibers remains constant, their activity enhances Ia afferent firing during dynamic stretch, resulting in bursts of Ia activity at the beginning and end of the dynamic phase. In contrast, activation of gamma static motor neurons has a substantial excitatory action on group Ia and II activity when muscle fibers are at constant length. They do this by increasing the group Ia and II resting firing rate activity prior to a muscle stretch, and thereby increase the muscle spindles sensitivity to that stretch (Macefield & Knellwolf, 2018).

How is information from the muscle spindle used during motor control? Muscle spindle information is used at many levels of the CNS hierarchy. At the lowest level, it is involved in reflex activation of muscles. However, as the information ascends the CNS hierarchy, it is used in increasingly complex and abstract ways. For example, it may contribute to our perception of our sense of effort. In addition, it is carried over different pathways to different parts of the brain, in this way contributing to the parallel-distributed nature of brain processing.

Stretch reflex loop. When a muscle is stretched, it stretches the muscle spindle, exciting the Ia afferents. Two types of reflex responses can be triggered by this Ia afferent excitation, a monosynaptic spinal reflex and a long-loop or transcortical reflex, as shown in Figure 3.4C. The spinal stretch reflex is activated by excitatory monosynaptic connections from the Ia afferent neurons to the alpha motor neurons, which activate their own muscle and synergistic muscles (Fig. 3.4B). The Ia afferents also excite Ia inhibitory interneurons, which then inhibit alpha motor neurons to the antagonist muscles (Fig. 3.4B). For example, if the gastrocnemius muscle is stretched, the muscle spindle Ia afferents in the muscle are excited, and they, in turn, excite the alpha motor neurons of the gastrocnemius, which cause it to contract. The Ia afferent also excites the Ia inhibitory interneuron, which inhibits motor neurons to the antagonist muscle, the tibialis anterior, so that if this muscle was contracting, it now relaxes. The group II afferents also excite their own muscle, but disynaptically (i.e., two neurons connected through an interneuron) (Patton et al., 1989; Pearson & Gordon, 2000). Experiments have shown that the strongest monosynaptic connections are found in type I motor units (i.e., fatigue-resistant slow twitch motor units) with Ia afferents that connect the alpha motoneuron with antigravity muscles during postural tasks (Windhorst, 2007). On the other hand, the long-loop or transcortical reflex (see Fig. 3.4C) is a more modifiable reflex, and therefore is often called a "functional stretch reflex." The gain of this reflex can be easily modified according to the environmental conditions or preparatory muscle set of the subject.

What is the purpose of gamma motor neuron activity, and when are these motor neurons to the muscle spindle active? Whenever there is a voluntary contraction, there is coactivation of both alpha (activating the main muscle, that is the extrafusal muscle fiber) and gamma (activating the spindle muscle, i.e., the intrafusal fiber) motor neurons. Without this coactivation, spindle sensory neurons would be silent during voluntary muscle contraction. With it, in addition to the regular extrafusal fibers of the muscle, the polar regions of the nuclear bag and chain fibers contract, and thus the central region of the muscle spindle (with the group Ia and II afferent endings) cannot go slack. Because of this coactivation, if there is unexpected stretch during the contraction, the group Ia and II afferents will be able to sense it and compensate.

Golgi Tendon Organs. Golgi tendon organs (GTOs) are spindle-shaped (1 mm long by 0.1 mm diameter) and are located at the muscle–tendon junction (Fig. 3.5A). They connect to 15 to 20 muscle fibers. Afferent information from the GTO is carried to the nervous system via the Ib afferent fibers. Unlike the muscle spindles, they have no efferent connections, and thus are not subject to CNS modulation.

The GTO is sensitive to tension changes that result from either stretch or contraction of the muscle. The GTO responds to as little as 2 to 25 g of force. The GTO reflex is an inhibitory disynaptic reflex, inhibiting its own muscle and exciting its antagonist (Fig. 3.5B). Note in the figure that joint receptors and cutaneous receptors may also contribute to this reflex.

Researchers used to think that the GTO was active only in response to large amounts of tension, so they hypothesized that the role of the GTO was to protect the muscle from injury. Current research has shown that these receptors constantly monitor muscle tension and are very sensitive to even small amounts of tension changes caused by muscle contractions. Another function of the GTO is that it modulates muscle output in response to fatigue. Thus, when muscle tension is reduced because of fatigue, the GTO output is reduced, lowering its inhibitory effect on its own muscle (Patton et al., 1989; Pearson & Gordon, 2000).

It has also been shown that the GTOs of the extensor muscles of the leg are active during the stance phase of locomotion and act to excite the extensor muscles and inhibit the flexor muscles until the GTO is unloaded (Pearson et al., 1992). This is exactly the opposite of what would be expected from the reflex when it is activated with the animal in a passive state. Thus, the reflex appears to have different properties under different task conditions.

Joint Receptors. How do joint receptors work, and what is their function? There are a number of different types of receptors within the joint itself, including Ruffini-type receptors or spray endings that respond to the mechanical stress and deformity of joint capsules, Paciniform corpuscles in joint capsules that respond to local compression, and others such as Golgi-type endings, in ligaments, in addition to free nerve endings. They are located in different portions of the joint capsule and are generally classified as type I (slowly adapting receptors) in the outer layers of the fibrous joint capsule, type II (rapidly adapting receptors) in the deeper layers of the joint capsule, and type III (slowly adapting receptors) embedded in the ligaments and terminal regions of the tendons near the joint capsule (Tuthill & Azim, 2018). Morphologically, they share the same characteristics as many of the other receptors found in the nervous system. For example, the ligament receptors are almost identical to GTOs, while the Paciniform endings are identical to Pacinian corpuscles in the skin.

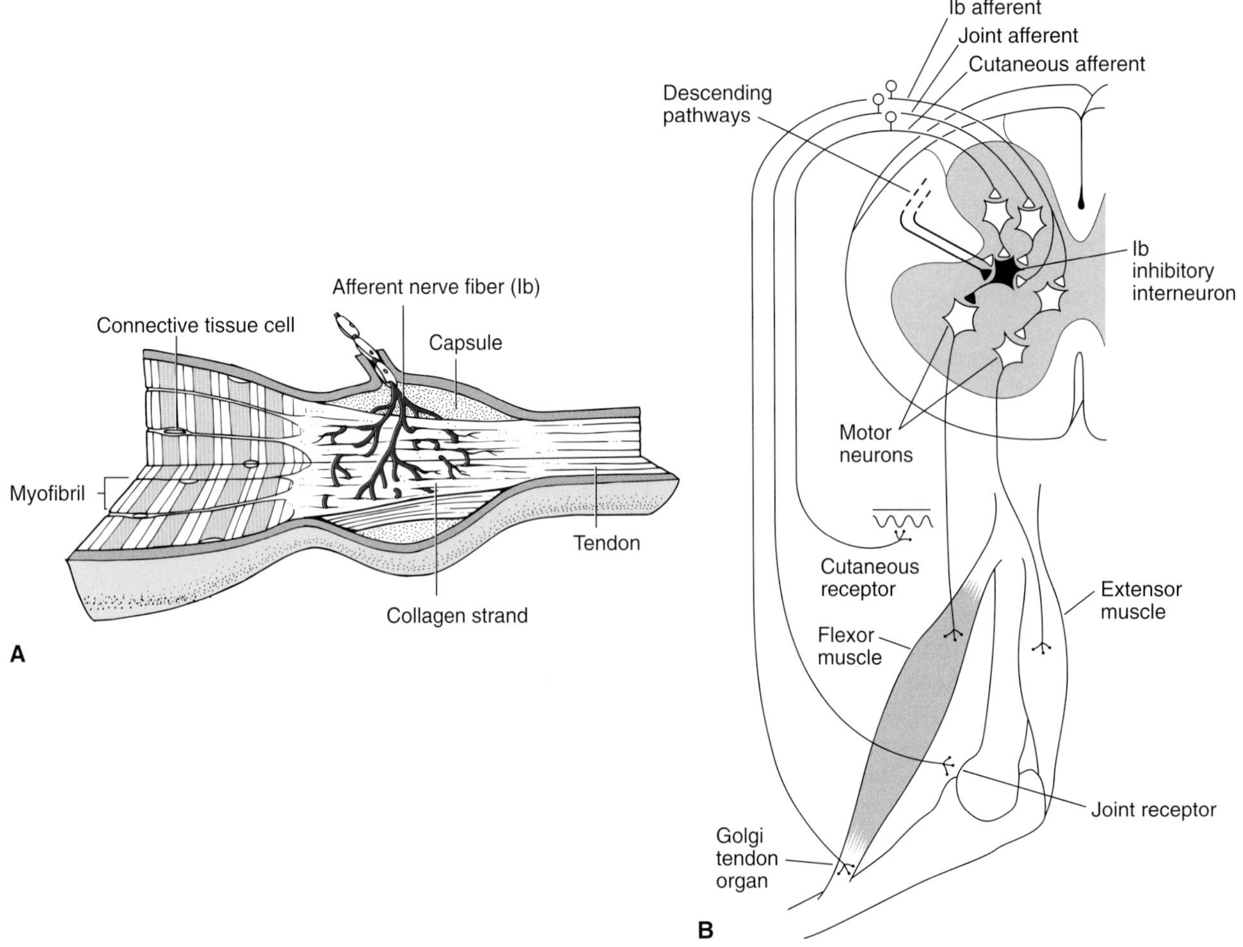

Figure 3.5 (A) Golgi tendon organ and its Ib afferent innervation. It is located at the muscle–tendon junction and is connected to 15 to 20 muscle fibers. **(B)** Neural circuitry of the Golgi tendon organ (GTO) reflex pathways, showing the GTO in the biceps muscle. Ib afferent information from the GTO synapses onto Ib inhibitory interneurons, which inhibit motor neurons to the agonist muscle and also disynaptically excite motor neurons in the antagonist triceps muscle. (Part **B** adapted from Kandel ER, Schwartz JH, Jessel TM, et al., eds. *Principles of neural science*, 5th ed. New York, NY: McGraw-Hill, 2013, with permission.)

There are a number of intriguing aspects of joint function. The joint receptor information is used at several levels of the hierarchy of sensory processing. Some researchers have found that a portion of joint receptors appear to be sensitive only to extreme joint angles, without being specific to any particular movement direction. The response of phasic joint receptors adapts rapidly to most joint angles but the response is sustained when maximal extension is combined with a twisting force (Burgess & Clark, 1969). Additionally, the concentration of mechanoreceptors is greater in the joint areas involved in extreme movements (Zimmy, 1988). Studies indicate that joint receptors signal movements but are not a critical component of the proprioceptive machinery to signal direction or joint position within a physiological range of motion in most joints. Researchers, however, have found that the combination of skin, joint, and muscle receptors is required for a complete and accurate detection of movements. For example, in the middle finger, when the muscle receptors are blocked, subjects cannot detect small and slow angular displacements. When the cutaneous and joint receptors are blocked, poor accuracy exists in the sensation of movements of low angular velocity (Proske & Gandevia, 2012). Altogether, the physiological and anatomical data suggest that joint receptors provide a danger signal about extreme joint motion as a mechanism of defense but not to accurately sense movements.

Cutaneous Receptors. There are also several types of cutaneous receptors: (a) mechanoreceptors, including Pacinian corpuscles, Merkel disks, Meissner corpuscles, Ruffini endings, and lanceolate endings around hair follicles, detecting mechanical stimuli; (b) thermoreceptors, detecting temperature changes; and (c) nociceptors, detecting potential damage to the skin. Figure 3.6 shows the location of these receptors in the skin. The number of receptors within the sensitive areas of the skin, such as the tips of the fingers, is very high, on the order of 2,500 cm^{-2} (Gardner et al., 2000).

Information from the cutaneous system is also used in hierarchical processing in several different ways. At lower levels of the CNS hierarchy, cutaneous

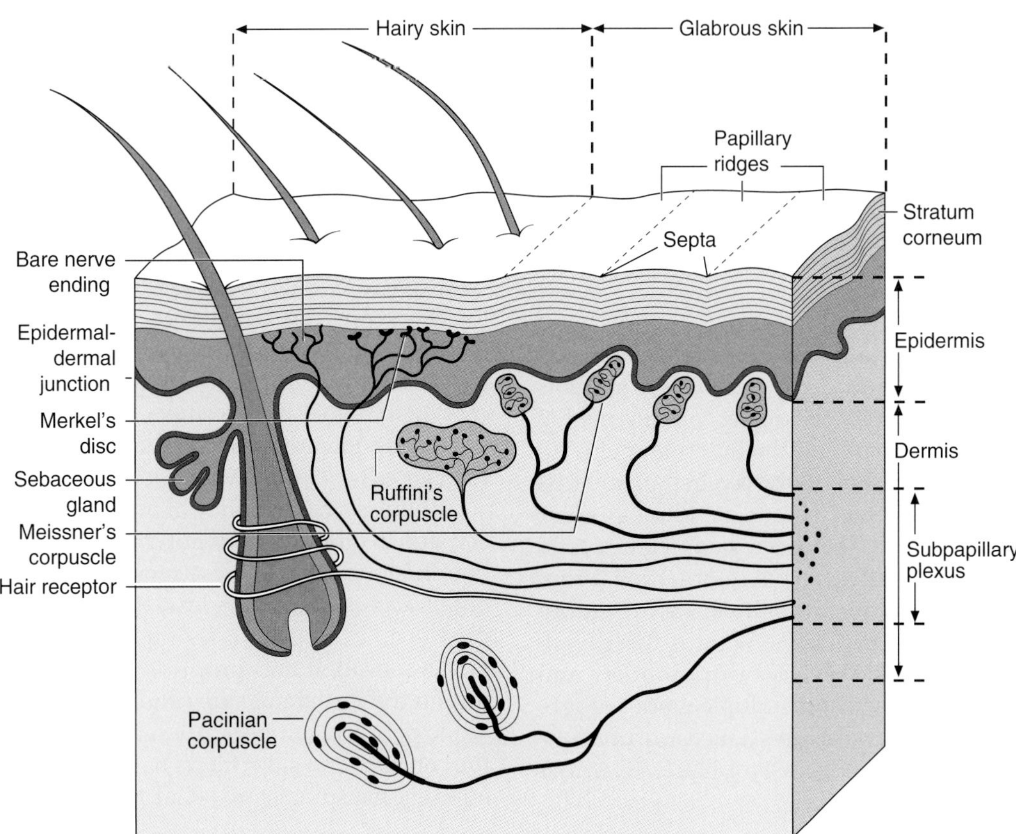

Figure 3.6 Location of cutaneous receptors in the skin. (Reproduced from Bear MF, Connors BW, Paradiso MA. *Neuroscience: Exploring the Brain*, 4th ed. Baltimore, MD: Lippincott Williams & Wilkins, 2015, with permission.)

information gives rise to reflex movements. Information from the cutaneous system also ascends and provides information concerning body position essential for orientation within the immediate environment.

The nervous system uses cutaneous information for reflex responses in various ways, depending on the extent and type of cutaneous input. A light, diffuse stimulus to the bottom of the foot tends to produce extension in the limb, as for example, when you touch the pad of a cat's foot lightly, it will extend it. This is called the "placing reaction," and it is found in human infants as well. In contrast, a sharp focal stimulus tends to produce withdrawal, or flexion, even when it is applied to exactly the same area of the foot. This is called the "flexor withdrawal reflex," and it is used to protect us from injury. The typical pattern of response in the cutaneous reflex is ipsilateral flexion and contralateral extension, which allows you to support your weight on the opposite limb (mediated by group III and IV afferents).

It is important to remember that even though we consider reflexes to be stereotyped, they are modulated by higher centers, depending on the task and the context. Remember our example of the flexor reflex, which typically causes withdrawal of a limb from a noxious stimulus. However, if there is more at stake than not hurting yourself, such as saving the life of your child, the CNS inhibits the activation of this reflex movement in favor of actions more appropriate to the situation.

Role of Somatosensation at the Spinal Cord Level

Information from muscles, cutaneous, and joint receptors modifies the output of circuits at the spinal cord level that control basic activities such as locomotion. In the late 1960s, Grillner and colleagues (Grillner, 1973, 1981) performed experiments in which they cut the dorsal roots to the spinal cord of cats to eliminate sensory feedback from the periphery and made lesions to eliminate inputs from higher brain centers. They stimulated the spinal cord and were able to activate the neural pattern generator for locomotor patterns. They found that low rates of repetitive stimulation gave rise to a walk and higher rates to a trot and then a gallop. This suggests that complex movements, such as locomotion, can be generated at the spinal cord level without supraspinal influences or inputs from the periphery.

If we do not need sensory information to generate complex movement, does that mean there is no role for sensory information in its execution? No. Hans Forssberg and his colleagues (1977) have shown that sensory information modulates locomotor output in a very elegant way. When he brushed the paw of a spinalized cat (the spinal cord was transected at level T12) with a glass rod during the swing phase of walking, it caused the paw to flex more strongly and get out of the way of the rod. But during stance, the very same stimulation caused stronger extension, in order to push off more quickly and avoid the rod in this way. Thus, he found that the same cutaneous input could modulate the step cycle in different functional ways, depending on the context in which it was used. Similar findings related to the modulation of the locomotor step cycle in response to phase-specific somatosensory input has been shown in humans as well (Stein, 1991).

Ascending Pathways

Information from the trunk and limbs is also carried to the sensory cortex and cerebellum. Two systems ascend to the cerebral cortex: the dorsal column–medial lemniscal (DC-ML) system and the anterolateral (AL) system. (Systems that ascend to the cerebellum are discussed later in this chapter.) These ascending systems are shown in Figure 3.7. They are examples of parallel ascending systems. Each relays information about somewhat different functions, but there is some redundancy between the two pathways. What is the advantage of parallel systems? They give extra subtlety and richness to perception, by using multiple modes of processing information. They also give a measure of insurance of continued function in case of injury (Gardner et al., 2000; Patton et al., 1989).

DC-ML System. The DCs (Fig. 3.7) are formed mainly by dorsal-root ganglion neurons, and thus they are first-order neurons. The majority of the fibers branch on entering the spinal cord, synapsing on interneurons and motor neurons to modulate spinal activity, and send branches to ascend in the DC pathway toward the brain. What are the functions of the DC neurons? They send information on cutaneous, muscle, tendon, and joint sensibility up to the somatosensory cortex and other higher brain centers. There is an interesting exception, however. Leg proprioceptors have their own private pathway to the brainstem, the lateral column. They join the DC pathway in the brainstem. The DC pathway also contains information from touch and pressure receptors, and codes especially for discriminative fine touch (Gardner et al., 2000).

Where does this information go, and how is it processed? The pathways synapse at multiple levels in the nervous system, including the medulla, where second-order neurons become the medial lemniscal pathway and cross over to the thalamus, synapsing with third-order neurons, which proceed to the somatosensory cortex. Every level of the hierarchy has the ability to modulate the information coming into it from below. Through synaptic excitation and inhibition, higher centers have the ability to shut off or enhance ascending information. This allows higher centers to selectively tune (up or down) the information coming from lower centers.

As the neurons ascend through each level to the brain, the information from the receptors is increasingly processed to allow meaningful interpretation of the information. This is done by selectively enlarging the receptive field (RF) of each successive neuron.

AL System. The second ascending system, shown in Figure 3.7, is the AL system. It consists of the spinothalamic, spinoreticular, and spinomesencephalic tracts. These fibers cross over upon entering the spinal cord and then ascend to brainstem centers. The AL system has a dual function. First, it transmits information on crude touch and pressure, and thus contributes in a minor way to touch and limb proprioception. It also plays a major role in relaying information related to thermal and nociception to higher brain centers. All levels of the sensory processing hierarchy act on the AL system in the same manner as for the DC-ML system (Gardner et al., 2000).

There is a redundancy of information in both tracts. A lesion in one tract does not cause complete loss of discrimination in any of these senses. However, a lesion in both tracts causes severe loss. Hemisection of the spinal cord (e.g., caused by a serious accident) would cause tactile sensation and proprioception in the arms to be lost on the ipsilateral side (fibers have not crossed yet), while pain and temperature sensation would be lost on the contralateral side (fibers have already crossed upon entering the spinal cord) (Gardner et al., 2000).

Thalamus

Information from both the ascending somatosensory tracts, like information from virtually all sensory systems, goes through the thalamus. In addition, the thalamus receives information from a number of other areas of the brain, including the basal ganglia and the cerebellum. Thus, the thalamus is a major processing center of the brain. In general, a lesion in this area will cause severe sensory (and motor) problems. The thalamus has become a target for treatments aimed at decreasing tremor in patients with Parkinson disease.

Somatosensory Cortex

The somatosensory cortex is a major processing area for all the somatosensory modalities, and marks the beginning of conscious awareness of somatosensation. The somatosensory cortex is divided into two major areas: primary somatosensory cortex (SI) (also called Brodmann areas 1, 2, 3a, and 3b); and secondary somatosensory cortex (SII). Figure 3.8A shows the location of areas SI and SII on the surface of the brain, while Figure 3.8B shows a coronal cross section of the brain indicating the location of Brodmann areas 1, 2, 3a, and 3b within SI. Figure 3.8C shows the input connections to SI, the internal connections between the various areas of SI, and the output to SII. In SI, kinesthetic and touch information from the contralateral side of the body is organized in a somatotopic manner and spans four cytoarchitectural areas, Brodmann areas 1, 2, 3a, and 3b.

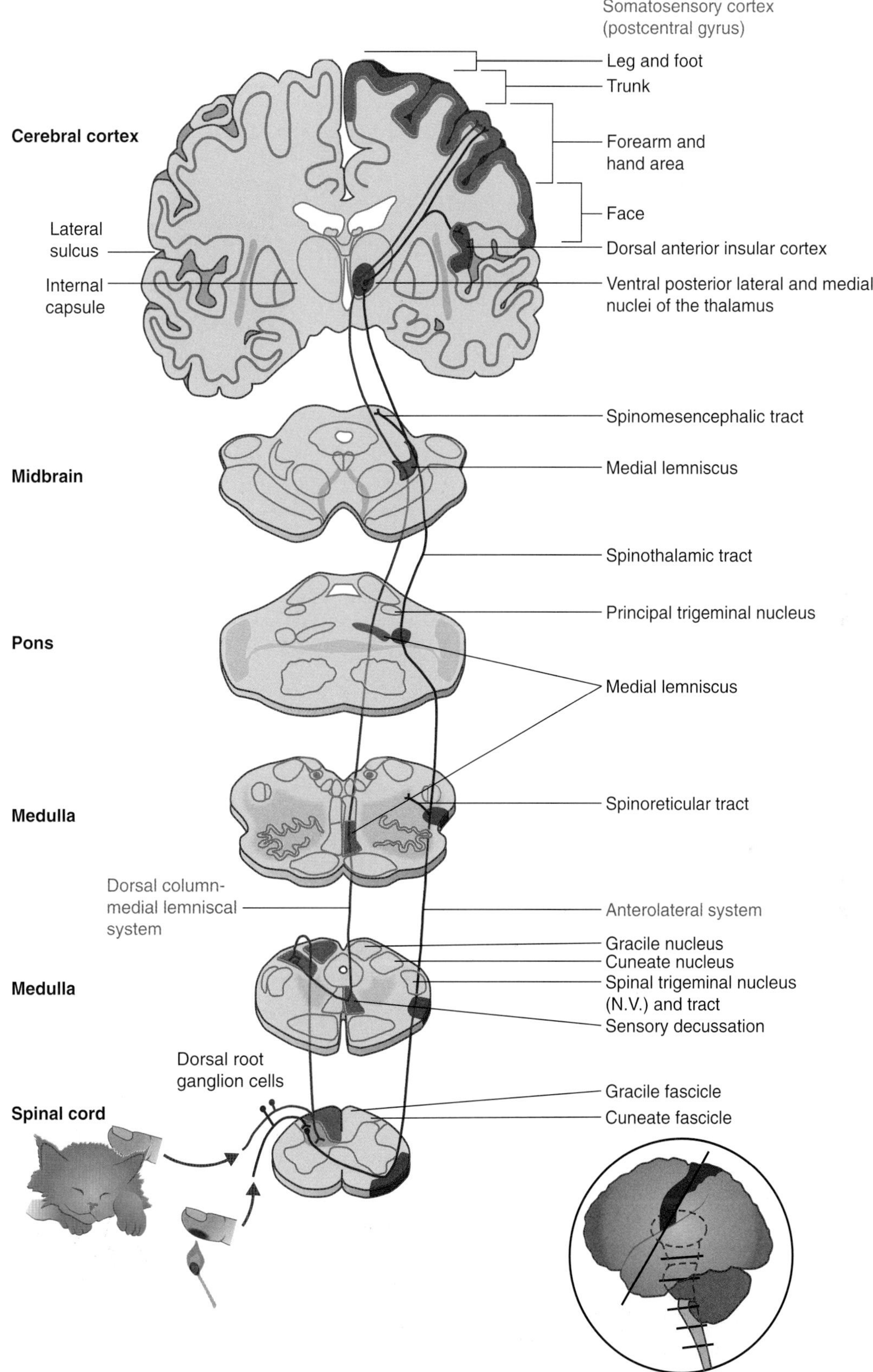

Figure 3.7 Ascending sensory systems, including the dorsal column–medial lemniscal pathway, which contains information from touch and pressure receptors, and the anterolateral system, which contains information on pain, temperature, crude touch, and pressure. The figure shows cross sections of the brain and spinal cord at six different levels, in order to see how the pathways change as you move upward toward the cortex. The positions of the cross-sectional cuts are shown in the circle at the bottom of the figure. The cutaneous receptor (fine touch) going to the dorsal-column pathway is shown being activated by lightly touching a kitten's head. The cutaneous pain receptor going to the anterolateral pathway is shown being activated by a match to a fingertip.

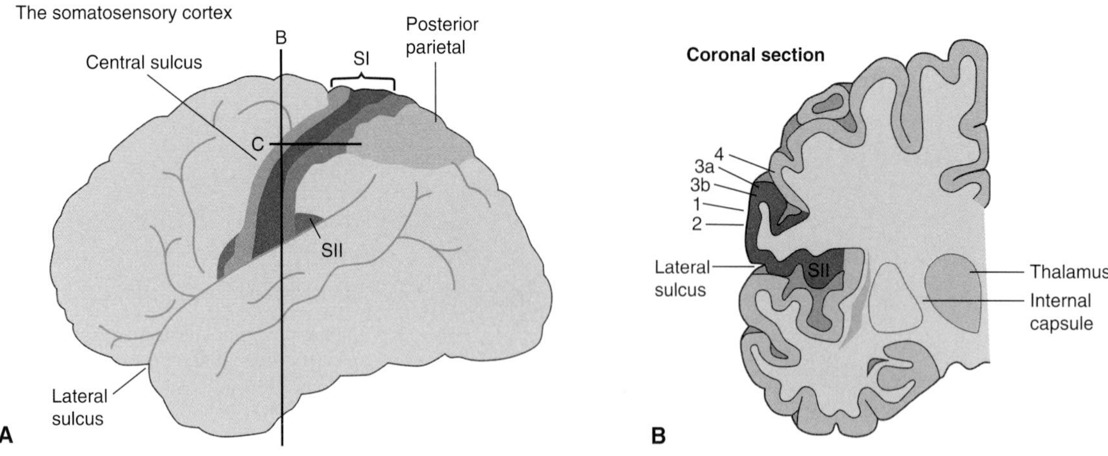

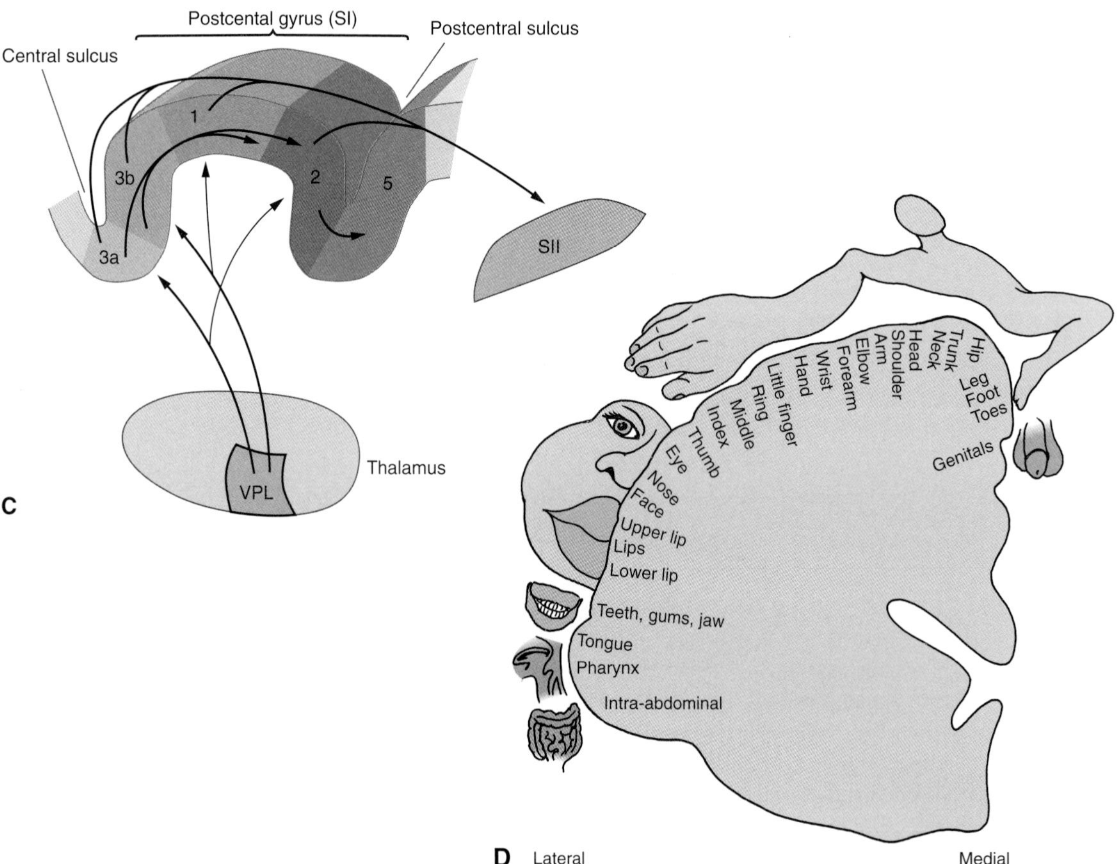

Figure 3.8 Somatosensory cortex and association areas. **(A)** Located in the parietal lobe, the somatosensory cortex contains three major divisions: the primary (SI) and secondary (SII) somatosensory cortices and the posterior parietal cortex. **(B)** Coronal section showing the location of Brodmann areas 1, 2, 3a, and 3b within SI. **(C)** Diagram showing the input to SI from the thalamus, internal connections within SI, and output to SII. **(D)** Sensory homunculus showing the somatic sensory projections from the body surface. VPL, ventral posterolateral nucleus. (**A, B**, and **C** are adapted from Kandel ER, Schwartz JH, Jessel TM, et al., eds. *Principles of neural science*, 5th ed. New York, NY: McGraw-Hill, 2013.)

It is in this area that we begin to see cross-modality processing. This means that information from joint receptors, muscle spindles, and cutaneous receptors is now integrated to give us information about movement in a given body area. This information is laid on top of a map of the entire body, which is distorted to reflect the relative weight given sensory information from certain areas, as shown in Figure 3.8D. For example, the throat, mouth, and hands are heavily represented because we need more detailed information to support the movements that are executed by these structures. This is the beginning of the spatial processing that is essential to the coordination of movements in space. Coordinated movement requires information about the position of the body relative to the environment and the position of one body segment relative to another (Gardner & Kandel, 2000).

Contrast sensitivity is very important to movement control, since it allows the detection of the shape and edges of objects. The somatosensory cortex processes incoming information to increase contrast sensitivity so that we can more easily identify and discriminate between different objects through touch. How does it do this? It has been shown that the RFs of the somatosensory neurons have an excitatory center and inhibitory surround. This inhibitory surround aids in two-point discrimination through lateral inhibition.

How does lateral inhibition work? The cell that is excited inhibits the cells next to it, thus enhancing contrast between excited and nonexcited regions of the body. The receptors themselves do not have lateral inhibition; it happens at the level of the DCs and at each subsequent step in the relay. In fact, humans have a sufficiently sensitive somatosensory system to perceive the activation of a single tactile receptor in the hand (Gardner & Kandel, 2000).

Different features of an object are processed in parallel in different parts of the somatosensory cortex. For example, neurons in Brodmann area 1 sense object size, having large RFs covering many fingers. Other cells, in area 2, respond best to moving stimuli and are sensitive to direction. One does not find this feature in the DCs or in the thalamus. These higher-level processing cells also have larger RFs than do the typical cells in the somatosensory cortex, often encompassing a number of fingers. These cells appear to respond preferentially when neighboring fingers are stimulated. This could indicate their participation in functions such as the grasping of objects.

It has been found that the RFs of neurons in the somatosensory cortex are not fixed in size. Both injury and experience can change their dimensions considerably. The implications of these studies are considered in the motor learning sections (Chapters 2 and 4) of this book. Somatosensory cortex also has descending connections to the thalamus, DC nucleus, and the spinal cord, and thus has the ability to modulate ascending information coming through these structures.

Many patients with neural pathology demonstrate somatosensory problems, including those who have had a stroke. Children with cerebral palsy including Thomas, our child with spastic diplegia, have somatosensory problems including loss of light touch and proprioception. Though Mike does not, many patients with Parkinson's disease do have problems with reduced proprioception. Finally, Bonnie, our balance-impaired older adult, has significant loss of somatosensation.

Association Cortices

It is in the many association cortices that we begin to see the transition from perception to action. It is here, too, that we see the interplay between cognitive and perceptual processing. The association cortices, found in parietal, temporal, and occipital lobes, include centers for higher-level sensory processing and higher-level abstract cognitive processing. The locations of these various areas are shown in Figure 3.9.

Within the parietal, temporal, and occipital cortices are association areas that are hypothesized to link

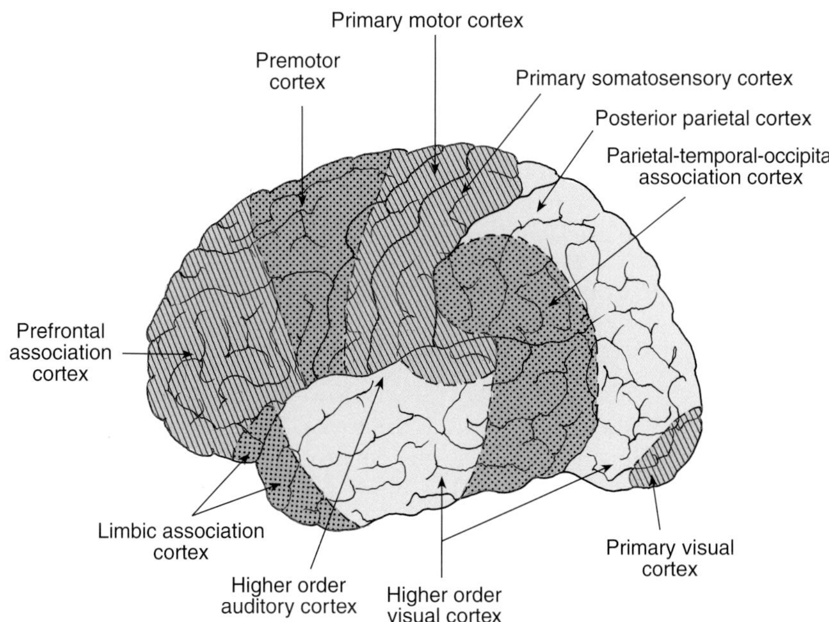

Figure 3.9 Locations of primary sensory areas, higher-level sensory association areas, and higher-level cognitive (abstract) association cortices. (Adapted from Kandel ER, Schwartz JH, Jessell TM, eds. *Principles of neural science*, 3rd ed. New York, NY: Elsevier, 1991:825.)

information from several senses. Brodmann area 5 of the parietal cortex is a thin strip posterior to the postcentral gyrus. After intermodality processing has taken place within area SI, outputs are sent to area 5, which integrates information between body parts. Area 5 connects to area 7 of the parietal lobe. Area 7 also receives processed visual information. Thus, area 7 combines eye–limb processing in most visually triggered or guided activities.

Lesions in Brodmann area 5 or area 7 in humans and other animals cause problems with learning skills that use information regarding the position of the body in space. In addition, certain cells in these areas are activated during visually guided movements, with their activity becoming more intense when the animal attends to the movement. These findings support the hypothesis that the parietal lobe participates in processes involving attention to the position and manipulation of objects in space.

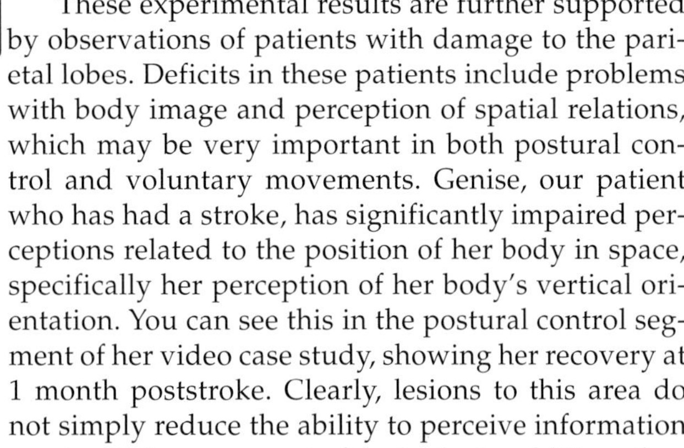

These experimental results are further supported by observations of patients with damage to the parietal lobes. Deficits in these patients include problems with body image and perception of spatial relations, which may be very important in both postural control and voluntary movements. Genise, our patient who has had a stroke, has significantly impaired perceptions related to the position of her body in space, specifically her perception of her body's vertical orientation. You can see this in the postural control segment of her video case study, showing her recovery at 1 month poststroke. Clearly, lesions to this area do not simply reduce the ability to perceive information coming in from one part of the body; in addition, they can affect the ability to interpret this information.

For example, people with lesions in the right angular gyrus (the nondominant hemisphere), just behind Brodmann area 7, show complete neglect of the contralateral side of body, objects, and drawings. This is called agnosia, or the inability to recognize. When their own arm or leg is passively moved into their visual field, they may claim that it is not theirs. In certain cases, patients may be totally unaware of the hemiplegia that accompanies the lesion and may thus desire to leave the hospital early since they are unaware that they have any problem (Kupfermann, 1991). Many of these same patients show problems when asked to copy drawn figures. They may make a drawing in which half of the object is missing. This is called "constructional apraxia." Larger lesions may cause the inability to operate and orient in space or the inability to perform complex sequential tasks.

When right-handed patients have lesions in the left angular gyrus (the dominant hemisphere), they show such symptoms as confusion between left and right; difficulty in naming their fingers, although they can sense touch; and difficulty in writing, although their motor and sensory functions are normal for the hands. Alternatively, when patients have lesions to both sides of these areas, they often have problems attending to visual stimuli, in using vision to grasp an object, and in making voluntary eye movements to a point in space (Kupfermann, 1991).

We have just taken one sensory system, the somatosensory system, from the lowest to the highest level of the CNS hierarchy, going from the reception of signals in the periphery to the integration and interpretation of those signals relative to other sensory systems. We have also looked at how hierarchical and parallel distributed processing has contributed to the analysis of these signals. We are now going to look at a second sensory system, the visual system, in the same way.

Visual System

Vision serves motor control in a number of ways. Vision allows us to identify objects in space and to determine their movement. When vision plays this role, it is considered an exteroceptive sense. But vision also gives us information about where our bodies are in space, the relation of one body part to another, and the motion of our bodies. When vision plays this role, it is referred to as "visual proprioception," which means that it gives us information not only about the environment but also about our own bodies. Later chapters show how vision plays a key role in the control of posture, locomotion, and manipulatory function. In the following sections, we consider the anatomy and physiology of the visual system to show how it supports these roles in motor control.

Peripheral Visual System

Photoreceptor Cells. Let us first look at an overall view of the eye. The eye is a great instrument, designed to focus the image of the world on the retina with high precision. As illustrated in Figure 3.10, light enters the eye through the cornea and is focused by the cornea and lens on the retina at the back of the eye. An interesting feature of the retina is that light must travel through all the layers of the eye and the neural layers of the retina before it hits the photoreceptors, which are at the back of the retina, facing away from the light source. Luckily, these layers are nearly transparent.

There are two types of photoreceptor cells: the rods and the cones. The cones are functional for vision in normal daylight and are responsible for color vision. The rods are responsible for vision at night, when the amount of light is very low and too weak to activate the cones. Right at the fovea, the rest of the layers are pushed aside so the cones can receive the light in its clearest form. The blind spot (where the optic nerve leaves the retina) has no photoreceptors, and therefore we are blind in this one part of the retina. Except for the fovea, there are 20 times more rods than cones in the retina. However, cones are more important than rods

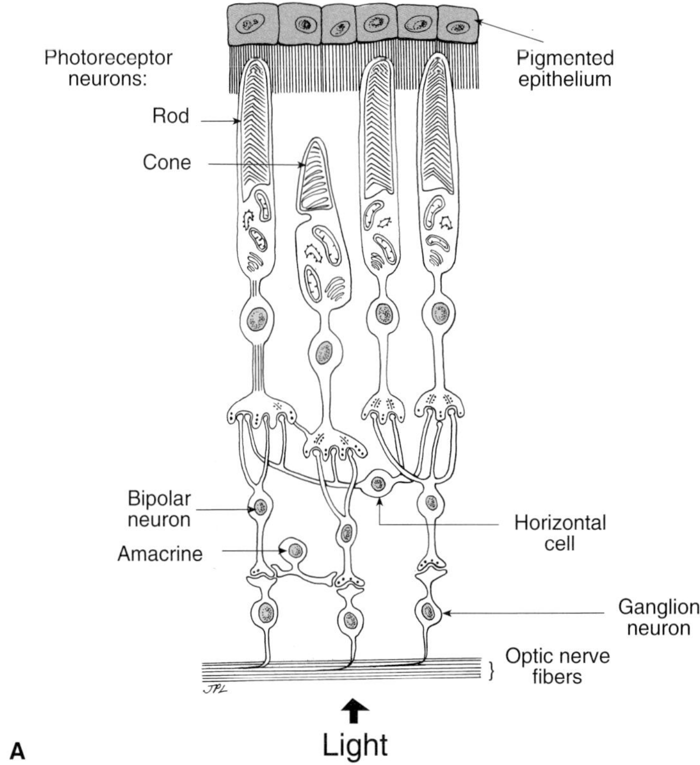

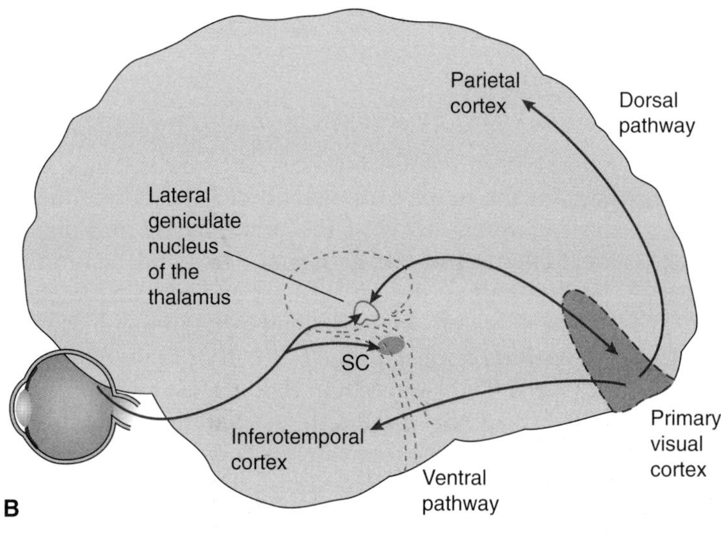

Figure 3.10 (A) The relationship among visual cells in the retina; **(B)** pathways from the retina in the eye through the superior colliculus and LGN to both primary visual cortex and the dorsal and ventral visual pathways.

for normal vision, because their loss causes legal blindness, while total loss of rods causes only night blindness (Tessier-Lavigne, 2000).

Remember that sensory differentiation is a key aspect of sensory processing that supports motor control. To accomplish this, the visual system has to identify objects and determine whether they are moving. So how are object identification and motion sense accomplished in the visual system? There are two separate pathways to process them. We will follow these pathways from the retina all the way up to the visual cortex. We will see that contrast sensitivity is used in both pathways to accomplish the goals of object identification and motion sense. Contrast sensitivity enhances the edges of objects, giving us greater precision in perception. As in the somatosensory system, all three processes are used extensively in the visual system. This processing begins in the retina. So, let us first look at the cells of the retina, so that we can understand how they work together to process information (Tessier-Lavigne, 2000).

In addition to the rods and cones, the retina contains bipolar cells and ganglion cells, which you might consider vertical cells, since they connect in series to one another but have no lateral connections (Fig. 3.10A).

For example, the rods and cones make direct synaptic contact with bipolar cells. The bipolar cells in turn connect to the ganglion cells. And the ganglion cells then relay visual information to the CNS by sending axons to the lateral geniculate nucleus (LGN) and superior colliculus as well as to brainstem nuclei (Dowling, 1987; Tessier-Lavigne, 2000).

There is another class of neurons in the retina, which modulate the flow of information within the retina by connecting the cells that are organized in series together laterally. These are called the horizontal and amacrine cells. The horizontal cells mediate interactions between the receptors and bipolar cells, while the amacrine cells mediate interactions between bipolar and ganglion cells. The horizontal cells and amacrine cells are critical for achieving contrast sensitivity. Although it may appear that there are complex interconnections between the receptor cells and other neurons before the final output of the ganglion cells is reached, the pathways and functions of the different classes of cells are straightforward.

Let us first look at the bipolar-cell pathway. There are two types of pathways that involve bipolar cells, a direct pathway and a lateral pathway. In the direct pathway, a cone, for example, makes a direct connection with a bipolar cell, which makes a direct connection with a ganglion cell. In the lateral pathway, activity of cones is transmitted to the ganglion cells lateral to them through horizontal cells or amacrine cells. Figure 3.10A shows these organizational possibilities (Dowling, 1987).

In the direct pathway, cones (or rods) connect directly to bipolar cells with either on-center or off-center RFs. The RF of a cell is the specific area of the retina to which the cell is sensitive, when that part of the retina is illuminated. The RF can be either excitatory or inhibitory, increasing or decreasing the cell's membrane potential. The RFs of bipolar cells (and ganglion cells) are circular. At the center of the retina, the RFs are small, while in the periphery RFs are large. The term on-center means that the cell has an excitatory central portion of the RF, with an inhibitory surrounding area. Off-center refers to the opposite case of an inhibitory center and excitatory surround (Dowling, 1987).

How do the cells take on their antagonistic surround characteristics? It appears that horizontal cells in the surround area of the bipolar-cell RF make connections onto cones in the center of the field. When light shines on the periphery of the RF, the horizontal cells inhibit the cones adjacent to them. Each type of bipolar cell then synapses with a corresponding type of ganglion cell: on-center and off-center, and makes excitatory connections with that ganglion cell.

On-center cells give very few action potentials in the dark, and they are activated when their RF is illuminated. When the periphery of the on-center cells' RF is illuminated, it inhibits the effect of stimulating the center. Off-center ganglion cells likewise show inhibition when light is applied to the center of their RF, and they fire at the fastest rate just after the light is turned off. They also are activated if light is applied only to the periphery of their RF.

Ganglion cells are also influenced by the activity of amacrine cells. Many of the amacrine cells function in a manner similar to that of horizontal cells, transmitting inhibitory inputs from nearby bipolar cells to the ganglion cell, increasing contrast sensitivity.

These two types of pathways (on- and off-center) for processing retinal information are two examples of parallel distributed processing of similar information within the nervous system. We talked about a similar center-surround inhibition in cutaneous-receptor RFs. What is the purpose of this type of inhibition? It appears to be very important in detecting contrasts between objects, rather than the absolute intensity of light produced or reflected by an object. This inhibition allows us to detect edges of objects very easily. It is very important in locomotion, when we are walking down stairs and need to see the edge of the step. It is also important in manipulatory function, in being able to determine the exact shape of an object for grasping.

The ganglion cells send their axons, via the optic nerve, to three different regions in the brain, the LGN, the pretectum, and the superior colliculus (Wurtz & Kandel, 2000a). Figure 3.10B shows connections to the LGN of the thalamus.

Central Visual Pathways

Lateral Geniculate Nucleus. To understand what parts of the retina and visual field are represented in these different areas of the brain, let us first discuss the configuration of the visual fields and hemiretina. The left half of the visual field projects on the nasal (medial—next to the nose) half of the retina of the left eye and the temporal (lateral) half of the retina of the right eye. The right visual field projects on the nasal half of the retina of the right eye and the temporal half of the retina of the left eye (Wurtz & Kandel, 2000a).

Thus, the optic nerves from the left and right eyes leave the retina at the optic disk, in the back. They travel to the optic chiasm, where the nerves from each eye come together, and axons from the nasal side of the eyes cross, while those from the temporal side do not cross. At this point, the optic nerve becomes the optic tract. Because of this resorting of the optic nerves, the left optic tract has a map of the right visual field. This is similar to what we found for the somatosensory system, in which information from the opposite side of the body was represented in the thalamus and cortex.

One of the targets of cells in the optic tract is the LGN of the thalamus. The LGN has six layers of cells, which map the contralateral visual field. The ganglion cells from different areas project onto specific points in the LGN, but just as we find for somatosensory maps of the body, certain areas are represented much more strongly than are others. The fovea of the retina, which we use for high-acuity vision, is represented to a far greater degree than is the peripheral area. Each layer of the LGN gets input from only one eye. The first two layers (most ventral) are the magnocellular (large cell) layers, and layers four through six are called the parvocellular (small cell) layers. The projection cells of each layer send axons to the visual cortex (Wurtz & Kandel, 2000a).

The RFs of neurons in the LGN are very similar to those found in the ganglion cells of the retina. There are separate on-center and off-center RF pathways. The magnocellular layers appear to be involved in the analysis of movement of the visual image (they have high temporal resolution, detecting fast pattern changes) and the coarse details of an object (they have low spatial resolution), with almost no response to color, while the parvocellular layers function in color vision and a more detailed structural analysis (high spatial resolution and low temporal resolution). Thus, magnocellular layers will be more important in motor functions such as balance control, for which movement of the visual field gives us information about our body sway, and in reaching for moving objects. The parvocellular layers will be more important in the final phases of reaching for an object, when we need to grasp it accurately.

Amazingly, only 10% to 20% of the inputs to the LGN come from the retina, with the rest coming from the cortex and reticular formation of the brainstem. These are feedback circuits, probably modulating the type of information moving from the retina to higher centers. This suggests that one of the most important aspects of sensory processing is choosing the inputs that are most important for an individual to attend to in a given moment and that each individual may have very different perceptions of a given event according to the sensory inputs his or her system allowed to move to higher perceptual centers (Wurtz & Kandel, 2000a).

Superior Colliculus. Ganglion-cell axons in the optic tract also terminate in the superior colliculus (in addition to indirect visual inputs coming from the visual cortex). The superior colliculus (labeled SC in Fig. 3.10B) is located posterior to the thalamus, in the roof of the midbrain. It has been hypothesized that the superior colliculus maps the visual space around us in terms of not only visual but also auditory and somatosensory cues. The three sensory maps in the superior colliculus are different from those seen in the sensory cortex. Body areas here are mapped not in terms of density of receptor cells in a particular area but in terms of their relationship to the retina. Areas close to the retina (the nose) are given more representation than are areas far away (the hand). For any part of the body, the visual, auditory, and somatosensory maps are aligned, in the different layers of the colliculus. This means that when a friend greets you as he or she bicycles by, the superior colliculus neurons will be activated, representing a particular spatial location within the visual field through which the friend is moving, and these same neurons in the superior colliculus will also be activated when the friend's voice is in the same spatial location (Wurtz & Kandel, 2000a).

In addition to these three maps, located in the upper and middle of the seven layers of the colliculus, there is a motor map in the deeper layers of the colliculus. Through these output neurons, the colliculus controls saccadic eye movements that cause the eye to move toward a specific stimulus. The superior colliculus then sends outputs to (a) regions of the brainstem that control eye movements; (b) the tectospinal tract, mediating the reflex control of the neck and head; and (c) the tectopontine tract, which projects to the cerebellum, for further processing of eye–head control.

Pretectal Region. Ganglion cells also terminate in the pretectal region, which is just anterior to the superior colliculus. The pretectal region is an important visual reflex center involved in pupillary eye reflexes, in which the pupil constricts in response to light shining on the retina.

Primary Visual Cortex

From the LGN, axons project to the primary visual cortex (V1, also called striate cortex) to Brodmann area 17, which is in the occipital lobe (Fig. 3.10B). The inputs from the two eyes alternate throughout the striate cortex, producing what are called ocular dominance columns. Output cells from primary visual cortex (V1) then project to Brodmann area 18 (V2). From area 18, neurons project to medial temporal (MT) cortex (Brodmann area 19) to inferotemporal cortex (Brodmann areas 20 and 21) and posterior parietal cortex (Brodmann area 7). In addition, outputs go to the superior colliculus and also project back to the LGN (feedback control). The primary visual cortex contains a topographic map of the retina. In addition, there are six other representations of the retina in the occipital lobe alone.

The RFs of cells in the visual cortex are not circular anymore, but linear: the light must be in the shape of a line, a bar, or an edge to excite them. These cells are classified as simple or complex cells. Simple cells respond to bars, with an excitatory center and an inhibitory surround, or vice versa. They also have a specific axis of orientation, for which the bar is most effective in exciting the cell. All axes of orientation for all parts of the retina are represented in the visual cortex. Results of experiments by Hubel and Wiesel (1959) suggest that this bar-shaped RF is created from many geniculate neurons with partially overlapping circular RFs in one line, converging onto a simple cortical cell. It has been suggested that complex cells have convergent input from many simple cells. Thus, their RFs are larger than simple cells, and have a critical axis of orientation. For many complex cells, the most useful stimulus is movement across the field.

The specific changes in the orientation axis across columns are interlaced with the presence of cells responding to color stimuli, organized in cylindrical shapes, known as "blobs."

In summary, we see that the visual cortex is divided into orientation columns, with each column consisting of cells with one axis of orientation, blobs, which are activated more by color than by orientation, and ocular dominance columns receiving input from the left versus the right eye. Hubel and Wiesel used the name hypercolumn to describe these sets of columns from one part of the retina, including color inputs and all orientation angles for the two eyes (Hubel & Wiesel, 1959).

These hypercolumns are connected horizontally to other columns with the same response properties, integrating visual inputs over broader areas of cortex. Depending on the inputs from these other areas, a cell's axis of orientation may change, showing the effect of context on a cell's output. Thus, the context in which a feature is embedded modulates the cell's response to that feature (McGuire et al., 1991).

Higher-Order Visual Cortex

Central visual processing pathways continue on to include cells in the higher-order visual cortices, located in the temporal and parietal cortex as well. Higher-order cortices are involved in the integration of somatosensory and visual information underlying spatial orientation, an essential part of all actions. This interaction between visual and somatosensory inputs within higher-order association cortices was discussed in the somatosensory section of this chapter.

The cells within the visual pathways contribute to a hierarchy within the visual system, with each level of the hierarchy increasing the visual abstraction (Hubel, 1988). In addition, Mishkin and Ungerleider (1982) have proposed a model of two visual systems, with parallel pathways through which visual information is processed. It has been proposed that these two pathways can be traced back to two main subdivisions of retinal ganglion cells, one of which synapses on the magnocellular layers (processing movement, depth, and coarse detail—processing where) and the other on the parvocellular layers (processing fine detail, contrast, contours, and color—processing what) of the LGN (Livingstone & Hubel, 1988; Wurtz & Kandel, 2000b).

One of these pathways, called the dorsal stream, terminates in the posterior parietal region. The second pathway, the ventral stream, terminates in the inferotemporal cortex. The authors noted that monkeys with lesions in the inferotemporal cortex were very impaired in visual pattern discrimination and recognition, but less impaired in solving tasks involving spatial visual cues. The opposite pattern of results was seen for monkeys with posterior parietal lesions (Milner et al., 1977; Ungerleider & Brody, 1977).

How do we sense motion? The magnocellular pathway continues to areas MT (middle temporal) and MST (medial superior temporal) and the visual motor area of the parietal lobe (the dorsal stream). In area MT, the activity in the neurons is related to the velocity and movement direction of objects. This information is then further processed in area MST for visual perception, pursuit eye movements, and guiding the movements of the body through space. Area MST has also been implicated in the processing of global motion or optic flow, which plays a role in posture and balance control, giving information on an individual's movement through space (Duffy & Wurtz, 1997).

Object vision, which depends on the ventral pathway to the inferior temporal lobe, includes separate subregions sensitive to different object characteristics. Experiments recording from neurons in the monkey have shown that cells in visual cortex area 2 (V2) analyze object contours, in a further level of abstraction beyond that of V1 in the visual hierarchy. Cells in V4 respond to color and form. A further abstraction occurs in the inferior temporal cortex, where cells have large RFs that recognize the same feature anywhere in the visual field, thus allowing us to recognize the same object wherever it is situated in space. Finally, some cells in this area respond only to specific complex inputs, such as faces or hands (Wurtz & Kandel, 2000b).

There is also interesting clinical evidence to support the existence of these parallel processing pathways. There is a perceptual deficit called movement agnosia, which occurs after damage to the MT or MST region of the cortex, which are part of the "dorsal stream." Patients show a specific loss of motion perception without any other perceptual problems. Other patients with damage to areas of the ventral stream lose color vision (achromatopsia) and the ability to identify forms (Wurtz & Kandel, 2000b).

Research by Goodale and Milner (1992; Goodale et al., 1991) suggests that there may be other functions for the dorsal and ventral streams. They suggest that the visual projection to the parietal cortex provides action-relevant information about the structure and orientation of objects and not just about their position. They also propose that projections to the ventral temporal lobe may provide our conscious visual perceptual experience.

Observations that support this model involve the fact that most neurons in the dorsal stream area show both sensory-related and movement-related activity (Andersen, 1987). In addition, patients with optic ataxia (due to lesions in the parietal areas) have problems not only with reaching in the right direction, but also with positioning their fingers or adjusting the orientation of their hand when reaching toward an object. They also have trouble adjusting their grasp to reflect the size of the object they are picking up. Goodale and colleagues note that damage to the parietal lobe can impair the ability of patients to use information about the size, shape, and orientation of an object to control the hand and fingers during a grasping movement, even though this same information can be used to identify and describe objects. This is the case for both Jean and Genise, whose problems with upper extremity function including grasp and manipulation are due to both motor impairments as well as sensory-related problems integrating information about objects to be grasped.

It is also interesting that the two cortical pathways are different with respect to their access to consciousness. One patient with ventral stream lesions had no conscious perception of the orientation or dimension of objects, but she could pick them up with great adeptness. Thus, it may be that information in the dorsal system can be processed without reaching conscious perception. As a result of their analysis of the above observations, the authors propose that the ventral stream of projections plays a major role in the perceptual identification of objects, while the dorsal stream mediates the required sensorimotor transformations for visually guided actions directed at those objects (Goodale & Milner, 1992).

How do we take the information processed by these parallel pathways and organize it into a perceptual whole? This process by which the brain recombines information processed in its different regions is called the binding problem. The recombination of this information appears to require attention, which may be mediated by subcortical structures such as the superior colliculus, as well as cortical areas, such as the posterior parietal and prefrontal cortex (see "Attentional Networks" section of this chapter for details). It has been hypothesized that the CNS takes information related to color, size, distance, and orientation and organizes it into a master map of the image (Treisman, 1999). Our attentional systems allow us to focus on one small part of the master map as we identify objects or move through space.

One neural mechanism hypothesized to contribute to binding everything into one cohesive experience is that information from neural events in many different parts of the cortex (visual, auditory, kinesthetic, memory, etc.) is integrated by the cortex to produce perceptual binding through synchronizing their neural activation patterns, leaving all other neural activations nonsynchronized (Dehaene & Changeux, 2004; Roskies, 1999; Treisman, 1999). This creates a global neuronal workspace.

According to this hypothesis, multiple inputs compete for access to an attentional network, and those that win become the contents of conscious experience (Baars, 1993; Delacour, 1997). Behaviorally, the experimenter knows the contents that won because they are the pieces of information that a person is able to report on among the many pieces that might be shown to him or her in an experiment.

This theory divides the brain into two separate computational spaces: network processors and a global neuronal workspace. According to this theory, there are many subcortical networks in the brain and also much of the cerebral cortex can be considered to be like modular processing networks for particular types of information (e.g., motion processors or visual word-form processors). But in addition to these processing networks, there is a special set of cerebral cortex neurons, the global workspace neurons, which have long-range axons and can send and receive information from modular processors in distant parts of the brain. The unconscious information from the modular processors would be temporarily made available (and therefore conscious) to the global workspace when these processors begin to fire in synchrony with these global neurons. This happens when either the signals from the modular processes become strong enough to "catch the attention" of the global neurons (a loud noise, for example) or the material they are conveying matches the "interest patterns" that the global workspace deems significant (you shift your focus to something, so the sensory input connected with it suddenly becomes relevant to the processing mechanism of the global workspace). At any moment in time, there would be a single global representation of workspace neurons and modular processors that are firing in synchrony and thus part of conscious awareness, with the rest of workspace neurons (neurons in the other processing modules) being inhibited (Woollacott, 2005).

Vestibular System

The vestibular system is sensitive to two types of information: the position of the head in space and sudden changes in the direction of movement of the head. Although we are not consciously aware of vestibular sensation, as we are of the other senses, vestibular inputs are important for the coordination of many motor responses, with inputs that help to stabilize the eyes and to maintain postural stability during stance and walking. Abnormalities within the vestibular system result in sensations such as dizziness or unsteadiness, which do reach our awareness, as well as problems with focusing our eyes and keeping our balance.

Diverse brain regions have been identified as cortical sites influenced by vestibular signals, including: posterior parietal cortex, posterior and anterior insula, temporo-parietal junction, somatosensory cortex, premotor cortex, precuneus, cingulate gyrus, hippocampus, and parahippocampal gyrus. Human and animal research also shows data indicating that vestibular information can be integrated at the cortex in conjunction with other sensory modalities (e.g., visual signals) to process self-motion perception, spatial navigation, internal models of gravity, one's body perception, and bodily self-consciousness (Lopez & Blanke, 2011; Ventre-dominey 2014).

Like other sensory systems, the vestibular system can be divided into two parts, a peripheral and a central component. The peripheral component consists of the sensory receptors and eighth cranial nerve, while the central part consists of the four vestibular nuclei as well as the ascending and descending tracts.

Peripheral Receptors

Let us first look at the anatomy of the vestibular system (Fig. 3.11A). The vestibular system is part of the membranous labyrinth of the inner ear (right side of figure). The other part of the labyrinth is the cochlea, which is concerned with hearing. The membranous labyrinth consists of a continuous series of tubes and sacs located in the temporal bone of the skull. The membranous labyrinth is surrounded by a fluid called perilymph and filled with a fluid called endolymph. The endolymph has a density greater than that of water, giving it inertial characteristics that are important to the way the vestibular system functions. The vestibular portion of the labyrinth includes five receptors: three semicircular canals, the utricle, and the saccule.

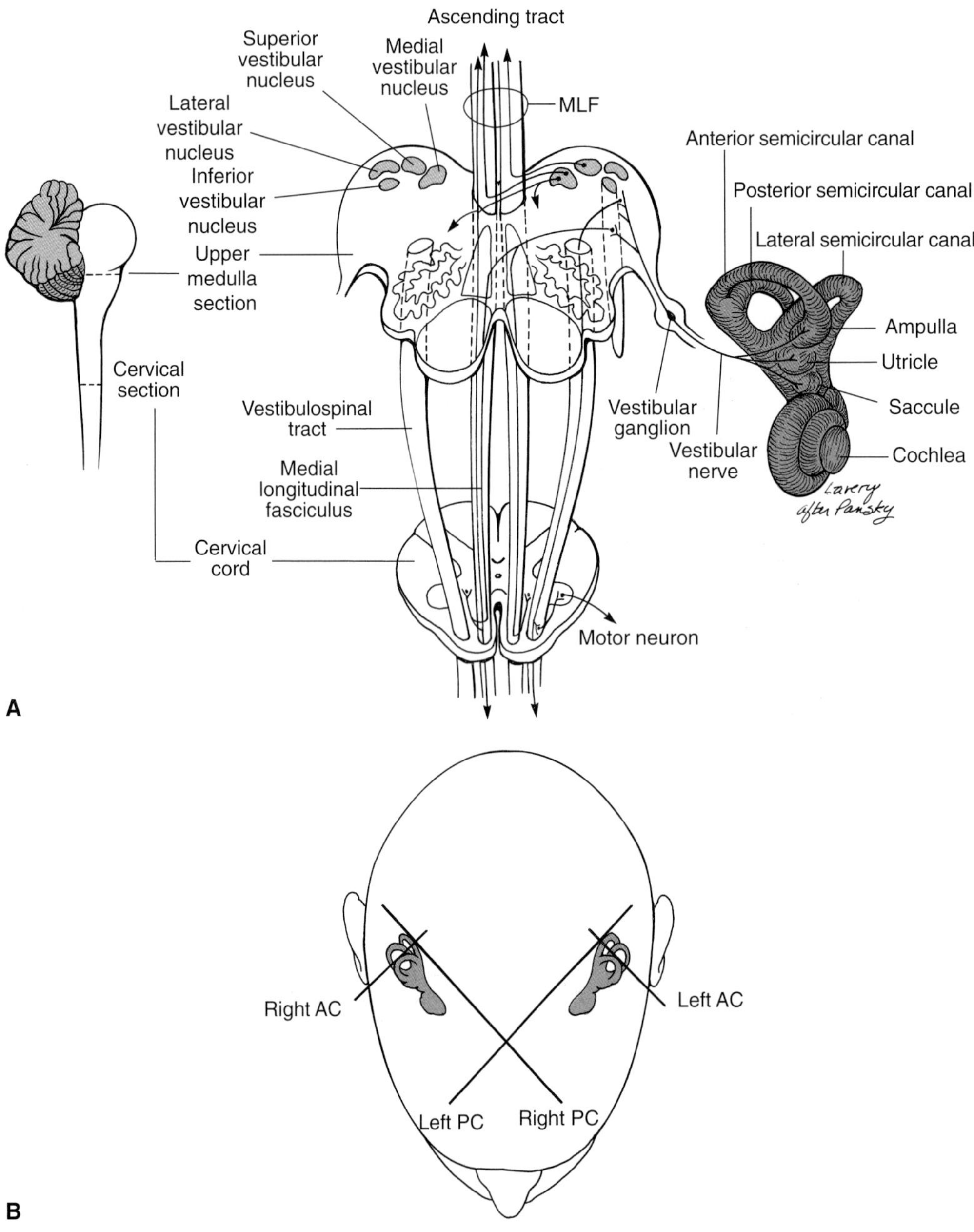

Figure 3.11 Vestibular system. **(A)** Membranous labyrinth (otoliths and semicircular canals) are shown on the right, and the central connections of the vestibular system are shown on the left. Two cross sections of the brain and spinal cord are shown, one at the upper medulla and one at the cervical spinal cord. The small figure of the brainstem and spinal cord on the far left shows the positions of these cross sections. The figure shows the ascending vestibular inputs to the oculomotor complex, important for stabilizing gaze, and the descending vestibulospinal system, important for posture and balance. **(B)** The paired semicircular canals within the temporal bone of the skull. Lines show their orientation. AC, anterior canal; PC, posterior canal; MLF, medial longitudinal fasciculus.

Semicircular Canals. The semicircular canals function as angular accelerometers. They lie at right angles to each other on either side of the head and are named the anterior, posterior, and horizontal (or lateral) canals (Fig. 3.11). At least one pair is affected by any given angular acceleration of the head or body. The sensory endings of the semicircular canals are in the enlarged end of each canal, which is called the *ampulla,* near its junction with the utricle. Each ampulla has an ampullary crest, which contains the vestibular hair cells. The hair cells project upward into the cupula (Latin for small inverted cup), which is made of gelatinous material and extends to the top of the ampulla, thus preventing movement of the endolymph past the cupula. The hair cells are the vestibular receptors and are innervated by bipolar sensory neurons, which are part of the eighth nerve. Their cell bodies are located in the vestibular ganglion (Baloh, 1984; Goldberg & Hudspeth, 2000).

How do the semicircular canals signal head motion to the nervous system? When the head starts to rotate, initially the fluid in the canals does not move because of its inertial characteristics. As a result, the cupula, along with its hair cells, bends in the direction opposite to head movement. When head motion stops, the cupula and hair cells are deflected in the opposite direction, that is, the direction in which the head had been moving.

When the hair cells bend, they cause a change in the firing frequency of the nerve, depending on which way the hair cells are bent. For each hair cell, there is a kinocilium (the tallest tuft) and 40 to 70 stereocilia, which increase in length, as they get closer to the kinocilium. Bending the hair cell toward the kinocilium causes a depolarization of the hair cell and an increase in the firing rate of the bipolar cells of the eighth nerve, and bending away causes hyperpolarization and a decrease in the firing rate of bipolar cells. At rest, the hair cells fire at 100 Hz, so they have a wide range of frequencies for modulation. Thus, increases or decreases in firing frequency of the neurons are possible because of this tonic resting discharge, which occurs in the absence of head motion (Baloh, 1984; Goldberg & Hudspeth, 2000).

Because canals on each side of the head are approximately parallel to one another, they work together in a reciprocal fashion. The two horizontal canals work together, while each anterior canal is paired with a posterior canal on the opposite side of the head, as shown in Figure 3.11B. When head motion occurs in a plane specific to a pair of canals, one canal will be excited, while its paired opposite canal will be hyperpolarized.

Thus, angular motion of the head, either horizontal or vertical, results in either an increase or decrease in hair-cell activity and an opposite change in the frequency of neuronal activity in paired canals. Receptors in the semicircular canal are very sensitive: they respond to angular accelerations of 0.1 degree per second^2, but do not respond to steady-state motion of the head. During prolonged motion of the head, the cupula returns to its resting position, and firing frequency in the neurons returns to its steady state.

Utricle and Saccule. The utricle and saccule provide information about body position with reference to the force of gravity and linear acceleration or movement of the head in a straight line. On the wall of these structures is a thickening where the epithelium contains hair cells. This area is called the *macula* (Latin for "spot") and is where the receptor cells are located. The hair cells project tufts or processes up into a gelatinous membrane, the otolith organ (Greek, from "lithos," meaning "stone"). The otolith organ has many calcium carbonate crystals called otoconia, or otoliths (Goldberg & Hudspeth, 2000).

The macula of the utricle lies in the horizontal plane when the head is held horizontally (normal position), so the otoliths rest upon it. But if the head is tilted, or accelerates, the hair cells are bent by the movement of the gelatinous mass. The macula of the saccule lies in the vertical plane when the head is positioned normally, so it responds selectively to vertically directed linear forces. As in the semicircular canals, hair cells in the otoliths respond to bending in a directional manner.

Central Connections

Vestibular Nuclei. Information from both the otoliths and the semicircular canals goes through the eighth cranial nerve (vestibulocochlear) and these neurons have their cell bodies in the vestibular ganglion (Scarpa ganglion). The axons then enter the brain in the pons, and most go to the floor of the medulla, where the vestibular nuclei are located, as shown in Figure 3.11A, center. There are four nuclei in the complex: the lateral vestibular nucleus (Deiters), the medial vestibular nucleus, the superior vestibular nucleus, and the inferior, or descending, vestibular nucleus. A certain portion of the vestibular sensory receptors goes directly to the cerebellum, the reticular formation, the thalamus, and the cerebral cortex.

The lateral vestibular nucleus receives input from the utricle, semicircular canals, cerebellum, and spinal cord. The output contributes to vestibulo-ocular tracts and to the lateral vestibulospinal tract, which activates antigravity muscles in the neck, trunk, and limbs.

Inputs to the medial and superior nuclei are from the semicircular canals. The outputs of the medial nucleus are to the medial vestibulospinal tract (MVST), with connections to the cervical spinal cord, controlling the neck muscles. The MVST plays an important role in coordinating interactions between head and eye movements. In addition, neurons from the medial and superior nuclei ascend to motor nuclei of the eye muscles and aid in stabilizing gaze during head motions.

The inputs to the inferior vestibular nucleus include neurons from the semicircular canals, utricle, saccule, and cerebellar vermis, while the outputs are part of the vestibulospinal tract and vestibuloreticular tracts.

Ascending information from the vestibular system to the oculomotor complex is responsible for the vestibulo-ocular reflex (VOR), which rotates the eyes in opposite direction to the head movement, allowing gaze to remain steady on an image even when the head is moving.

Vestibular nystagmus is the rapid alternating movement of the eyes in response to continued rotation of the body. One can create vestibular nystagmus in a subject by rotating the person seated on a stool to the left: when the acceleration first begins, the eyes go slowly to the right, to keep the eyes on a single point in space. When the eyes reach the end of the orbit, they "reset" by moving rapidly to the left; then they move again slowly to the right.

This alternating slow movement of the eyes in the direction opposite head movement, and rapid resetting of the eyes in the direction of head movement, is called nystagmus. It is a normal consequence of acceleration of the head. However, when nystagmus occurs without head movement it is usually an indication of dysfunction in the peripheral or CNS.

Postrotatory nystagmus is a reversal in the direction of nystagmus; it occurs when a person who is spinning stops abruptly. Postrotatory nystagmus has been used clinically to evaluate the function of the vestibular system.

The vestibular apparatus has both static and dynamic functions. The dynamic functions are controlled mainly by the semicircular canals, allowing us to sense head rotation and angular accelerations, and allowing the control of the eyes through the VORs. The static functions are controlled by the utricle and saccule, allowing us to monitor absolute position of the head in space, and are important in posture. (The utricle and saccule also detect linear acceleration, a dynamic function.)

ACTION SYSTEMS

The action system includes areas of the nervous system such as motor cortex, brainstem, cerebellum, and basal ganglia, which perform processing essential to the coordination of movement.

In our example presented in the beginning of this chapter, you are thirsty and want to pour some milk from the carton in front of you into a glass. We have already seen how sensory structures help you form the map of your body in space and locate the milk carton relative to your arm. Now you need to generate the movements that will allow you to pick up the carton and pour the milk. You will need a plan to move, you will need to specify specific muscles (both timing and force), and you will need a way to modify and refine the movement. So, let us look at the structures that allow you to do that.

Motor Cortex

Primary Motor Cortex and Corticospinal Tract

The motor cortex is situated in the frontal lobe and consists of a number of different processing areas, including the primary motor cortex (MI) and two premotor cortical areas, including the supplementary motor area (SMA), (occasionally called MII), and the premotor cortex, shown in Figure 3.12A. These areas interact with sensory processing areas in the parietal lobe and also with basal ganglia and cerebellar areas to identify where we want to move, to plan the movement, and finally, to execute our actions (Krakauer & Ghez, 2000).

All three of these areas have their own somatotopic maps of the body, so if different regions are stimulated, different muscles and body parts move. The primary motor cortex (Brodmann area 4) contains a very complex map of the body. Early experiments suggested a one-to-one correspondence between cells stimulated in the primary motor cortex and the activation of individual alpha motor neurons in the spinal cord; however, more recently it has been shown that the same muscles can be activated from several sites in the cortex, suggesting that neurons from several motor cortex areas project to the same muscle. In addition, it has been found that most stimuli from the primary motor cortex activate many muscles. However, stimulations tend to activate simple movements of single joints. In contrast, stimulation of neurons in the premotor areas typically activates multiple muscles at multiple joints, giving rise to more coordinated movements. The motor map, or motor homunculus (shown in Fig. 3.12B), is similar to the sensory map in the way it distorts the representations of the body. In both cases, the areas that require the most detailed control (the mouth, throat, and hand), allowing finely graded movements, are most highly represented (Penfield & Rassmussen, 1950).

Inputs to the motor areas come from the basal ganglia, the cerebellum, and sensory areas, including the periphery (via the thalamus), SI, and sensory association areas in the parietal lobe. Interestingly, MI neurons receive sensory inputs from their own muscles and also from the skin above the muscles. It has been suggested that this transcortical pathway (see Fig. 3.4) might be used in parallel with the spinal reflex pathway to give additional force output in the muscles when an unexpected load is encountered during a movement. This pathway has also been hypothesized to be an important proprioceptive pathway functioning in postural control.

Outputs from the primary motor cortex contribute to the corticospinal tract (also called the pyramidal tract) and often make excitatory monosynaptic connections onto alpha motor neurons via the corticomotoneuronal component of the tract. Animal models show that the loss of corticomotoneuronal fibers result in poor fractionation of distal muscles and inability to move the fingers independently (Porter, 1985). In addition, the

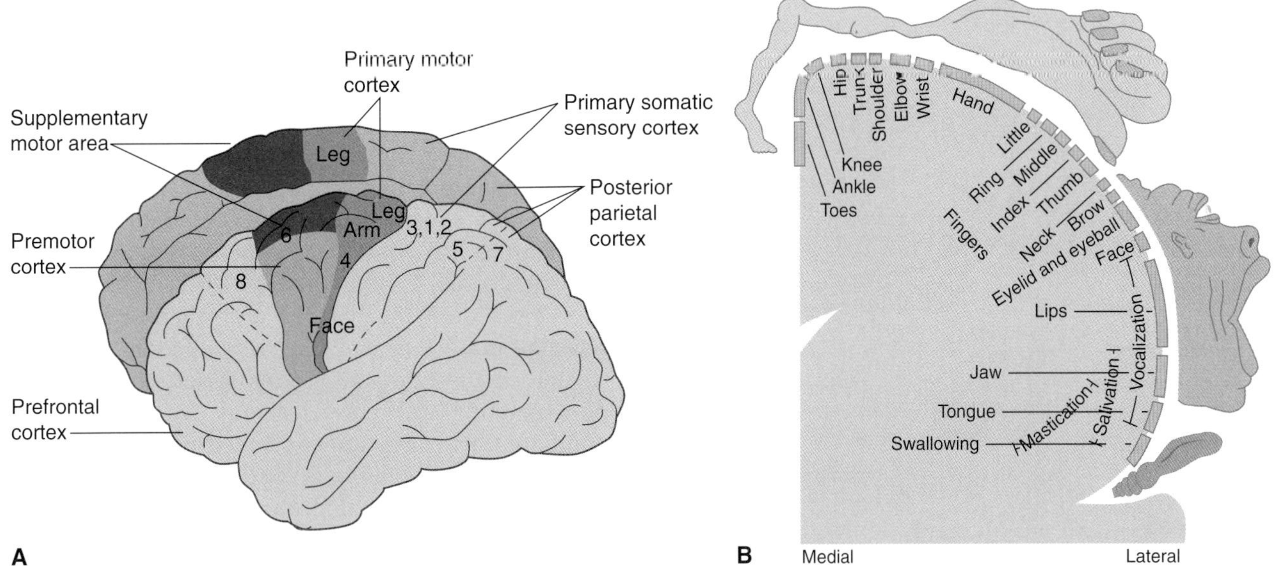

Figure 3.12 Motor cortex. **(A)** Lateral view of the brain showing the location of the primary motor cortex, supplementary motor area, and premotor cortex. **(B)** Motor homunculus. (Adapted from Kandel ER, Schwartz JH, Jessel TM, et al., eds. *Principles of neural science*, 5th ed. New York, NY: McGraw-Hill, 2013.)

corticospinal tract sends polysynaptic connections to gamma motor neurons, which control muscle spindle length, and to propriospinal interneurons in the spinal cord, which receive sensory inputs from other sources and send their axons to adjacent (short propriospinal) or distal (long propriospinal) spinal levels with the goal of coordinating movements such as locomotion (Laliberte et al., 2019). Moreover, animal research indicates that cervical propriospinal interneurons may play a critical role during the recovery of dexterous hand movements after damage of the corticospinal tract (Tohyama et al., 2017).

The corticospinal tract, shown in Figure 3.13, includes neurons from primary motor cortex (about 50%), and premotor areas including supplementary motor cortex, dorsal and ventral premotor cortex, and even somatosensory cortex. The fibers descend ipsilaterally from the cortex through the internal capsule, the midbrain, and the medulla. In the medulla, the fibers concentrate to form "pyramids," and near the junction of the medulla and the spinal cord, most (90%) cross to form the lateral corticospinal tract, controlling precise movements of the distal muscles of the limbs. The remaining 10% continue uncrossed to form the anterior (or ventral) corticospinal tract, controlling less precise movements of the proximal muscles of the limbs and trunk. The majority of the anterior corticospinal neurons cross just before they terminate in the ventral horn of the spinal cord. Most axons enter the ventral horn and terminate in the intermediate and ventral areas on interneurons and motor neurons.

What is the specific function of the primary motor cortex and the corticospinal tract in movement control? Evarts (1968) recorded the activity of corticospinal neurons in monkeys while they made wrist flexion and extension movements. He found that the firing rate of the corticospinal neurons codes (a) the force used to move a limb and (b) in some cases, the rate of change of force. Thus, both absolute force and the speed of a movement are controlled by the primary motor cortex and its connections to the spinal cord via the corticospinal tract.

Now, think about a typical movement that we make—reaching for the carton of milk, for example. How does the motor cortex encode the execution of such a complex movement? Georgopoulos et al. (1982) performed experiments in which a monkey made arm movements to many different targets around a central starting point. They found that there were specific movement directions for which each neuron was activated maximally, yet each responded for a wide range of movement directions. To explain how movements could be finely controlled when neurons are so broadly tuned, these researchers suggested that actions are controlled by a population of neurons. The activity of each of the neurons can be represented as a vector, whose length represents the degree of activity in any direction. The sum of the vectors of all the neurons would then predict the movement direction and amplitude.

If this is the case, does it mean that whenever we make a movement, for example, with our hand, the exact same neurons are activated in the primary motor cortex? No. It has been shown that specific neurons in the cortex, activated when we pick up an object, may remain totally silent when we make a similar movement, such as a gesture in anger. This is a very important point to understand because it implies that there are many parallel motor pathways for carrying out an action sequence, just as there are parallel pathways for sensory processing. Thus, simply by training a patient to utilize a specific set of muscles to make a particular movement in

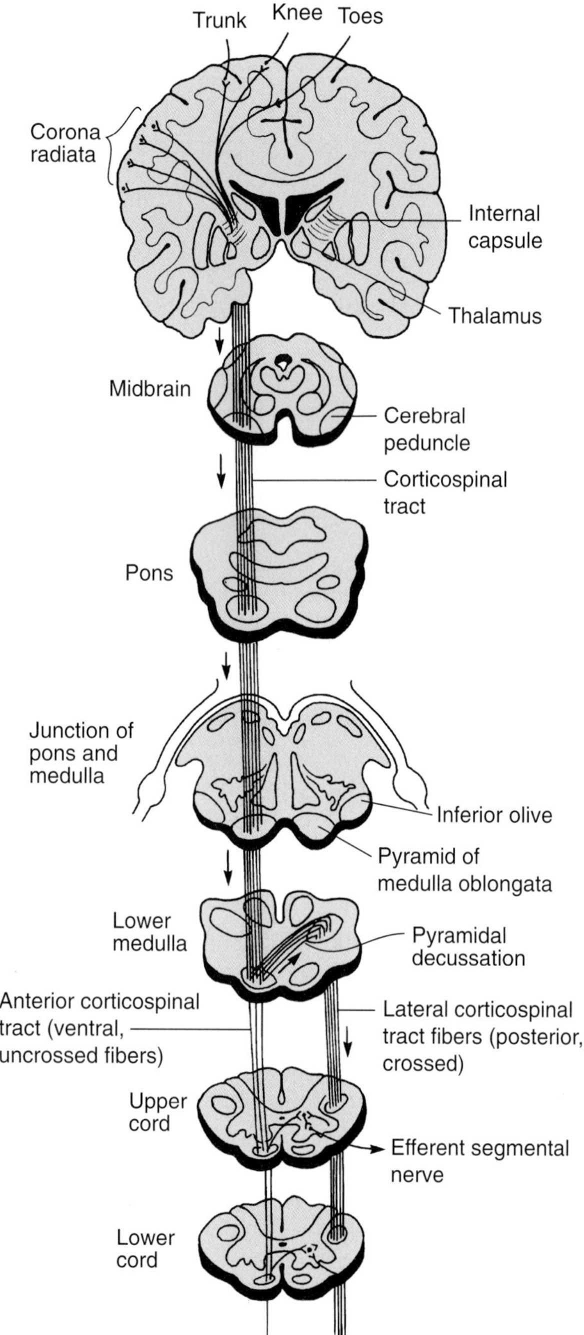

Figure 3.13 Pyramidal (corticospinal) tract, including lateral (crossed) and ventromedial (uncrossed) pathways.

one situation, it does not automatically mean that the training will transfer to all other activities requiring the same set of muscles (Krakauer & Ghez, 2000).

A stroke that compromises the motor cortex and or corticospinal tract results in loss of descending inputs to the spinal cord and depending on the size of the lesion is associated with paralysis (complete loss of movement) or paresis (partial loss of movement) in the contralateral limbs. Paresis of the right limbs is a primary problem affecting functional movement control in both Jean and Genise following their left cerebral strokes.

Supplementary Motor and Premotor Areas

What are the functions of the SMA, and the premotor area? These areas comprise Brodmann area 6 and send projections to the primary motor cortex and also to the spinal cord. Surprisingly, there are direct monosynaptic connections from premotor neurons to motor nuclei of the hand and proximal limb muscles, suggesting that these neurons can control movements separately from the primary cortex. In addition, these areas receive largely distinct inputs from the thalamus and other cortical areas. This suggests that they may have very different functions.

Each of these areas controls different aspects of motor planning and motor learning. Movements that are initiated internally are controlled primarily by the SMA. (In fact, the negative preparatory or Bereitschafts potential electroencephalogram recorded when subjects are getting ready to make a movement appears to be associated with activity in the SMA.) This area also contributes to activating the motor programs involved in learned sequences. The learning of sequences themselves also involves the presupplementary motor area. The presupplementary motor area is the rostral extension of the SMA. However, when sequences become overlearned with extensive training, the control of the movement sequence can be transferred to the primary motor cortex (Krakauer & Ghez, 2000).

Movements that are activated by external stimuli (e.g., a visual cue such as a traffic light changing from red to green) are controlled primarily by the lateral premotor area (dorsal and ventral premotor cortex). These areas control how stimuli are to be used to direct the action, specifically associating a given sensory event with a movement to be made. This is defined as associative learning (see Chapters 2 and 4 for more details). Monkeys that have lesions in this area are unable to learn new tasks involving associating a specific stimulus with a movement they are to make, although they can execute the movements without a problem.

Research by Mushiake et al. (1991) supports the hypothesis that premotor and SMAs differ in their activity depending on how the movement is initiated and guided. They found that premotor neurons were more active when a sequential task was visually guided, while SMA neurons were more active when the sequence was remembered and self-determined.

Previous researchers had proposed a hypothesis about the functional specialization of the SMA and premotor cortex based on different phylogenetic origins, with the SMA being specialized for controlling internally referenced motor output and the premotor area specialized for control of externally referenced motor acts (Passingham, 1985; Roland et al., 1980). Studies also indicate that premotor lesions cause impairment of retrieval of movements in accordance with visual cues, while SMA lesions disrupt retrieval of self-initiated movements (Passingham, 1985; Passingham et al., 1989).

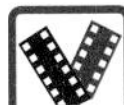

Interestingly, the SMA receives inputs from the putamen of the basal ganglia complex, while the premotor area receives inputs from the cerebellum. In Parkinson disease, there is massive depletion of dopamine in the putamen, and patients, such as our patient Mike, with Parkinson disease have difficulty with self-initiating movements (akinesia) such as walking. Gait impairments common to persons with Parkinson disease can be seen in the mobility section of Mike's video case study. Thus, Parkinson disease may cause impaired input to the supplementary cortex, and nearby motor areas, which results in difficulty in initiating movements (akinesia) and/or slowness in performing movements (bradykinesia) (Berardelli et al., 2001; Marsden, 1989).

Studies by Roland and others (Lang et al., 1990; Roland et al., 1980) have examined the role of the supplementary cortex in humans and have begun to clarify its functions. Roland et al. (1980) asked subjects to perform tasks ranging from very simple to complex movements, and while they were making the movements, the investigators assessed the amount of cerebral blood flow in different areas of the brain. (To measure blood flow, one injects short-lived radioactive tracer into the blood, and then measures the radioactivity in different brain areas with detectors on the scalp.)

As shown in Figure 3.14, when subjects were asked to perform a simple task (simple repetitive movements of the index finger or pressing a spring between the thumb and index finger) the blood flow increase was only in primary motor and sensory cortex. In contrast, when they were asked to perform a complex task (a sequence of movements involving all four fingers, touching the thumb in different orders), subjects showed a blood flow increase in the SMA, bilaterally, and the primary motor and sensory areas. Finally, when they were asked to rehearse the task but not perform it, the blood flow increase was only in the SMA, not the primary sensory or motor cortex. Roland et al. concluded that the supplementary area is active when a sequence of simple ballistic movements is planned. Thus, they proposed that it participates in the assembly of the central motor program or forms a motor subroutine.

Research suggests that two separate pathways from the parietal cortex to the premotor areas control reaching and grasping. The reaching pathway originates in the parieto-occipital area and terminates in the dorsal premotor area, with some neurons synapsing in other areas en route. This pathway uses visual information about object location in three-dimensional space to control the direction of reaching movements. The grasping pathway originates in the dorsal extrastriate area of the occipital cortex and terminates in the ventral premotor area, with relays to other areas. This pathway uses visual information about object characteristics (shape, size, etc.) to control hand shaping for grasping (Krakauer & Ghez, 2000).

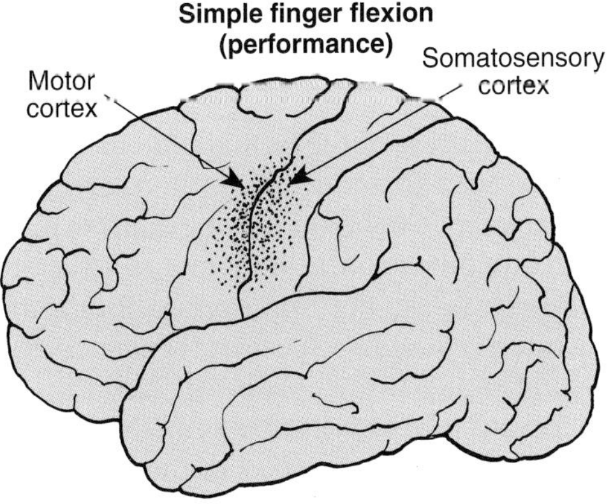

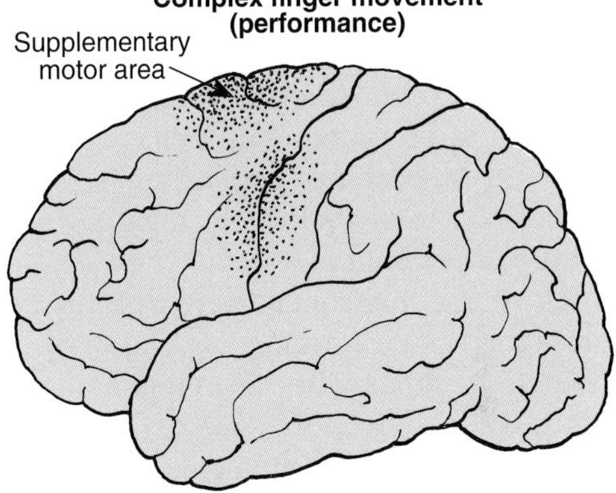

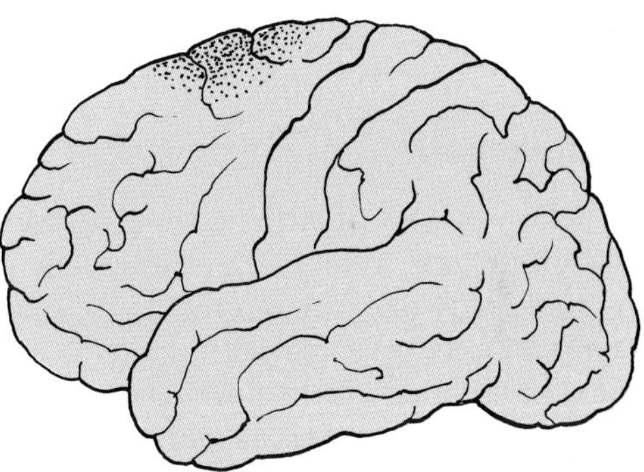

Figure 3.14 Changes in blood flow during different motor behaviors, indicating the areas of the motor cortex involved in the behavior. (Adapted from Roland PE, Larsen B, Lassen NA, et al. Supplementary motor area and other cortical areas in organization of voluntary movements in man. *J Neurophysiol.* 1980;43:118–136, with permission.)

Work by Rizzolatti et al. (1988) suggests an interesting function of the ventral premotor area (F5) in reaching. They recorded from single neurons in F5 in monkeys during reaching. They found that an important property of most (85%) of these neurons was their selectivity for different types of handgrip: precision grip (most common), finger prehension, and whole-hand prehension. Interestingly, precision grip neurons were activated only by small visual objects (Jeannerod et al., 1995; Taira et al., 1990).

Higher-Level Association Areas

Association Areas of the Frontal Regions

The association areas of the frontal regions (areas rostral to Brodmann area 6) are important for motor planning and other cognitive behaviors. For example, these areas have been hypothesized to integrate sensory information and then select the appropriate motor response from the many possible responses (Fuster, 1989).

The prefrontal cortex may be divided into the principal sulcus and the prefrontal convexities. Experiments have indicated that the neurons of the principal sulcus are involved in the strategic planning of higher motor functions. For example, monkeys with lesions in this area had difficulty performing spatial tasks in which information had to be stored in working memory in order to guide future action. This area is densely interconnected with the posterior parietal areas. These areas are hypothesized to work closely together in spatial tasks that require attention.

Lesions in the prefrontal convexity, in contrast, cause problems in performing any kind of delayed response task. Animals with these lesions have problems with tasks for which they have to inhibit certain motor responses at specific moments. Lesions in adjacent areas cause problems with a monkey's ability to select from a variety of motor responses when given different sensory cues (Kupfermann, 1991).

Attentional Networks

There is also a widely distributed set of attentional networks within the cortex. One framework for categorizing these networks divides them into three separate attentional networks: alerting (bilateral thalamus, brainstem), orientation (right pulvinar and temporoparietal regions), and conflict resolution or executive attention (anterior cingulate cortex, frontoparietal cortex) (Petersen & Posner, 2012). A second framework for characterizing attention categorizes attention, slightly differently, into two separate but interacting networks. The first is the dorsal frontoparietal network that controls spatial attention and eye movements and controls the top–down voluntary allocation of attention to locations or features of objects; the second is a ventral frontoparietal network involved in nonspatial behaviors such as arousal, reorienting or shifting attention, and detection of unexpected or novel events (Corbetta & Shulman, 2011).

Both these frameworks are consistent in suggesting that attentional networks are of fundamental importance in our ability to perceive sensory stimuli. Lesions in these networks are also the basis for certain perceptual impairments associated with stroke, such as spatial neglect. The section above titled Higher-Order Visual Cortex discusses these perceptual–attentional interactions in more detail.

Cerebellum

The cerebellum is considered one of the three important brain areas contributing to coordination of movement, in addition to the motor cortex and basal ganglia. Yet, despite its important role in the coordination of movement, the cerebellum does not play a primary role in motor function, in the sense that it has no direct pathway to the alpha motor neurons in the spinal cord. If the cerebellum is destroyed, we do not lose sensation or become paralyzed. However, lesions of the cerebellum do produce devastating changes in our ability to perform movements, from the very simple to the most elegant. The cerebellum receives afferent information from almost every sensory system, consistent with its role as a regulator of motor output (Ghez & Thatch, 2000; Ito, 1984).

How does the cerebellum adjust the output of the motor systems? Its function is related to its neuronal circuitry. Through this circuitry and its input and output connections, it appears to act as a comparator, a system that compensates for errors by comparing intention with performance.

The cerebellum's input and output connections are vital to its role as error detector, and they are summarized in Figure 3.15. The cerebellum receives information from other parts of the brain related to the programming and execution of movements (corticopontine areas). Information from the primary motor cortex regarding a motor plan is sent to the spinal cord while a copy of the plan is sent to the cerebellum; this copy is referred to as efference copy or corollary discharge. The cerebellum also receives sensory feedback information (reafference) from the receptors about the movements as they are being made (spinal or trigeminal somatosensory input, visual, auditory, and vestibular inputs). After processing this information, outputs (Fig. 3.15) from the cerebellum go to the motor cortex and other systems within the brainstem to modulate their motor output. In addition to its role in motor control processes, research has also suggested that the cerebellum may have important nonmotor functions, including cognition, which will be discussed below (Fiez et al., 1992).

Anatomy of the Cerebellum

An understanding of the anatomy of the cerebellum is helpful in explaining its function. The cerebellum consists of an outer layer of gray matter (the cortex), internal white matter (input and output fibers), and three pairs of deep nuclei: the fastigial nucleus, the interposed nucleus, and the dentate nucleus. All the inputs to the cerebellum go first to one of these three deep cerebellar nuclei and then go on to the cortex. All the outputs of the cerebellum go back to the deep nuclei, before going on to the cerebral cortex or the brainstem (Ghez & Thatch, 2000; Ito, 1984).

The cerebellum can be divided into three phylogenetic zones (see Fig. 3.15). The oldest zone corresponds

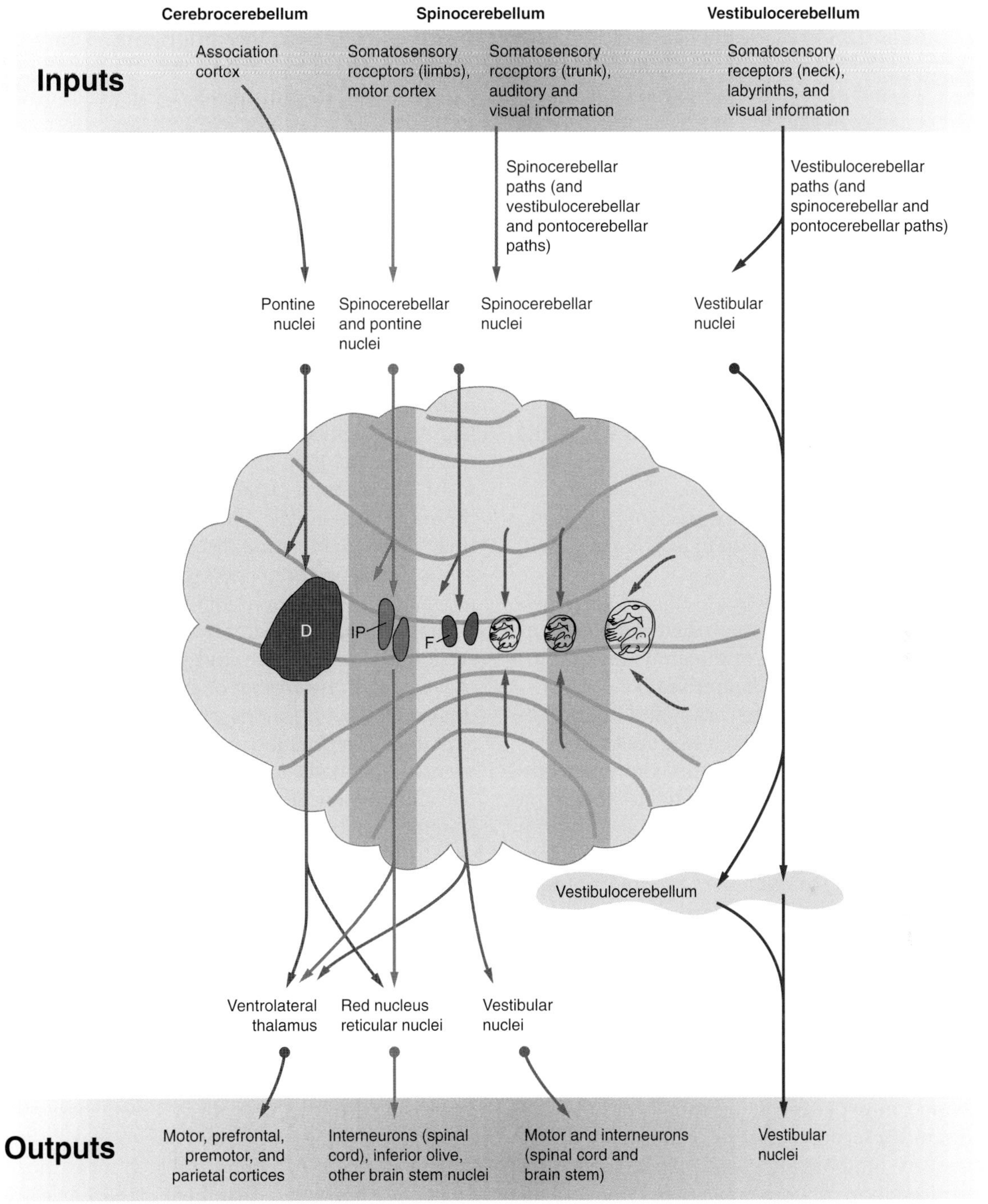

Figure 3.15 The three functional regions of the cerebellum (cerebrocerebellum, spinocerebellum, vestibulocerebellum), including input and output pathways. D, dentate nucleus; IP, interposed nucleus; F, fastigial nucleus.

to the flocculonodular lobe and is functionally related to the vestibular system. The phylogenetically more recent areas to develop are (a) the vermis and intermediate part of the hemispheres and (b) the lateral hemispheres, respectively. These three parts of the cerebellum have distinct functions and distinct input–output connections, as you see in Figure 3.15.

Flocculonodular Lobe. The flocculonodular lobe, often referred to as the vestibulocerebellum, receives inputs from the visual, somatosensory, and vestibular systems, and its outputs return to the vestibular nuclei. It functions in the control of the axial muscles, which are used in equilibrium control. If a patient experiences dysfunction in this system, one observes an ataxic gait, wide-based stance, and nystagmus. You can see examples of these problems in the video case study of John, our patient with spinocerebellar degeneration.

Vermis and Intermediate Hemispheres. The vermis and intermediate hemispheres, often referred to as the spinocerebellum, receive proprioceptive and cutaneous inputs from the spinal cord (via the spinocerebellar tracts), in addition to visual, vestibular, and auditory information. Researchers used to think that there were two maps of the complete body in the cerebellum, but now it has been shown that the maps are much more complex and can be divided into many smaller maps. This has been called fractured somatotopy. These smaller maps appear to be related to functional activities; thus, in the rat, the mouth and paw RFs are positioned close together, possibly to contribute to the control of grooming behavior. Inputs to this part of the cerebellum go through the fastigial nucleus (vermis) and interposed nucleus (intermediate lobes) (Shambes et al., 1978).

There are four spinocerebellar tracts that relay information from the spinal cord to the cerebellum. Two tracts relay information from the arms and the neck, and two relay information from the trunk and legs. Inputs are also from the spino-olivocerebellar tract, through the inferior olivary nucleus (climbing fibers). These inputs are important in learning and will be discussed later.

What are the output pathways of the spinocerebellum? The outputs go to the (a) brainstem reticular formation, (b) vestibular nuclei, (c) thalamus and motor cortex, and (d) red nucleus in the midbrain.

What are the functions of the vermis and intermediate lobes (spinocerebellum)? First, they appear to function in the control of the actual execution of movement: they correct for deviations from an intended movement through comparing feedback from the spinal cord with the intended motor command. They also modulate muscle tone. This occurs through the continuous output of excitatory activity from the fastigial and interposed nucleus, which modulates the activity of the gamma motor neurons to the muscle spindles. When there are lesions in these nuclei, there is a significant drop in muscle tone (hypotonia) (Ghez & Thatch, 2000).

Finally, the spinocerebellum is involved in feedforward mechanisms to regulate movements. This was discovered in experiments on monkeys in which the dentate and interposed nuclei of this part of the cerebellum were temporarily cooled while they were making precise elbow flexion movements (by activating the biceps muscle) back to a target after the arm was moved. When the cerebellar nuclei were cooled, the triceps muscle, used to keep the arm from overshooting its target, was no longer activated in a feedforward manner, but only in a feedback manner, after being stretched when the biceps moved the elbow too far (Ghez & Thatch, 2000; Vilis & Hore, 1980).

Lateral Hemispheres. The last part of the cerebellum, and the newest phylogenetically, is the lateral zone of the cerebellar hemispheres, often called the cerebrocerebellum (see Fig. 3.15). It has undergone a marked expansion in the course of human evolution, which has added many nonmotor functions to its repertoire. It receives inputs from the pontine nuclei in the brainstem, which relay information from wide areas of the cerebral cortex (sensory, motor, premotor, and posterior parietal). Its outputs are to the thalamus and then to the motor, premotor, parietal, and prefrontal cortex (Kandel et al., 2013; Middleton & Strick, 1994).

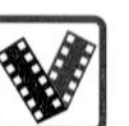

What is the function of the lateral hemispheres? This part of the cerebellum appears to have a number of higher-level functions involving both motor and nonmotor skills. First, research suggests that it is involved in the planning or preparation of movement and the evaluation of sensory information for action as a part of the motor learning process. In contrast, the intermediate lobes function in movement execution and fine-tuning of ongoing movement via feedback information. It appears that the lateral hemispheres of the cerebellum participate in programming the motor cortex for the execution of movement. For example, lateral cerebellar lesions disrupt the timing of movements, so that joints are moved sequentially rather than simultaneously. This deficit is referred to as decomposition of movement. Decomposition of movement is very apparent in John, our patient with cerebellar degeneration, and can be seen in the impairment section of his video case study. During a reach-and-grasp movement, grasp formation begins during the transport phase. However, lesions of the cerebrocerebellum disrupt this coordination so that reaching and grasping occur sequentially instead of simultaneously. The cerebellar pathways are a part of many parallel pathways affecting the motor cortex.

Cerebellar Involvement in Nonmotor Tasks

In addition to its role in motor control processes, research has suggested that the lateral cerebellum may have important nonmotor functions, including cognition (Fiez et al., 1992). It is interesting to note that neuroanatomical experiments have shown projections from the lateral dentate nucleus of the cerebellum to frontal association areas known to be involved in higher-level cognitive processing (Middleton & Strick, 1994). These connections suggest that subjects do not have to make a movement to activate the cerebellum; research measuring cerebral blood flow has shown that there is an increase in cerebellar activity when subjects are asked only to imagine making a movement (Decety et al., 1990).

Ivry and Keele (1989) have shown that the cerebellum has important timing functions, with patients with cerebellar lesions showing problems in both timing production and perception. Patients with lateral hemisphere lesions showed errors in timing related to perceptual abilities, which researchers think may be related to a central clock-like mechanism. In contrast, patients with intermediate-lobe lesions made errors related to movement execution.

Many parts of the cerebellum, including the lateral cerebellum, seem to be important in both motor and nonmotor learning. The unique cellular circuitry of the cerebellum has been shown to be perfect for the long-term modification of motor responses, including simple types of learning, such as adaptation. Experiments have shown that as animals learn a new task, the climbing fiber (which detects movement error) changes the effectiveness of the synapse between the granule-cell parallel fiber and the Purkinje cells (the main output cells of the cerebellum) (Gilbert & Thatch, 1977).

This type of cerebellar learning also appears to occur in the VOR circuitry, which includes cerebellar pathways. The VOR keeps the eyes fixed on an object when the head turns. In experiments in which humans wore prismatic lenses that reversed the image on the eye, adaptation of the gain of the VOR occurred over time, with the size of the reflex progressively reducing and then reversing in direction. This modification of the reflex did not occur in patients with cerebellar lesions (Gonshor & Melville-Jones, 1976). This inability to modulate the VOR can be seen in the impairment section of the video case study on John, our patient with cerebellar degeneration. The cerebellum may also contribute to associative learning, and specifically, classical conditioning, as lesions to the cerebellum constrain the ability of animals to acquire and retain the eye-blink reflex (Ghez & Thatch, 2000).

Studies have shown that the right lateral cerebellum becomes active when subjects read verbs aloud, but not when they read nouns, implying that something about the cognitive processing of verb generation requires the cerebellum, whereas the same processing of other words does not. Correlated with this, certain patients with cerebellar deficits also showed difficulty in these verb-generation tasks and in learning and performing a variety of tasks involving complex nonmotor (cognitive) cortical processing. This is the case even though scores on intelligence, language, "frontal function," and memory were normal. For example, patients showed problems in detecting errors they made in nonmotor as well as motor tasks. This implies that they had problems with both perception and production processes in higher-order analyses, including those involving language (Fiez et al., 1992).

Research on learning problems in patients with cerebellar lesions has shown that while they had normal scores on the Wechsler Memory Scale, they had problems with some types of learned responses. In particular, problems were found in recalling habits, defined as automatic responses learned through repetition. This is opposite to the learning problems seen in patients with severe amnesia (resulting from hippocampal and/or midline diencephalic damage), who do not learn tasks that rely on conscious recall of previous experience but show normal improvement on a variety of skill-learning tasks that involve repetition (Fiez et al., 1992; Squire, 1986).

It is interesting to note that certain neurons in the dentate nucleus of the cerebellum are preferentially involved in the generation and/or guidance of movement based on visual cues. As mentioned earlier, these neurons project to the premotor areas of the cerebral cortex (Mushiake & Strick, 1993). Experiments have shown that patients with cerebellar deficits showed improved motor performance when their eyes were closed or when visual feedback was reduced. In fact, Sanes et al. (1988) noted that cerebellar tremor was greatest when patients used visual cues to guide movements.

Basal Ganglia

The basal ganglia complex consists of a set of nuclei at the base of the cerebral cortex, including the putamen, caudate nucleus, GP, subthalamic nucleus (STN), and SN that is subdivided into pars compacta (SNc) and pars reticulata (SNr). Basal literally means at the base, or in other words, just below the cortex. As with patients with cerebellar lesions, patients with damage to the basal ganglia are not paralyzed, but have problems with the coordination of movement. Advancement in our understanding of the function of basal ganglia first came from clinicians, especially James Parkinson, who in 1817 first described Parkinson disease as "the shaking palsy" (Cote & Crutcher, 1991).

The basal ganglia were once believed to be part of the extrapyramidal motor system, which was believed to act in parallel with the pyramidal system (the corticospinal tract) in movement control. Thus, clinicians defined pyramidal problems as relating to spasticity and paralysis, while extrapyramidal problems were defined as involuntary movements and rigidity. As we have seen in this chapter, this distinction is no longer valid, since many other brain systems also control movement. In addition, the pyramidal and extrapyramidal systems are not independent but work together in controlling movements.

Anatomy of the Basal Ganglia

The major connections of the basal ganglia are summarized in Figure 3.16, including the major afferent, internal and efferent connections. The excitatory connections are shown in red, while inhibitory pathways are shown in gray. The main input nuclei of the basal ganglia complex are the caudate and the putamen. The caudate and the putamen develop from the same structure and are often discussed as a single unit, the *striatum*. Their primary inputs (the arrows labeled cortical inputs in Fig. 3.16) are from widespread areas of the neocortex, including sensory, motor, and association areas (Alexander & Crutcher, 1990).

The GP has two segments, internal and external (GPi and GPe, respectively), and is situated next to the putamen, while the SN is situated a little more caudally, in the midbrain, as shown in the top half of Figure 3.16. The GPi and the SNr are the major output areas of the basal ganglia, which send inputs to the

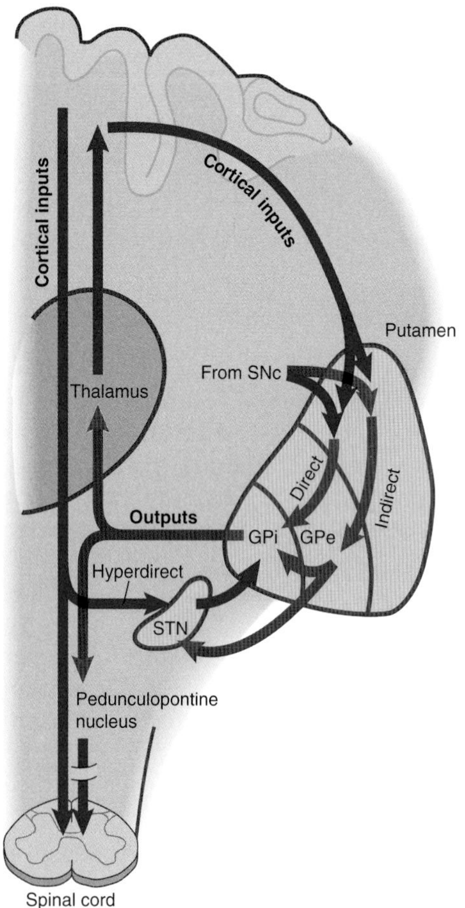

Figure 3.16 The basal ganglia circuitry, including internal, input and output pathways. Cortical inputs go to the striatum (represented in the figure by one of its parts, the putamen) and subthalamic nucleus. Basal ganglia output goes to the thalamus and the pedunculopontine nucleus. Excitatory pathways are shown in *red*, while inhibitory pathways are shown in *gray*. GPe and GPi, globus pallidus internal and external segments; SNc, substantia nigra.

thalamus (ventral anterior, ventrolateral, and intralaminar nuclei) and brain stem regions. The thalamic projections send information from the basal ganglia to the same areas in the frontal lobe that send inputs to the basal ganglia. Projections from GP and SN are also sent to the pedunculopontine nucleus and superior colliculus. Thus, these pathways may directly influence brain stem and spinal motor circuits, especially those related to gait and balance, and allow the brain stem nuclei to integrate basal ganglia inputs with cerebellar inputs.

Additionally, outputs from the SNr are directed to the superior colliculus for the control of head and eye movements (Wichman & DeLong, 2013). As shown in Figure 3.16, the connections within the basal ganglia are complex. The striatum receives direct excitatory cortical inputs and projects to the output nuclei of the basal ganglia (the GPi) and the SNr through two major projection systems: direct and indirect pathways (Nambu et al., 2002). A more detailed description of the direct and indirect pathways can be found in Extended Knowledge 3.1. Furthermore, the STN, which is located between the thalamus and the SN, receives inputs from several brain areas (GPe, cortex, thalamus, and brain stem centers) and sends outputs to the GP and SNr. A third pathway, called the "hyperdirect pathway" (cortico-subthalamo-pallidal) of the basal ganglia circuitry has been recently described (refer to Fig. 3.16). The STN was for many years considered part of the "indirect" pathway, but it has recently been shown to also receive direct signals from the cerebral cortex. The hyperdirect pathway sends direct projections from motor-related cortical areas to the STN and then to the GPi. The conduction velocity of this information is fast since it bypasses the striatum and seems to have a critical role in holding back movements (Milardi et al., 2019; Wichman & DeLong, 2013).

Extended Knowledge 3.1

Direct and Indirect Pathways in the Basal Ganglia

The direct pathway begins with projections from the cortex to the striatum, which project monosynaptically to the GPi/SNr. The GPi projects to the thalamus, which then projects back to the cortex. The connections from the cortex to the striatum are excitatory, while the connections from the striatum to the GPi and from the GPi to the thalamus are inhibitory. The connections from the thalamus back to the cortex are excitatory. How does activity in the direct pathway facilitate movement? The cortex excites the striatum, which then inhibits the GPi through the direct pathway. The GPi is normally tonically active and inhibitory to the thalamus. When the GPi is inhibited, this reduces the tonic inhibitory influence of the thalamus (this is called "disinhibition"), increasing excitatory drive to the cortex and reinforcing the desired movement.

The indirect pathway begins with projections from the cortex to the striatum, from the striatum to the external segment of the GPe, which projects to the STN, and then to the GPi. The GPi projects to the thalamus, which projects back to the cortex. The projections from the striatum to the GPe and from GPe to STN are inhibitory, while the projections from the STN to the GPi are excitatory. How does activity in the indirect pathway inhibit unwanted movement? Input from the cortex excites the striatum, which then inhibits GPe. Since GPe is inhibitory to the STN, the STN becomes more active and excites the GPi. Increased activation of the GPi inhibits the thalamus, and as a result the thalamus does not excite the cortex. In this way, activation of the indirect pathway by the striatum causes a relative inhibition of movement.

A third "hyperdirect" pathway has also been proposed, whereby the STN receives inputs from the cerebral cortex and, in turn, sends outputs to the GPi/SNr. The cortico-STN-pallidal "hyperdirect" pathway has a powerful excitatory effect on the output nuclei of the basal ganglia, which results in inhibition of large areas of the thalamus and cerebral cortex (Nambu et al., 2002).

The STN is a frequent anatomical site used for neurosurgical deep brain stimulation in people diagnosed with Parkinson disease. This treatment has been shown to be effective in improving quality of life, motor deficits (tremor, rigidity, bradykinesia, gait, and postural instability) during off-medication, decreasing on-mediation dyskinesias, and reducing the intake of Parkinson-related medication (e.g., L-dopa) (Hamani et al., 2005; Kleiner-Fisman et al., 2006).

The basal ganglia consist of four different functional circuits that also include the thalamus and the cortex. These comprise the motor circuit (including the premotor cortex, supplementary motor cortex and primary motor cortex), the oculomotor circuit (including the frontal and supplementary eye fields of the cortex), the executive/associative circuit, and the emotion/motivation circuit. These circuits are shown in Figure 3.17. The existence of these different functional circuits explains the variety of movement disorders involving the dysfunction of basal ganglia (DeLong, 2000).

Role of the Basal Ganglia

The cortico-basal ganglia-thalamocortical motor projections show a high topographical distribution and the circuit ends on cortical areas related to movements. In general, the basal ganglia motor circuit is involved in a wide variety of motor behaviors such as action selection, preparation for movement, movement execution, sequencing of movement, self-initiated or remembered movements, movement control parameters, and reinforcement motor learning. In this last function, the projections from the dopaminergic neurons in the SNc to the striatum, and cholinergic interneurons in the striatum, are critically active during behavioral reinforcement cues and rewarded behaviors (Wichman & DeLong, 2013).

The motor circuit contributes to both the preparation for and execution of movement. For example, it has been shown that many neurons in the premotor areas and in the basal ganglia motor circuitry show changes

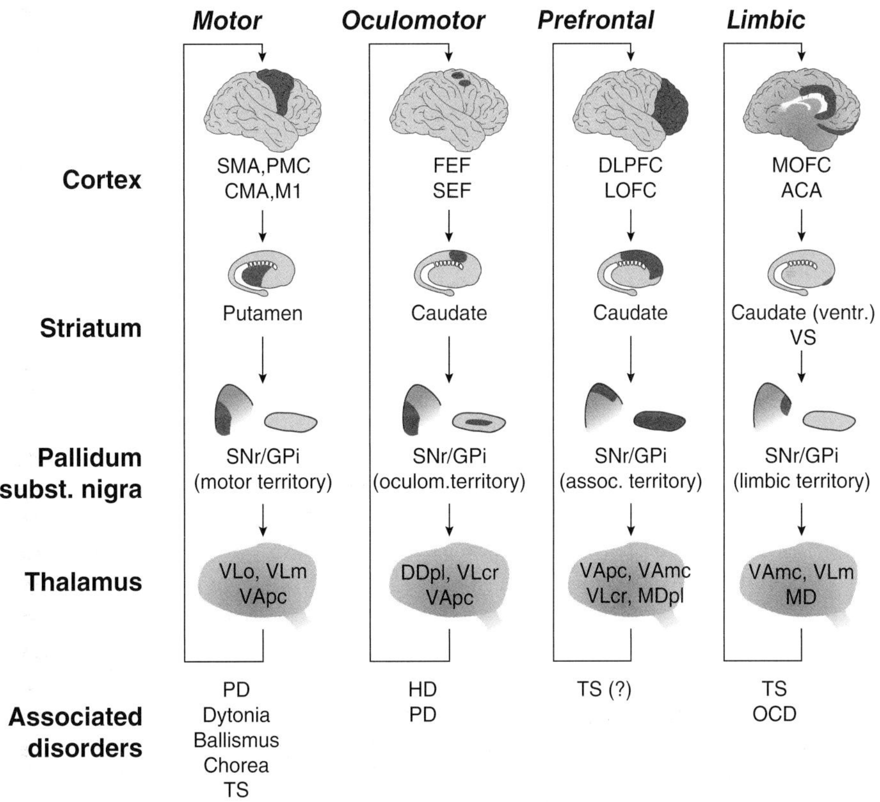

Figure 3.17 The four functional circuits of the basal ganglia that also include the thalamus and the cortex. These include the motor circuit, the oculomotor circuit and the executive/associative (prefrontal) and the emotion/motivation (limbic) circuits. ACA, anterior cingulate area; CMA, cingulate motor area; DLPFC, dorsolateral prefrontal cortex; FEF, frontal eye field; GPi, internal segment of the globus pallidus; LOFC, lateral orbitofrontal cortex; M1, primary motor cortex; MDpl, mediodorsal nucleus of the thalamus, lateral part; MOFC, medial orbitofrontal cortex; PMC, premotor cortex; *SEF*, supplementary eye field; *SMA*, supplementary motor area; SNr, substantia nigra pars reticulata; VAmc, ventral anterior nucleus of thalamus; magnocellular part; VApc, ventral anterior nucleus of thalamus, parvocellular part; VLcr, ventrolateral nucleus of thalamus, caudal part, rostral division; VLm, ventrolateral nucleus of thalamus, medial part; VLo, ventrolateral nucleus of thalamus, pars oralis; PD, Parkinson Disease, HD, Huntington Disease, OCD, Obsessive-Compulsive Disease, TS, Tourette's Syndrome. (Adapted from Wichmann T, Delong MR. Deep brain stimulation for neurologic and neuropsychiatric disorders. *Neuron*. 2006;52:197–204, with permission.)

in activity after the presentation of a cue that gives information on a movement to be made later. The activity continues until the movement is made. This is referred to as "motor set." Other subsets of neurons in the motor circuitry show only movement-related responses, indicating that there are separate populations of neurons for these two functions (DeLong, 2000).

It has been hypothesized that the circuitry of the basal ganglia selectively facilitates some movements patterns as it suppresses others (Alexander & Crutcher, 1990; Nambu et al., 2002). In this sense, the motor cortexes would generate a motor pattern that is sent to the basal ganglia where the selected pattern is released while suppressing unintended motor patterns (Milardi et al., 2019; Yanagisawa, 2018). The cortical activation of striatal neurons that contribute to the direct pathway transiently suppresses the high spontaneous discharge rate of movement-related neurons in the output nuclei of the basal ganglia (GPi/SNr), which in turn removes the inhibition from the thalamocortical neurons. The result of this disinhibition is the activation of cortical areas and the facilitation of the selected movement. In contrast, the activation of the striatal neurons that contribute to the indirect pathway (striatum-|GPe-STN-GPi/SNr), or from the motor-related cortexes that comprise the hyperdirect pathway (STN-GPi/SNr), transiently increases the inhibition of thalamocortical neurons and thereby inhibits movements. The synchronous and coordinated activation of these pathways during self-triggered movements would facilitate intended movements and suppress competing ones (Milardi et al., 2019; Wichman & DeLong, 2013; Yanagisawa, 2018).

The basal ganglia also play an important role in eye movements. The oculomotor circuit is involved in the control of saccadic eye movements. The executive/associative and the emotion/motivation circuits are involved in nonmotor functions. The executive functions include organizing behaviors using verbal skills in problem solving and mediating socially appropriate responses. Lesions in this area contribute to obsessive–compulsive disorder. The emotion/motivation circuit is involved in the control of motivated behavior (involving circuits for reinforcing stimuli for behaviors) and procedural learning.

Most disorders of the basal ganglia involve problems with action rather than perception. They may involve either hyperactivity/impulsivity (e.g., Huntington disease or obsessive–compulsive disorder) or reduced activity and flat affect (e.g., Parkinson disease, depression) (DeLong, 2000).

For example, certain diseases of the basal ganglia may produce poor and slow movements and disorders of muscle tone and postural reflexes. As can be seen in his video case study, Mike, our patient with Parkinson disease, demonstrates symptoms that include resting tremor, increased muscle tone or rigidity, and slowness in the initiation of movement (akinesia) as well as in the execution of movement (bradykinesia). The site of the lesion for Parkinson disease is in the dopaminergic pathway from the SN to the striatum. The tremor and rigidity may be due to loss of inhibitory influences within the basal ganglia. On the other hand, other diseases of the basal ganglia produce involuntary movements (dyskinesia). For example, Huntington disease characteristics include chorea and dementia. Symptoms appear to be caused by loss of cholinergic neurons and gamma aminobutyric acid-ergic neurons in the striatum (Alexander & Crutcher, 1990; Cote & Crutcher, 1991).

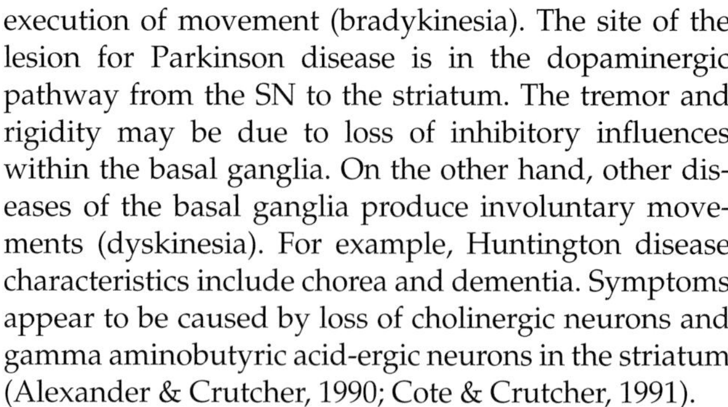

What are the functional differences between the basal ganglia and the cerebellum? Research suggests that the basal ganglia may be particularly concerned with internally generated movements, while the cerebellum is involved in visually triggered and guided movements. For example, experiments have shown that in the internal GPi, cells that project to the SMA are activated during internally generated movements (Mushiake & Strick, 1993). This is consistent with clinical data demonstrating that patients with Parkinson disease have a great deal of difficulty with internally generated movements (Georgiou et al., 1993; Morris et al., 1996). It is interesting to note that patients like Mike, with Parkinson disease with frozen gait syndrome (difficulty initiating or maintaining gait) are able to use visual cues to improve their walking abilities. The above research suggests that this may be due to the use of alternative pathways from the cerebellum to trigger and guide the movements.

Mesencephalon and Brainstem

The nuclei and pathways from the mesencephalon and brainstem to the spinal cord mediate many aspects of motor control as part of descending pathways from the cerebral cortex, cerebellum, and basal ganglia. This includes the generation of locomotor rhythms, the regulation of postural tone, the integration of sensory information for posture and balance, as well as contributions to anticipatory postural control accompanying voluntary movements.

Stimulation of the mesencephalic locomotor region (and also the subthalamic locomotor region) initiates locomotion and adjusts stepping movements. Signals from this system are relayed to the spinal cord central pattern generators for locomotion via the medial reticular formation and reticulospinal pathways (including the pontomedullary locomotor strip). These pathways and brainstem centers are shown in Figure 3.18A. The brainstem has important centers for controlling the facilitation and inhibition of muscle tone important for the control of posture. These muscle tone facilitatory and inhibitory systems within the brainstem are shown in Figure 3.18A,B. It is interesting to note that when the brainstem reticular formation is inactivated by pharmacologic means, anticipatory postural adjustments that would normally be activated to stabilize a

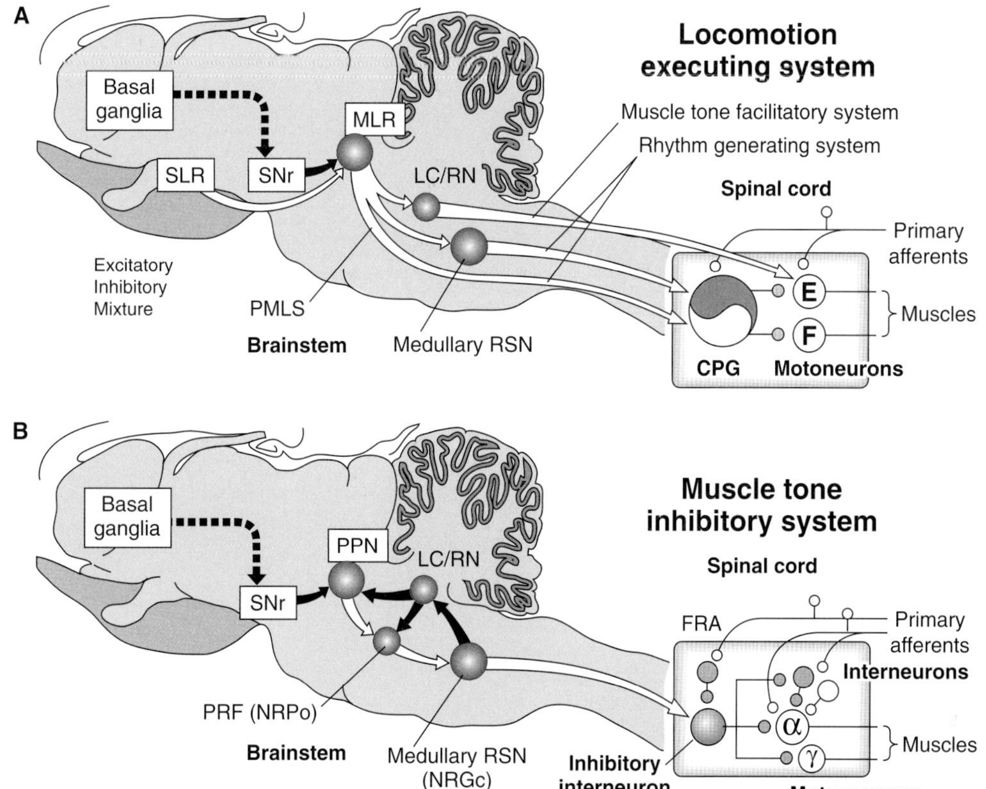

Figure 3.18 Important connections between the basal ganglia, brainstem, and spinal cord for regulation of locomotion and muscle tone. **A.** Circuitry involved in the locomotor executing systems, including the muscle tone facilitatory system and the rhythm-generating system, with its connections to the central pattern generators for locomotion in the spinal cord. **B.** Circuitry for the muscle tone inhibitory system. E, extensor motor neurons; F, flexor motor neurons; FRA, flexion reflex afferents; LC, locus coeruleus; MLR, mesencephalic locomotor region; NRGc, nucleus reticularis gigantocellularis; PMLS, pontomedullary locomotor strip; PPN, pedunculopontine tegmental nucleus; PRF, pontine reticular formation; RN, raphe nuclei; RSN, reticulospinal neuron; SLR, subthalamic locomotor region; *SNr*, substantia nigra. (Adapted from Takakusaki K, Saitaoh K, Harada H, et al. Role of the basal ganglia-brainstem pathways in the control of motor behaviors. *Neurosci Res*. 2004;50:141, Fig. 3, with permission.)

voluntary movement initiated through activation of the motor cortex are no longer activated (Takakusaki et al., 2004). This indicates the importance of brainstem nuclei in anticipatory postural control.

Thus, as shown in Figure 3.19, basal ganglia–cortical–spinal pathways are important to the control of voluntary movements, while basal ganglia–brainstem–spinal cord pathways contribute to automatic control of movements such as locomotion and postural tone mainly via pathways originating in the SN. Figure 3.19 shows both the locomotor execution system and the muscle-tone facilitation and inhibition system pathways from the basal ganglia through the spinal motor neurons (Takakusaki et al., 2004).

In addition to the corticospinal (or pyramidal) tract (the direct pathway from motor cortex to the spinal cord), there are additional indirect pathways (the medial and lateral descending motor system tracts) that synapse or originate in brainstem nuclei. All of these tracts are shown in Figure 3.20. They include the corticorubrospinal tract, which synapses in the red nucleus and is part of the lateral system, and the tracts that make up the medial system including the corticoreticulospinal tract, which synapses in the reticular nucleus; the tectospinal tract, which originates in the superior colliculus; and the vestibulospinal tract, which originates in the vestibular nucleus. As also shown in Figure 3.20, the lateral system plus the pyramidal (corticospinal) tract controls the distal muscles; in contrast, the medial system controls proximal and axial muscles.

This concludes our review of the physiologic basis for motor control. In this chapter, we have tried to show you the neural substrates for movement. This has involved a review of the perception and action systems and the higher-level cognitive processes that play a part in their elaboration. We have tried to show the importance of both the hierarchical and distributed nature of these systems. The presentation of the perception and action systems separately is somewhat misleading. In real life, as movements are generated to accomplish tasks in varied environments, the boundaries between perception, action, and cognition are blurred.

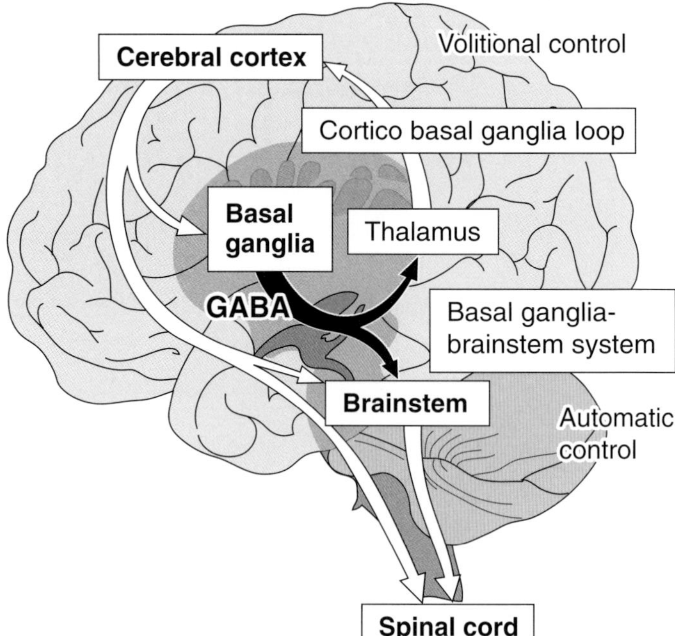

Figure 3.19 Hypothetical model for the control of movements by the basal ganglia, showing cortical–basal ganglia–spinal pathways important for volitional control, and basal ganglia–brainstem–spinal pathways important for automatic control of muscle tone and locomotion. (Adapted from Takakusaki K, Saitaoh K, Harada H, et al. Role of the basal ganglia-brainstem pathways in the control of motor behaviors. *Neurosci Res.* 2004;50:139, Fig. 3, with permission.)

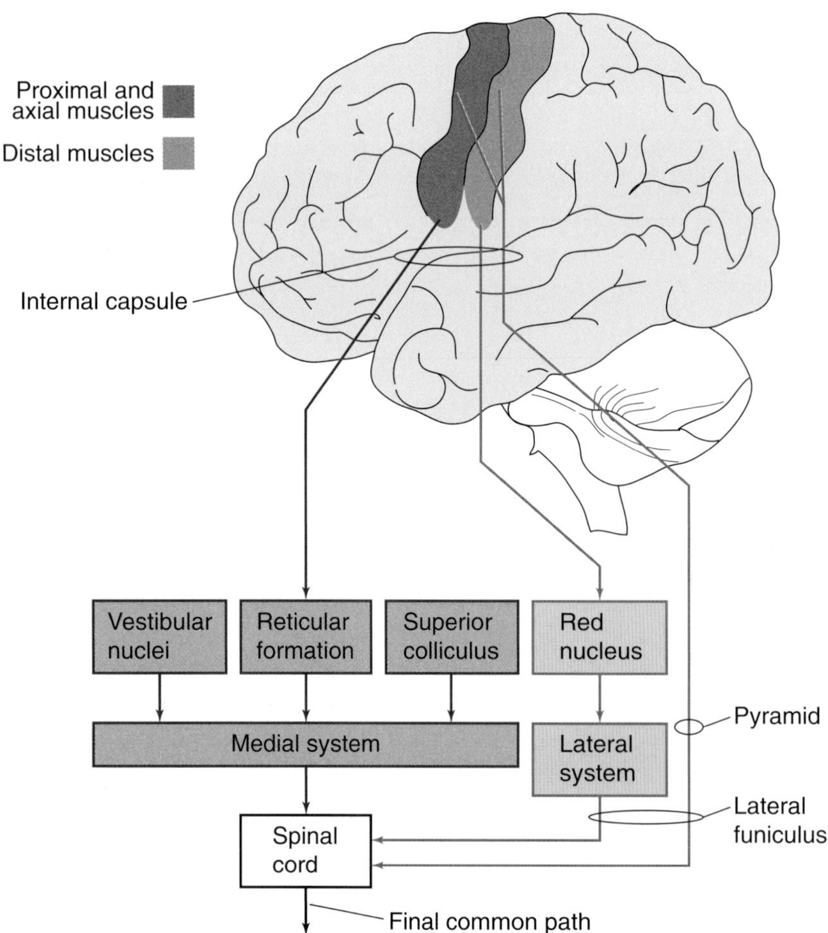

Figure 3.20 The medial and lateral motor system pathways. The medial system, including the vestibulospinal, reticulospinal, and tectospinal pathways, which activate proximal and axial muscles. The lateral system includes the rubrospinal pathway, and along with the pyramidal pathway activates the distal muscles. (Adapted from Brooks DC. The Pixelated Brain, 2011, with permission.)

SUMMARY

1. Movement control is achieved through the cooperative effort of many brain structures, which are organized both hierarchically and in parallel.
2. Sensory inputs perform many functions in the control of movement. They (a) serve as the stimuli for reflexive movement organized in the spinal cord; (b) modulate the output of movement that results from the activity of pattern generators in the spinal cord; (c) modulate commands that originate in higher centers of the nervous system; and (d) contribute to the perception and control of movement through ascending pathways in much more complex ways.
3. In the somatosensory system, muscle spindles, GTOs, joint receptors, and cutaneous receptors contribute to spinal reflex control, modulate spinal pattern generator output, modulate descending commands, and contribute to perception and control of movement through ascending pathways.
4. Vision: (a) allows us to identify objects in space and to determine their movement (exteroceptive sensation) and (b) gives us information about where our body is in space, about the relation of one body part to another, and about the motion of our body (visual proprioception).
5. The vestibular system is sensitive to two types of information: the position of the head in space and sudden changes in the direction of movement of the head.
6. As sensory information ascends to higher levels of processing, every level of the hierarchy has the ability to modulate the information coming into it from below, allowing higher centers to selectively tune (up or down) the information coming from lower centers.
7. Information from sensory receptors is increasingly processed as it ascends the neural hierarchy, enabling meaningful interpretation of the information. This is done by selectively enlarging the receptive field of each successively higher neuron.
8. The somatosensory and visual systems process incoming information to increase contrast sensitivity so that we can more easily identify and discriminate between different objects. This is done through lateral inhibition, in which the cell that is excited inhibits the cells next to it, thus enhancing contrast between excited and nonexcited regions of the body or visual field.
9. There are also special cells within the somatosensory and visual systems that respond best to moving stimuli and are directionally sensitive.
10. In the association cortices, we begin to see the transition from perception to action. The parietal lobe participates in processes involving attention to the position of and manipulation of objects in space.
11. The action system includes areas of the nervous system such as the motor cortex, the cerebellum, the basal ganglia, and brainstem.
12. The motor cortex interacts with sensory processing areas in the parietal lobe and also with basal ganglia and cerebellar areas to identify where we want to move, to plan the movement, and, finally, to execute our actions.
13. The cerebellum appears to act as a comparator, a system that compensates for errors by comparing intention with performance. In addition, it modulates muscle tone, participates in the programming of the motor cortex for the execution of movement, and contributes to the timing of movement and to motor and nonmotor learning. It is involved in the control of visually triggered and guided movements.
14. The function of the basal ganglia is related to the planning and control of complex motor behavior, including modulating the central set for a movement and controlling self-initiated movements through outputs to premotor and supplementary motor areas. In addition, it may play a role in selectively activating some movements and suppressing others.
15. The brainstem mediates many aspects of motor control as part of descending pathways from the cerebral cortex, cerebellum, and basal ganglia. This includes the generation of locomotor rhythms, the regulation of postural tone, and the integration of sensory information for posture and balance.

CHAPTER 4

Physiological Basis of Motor Learning and Recovery of Function

Learning Objectives

Following completion of this chapter, the reader will be able to:

1. Define plasticity and discuss its relationship to recovery of function.
2. Describe the neural mechanisms that underlie implicit forms of learning, including nonassociative, associative, and procedural learning.
3. Discuss the neural mechanisms underlying explicit forms of learning, including declarative learning, and describe how they differ from implicit forms of learning.
4. Describe the neural mechanisms involved in the shift from implicit to explicit knowledge.
5. Describe the transient events that occur following central nervous system (CNS) injury and discuss their contribution to early recovery of function.
6. Describe the different forms of synaptogenesis and discuss their role in recovery of function.
7. Summarize the changes in cortical reorganization that occur in both acquired and degenerative neural pathology including changes in the affected and contralateral hemispheres.
8. Briefly describe some of the emerging strategies designed to enhance neural plasticity and optimize recovery of function in both acquired brain injury and neurodegenerative conditions.

INTRODUCTION

In Chapter 2, we defined *learning* as the process of acquiring knowledge about the world and *motor learning* as the process of the acquisition and/or modification of skilled action. We also mentioned that, just as motor control must be seen in light of the interaction between the individual, the task, and the environment, this also applies to motor learning.

In this chapter, we examine the physiological basis of motor learning. We show that the physiological basis for motor learning, like motor control (see Chapter 3), is typically distributed among many brain structures and processing levels, rather than being localized to a particular learning site of the brain. Likewise, the physiological basis for the recovery of function is similar to learning, in that recovery involves processes occurring throughout the nervous system and not just at the lesioned site. These processes have many properties in common with those occurring during learning.

This chapter focuses on the physiological basis of motor learning and recovery of function, showing the similarities and differences between these important functions. The material in this chapter builds on material presented in Chapter 2 on motor learning and recovery of function. Since we assume that the reader has a basic familiarity with the concepts presented in Chapters 2 and 3, these concepts will not be reviewed in this chapter.

Integral to a discussion of the physiological basis of motor learning are issues related to neural plasticity.

A fundamental question addressed in this chapter is as follows: What is the relationship between neural plasticity and motor learning? Specifically, we want to know how learning modifies the structure and function of neurons in the brain. Of equal concern is understanding the relationship between neural plasticity and recovery of function. Specifically, we want to know what changes in the structure and function of neurons underlie the recovery of function following injury or in the face of neurodegenerative conditions.

We will also look at research that explores whether physiological plasticity associated with recovery of function following neural pathology is the same as or different from that involved with normal development and learning, that is, in the absence of neural pathology. Previous views have typically held that recovery of function and learning are served by different neural mechanisms. More recent physiological studies suggest that the same mechanisms of neural plasticity underlie recovery of function as well as normal development and learning. Finally, in this chapter, we consider how developmental processes modify the neural mechanisms underlying both learning and recovery of function. During development, synaptic connectivity develops and is fine-tuned during critical periods because of interacting environmental and genetic factors. Thus, developmental factors play a significant role in how plasticity manifests throughout life.

Defining Neural Plasticity

Plasticity is a general term describing the ability of a structure to show modification. Throughout this book, we use the term *plasticity* in reference to mechanisms related to neural modifiability. The term *neural plasticity* (or neural modifiability) has been long used by pioneer researchers such as Ioan Minea, Santiago Ramón y Cajal, and Jerzy Konorski (Bijoch et al., 2019; Stahnisch et al., 2002). Overall, neural plasticity may be seen as a continuum from short-term changes in the efficiency or strength of synaptic connections to long-term structural and functional changes in the organization and numbers of connections among neurons. Neural plasticity may also coexist at many different levels, including the following:

- Brain level (glial and vascular support)
- Network level (changes in patterns of neural activation and cortical remapping)
- Intercellular level (changes between neurons at the synaptic level, including synaptic sprouting)
- Intracellular level (mitochondrial and ribosomal function)
- Biochemical level (protein conformation, enzyme mobilization)
- Genetic level (transcription, translation, and posttranslation modifications)

Neural plasticity is present in our nervous system when we are born and remains present throughout our life. Despite being always present, there exist certain restrictive time windows known as sensitive, or critical, periods when the plasticity of the nervous system is heightened, that is more open to modification. The embryonic circuits we are born with undergo refinement in response to both genetics and experience. In humans, experience-dependent neural modifications are associated with long-lasting behavioral changes (Sanes & Jessell, 2013). Evidence for critical time windows in neuroplasticity is based on research examining exposure to different stimuli before, during, or after a sensitive (or critical) period. For example, Elbert and colleagues (1995) used string players (e.g., guitarist, violinist, or cellist) as a model to investigate how the different sensorimotor inputs coming from the left hand (continuous fingering activity to change the pitch of notes) and right hand (less active fingering activity, e.g., during bowing) could modify the cerebral cortices. Compared to nonmusicians, the string players had an extended cortical network of the hand area (more for the fifth than the first finger) in response to tactile stimulation. Most importantly, the authors found that the subject's age of exposure to practice of the string music instrument was significantly correlated to the observed somatosensory area increase; whereas the amount of practice was not significantly correlated (Elbert et al., 1995). These types of results demonstrate the importance of critical periods of neuroplasticity. It is also noteworthy to mention that neuromaturation of brain structures continues through childhood and adolescence. For instance, postnatal myelination of sensorimotor (internal capsule) and left-hemisphere speech-related tracts (arcuate fasciculus) continue, at least, through adolescence (Paus, 1999).

Learning also can be seen as a continuum of short-term to long-term changes in the ability to produce skilled actions. The gradual shift from short-term to long-term learning reflects a move along the continuum of neural modifiability, as increased synaptic efficiency gradually gives way to structural changes, which are the underpinnings of long-term modification of behavior. This relationship is shown in Figure 4.1.

Like learning, recovery of function can also be characterized by a continuum of changes from short-term functional changes that occur immediately following injury (like unmasking of existing but weak connections) to long-term structural changes such as remapping of the sensory or motor cortex.

Learning and Memory

Learning is defined as the acquisition of knowledge or ability; memory is the outcome of learning, including the retention and storage of that knowledge or ability (Kandel et al., 2000a). Learning reflects the *process* by which we acquire knowledge; memory is the *product* of that process. Remember, from Chapter 2, that memory is not a single process but has two major forms. The first is implicit memory, which operates unconsciously and automatically, as, for example, in the memory for habits as well as perceptual and motor skills. The second is explicit memory, which operates consciously, as, for example, in the memory for people, places, and objects (Kandel & Siegelbaum, 2013). Figure 4.2 summarizes the forms of long-term memory (Fig. 4.2, bottom) and in addition shows the neural structures associated with these different forms of memory (Fig. 4.2, top).

Memory storage is often divided into short- and long-term components. Short-term memory refers to working memory, which has a limited capacity for information and lasts for only a few moments. Short-term memory reflects a momentary attention to something, such as when we remember a phone number only long enough to dial it and then forget it.

Long-term memory is intimately related to the process of learning. Long-term memory can also be seen as a continuum. Initial stages of long-term memory

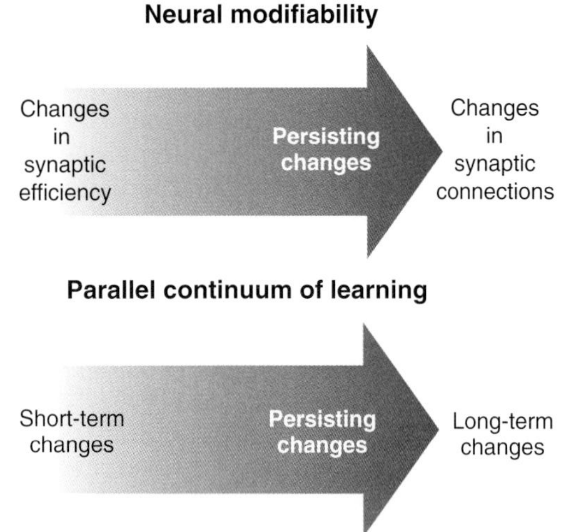

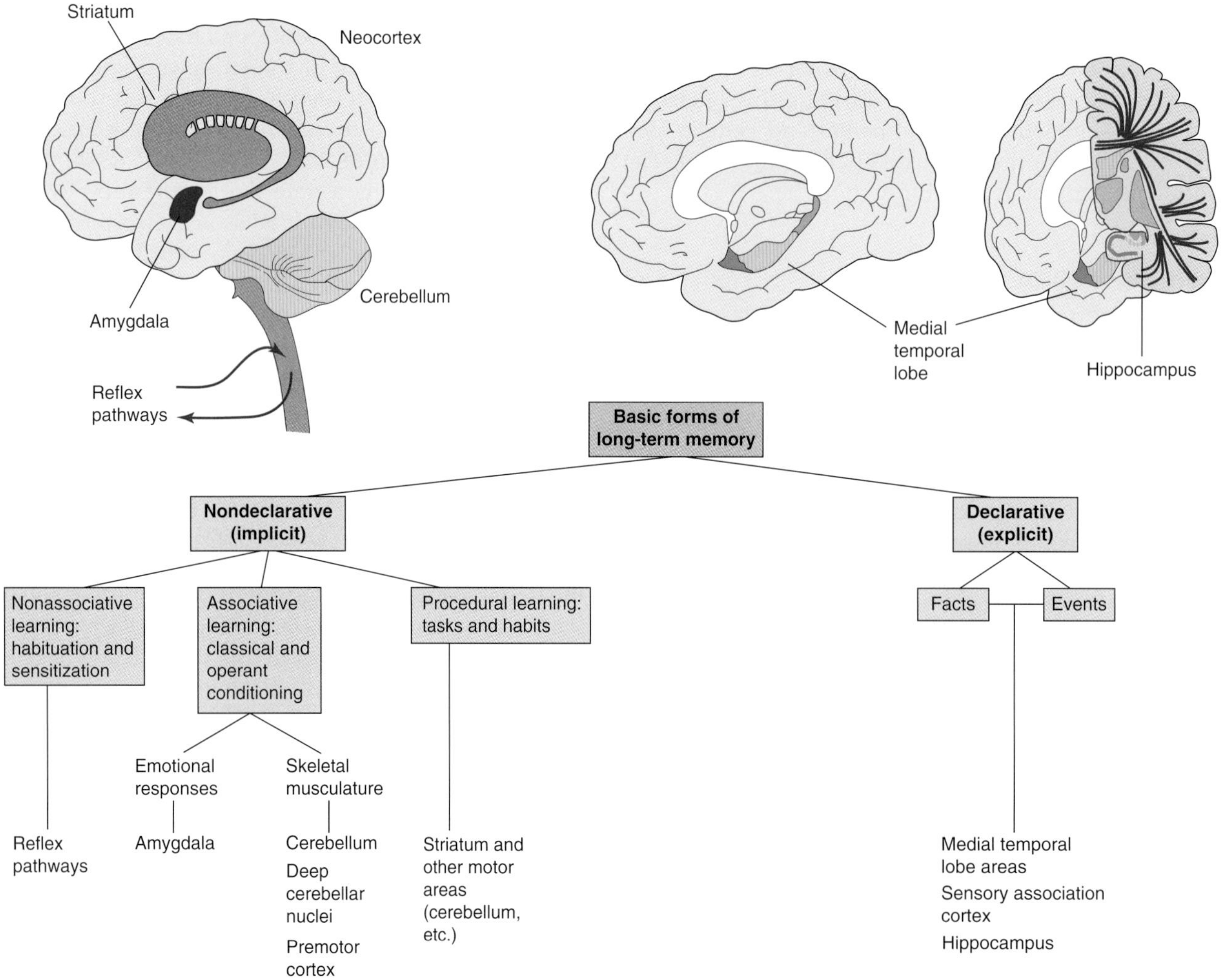

Figure 4.1 The gradual shift from short-term to long-term learning is reflected in a move along the continuum of neural modifiability. Short-term changes, associated with an increased synaptic efficiency, persist and gradually give way to structural changes, the underpinning of long-term learning.

Figure 4.2 A summary of the various forms of long-term memory **(bottom)** and the neural structures associated with these different forms of memory **(top)**. Nondeclarative (implicit) memory involves the neocortex, striatum, amygdala, cerebellum, and in the simplest cases, the reflex pathways. Declarative (explicit) memory requires the medial temporal lobe, the sensory association cortex, and the hippocampus, as well as certain areas of the neocortex (not shown).

formation reflect functional changes in the efficiency of synapses. Later stages of memory formation reflect structural changes in synaptic connections. These memories are less subject to disruption.

Localization of Learning and Memory

Are learning and memory localized in a specific brain structure? As noted in Chapter 3, and illustrated in Figure 4.2, they are not. In fact, learning can occur in all parts of the brain. Learning and the storage of that learning, memory, appear to involve both parallel and hierarchical processing within the CNS. Even for relatively simple learning tasks, multiple parallel channels of information are used.

We could distinguish three main types of learning based on the computational learning methods used by the brain: unsupervised, reinforcement, and supervised. The learning-related information of goal-oriented behaviors are processed differently and also occur in different areas and circuits of the brain—cortex, basal ganglia, and cerebellum (Fig. 4.3). In unsupervised learning (highlighted in Fig. 4.3A), the features of the input itself guide the learning. The cerebral cortex provides a representation of the sensory state, context, and action; and this information is represented as different modalities and frames of references in diverse cortical areas. In general, cortical neurons show a response tuning that is highly dependent on sensory experience, and their synapses follow a Hebbian-type plasticity rule (synapses are potentiated or depressed when presynaptic and postsynaptic responses are or are not associated, respectively) (Doya, 1999, 2000). In reinforcement learning (highlighted in Fig. 4.3B), the basal ganglia contribute to processing the current situation, predict the reward, and then select the most suitable action across different options (Doya, 2000). In this regard, Nakahara and colleagues (2001) presented a model to explore how a visual loop—including the dorsolateral prefrontal cortex and anterior region of basal ganglia—and a motor loop—including the supplementary motor area and posterior basal ganglia—presumably coordinated by the pre-supplementary region promote the learning of a sequential visuomotor task. The concurrent learning in the visual and motor loops depends on reinforcement signals mediated by divergent dopaminergic connections. The authors propose that this coordinated network allows visually guided discrete movements to progressively become a gross motor skill (Nakahara et al., 2001). Finally, in supervised learning (highlighted in Fig. 4.3C), the cerebellum may serve as a neural structure to create internal models of the body and the environment (dynamics and kinematics) for the implementation of feedforward and feedback modes of control of movements (Kawato, 1999). The cerebellar circuitry promotes trial-and-error learning (i.e., supervised learning) by encoding movement-error signals via climbing fibers from the inferior olive to Purkinje cells and via climbing-fiber–induced long-term potentiation (LTP) and depression in coordination with parallel fibers (Doya 1999, 2000; Kitazawa et al., 1998; Kobayashi et al., 1998; Zang & Schutter, 2019).

Apparently, mechanisms underlying learning and memory are the same whether the learning is occurring in fairly simple circuits or involves very complex circuits incorporating many aspects of the CNS hierarchy. Thus, current neuronal models of memory suggest that a memory consists of a pattern of changes in synaptic connections among networks of neurons distributed in

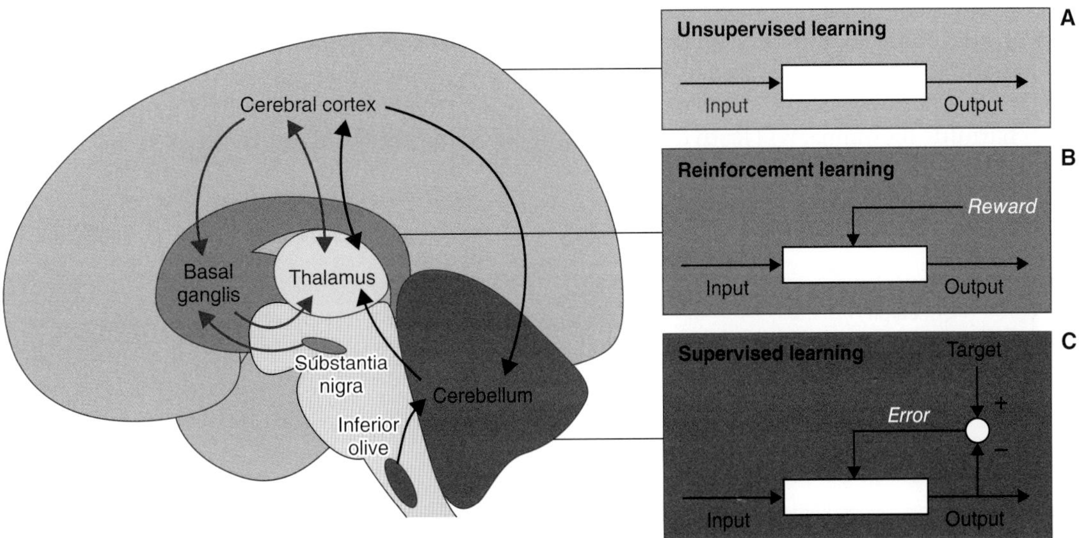

Figure 4.3 Brain diagram that depicts the three proposed brain areas and networks for unsupervised, reinforcement, and supervised types of learning. Unsupervised learning in the cortex **(A)**; reinforcement, or reward-based learning, in the basal ganglia **(B)**; and supervised, or error-based learning, in the cerebellum **(C)**. (Adapted with permission from Doya K. Complementary roles of basal ganglia and cerebellum in learning and motor control. *Curr Opin Neurobiol* 2000;10:732–739.)

many parts of the brain. It is interesting to note that in 1929, Lashley was the first to hypothesize that memory was stored throughout the nervous system (Lashley, 1929). In order to try to find the location of memory storage, he performed experiments in which he made lesions to many areas of the cortex of animals. To his surprise, he found that loss of memory abilities was related not to the site of the lesion but to the amount of cortex in which lesions were made.

This chapter describes the continuum of plasticity within the nervous system that represents learning and, specifically, motor learning. The processes underlying learning in the nervous system, as well as those that underlie recovery of function, are described. In this, and later chapters, we explore the implications of principles of plasticity related to learning and recovery of function to rehabilitation of patients with neural pathology.

PLASTICITY AND LEARNING

Many factors potentially modify synaptic connections. We are concerned in this chapter with activity-dependent modifications of synaptic connections, that is, both the transient and long-term modulation of synapses resulting from experience. Learning alters our capability for acting by changing both the effectiveness and anatomic connections of neural pathways. We discuss modifications of synaptic connections at both the cellular level and at the level of whole networks of neurons.

Plasticity and Nondeclarative (Implicit) Forms of Learning

Remember that nonassociative learning is a form of implicit learning, where the subject is learning about the properties of a stimulus that is repeated. The learned suppression of a response to a nonnoxious stimulus is called habituation. For example, an animal will orient to a novel stimulus. If, however, the stimulus is neither beneficial nor harmful, the animal will learn to ignore the stimulus with repeated exposure (Kandel & Siegelbaum, 2013). In contrast, an increased response to one stimulus that is consistently preceded by a noxious stimulus is called sensitization. Keep in mind that nonassociative forms of learning can be short term or long term. What are the neural mechanisms underlying these simple forms of learning, and do the same neural mechanisms underlie both short- and long-term changes?

Habituation

Habituation, the simplest form of implicit learning, was first studied by Sherrington, who found that the flexion reflex habituated with many stimulus repetitions. More recent research examining habituation in relatively simple networks of neurons in invertebrate animals has shown that habituation is related to a decrease in synaptic activity between sensory neurons and their connections to interneurons and motor neurons (Kandel et al., 2000a; Sherrington, 1906).

During habituation, there is a reduction in the amplitude of synaptic potentials (a decreased excitatory postsynaptic potential [EPSP]) produced by the sensory neuron on the interneuron and motor neuron. This short-term change in EPSP amplitude during habituation is illustrated in Figure 4.4, showing the synapses before habitation (A) and the reduced EPSP amplitude associated with short-term habituation (B). During initial stages of learning, the decreased size of the EPSP may last for only several minutes. With continued presentation of the stimulus, persisting changes in synaptic efficacy occur, representing longer-term memory for habituation.

During the course of learning, continued presentation of the stimulus results in structural changes in the sensory cells themselves. Structural changes include a decrease in the number of synaptic connections between the sensory neuron and interneurons and motor neurons, shown diagrammatically in Figure 4.4C. In addition, the number of active transmitting zones within existing connections decreases. As a result of these

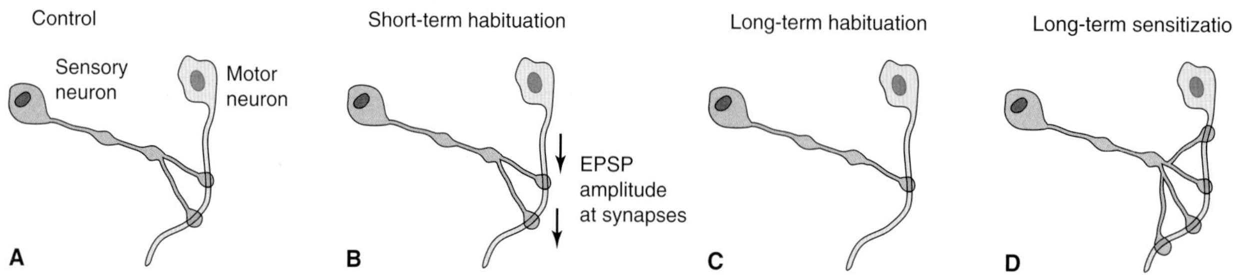

Figure 4.4 Neuronal modifications underlying short- and long-term nonassociative learning. **(A)** Synapse prior to nonassociative learning (labeled control). **(B)** Short-term habituation results from a decrease in excitatory postsynaptic potential (EPSP) amplitude at the synapse between the sensory and motor neuron, but no change in the synaptic structure. **(C)** Long-term habituation results in a decrease in the numbers of connections. **(D)** Long-term sensitization results in an increase in the numbers of connections. (Adapted from Kandel ER. Cellular mechanisms of learning and the biological basis of individuality. In: Kandel ER, Schwartz JH, Jessell TM, eds. *Principles of neural science*, 3rd ed. New York, NY: Elsevier, 1991:1009–1031.)

structural changes, habituation persists over weeks and months, representing long-term memory for habituation. Thus, the process of habituation does not involve specific memory storage neurons found in specialized parts of the CNS. Rather, memory (retention of habituation) results from a change in the neurons that are normal components of the response pathway.

Different synapses have different levels of adaptability. For example, some synapses show little habituation, even with high levels of activation, while others, especially synapses between sensory and motor neurons and some interneurons, show large habituation with a small amount of training. In addition, if the habituating stimulus is massed without rest between sessions, there is a large short-term effect but very little long-term effect (Kandel et al., 2000a).

How might this research apply to intervention strategies used by therapists in the clinic? As discussed in detail in Chapter 5, habituation exercises are given to patients who have certain types of inner ear disorders that result in reports of dizziness when they move their head in certain ways. To decrease movement-provoked dizziness, patients are given habituation exercises in which they are asked to repeat the provocative movements, in order to habituate the dizziness response. When patients begin therapy, they may experience an initial decline in the intensity of their dizziness symptoms during the course of one session of habituation exercise. But the next day, dizziness is back at the same level. Gradually, over days and weeks of practicing the exercises, the patient begins to see decreases in dizziness persist across sessions (Herdman, 2007; Shumway-Cook & Horak, 1990).

Application of Kandel's research to patients with inner ear disorders would suggest that the initial repetition of the provocative movements results in a temporary decrease in the synaptic effectiveness of certain vestibular neurons and their connections, due to a decrease in the size of the EPSPs. Continued repetitions of these movements would result in more permanent changes in synaptic effectiveness. In addition, structural changes, including a reduction in the number of vestibular neuron synapses connecting to interneurons, would occur. With the advent of structural changes, the decline in dizziness in response to the repeated head movement would persist, allowing the patient to discontinue the exercise without reexperiencing symptoms of dizziness. It is possible that if exercises were discontinued too soon, or practiced within a single session rather than over many separate sessions, structural changes in the sensory connections would not occur and dizziness symptoms would recur because of the absence of long-term structural changes underlying persisting habituation.

Sensitization

As we mentioned in Chapter 2, sensitization, another form of implicit learning, is caused by a strengthening of a response to a stimulus that is preceded by an intense or noxious stimulus. Sensitization may also be short or long term, and it may involve the exact set of synapses that shows habituation. However, the mechanisms involved in sensitization are a little more complex than are those involved in habituation. One way that sensitization may occur is by prolonging the action potential through changes in potassium conductance. This allows more transmitters to be released from the terminals, giving an increased EPSP. It also appears to improve the mobilization of transmitter, making it more available for release. Surprisingly, the same synapse can participate in both habituation and sensitization, with synaptic efficacy being depressed in one situation and enhanced in another, since the different types of learning use different cellular mechanisms (Kandel et al., 2000a).

Sensitization, like habituation, can be short or long term. Mechanisms for long-term memory of sensitization involve the same cells as short-term memory but now reflect structural changes in these cells (Kandel & Schwartz, 1982; Sweatt & Kandel, 1989). Kandel (1989) has shown that in invertebrates, short-term sensitization involves changes in preexisting protein structures, while long-term sensitization involves the synthesis of new protein. This synthesis of new protein at the synapse implies that long-term sensitization involves changes that are genetically influenced.

This genetic influence also encompasses the growth of new synaptic connections, as illustrated in Figure 4.4D. Animals that showed long-term sensitization were found to have twice as many synaptic terminals as did untrained animals, increased dendrites in the postsynaptic cells, and an increase in the numbers of active zones at synaptic terminals, from 40% to 65% (Bailey & Chen, 1983).

In summary, the research on habituation and sensitization suggests that short-term and long-term memory may not be separate categories but may be part of a single-graded memory function. With sensitization, as with habituation, long-term memory and short-term memory involve change at the same synapses. While short-term changes reflect relatively temporary changes in synaptic effectiveness, structural changes are the hallmark of long-term memory (Kandel et al., 2000a).

Associative Learning

Associative learning, also known as Hebbian learning, involves the association between two factors (Kussmierz et al., 2017). Remember that during associative learning, a form of implicit learning, a person learns to predict relationships, either relationships of one stimulus to another (classical conditioning) or the relationship of one's behavior to a consequence (operant conditioning). Through associative learning, we learn to form key relationships that help us adapt our actions to the environment. Refer back to Figure 4.2.

Researchers examining the physiological basis for associative learning have found that it can take place through simple changes in synaptic efficiency without requiring complex learning networks. Associative learning, whether short-term or long-term, uses common cellular processes. Initially, when two neurons are active at the same time (i.e., in association), there is a modification of existing proteins within these two neurons that produces a change in synaptic efficiency. Long-term association results in the synthesis of new proteins and the subsequent formation of new synaptic connections between the neurons.

Classical Conditioning

During classical conditioning, an initially weak stimulus (the conditioned stimulus) becomes highly effective in producing a response when it becomes associated with another stronger stimulus (the unconditioned stimulus). It is similar to, although more complex than, sensitization. In fact, it may be that classical conditioning is simply an extension of the processes involved in sensitization.

Remember that in classical conditioning, timing is critical. When conditioned and unconditioned stimuli converge on the same neurons, facilitation occurs if the conditioned stimulus causes action potentials in the neurons just before (usually about 0.5 s) the unconditioned stimulus arrives. This is because action potentials allow Ca^+ to move into the presynaptic neuron, and this Ca^+ activates special modulatory transmitters involved in classical conditioning. If the activity occurs after the unconditioned stimulus, Ca^+ is not released at the right time, and the stimulus has no effect (Abrams & Kandel, 1988; Kandel et al., 2000a).

Operant Conditioning

Although operant conditioning and classical conditioning may seem like two different processes, in fact, the laws that govern the two are similar, indicating that the same neural mechanisms may control them. In each type of conditioning, learning involves the development of predictive relationships. In classical conditioning, a specific stimulus predicts a specific response. In operant conditioning, we learn to predict the outcome of specific behaviors. However, the same cellular mechanisms that underlie classical conditioning are also responsible for operant conditioning.

Procedural Learning (Skills and Habits)

Procedural learning is one of the more complex forms of nondeclarative or implicit learning and is responsible for the acquisition of many skills and habits. It includes the learning and execution of both motor and nondeclarative cognitive skills, especially those involving sequences. It occurs only when a movement is performed by learners themselves through trial-and-error practice and within the context of actions that will be carried out in a normal setting. Many habits, such as learning to navigate through the world, avoiding objects including people in our path, are habitual movement patterns that are learned early and retained throughout life (Kandel & Siegelbaum, 2013).

Habit learning (procedural learning) depends on a neural system distinct from that of explicit or declarative learning, described in the following section. The implicit system underlying procedural learning is composed of a network of specific frontal regions (including sensorimotor cortex), four nuclei in the basal ganglia, parietal regions, and cerebellar structures. As will be noted in the next section on declarative learning, the neural pathways underlying the explicit system include frontal brain areas such as the anterior cingulate, prefrontal cortex (PFC), head of the caudate nucleus, hippocampus, and other medial temporal lobe structures (Maddox & Ashby, 2004; Ullman, 2004). Experiments that demonstrate the role of the cerebellum in procedural learning are discussed in Extended Knowledge 4.1.

Plasticity and Declarative (Explicit) Forms of Learning

Remember that associative learning can also be thought of in terms of the type of knowledge acquired. As already discussed, nondeclarative learning and, specifically, *procedural learning* (resulting in implicit knowledge) refer to learning tasks that can be performed automatically without attention or conscious thought (e.g., many of our daily habits). In contrast, *declarative learning* (resulting in explicit knowledge) requires conscious processes such as awareness and attention and results in knowledge that can be expressed consciously. Procedural learning is expressed through improved performance of the task learned, while declarative learning can be expressed in a form other than that in which it was learned. As shown in Figure 4.2, the neural pathways underlying declarative or explicit learning include frontal brain areas such as the anterior cingulate, PFC, and head of the caudate nucleus as well as the medial temporal lobes and hippocampus.

Wilder Penfield, a neurosurgeon, was one of the first researchers to understand the important role of the temporal lobes in memory function. While performing temporal-lobe surgery in patients with epilepsy, he stimulated the temporal lobes of the conscious patients, in order to determine the location of the diseased versus the normal tissue. When the temporal lobes were stimulated, the patients experienced memories from the past as if they were happening again. For example, one patient heard music from an event long ago and saw the situation and felt the emotions that surrounded the singing of that music, with everything happening in real time (Penfield, 1958).

Extended Knowledge 4.1

The Role of the Cerebellum in Procedural Learning

The following experiments support the hypothesis that procedural learning involves the cerebellum and/or the motor cortex. Gilbert and Thatch (1977) examined the involvement of the cerebellum in a very simple form of procedural learning, involving increasing or decreasing the gain of a response when increased or decreased forces are required, a form of **adaptation**. You will recall from Chapter 3 that the cerebellum has two types of input fibers, the climbing fibers and the mossy fibers, and one type of output fiber, the Purkinje cells. Climbing-fiber inputs to the Purkinje cells typically signal error and are important in the correction of ongoing movements. In contrast, mossy-fiber inputs to the Purkinje cells provide kinesthetic information about ongoing movements and are important in the control of those movements. Figure 4.5B reviews the relationship of these fibers. It has been shown that the climbing-fiber inputs signaling error to the Purkinje cells may increase or decrease the strength of mossy-fiber synapses onto the same Purkinje cells. This produces a long-term change in Purkinje cell output, which contributes to motor learning.

Gilbert and Thatch (1977) examined the role of the cerebellum in motor learning during experiments in which monkeys were trained to return a handle to a central position whenever it was moved to the left or right. During the sessions, they recorded the activity of Purkinje neurons in the arm area of the anterior lobe of the cerebellum. Once the task was learned and repeatedly performed in the same way, the arm movement was accompanied by predictable changes occurring primarily in mossy-fiber inputs reporting the proprioceptive effects of the movement, with occasional climbing-fiber input. Figure 4.5A1 shows the activity of the mossy fibers (simple spikes) and climbing fibers (complex spikes) during the wrist flexion movements when the monkeys were moving against an expected force or load.

Then the experimenters modified the task, requiring the monkeys to use more force to return the handle to the original position. At first, the animal was not able to return the handle in one simple movement. But gradually, the animal learned to respond correctly. During the first few trials of the new task, there was a sudden increase in activity in the climbing fibers, signaling the error, as shown in Figure 4.5A2.

This increase in climbing-fiber activity was associated with a reduction in the efficiency of the mossy-fiber connections to the Purkinje cells. The reduction in Purkinje cell output then was associated with an increase in force generation, allowing the monkey to complete the task successfully, as shown in Figure 4.5A3. Thus, it appears that changes in synaptic efficiency between these neurons in the cerebellum are an important link in the modification of movements through procedural learning.

This type of cerebellar learning may also occur in the vestibuloocular reflex circuitry, which includes cerebellar pathways. This reflex keeps the eyes fixed on an object when the head turns. In experiments in which humans wore prismatic lenses that reversed the image on the eye, the vestibuloocular reflex was reversed over time. This modification of the reflex, another form of adaptation, did not occur with cerebellar lesions (Melville-Jones & Mandl, 1983).

In humans, lesions in the temporal lobe of the cortex and the hippocampus may interfere with the laying down of declarative memory. A few patients have been studied after having the hippocampus and related temporal lobe areas removed because of epilepsy. After surgery, the patients were no longer able to acquire long-term declarative memories, although they remembered old memories. Their short-term memory was normal, but if their attention was distracted from an item held in short-term memory, they would forget it completely. However, skill learning was unaffected in these patients. They would often learn a complex task but be unable to remember the procedures that made up the task or the events surrounding learning the task (Milner, 1966). This work suggests that the temporal lobes and hippocampus may be important to establishing memory but are not a part of the memory storage area.

The hippocampus, which is a subcortical structure, and part of the temporal lobe circuitry, is critical for declarative learning, as shown again in Figure 4.2. Research has shown evidence of plastic changes in hippocampal neurons similar to those found in neural circuits of simpler animals when learning takes place.

Researchers have shown that pathways in the hippocampus show a facilitation that has been called *long-term potentiation*, which is similar to the mechanisms causing sensitization (Bliss & Lomo, 1973). For example, in one region of the hippocampus, LTP occurs when a weak and a strong input arrive at the same region of a neuron's dendrite. The weak input will be enhanced if it is activated in association with the strong one. This process is shown in Figure 4.6, which shows the size of the response to the first stimulus and the response to the same stimulus after LTP was induced. LTP appears to require the simultaneous firing of both presynaptic and postsynaptic cells. After this occurs, LTP is maintained through an increase in presynaptic transmitter release. There also exists *long-term depression* (LTD) in which the neural connection is weakened and the postsynaptic action potentials precedes the presynaptic action potentials. Both LTP and LTD are biologically complex and can be influenced by neuromodulators (dopamine, noradrenaline, acetylcholine, and serotonin), inhibition of the gamma-aminobutyric acid (GABA) neurotransmitter, and other neurochemical processes such as calcium-based plasticity (Kussmierz et al., 2017).

There are both a short-term early phase to LTP (1–3 hours) that does not require protein synthesis and a longer late phase that lasts at least 24 hours and requires cyclic adenosine monophosphate (cAMP)-induced and cAMP-responsible element-binding protein (CREB)-mediated gene expression, accompanied by protein synthesis. The early phase involves a functional change, with no new synapses, while the late phase involves a structural change, involving new synaptic release sites (Kandel et al., 2000a).

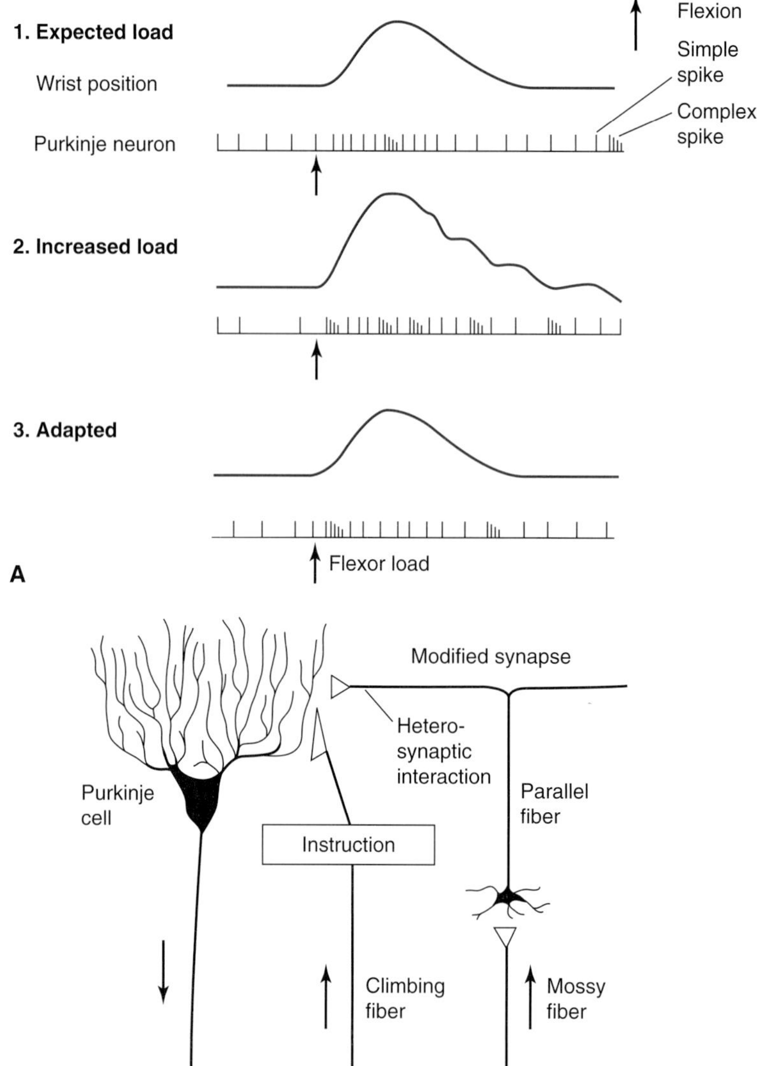

Figure 4.5 **(A)** Activity of mossy fibers (simple spikes) and climbing fibers (complex spikes) during wrist flexion movements when monkeys were moving against (1) an expected load, (2) an unexpectedly increased load, and (3) the increased load, after practice (adapted). Note that climbing-fiber (complex spike) activity increased with the increase in load, signaling an error in returning the handle to its original position and reducing the efficiency of the mossy-fiber/Purkinje cell synapse. After adaptation, the simple spike activity is reduced and complex spike activity is back to low levels. **(B)** Cerebellum, showing the relationship between mossy-fiber input (via parallel fibers) and climbing-fiber input important to learning. (Adapted from Ghez C. The cerebellum. In: Kandel ER, Schwartz JH, Jessell TM, eds. *Principles of neural science*, 3rd ed. Norwalk, CT: Appleton & Lange, 1991:643.)

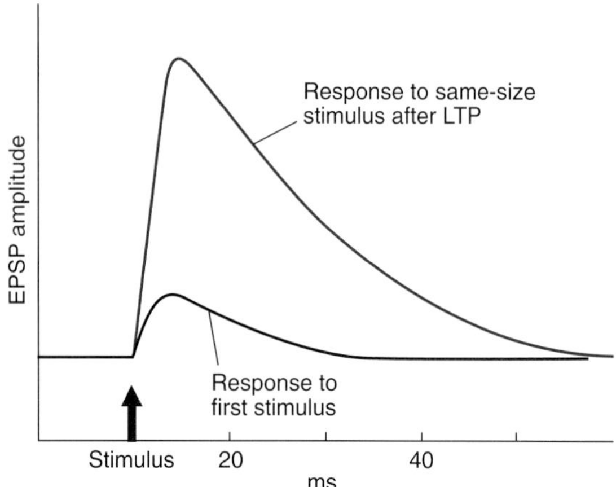

Figure 4.6 Cellular basis for long-term potentiation (LTP), showing small excitatory postsynaptic potentials (EPSPs) to first stimulus and large EPSPs to the same-size stimulus after LTP.

In the 1970s, it was discovered that the hippocampus codes a cognitive map of the spatial areas in which we move. The cells that code these spatial characteristics have been called place cells, and each cell is activated optimally when an animal moves in a given part of its environment. In this way, the animal creates a place field or an internal representation of the space in which it lives. These place fields are created very quickly (e.g., minutes) when animals enter a new space and are often present for months. The same neurons may be active as part of different place fields, so they can be used in multiple maps (Kandel et al., 2000a; O'Keefe & Dostrovsky, 1971).

In order to determine whether LTP was important in forming place fields, scientists determined the ability of mice with genetic mutations affecting LTP to create place fields. They found that the two mutations only made the place fields fuzzier than normal, showing that LTP was not required for the basic sensory process of creating place fields. However, the place fields were no longer stable over time, suggesting that the mice had a long-term problem with the retention of these place fields. Inability to form and retain stable place fields, allowing navigation through the environment, is common among patients with medial temporal lobe lesions (Kandel et al., 2000a).

In addition to being important for the formation of long-term memory of spatial maps, LTP within the hippocampus has also been shown to be critical for spatial memory (Kandel et al., 2000a). For example, Morris et al. (1986) performed an experiment in which rats swam a water maze to find a platform under the water. The water was made opaque in order to block the use of vision in finding the target. The rats were released in different parts of the maze and were required to use spatial cues related to the position of the walls to find the target. They also performed a nonspatial task in which the platform was above the water and the rat could simply use visual cues to swim to the target.

These experimenters showed that blocking specific receptors (*N*-methyl-d-aspartate [NMDA] receptors) in hippocampal neurons caused the rats to fail to learn the spatial version of the task. This finding suggests that certain hippocampal neurons are involved in spatial learning through LTP. Mice with genetic mutations affecting NMDA receptors, which disrupted LTP, showed a profound deficit in spatial memory on the water maze. Animals with genetic deficits affecting only late LTP showed normal learning and short-term memory but had defective long-term memory (Kandel et al., 2000a).

In comparing the results of experiments on short- and long-term learning, it is noteworthy that simple forms of nondeclarative implicit learning involving habituation or sensitization have much in common with complex declarative explicit learning, although different brain structures may be involved. Both show a short-term memory phase involving only functional changes in synaptic output, followed by a long-term memory phase involving structural changes in synapses. In both implicit and explicit learning, long-term changes are activated by cAMP-responsive genes and the CREB gene expression, which are accompanied by protein synthesis and new synapses (Bailey & Kandel, 2004).

The Shift from Implicit to Explicit Knowledge

Pascual-Leone and colleagues (1994) have shown that modulation of motor cortex outputs occurs when explicit knowledge is associated with improved motor performance. In addition, they have now explored the changes in motor cortical outputs when implicit knowledge is transformed into explicit knowledge.

They used a sequential finger movement task, in which the subject sat in front of the computer with a response pad with four buttons, to be pressed by the four fingers of the hand. When a number was displayed on the screen, the subject was to press the appropriate button as quickly as possible. A group of experimental subjects was given a repeating sequence of cues but not told of the repetitive nature. Their performance was compared with that of a control group given a random sequence. Subjects were asked whether the sequence was random or repeating at the end of each block of 10 repetitions of the sequence.

Pascual-Leone et al. (1994) found that during the course of learning, the sequence of finger movement reaction times became shorter, and the cortical maps representing the finger muscles involved in the movement became progressively larger (measured by transcranial magnetic stimulation [TMS]). After four blocks of trials, reaction time was significantly shorter, and peak amplitudes and sizes of the cortical outputs to the muscles were significantly higher. At this point, all subjects in the experimental group knew that the sequences being presented were not random but did not yet know the entire sequence. The maps of cortical output to the muscles continued to enlarge until the subjects attained explicit knowledge of the sequence (six to nine blocks). At this point, the motor cortex maps returned to baseline size within three additional blocks of trials, as subjects also began to anticipate the cues for the finger presses. The authors suggest that after explicit learning of a sequence has occurred, the contribution of the motor cortex is attenuated and other brain structures begin to assume a more active role in task execution (Pascual-Leone et al., 1994).

The Shift from Explicit to Implicit Memory

We have seen that practice can result in a shift of implicit memory to explicit memory, as a person becomes conscious of the rules or procedures of the skilled action. It is also the case that constant repetition of a task can result in a shift from explicit to implicit memory. A good example of this is learning to drive a car. Initially, driving a car requires much conscious effort to recall the rules and procedures of driving (explicit memory). With continued practice, many aspects of driving become automatic and unconscious (implicit memory) (Kandel & Siegelbaum, 2013).

It is important to remember that the use of the two memory systems together (implicit and explicit) is the rule, not the exception. The two systems overlap and are used together in most learning experiences.

Complex Forms of Motor Learning

Motor learning includes both simple forms, such as operant and classical conditioning, as well as more complex forms involving the acquisition of skilled movements. Asanuma and Keller (1991) examined the neural mechanisms underlying the procedural learning of more complex motor skills. They hypothesized that one mechanism underlying procedural learning of skilled actions involved LTP of specific cells in the motor cortex by cells in the somatosensory cortex.

To test this hypothesis, Asanuma and Keller (1991) carried out the following experiments. A cat was placed in a clear plastic box with a small opening in the front (Fig. 4.7). In front of the box was a rotating beaker, in which a food pellet was placed. There was a gap between the beaker and the box, so the cat would drop the food unless it learned a new technique of supinating the wrist while picking up the food. Prior to training, the somatosensory cortex in one hemisphere was removed. Acquisition of the skill by the contralateral limb to the lesion was severely affected, suggesting the importance of the somatosensory cortex to acquiring this skill. In contrast, learning in the control limb, with an intact somatosensory cortex, was normal. In Figure 4.7A, the cat reaches through a slit with the contralateral limb to retrieve the food pellet, but as expected, because of the absence of somatosensory cortex, the cat does not learn to supinate, and the pellet drops between the beaker and the box (Fig. 4.7B). After training both limbs, the other somatosensory cortex was removed. Interestingly, the previously learned skill, involving supination of the limb to retrieve the pellet, was not affected. Thus, the trained cats were able to supinate and flex the paw to retrieve the food pellet (Fig. 4.7C). This suggests that the somatosensory cortex participates in the learning of motor skills, through LTP. However, after learning the skilled action, other areas, such as the thalamocortical pathways, may take over.

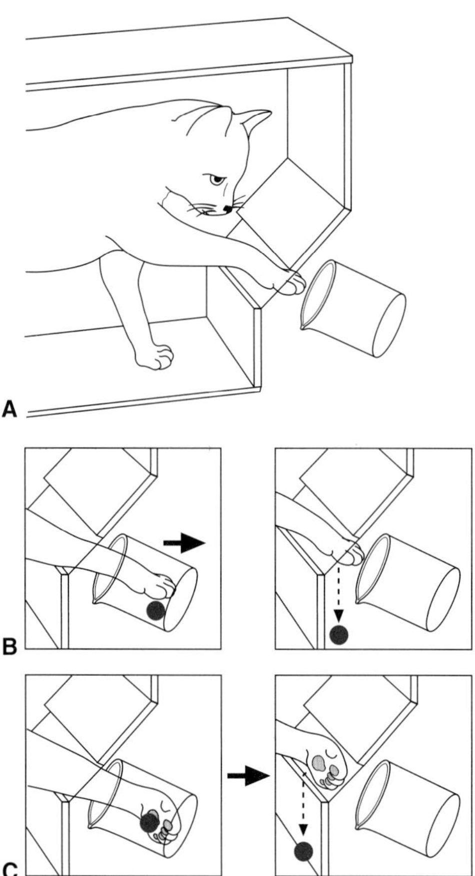

Figure 4.7 **(A)** Paradigm used to study the role of the somatosensory cortex in learning complex motor skills in the cat. **(B)** After removal of the ipsilateral somatosensory cortex, the cat reaches through a slit with the contralateral limb to retrieve the food pellet, but the cat does not learn to supinate the limb, and the pellet drops between the beaker and the box. **(C)** After training both limbs, the other somatosensory cortex was removed. The trained cat was able to supinate and flex the paw to retrieve the food pellet with the ipsilateral limb, because it had been trained before the contralateral somatosensory cortex was removed. (Adapted from Sakamoto T, Arissian K, Asanuma H. Functional role of the sensory cortex in learning motor skills in cats. *Brain Res.* 1989;503:258–264.)

These results suggest that with practice, changes in the sensorimotor cortical pathways also increase the efficiency of the thalamocortical pathways that are coactivated during the learning process. Thus, with training, these alternative pathways (e.g., the thalamocortical pathways) could take over activation of the motor cortex. The efficiency of the thalamic input to the motor cortex was retained, even when sensorimotor cortical inputs were no longer activated (Asanuma & Keller, 1991). This could thus explain the lack of sensory input required in making movements after learning, since the somatosensory cortex could be bypassed and other pathways could take over.

What are the clinical implications of this research? First, it underscores the importance of the development of parallel pathways during the motor learning process. For example, with practice, neurons in the motor cortex are potentiated by neurons in the somatosensory cortex. In addition, with learning, pathways from the thalamus to the motor cortex develop, such that neurons in the motor cortex can now also be activated directly by the thalamus, reducing the need for sensory input to the motor cortex. A person who is very active in learning a variety of skilled actions is likely to have developed these parallel pathways. These parallel pathways then will have important implications to the recovery of function, when neural pathology interrupts the primary pathways. In this case, parallel or alternative pathways can be utilized to activate motor cortex.

Acquisition of Skill: The Shift to Automaticity

The development of a motor skill has been characterized as a shift toward automaticity (Fitts & Posner, 1967). One of the important steps on the road to becoming expert in a motor skill occurs when the individual can perform the movements in an apparently effortless and automatic fashion (Milton et al., 2004). Automation with skill development allows general attentional resources to become available for other tasks. Thus, as automaticity increases, it becomes easier to perform a second, attention-demanding task simultaneously. Many activities of daily living, such as speaking, writing, and pointing at a target, are examples of automatic skilled voluntary movements (Fitts & Posner, 1967). Neurological diseases affecting the control of movement frequently alter motor automaticity; thus, tasks that were previously performed automatically, that is, without exerting full attention, now require attentional resources.

A number of research studies have investigated the changes in neural activity associated with the shift to automaticity that occurs when learning a new movement skill in healthy adults (Floyer-Lea & Matthews, 2004; Poldrack et al., 2005; Wu et al., 2004a) and explored changes in activity patterns during learning in older adults (Wu & Hallet, 2005) and in persons with neurologic pathology (Wu & Hallet, 2008).

Floyer-Lea and Matthews (2004) used functional magnetic resonance imaging (fMRI) to examine changes in the level and pattern of brain activity in healthy young adults during short-term learning of a visuomotor skill. A separate experiment was carried on outside the fMRI to evaluate stages of development of automaticity; interference during dual-task performance of the visual tracking task (a serial subtraction task was the secondary task) was used to determine shifts in automaticity during learning. When a new level of automaticity was reached, subjects were again asked to perform the visual motor tracking task by itself in the fMRI. The study found two distinct, time-dependent patterns of functional changes in the brain associated with learning this task. The initial phase of learning, when performance of the task was more attentionally demanding, was associated with activity in widely distributed, predominantly cortical regions, including prefrontal, bilateral sensorimotor, and parietal cortices. Specifically, the dorsolateral PFC, the caudate nucleus, and the ipsilateral cerebellar hemisphere showed significant activity during initial stages of learning. There was a progressive decrease in neural activity in certain brain regions as performance improved and a shift in the pattern of brain activity. Later stages of learning were associated with a decrease in primary motor cortex but an increase in activity in subcortical motor regions, including that of the cerebellar dentate nucleus, the thalamus, and the putamen. The authors suggest that motor skill learning is associated with a progressive reduction of widely distributed activation in cortical regions responsible for executive functions, processing somatosensory feedback, and motor planning. Performance gains during early learning strongly rely on prefrontal–caudate interactions, while later learning improvements in performance involve increased activity in a subcortical circuit involving the thalamus, cerebellar nuclei, and basal ganglia as the task becomes more automatic.

Wu and Hallet (2005) also examined age-related changes in neural activity associated with the shift to automaticity during acquisition of a simple motor skill (sequence of 4 finger movements) and a more complex one (sequence of 12 finger movements) in healthy older adults as compared with younger adults. They found that older adults were able to achieve automaticity in both simple and more complex learning tasks but required significantly more training than did the young adults. In addition, fMRI results showed that while the pattern of brain activity was similar between the two groups before and after training, significantly greater amounts of brain activity were necessary to achieve the same level of automaticity in older adults as compared with young adults.

What are the clinical implications of this research? They suggest that older adults, such as our balance-impaired older adult Bonnie, when learning a new task, can achieve the same level of automaticity as young adults but will require lots more practice. In addition, automaticity will require more brain activity in Bonnie, compared with young adults.

In a study using similar methods, Wu and Hallet (2005, 2008) studied neural correlates of dual-task performance in persons with Parkinson's disease (PD). They found that many of the individuals with PD were able to learn to perform simple tasks automatically; however, many were unable to perform complex tasks automatically, and thus, complex dual-task performance was impaired, even with extended practice. Results from the fMRI showed that for both groups, simple sequential movements activated similar brain regions before and after automaticity was achieved. However, whereas normal subjects reduced brain activity at the automatic stage, the individuals with PD had greater activity in the cerebellum, premotor area, parietal cortex, precuneus, and PFC as compared with normal subjects while performing automatic movements. The authors suggest that persons with PD require more brain activity to compensate for basal ganglia dysfunction in order to perform automatic movements. In addition, some skilled movements may never be performed completely automatically.

This research suggests that the shift to automaticity during skill acquisition is associated with a reduction of brain activation in several regions, such as the cerebellar hemispheres, premotor area, and dorsolateral PFC. In addition, there is some evidence that activity in specific regions like the basal ganglia increases with automaticity. Finally, aging and neurologic pathology can affect the ability of the brain to control movements automatically, and this can impair dual-task performance in these populations.

Summary of Forms of Learning

In summary, as you can see, there are many forms of learning, from simple to complex, and many parts of the CNS are involved in learning and memory. A characteristic trait of implicit or procedural memory storage is that the recall of the memory is accomplished without conscious thought. Much of what we do in daily life is guided by implicit memory (i.e., daily life habits). Implicit memory comprises several processes, which are controlled by different brain systems. Formation of new motor (and perhaps cognitive) habits requires the neostriatum. Learning new skilled motor behavior requires the cerebellum. Finally, simple reflex learning occurs directly in sensory and motor pathways. However, in different learning conditions, implicit memory formation requires different combinations of neural activity.

Implicit memory systems work in parallel with the explicit memory systems (Kandel & Siegelbaum, 2013). A characteristic trait of the explicit (declarative) memory system is the conscious recall of factual knowledge about people, places, and things. The medial temporal lobe, especially the hippocampus, mediates the storage of explicit memory. Thus, implicit memory is "recalled" only through performance, while explicit memory involves conscious recall.

NEURAL PLASTICITY AND RECOVERY OF FUNCTION

In the early part of this century, the Spanish neuroscientist Ramon y Cajal (considered by many to be the "father of neuroscience"), performed many histological studies on the degeneration and regeneration of neural tissue. He concluded that "once development was ended, the founts of growth and regeneration of the axons and dendrites dried up irrevocably" (Ramon y Cajal et al., 1991; Stahnisch & Nitsch, 2002). This conclusion by Ramon y Cajal led to the view that the adult nervous system is a static structure with rigid and unalterable connections (Gordon, 1987; Stein et al., 1995). This perspective within the field of neuroscience persisted until the late 1960s and 1970s, when researchers began to discover growth and reorganization of neurons in the adult CNS after injury. This research has revealed that the brain is not structurally static but continuously changes in structure and function.

This section of the chapter first considers injury-induced plasticity and its relationship to recovery of function. We examine this from two levels, intercellular (changes at the synaptic level) and network (cortical reorganization) levels and consider the implications of this research for our patient Genise who has had a stroke. We then briefly consider neural plasticity in relationship to neurodegenerative diseases such as PD and multiple sclerosis (MS) and consider the clinical implications of this research for our patient Mike, who has PD.

Conceptualizing Recovery

The term *recovery of function* is used in several ways. Clinicians often use the term *recovery of function* to describe the emergence of functional behavior observed in patients across time. This includes both "spontaneous recovery" (initial or early recovery that occurs independent of external interventions) and activity-induced recovery of function (improvements associated with specific activities and training). Recovery is also a term used to describe changes in the underlying neural structures that are occurring in the same time frame (Levin et al., 2009). The ability to relate changes in the underlying neural structures with observed behavioral change can be very difficult as there is not always a simple one-to-one relationship between these two levels of change. Thus, it is not a simple task to relate an observable behavioral change to a specific alteration in underlying neural process (Levin et al., 2009; Nudo, 2011).

Mechanisms underlying recovery of function after neural injury have been categorized as either restorative (direct) or compensatory (indirect) (Friel & Nudo, 1998). Direct or restorative mechanisms involve the resolution of temporary changes and recovery of the injured neural tissue itself. In addition, nearby neural tissue takes over identical neural functions to the original damaged tissue, resulting in restitution of function. In indirect, or compensatory, recovery, completely different neural circuits enable the recovery of lost or impaired function. Compensatory neural reorganization can include both function-enabling and function-disabling plasticity. Examples of function-enabling plasticity include changes in cortical representation associated with forced-use paradigms that improve motor function. Examples of function-disabling plasticity include changes in cortical representation associated with disuse that reduce motor capabilities and phantom limb sensation after amputation that is attributed to cortical reorganization and sensory-disabling plasticity.

We begin our discussion of injury-related neural plasticity with a discussion of mechanisms underlying axonal damage.

Axonal Damage: Effects on Neurons and Neighboring Cells

Injury to the CNS can affect function through direct damage to the neurons themselves. Because neurons have long axons and relatively smaller cell bodies, most injuries to both the central and peripheral nervous systems involve damage to the axons (Sanes & Jessell, 2013). An injury that divides an axon into two parts (called an axotomy) has a proximal segment still attached to the cell body and a distal segment that is no longer attached. The sequence of physical degeneration of the axon begins after a short delay, proceeds relatively rapidly, and results in loss of synaptic transmission at the severed nerve terminals. This eight-step process is shown in Figure 4.8 (bottom). A normal neuron with intact axon and its synaptic connections are shown in Figure 4.8 (top). After axotomy (Fig. 4.8, bottom), the nerve terminal of the injured neuron begins to degenerate (step A).

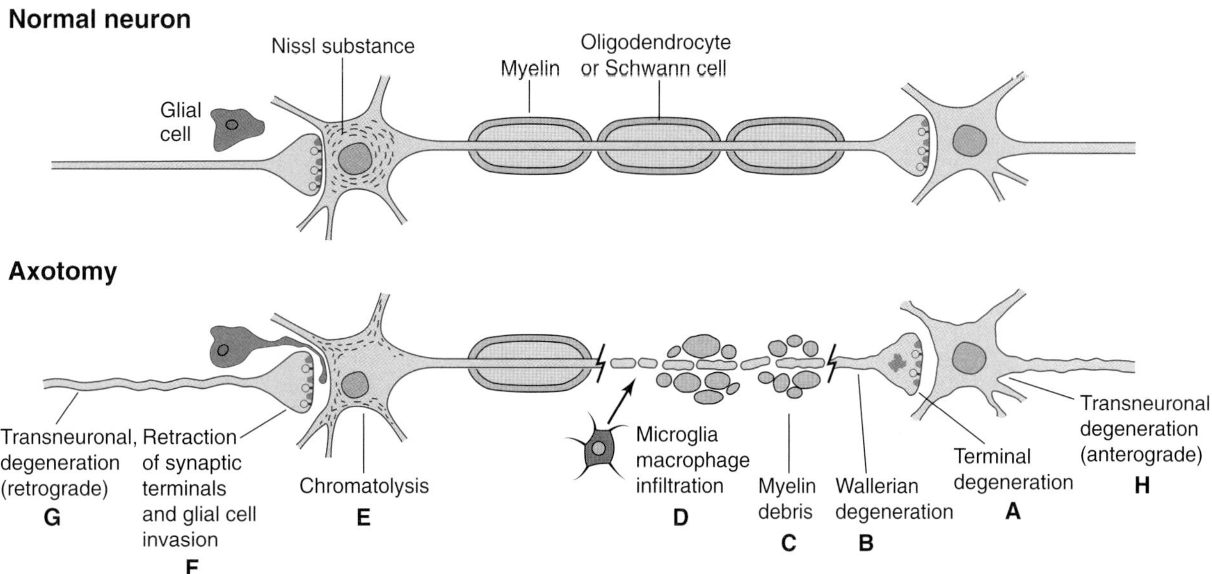

Figure 4.8 The sequence of physical degeneration of an injured axon. A normal neuron **(top)** with intact axon and its synaptic connections. After axotomy **(bottom)**, the nerve terminal of the injured neuron begins to degenerate **(A)**. The distal axonal stump separates from the parental cell body and undergoes wallerian degeneration **(B)**. Myelin begins to fragment **(C)**, and the lesion site is invaded by phagocytic cells **(D)**. The cell body of the damaged neuron undergoes chromatolysis (the cell body swells and the nucleus moves to an eccentric position) **(E)**. Synaptic terminals that are in contact with the damaged neuron withdraw and the synaptic cleft is invaded by glial cells **(F)**. The injured neuron's inputs **(G)** and targets **(H)** atrophy and degenerate (retrograde **[G]** and anterograde **[H]** degeneration).

The distal axonal stump separates from the parental cell body and undergoes Wallerian degeneration (step B). Myelin begins to fragment (step C), and the lesion site is invaded by phagocytic cells (step D). The cell body of the damaged neuron undergoes chromatolysis (the cell body swells and the nucleus moves to an eccentric position) (step E). An axotomy not only results in degeneration of the injured neuron but also causes damage to adjacent neurons. Presynaptic terminals that are in contact with the damaged neuron withdraw, and the synaptic cleft is invaded by glial cells (step F). In addition, the presynaptic neurons atrophy and degenerate (retrograde degeneration) (step G), as do the postsynaptic neurons (anterograde degeneration) (step H) (Sanes & Jessell, 2013). So, as you can see, loss of a neuron at the site of injury has a cascading effect, causing degeneration along neuronal pathways, increasing the extent of neuronal disruption with time (Steward, 1989).

Damaged axons within the CNS can also affect function. For example, the motor and functional outcomes after a traumatic brain injury (TBI) will be dependent upon the location, the type, and the severity of the brain lesion. However, high-speed impacts with acceleration–deceleration and rotational forces may cause diffuse axonal injury, which also contribute to functional deficits. The extent of axonal injury also determines the prognosis after a TBI. In a systematic review, van Eijck and colleagues (2018) found that people who experienced a TBI associated with diffuse axonal injury, as diagnosed by MRI, demonstrated a greater risk for unfavorable functional outcomes compared to people with TBI but without diffuse axonal injury (van Eijck et al., 2018). This finding highlights the particular role of axons in injury and recovery after acquired brain injury.

Early Transient Events That Depress Brain Function

Before discussing intercellular responses to CNS injury, we will review other events that occur within the nervous system following injury that produce transient disruption of brain tissue not directly due to the injury. These events may contribute to initial loss of function, and their resolution produces early recovery of function.

Diaschisis

The term *diaschisis*, described by von Monakow in 1914, is one of the first events following nervous system injury (Feeney, 1991; von Monakow, 1914). Diaschisis is a transient CNS disorder in which a part of the brain that is structurally intact loses function because of a loss of inputs from an anatomically connected area of the brain that is injured (Feeney & Baron, 1986). A detailed discussion of diaschisis and its subtypes is presented in the review by Carrera and Tononi (2014). The sudden functional depression of brain regions distant from the primary site of injury can be due to a reduction in blood flow and/or metabolism. Research using positron emission tomography (PET) scans (to measure blood flow to various parts of the brain and thus infer neural activity) indicates that in many cases, there is recovery of normal activity levels with time (Stein et al., 1995). It has been proposed that early recovery of function following stroke is due to the resolution of diaschisis.

In conflict with this theory is research by Bowler et al. (1995), who found no correlation between diaschisis (identified as regions of decreased cerebral blood flow seen on single-photon emission computed tomography) and measures of early functional recovery following stroke. In addition, diaschisis persisted during the 3-month follow-up period, though functional recovery of behavior was observed. The authors conclude that diaschisis does not independently add to the clinical deficit after stroke, nor does its resolution contribute significantly to early recovery (Bowler et al., 1995).

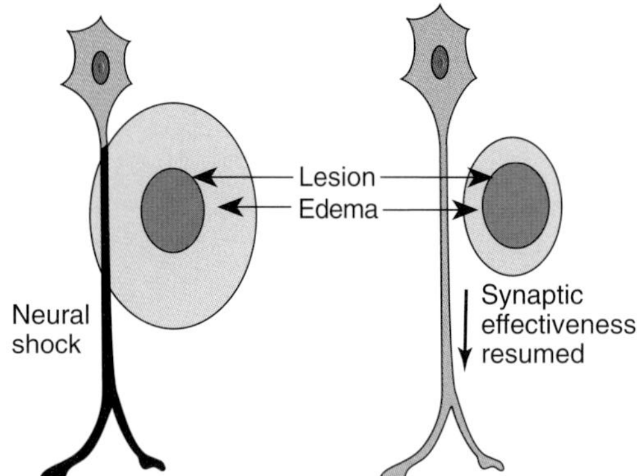

Figure 4.9 Recovery of synaptic effectiveness due to the resolution of edema, allowing nerve conduction to resume. (Adapted from Craik RL. Recovery processes: maximizing function. In: Contemporary management of motor control problems. *Proceedings of the II Step Conference*. Alexandria, VA: American Physical Therapy Association, 1992:165–173, with permission.)

Edema

Cerebral edema, commonly associated with brain injury, is a space-occupying lesion that can cause an increase in intracranial pressure. Brain edema can be *local* (i.e., adjacent to the primary injury site due to contusion, infarction, or tumor) or *generalized*. Cerebral edema produces a functional depression in brain tissue that may not be part of the primary injury (Goldstein, 1993). For example, local brain edema can result in herniation of brain tissue in the relatively noncompliant membranes that surround the brain (Laterra & Goldstein, 2013). Large cerebrovascular infarcts involving the middle cerebral artery can cause edema that appears 2to 5 days after the stroke. During a stroke, the size of infarction, the presence of perfusion deficits, and involvement of additional brain vascular sites all determine the extent of potentially life-threatening brain edema (Hofmeijer et al., 2008).

Cytotoxic cerebral edema involves the accumulation of intracellular fluid and swelling—as it is usually observed in asphyxia, global cerebral ischemia or water intoxication (overhydration causing electrolyte imbalance). Vasogenic edema, however, is due to increased permeability of capillary endothelial cells with leakage of proteins and fluid from damaged blood vessels into the extracellular space—a situation that can impact the long axons that form the white matter (Laterra & Goldstein, 2013).

Edema at the site of neuronal injury may lead to a compression of axons and physiological blocking of neuronal conduction as is shown in Figure 4.9 (left) (Craik, 1992). Reduction of the edema would then restore a portion of the functional loss (Fig. 4.9, right).

Axonal Regeneration: Difference in the Peripheral versus Central Nervous Systems

There is a considerable difference in the ability of central versus peripheral nerves to regenerate after injury. Why can peripheral nerves recover following injury but central nerves cannot? The differences in regenerative capacity are explained and shown in Figure 4.10. On the left is an intact nerve from the peripheral nervous system (top), and one that has undergone an axotomy (middle). Following the axotomy, the perineural sheath reforms rapidly, and Schwann cells produce trophic factors and adhesive proteins that promote axonal growth (lower figure). In contrast, in the CNS (shown on the right) after axotomy (middle figure), the distal segment of the axon degenerates and the surrounding myelin fragments. Reactive astrocytes and macrophages are attracted to the lesion site, forming a glial scar that inhibits axonal regeneration.

Thus, there are significant differences in the degenerative process in the peripheral versus the CNS. Axons within all three parts of the peripheral nervous system, motor, sensory, and autonomic, are capable of regeneration. Once the peripheral axon regenerates and reaches its intended target neurons, new functional nerve endings are formed, myelin sheaths are remyelinated, and cell bodies return to their normal position. Function is recovered though not always as it was prior to injury.

In contrast, axons in the CNS do not regenerate. Interestingly, researchers have found that the same central nervous axon, when transplanted to the peripheral nervous system, will not regenerate. This suggests that something internal to the CNS axons contributes to this inability to regenerate.

CNS Response to Injury

The CNS responds to neural insult at many levels; this includes changes at the neuronal level (the level of the cell) and also at the level of the cortex. We begin by discussing intercellular responses to injury at the neuronal level and then consider injury-induced changes at the cortical level.

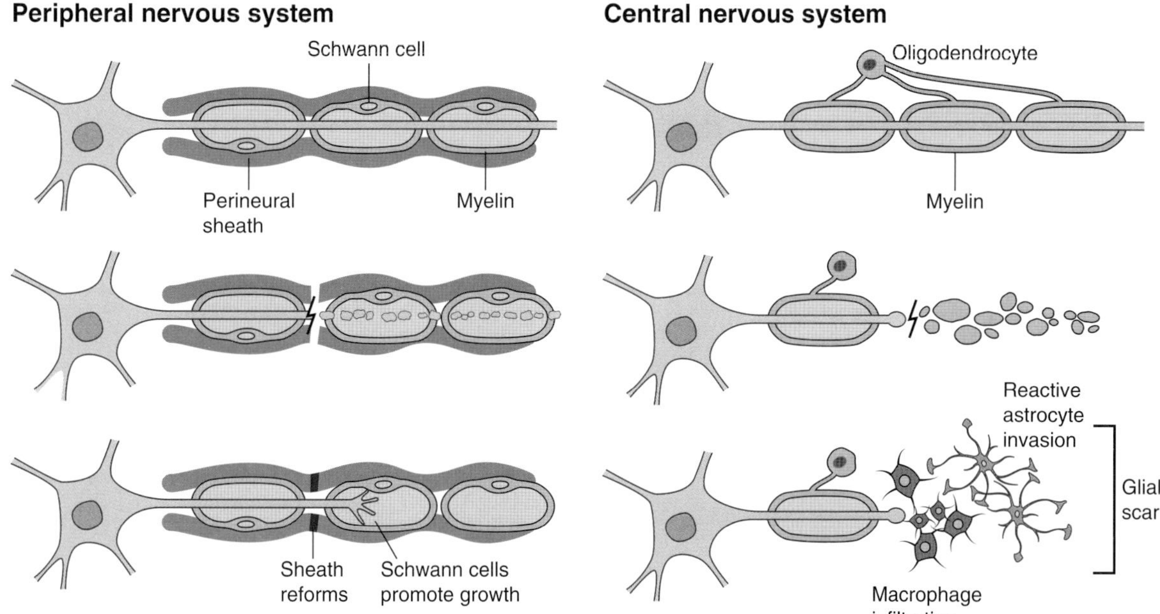

Figure 4.10 Differences in regenerative capacity in the peripheral versus central nervous system. On the left is an intact nerve from the peripheral nervous system **(top)** and one that has undergone axotomy **(middle)**. Following the axotomy, the perineural sheath reforms rapidly, and Schwann cells produce trophic factors and adhesive proteins, which promote axonal growth **(bottom)**. In contrast, in the central nervous system (shown on the right) after axotomy, the distal segment of the axon degenerates and myelin fragments. In addition, reactive astrocytes and macrophages are attracted to the lesion site, forming a glial scar that inhibits axonal regeneration.

Intercellular Responses to Injury

Intercellular response to injury reflects the formation and regeneration of synapses (synaptogenesis).

Denervation Supersensitivity. Denervation supersensitivity can occur when neurons show a loss of input from another brain region. In this case, the postsynaptic membrane of a neuron becomes hyperactive to a released transmitter substance. For example, PD causes a loss of dopamine-producing neurons in the substantia nigra of the basal ganglia. In response to this disease-induced denervation, the postsynaptic target neurons in the striatum become hypersensitive to the dopamine that is released by the remaining substantia nigra neurons. This occurs through the postsynaptic cells forming more receptors to capture more dopamine. It is interesting that this denervation supersensitivity occurs only when at least 90% of the nerve fibers in the substantia nigra are gone. Thus, it occurs only when a critical number of neurons have been destroyed (Stein et al., 1995).

Unmasking of Silent Synapses. Recruitment of previously silent synapses also occurs during recovery of function. This suggests that structural synapses are present in many areas of the brain that may not normally be functional because of competition within neuronal pathways. However, experiential factors or lesions may lead to their being unmasked when they are released from these previous effects. Certain drugs, such as amphetamines, may promote recovery of function by facilitating unmasking (Goldstein, 1990).

Neural Regeneration (Regenerative Synaptogenesis). Neural regeneration or regenerative synaptogenesis occurs when injured axons begin sprouting. An example of regenerative synaptogenesis is shown in Figure 4.11, top left (Craik, 1992; Held, 1987). Bjorklund, a neurologist from Sweden, was one of the first scientists to perform research that provided evidence that neural growth and regeneration were possible after brain damage. Bjorklund and his colleagues made lesions in nigrostriatal pathways within the basal ganglia of rats, trying to simulate the degeneration of the pathway that occurs with PD. They then examined the brains with special histologic fluorescence techniques at different times after the lesions. They found that within 3 to 7 days, neurons had begun to grow across the cut area and eventually reestablished their connections with their target neurons in the caudate nucleus of the basal ganglia (Bjorklund, 1994).

Collateral Sprouting (Reactive Synaptogenesis). Collateral sprouting, or reactive synaptogenesis, occurs when neighboring normal axons sprout to innervate synaptic sites that were previously activated by the injured axons. This process is shown in Figure 4.11 (right), in which the neuron on the right is growing a collateral sprout to create a functional synapse with a

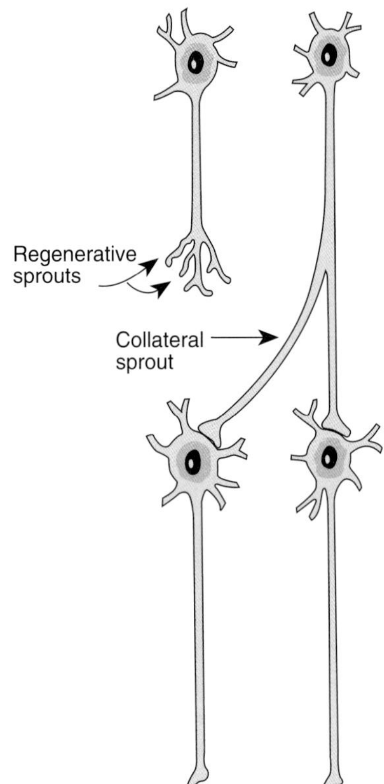

Figure 4.11 Regenerative and reactive synaptogenesis in related neurons following injury. (Figure 4.2 [Adapted]. Carr JH, Shepherd RB. *Movement science: Foundation for physical therapy in rehabilitation,* 2nd ed. (p. 160). Austin, TX: PRO-ED, 2000. Copyright 2000 by PROED, Inc. Adapted with permission. No further duplication allowed.)

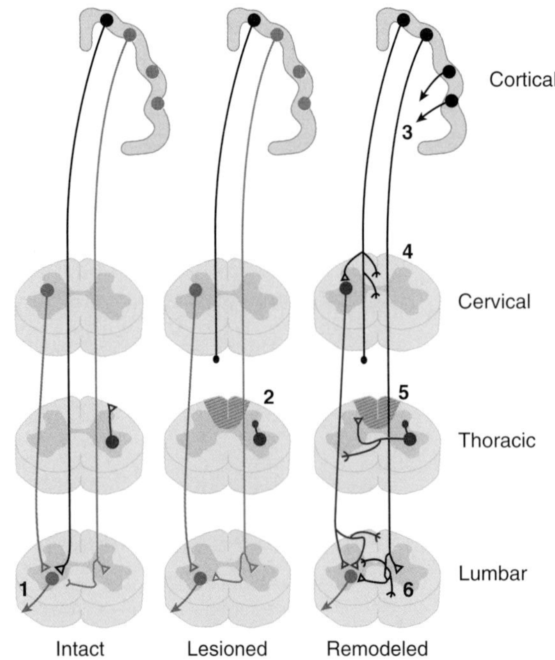

Figure 4.12 An illustration of the process of axonal remodeling that occurs following a lesion to the dorsal column at the thoracic level of the spinal cord. See text for a detailed explanation of this figure. (Adapted from Kerschensteiner M, Bareyre FM, Buddeberg BS, et al. Remodeling of axonal connections contributes to recovery in an animal model of multiple sclerosis. *J Exp Med*. 2004;200(8):1027–1038, with permission.)

nearby postsynaptic neuron that has been denervated. Typically, the axons that begin to sprout belong to the same neural system that originally innervated the synaptic sites. Steward (1989), working with rats, decided to determine whether collateral sprouting could occur in the entorhinal–hippocampal circuitry, which is involved in short-term memory. He showed that when lesions were made in the entorhinal cortex on one side of the brain, fibers from the intact entorhinal cortex on the opposite side of the brain sprouted branches that crossed over and innervated the hippocampal sites damaged by the lesion. The new connections were similar in organization to the original ones. Steward (1989) and Stein et al. (1995) also noted that the time for the fibers to sprout and make connections was about the same as the time for the return of the behaviors used to indicate the return of short-term memory.

As you can see, following neural injury, many mechanisms interact to promote the recovery of function. Figure 4.12 illustrates one example of the process of axonal remodeling that occurs following a lesion to the dorsal column at the thoracic level of the spinal cord. The intact system is shown on the far left, with its intact corticospinal tract (shown in black) to the lumbar motor neurons (1). In the intact system, in addition to the corticospinal tract, are weak or masked connections from both the cervical cord to the same lumbar motor neurons (shown as a pale red tract) and another weak or masked corticospinal connection (shown in gray). When a lesion occurs (shown in the middle) (2), there is a disruption to the direct descending corticospinal tract. Extensive remodeling contributes to partial recovery of function as shown in the far right. Near the lesion, interneurons sprout (shown in red and labeled [5]). Spared and previously masked corticospinal fibers become unmasked (shown now as black) and increase their collateral sprouting, which contact more target motor neuron cells (6). Above the lesion, damaged corticospinal fibers (also black) extend new collaterals to contact preserved interneurons. Thus, previously masked propriospinal pathways (shown in red), which connect with lumbar motor neurons, become more strongly activated. Finally, this interspinal remodeling is complemented by cortical reorganization (3) (Kerschensteiner et al., 2004). Cortical reorganization will be discussed in more detail in the next section.

Previous research had suggested that early recovery was due to resolution of temporary factors interfering with neural function, such as diaschisis and reduction of edema, and that later recovery was due to plastic changes involving synaptic modulation and cortical reorganization. More recently, it has been documented that plastic changes, including synaptic potentiation, pruning, and sprouting, and dendritic arborization occur within milliseconds to hours following injury (Zucker & Regehr, 2002).

Neuronal Regeneration: The Birth of New Neurons

Up to now, we have been discussing the underlying mechanisms associated with axonal remodeling in response to injury in both the peripheral and CNS. Now, we turn to a discussion of the genesis of new neurons in response to injury. Because damage to axons can lead to death of the cell itself, mechanisms designed to support neuronal survival as well as axonal regeneration are critical. In addition, since neuronal death is a common consequence of severe neural insults, such as stroke or neurodegenerative disease, mechanisms supporting the retention or replacement of neurons are critically important (Sanes & Jessell, 2013).

Can new neurons develop? As discussed in the beginning of this chapter, from the time of Ramon y Cajal (early 1920s), scientists had believed that the generation of neurons was complete by birth and neurogenesis (the creation of new cells) was not possible in the adult mammalian nervous system. This long-held belief was challenged by Joseph Altman's research in the 1960s, demonstrating the growth of new neurons in the hippocampus and olfactory bulb of postnatal rats. Interestingly, the findings were treated with skepticism for three decades (Sanes & Jessell, 2013).

Recent research has confirmed Altman's results, demonstrating the development of new neurons in nonhuman primates, and even in humans, though this neurogenesis is limited to the hippocampus and olfactory bulb (Sanes & Jessell, 2013). New neurons develop, extend axons and dendrites, form new synapses, and become integrated into existing functional circuits. It is not entirely clear how these new neurons function. When the generation of new neurons in the adult animal is prevented, certain behaviors that are mediated by either the olfactory bulb or the hippocampus deteriorate. Interestingly, neurogenesis in adult mammals can be decreased in the presence of depression or stress or, alternatively, increased when the animal is exposed to either an enriched environment or increased physical activity. In addition, traumatic or ischemic injury (such as stroke) can stimulate the generation of new neurons even in areas such as the cerebral cortex; however, despite this neurogenesis, recovery of function remains poor. Many scientists are looking at how injury-induced neurogenesis can be improved through such things as administration of neural growth factors.

Research has confirmed that stem cells are the source of neurons in both the adult and the embryo. This has led to the experimental use of transplanted developing neurons or, alternatively, neural precursors, such as stem cells, into experimental animals to see if these new neurons could reverse the effects of injury or disease. A well-known example of this research in humans is the use of transplanted embryonic mesencephalic dopaminergic neurons into the putamen in PD to compensate for the loss of dopaminergic neurons in the substantia nigra. These new cells enable the reactivation of globus pallidus output pathways (Sanes & Jessell, 2013). This research, while still very experimental, holds promise for recovery from significant neural insult.

Changes in Cortical Maps after Lesions and during Recovery of Function

There is a growing body of evidence demonstrating that cortical representation of the body is continuously modified in healthy adults in response to activity, behavior, and skill acquisition. Cortical reorganization also occurs after a peripheral injury (such as amputation) or CNS injury (such as stroke or traumatic brain injury). Research on cortical reorganization following neural injury suggests that a focal lesion opens a window of increased plasticity in the CNS. This early lesion–induced cortical hyperexcitability facilitates cortical plasticity (Ward & Cohen, 2004). Of particular interest to professionals in neurologic rehabilitation is the research on activity-dependent changes in structure and function that occur following injury.

If you are unfamiliar with the technology used to study neural plasticity during recovery of function, see Technology Tool 4.1 for a brief review of some of these methods.

Remapping Following Peripheral Lesions

What have researchers learned about how cortical maps change during recovery of function? When the median nerve (which innervates the radial part of the glabrous [nonhairy] regions of the hand) of the monkey is severed, one might expect that corresponding parts of the somatosensory cortex would become silent, since there would be no input coming into them. In studies examining this issue, Merzenich and colleagues (1983a, 1983b) found that immediately after the lesion, much of the deprived cortex did not respond to light cutaneous stimulation, but over the next days and weeks, the neurons began to respond again. Now, they responded when the hairy dorsal surface was stimulated.

When experiments were performed to test the mapping of the cortex after surgery, it was found that neighboring maps had expanded their receptive fields to cover much of the denervated region. These representations increased even further in the weeks following denervation (Merzenich et al., 1983a, 1983b). Since the extent of the reorganization of the cortex was a few millimeters, it was assumed that it occurred because of the increased responsiveness of existing, previously weak connections.

However, if nerves to matching parts of the back and front of the hand were cut, there were zones of the cortex that remained unresponsive even months after

TECHNOLOGY TOOL 4.1 Methods Used to Study Neural Plasticity

Many methods have evolved to assist researchers in studying neural plasticity and cortical reorganization underlying the recovery of function following CNS injury, including neuroimaging techniques with different temporal and spatial resolution. PET has a temporal resolution of minutes, while the resolution of fMRI is seconds and the resolution using magnetoencephalography (MEG) is milliseconds, allowing researchers to determine where and when activation starts and to track its temporal spread to other brain regions (Johansson, 2004).

TMS is another noninvasive method for studying brain function. A pulsed magnetic field creates a current flow in the brain and can temporarily excite or inhibit synaptic efficiency and alter brain function (Hallet, 2000). MEPs are recorded and used to determine changes in representation and excitability of the motor system (Chen et al., 2002). For example, a researcher may use TMS to activate pyramidal tract neurons and record the MEP amplitude of muscles proximal to the amputation to determine the extent of cortical reorganization that occurs following amputation.

PET scans, which plot regional cerebral blood flow and infer the level of neural activity from the level of blood flow to specific brain areas, can be used to examine changes in activation patterns following injury.

the lesion (Garraghty et al., 1994; Kaas et al., 1997). These studies support the proposal that the reactivation of the cortex was due to the increased responsiveness of weak inputs from neighboring areas, and if the denervation exceeded a certain distance, silent areas would remain (Kaas et al., 1997).

Other related work suggests that there can be reactivation of cortex in areas that are too large to be explained by the strengthening of existing connections. For example, Taub (1976) showed that at least 12 years after a dorsal rhizotomy to eliminate sensory input from the arm of a monkey, the somatosensory cortex had been completely reactivated by remaining inputs, mainly from the face. Since this area covered more than 10 mm of Brodmann's area 3b, it was too large to have occurred through the increased effectiveness of previously weak connections. Thus, new connections had formed somewhere in the nervous system.

To determine where these connections occurred, Florence and Kaas (1995) studied the reorganization of the spinal cord, brainstem, and cortex in monkeys with a history of amputation of the hand or forearm. They found that the central termination of the nerves that had not been injured by the amputation had sprouted into territories of the spinal cord and brainstem that were no longer in use because of the amputation. They believed that the expansion of the arm representation in the cortex after amputation was due to the growth of axons that relayed information about the arms into the parts of the spinal cord and brainstem previously occupied by the hand. Thus, the researchers hypothesized that the key to the large-scale reorganization following amputations and dorsal root damage is due to sensory neuron loss and the creation of space in the spinal cord and cuneate nucleus, allowing new growth that leads to reactivation of the cortex (Kaas et al., 1997).

In humans, reorganization of the somatosensory and motor systems also occurs following amputation. Researchers used TMS to map motor responses of different muscles activated by cortical areas. They found that muscles proximal to the amputation showed evoked potentials that were larger than those of the equivalent muscles on the opposite side of the body. These muscles were also activated at lower stimulation levels and over a wider area of the cortex than were those on the opposite side (Cohen et al., 1991, 1993; Lee & van Donkelaar, 1995). Researchers have found that stimulation of the face and upper body in patients who have had their upper limbs amputated can elicit phantom-limb sensation, suggesting that after upper-limb amputation, the somatosensory representation of the face and upper body expanded to occupy the arm and hand area (Chen et al., 2002; Ramachandran et al., 1992). The extent of shift in cortical representation was correlated with the amount of phantom sensation (Chen et al., 2002). This research demonstrates that alterations in cortical mapping occur following peripheral-nerve lesions or amputation.

Remapping Following Central Lesions

In addition to peripheral injury, damage to central neural structures also results in alterations to cortical maps and changes in neural activation patterns. Focal damage to the CNS can increase the capacity for structural and functional changes within the CNS, such as happens in development during critical periods (Ward & Cohen, 2004). Researchers are examining the relationship between cortical reorganization and recovery of function using longitudinal studies to understand processes associated with complete versus incomplete recovery of function. In addition, studies are exploring how neural plasticity following injury can be enhanced through various manipulations, including environmental modifications, behavioral training, and pharmacology. Studies on recovery of function and cortical reorganization have used both animal models and studies of humans recovering from neurologic injury such as stroke and traumatic brain injury.

Reorganization of the Affected Hemisphere during Recovery of Function. Motor recovery following damage to the primary motor cortex may be mediated by other cortical areas in the damaged hemisphere, through the use of either redundant pathways or new regions that take over the function of the damaged area (Chen et al., 2002; Nudo, 2006, 2007). Jenkins and Merzenich (1987) were some of the earliest scientists to suggest that reorganization of cortical representation after brain injury could be a model for the basis for recovery from cortical lesions. They performed a study in the monkey, in which they made ablations in the sensory cortex area representing one of the fingers. They found that skin surfaces originally represented in the ablated area were now represented in the nearby intact somatosensory areas. Studies of human subjects with infarcts in the internal capsule have shown that recovery of hand function was associated with a ventral extension of the hand area of the cortex into the area normally controlled by the face (Weiller et al., 1993). In another study, Pons et al. (1988) selectively removed the hand area of primary somatosensory cortex (SI), which is the input to the secondary somatosensory area (SII). They found that the hand areas of SII no longer responded to cutaneous stimulation of the hand, but after a number of weeks of recovery, the area became responsive to light touch of the foot. These results demonstrate that the nervous system is capable of reorganization following central as well as peripheral lesions.

Damage to primary motor areas also results in reorganization of neural activity during recovery of function. Primary motor cortex lesions result in activation of secondary motor areas, including premotor and supplementary motor cortex as well as the cingulate cortex. Thus, recovery of function related to small lesions to the internal capsule may be mediated by undamaged parallel motor pathways (Alexander & Crutcher, 1990; Chen et al., 2002; Fries et al., 1993; Lee & van Donkelaar, 1995; Strick, 1988).

Is activation of secondary motor areas associated with good recovery of function following stroke? Longitudinal studies using neural imaging technology to study the relationship between reorganized neural activation patterns and levels of recovery of function following stroke are beginning to answer this question. These studies support findings that after damage to primary motor cortex, there is recruitment of secondary motor regions as described previously. However, among individuals demonstrating good motor recovery, these initial patterns of overactivation in secondary motor regions are replaced by focused and more normal activation patterns. Normalization of activation patterns is associated with better motor recovery, while continued activation of secondary areas appears to be associated with less than optimal recovery of function (Ward et al., 2003).

There is also evidence that adjacent cortex takes over the function of damaged areas. For example, following stroke, recovered hand movements were associated with activation of motor cortex that extended into the face area, suggesting that the hand representation shifted toward the face area (Weiller et al., 1993).

Contributions of Ipsilateral (Uncrossed) Motor Pathways to Recovery of Function. Do uncrossed pathways play an important role in recovery of function? This appears to be the case in many patients. For example, a complete cerebral hemisphere was removed in certain patients to control intractable epilepsy, but no significant hemiplegia was seen. This unusual occurrence may have been due to the fact that the hemisphere had been abnormal since early childhood, and thus, there had been many years during which the ipsilateral hemisphere could gradually take over control of the limbs (Lee & van Donkelaar, 1995).

Weiller et al. (1992) used PET scans to examine ipsilateral motor activity in patients who had a capsular infarct and eventually recovered from the resulting paresis. The patients were asked to sequentially touch their thumbs to the different fingers of the same hand, while regional blood flow was measured. The investigators found that in control subjects and for the unaffected hand of the patients, the contralateral motor cortex and premotor areas were active during the task. But when the previously paretic hand was used, both ipsilateral and contralateral motor areas showed increased blood flow, indicating that ipsilateral pathways were now contributing to the control of this movement (Weiller et al., 1993).

However, the role of contralesional primary motor cortex (motor cortex in the side opposite to the affected cortex) to the recovery of function is not clear. Although researchers have demonstrated activation of contralesional primary motor cortex during hand movements on the paretic side, disruption of this activity using TMS did not impair hand movements. There is also some evidence that recruitment of contralesional primary motor cortex can impede recovery through increased intracortical inhibition (Hummel et al., 2005; Ward & Cohen, 2004).

Cerebellar Contributions to Recovery from Cortical Injury. New longitudinal studies have reported the importance of the cerebellum to motor recovery after lesions to the primary motor cortex, with the cerebellar hemisphere opposite to the damaged corticospinal tract appearing to have a more important role (Small et al., 2002). These studies suggest that the role of the cerebellum in recovery of function may be related to its role in motor learning. Specifically, the cerebellum is thought to play a role in the improvement of motor performance through the establishment of automatic motor skills. It appears that cerebellar involvement in motor recovery begins 2 to 3 months poststroke and persists for 6 months, supporting researchers' belief that the role of the cerebellum in recovery of function is through learning (Kleim et al., 1997, 1998).

Activation of Brainstem Pathways. Following stroke-related damage to the corticospinal system, strengthening of brainstem inputs to spinal cord motor neurons both contributes to and constrains recovery of function following stroke. Zaaimi et al. (2012) found that in adult monkeys, functional recovery following corticospinal lesions was associated with an increase in the EPSPs in reticulospinal pathways. These pathways originated in the medial brainstem and synapsed on spinal cord motor neurons innervating forearm and hand flexor, but not extensor muscles. This imbalanced strengthening of brainstem connections to flexor, but not extensor, motor neurons may explain why this pattern of recovery (flexor activity in conjunction with extensor weakness) is commonly found in stroke survivors (Zaaimi et al., 2012). Thus, recruitment of reticulospinal pathways following a corticospinal lesion not only supports functional recovery by increasing recruitment of flexor motor neurons but also constrains functional recovery due to the absence of extensor neuron activation.

What is the effect of damage to the corticospinal system and recruitment of reticulospinal pathways to finely controlled, individuated movements of the hand? Within the spinal cord, corticospinal axons branch only to a small number of motor neuron pools, allowing control of small groups of synergistic muscles, insuring independent control of the digits (individuation or fractionated control). Thus, damage to the corticospinal system results in loss of individuated movements of the hand. Reticulospinal axons branch extensively within the spinal cord and contact many motor neuron pools. In addition, the reticulospinal tract is a bilaterally organized system with a single axon innervating motor neurons on both sides of the cord. Thus, activation of the reticulospinal pathway results in broad, bilateral activation of muscles in the hand and arm, rather than fine fractionated control of the hand. In a normal intact system, the corticospinal system suppresses activity in the reticulospinal system; with a lesion in the corticospinal system, this suppression of reticulospinal activity is lost. It is thought that this release of reticulospinal activity may explain why, when a person who has had a stroke attempts unilateral movements of the affected arm, bilateral movements occur (Ortiz-Rosarioa et al., 2014).

Cross-Modality Plasticity. *Cross-modality plasticity* refers to the idea that when deprived of its usual input, the part of the cortex normally responsive to that input may now be responsive to inputs from other sensory modalities (Chen et al., 2002). Cross-modality plasticity has been most often studied in the visual system. The visual system projects to the visual cortex, while the auditory system projects to the auditory cortex. Experiments in ferrets by Sur et al. (1990) have shown that retinal cells may be induced to project into the medial geniculate nucleus, which projects onto the auditory cortex. When this occurs, the primary auditory cortex also responds to visual stimulation, with both orientation- and direction-selective neurons. Other researchers have performed similar experiments to induce visual neurons to project onto the somatosensory thalamus, and they have then found somatosensory cells responding to visual stimulation. This suggested that the different primary sensory areas had many characteristics in common, which allowed sensory inputs from one modality to activate cortical areas of others. However, although these new connections were functional, there were many abnormalities, indicating that prior specification had already occurred in these primary cortical areas (Sur et al., 1990). In humans, Braille readers have expanded sensory and motor representation for the reading finger, again showing that cortical representations are dynamically modulated based on learning and experience (Donoghue, 1995; Pascual-Leone et al., 1993).

Neuroimaging research has shown task-dependent activation of the occipital cortex during tactile-, auditory-, memory-, and language-related neural processing in subjects blind from an early age. Both PET and fMRI studies have shown that auditory spatial processing and auditory motion occur over the same areas that would normally process visual spatial and visual motion information in sighted individuals, suggesting that areas keep their function and neural coding abilities when a new modality takes over cortical areas. There has been considerable debate about the extent of plastic changes that can occur in the cortex of subjects blinded later in life. It has now been shown that these individuals do show altered functioning of their deafferented visual cortices. However, the extent of plasticity and the regions recruited for auditory tasks is affected by the age of onset (Collignon et al., 2009).

Behavioral and cortical reorganization can also occur in visually normal individuals when deprived of vision for short periods. For example, Pascual-Leone et al. (2005) showed a significant increase in occipital responses to sounds in sighted subjects blindfolded for 5 days, while Lewald (2007) showed reversible improvements in accuracy during sound localization after 90 minutes of blindfolding, a smaller but similar effect to those seen in blind subjects. How could this occur in such a short period of time? It has been shown that even in sighted individuals, there is involvement of the visual cortex in the processing of sounds (Collignon et al., 2008).

Strategies to Enhance Neural Plasticity and Cortical Reorganization

These studies have demonstrated the incredible plasticity of the nervous system and have shown the importance of this plasticity to the recovery of function following neural injury. Even more exciting is research exploring the effect of strategies to enhance neural plasticity and drive CNS reorganization in order to optimize recovery.

Effect of Training

Studies by Merzenich and colleagues looked at the effect of experience on reorganization of somatotopic maps in normal monkeys (Jenkins et al., 1990). In one experiment, monkeys were able to reach for food by using a strategy that involved use of their middle three fingers only (fingers 2, 3, and 4 in Fig. 4.13). After considerable experience with this task (i.e., several thousand trials!), the monkeys' cortical map showed a significant increase in the area for those three fingers only. This training-induced reorganization in the somatosensory cortex is shown in Figure 4.13, with the top of the figure showing the size of the cortical finger areas before stimulation and the bottom of the figure showing the size of the areas after stimulation. The right hand side of the figure shows the receptive fields of the cutaneous receptors of the finger. Note that after training, the receptive fields of the three middle fingers (fingers 2, 3, and 4) are larger. Later experiments found that once a new task is learned, there are certain aspects of central mapping changes that persist for long periods (Nudo, 2006, 2007; Nudo et al., 1996).

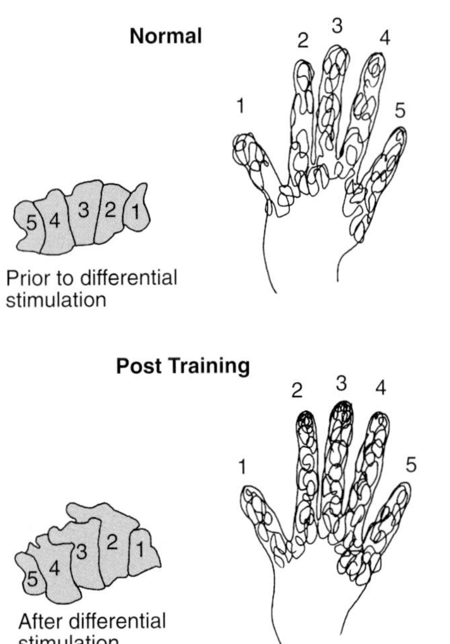

Figure 4.13 Monkeys were trained to reach for food using a strategy involving use of their middle three fingers only (fingers 2, 3, and 4). The top of the figure shows the cortical map for the 5 fingers of the hand before training **(left)** and the size of the receptive field for the cutaneous receptors of the fingers **(right)**. The bottom of the figure **(left)** shows the increased size of the monkeys' cortical map for the three middle fingers, after considerable experience with this task. The right-hand side shows the increased receptive fields of the three middle fingers after training. (Adapted from Jenkins WM, Merzenich MM, Och MT, et al. Functional reorganization of primary somatosensory cortex in adult owl monkeys after behaviorally controlled tactile stimulation. *J Neurophysiol.* 1990;63:82–104, with permission.)

Cortical remapping following training has also been shown in humans, specifically cortical reorganization following training in persons with stroke. Using TMS, Leipert and colleagues demonstrated increased cortical hand representation in the affected hemisphere in 13 persons with stroke following 12 days of intensive training of the affected upper extremity. They reported that the increased size of the motor output area in the affected hemisphere was associated with significant improvements in motor function of the hand. Functional improvements were still present 6 months after training; in addition, the size of the cortical area representing hand function was identical in the two hemispheres, suggesting a return to a balance of excitability between the hemispheres (Leipert et al., 2000).

Research has also demonstrated the existence of neuroplastic changes in children with cerebral palsy (CP) after motor learning–based therapies involving both the upper and lower extremities (Hand-Arm Bimanual Intensive Training [HABIT] or HABIT-ILE, involving the lower extermities). In a group of children with spastic hemiplegic CP, Friel and colleagues (2016) showed that a structured skill training program characterized by three key parameters (progression of task difficulty, repeated practice of isolated movements that include complex motor tasks, and repetition of functional goals) promoted neural plasticity within the motor system. They found an increase in the size of the affected hand motor map and greater amplitude in motor-evoked potentials (MEPs), which was measured with TMS and surface electromyography. Similarly, a study involving children with unilateral CP used diffusion tensor imaging (DTI) to demonstrate that intensive motor skill trainings such as HABIT-ILE improved hand function as well as the anatomical integrity of the corticospinal tract from both the lesioned and nonlesioned brain hemispheres (Bleyenheuft et al., 2020).

Does all training induce cortical reorganization? The answer appears to be no. Research is beginning to clarify the optimal timing and intensity of training to maximize neural plasticity. In animal models, skill learning was associated with cortical reorganization; however, strength training was not (Maldonado et al., 2008; Remple et al., 2001). Exercise, independent of skill acquisition, affected angiogenesis (blood vessel formation) but did not alter movement representation in the rat cortex (Kleim & Jones, 2008; Kleim et al., 2002). Early and intense forced motor behavior after a neural lesion can lead to undesirable neurodegeneration in vulnerable neural tissue (Kozlowski et al., 1996; Schallert et al., 2000). However, training in combination with other interventions, such as pharmacological treatment or neural transplantation, improved outcomes beyond that associated with an individual intervention (Dobrossy & Dunnett, 2001). Cortical stimulation has also been used to facilitate motor recovery. For more on this research, see Extended Knowledge 4.2.

Details on the specific types of rehabilitative training that are associated with changes in neural plasticity in humans are discussed in more detail in later chapters.

What do all these studies tell us? They suggest that we have multiple pathways innervating any given part of the sensory or motor cortex, with only the dominant pathway showing functional activity. However, when a lesion occurs in one pathway, the less dominant pathway may immediately show functional connections. This leads us to the conclusion that even in adults, cortical maps are very dynamic. There appears to be use-dependent competition among neurons for synaptic connections. Thus, when one area becomes inactive, a neighboring area can take over its former targets and put them to functional use.

Extended Knowledge 4.2

The Effect of Cortical Stimulation on Motor Recovery

Cortical stimulation is also being used to facilitate motor recovery. Researchers have shown that transcranial stimulation to the motor cortex enhances the effects of motor training on cortical plasticity in healthy adults (Antal et al., 2004; Bütefisch et al., 2004; Nitsche et al., 2003). Does cortical stimulation enhance function following a stroke? Stimulation of the contralateral intact hemisphere has been used to decrease cortical activity, reducing abnormal inhibition of the affected hemisphere by the intact hemisphere (Kobayashi et al., 2004). Hummel and colleagues (2005) examined the effects of cortical stimulation on hand function in individuals with chronic stroke. They examined performance of paretic hand function using the Jebsen–Taylor hand-function test (JTT) before and during cortical stimulation of the affected hemisphere. Performance on the JTT improved by about 12% during stimulation, and improved hand function persisted for about 25 minutes after stimulation ended.

While transcranial cortical stimulation applied during or shortly before skill training has been shown to enhance motor learning, cortical stimulation given after training reduced the training-dependent increases in cortical excitability (Rosenkranz et al., 2000). It has been suggested that synchronizing training with stimulation improves performance because the behavioral signals driving plasticity during training are augmented by the presence of the extra stimulation. In contrast, when stimulation is applied outside the training experience, it disrupts the memory consolidation process and may induce plasticity that is not shaped by behavioral signals and is, therefore, detrimental to performance (Kleim & Jones, 2008).

These experiments also suggest that our sensory and motor maps in the cortex are constantly changing in accordance with the amount to which they are activated by peripheral inputs. Since each of us has been brought up in a different environment and has practiced very different types of motor skills, the maps of each of our brains are unique and constantly changing as a result of these experiences.

Based on an extensive review of relevant research on activity-dependent neural plasticity, Kleim and Jones (2008) suggested 10 principles that potentially impact neurorehabilitation practices. These principles are summarized in Table 4.1:

- Principle 1, "use it or lose it", suggests that neural circuits not actively engaged in task performance for an extended period of time begin to degrade.
- Principle 2, "use it and improve it", suggests that training can protect neurons and networks that would otherwise be lost after the injury.
- Principle 3, "specificity", indicates that while practice associated with acquisition of a novel or reacquisition of a lost skill is associated with changes in motor cortex, repetition of a movement already learned is not. Research suggests that specific forms of neural plasticity are dependent upon specific kinds of experience. Neural plasticity is facilitated during practice related to acquisition of skill, not just repetition of an already learned or nonrelevant movement.
- Principle 4, "repetition matters", reflects the importance of repetition to neural reorganization. Repetition of a newly learned (or relearned) behavior is required to induce lasting neural changes, making repetition an important principle in neurorehabilitation. Kleim and Jones (2008) suggest that repetition of a skilled movement is needed to obtain a level of brain reorganization sufficient to allow the patient to continue to use the affected function outside of therapy and to maintain and make further functional gains.
- Principle 5, "intensity", suggests that training must be sufficiently intense to stimulate experience-dependent neural plasticity. This also requires that training be progressively modified to match the dynamic and changing skill level of the patient, thus maintaining a level of training intensity that ensures continued neural adaptation throughout recovery and rehabilitation. However, the effect of intensity of training may be dependent on the timing of that intervention. A study supporting the interactions between timing and intensity may be found in Extended Knowledge 4.3.
- Principle 6, "time matters", reflects the fact that neural plasticity underlying learning and recov-

TABLE 4.1 Principles of Experience-Dependent Plasticity

Principle	Description
1. Use it or lose it.	Failure to drive specific brain functions can lead to functional degradation.
2. Use it and improve it.	Training that drives a specific brain function can lead to an enhancement of that function.
3. Specificity.	The nature of the training experience dictates the nature of the plasticity.
4. Repetition matters.	Induction of plasticity requires sufficient repetition.
5. Intensity matters.	Induction of plasticity requires sufficient training intensity.
6. Time matters.	Different forms of plasticity occur at different times during training.
7. Salience matters.	The training experience must be sufficiently salient to induce plasticity.
8. Age matters.	Training-induced plasticity occurs more readily in younger brains.
9. Transference.	Plasticity in response to one training experience can enhance the acquisition of similar behaviors.
10. Interference.	Plasticity in response to one experience can interfere with the acquisition of other behaviors.

Adapted from Kleim JA, Jones TA. Principles of experience-dependent neural plasticity: Implications for rehabilitation after brain damage. *J Speech Lang Hear Res*. 2008;51:S225–S239.

Extended Knowledge 4.3

The Interaction between Timing and Intensity during Training

The interaction between timing and intensity of training is illustrated in the VECTORS study. The Very Early Constraint-Induced Movement during Stroke Rehabilitation (VECTORS) study compared recovery of arm function recovery in a population of acute (within 14 days after stroke) patients with stroke in response to three types of training: constraint-induced movement therapy (CIMT) (2-hour task-specific training, 6 hours per day constraint of the noninvolved hand), conventional training (2-hour traditional occupational therapy), and a high-intensity dose of CIMT (3-hour shaping, 90% waking hours constraint of noninvolved hand) (Dromerick et al., 2009). Recovery of arm function measures using the Action Research Arm Test (ARAT) at 90 days after randomization was best in the groups receiving CIMT and conventional therapy, with no difference between the two. Most surprising was the finding that the group that received the high-intensity CIMT training had the poorest arm function at 90 days. Thus, the VECTORS study did not support the hypothesis that more intense therapy in the acute stage would lead to better outcomes. Instead, a *higher dose* of CIMT was associated with *less motor recovery*, at least in the acute stage of recovery (Dromerick et al., 2009). This study reminds us that the benefits of using a highly intense training schedule may vary depending on where the patient is in the recovery process. In early recovery, less may actually be more.

ery of function is a process, with later types of plasticity often dependent on those that occur earlier in the process. For example, during motor skill training, gene expression precedes synapse formation, which in turn precedes motor map reorganization (Kleim & Jones, 2008). The importance of time in the recovery process is also supported by research demonstrating that specific types of interventions may be more or less effective depending on the time at which they are introduced. For example, Biernaskie et al. (2004) found that a 5-week period of rehabilitation initiated 30 days after cerebral infarct was far less effective in improving functional outcome and in promoting growth of cortical dendrites than the same regimen initiated 5 days after infarct.

- Principle 7, "salience matters", suggests that in order to maximize activity-dependent neural plasticity, training must be functionally relevant and significant to the individual. For an activity to be salient, it must reflect an activity that the person wants to do (Hadders-Algra & Gramsberg, 2007; Kleim & Jones, 2008). Simply repeating an activity that is not functionally relevant will not induce neural plasticity and reorganization after brain damage; instead, activity related to plasticity has to be salient, that is, make some sense to the person being trained. Thus, the desire and motivation of the patient to do a task increases the likelihood for neural adaptation associated with task-specific training.
- Principle 8, "age matters", suggests that experience-dependent synaptic potentiation, synaptogenesis, and cortical map reorganization are all reduced with aging, suggesting that age matters

when it comes to activity-dependent neural plasticity (Kleim & Jones, 2008). However, researchers have shown that the aging brain demonstrates experience-dependent reorganization, though brain changes may be less profound and/or slower to occur than those observed in younger brains (Kleim & Jones, 2008).

- Principle 9, "transference", refers to the ability of plasticity within one set of neural circuits to promote concurrent or subsequent plasticity in other circuits. Thus, one training experience can enhance the acquisition of similar behaviors (Kleim & Jones, 2008).
- Principle 10, "interference", refers to the possibility of plasticity within a given neural circuit impeding the induction of new or expression of existing plasticity within the same or other circuits, which can impair learning. For example, as we have seen, transcranial cortical stimulation has been shown to improve plasticity when applied during or shortly before training but impede plasticity (interference) when given after training (Bütefisch et al., 2004; Floel & Cohen, 2006; Rosenkranz et al., 2000).

In summary, a wealth of research overwhelmingly supports neural plasticity as the basis for both motor learning in the intact brain and relearning in the damaged brain. Principles derived from research on activity-dependent neural plasticity can inform and guide the application of interventions designed to facilitate neural adaptation and promote the recovery of function in patients with impaired motor control.

Clinical Implications of Research on Neural Plasticity and Recovery of Function in Acquired Brain Injury

What are the clinical implications of the research on injury-induced neural mechanisms contributing to recovery of function, including both the intercellular response and cortical remapping? First, it can help us to

understand some of the neural changes that occur following an injury. Let's take, for example, Genise, our 53-year-old woman who has had an ischemic stroke in the internal capsule in her left hemisphere. First, let's consider what the research on intercellular response to neural injury tells us about the events that are likely to be taking place in Genise's brain following her stroke. One of the immediate but transitory events that occurs is diaschisis, a transient loss of function controlled by intact brain regions due to the loss of input from the parts of her brain affected by the stroke. The degree to which the resolution of diaschisis contributes to Genise's early recovery of function is still somewhat unclear.

In addition, unmasking of previous silent neurons (and pathways) begins to occur and contribute to recovery of function. Adjacent to the damaged neurons, intact neurons will begin to demonstrate both regenerative and reactive synaptogenesis, so collateral pathways to target neurons previously innervated by the damaged neurons begin to develop. It is possible that neurogenesis (the creation of new neurons) will occur in the motor cortex, though whether these new cells will contribute to her functional recovery is not clear.

In addition to the intracellular responses, Genise's stroke will also result in almost immediate alterations to cortical maps and changes in neural activation patterns in both the affected and unaffected hemisphere. In the affected hemisphere, her damage to the primary motor cortex will result in activation of secondary motor areas and undamaged parallel motor pathways, including premotor and supplementary motor cortex as well as the cingulate cortex. In addition, ipsilateral (uncrossed) descending motor pathways become more active in controlling movement. However, in order for recovery to be optimal, these initial patterns of overactivation in secondary motor regions must be replaced by focused and more normal activation patterns. It is probable that neural activity in the contralesional hemisphere may increase; however, this may be detrimental to her recovery. In addition, pathways that descend from the brainstem to spinal motor neurons, such as the reticulospinal pathway, may be strengthened. These descending brainstem pathways may contribute to recovery of movement, though this may be reflected in more synergistic mass patterns of movement.

Finally, research tells us that experience will strongly influence the neural mechanisms associated with recovery of function. Early, intense, and focused training, particularly training focused on skill acquisition, will have a powerful effect on shaping her cortical maps. If rehabilitation training is delayed following her stroke, Genise's brain will show changes in organization, reflecting disuse, which will be detrimental to recovery of function. However, if Genise is engaged in training for skill reacquisition, cortical reorganization underlying recovery of function will occur and be retained long after her training ends.

NEURAL PLASTICITY AND NEURODEGENERATIVE DISEASE

What does neural plasticity mean in the context of a neurodegenerative disease? In a chronic, progressive neurologic condition, such as PD or MS, do changes in the nervous system result only in degradation of function, or are there also nervous system changes that help to maintain or enable function? Importantly, if function-enabling plasticity can occur, what types of rehabilitative training will promote this? While the previous section of this chapter examined neural plasticity associated with an acquired brain injury, this section discusses neural mechanisms that may modify function and disease progression in the context of a neurodegenerative condition, using PD as an example. Neural plasticity in MS is discussed in detail in Extended Knowledge 4.4. As stated previously, there is a complex relationship between observed behavioral changes and underlying structural and functional changes in the nervous system. Thus, as was noted in the case of acquired brain injury, there is not a simple one-to-one relationship between functional changes and mechanisms of neural plasticity in degenerative neurologic conditions.

Neural Plasticity and Parkinson's Disease

PD is a slowly progressive disorder, with motor symptoms that include slow, small amplitude movements,

Extended Knowledge 4.4

Neuroplasticity and Multiple Sclerosis

MS is a debilitating neuroimmunological disorder that commonly begins in early adulthood and affects 2.5 million people worldwide (Kingwell, 2012). Axonal damage is the primary pathological feature of MS and is most severe in new inflammatory demyelinating lesions and occurs at a slower rate during progressive disease, resulting in permanent loss of function. The precise cause of MS remains unknown, and the clinical course is highly heterogeneous between patients. Relapsing–remitting MS (RRMS) is the most common form of the disease and involves alternating periods of clinical worsening and abatement, commonly followed by sustained deterioration during secondary progressive MS (SPMS). Each of these stages involves numerous disease mechanisms; thus, MS represents a multifaceted disease process.

Functional recovery in MS is achieved and sustained by repair of damage through resolution of inflammation and remyelination and also through adaptive neural reorganization. Remyelination is an important mechanism of restoration of axonal function after acute inflammatory demyelination. Remyelination occurs when adult oligodendrocyte progenitor cells respond to injury by dividing and migrating and finally differentiating into oligodendrocytes that provide the demyelinated axon with new myelin sheaths. Neural reorganization relies on molecular and cellular mechanisms that produce changes in systems-level functional connections. Therapeutic interventions to promote adaptive neural plasticity and enhance functional recovery are being developed in MS and include both pharmacological approaches and activity-dependent strategies.

Pharmacological approaches in MS are aimed at (1) reducing the incidence and intensity of new lesions by limiting the activity of immune cells, (2) enhancing remyelination to slow or prevent axonal loss, and (3) enhancing adaptive functional reorganization of intracortical connections.

Functional neural reorganization (adaptive neural plasticity) in MS can be compensatory to the disease process itself or externally driven by activity and training. In addition, functional neural reorganization can be adaptive or maladaptive. In MS, a common form of maladaptive neural reorganization is associated with learned disuse, similar to that reported following stroke.

Neural reorganization following episodes of acute demyelinization can be seen in perceptual, motor, and cognitive systems. For example, visual recovery after acute demyelinating optic neuritis typically occurs within weeks despite permanent axonal loss. fMRI studies in patients after onset of optic neuritis show reduced activation in the visual cortex in response to visual stimulation of the affected eye. However, within 2 to 6 weeks of disease onset, activity in the visual cortex increases but remains below that of the unaffected eye. Recovery of activity in the visual cortex is associated with adaptive functional reorganization that occurs at many levels along the visual pathways, including remyelination of the optic nerve to partially restore visual function, functional reorganization within the lateral geniculate nucleus that compensates for an impaired optic nerve input to the primary visual cortex, adaptive changes within the primary and secondary visual cortex, and cortical reorganization within extrastriate visual areas.

In the motor system, changes in functional patterns of sensorimotor activation are consistently reported in all forms of MS. Persons with MS show more widespread recruitment of sensorimotor networks than do healthy volunteers. As the disease progresses, patterns of functional reorganization show an increasingly bilateral distribution and higher control sensorimotor areas, normally only recruited for novel or complex tasks. With functional recovery following a relapse, bilateral patterns of sensorimotor recruitment relateralize to the contralateral (affected) hemisphere. In fact, persistent recruitment of the ipsilateral (unaffected) sensorimotor cortex is associated with poor clinical recovery (Tomassini et al., 2012a).

Finally, cognitive processes such as memory, efficiency of information processing, attention, and executive functions are also associated with the activity of wider and more bilateral networks of task-specific regions in patients with MS than in healthy individuals. The extent of cognitive recruitment increases with increased cognitive load and becomes more prominent as MS progresses (Tomassini et al., 2012a).

Activity-dependent cortical plasticity also contributes to functional recovery in persons with MS. Research has shown that functional impairments in persons with MS can be reduced with practice, even in persons with considerable brain damage and disability. Tomassini and colleagues (2012b) reported that when performing a visuomotor tracking task unlike healthy controls, persons with MS recruit ipsilesional sensorimotor areas to limit the behavioral impact of brain pathology. Short-term practice of a visuomotor task in persons with MS resulted in improved performance and was associated with functional reorganization of ipsilateral sensorimotor regions (Tomassini et al., 2012b).

In contrast to this work, Morgen et al. (2004) reported that, unlike healthy subjects, persons with MS did not show a decrease in motor activation in the contralateral primary motor and parietal cortices, after motor training. The authors suggest that in healthy volunteers, reductions in cortical activity reflect a form of training-dependent neural plasticity that reflects either a shift from effortful to more automated performance or, alternatively, a form of perceptual learning (a decrease in the monitoring effort required to maintain proper output). In contrast, in persons with MS, the absence of training-dependent reductions in cortical activity suggests a decreased capacity to optimize recruitment of the motor network with practice (Morgen et al., 2004).

increased muscle tone (rigidity), tremor, and impairments in balance and gait. The pathology of PD is widespread, with degeneration that is proposed to begin many years prior to the onset of motor symptoms. Pathological changes can affect brainstem, subcortical, and cortical structures, but a characteristic feature of PD is degeneration of dopamine-producing neurons in the substantia nigra pars compacta, leading to limited availability of the neurotransmitter dopamine. Thus, the preservation of dopamine production, availability, and uptake is a primary target of therapeutic interventions, both pharmacological and rehabilitative. This section will focus specifically on the role of physical activity and exercise as a means to mediate dopamine availability and improve function (Kelly, *personal communication*, 2015).

Do physical activity and exercise impact behavioral deficits and underlying neurodegenerative processes? The answer appears to be yes. Animal models of PD have examined this question by studying the effects of physical activity or exercise at two levels—changes in behavior and changes in underlying neurophysiology as indicated by measures of dopamine production, metabolism, and uptake. In animal models of PD, restricting use of the affected limb by casting it for 7 days resulted in increased behavioral deficits and increased dopamine loss compared to animals that did not receive casting. This effect was independent of the severity of the dopamine loss and was found for animals with both mild and severe dopaminergic lesions (Tillerson et al., 2001). In contrast, when forced to use the affected limb, animals showed preservation of limb function and dopamine sparing. Behavioral and physiological benefits were greatest when forced use was initiated immediately after the experimental lesion. Partial behavioral and physiological benefits were observed if forced use was initiated 3 days after the experimental lesion, but no behavioral or physiological benefits were found when forced use was initiated 7 days after the experimental lesion (Tillerson et al., 2001). This suggests that the benefits of forced use are greatest when begun early.

Research in animal models of PD has also demonstrated that high-intensity aerobic exercise can improve behavior and dopamine availability. Exercise initiated before or during experimental lesions is protective and reduces striatal dopamine loss, whereas exercise initiated soon after experimental lesions results in compensatory changes that improve dopamine availability despite the loss of dopamine-producing cells. For example, animals that initiated intensive exercise within 5 days of the experimental lesion demonstrated improved movement speed and better motor performance on balance tests compared to animals that did not exercise. Although loss of striatal dopamine was similar between the two groups, animals that exercised also showed a number of changes that increased the availability of synaptic dopamine, including increased release, reduced uptake, and a reduced rate of decay of dopamine (Petzinger et al., 2007).

Why might aerobic exercise such as treadmill training impact dopamine availability? Findings in animal models support the proposal that exercise may protect dopaminergic cells by inducing mild cellular stress that triggers increases neurotrophic factors and elevates the intracellular response to stress (Zigmond et al., 2009). Thus, it has been suggested that exercise, and specifically intensive forms of exercise, may be neuroprotective in PD. Consistent with this idea, epidemiological studies have shown that the risk of developing PD is reduced in people with a history of moderate-to-vigorous physical activity (Chen et al., 2005; Thacker et al., 2008). Indeed, exercise has been proposed as critical to neuroprotection in PD (Petzinger et al., 2013; Zigmond & Smeyne, 2014), and ongoing clinical trials are examining the feasibility of using high-intensity exercise to modify the motor symptoms of PD (Moore et al., 2013).

In humans with PD, therapeutic aerobic exercise can improve cardiorespiratory fitness, motor performance during walking, executive function, and functional capability. In line with the animal studies previously described, diverse mechanisms have been proposed to explain these gains such as increased cerebral blood flow, neurotransmitter release, structural changes in the nervous system, enhanced arousal levels, and the overexpression of neurotrophic factors like the Brain-Derived-Neurotrophic Factor (BDNF). The current literature indicates that an upregulation of BDNF associated with aerobic exercise programs (i.e., multiple sessions of exercise that are regularly implemented over a planned period of weeks) is beneficial in CNS disorders like PD because it enhances plasticity-related processes (dendritic growth and sprouting and LTP of neurons) (Mackay et al., 2017).

Clinical Implications of Research on Neural Plasticity and Recovery of Function in PD

What are the clinical implications of this research for people with PD? What are the underlying neural processes that might mediate behavioral change in people with PD, such as Mike? Given the slowly progressive nature of PD, it is likely that neurodegenerative changes were occurring for several years before Mike noticed the onset of motor symptoms. There is a possibility that Mike's history of vigorous physical activity, such as biking and mountaineering, may have conferred some protective effects prior to the onset of motor symptoms, resulting in spared dopamine-producing neurons and delaying the onset of tremor, rigidity, and bradykinesia. After his diagnosis, continued aerobic activity, including biking, walking, and cross-country skiing, early in the disease process may have led to increased availability of dopamine through increased release from remaining dopamine-producing neurons, an increase in the number of dopamine receptors, and changes in dopamine metabolism that prolonged the availability of dopamine within the synapse.

In combination with aerobic activity, Mike's early engagement in rehabilitation therapies, such as physical therapy, may have prevented many secondary musculoskeletal complications such as deconditioning and loss of strength and range of motion. Maintaining consistent and regular engagement in an exercise program may be challenging due to the effects of PD on motivation and the potential need to adapt exercises to maintain safety. Mike was particularly determined to continue exercising, and his very supportive family and active lifestyle have helped him to remain active over the 15-year course of his disease. He was also referred to rehabilitative services early in the disease process, allowing him to further refine an exercise program that was individualized to his presentation. Rehabilitation therapies and a physically active lifestyle can continue to benefit Mike through preservation of functional abilities, minimization of secondary complications as he continues to live well with PD (Kelly, *personal communication*, 2015).

As you can see, the CNS adapts to neural pathology, whether it occurs quickly (as in stroke) or slowly (as in neurodegenerative diseases), with evidence of plasticity at many levels within the nervous system. In addition, experience leads to plasticity; this can be maladaptive plasticity as in the case of disuse or adaptive in response to activity and training. Finally, we see that the principles of activity-dependent neural plasticity presented by Kleim and Jones (2008) and summarized earlier in this chapter apply to patients like Genise, with acquired brain injury, as well as to patients like Mike, with a neurodegenerative disease.

SUMMARY

1. The brain is incredibly plastic, and it has great capacity to change; this includes not just the immature brain but also the mature adult brain.
2. The most important way in which the environment changes behavior in humans is through learning.
3. CNS structural changes occur as a result of the interaction of genetic, experiential, and environmental factors.
4. A key factor in experience is the concept of active competition, and this may be summed up in the phrase "the squeaky wheel gets the oil", or in this case, it gets the new synaptic connections. This concept is applicable from simple circuits to complex neural pathways.
5. Research suggests that short-term and long-term memory may not be separate categories but instead may be part of a single-graded memory function involving the same synapses.
6. Short-term changes reflect relatively temporary changes in synaptic effectiveness; structural changes are the hallmark of long-term memory.
7. Scientists believe that the circuits involved in the storage of procedural and declarative learning are different, with procedural memory involving the neocortex, striatum, amygdala, cerebellum, and in the simplest cases the reflex pathways and declarative memory involving the medial temporal lobe and the hippocampus, as well as certain areas of the neocortex.
8. Principles derived from research on activity-dependent neural plasticity can inform and guide rehabilitation practices to promote neural adaptation and functional recovery in patients with impaired motor control.

CHAPTER 5

Constraints on Motor Control: An Overview of Neurologic Impairments

Learning Objectives

Following completion of this chapter, the reader will be able to:

1. Define the following terms used to classify impairments associated with central nervous system (CNS) pathology: signs versus symptoms, positive versus negative symptoms, primary versus secondary effects.
2. Define and describe impairments associated with pathophysiology of the motor cortex, including motor weakness (paresis), abnormal muscle tone (spasticity), and coordination problems, including loss of individuation and presence of abnormal synergies of movement. Discuss methods for assessing and treating these impairments.
3. Compare and contrast impairments in persons with pathology in the cerebellum versus the basal ganglia. Discuss the assessment and treatment of impairments associated with these subcortical structures, including abnormal muscle tone, tremor, and coordination problems affecting the timing and scaling of muscle activity.
4. Discuss the relationship between secondary musculoskeletal impairments and primary neuromuscular impairments. Describe the management of musculoskeletal impairments in persons with neurologic pathology.
5. Discuss the primary impairments associated with deficits in the visual, somatosensory, and vestibular systems, and describe some clinical strategies for assessing and managing these impairments.
6. Discuss the relationship between attention and spatial and nonspatial deficits. Briefly describe some of the clinical strategies for assessing and managing perceptual/cognitive deficits.

INTRODUCTION: SIGNS AND SYMPTOMS OF PATHOPHYSIOLOGY OF MOTOR CONTROL

Clinical treatment of the patient with motor control problems requires both knowledge and skill. Part of an essential knowledge base in treating patients with movement problems is understanding the physiology and pathophysiology of motor control. This information enables the therapist to form initial hypotheses regarding the pattern of impairments likely to be found in patients with a specific neural pathology. Understanding the impairments constraining movement allows the clinician to form initial hypotheses regarding the probable functional limitations and restrictions to participation, that are likely to be affecting a patient's life.

The formation of initial hypotheses regarding likely impairments, functional limitations, and reduced participation, guides the selection of appropriate tests and measures that are used to examine initial assumptions relative to a specific patient. Through examination procedures, the clinician determines the impairments and functional limitations in a specific patient and identifies how these influence the capacity of the patient to participate in their daily life. This then leads to the selection of interventions appropriate to that patient. This therapeutic plan includes strategies that focus on changing modifiable factors and strategies designed to help patients learn to adapt to non-modifiable factors, in this way maximizing functional capacity and participation in society.

Since movement arises from the interaction of multiple processes, including those related to sensory/perceptual, cognitive, and action or motor systems, pathology within any of the systems will result in impairments that potentially constrain functional movement. A comprehensive discussion of the pathophysiology of motor control is beyond the scope of this chapter. Rather, in the first half of this chapter, we focus on an overview of pathophysiology and associated impairments within the action (motor), sensory/perceptual, and cognitive systems. We begin with a discussion of issues related to classifying or categorizing impairments in persons with neurologic pathology. The last half of the chapter reviews common approaches to clinical examination and treatment of impairments in each of these systems. The impairment section in each of the video case studies accompanying this book is designed to provide a visual image of the types of impairments discussed in this chapter, as well as an idea of the types of clinical tests used to examine these impairments. The focus then of this chapter is on understanding common underlying impairments potentially constraining function and participation in patients with specific types of neural pathology. The relationships between underlying impairments and both function and participation are discussed in later chapters of the book, which also describe approaches to assessing and treating functional limitations and restricted participation.

CLASSIFYING IMPAIRMENTS ASSOCIATED WITH CENTRAL NERVOUS SYSTEM LESIONS

Signs versus Symptoms

Brain pathology produces a unique pattern of behavioral signs and symptoms associated with the destruction of specific neuronal populations. Signs of neurologic dysfunction represent objective findings of pathology that can be determined by physical examination (e.g., the presence of nystagmus suggests that a patient has a vestibular disorder). In contrast, symptoms are subjective reports associated with pathology that are perceived by the patient but may not necessarily be objectively documented on examination. Dizziness is a common symptom associated with vestibular pathology.

Positive versus Negative Signs and Symptoms

Hughlings Jackson described upper motor neuron lesions as damage to cortical and subcortical structures producing motor dyscontrol because of either (a) the release of abnormal behaviors, called "positive symptoms," or (b) the loss of normal behaviors, called "negative symptoms" (Foerster, 1977). Positive symptoms might include the presence of abnormal reflexes such as the extensor plantar (or Babinski) reflex or hyperactive stretch reflexes resulting in spasticity. Paresis, the loss of descending control of lower motor neurons, is an example of a negative symptom. In the rehabilitation environment, attempts to understand functional deficits in the patient with neurologic pathology often emphasize positive symptoms, such as increased muscle tone, at the expense of negative symptoms, such as loss of strength (Gordon, 1987; Katz & Rymer, 1989).

Primary versus Secondary Effects

Central nervous system (CNS) lesions can result in a wide variety of primary impairments affecting motor (neuromuscular), sensory/perceptual, and/or cognitive/behavioral systems. In addition to primary impairments such as paresis or spasticity, secondary effects also contribute to motor control problems. Secondary impairments do not result from the CNS lesion directly but rather develop as a result of the original problem (Schenkman, 1990). For example, as shown in Figure 5.1, an upper motor neuron (motor cortex) lesion results in primary impairments of paresis and spasticity. These impairments limit movement capabilities in the patient, and this immobility may result in the development of a secondary musculoskeletal impairment, such as changes in the structure and function of muscles, muscle

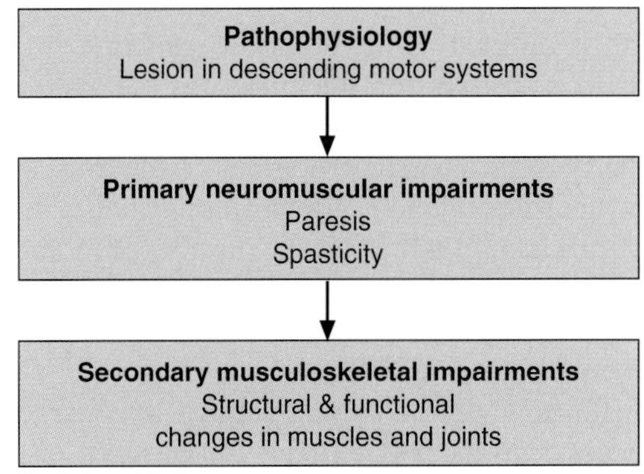

Figure 5.1 Pathophysiology within the CNS can result in both primary impairments and secondary impairments. For example, a CNS lesion produces primary neuromuscular impairments such as paresis and spasticity. These impairments, which limit movement, can result in the development of secondary musculoskeletal system impairments, such as changes in the structure and function of muscles and joints, which further constrain the person's ability to move.

contractures, and decreased joint range of motion, which further constrain the person's ability to move.

With this overview of methods for classifying impairments associated with CNS lesions, we can now turn our attention to the heart of this chapter, an overview of the pathophysiological basis for deficits in motor control in the patient with neurologic pathology.

IMPAIRMENTS IN THE ACTION SYSTEMS

The action system includes areas of the nervous system such as motor cortex, cerebellum, and basal ganglia, which perform processing essential to the control of movement.

Motor Cortex Deficits

A neurological insult to the motor cortex neurons (first-order motor neurons) and/or the descending corticospinal pathway (the descending motor system) results in an upper motor neuron syndrome, which is associated with a wide range of neuromuscular impairments that constrain functional movement in the person with neurologic dysfunction (Emos & Rosner, 2020). In the initial stage, there exists a period of hypotonia and muscle flaccidity—a spinal shock due to the sudden lack of cortical inputs to the spinal cord. This general flaccid status is followed by a group of characteristic motor signs and symptoms, which are reviewed later in this chapter. Several of our patient case studies, for example, Genise, our patient with acute stroke; Jean, our patient with chronic stroke; and both Thomas and Malachi, our children with cerebral palsy (CP), demonstrate a range of impairments associated with neural pathology affecting the descending motor systems.

Motor Strength and Weakness (Paresis)

Strength is defined as the ability to generate sufficient tension in a muscle for the purposes of posture and movement (Smidt & Rogers, 1982). Strength results from both the musculoskeletal properties of the muscle itself and the neural activation of that muscle. Neural aspects of force production reflect (a) the number of motor units recruited, (b) the type of units recruited, and (c) the discharge frequency (Buchner & DeLateur, 1991; Duncan & Badke, 1987; Rogers, 1991).

Weakness is defined as an inability to generate normal levels of force; it is a major impairment of motor function in many patients with motor cortex and descending pathway lesions. Depending on the extent of the lesion, weakness (a reduced ability to generate force) in the patient with a cerebral cortex lesion can vary in severity from total or severe loss of muscle activity, called "paralysis" or "plegia," to mild or partial loss of muscle activity, called "paresis."

Paralysis or paresis (a negative sign of CNS pathology) results in an inability or difficulty in recruiting and/or modulating skeletal motor units, particularly high-threshold motor units, to generate torque or movement, and is one component of the upper motor neuron syndrome (Gracies, 2005a, 2005b). Paresis and plegia are often referred to by their distribution: hemiplegia (or hemiparesis) is weakness affecting one side of the body, paraplegia affects the lower extremities, and tetraplegia affects all four limbs.

Many studies have documented problems in motor unit recruitment and discharge behavior in patients with cerebral cortex lesions (Frascarelli et al., 1998; Yan et al., 1998a, 1998b). Reduced descending drive is associated with a failure to recruit high-threshold motor units and a reduced ability to modulate or increase motor unit discharge rate when trying to increase voluntary force (Gracies, 2005a, 2005b).

Research has also improved our understanding of the intensity and distribution of strength impairments in persons with CNS lesions. Andrews and Bohannon (2000) quantified the distribution of strength impairments following stroke in 48 patients with acute stroke. Strength was impaired on both sides of the body, suggesting the bilateral effects of a cerebral cortex lesion. Interestingly, contrary to what was expected, distal muscles were less impaired than proximal muscles on the nonparetic side, and extensor muscle activity was less affected than flexor activity bilaterally. Other studies have also shown the bilateral effects of ipsilateral lesions of the cerebral cortex (Hermsdorfer et al., 1999; Marque et al., 1997; Winstein & Pohl, 1995). Wiley and Damiano (1998) compared strength profiles in lower-extremity muscles in 30 children with CP (15 children with spastic diplegia and 15 with spastic hemiplegia) with 16 age-matched peers. Using a handheld dynamometer, they quantified isometric strength in major lower-extremity muscle groups bilaterally. The results of this study are summarized in Figure 5.2A and B, which compare strength values normalized by body weight in the three groups of children, across a variety of muscles, as shown along the *x*-axis. Significant results from the study included the following: (a) children with CP were weaker than age-matched peers in all muscles tested; (b) the children with hemiplegia showed significant weakness on both the involved and noninvolved limbs; (c) weakness was greater in the distal muscles as compared with proximal muscles; and (d) hip flexors and ankle plantar flexors were stronger than their antagonist muscles. In trying to explain the basis for weakness in these children, the authors collected electromyographic (EMG) data during strength testing on several of their subjects. These data are shown in Figure 5.3A and B. Shown are the rectified EMG recordings of the agonist and antagonist muscles during a strength test in a normally developing 8-year-old (Fig. 5.3A) and a child with CP. When asked to maximally contract her hamstrings,

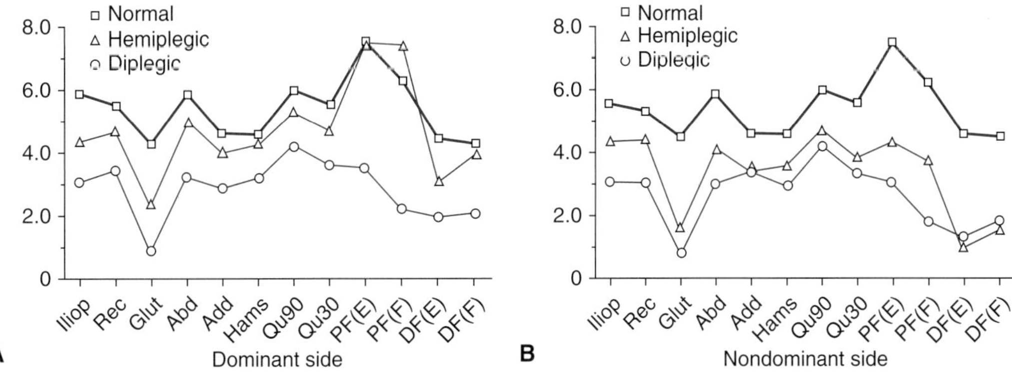

Figure 5.2 A comparison of strength profiles in lower-extremity muscles (normalized to body weight) in children with spastic hemiplegia and diplegia and age-matched peers ("normal"). Strength in the muscles of the dominant side is shown in **(A)** and the nondominant side in **(B)**. (Adapted from Wiley ME, Damiano DL. Lower-extremity strength profiles in spastic cerebral palsy. *Dev Med Child Neurol.* 1998;40:104, with permission.)

the normally developing child shows a phasic burst of activity in the left hamstrings with no activation of the antagonist quadriceps. Similarly, a maximal contraction of the quadriceps (Fig. 5.3B) was not associated with activation of the antagonist hamstrings. In contrast, when the child with CP was asked to activate the quadriceps (Fig. 5.3D), there was a concomitant activation of the antagonist hamstrings. Interestingly, there was poor activation of the hamstring muscle when this child was trying to activate it for a maximal contraction (Fig. 5.3C). Thus, the studies suggest that weakness in children with CP appears to have both a neurophysiological and a biomechanical basis.

Thus, paresis and weakness appear to be primary negative signs of pathology in the descending motor system. An example of profound hemiparesis following an acute stroke can be seen in the impairment section of the video case study on Genise. In addition, prolonged paresis/weakness, a primary neuromuscular impairment, leads to the development of secondary musculoskeletal weakness, defined by peripheral changes in the muscle itself. This type of weakness is discussed in detail in later sections of this chapter.

Abnormal Muscle Tone: Spasticity

In this chapter, we typically use the term "lesion in the descending motor systems" instead of "upper motor neuron lesion." A lesion in the descending motor systems could reflect pathology in the pyramidal tract or other nearby descending motor pathways such as the corticoreticulospinal tract. Damage to these tracts results in increased alpha motor neuron excitability, with a resulting increase in muscle tone (hyperactivity of tonic stretch reflexes) and exaggerated tendon jerks (phasic stretch reflexes) (Mayer, 1997).

Muscle tone is characterized by a muscle's resistance to passive stretch, and a certain level of tone is typical in normal muscles. On the upper end of the tone spectrum (Fig. 5.4) is hypertonicity, manifested by spasticity or rigidity (a positive sign of CNS pathology). At the other end are disorders of hypotonicity (a negative sign). The presence of abnormalities of muscle tone in persons with CNS pathology is well known. However, the exact contributions of abnormalities of muscle tone to functional deficits are not well understood.

Spasticity is defined as "a motor disorder characterized by a velocity-dependent increase in tonic stretch reflexes (muscle tone) with exaggerated tendon jerks, resulting from hyperexcitability of the stretch reflex, and is one component of the upper motor neuron syndrome" (Lance, 1980, p. 485). We should keep in mind that the excitability of reflex circuits is different at rest (when muscle tone is frequently examined) than during movement (Burke et al., 2013). Understanding spasticity is difficult in part because the term is used clinically to cover a wide range of abnormal behaviors. It is used to describe (a) hyperactive stretch reflexes, (b) abnormal posturing of the limbs, (c) excessive coactivation of antagonist muscles, (d) associated movements, (e) clonus, and (f) stereotyped movement synergies, which are motor defects that are associated with a wide variety of pathological mechanisms. Thus, the word *spasticity* is used to describe many abnormal behaviors often seen in patients with CNS pathology.

A key sign of spasticity is a velocity-dependent increase in resistance of a muscle or muscle group to passive stretch. Examples of velocity-dependent resistance to quick stretch indicating the presence of spasticity can be seen in several video case studies including Jean and Genise, our patients with stroke, as well as Thomas, our child with CP. The neural mechanism underlying spasticity is abnormality within the segmental stretch reflex. Disorders in the stretch reflex mechanism could reflect alterations in the threshold and/or the gain of the stretch reflex in response to stretch. Several studies have been consistent in demonstrating changes in threshold, rather than gain, of the stretch reflex, in muscles with spastic hypertonus. This is because the alpha motor neuron pool at the segmental level is hyperexcitable, due to loss of descending inhibitory input, postsynaptic denervation supersensitivity,

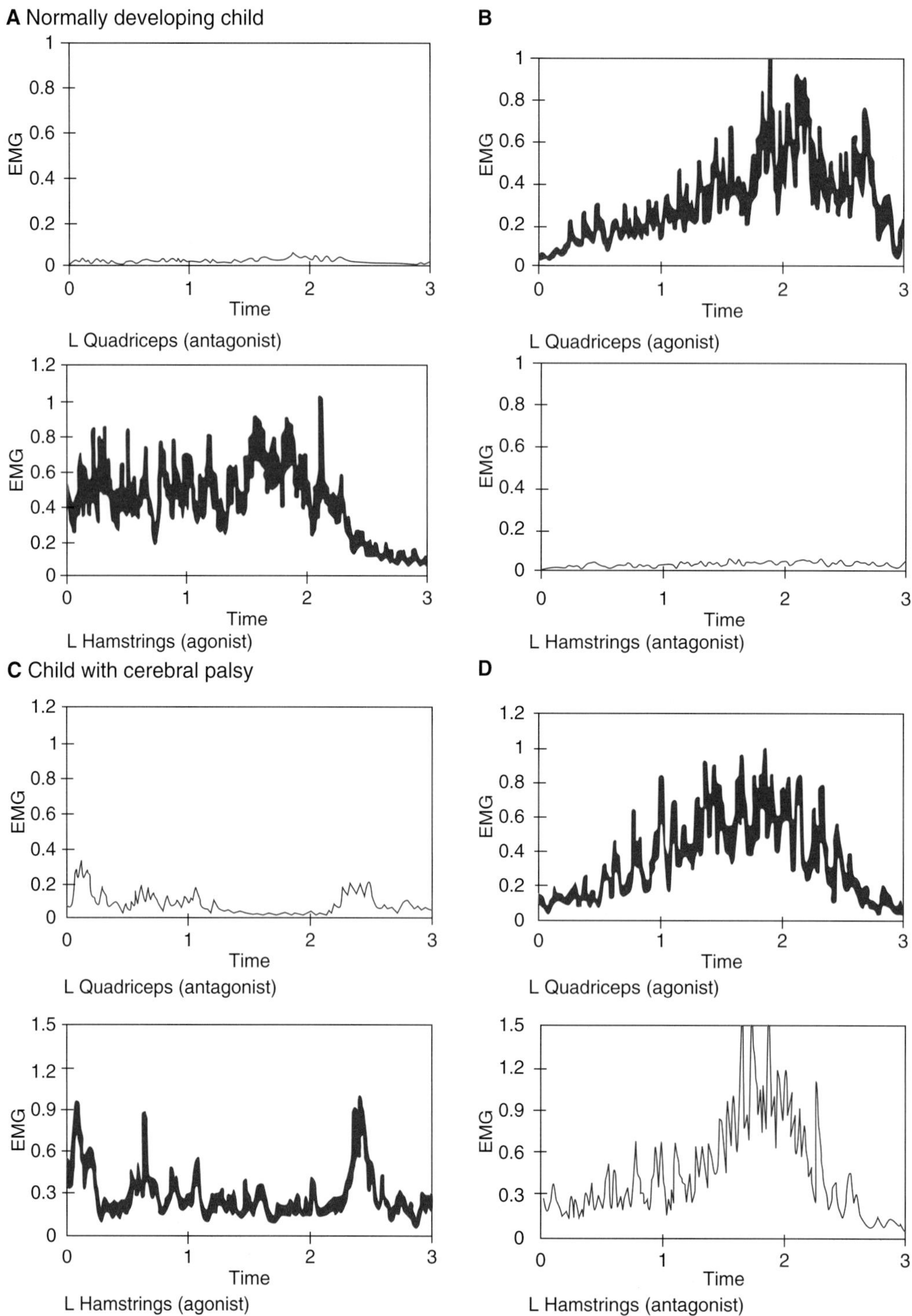

Figure 5.3 Rectified integrated EMG activity of the agonist and antagonist muscles in a normally developing 8-year-old child during isometric strength test of the left hamstrings **(A)** and quadriceps **(B)**. EMG activity in the same set of muscles in an 8-year-old child with spastic cerebral palsy **(C** and **D)**. (Adapted from Wiley ME, Damiano DL. Lower-extremity strength profiles in spastic cerebral palsy. *Dev Med Child Neurol.* 1998;40:105, with permission.)

collateral sprouting of the dorsal root afferents, and changes in the intrinsic motoneuron properties—persistent inward currents of calcium and sodium result in a plateau of motoneuron potentials, amplified motoneurons inputs (reflex gain), and self-sustained firing potentials (Burke et al., 2013; Katz & Rymer, 1989; Latash et al., 1998; Powers et al., 1989; Thilmann et al., 1991).

Although we have greater understanding of the neural mechanisms underlying spastic hypertonicity, there is still no agreement on the role of spasticity in the loss of functional performance (Rymer & Katz, 1994). It has been suggested that spasticity limits a patient's ability to move quickly, since activation of the stretch reflex is velocity-dependent. While excessive activation of the stretch

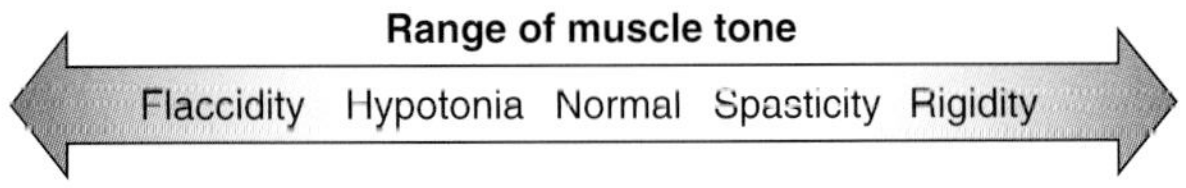

Range of muscle tone

Flaccidity Hypotonia Normal Spasticity Rigidity

Figure 5.4 Continuum of muscle tone. The center of the graph illustrates the range of normal muscle tone. A decrease in muscle tone compared with normal is referred to as "hypotonia." In contrast, an increase in muscle tone compared with normal is referred to as "hypertonia" and manifests as either spasticity or rigidity.

reflex mechanism in an antagonist muscle could serve to prevent lengthening of that muscle during a shortening contraction of the agonist, researchers have shown that it is inadequate recruitment of agonist motor neurons (a negative sign), not increased activity in the antagonist (a positive sign), that is the primary basis for disorders of motor control following a CNS lesion (Bohannon & Andrews, 1990; Dietz et al., 1991; Gowland et al., 1992; Sahrmann & Norton, 1977; Tang & Rymer, 1981). Thus, other problems such as inability to recruit motor neurons (paresis), abnormal reciprocal inhibition between agonist and antagonist, and impaired coordination of muscle synergists may be more disabling in relation to motor control than simple hypertonicity (Katz & Rymer, 1989). In fact, research has shown that the reduction of spasticity does not always improve function and may even be counterproductive. In some patients with a CNS lesion, a spastic quadriceps can assist locomotion, and as such, therapeutic measures to reduce spasticity may negatively impact the ability to walk (Burke et al., 2013).

This research has tremendous implications for clinical practice. It suggests that treatment practices directed primarily at reducing spastic hypertonicity (a positive sign) as the major focus in regaining motor control may have limited impact on helping patients regain functional independence. This is because loss of functional independence is often the result of many factors that limit the recovery of motor control and is not limited to the presence of abnormal muscle tone.

Loss of Selective Muscle Activation and Abnormal Synergies

Pathology within the descending motor system (motor cortex and corticospinal tract) results in loss of individuation (a negative sign). *Individuation* (also called "fractionation of movement") refers to the ability to selectively activate a muscle (or limited set of muscles), allowing isolated joint motion. Impaired individuation is characterized by the abnormal coupling between related muscles. When individuation is lost, activation of one muscle is abnormally coupled with other related muscles. Thus, during a voluntary movement, rather than selectively activating only those muscles necessary, the attempt to activate one muscle results in the activation of abnormally coupled muscles (Zackowski et al., 2004). For example, following stroke, abnormal coupling has been shown between shoulder and elbow flexors (Dewald & Beer, 2001; Lum et al., 2003; Zackowski et al., 2004). When a person with hemiparesis generates a flexor torque at the shoulder, a secondary flexor torque at the elbow is also generated (Dewald & Beer, 2001). Within reaching tasks, animal and non-human primate research has demonstrated the relevance of cervical propriospinal neurons in coordinating descending motor commands from higher center regions (Pierrot-Deseilligny & Burke 2009). Specifically, the C3-4 propriospinal system receives corticospinal, reticulospinal, and tectospinal signals as well as afferent information from the limb that may facilitate the activation of selective muscle synergies (Alstermark et al, 1999; Isa et al., 2006, 2007; Lemon 2008). For example, in the impairment segment of Genise's video case study, efforts to flex her shoulder are accompanied by flexion at the elbow and fingers. This loss of selective activation of muscles and the consequent decrease in individuation of joint movement are associated with decreased function (Lang & Schieber, 2004).

In the rehabilitation field, abnormal coupling of muscles and joints into characteristic patterns of movement has historically been referred to as "abnormal synergies" or "massed patterns of movement" (Brunnstrom, 1966; Fugl-Myer et al., 1975; Twitchell, 1951). In the rehabilitation literature, the term *synergy* has often been used to describe abnormal or disordered motor control (Bobath, 1990; Brunnstrom, 1970).

Abnormal synergies are stereotypical patterns of movement that cannot be changed or adapted to changes in task or environmental demands. Because muscles in an abnormal synergy are so strongly linked, movement outside the fixed pattern is often not possible.

Twitchell's 1951 classic paper described the role of synergies as part of the stepwise sequence of motor recovery following stroke. He suggested that stroke recovery begins with an initial areflexia or flaccid paralysis. Voluntary movement appears first as stereotyped flexor and extensor muscle synergies. As recovery continues, voluntary movement out of synergies emerges, and finally, the ability to move normally returns. Twitchell described the process of recovery proceeding from proximal to distal, with flexor movements occurring first in the upper extremity and extensor movements occurring first in the lower extremity.

The flexion synergy of the upper extremity, shown in Figure 5.5, is characterized by scapular retraction and elevation, shoulder abduction and external rotation, elbow flexion, forearm supination, and wrist and finger flexion. The extensor synergy in the lower extremity involves hip extension, adduction and internal rotation, knee extension, ankle plantar flexion and inversion, and toe plantar flexion. Consistent with Twitchell's proposal, Signe Brunnstrom (1970) characterized the process of stroke recovery relative to the emergence and dissolution of abnormal synergies. Additional examples of abnormal synergies can be seen in both Jean and Genise's video case studies.

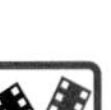

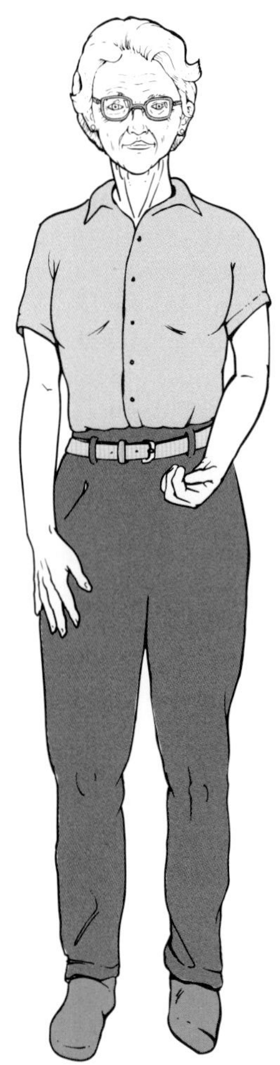

Figure 5.5 Flexion synergy of the upper extremity.

What is the underlying neural mechanism of abnormal synergies? There is no relationship between either weakness or spasticity and the presence of abnormal synergies (Zackowski et al., 2004). Research demonstrates that abnormal synergies result from increased recruitment of descending brainstem pathways (Krakauer, 2005; Ortiz-Rosarioa et al., 2014; Zaaimi et al., 2012).

Coactivation

As discussed in the abnormal synergy section, normal, skilled movement entails the activation of only those muscles necessary to the task being completed. *Coactivation* is characterized by the simultaneous activation of additional muscles (most often agonist and antagonist muscles) during functional movements and is present in both neurologically intact individuals just learning a skill as well as individuals with neurologic pathology. Thus, coactivation is not always the result of neural pathology, but can, in some cases, represent a normal control strategy. For example, coactivation can be used when controlling the mechanical stiffness of joints during complex multi-joint movements, or when selectively regulating joint amplitudes during movements.

Muscle agonist–antagonist interactions change the non-linear dynamics of skeletal muscles contractions, which depend upon instantaneous current and previous neural activation, external load, and direction of previous movements. Thus, deficits in the reflexive mechanisms that regulate these agonist–antagonist interactions can accentuate the effects of cortically misdirected motor commands that result from injured sensorimotor areas of the brain (Burke et al., 2013; Gorkovenko et al., 2012; Latash, 2018; Yamazaki et al., 1994).

We now turn to our case studies to summarize the impairments present in persons with pathology in the descending motor system (cortex and corticospinal tract).

Clinical Case Studies

Jean J. and Genise T: Motor Impairments Associated with Cerebral Vascular Accident. Jean is an 82-year-old woman who has had a cerebral vascular accident (CVA) of the middle cerebral artery (MCA) 6 years ago. Genise is a 53-year-old woman who also had a CVA of the MCA 4 days ago. Stroke, or CVA, is defined as a sudden, focal, neurologic deficit resulting from disruption to the blood supply in the brain that persists for at least 24 hours. There are two main categories of CVA: ischemia (a lack of blood flow) and hemorrhage (release of blood into the extravascular space).

The impairments resulting from a stroke vary depending on the site and extent of vascular damage. Genise and Jean have neuromuscular impairments that include right-sided weakness (paresis), which significantly limits the ability to activate muscles in the hemiparetic arm and leg, as well as the trunk. In the impairment section of their videos, this can be seen in their limited ability to voluntarily move the right arm and leg. In addition to paresis, both Genise and Jean have abnormal muscle tone (spasticity), which can be seen in the resistance to quick stretch of muscles in both the hemiparetic arm and leg. The ability to activate individual muscles (individuation) in the hemiparetic limbs is significantly impaired in both women. Voluntary movement is characterized by abnormal synergies, with a flexor synergy present in the hemiparetic arm (as seen in the resting posture of the right arm, and an inability to flex the shoulder without also flexing the elbow and fingers). In addition, in the lower extremity, both patients demonstrate a flexor synergy (as indicated by an inability to flex the knee without also flexing the hip) and an extensor synergy (more apparent in gait) in the hemiparetic leg. Jean, who had her stroke 6 years ago, has developed significant musculoskeletal problems, including reduced range of motion that limits her functional movement. At 4 days poststroke, Genise had not developed secondary musculoskeletal problems. However, at 1 month poststroke, she was already demonstrating increased tightness in the finger and wrist flexors as well as in the ankle plantar flexors in her hemiparetic limbs.

Thomas: Motor Impairments Associated with Spastic Diplegia Cerebral Palsy. Thomas is a 7-year-old with a spastic diplegia form of CP. CP is a nonprogressive disorder that results from prenatal or perinatal damage to the CNS. The site and extent of damage to the developing CNS determine the continuum of impairments seen in a patient diagnosed with CP. Classification is based on the type of motor disorder found and the extremities involved. Spastic CP (hemiplegia, diplegia, and quadriplegia) represents 50% to 60% of the cases. Because Thomas has spastic diplegia, his impairments affect his lower extremities more than his upper extremities.

His neuromuscular impairments (see the impairment section of Thomas's video) include hypertonicity (spasticity) (evidenced by his resistance to quick stretch), hyperreflexia (not shown), and poor individuation during voluntary movements, in conjunction with the presence of abnormal synergies particularly in his lower extremities (evidenced by his inability to flex his knee without also flexing his hip). He has significant weakness in his lower extremities, which reflects both problems with neural recruitment and underlying musculoskeletal problems. His other musculoskeletal problems, including reduced range of motion, have developed secondary to his primary neuromotor pathology but are a major factor limiting his functional ability.

Motor Impairments Associated with Subcortical Pathology

Motor Impairments Associated with Cerebellar Pathology

Disorders of the cerebellum result in distinctive symptoms and signs, as described by Babinski in 1899 and Gordon Holmes in the 1920s and 1930s (Kandel et al., 2000b). Holmes grouped signs and symptoms of cerebellar pathology into three categories: (a) hypotonia, (b) ataxia or discoordination of voluntary movement, and (c) action or intention tremor. Other cerebellar motor signs are dyssynergia (decomposition of movement), dysdiadochokinesia (impaired ability to perform rapid alternating movements), dysarthria (deficits in articulating words), and impaired oculomotor control (Fahn et al, 2011; Schmahmann et al., 2019). Because the cerebellum is related to areas of the brain regulating cognition, emotion, and autonomic functions; these may also be affected by cerebellar damage. Lesions to specific sites within the cerebellum result in specific impairments. For example, lesions of the vermis and fastigial nuclei produce disturbances in the control of axial and trunk muscles affecting postural control and balance and characteristic speech deficits. In contrast, damage to the intermediate cerebellum or interposed nuclei produces action tremor in the limbs, while disorders in the lateral cerebellar hemispheres primarily cause delays in initiating movement and impaired control of multijoint movements. A lesion of the posterior cerebellar lobe may result in cerebellar cognitive affective syndrome, which is characterized by deficits in executive function, visual spatial processing, linguistic skills, and regulation of affect (Schmahmann et al., 2019). Our case study of John, our patient with spinocerebellar degeneration (as seen in the impairment section of John's video), demonstrates some of the underlying impairments that manifest with cerebellar pathology.

Hypotonia. We previously described deficits related to increased tone, specifically spasticity, associated with motor cortex deficits. At the other end of the tone spectrum is hypotonicity, defined as a reduction in the stiffness of a muscle to lengthening. Hypotonia is characteristically associated with deficits in the cerebellum; however, hypotonicity is described in many different kinds of patients, including those with spinocerebellar lesions (Ghez, 1991), and in many developmentally delayed children, such as children with Down syndrome (Shumway-Cook & Woollacott, 1985b). Acute damage of the cerebellum is associated with transient hypotonia that tends to improve gradually in parallel to the recovery of muscle spindle sensitivity, which is acutely depressed by loss of cerebellar fusimotor facilitation, principally through vestibulospinal and reticulospinal pathways. Animal models have helped to explain how cerebellar damage, mainly involving the anterior lobule, results in disrupted regulation of muscle spindle sensitivity, reactions to labyrinthine or cutaneous stimuli, and proprioceptive supporting reactions (Bodranghien et al., 2016; Gilman, 1969; Gilman & Ebel, 1970; Manto, 2018; Mukherjee & Chakravarty, 2010). Hypotonia in patients with cerebellar pathology is often associated with pendular reflexes. In patients with cerebellar disease, a knee-jerk response to a brief tendon tap may result in prolonged oscillations of the leg (Kandel et al., 2000b; Manto, 2018).

Coordination Problems Associated with Cerebellar Pathology. Problems in the coordination of movements are considered a hallmark of pathology within the cerebellum. Coordinated movement involves multiple joints and muscles that are activated at the appropriate time and with the correct amount of force so that smooth, efficient, and accurate movement occurs. Thus, the essence of coordination is the sequencing, timing, and grading of the activation of multiple muscle groups. Because of the synergistic nature of coordination, the capacity to generate force in an isolated muscle does not predict the ability of that muscle to work in concert with others in a task-specific way (Giuliani, 1991).

In healthy individuals, movements involving more than one joint are associated with movement trajectories that have bell-shaped velocity profiles (Hogan et al., 1987). In contrast, movement trajectories in patients with cerebellar pathology are often uneven and lack a bell-shaped profile because of the loss of coordinated coupling between synergistic muscles and joints. Cerebellar discoordination can manifest in a number of ways, including delays in the onset of movements (delayed reaction time), errors in the range and direction of movement (called "dysmetria"), and an inability to sustain regular rhythmic movements (called "dysdiadochokinesia"). Movement trajectories are characterized by decomposition (e.g., moving one joint at a time) (Bastian et al., 1996). Cerebellar coordination deficits are illustrated in Figure 5.6. Since single-joint control appears to be better than multijoint control, patients with cerebellar lesions may decompose movements into sequential movement at individual joints as a strategy to minimize the impact of multijoint discoordination.

Patients with cerebellar pathology often have difficulty terminating a movement, which can manifest as an inability to stop a movement, but also as inability to change the direction of a movement. Problems terminating a movement can manifest as difficulties in checking or halting a movement, resulting in a "rebound" phenomenon. Rebound phenomena can be seen as involuntary movements of a limb when resistance to an isometric contraction is suddenly removed (Fredericks & Saladin, 1996).

In addition to appropriate timing of muscle activation, coordinated functional movement requires the scaling, or grading, of forces appropriate to the metrics of the task. Hypometria is underestimation of the required force or range of movement, while hypermetria is overestimation of the force or range of movement needed for a specific task. Inability to scale or grade forces appropriately can be seen as undershooting or overshooting in tasks such as reaching or pointing (Bastian et al., 1996; Hore et al., 1991).

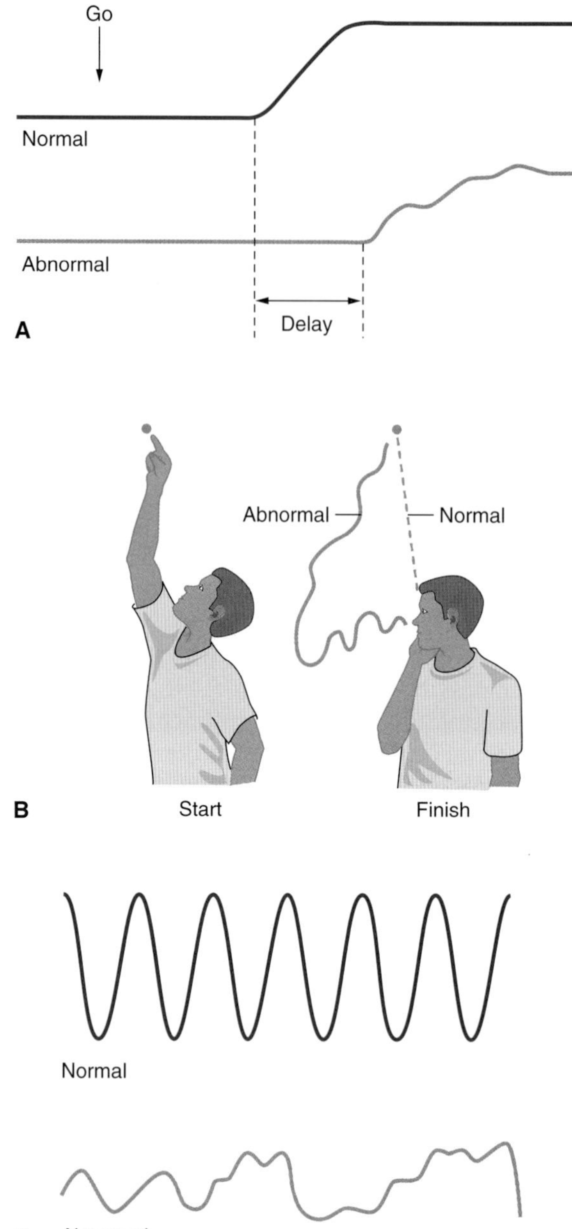

Figure 5.6 (A) Movement deficits observed in persons with cerebellar disease. Delay in the onset of movement following the signal to "go" can be seen in the bottom trace as compared with the normal reaction time shown in the upper trace. **(B)** Dysmetria, a disorder in the range and direction of movement, is seen when the person is asked to move his arm from the target to his nose. Intention tremor can be seen when the arm approaches the nose. **(C)** Dysdiadochokinesia, an irregular pattern of alternating movement, can be seen in the abnormal position trace made when the person with cerebellar pathology alternately pronates and supinates the forearm, compared with a normal position trace. (Adapted from Kandel ER, Schwartz JH, Jessell TM, eds. *Principles of neural science*, 3rd ed. New York, NY: Elsevier, 1991:849, Fig. 42.16.)

Intention Tremor. Tremor is defined as a rhythmic, involuntary oscillatory movement of a body part (Deuschl et al., 1998). Intention tremor is tremor that occurs during the performance of a voluntary movement and is characteristic of pathology of the cerebellum and its afferent or efferent pathways. Intention tremor has a frequency range of less than 5 Hz and is most marked at the end of a movement.

Impaired Error Correction Affecting Motor Learning. The cerebellum plays a critical role in error correction, an essential part of motor learning. Within the cerebellum, internal feedback signals reporting intended movements are compared with external feedback signals that report actual movement. The cerebellum generates a corrective signal used in feedforward control to reduce errors in subsequent movements. Thus, in addition to their role in the control of movement, cerebellar structures also are important in practice-dependent motor adaptation and learning in many different systems (Morton & Bastian, 2004, 2007). Damage to the cerebellum affects the extent and rate at which individuals adapt movements to new contexts (Morton & Bastian, 2004, 2007). This suggests that the training of individuals with cerebellar pathology may require a longer duration or intensity of practice to improve motor function.

Goal-oriented movements are frequently preprogrammed and thus, do not rely solely on sensory feedback. Recent studies on the neural control of movements hypothesize that the brain can create neural models with the internal representations of the sensorimotor transformations required to execute a desired movement. There exist two conceptual models: forward and inverse. While the *forward model* predicts the sensory consequences of the movement based on motor commands, the *inverse model* uses the desired goal and sensory consequences of movements to compute motor commands (Stein, 2009). Thus, motor behaviors rely on *prediction errors* (i.e., discrepancy between predicted and actual sensorimotor information). Within the motor system, the cerebellum—principally Purkinje cells—seems to be the key to represent forward internal models to predict sensory consequences related to motor commands and to compute sensory prediction errors by comparing predictions and sensory feedback (Popa & Ebner, 2019). In a recent review by Therrien and Bastian (2019), the cerebellum is understood as a "type of movement sensor" that can generate adaptable and predictive information about the sensory consequences secondary to motor outputs. The sensory estimates may serve as a readily available internal feedback model to the motor system. The brain uses peripheral sensory feedback to determine whether a desired movement, or body state, has been achieved. However, if the brain just relies on sensory feedback to correct for the mismatch between sensory-motor events during ongoing movements, such motor corrections would result in poor motor control due to delays in sensory processing. New research now emphasizes that the brain may predict the future sensory state of the body with forward internal models that act as an internal sensory feedback signal and convey current sensory information with a copy of the motor command. For this purpose, it is hypothesized that forward model predictions need to learn and update body dynamics within the features of the surrounding environment (Therrien & Bastian, 2019).

Research on cerebellar damage support the role of the cerebellum in the composition of forward models to predict sensory consequences so that the motor system can accurately evaluate and carry the most appropriate movement in each context. In this sense, an impaired ability to predict the effects of the inertial properties of the limbs during motion can derive in dysmetria. In motor tasks that involve multiple joints, the lack of sensory prediction of limb inertia or interactive torques among the joints may result in the characteristic dyssynergia observed in patients with damaged cerebellum. Therefore, the decomposition of multijoint movements into small sub-movements controlled by single joints could be understood as a compensatory strategy to control the limbs. Similarly, impaired sensory predictions could be the cause of the typical intention tremor observed in patients with cerebellar pathology since during goal-oriented tasks the absence of the current predictive body sensory state would make the motor system highly dependent on outdated peripheral sensory feedback with subsequent delayed motor corrections. That is, the motor correction is based on sensory feedback that matches the previous sensory body state and not the current one. Differently from healthy individuals, who can proactively scale the time and the magnitude of forces during grasping or catching tasks, people with cerebellar injury show deficits in scaling hand forces due to an inability to predict the inertial properties of objects. Specifically, individuals with cerebellar problems tend to re-adjust gripping forces approximately 100 ms after the object contacts the hands in catching tasks; which is indicative of the execution of motor commands based on sensory feedback more than sensory prediction (Therrien & Bastian, 2019).

Clinical Case Study

John C.: Impairments Associated with Cerebellar Degeneration. John is our patient with spinocerebellar ataxia type 2, a genetic disorder causing slow degeneration of the cerebellum. John has significant problems in coordination. He evidences dysmetria and dyssynergia (errors in the timing and metrics of multijoint movements). This can be seen in the impairment section of his video, when he is asked to alternate touching his nose and the tester's finger and in his legs when he is asked to slide the heel of one leg down the shin of the other (heel-to-shin test). In both cases, his movements are slow, jerky, and erratic, and the trajectory of his movement is not smooth. He also has dysdiadochokinesia, which can be seen by his inability to sustain a rapid alternating rhythmic movement, including pronation and supination of his hands. He has difficulty terminating a movement as seen by the rebound of his arm when it is released from resistance. Though some persons with cerebellar pathology evidence hypotonia, John does not. In addition, his underlying strength is excellent.

Sue D.: Impairments Associated with Multiple Sclerosis. Sue is our 66-year-old woman diagnosed with relapsing remitting multiple sclerosis (MS). MS is a degenerative neurological disease affecting approximately 350,000 people in the United States and as many as 2 million worldwide (Noseworthy et al., 2000). MS is an immune-mediated disease that causes demyelination and degeneration within the brain and spinal cord. Symptoms depend on the location and severity of demyelination, are highly variable, but typically include sensory, cognitive, and motor impairment. MS is a progressive disease resulting in progressive disability, which is measured clinically by the Expanded Disability Status Scale (Kurtzke, 1983), a 0 to 10 scale in which 0.0 represents no impairment due to MS, 4.0 indicates the onset of significant walking impairment, 7.5 indicates wheelchair dependence, and 10.0 represents death due to MS. Sue also has significant cerebellar involvement. This can be seen in the impairment segment of her video case study. When she is asked to alternate touching her nose and the tester's finger, she demonstrates mild difficulty with end point accuracy. Her cerebellar coordination problems are much more apparent in her lower extremities. When she is asked to slide the heel of one leg down the shin of the other (heel-to-shin test), she has considerable difficulty placing her heel and cannot slide it smoothly down her shin.

Motor Impairments in Basal Ganglia Pathology

Pathology in the basal ganglia can result in either "hypokinetic disorders," such as Parkinson's disease (PD), which is characterized by diminished movement, or hyperkinetic disorders, such as Huntington's disease (HD) or athetoid CP, which is characterized by excessive movement. Our case study, Malachi, is an example of a child with damage to the basal ganglia resulting in athetoid CP. Because of complex connections with the cerebral cortex, damage to the basal ganglia is often associated with cognitive and behavioral disturbances in addition to motor deficits.

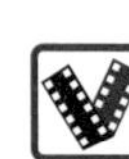

Hypokinetic Disorders: PD. PD was first described by James Parkinson in 1817 (Kandel et al., 2000b; Parkinson, 1817). The PD-related movement disorders are due to a dysfunction of the basal ganglia-thalamocortical motor circuit (Wichmann & DeLong, 2013). Cardinal signs of PD include paucity of spontaneous movement (akinesia), voluntary movements that are slow and reduced in amplitude (bradykinesia), increased muscle tone (rigidity), and a resting tremor. Also, characteristics of PD are flexed posture and impaired balance and gait. PD results from degeneration of dopaminergic neurons in the substantianigra pars compacta.

Bradykinesia and akinesia. In patients with PD, there is a complex constellation of motor, sensory, cognitive–emotional, and sleep alterations that impair activities of daily living. *Akinesia* is the inability to initiate or execute movements. *Hypokinesia* is a reduced frequency and amplitude of spontaneous or automatic movements (i.e., blinking, facial movements that result in a mask-like expression, or reduced arm swinging during gait). Micrographia is a functional outcome of hypokinesia in which there is a reduction in the amplitude and speed of automatized (well-learned) wrist movements during writing. *Bradikinesia* is characterized by slow initiation and execution of movements; and during repetitive voluntary movements, the amplitude tends to progressively diminish until there is no motion. All these hypokinetic features in PD significantly impair the ability to perform sequential movements and carry out simultaneous tasks—which likely reflect an impairment of procedural learning processes, as the basal ganglia play an important role in such type of learning (Gordon et al., 1997; Horak, 1990; Rodriguez-Oroz et al., 2009; Shukla et al., 2012; Teulings et al., 1997; Wichmann & DeLong, 2013). A study has found an association between functional deficits such as micrographia and bradykinesia and hypophonia—a characteristic soft and reduced speech volume of people with PD (Shukla et al., 2012). While bradykinesia is characteristic of pathology in the basal ganglia, prolonged movement time is a commonly reported impairment associated with a wide variety of neural pathologies, including stroke (Levin et al., 1993; Levin, 1996), CP (Steenbergen et al., 1998), and cerebellar dysfunction (Van Donkelaar & Lee, 1994).

Rigidity. Rigidity is characterized by a heightened muscle resistance to passive movement of joints. Shortening reactions, which are significantly influenced by joint afferents and mediated by long-lasting stretch reflexes, have been proposed to mediate muscle rigidity in PD (Katz & Rondot, 1978; Xia & Rymer, 2004). Parkinsonian muscle tone does not manifest as spasticity, which is a velocity-dependent pathological reflex. However, some studies and authors report that PD-related muscle rigidity can be velocity- and amplitude-dependent during large-amplitude passive joint movements. Velocity-dependent changes in PD-related rigidity could be due to the interaction between the velocity-dependent increases in the stretch reflex of the antagonist muscle (stretched muscle) and unchanged contributions of the velocity-independent activity of the shortening reaction found in the agonist muscles (shortened muscle) (Andrews et al., 1972; Powell et al., 2012; Xia et al., 2009). Moreover, muscle rigidity in PD has been proposed to be the result of hyperactivity in the fusimotor system and it tends to be predominant in flexor muscles (Noth, 1991). Presently, there is no clear evidence on how dopamine-induced basal ganglia impairments can affect reflexive mechanisms. Another neural observation is that while premotor and prefrontal areas are hypoactive in PD, there is enhanced primary cortical excitability (Brodmann area 4) that may hyperactivate the subthalamic nucleus and subsequently increase reflex gains (Obeso et al., 2008). There are two well-defined types of rigidity, lead pipe (plastic-like feeling) and cogwheel. Lead pipe rigidity is characterized by a constant resistance to movement throughout the entire range of motion. Cogwheel rigidity is characterized by alternating episodes of resistance and relaxation, so-called catches, as the extremity is passively moved through its range of motion (Rodriguez-Oroz et al., 2009).

Tremor. Resting tremor is a cardinal impairment in people with PD. It consists of an involuntary 4 to 6 Hz limb oscillation with certain predominance in distal segments. The "pill-rolling" tremor is owed to the continuous oscillatory motion of fingers. In line with this clinical observation, research has also found a rhythmical 4 to 6 Hz firing rate in neuronal recordings of the basal ganglia nuclei (globuspallidus and subthalamic nucleus) and thalamus (ventralis intermedius nucleus). Jaw muscles and tongue may also be involved (Obeso et al., 2008; Rodriguez-Oroz et al., 2009). Resting tremor occurs in a body part that is not voluntarily activated and is supported against gravity. However, the amplitude of resting tremor increases during mental stress or during movements of another body part (especially the movements involved in walking). Postural tremor is present in PD patients when voluntarily maintaining a position against gravity. Kinetic tremor occurs during a voluntary movement and can vary from a simple kinetic tremor (not target related) to an intention tremor (those occurring during a target-directed movement). A complete discussion of this complex topic is provided in reviews by Deuschl et al. (1998) and Hallett (1998).

Hyperkinetic Disorders. Hyperkinetic disorders of the basal ganglia, such as HD, hemiballismus, and athetoid CP, are characterized by excessive and involuntary movements and decreased muscle tone (hypotonia). Chorea or choreiform movements are involuntary, rapid, irregular, and jerky movements that result from basal ganglia lesions. Chorea is one type of dyskinesia that is often observed as a side effect of antiparkinsonian medications in people with PD. Choreiform dyskinesias typically emerge after prolonged use of antiparkinsonian medications and are typically observed at the peak or at the end of a dose of antiparkinsonian medications. Athetosis, or athetoid movement, consists of slow involuntary writhing and twisting movements, usually involving the upper extremities more than the lower extremities; however, they may also involve the neck, face, and tongue. Athetoid CP is the second most common form of CP (Jellinger, 2019).

Dystonia. The term "dystonia" was first used in 1911 by the neurologist Hermann Oppenheim (cited in Marsden & Quinn, 1990). *Dystonia* is a syndrome dominated by sustained or intermittent muscle contractions, frequently causing hypertonia, twisting and repetitive movements, and abnormal postures (Fahn et al., 1987). Dystonia is often initiated or worsened by voluntary action and it is associated with overflow muscle activation, defined as unintentional muscle contractions that are different from those involved in the primary dystonic pattern (Albanese et al., 2013; Sanger, 2018). The abnormal movements associated with dystonia are diverse and range from slow athetotic to quick myoclonic dystonia (Fahn et al., 1987).

Dystonic movements are often characterized by cocontraction of agonist and antagonist muscles (Hallett, 1993; Rothwell, 1995–1996). While dystonia is thought to be primarily a disorder of the basal ganglia, animal models and human data suggest that dystonia may also result from lesions in the thalamus, cerebellum, and brainstem as well (Sanger, 2018).

Clinical Case Studies

Mike M.: Motor Impairments Associated with PD (Hypokinetic Disorder). Mike is our patient with PD. As seen in the impairment section of his video, Mike's primary neuromuscular impairments include rigidity, bradykinesia, resting and postural tremor, and impairments of postural control and gait. Mike has a mild resting tremor, moderate postural tremor, and mild kinetic tremor when on medication. Off medication, resting tremor remains mild but postural and kinetic tremor increase substantially. His bradykinesia (or slowed movement) on both the finger-to-nose test and when asked to repeatedly tap his finger or his foot are worse off medication compared to on medication. Mike has rigidity, which is felt as resistance to passive motion of his arms, legs, and neck. All of his impairments are much worse when he is off medication compared to when on.

Malachi: Athetoid CP (Hyperkinetic Disorder). Malachi is our 3.5-year-old child with mixed-type CP. He has significant athetoid and dystonic components affecting control of his facial muscles and upper-extremity movements. These impairments are particularly evident in the upper-extremity segment of his video case study. Note the finger and hand posturing he does when reaching and grasping. Also, note his rapid dystonic movements, particularly when he is excited.

Secondary Musculoskeletal Impairments

In the patient with CNS lesions, musculoskeletal disorders develop most often secondary to the primary lesion. Since physical activity is necessary to the maintenance of both muscle and the bony skeleton, the limitations in movement associated with neurologic pathology can lead to a wide range of musculoskeletal problems, including muscle atrophy and deconditioning, contractures, degenerative joint disease, and osteoporosis (Fredericks & Saladin, 1996).

In CNS pathologies like PD, the loss of skeletal muscle tissue because of neuromuscular factors and aging (sarcopenia) causes a decline in strength and function (Lima et al., 2020; Waltson, 2012). Lima and colleagues (2020) investigated in 218 patients with PD the relationship between the presence of sarcopenia (SARC-F questionnaire) and low muscle strength with the risk of falls. The authors found that 55.5% of the patients with PD tested positive in the SARC-F and the presence of falls was more frequent in these patients compared to those that screened negative for sarcopenia. This is yet another example of how muscle weakness can increase the likelihood of falling in PD. However, as we saw before in this chapter, there may be many other neurological and musculoskeletal factors involved in the risk of falls in this population. Spasticity is associated with changes in the physical properties of the muscle, including increased fiber-size variability (Ito et al., 1996), and in other tissues, including the amount and composition of extracellular matrix material (Lieber et al., 2003). Researchers analyzing gait in children with CP have found that increased tension in the gastrocnemius muscle is not always associated with increased muscle activity in that muscle, supporting the concept that spastic patterns of movement are partly due to changes in intrinsic muscle characteristics (Berger et al., 1984a).

In stroke, impaired muscle recruitment and cortical activation are predominately responsible for muscle paresis and weakness with subsequent muscle atrophy (loss of muscle mass), which in turn correlates with decreased gait speed and reduced physical fitness (Hunnicut et al., 2017). Paresis is therefore another primary neuromuscular impairment that results in underlying structural changes to the muscle. Positioning a paretic muscle in a shortened position results in muscle unloading (a reduction in longitudinal tension), which is the first step in the development of muscle contracture (Gracies, 2005a, 2005b). Furthermore, muscle unloading results in atrophy, a reduction in muscle cross-sectional area, loss of sarcomeres (shortening), an accumulation of connective tissue, and an increase in fat deposits in the tendons (Gracies, 2005a, 2005b). Immobilization of a muscle at a shortened range also results in changes in the joint, including proliferation of connective tissue into the joint space, adherence of connective tissue to cartilage surfaces, atrophy of the cartilage, and disorganization of ligament alignment (Liebesman & Carafelli, 1994). Immobilization also results in a reduction in bone mineralization leading to regional osteopenia or osteoporosis (Alzghoul et al., 2004).

Thus, primary neuromuscular impairments result in secondary musculoskeletal impairments, which are a significant constraint on functional movements.

IMPAIRMENTS IN SENSORY SYSTEMS

As discussed in Chapter 3, sensation plays multiple roles in the control of normal movement. Thus, it should not be surprising that sensory deficits are a major factor contributing to motor control problems in patients with CNS lesions. The type of sensory problem will depend on the location of the lesion (i.e., where in the sensory pathway the lesion is) as well as the size of the lesion. The following sections discuss the effect of CNS pathology on sensory and perceptual aspects of motor control.

Somatosensory Deficits

Both researchers and clinicians alike have shown a strong association between impaired somatosensation and recovery of motor function following CNS damage, with most of the research related to stroke. The prevalence rates of somatosensory impairment following stroke range from 11% to 85%; the specific deficits depend on the location and extent of damage (Yekutiel, 2000). Research examining sensory deficits in human patients is complicated because damage is rarely localized to a specific brain area.

Damage to the primary somatosensory cortex (S-I) results in contralesional loss of touch and proprioception, but not often to loss of temperature or nociception. Specific and localized lesions in the anterior parietal cortex lead to severe difficulties with touch threshold, vibration, joint position sense, and two-point discrimination tasks. More complex functions such as texture discrimination and stereognosis are also impaired; however, patients have relatively little impairment of exploratory and skilled movement tasks, such as catching a ball or pinching small objects between the fingertips (Gardner & Johnson, 2013a).

The posterior parietal cortex is a region for multimodal integration, which enables the representation of the surrounding environment important to the planning and execution of object-centered movements. Specifically, the intraparietal sulcus serves as an interface between motor and perceptual systems critical to controlling functionally oriented visuomotor and object manipulation tasks, and visual spatial attention (Giacomo & Kalaska, 2013; Grefkes & Fink, 2005). Lesions in the posterior parietal cortex lead to mild difficulty with simple tactile tests, but profound difficulty with complex tactile recognition tasks, as well as significant problems with exploratory and skilled movements. Patients also have difficulty shaping the hand to the orientation and shape of objects and often misdirect the arm during reaching. Finally, patients with localized lesions in secondary SS cortex (S-II) have difficulty with complex tactile discrimination tasks, such as stereognosis (Gardner & Johnson, 2013b).

Stroke-related impairments in the somatosensory system are associated with significant loss of function. In general, impaired somatosensory function has been related to a longer hospital length of stay following stroke (Sommerfeld & Von Arbin, 2004; Tyson et al., 2008). Specific impairments are also predictive of recovery of function. For example, impaired two-point discrimination was associated with poor recovery of upper limb dexterity (Au-Yeung & Hui-Chan, 2009), while impaired proprioception was associated with poor recovery of functional upper-extremity movement (Desrosiers et al., 2002). Combined impairment of light touch and proprioception was related to poor recovery of activities of daily living (ADL) function in some studies (Park et al., 2008) but not in others (Paci et al., 2009). Finally, stroke-related somatosensory deficits are related to impaired motor learning (Vidoni & Body, 2009). Both Genise and Jean, our patients with stroke, have significantly impaired somatosensation, including reduced light touch and two-point discrimination. Sue, our patient with MS, also has impaired light touch and two-point discrimination.

Impaired proprioception has also been reported in patients with PD, especially those who rely on visual guidance to control voluntary movements. While clinical examination rarely reveals sensory system impairments in patients with HD, somatosensory-evoked potential studies reveal abnormal responses to sensory nerve stimulation, suggesting a possible role of impaired sensorimotor integration in HD voluntary movement control. Thus, research suggests that abnormalities in the brain's ability to integrate sensory information, particularly somatosensory information, may interfere with the processing of motor programs in the cortical motor areas and contribute to movement disorders in patients with basal ganglia pathology (Abbruzzese & Berardelli, 2003).

As you can see, pathology in the somatosensory system can result in a wide range of sensory impairments depending on the location and size of the lesion. Damage to the parietal cortex, including primary, secondary, and associative areas, does not simply reduce the ability to perceive information coming in from somatosensory inputs in one part of the body but affects the ability to integrate somatosensory inputs with other sensory modalities from multiple parts of the body and interpret this information, so it can be used in complex ways.

Visual Deficits

As discussed in Chapter 3, vision gives us information on the position and movement of objects in space (vision as an exteroceptive sense) as well as the position and movement of our own bodies (visual proprioception). As was true for the somatosensory system, disorders of the visual system will vary according to the location of the lesion (Fig. 5.7). A person who has a stroke to the right occipital lobe will have a visual field defect, homonymous hemianopsia, or the loss of visual information for one hemifield. A stroke on the right side of the brain (especially parietal lobe), in addition to producing a homonymous hemianopsia, may also lead to the syndrome of hemispatial neglect. Because their strokes were in the left hemisphere, neither Jean nor Genise has a visual field defect. In addition, neither one has hemispatial neglect.

In addition, interruptions of the dorsal versus ventral stream—coming from the visual cortex—result in different types of impairments. Dysfunction of the dorsal stream in the posterior parietal cortex may result in visuomotor disorders such as optic ataxia. People who suffer optic ataxia show problems with reaching in the contralesional visual field, impaired preshaping of the hand while grasping, and inability to correct reaching movements online (Andersen et al., 2014). In contrast, the ventral stream, which projects to the temporal lobe, provides detailed information about the world for cognitive tasks such as recognition, identification, and planning. A dysfunction of the ventral stream causes visual agnosia (impaired recognition of visual stimuli) (Goddale et al., 2005).

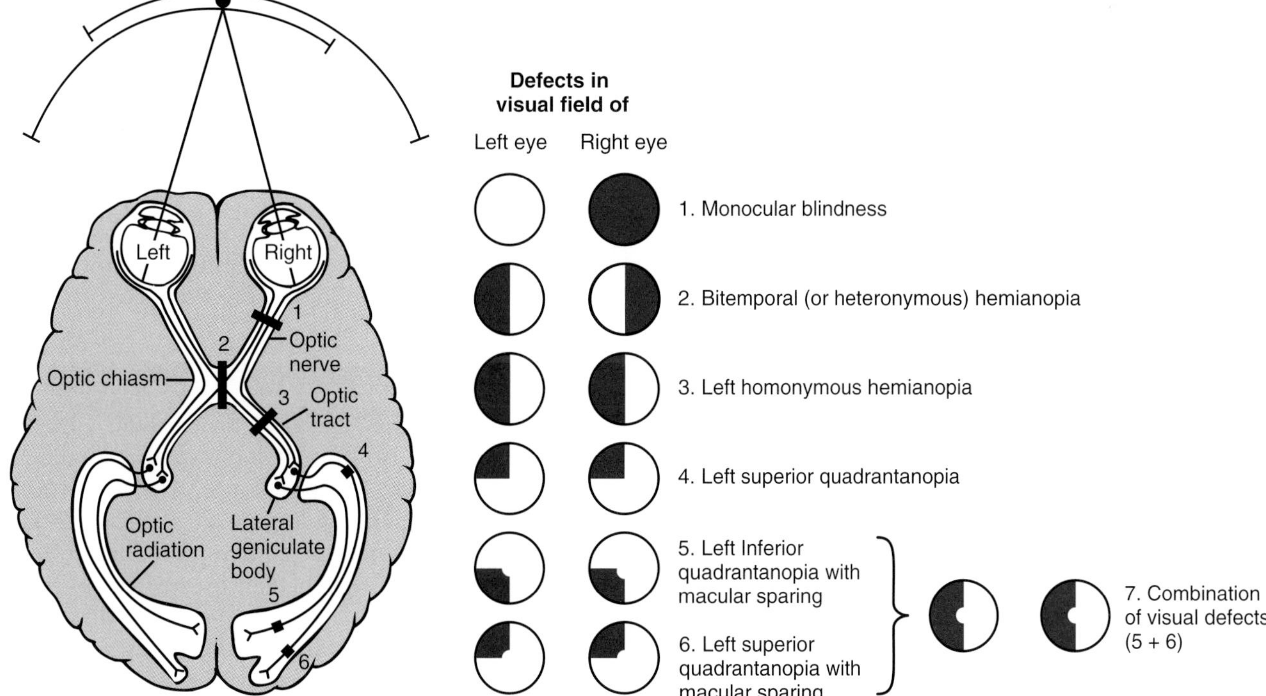

Figure 5.7 Visual deficits produced by lesions at various locations in the visual system.

Vestibular Deficits

The vestibular system provides sensory information regarding head movements and position with reference to gravity. Vestibular afferent information is used for gaze stabilization, posture, and balance, and it contributes to our conscious sense of orientation in space. Thus, pathology within the vestibular system can produce problems related to (a) gaze stabilization, including blurred vision or oscillopsia (oscillating vision), due to the disruption of the vestibuloocular reflex; (b) posture and balance; and (c) vertigo or dizziness (Herdman, 2007; Shumway-Cook & Horak, 1989, 1990).

The term *dizziness* is often used by patients to describe a variety of sensations, including spinning of the environment relative to themselves (referred to as "vertigo"), rocking, tilting, unsteadiness, and lightheadedness. The specific types of symptoms found depend on the type and location of pathology within the vestibular system and are discussed in more detail in the section on clinical management of vestibular disorders.

PATHOLOGY OF HIGHER-ORDER ASSOCIATION CORTICES: SPATIAL AND NONSPATIAL IMPAIRMENTS

Peter is a 68-year-old man who has had a stroke. On examination, his visual fields are normal, but his gaze tends to deviate to the right. When presented with two objects, one in each visual field, he always looks to the right object and denies the presence of the object presented on the left. However, when he is asked to move his eyes to the left, he can report seeing that object. When presented with objects scattered on a table, he explores mainly on the right side of the table, and only searches on the left when directed. Touches on his right hand are easily detected but he fails to consistently detect touches on his left side. Though his motor function is normal with respect to strength, coordination, and dexterity on both sides, he is reluctant to use his left hand unless specifically asked to. This clinical picture illustrates some of the key features of unilateral spatial neglect, a common outcome of a stroke in the right parietal lobe.

What are the factors that contribute to spatial neglect and other behavioral disorders in this patient? Is it the result of a focal lesion producing a specific perceptual problem? Or, is it the result of an interruption in a complex distributed network of attention processes that affect perceptual function? Traditionally, the clinical approach to understanding neglect and other types of spatial and nonspatial deficits has been to examine the relationship between focal lesions in specific areas of the CNS and their associated impairments, or to subcategorize different types and forms of spatial and nonspatial impairments based on performance of different behavioral tests.

More recently, a new framework for understanding spatial disorders, such as neglect, and nonspatial disorders has been proposed. In this framework, the core deficit underlying these disorders is disruption in a one of several distributed attentional networks. These include the dorsal–frontal–parietal network that controls spatial attention and eye movements and the ventral–frontal–parietal network involved in nonspatial behaviors such as arousal, reorienting, and detection of novel events. There is a great deal of interaction between these two networks, such that a deficit in ventral network affecting nonspatial processing directly affects processing in the dorsal network and spatial attention (Corbetta & Shulman, 2011).

A second framework for examining attention and subsequent impairments related to CNS pathology categorizes attention, slightly differently, according to a set of three separate attentional networks: alerting (bilateral thalamus, brainstem), orientation (right pulvinar and temporoparietal regions; the dorsal and ventral networks described above are part of this orienting network), and conflict resolution or executive attention (anterior cingulate cortex, frontoparietal cortex) (Petersen & Posner, 2012). Both these frameworks are consistent in suggesting an attentional basis for both spatial and nonspatial deficits.

Right Hemisphere Spatial Deficits

The primary spatial impairment in patients who have hemineglect is an inability to attend to stimuli in contralesional egocentric space (De Haan et al., 2012). Extinction, a condition similar to neglect, represents a failure to identify a contralesional stimulus only when it is presented simultaneously with an ipsilateral stimulus (De Haan et al., 2012). Hemineglect and extinction can occur in any sensory modality (e.g., auditory, visual, or somatosensory). Visual neglect (VN) can be either egocentric, which is related to the body itself, or allocentric, related to the environment. In the clinic, the term "visual neglect" or "unilateral neglect" primarily refers to egocentric VN, which is the most common form of neglect. Spatial deficits such as hemineglect are related to disruption within the dorsal attention network.

Right Hemisphere Nonspatial Deficits

Damage to the right ventral frontoparietal cortex in neglect patients also impairs nonspatial functions including an inability to reorient attention, to attend to novel stimuli, and to maintain arousal and vigilance.

Patients with neglect are also impaired in reorienting their attention to unexpected events (Petersen & Posner, 2012). Patients demonstrate larger deficits in detecting contralesional targets when they expect an ipsilesional target; this suggests the existence of a deficit in disengaging attention from the ipsilesional field (Corbetta & Shulman, 2011).

Patients with right hemisphere lesions, including those with neglect, also show deficits in target detection, as indicated by slowed reaction times. Auditory reaction time is much slower in patients with right hemisphere damage compared to those with left hemisphere damage (Corbetta & Shulman, 2011; Howes & Boller, 1975). Slowed reaction times in these patients are not the result of motor deficits but instead appear to reflect deficits in arousal and processing capacity (Duncan et al., 1999). Finally, deficits in arousal and vigilance are also common among patients with spatial neglect (Corbetta & Shulman, 2011).

This concludes review of pathophysiology in the motor, sensory, and cognitive systems. We now turn to a discussion of clinical methods for examining and treating these impairments.

CLINICAL MANAGEMENT OF IMPAIRMENTS IN THE ACTION (MOTOR) SYSTEMS

Motor Cortex and Corticospinal Tract Impairments

Pathology in the descending motor system (motor cortex and medial and lateral corticospinal tracts) is characterized by paresis and abnormalities of muscle tone. Clinical assumptions regarding the relative importance of each of these impairments to functional limitations are changing in response to research examining this question, and this in turn has had an impact on clinical practice.

Motor Paresis/Weakness

Examination. Paresis/weakness is a hallmark of lesions in the descending motor system and is clinically assessed in a number of ways. Resting posture of the limbs and trunk is noted, as is the extent and distribution of voluntary movement. Examples of this may be seen in the impairment segment of the video case studies related to Genise and Jean. In the clinic, manual muscle testing (assessing a subject's ability to move a body segment through its range of motion against gravity, or against externally applied resistance) is the most common approach to measuring strength (Andrews, 1991; Buchner & DeLateur, 1991). However, whether strength should be tested in a person with a CNS lesion remains controversial.

Traditionally, clinicians believed that an accurate measurement of strength in individuals with CNS pathology was neither possible nor appropriate. This was based on the assumption that the primary impairment affecting functional performance was not weakness, but spasticity. In addition, strength training in the person with a CNS lesion was considered contraindicated, since it was believed that strength training would increase tone problems (Bobath, 1990). However, this view has changed in the last years, as shown by the research presented earlier in this chapter, which demonstrates that weakness (a negative sign) is as important and, in some cases, more important in determining functional performance than spasticity (a positive sign) (Andrews & Bohannon, 2000; Bohannon & Walsh, 1992; Katz & Rymer, 1989; Powell et al., 1999; Smith et al., 1999; Wiley & Damiano, 1998). Thus, measuring strength, whether tested isometrically, isotonically, or isokinetically, is an important part of examination of the patient with motor system pathology.

The gold standard equipment to measure muscle strength is isokinetic dynamometers. In most instances, clinicians evaluate muscle strength following manual muscle tests such as those described by authors like Kendall (Kendall et al., 2005) or Daniels and Worthingham (Avers & Brown, 2019). In manual muscle testing, patients are instructed to elicit specific movements in standardized positions while the examiner offers specific hand placements to resist a muscle or a muscle group. The use of gravity and the intensity of external resistance offered by the examiner are of critical importance to grade muscle strength (Avers & Brown, 2019; Kendall et al., 2005). For example, the Medical Research Council Manual Muscle Testing scale grades muscle strength on a 0 to 5 scale (Table 5.1) (Ciesla et al., 2011). A digital hand-held dynamometer is practical, affordable, and it can be a reliable and valid tool to obtain objective and accurate muscle strength measurements. Generally, there are two techniques. In the *make-technique*, the patient exerts maximal isometric contraction while the examiner holds the dynamometer in a fixed position; whereas, in the *break-technique*, the examiner tries to overpower the maximal effort generated by the patient (Burns & Spanier, 2005). One complication of using a hand-held dynamometer is the lack of standardized method describing how to perform manual muscle tests using this device (Mentiplay et al., 2015; Stark et al., 2011).

Treatment: Recruiting Paretic Muscles. A number of clinical strategies have been suggested to improve recruitment of paretic muscles. Biofeedback and functional electrical stimulation (FES) are interventions typically used to assist patients in recruiting paretic muscles for functional activities. For example, electrical stimulation of the peroneal nerve is commonly performed in patients with hemiplegia to improve control over the anterior tibialis muscle during a voluntary contraction or during gait. FES has been used to improve recruitment of paretic upper-extremity muscles following stroke.

Powell et al. (1999) used FES of the wrist extensors in 60 patients with hemiparesis 2 to 4 weeks after stroke. Subjects were randomly assigned to a control group who received standard treatment or to an experimental group who received standard treatment in addition to

TABLE 5.1 Grading Scale to Measure Strength Following the Medical Research Council System

Grade	Resistance
5	Movement against gravity plus full resistance
4	Movement against gravity plus some resistance
3	Completes the available test range of motion against gravity, but tolerates no resistance
2	The patient completes full or partial range of motion with gravity eliminated
1	Slight contractility without any movement
0	No evidence of contractility (complete paralysis)

Reprinted with permission from Ciesla N, Dinglas V, Fan E, Kho M, Kuramoto J, Needham D. Manual muscle testing: A method of measuring Extremity muscle strength applied to critically ill patients. *J Vis Exp*. 2011;50:2632.

FES of the wrist extensors (30 minutes 3 times a day for 8 weeks). They found that the FES group had significantly greater isometric strength of the wrist extensors as compared with the control group, suggesting that FES is a viable therapeutic intervention to improve strength in wrist extensors in patients after stroke.

Case reports have been published on the integration of FES into functional task training of the upper extremity following stroke (Brown et al., 2000; Sullivan & Hedman, 2004). Sullivan and Hedman (2004) used a combination of sensory stimulation and FES to improve upper limb function in a 67-year-old man 5 years after stroke. Sensory stimulation over the hemiparetic wrist extensors (electrical stimulation [10 seconds on and 10 seconds off] that was perceived but resulted in no observable or palpable muscle contraction) was carried out for 2 hours per day. FES was delivered to the wrist extensors while the patient practiced a lifting task for 15 minutes twice a day (Fig. 5.8). After 18 weeks of home exercise that included six physical therapy home visits, there was a significant improvement on scores on the Action Research Arm Test (Fig. 5.9) and the Stroke Rehabilitation Assessment of Movement. In addition, the patient reported improved functional ability to button clothing, use a knife and fork, and tie fishing knots (Sullivan & Hedman, 2004).

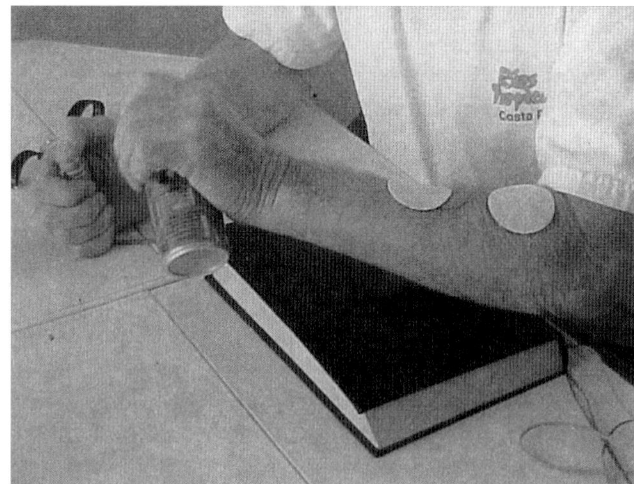

Figure 5.8 Use of neuromuscular electrical stimulation to facilitate recruitment of paretic muscles during a functional lifting task following stroke. (Adapted with permission from Sullivan JE, Hedman LD. A home program of sensory and neuromuscular electrical stimulation with upper limb task practice in a patient 5 years after stroke. *Phys Ther*. 2004;84:1048, with permission of the American Physical Therapy Association. This material is copyrighted, and any further reproduction or distribution requires written permission from APTA.)

Several researchers have suggested the use of bimanual training to improve the recovery of paretic limb function. The rationale for this approach is based on interlimb coordination studies by Kelso et al. (1981), who demonstrated that when the two hands perform identical tasks, there is a tight phasic relationship observed in which one limb "entrains" the other, causing them to function as a unit. Kelso also found that when the two limbs are performing asymmetric tasks, the limb performing the more difficult task has an impact on the limb performing the easier task. This has also been found for the performance of bilateral movements in patients with stroke hemiparesis. Following hemiparetic stroke, bilateral movement tasks resulted in slowed movement times in the nonhemiparetic limb (Lewis & Byblow, 2004; Rice & Newell, 2001, 2004) and improved movement characteristics (specifically smoother kinetic profiles) in the hemiparetic limb (Rose & Winstein, 2004). Rose and Winstein (2004) suggest that in addition to the bimanual requirement, other task requirements may be important to enhancing paretic limb function. For example, they found an increase in peak velocity in the paretic limb of subjects with stroke during asymmetric rapid aiming tasks when the paretic limb aimed at a far target.

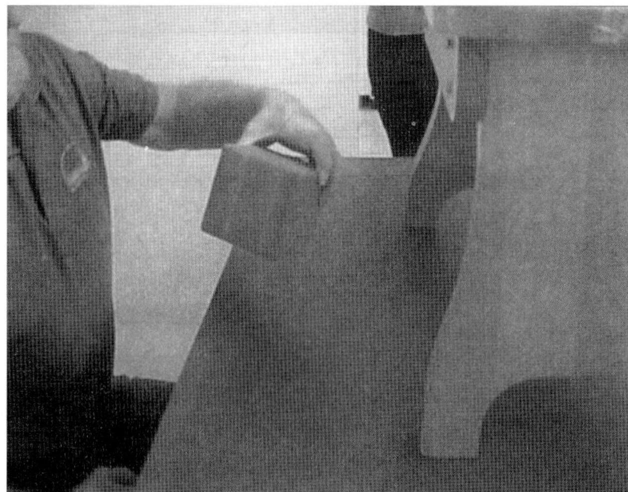

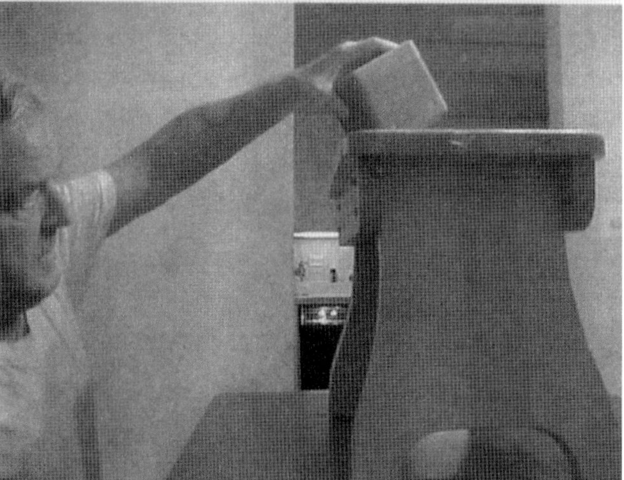

Figure 5.9 Effect of 18 weeks of FES on the Action Research Arm Test. **(A)** When the person attempts to lift a block, the wrist remains flexed. **(B)** Following FES treatment, the person lifts a block with the wrist in neutral position. (Adapted with permission from Sullivan JE, Hedman LD. A home program of sensory and neuromuscular electrical stimulation with upper limb task practice in a person 5 years post stroke. *Phys Ther.* 2004;84:1050, with permission of the American Physical Therapy Association. This material is copyrighted, and any further reproduction or distribution requires written permission from APTA.)

Task-specific effects were also reported by Lewis and Byblow (2004), who found that movement tasks involving proximal muscles benefited most from bilateral training. Research on the use of bimanual training to improve paretic limb function has been mixed. In CP, therapeutic strategies based on motor learning principles such as task-oriented practice using structured and progressive task-complexity, high number of repetitions, high intensity, and movement variability have been shown to promote neural plasticity and long-lasting functional improvements. Examples of this type of training include, Hand Arm Bilateral Intensive Training (HABIT) or HABIT involving lower extremities (Bleyenheuft et al., 2015; Friel et al., 2016; Gordon et al., 2011). A more complete review on these topics is presented in Rose and Winstein (2004); Sakzewski et al. (2014); and in Chapter 20 of this book.

Visual mirror feedback combined with movement training in the nonparetic limb has also been shown to increase recruitment of paretic muscles in both the upper and lower extremities (Ji & Kim, 2015; Sütbeyaz et al., 2007; see Thieme et al. [2012] for a review). This approach is discussed in more detail in Chapters 16 and 20 of this book and is shown in Genise'streatment video.

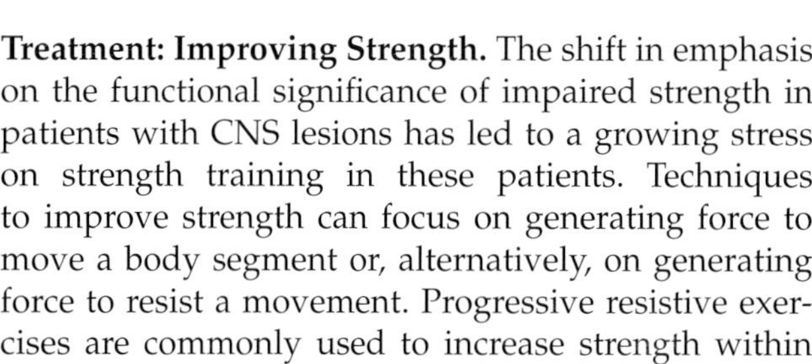

Treatment: Improving Strength. The shift in emphasis on the functional significance of impaired strength in patients with CNS lesions has led to a growing stress on strength training in these patients. Techniques to improve strength can focus on generating force to move a body segment or, alternatively, on generating force to resist a movement. Progressive resistive exercises are commonly used to increase strength within individual muscles.

Isokinetic equipment can also be used to improve a patient's ability to generate force throughout the range of motion, at different speeds of motion, and through repeated efforts within individual and groups of muscles (Duncan & Badke, 1987). There have been numerous articles examining the effects of strength training in various patient groups. In addition, there are several good review articles on strength training in persons with CP (Dodd et al., 2002; Mockford & Caulton, 2008; Scianni et al., 2009) and stroke (Morris et al., 2004; Riolo & Fisher, 2003). These reviews suggest fairly strong evidence related to the effect of strength training on improving muscle strength; however, the evidence for improving functional activities including gait was less compelling.

Individuation and Abnormal Synergies

Examination. The clinical examination of individuated movement and the presence of abnormal synergies of movement often begin with the observation and description of the resting posture of the arm and leg. In addition, the patient is asked to perform volitional isolated movements of a joint, and the quality and nature of those movements with reference to the presence of additional movement at other joints are described.

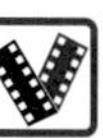

The Fugl–Meyer Assessment (FMA) is a stroke-specific test of impairments designed to evaluate recovery in the patient with poststroke hemiplegia (Fugl-Meyer et al., 1975; Gladstone et al., 2002). An example of one of the lower-extremity tasks used in this test is shown in the impairment segment of Jean's case study. The test is based on Twitchell's description of the natural history of motor recovery following stroke and Brunnstrom's stages of motor recovery and was designed as a measure of neurologic recovery at the impairment level (Gladstone et al., 2002; Poole & Whitney, 1988). The scale is organized into five domains: motor function in the upper and lower extremities, sensory functioning including light touch and joint position sense, balance, joint range of motion, and joint pain. Items are scored using a 3-point ordinal scale, where 0 = cannot perform, 1 = performs partially, and 2 = performs fully. Motor scores range from 0 (hemiplegia) to 100 (normal motor performance) points, with 66 points for the upper extremity and 34 points for the lower extremity. Training in the correct administration of the FMA is recommended; the test takes approximately 30 minutes to administer.

The psychometric properties of the FMA, particularly the Motor Subscale, have been studied extensively and shown to have good reliability (Duncan et al., 1983; Sanford et al., 1993). Several studies have established construct validity with measures of performance of activities of daily living (Fugl-Meyer et al., 1975; Wood-Dauphinee et al., 1990) and other measures of arm and hand function in stroke (De Weerdt & Harrison, 1985; Malouin et al., 1994; Rabadi & Rabadi, 2006; van der Lee et al., 2001). Rasch analysis of the upper-extremity subscale has suggested removal of the three reflex items, leaving a 30-item unidimensional measure of volitional movement (Woodbury et al., 2007). In addition, research has described and validated a short form of the Motor Scale (Hsieh et al., 2007). Another research examining the hierarchical properties of the Fugl–Meyer Motor Scale has suggested that it can be administered in a shortened manner and a summary score used (Crow et al., 2008).

Spasticity

Examination. Both clinical scales and instrumented measures have been developed to evaluate muscle tone. Muscle tone is assessed clinically by describing a muscle's resistance to quick stretch. Examples of this type of testing can be seen in the impairment segments of the case studies on Mike, our patient with PD, and both Jean and Genise, our two patients with stroke.

Subjective rating scales, such as the modified Ashworth scale (MAS) shown in Assessment Tool 5.1, are often used to describe alterations in muscle tone (Bohannon & Smith, 1987; Snow et al., 1990). The Ashworth scale has been shown to have good interrater and intrarater reliability in patients with stroke (Brashear et al., 2002; Gregson et al., 1999), but its reliability in children with CP was poor to moderate (Mutlu et al., 2008). In addition, questions have been raised as to the validity and psychometric properties of both the Ashworth and the MAS (Damiano et al., 2002; Haugh et al., 2006; Johnson, 2002; Patrick & Ada, 2006; Scholtes et al., 2006). Johnson points out that the addition of the 1+ to the scoring system raises questions as to whether it is now an ordinal scale, since it is not clear that the distances between 1 and 1+ and 1+ and 2 are equal and hierarchical in nature (Johnson, 2002). In addition, since soft tissue changes associated with muscle contractures in spastic muscles also contribute to resistance to passive movement, resistance felt to passive movements cannot be attributed solely to spasticity (Haugh et al., 2006; Patrick & Ada, 2006; Scholtes et al., 2006). Gracies (2005a, 2005b) suggest's that to assess muscle stiffness accurately, the muscle should be stretched no more than once, if possible, as subsequent stretches reduce stiffness by 20% to 60% as compared with the initial stretch. In addition, it is important that the muscle is at rest, as muscle contraction will also contribute to increased resistance to stretch.

The pendulum or drop test, first reported by Wartenberg in the early 1950s, is a clinical method for assessing hypertonicity in the lower extremities (Wartenberg, 1951). In this test, the patient sits (or is supine) with legs dangling over the edge of a table. As shown in Figure 5.10, the relaxed leg is passively straightened and released so the leg swings by gravity alone. In subjects with normal muscle tone, the leg flexes to about 70 degrees and oscillates back and forth in a pendular motion about 6 times. In a patient with quadriceps or hamstrings spasticity, the leg may not reach vertical and swings with fewer repetitions than a noninvolved leg. Leg motion can be quantified using isokinetic exercise equipment, an electrogoniometer, or computerized video equipment that measures leg kinematics (Stillman & McMeeken, 1995). The drop test has been shown to be a relatively simple, reliable, and practical objective measure of abnormal muscle tone (Brown, 1993; Katz et al., 1992). Measures of spasticity, whether clinical or instrumented, are not always

Assessment Tool 5.1

Modified Ashworth Scale for Grading Abnormal Tone

0 = No increase in muscle tone
1 = Slight increase in muscle tone, manifested by a slight catch and release or by minimal resistance at the end of the range of motion when the affected part is moved in flexion or extension
1+ = Slight increase in muscle tone, manifested by a catch, followed by minimal resistance throughout the remainder (less than half) of the range of motion
2 = More marked increase in muscle tone, passive movement difficult
3 = Considerable increase in muscle tone, passive movement difficult
4 = Affected part(s) rigid in flexion or extension

Adapted from Bohannon RW, Smith MB. Interrater reliability of a modified Ashworth scale of muscle spasticity. *Phys Ther.* 1987;67:206, with permission of the American Physical Therapy Association. This material is copyrighted, and any further reproduction or distribution requires written permission from APTA.

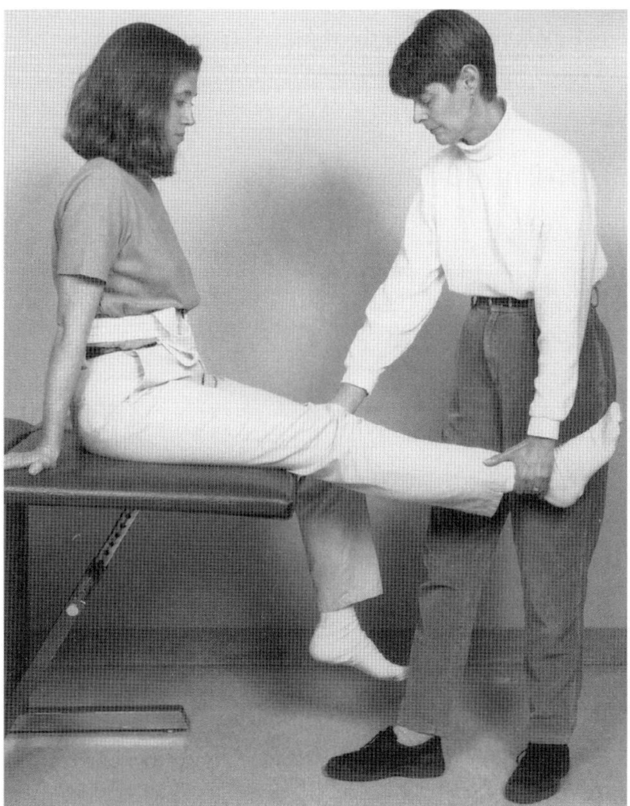

Figure 5.10 The pendulum test for spasticity in the lower extremity. The leg is passively extended then released so it swings by gravity alone. A reduction in the number of oscillations is indicative of spasticity.

good predictors of motor performance and disability, suggesting the importance of other factors.

Clinicians should be able to objectively differentiate between spasticity, hypertonia, and rigidity. For this purpose, the Hypertonia Assessment Tool (HAT) is a validated 7-item instrument that guides clinicians to discriminate among spasticity, dystonia, and rigidity in each extremity (Assessment Tool 5.2). It also helps identify in which extremity the muscle tone dysregulation occurs through scoring—two spasticity items, two rigidity items, and three dystonia items in a yes/no format (Jethwa et al., 2010; Marsico et al., 2017; Sanger et al., 2003). HAT manual and instructional videos can be found online at the Holland Bloorview Kids Rehabilitation Hospital Foundation website.

There is considerable discussion and disagreement among clinicians and researchers alike as to the validity, reliability, and clinical utility of various methods used to measure spasticity (see reviews by Burridge et al., 2005; Pandyan et al., 2001; Platz et al., 2005; Scholtes et al., 2006; Wood et al., 2005). Often, methods appropriate for use by researchers are not useful to clinicians; thus, at this time, it is difficult to identify a best practice related to the assessment of abnormalities of muscle tone.

Treatment. A number of therapeutic interventions have been developed to manage spasticity, including pharmacologic, surgical, and physical approaches. The type of treatment chosen will depend on a number of factors, including the distribution, severity, and chronicity of spasticity (Ward, 2002). For example, mild spasticity may be treated with a combination of therapeutic exercise, splinting, orthotics, and oral medication. In contrast, severe spasticity may require chemodenervation (nerve blocks or injection with botulinum toxin) and/or surgery to reduce contracture and improve motor control (Gormley et al., 1997; Ward, 2002).

Some physical approaches to managing abnormal muscle tone are based on neurophysiological rationales, while others are biomechanically based (Richardson, 2002). Neurophysiological approaches use techniques designed to alter muscle tone by changing the background level of activity in the motor neuron pool of the muscle. As the background level of activity in the motor neuron pool increases, so does the likelihood that the muscle will respond to any incoming stimulus, whether from the periphery or as part of a descending command. The opposite is also true; as background levels of activity decrease, the muscle is less likely to be activated. What techniques can be used to alter the background activity of motor neuron pools and thereby influence muscle tone?

Neurophysiological approaches, including the use of sensory stimulation techniques (sensory modalities), have traditionally been used to facilitate or inhibit muscle tone, depending on the type of stimulus and how it is applied. However, the research to support the efficacy of these techniques in altering muscle tone in patients with neural pathology is lacking. Many therapists use ice to increase muscle tone in patients with hypotonia. Alternatively, prolonged icing is considered inhibitory and is used to decrease hypertonia. Vibrators have also been used to either facilitate or inhibit activity in a muscle. High-frequency vibration tends to facilitate muscle activity, while low-frequency vibration inhibits muscle activity levels (Bishop, 1974). In the same way, a quick stretch to a muscle facilitates activation of the muscle through the stretch reflex.

Techniques, such as approximation, that activate joint receptors have also been used to facilitate muscle activity in patients with neurologic impairments. Joint approximation involves compressing a joint either manually or through the application of weights. Manual techniques that apply traction to a joint are also used to facilitate muscle activity (Voss et al., 1985).

Biomechanical approaches to managing hypertonicity focus on altering muscle length through prolonged stretching (manually or through the use of casts, splints, or orthoses). A systematic review by Bovend'Eerdt and colleagues (2008) suggested that the clinical benefit of stretching for spasticity is uncertain; while research supported the immediate effects of a single stretching session, the functional benefits and long-term consequences of stretching were unclear.

Assessment Tool 5.2

Hypertonia Assessment Tool (HAT)—Scoring Chart

HYPERTONIA ASSESSMENT TOOL (HAT) – SCORING CHART

Name: ______________________ **Chart/File #:** ______________________

Clinical Diagnosis: ______________________ **Date of Birth:** ______________________

Limb Assessed: **Gender:** ☐ Male ☐ Female

☐ Arm ☐ Left ☐ Right **HAT Assessor:** ______________________

☐ Leg ☐ Left ☐ Right **Date of Assessment:** ______________________

HYPERTONIA ASSESSMENT TOOL (HAT)

HAT ITEM	SCORING GUIDELINES (0=negative or 1=positive)	SCORE 0=negative 1=positive *(circle score)*	TYPE OF HYPERTONIA
1. Increased involuntary movements/postures of the designated limb with tactile stimulus of another body part	0 = No involuntary movements or postures observed	0	DYSTONIA
	1 = Involuntary movements or postures observed	1	
2. Increased involuntary movements/postures with purposeful movements of another body part	0 = No involuntary movements or postures observed	0	DYSTONIA
	1 = Involuntary movements or postures observed	1	
3. Velocity dependent resistance to stretch	0 = No increased resistance noticed during fast stretch compared to slow stretch	0	SPASTICITY
	1 = Increased resistance noticed during fast stretch compared to slow stretch	1	
4. Presence of a spastic catch	0 = No spastic catch noted	0	SPASTICITY
	1 = Spastic catch noted	1	
5. Equal resistance to passive stretch during bi-directional movement of a joint	0 = Equal resistance not noted with bi-directinoal movement	0	RIGIDITY
	1 = Equal resistance noted with bi-directional movement	1	
6. Increased tone with movement of another body part	0 = No increased tone noted with purposeful movement	0	DYSTONIA
	1 = Greater tone noted with purposeful movement	1	
7. Maintenance of limb position after passive movement	0 = Limb returns (partially or fully) to original position	0	RIGIDITY
	1 = Limb remains in final position of stretch	1	

SUMMARY SCORE – HAT DIAGNOSIS

			Check box:	
DYSTONIA	→	Positive score (1) on at least one of the Items #1, 2, or 6	☐ Yes	☐ No
SPASTICITY	→	Positive score (1) on either one or both of the Items #3 or 4	☐ Yes	☐ No
RIGIDITY	→	Positive score (1) on either one or both of the Items #5 or 7	☐ Yes	☐ No
MIXED TONE	→	Presence of 1 or more subgroups (e.g., dystonia, spasticity, rigidity)	☐ Yes	☐ No

HAT DIAGNOSIS:
(Fill in all that apply) ______________________

Adapted with permission from Fehlings D, Switzer L, Jethwa A, Mink J, Macarthur C, Knights S, & Fehlings T. Development of the Hypertonia Assessment Tool (HAT): *Dev Med & Child Neurol*. 2020;52:e83–e87.

Uncertainty regarding the benefits of stretching was in part due to the diversity of research methods used, making comparisons across studies difficult.

Casts, splints, and orthoses have been used to manage hypertonia, maintain or increase the passive range of motion, and improve function in patients with neural pathology. Mortenson and Eng (2003) did a systematic review and graded the evidence for the use of casts in these three areas. They concluded that the evidence did support the use of casts for improving passive range of motion, but more research was needed to determine the efficacy of casts in managing muscle tone and improving functional outcomes.

Altering a patient's position has also been suggested as a technique that can be used to alter muscle tone. The use of positioning has been argued from both neurophysiological and biomechanical perspectives. Biomechanically, positioning patients is used to improve muscle length. A neurophysiological rationale for positioning patients is based on the assumption that placing patients in certain positions will alter the distribution of muscle (and postural) tone, primarily through the changes in reflex activity. For example, it has been suggested that placing a patient in the supine position will facilitate extensor tone, while flexor tone is facilitated when the patient is prone, because of the presence of released tonic labyrinthine reflexes in the patient with lesions to motor cortex neurons. The use of a side-lying position is often suggested as an approach to inhibiting the effects of the asymmetrical tonic neck reflex on muscle tone, facilitating bilateral symmetrical activities (Bobath & Bobath, 1984).

Effect of Strength Training on Spasticity. Does training to improve strength increase spasticity as well? Teixeira-Salmela et al. (1999) examined the effects of strength training on spasticity in subjects with chronic (>9 months) stroke after a 10-week (3 days/week) program consisting of warm-up, aerobic exercise, lower-extremity muscle strengthening, and a cooldown. Changes in peak isokinetic torque production of the major muscle groups in the paretic lower limb, quadriceps and ankle plantar flexor spasticity, gait speed, and the rate of stair climbing were examined before and after training. The researchers found a significant improvement in strength in the affected muscle groups, as well as an increase in gait speed and rate of stair climbing after training. Improvements in strength were not associated with an increase in either quadriceps or ankle plantar flexor spasticity.

Damiano and Abel (1998) also investigated the effects of strength training in a group of adolescents with various forms of spastic CP. They found that training significantly improved strength in the affected muscles without increasing the severity of spasticity. Similar results were found by Scholtes and collaborators (Scholtes et al., 2010), who carried out a randomized controlled trial in 51 children with unilateral and bilateral CP. The intervention group received a functional progressive resistance muscular training (3× week, for 12 weeks). The authors found increased muscle strength of up to 14% without changes in spasticity (Scholtes et al., 2010). In summary, research has demonstrated that improving strength in the patient with descending motor system pathology is not associated with increased spasticity.

Clinical Management of Cerebellar and Basal Ganglia Impairments

Coordination

Examination. The most common approach to examining coordination is to observe patients performing functional movements and noting the characteristics of the movements used. Does the patient have difficulty initiating or terminating the functional movement? Is the movement slow? Is the movement trajectory smooth and fluid or jerky? More formal tests of coordination have been proposed and are divided into nonequilibrium and equilibrium subcategories (Schmitz, 2001). Equilibrium tests of coordination generally reflect the coordination of multijoint movements for posture and gait and will be discussed in later chapters. Nonequilibrium tests are summarized in Table 5.2 and are often used to indicate specific pathology within the cerebellum (Schmitz, 2001). Performance is graded subjectively using the following ordinal scale: 5, normal; 4, minimal impairment; 3, moderate impairment; 2, severe impairment; and 1, cannot perform. Examples of coordination tests, including finger to nose and heel to shin, may be seen in the impairment segment of two case studies, John, our patient with cerebellar pathology, and Sue, our patient with MS.

It is important to remember that coordination deficits can be caused by other factors besides neuromuscular impairments. For instance, a study has shown that children with visual defects—such as strabismus or lack of binocular vision—may present with developmental motor coordination problems compared to age-matched controls (Vagge et al., 2021). Thus, clinicians should consider a range of motor and sensory impairments that may be contributing to coordination problems.

Treatment. There are many therapeutic techniques used to treat coordination problems in patients with neurologic deficits. Some techniques can be considered "general" approaches to discoordination, while others more specifically target problems in timing, sequencing, or grading synergistic muscle activity.

Probably, the most frequently used technique to improve coordinated movement is repetition and practice of a functional task-specific movement. For example, in children with developmental coordination disorders, the use of task-oriented therapy shows substantial

TABLE 5.2 Nonequilibrium Tests of Coordination

Test	Description
1. Finger to nose	The shoulder is abducted to 90 degrees with the elbow extended. The patient is asked to bring the tip of the index finger to the tip of the nose. Alterations may be made in the initial starting position to assess performance from different planes of motion.
2. Finger to therapist's	The patient and therapist sit opposite each other. The therapist's index finger is held in front of finger of the patient. The patient is asked to touch the tip of the index finger to the therapist's index finger. The position of the therapist's finger may be altered during testing to assess ability to change distance, direction, and force of movement.
3. Finger to finger	Both shoulders are abducted to 90 degrees with the elbows extended. The patient is asked to bring both hands toward the midline and approximate the index fingers from opposing hands.
4. Alternate nose to finger	The patient alternately touches the tip of the nose and the tip of the therapist's finger with the index finger. The position of the therapist's finger may be altered during testing to assess ability to change distance, direction, and force of movement.
5. Finger opposition	The patient touches the tip of the thumb to the tip of each finger in sequence. Speed may be gradually increased.
6. Mass grasp	An alternation is made between opening and closing fist (from finger flexion to full extension). Speed may be gradually increased.
7. Pronation/ supination	With elbows flexed to 90 degrees and held close to body, the patient alternately turns the palms up and down. This test also may be performed with shoulders flexed to 90 degrees and elbows extended. Speed may be gradually increased. The ability to reverse movements between opposing muscle groups can be assessed in many joints. Example includes active alternation between flexion and extension of the knee, ankle, elbow, fingers, and so forth.
8. Rebound test	The patient is positioned with the elbow flexed. The therapist applies sufficient manual resistance to produce an isometric contraction of biceps. Resistance is suddenly released. Normally, the opposing muscle group (triceps) will contract and check movement of the limb. Many other muscle groups can be tested for this phenomenon, such as the shoulder abductors or flexors, elbow extensors, and so forth.
9. Tapping (hand)	With the elbow flexed and the forearm pronated, the patient is asked to tap the hand on the knee.
10. Tapping (foot)	The patient is asked to tap the ball of one foot on the floor without raising the knee; the heel maintains contact with floor.
11. Pointing and past pointing	The patient and therapist are opposite each other, either sitting or standing. Both patient and therapist bring shoulders to a horizontal position of 90 degrees of flexion with elbows extended. Index fingers are touching or the patient's finger may rest lightly on the therapist's. The patient is asked to fully flex the shoulder (fingers will be pointing toward ceiling) and then return to the horizontal position such that index fingers will again approximate. Both arms should be tested, either separately or simultaneously. A normal response consists of an accurate return to the starting position. In an abnormal response, there is typically a past pointing, or movement beyond the target. Several variations to this test included movements in other directions such as toward 90 degrees of shoulder abduction or toward 0 degrees of shoulder flexion (fingers will point toward the floor). Following each movement, the patient is asked to return to the initial horizontal starting position.

TABLE 5.2 Nonequilibrium Tests of Coordination (*continued*)

12. Alternate heel to knee; heel to toe	From a supine position, the patient is asked to touch the knee and big toe alternately with the heel of the opposite extremity.
13. Toe to examiner's finger	From a supine position, the patient is instructed to touch the great toe to the examiner's finger.
	The position of the finger may be altered during testing to assess ability to change distance, direction, and force of movement.
14. Heel on shin	From a supine position, the heel of one foot is slid up and down the shin of the opposite lower extremity.
15. Drawing a circle	The patient draws an imaginary circle in the air with either upper or lower extremity (a table or the floor alone may be used). This also may be done using a figure-eight pattern. This test may be performed in the supine position for lower-extremity assessment.
16. Fixation or position holding	Upper extremity: the patient holds arms horizontally in front. Lower extremity: the patient is asked to hold the knee in an extended position.

Tests should be performed first with eyes open and then with eyes closed. Abnormal responses include a gradual deviation from the "hold" position and/or a diminished quality of response with vision occluded. Unless otherwise indicated, tests are performed with the patient in a sitting position.

Reprinted from Schmitz TJ. Coordination assessment. In: O'Sullivan S, Schmitz TM, eds. *Physical rehabilitation: assessment and treatment*, 4th ed. Philadelphia, PA: FA Davis, 2001:212, with permission.

motor benefits (Smits-Engelsman et al., 2013). It is noteworthy to mention that the requirement for accuracy creates increasing demands for coordination. Thus, therapists can select functional tasks with increasing accuracy demands when training the patient on motor performance and giving attention to motor learning and control parameters, and ecological principles (i.e., the relative weight of task and environmental constraints on the action being practiced). To assist the patient in recognizing errors in performance of coordinated movement, the therapist can provide feedback (either knowledge of results or knowledge of performance). Remember from Chapter 2 that intermittent feedback facilitates learning better than constant feedback.

Use of weight-bearing activities has also been recommended for improving coordinated action in the lower extremities. In addition to functional movements, therapists often have patients practice nonfunctional movements to improve coordination. Examples of nonfunctional movements are rapid alternating movements, reciprocal movements of the hands or feet, and tracing shapes and numbers, such as Figure 8, with a limb.

A number of different therapeutic strategies can have an impact on timing components (reaction time, movement time, and termination time) of functional movement. Practicing a functional movement under externally imposed time constraints is one approach. For example, having a patient perform functional movements to music or in time with a metronome can be used to influence the timing of movement. Timing a patient while he or she performs a functional task and using the time taken to complete the task as external feedback (knowledge of results) is another approach. Verbal, visual, or manual feedback regarding speed of performance can also be used. Sensory stimulation such as brisk icing or tapping to facilitate recruitment of motor neurons may improve reaction time. Although these are common techniques used by therapists to treat coordination problems, few (if any) of these techniques have been subjected to experimental testing.

Scaling problems represent an inability to grade forces appropriately to the demands of the task. Treatment focuses on having patients practice a wide variety of tasks that require precise grading of force and providing external feedback through knowledge of results and/or performance. Functional movements performed quickly will require less precision of force control than those performed slowly. In addition, functional tasks demanding a high degree of accuracy require more precise grading of forces than those demanding limited accuracy. For example, moving to a large target will require less force control than moving to a small target. Picking up a paper cup full of water will require more precision than lifting a paper cup that is empty. Therapeutic interventions directed at remediating coordination problems during tasks related to postural control, mobility, and upper-extremity functions are presented in sections of the book related to these functions.

Involuntary Movements

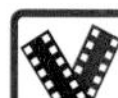

Examination. Involuntary movements, including tremor, are identified primarily through systematic clinical observation, describing the body parts affected and the conditions under which tremor is activated. Electrophysiological techniques can be further applied to determine the rhythmic oscillation of tremor (Gövert & Deuschl, 2015; Kamble & Pal, 2018). For example, a clinician might observe whether a tremor is resting versus associated with activity (action tremor). The intensity of the tremor can be graded on an ordinal scale. Conditions that increase versus decrease the severity of tremor are also noted. Tremor associated with PD can be seen in the impairment segment of Mike's video case study.

Treatment. Rehabilitation strategies for treating involuntary movement focus primarily on strategies to compensate for the movement, rather than on changing the movement itself. For example, since increased effort tends to magnify involuntary movements, patients can be taught to perform functional movements with reduced effort. Patients often tend to develop compensatory strategies on their own, such as walking with hands in pockets or grasping objects to decrease resting tremor.

Weight bearing and approximation—types of sensory integration techniques—have been recommended as a method to increase joint stability in patients with chorea or athetosis. Distal fixation is another method used to control involuntary movements and can be achieved by providing external handholds on wheelchairs, lapboards, or desks (Fig. 5.11). The use of limb weighting in the management of involuntary movement is somewhat controversial. Application of a weight to the distal portion of a limb segment increases the overall mass of the limb and results in reduced motion. However, there is some evidence that limb motion is worse when the weight is removed.

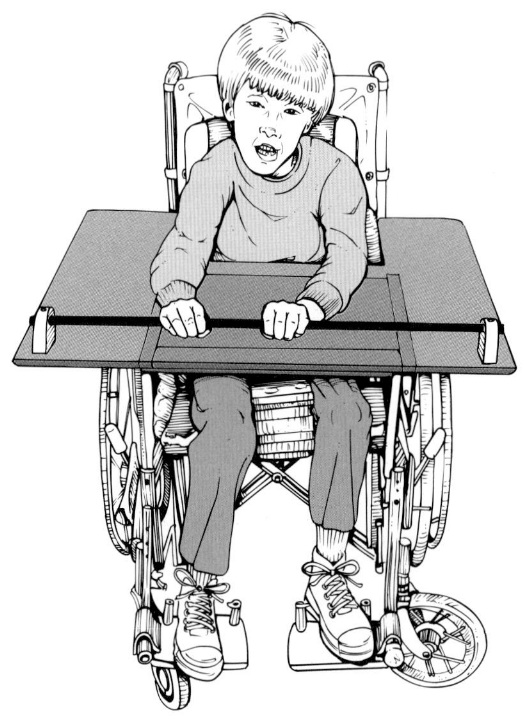

Figure 5.11 A horizontal dowel on a lapboard is used for distal fixation to control athetoid movements. (Adapted from Kandel ER, Schwartz JH, Jessell TM, eds. *Principles of neuroscience*, 4th ed. New York, NY: McGraw-Hill, 2000:544, with permission.)

These treatment approaches have also been used in the neurorehabilitation of patients who have dyskinetic disorders. However, to date there is only limited research examining the efficacy of physical and/or occupational therapy to improve the course of dyskinetic movements. Most of the available research has examined the effectiveness of medical treatments—botulinum toxin injections, therapeutic drugs (e.g., dopamine-depleting agents) or deep brain stimulation—in the treatment of dystonia or dyskinesia (Jinnah & Factor, 2015; Monbaliu et al., 2017).

Clinical Management of Musculoskeletal Impairments

Examination and treatment of impairments in the musculoskeletal system is covered in detail in other books and will not be addressed in this chapter (Kendall & McCreary, 1983; Kessler & Hertling, 1983; Magee, 1987; Saunders, 1991).

CLINICAL MANAGEMENT OF IMPAIRMENTS IN THE SENSORY SYSTEMS

The literature on examination and treatment of impairments in sensory systems including the somatosensory, visual, and vestibular system is vast. The following is a brief review, and readers are encouraged to explore other sources for a more detailed discussion of this important topic.

Somatosensory Impairments

Evaluation of somatosensation is complex, and many methods have been suggested. Sensory testing can vary from simple screening tests to complex assessment of the type and distribution of sensory function. Fess (1990) has described a hierarchy of sensory functioning. Detection, defined as the ability to distinguish a single point stimulus from background stimulation, is the lowest level of the hierarchy. Discrimination, the ability to distinguish the difference between stimulus a and stimulus b, is next. Quantification, the ability to organize tactile stimuli according to degree (e.g., roughness or weight), is the next level. Finally, cortical sensation is the highest level. It can be examined by having the patient, with eyes closed, identify letters or numbers traced on the hand palms (graphesthesia) or fingertips, or asking the patient to recognize objects by touch with one hand (stereognosis) (Blumenfeld, 2010).

Sensory tests associated with these levels within the hierarchy are summarized in Table 5.3. Fess's hierarchy suggests that it may not be necessary to test every sensory modality in a patient. If the patient is able to discriminate stimuli, sensory detection tests need not be performed. In addition, researchers have shown a high correlation among sensory tests, so that results from one test (such as two-point discrimination) can be used to

TABLE 5.3 A Summary of Methods for Testing Somatosensation[a]

Sensory modality	Stimulus	Response	Score
Discriminative Touch			
Touch awareness	Light touch to skin with cotton ball.	With vision occluded, patient says "yes" or signals when stimulus is felt.	% of correct responses out of total (e.g., 50% correct touches felt).
Touch localization	Lightly touch skin with cotton ball or monofilament number 4.17.	With vision occluded, patient points to location of touch.	Record error in accuracy of location.
Bilateral touch (sensory extinction)	Touch patient on one vs. both sides of the body with fingertips.	With vision occluded, patient says "one" or "two" to indicate number of stimuli felt.	Record presence of sensory extinction.
Touch pressure threshold	Use range of Semmes–Weinstein monofilaments.	With vision occluded, patient indicates when he or she feels stimulus.	Score the number of the thinnest filament felt (normal is perception of filament 2.83).
Two-point discrimination	Using two paper clips,apply the two points to the skin; start 5 m apart; gradually bring points together.	Patient responds "one," "two," or "can't tell."	Percentage of correct responses out of total.
Proprioception			
Vibration	Apply tuning fork or vibrometer to skin.	Patient indicates when he or she feels stimulus.	Percentage of correct responses out of total.
Joint position	Passively position joint in flexion or extension.	With vision occluded, patient mimics position with contralateral limb	Percentage of correct responses out of total.
Joint motion	Passively move the joint into flexion or extension.	With vision occluded, patient reports whether joint is bending or straightening.	Percentage of correct responses out of total.
Stereognosis	Place a series of small objects in patient's hand.	Patient names object (may manipulate object first).	Percentage of correct responses out of total.
Pain			
Pain: Sharp/dull	Randomly apply sharp and blunt end of safety pin to skin.	With vision occluded, patient indicates "sharp" or "dull."	Percentage of correct responses out of total.
Temperature			
Temperature	Apply cold (40°F) or hot (115°F) to patient's skin.	Patient indicates "hot" or "cold."	Percentage of correct responses out of total.

[a]Based on material from Bentzel K. Evaluation of sensation. In: Trombly CA, ed. *Occupational therapy for physical dysfunction,* 4th ed. Baltimore, MD: Williams & Wilkins, 1995.

predict results on other tests, such as finger proprioception (Moberg, 1991). Thus, it may be possible to select a sample of sensory tests to predict overall somatosensory functioning. Examples of various types of sensory testing including light touch, two-point discrimination, and proprioception can be seen in the impairment segment of all the video case studies.

Results from sensory testing can be interpreted in relationship to established norms—expected performance based on anatomy and pathology—or in comparison to noninvolved areas. The relationship between sensory loss and function, however, is not clear. Dellon and Kallman (1983) found that tests that best predict hand function are static and moving two-point discrimination tests.

Often, clinicians tend to view sensory impairments such as loss of limb position sense or somatosensory deficits leading to decreased object recognition as being permanent or not modifiable by treatment. However, a number of interesting studies suggest that treatment can affect the patient's ability to process sensory stimuli. Based on some studies examining the reorganization of the somatosensory cortex in primates (Merzenich et al., 1983a, 1983b), which were discussed in Chapter 4, a number of researchers have developed structured sensory reeducation programs to improve the patient's ability to discriminate and interpret sensory information (Carey et al., 1993; Dannenbaum & Dykes, 1988; DeJersey, 1979). The goal of these interventions is to improve a patient's ability to detect and process information in the environment and thereby improve motor performance. Suggestions for retraining sensory discrimination are presented in more detail in Chapter 20, which outlines methods for retraining upper-extremity control.

Visual Impairments

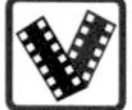

Visual testing includes information on visual acuity, depth perception, visual fields, and oculomotor control. Visual acuity can be tested directly or determined via self-report. Depth perception is critical for functional skills such as mobility or driving. It can be tested by holding two identical objects at eye level and moving one in relation to the other, asking the patient to indicate which is closer (Quintana, 1995). Visual field deficits are identified using the Visual Field Confrontation Test. The patient is told to look forward at the therapist, who sits in front of the patient. The patient is asked to indicate when he or she detects a visual stimulus (often the therapist's finger) presented in the periphery; all four visual quadrants are tested. Oculomotor tests examine the control of eye movements. These are discussed in Chapter 20, under examination of visual regard, a component of reach and grasp. Examples of visual testing can be seen in the impairment segment of the video case study of John, our patient with cerebellar degeneration.

Vestibular Impairments

Examination of vestibular function includes tests of gaze stabilization, posture and balance control, and dizziness. Treatment varies, depending on the underlying cause. Specific procedures for assessing gaze stabilization are discussed in Chapter 20, while those for assessing posture and balance are presented in Chapter 11. Thus, the following section gives a brief overview of the examination and treatment of dizziness.

Examination begins with taking a careful history to determine the patient's perceptions of whether dizziness is constant or provoked and the situations or conditions that stimulate dizziness. The Vertigo Positions and Movement Test (Shumway-Cook & Horak, 1990) examines the intensity and duration of dizziness in response to movement and/or positional changes of the head while sitting, standing, and walking. The patient is asked to rate the intensity of dizziness on a scale of 0 (no dizziness) to 10 (severe dizziness). In addition, the duration of symptoms is timed and recorded, as are the presence of nystagmus and autonomic nervous system symptoms including nausea, sweating, and pallor. The Dix–Hallpike maneuver (Fig. 5.12) is used to test for posterior semicircular canal benign paroxysmal positional vertigo (BPPV). BPPV is the most common cause of vertigo (Fetter, 2000). Most often, patients describe a spinning vertigo associated with head positions involving rapid extension of the neck (such as looking up into a high shelf) or when lying down and rolling to the affected side. Key to the diagnosis of BPPV is the Dix–Hallpike maneuver. In response to this rapid position change, the patient describes vertigo lasting from 30 seconds to 1 minute, and torsional nystagmus in the direction of the downward ear is present. The pathophysiology of BPPV is thought to be displacement of otoconia into the posterior semicircular canals (SCCs). For a detailed description of examination of dizziness, the reader is referred to other sources (Herdman, 2007; Shumway-Cook & Horak, 1989, 1990).

Treatment of vestibular pathology, referred to as "vestibular rehabilitation," uses exercises to treat symptoms of dizziness and imbalance that result from pathology within the vestibular system. Since there are many potential causes of dizziness, including metabolic disturbances; side effects of medication; cardiovascular problems, such as orthostatic hypotension; and pathology within peripheral or central vestibular structures, it is essential that the therapist know the underlying diagnosis prior to beginning an exercise-based approach.

The type of exercise used to treat dizziness depends on the specific type of pathology causing the dizziness. Vertigo secondary to posterior SCC BPPV is most often treated with a repositioning maneuver designed to mechanically move displaced otoconia from the SCC(s) (Herdman, 2007). This procedure is shown in Figure 5.13A–E.

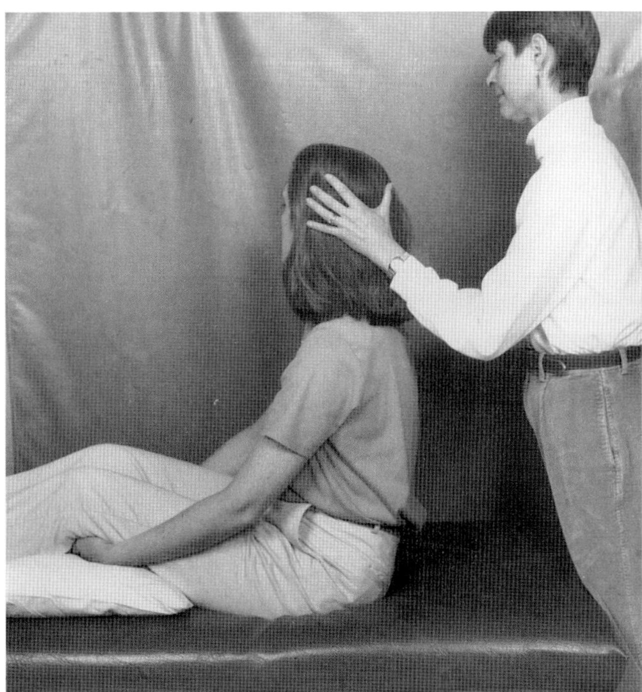

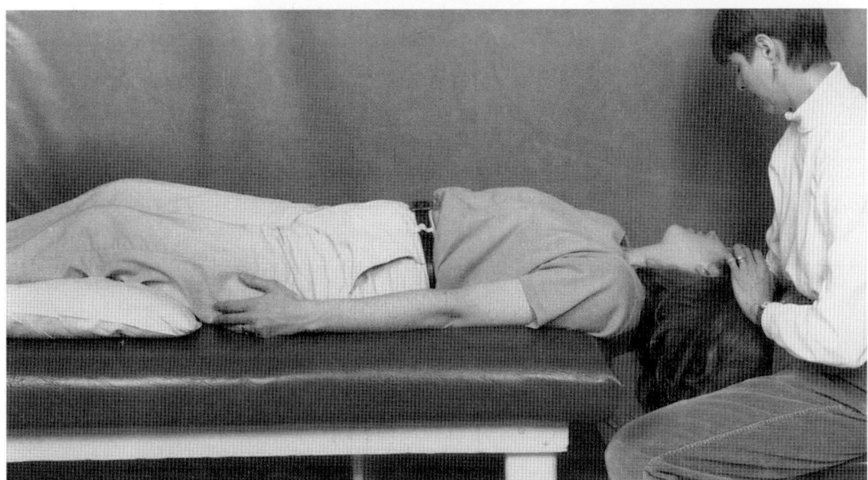

Figure 5.12 **(A)** The Dix–Hallpike position, a specific test for benign paroxysmal positional vertigo. The test is begun with the patient in the seated position. **(B)** The person is quickly assisted into a position in which the head is hanging off the edge of the supporting surface.

In contrast to treatment of positional vertigo, dizziness associated with asymmetric vestibular loss is treated with habituation exercises. The patient is instructed to repeat the position or movements that provoke dizziness 5 to 10 times in a row, 2 to 3 times per day. Exercises are progressive in nature. The patient begins with fairly simple exercises, such as horizontal head movements in the seated position, and progresses to more difficult tasks, such as horizontal head movements integrated into gait. This approach is discussed in more detail elsewhere (Herdman, 2007; Shumway-Cook & Horak, 1989, 1990). A Cochrane review suggests strong evidence for the safety and effectiveness of vestibular rehabilitation in patients with unilateral peripheral vestibular dysfunction. In the case of BPPV, the review suggests that physical maneuvers are more effective in the short-term than exercise-based vestibular rehabilitation (McDonnell & Hillier, 2015).

CLINICAL MANAGEMENT OF IMPAIRMENTS IN THE PERCEPTUAL AND COGNITIVE SYSTEMS

As discussed earlier, pathology in higher-order association cortices is associated with a wide variety of interacting perceptual and cognitive impairments. A clinical summary of some of these impairments may be found in Table 5.4. A complete discussion of the clinical management of these diverse perceptual and cognitive impairments is beyond the scope of this book; thus, only a brief review of selected spatial and nonspatial impairments follows.

Spatial Deficits: Hemineglect

Unilateral spatial neglect (in either the somatosensory or visual systems) can be assessed using formal

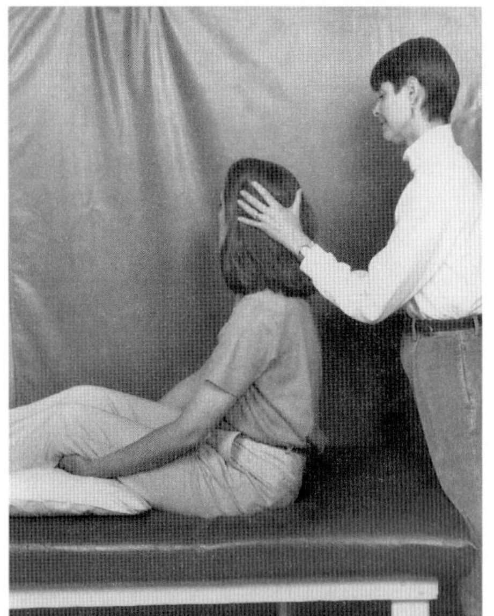
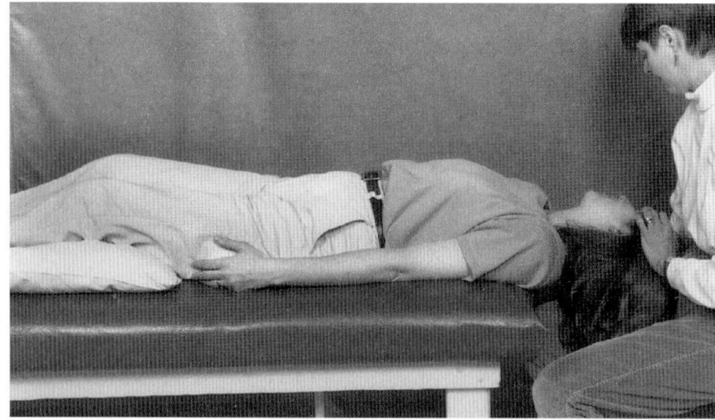
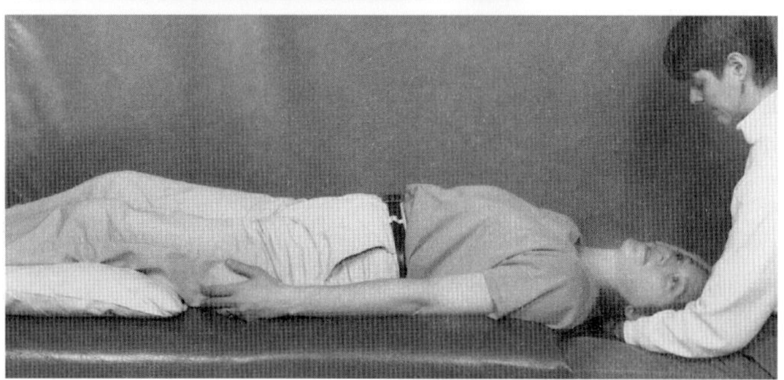
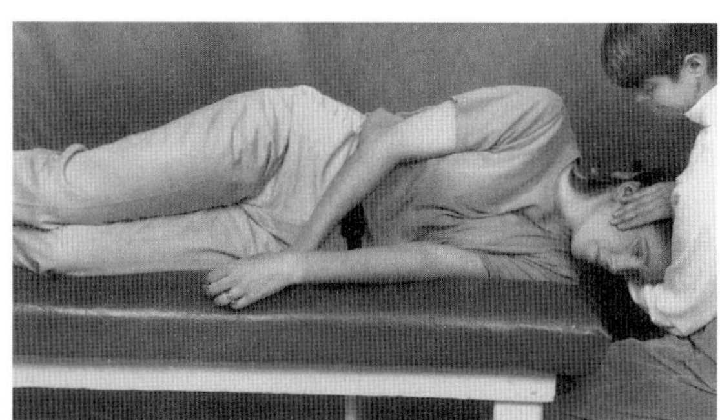
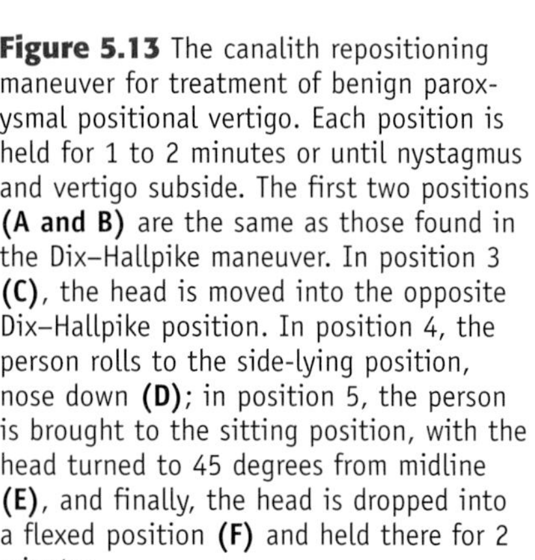
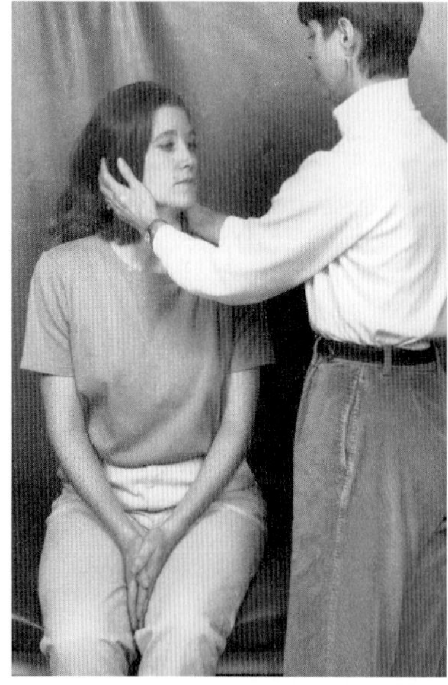
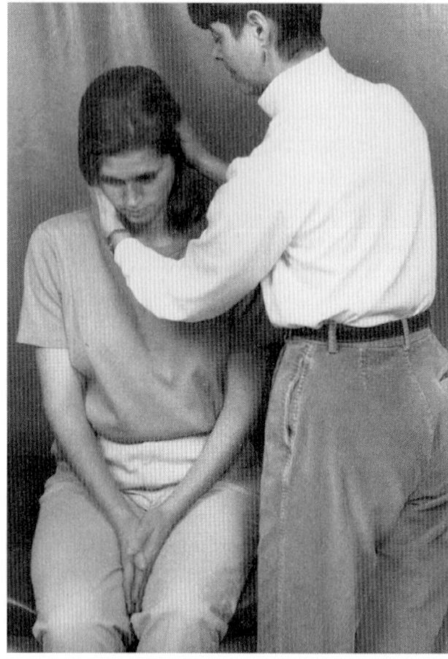

Figure 5.13 The canalith repositioning maneuver for treatment of benign paroxysmal positional vertigo. Each position is held for 1 to 2 minutes or until nystagmus and vertigo subside. The first two positions **(A and B)** are the same as those found in the Dix–Hallpike maneuver. In position 3 **(C)**, the head is moved into the opposite Dix–Hallpike position. In position 4, the person rolls to the side-lying position, nose down **(D)**; in position 5, the person is brought to the sitting position, with the head turned to 45 degrees from midline **(E)**, and finally, the head is dropped into a flexed position **(F)** and held there for 2 minutes.

standardized testing or through observation of the patient performing functional tasks. The disorder may manifest functionally as eating food on one-half of the plate, shaving one side of the face, or walking into objects present in contralesional space.

A variety of tests, for example, the cancellation test and the line bisection test (shown in Fig. 5.14), have been recommended as screening tools for all patients with hemispheric stroke in order to determine the presence of VN (for a more detailed discussion, see Plummer et al., 2003). The cancellation task (Fig. 5.14A) requires the patient to delete multiple identical visual target symbols on a paper sheet. Incomplete or disproportionate deletion on one side indicates VN. In addition to the quantitative score, qualitative information is gathered, including the location of the initial point at which the

TABLE 5.4 Clinical Typology of Perceptual and Cognitive Deficits

Deficit	Definition	Function effects
Perceptual Impairments		
Body scheme	Awareness of body parts, position of body in relationship to environment	Difficulty dressing, unsafe transfers
Right–left discrimination	Ability to understand concepts of right and left	Difficulty with dressing, transfers, mobility, following directions that include right/left
Body part identification	Ability to identify body parts of self and others	Incorrect response to instructions to move a body part
Anosognosia	Unawareness or denial of deficits	Unsafe in functional activities
Unilateral neglect	Neglect of one side of body or extrapersonal space	Activities of daily living limited to one-half of body, transfers and mobility unsafe
Position in space	Ability to understand concepts like over, under, around, above, and below	Difficulty with mobility, following directions that include these terms
Spatial relations	Ability to perceive self in relation to other objects	Transfers and mobility unsafe
Topographic orientation	Ability to find one's way from one place to another	Mobility unsafe
Figure ground perception	Ability to distinguish foreground from background	Unable to find objects in cluttered drawing
Limb apraxia	Inability to carry out purposeful movement in the presence of intact sensation	ADL affected due to difficulty in using objects
Constructional apraxia	Deficit in constructional activities	ADL apraxia
Dressing apraxia	Inability to dress oneself	Puts clothing on incorrectly
Cognitive Impairments		
Attention	Ability to focus on a specific stimulus without being distracted	Inability to follow direction
Orientation	Knowledge related to person, place, and time	Disoriented
Memory	Registration, encoding, storage, recall, and retrieval of information	Appears disoriented; will forget names, schedules, etc.; decreased ability to learn
Problem solving	The ability to manipulate a fund of knowledge and apply this information to new or unfamiliar situations	Difficulty with ADL, socially inappropriate, inability to recognize threats to safety

ADL, activities of daily living.

Adapted from Quintana LA. Evaluation of perception and cognition. In: Trombly CA, ed. *Occupational therapy for physical dysfunction*, 4th ed. Baltimore, MD: Williams & Wilkins, 1995, with permission.

individual begins the pattern of cancellation (deemed to be the most sensitive measure), the scanning pattern, the search time, and the number of recancellations of the same target. The line bisection test (LBT) (Fig. 5.14B) requires the patient to estimate and bisect the midline, thereby determining leftward/rightward orientation bias. Research supporting the sensitivity of the LBT as a measure of neglect is mixed (Ferber & Karnath, 2001; Molenberghs & Sale, 2011).

Kerkhoff and Schenk (2012) offer a review on rehabilitation of spatial hemineglect and the diverse sensory deficits that accompany this high-order brain impairment. Some treatment strategies include Visual Scanning Therapy (teaching patients to consciously

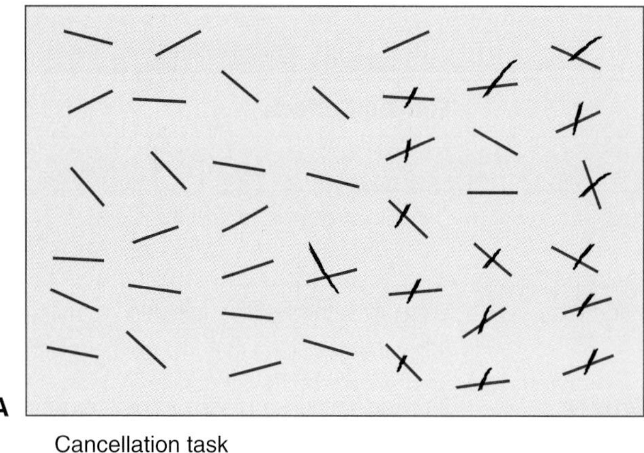

A Cancellation task

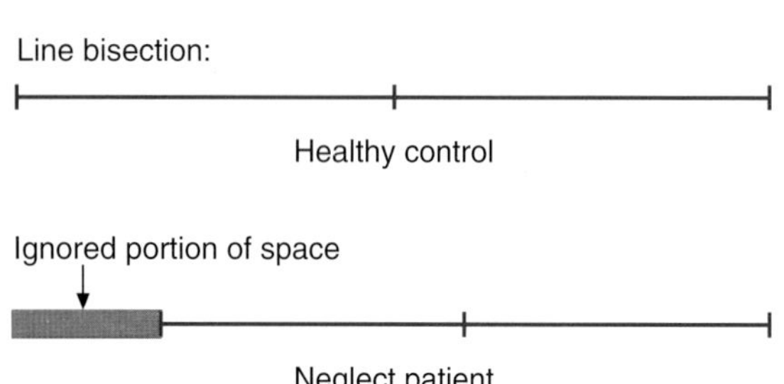

B Line bisection task

Figure 5.14 Clinical tests to identify visual neglect. The cancellation test **(A)** requires patients to delete multiple identical visual target symbols on a paper sheet. Incomplete or disproportionate deletion on one side indicates VN. The line bisection test **(B)** requires the patient to estimate and bisect the midline, thereby determining leftward/rightward orientation bias.

scan the environment), use of sensory stimulation to increase awareness, or modifying the environment to accommodate the impairment (Quintana, 1995).

New technologies are also being investigated to assist people with hemineglect. The application of lightweight bracelets that provide continuous sensory visuo-acoustic feedback in response to a motor mismatch during bimanual activities of daily living (e.g., carrying a tray, buttoning a shirt or using a fork and knife) improves motor performance when the person wears the bracelets (Trejo-Gabriel-Galan et al., 2016).

Nonspatial Cognitive Deficits

Nonspatial cognitive impairments related to arousal, attention, memory, and learning are quite common in patients with CNS lesions. Behavioral problems are also common and may include apathy, aggression, low frustration tolerance, emotional lability, and loss of behavioral inhibition that result in impulsivity. This combination of cognitive and behavioral deficits can seriously affect decision-making processes in people with neurologic disorders, and affect their ability to socialize and interact appropriately with their surroundings.

Arousal/Level of Consciousness

Alertness is a basic arousal process allowing the patient to respond to stimuli in the environment. The Rancho Los Amigos Scale is probably the most well-known approach to quantifying level of consciousness in the patient with neurologic impairments. This scale is shown in Assessment Tool 5.3. Assessment of level of

Assessment Tool 5.3

Rancho Los Amigos Scale of Level of Consciousness

I. **No response:** unresponsive to any stimulus.
II. **Generalized response:** limited, inconsistent, nonpurposeful responses, often to pain only.
III. **Localized response:** purposeful responses; may follow simple commands; may focus on presented object.
IV. **Confused, agitated:** heightened state of activity; confusion, disorientation; aggressive behavior; unable to do self-care; unaware of present events; agitation appears related to internal confusion.
V. **Confused, inappropriate:**nonagitated; appears alert; responds to commands; distractible; does not concentrate on task; agitated response to external stimuli; verbally inappropriate; does not learn new information.
VI. **Confused, appropriate:** good directed behavior; needs cueing; can relearn old skills as activities of daily living; serious memory problems; some awareness of self and others.
VII. **Automatic, appropriate:** appears appropriate, oriented; frequently robot-like in daily routine; minimal or absent confusion; shallow recall; increased awareness of self, interaction in environment; lacks insight into condition; decreased judgment and problem solving; lacks realistic planning for future.
VIII. **Purposeful, appropriate:** alert, oriented; recalls and integrates past events; learns new activities and can continue without supervision; independent in home and living skills; capable of driving; defects in stress tolerance, judgment, and abstract reasoning persist; many function at reduced levels in society.

(Reprinted with permission from Hagen, C., Malkmus, D., Durham, P. (1979). *Levels of Cognitive Functioning, Rehabilitation of the Head Injured Adult; Comprehensive Physical Management,* Downey, CA: Professional Staff Association of Rancho Los Amigos National Rehabilitation Center.)

1. Reduce confusion—make sure the task goal is clear to the patient.
2. Improve motivation—work on tasks that are relevant and important to the patient.
3. Encourage consistency of performance—be consistent in your goals and reinforce only those behaviors that are compatible with those goals.
4. Reduce confusion—use simple, clear, and concise instructions.
5. Improve attention—accentuate perceptual cues that are essential to the task, and minimize the number of irrelevant stimuli in the environment.
6. Improve problem-solving ability—begin with relatively simple tasks, and gradually increase the complexity of the task demands.
7. Encourage declarative as well as procedural learning—have a patient verbally and/or mentally rehearse sequences when performing a task.
8. Seek a moderate level of arousal to optimize learning—moderate the sensory stimulation in the environment; agitated patients require decreased intensity of stimulation (soft voice, low lights, slow touch) to reduce arousal levels; stuporous patients require increased intensity of stimulation (use brisk, loud commands, fast movements; work in a vertical position).
9. Provide increased levels of supervision, especially during the early stages of retraining.
10. Recognize that progress may be slower when working with patients who have cognitive impairments.

Figure 5.15 Strategies for modifying treatment to accommodate a cognitive impairment.

consciousness, arousal, or state is an essential part of examining motor control, since motor behavior is very dependent on arousal level (Duncan & Badke, 1987).

Many patients with CNS lesions demonstrate significant cognitive or behavioral impairments that affect the patient's ability to participate fully in a retraining program. For example, depression is estimated to occur in 31% of people who suffer a stroke within 5 years after the cerebrovascular accident (Hackett et al., 2014). Poststroke depression is related to motor recovery, performance in ADLs, and cognitive function (Robinson & Jorge, 2016). With this in mind, Figure 5.15 provides a few suggestions for modifying treatment strategies when working with a patient who has cognitive problems.

Attention

As we saw in Chapter 2, attention is a fundamental cognitive process with a complex neural substrate that is essential to the ability to react to external stimuli and to generate goal-oriented actions in diverse environments. Thus, attentional deficits have a profound impact on both sensory/perceptual and motor functions and, thus, are a critical part of examination in patients with CNS pathology. But there are many different approaches based on the underlying framework used to understand attention. Clinical models of attention are not specifically tied to neural processing modules in the brain but rather describe subtypes (Sohlberg & Mateer, 2001). These include the following:

- Focused attention: the ability to respond discretely to specific visual, auditory, or tactile stimuli.
- Sustained attention (vigilance): the ability to maintain a consistent behavioral response during continuous and repetitive activity.
- Selective attention: the ability to maintain a behavioral or cognitive set in the face of distracting or competing stimuli. Therefore, it incorporates the notion of "freedom from distractibility."
- Alternating attention: the ability of mental flexibility that allows individuals to shift their focus of attention and move between tasks having different cognitive requirements.
- Divided attention: the ability to respond simultaneously to multiple tasks or multiple task demands.

Specific tests have been developed to examine these different aspects of attention. For example, the Random Letter Test is used as a test of sustained attention, while the Stroop test is used for testing selective attention, and the Trail-Making Test parts A and B are used to examine the ability to alternate attention between two tasks (Sohlberg & Mateer, 2001).

The attention network test (ANT) developed by Posner and colleagues (Fan et al., 2002) is designed to test the three attentional networks: alerting, orienting, and executive control. The alerting network is examined by changes in reaction time resulting from a presentation of a warning signal. The orienting network is examined by changes in the reaction time that accompany cues indicating where the target will occur. The executive control network is examined by requiring the participant to respond by pressing two keys indicating the direction (left or right) of a central arrow surrounded by congruent, incongruent, or neutral arrows (called flankers).

Using the ANT test, researchers examined the prevalence of the three types of attentional deficits in 110 persons with acute stroke and related performance on the ANT to lesion location using MRI (Rinne et al., 2013). More than half of the subjects with stroke had a deficit in one of the three attentional networks. Alerting deficits were present in 17% of subjects and were associated with lesions in the thalamus and upper brainstem; 15% had orienting impairments associated with lesions to the right pulvinar and right temporoparietal cortex;

and 23% had problems with executive function/conflict resolution, associated with lesions in the bilateral prefrontal and premotor areas (Rinne et al., 2013).

The many approaches developed to test the complex concept of attention underscore its importance to understanding movement disorders in the patient with CNS pathology.

Memory

Like attention, memory is a complex concept involving many facets. Memory is the ability to process, store, and retrieve information. After brain injury, deficits in both short-term memory (STM) and long-term memory (LTM) have been reported. Assessment of STM and LTM involves asking patients to remember four words and then testing their immediate recall and their recall after 5, 10, and 30 minutes (Strub & Black, 1977).

Explicit and Implicit Motor Learning

Therapists rely on both implicit (repetition of movement to promote learning) and explicit (instructions on how to perform a task) motor learning strategies to guide recovery of motor skills in patients with CNS pathology. Understanding the effect of CNS pathology on explicit and implicit learning is very important because of its impact on the therapeutic interventions we use when assisting patients to acquire functional motor skills.

Several studies have explored the effect of unilateral CNS pathology on implicit and explicit learning, with varied results. Explicit learning is impaired in patients with medial temporal lobe damage; however, implicit learning is retained (Reber & Squire, 1998). Lesions in the prefrontal cortex appear to impair both implicit and explicit learning of visuomotor sequencing tasks (Beldarrain et al., 2002). Patients with MCA stroke affecting the sensorimotor cortex appear to retain the capacity for implicit motor sequence learning (Boyd & Winstein, 2001; Pohl et al., 2001; Winstein et al., 1999), as do patients with cerebellar lesions (Boyd & Winstein, 2003). This research underscores the concept that the neural systems underlying implicit and explicit memory and learning are anatomically separate, and therefore, the effects of CNS pathology on learning are in part lesion-dependent. In addition, because control of implicit learning is distributed among many brain structures, the research suggests that no single lesion completely eliminates the capacity for implicit learning (Boyd & Winstein, 2003).

Does providing explicit information improve implicit learning of a motor skill? It is generally assumed by therapists that it does, so we routinely provide explicit instructions to patients while they are practicing a motor skill. However, results from current research examining the effect of explicit

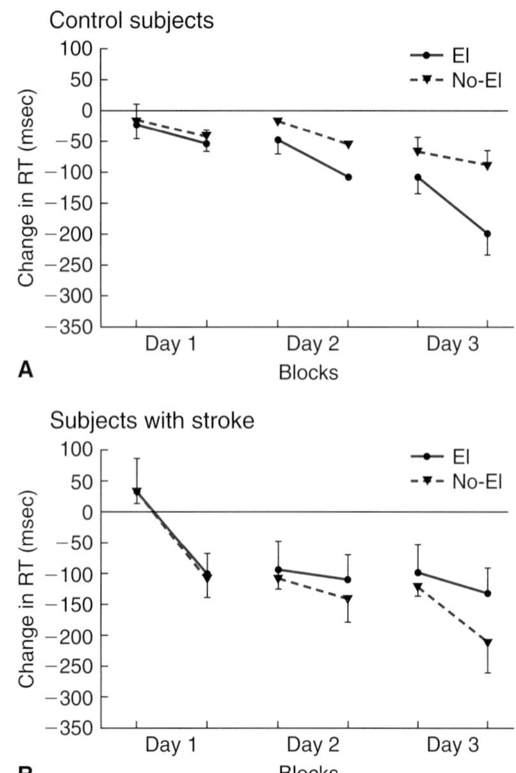

Figure 5.16 Effect of explicit instructions on implicit motor sequence learning in persons with stroke. Both control subjects **(A)** and subjects with stroke **(B)** demonstrate implicit learning, as indicated by a change in reaction time over the 3 days of practicing an implicit motor sequence task. Explicit instruction improved implicit learning in the control subjects who receive it (shown by the *solid lines*) compared to subjects who did not receive it (shown by the *dashed lines*). In contrast, subjects with stroke who received explicit instructions (*solid line*) had less improvement in reaction time as compared with subjects who did not receive it (*dashed line*), suggesting that explicit instruction impeded implicit learning after stroke. (Adapted with permission from Boyd LA, Winstein CJ. Impact of explicit information on implicit motor sequence learning following middle cerebral artery stroke. *Phys Ther.* 2003;83:983, with permission of the American Physical Therapy Association. This material is copyrighted, and any further reproduction or distribution requires written permission from APTA.)

instructions on implicit learning suggest a need to re-examine these assumptions. A number of studies have examined the effect of explicit instructions on implicit motor skill learning in patients with various CNS pathologies. Boyd and Winstein (2003) examined this in 10 patients with MCA stroke affecting the sensorimotor cortex and 10 nonimpaired controls (some of the results of this study are shown in Fig. 5.16). This study found that implicit learning did occur in the patients with MCA stroke. Similar to the control group, the subjects with stroke (shown in Fig. 5.16B) reduced reaction time over the 3 days of practicing the repeated sequence motor task (reaction time did not change when practicing a random sequence motor task). This figure also shows the differential effects of explicit instruction on implicit learning in the two groups. Explicit instruction improved implicit learning in the control group (Fig. 5.16A, steeper drop in reaction time in the control subjects who received explicit instructions [solid line] compared with those who did not [dashed line]).

In contrast, explicit instruction had a detrimental effect on learning in the subjects with stroke. This can be seen in Figure 5.16B, which shows that the subjects with stroke who received explicit information (solid line) had less improvement in reaction time compared with subjects with stroke who did not receive explicit information (dashed line). The finding that explicit instruction impairs implicit learning was also found for patients with basal ganglia stroke (Pohl et al., 2006). In contrast, in patients with cerebellar stroke, explicit instruction improved implicit learning (Molinari et al., 1997). These results suggest that the impact of explicit instruction on implicit learning depends on a number of factors, including the type, timing, and meaningfulness of instructions, as well as the location of CNS pathology.

SUMMARY

1. Knowledge regarding both the physiology and pathophysiology of motor control is essential to examining and treating the patient with movement problems. This knowledge enables the therapist to form initial assumptions regarding the types of functional problems and underlying impairments likely to be present in a particular patient, thus guiding the selection of appropriate tests and measurements, as well as suitable intervention methods.
2. Brain injury produces a unique pattern of behavioral signs and symptoms associated with the destruction of specific neuronal populations. Hughlings Jackson divided abnormal behaviors associated with CNS lesions into either positive signs and symptoms (i.e., the presence of abnormal behaviors) or negative signs and symptoms (i.e., the loss of normal behaviors). In the rehabilitation environment, emphasis is often placed on positive signs and symptoms (such as abnormalities of muscle tonus) at the expense of negative signs and symptoms (such as loss of strength) when attempting to understand performance deficits in persons with a neurologic dysfunction.
3. Pathophysiology within the action system including the motor cortex and subcortical structures such as the cerebellum, and basal ganglia, results in a wide range of impairments affecting the control of movement.
4. Impairments associated with pathophysiology of the motor cortex include motor weakness (paresis), abnormal muscle tone (spasticity), and coordination problems including abnormal synergies of movement.
5. Pathophysiology of subcortical structures, such as the cerebellum and basal ganglia, produces a range of impairments including abnormal muscle tone (rigidity), tremor, dyskinesia, and problems with the timing and scaling of muscle activity that significantly affect movement coordination.
6. In the person with neurologic pathology, musculoskeletal impairments develop secondary to neuromuscular impairments, but they can significantly constrain functional movement.
7. Sensory deficits are a major factor contributing to motor dyscontrol in persons with CNS lesions. Sensory deficits can result in a disruption of sensory information in somatosensory, visual, or vestibular systems.
8. Perceptual problems including spatial deficits also constrain functional movement in a person with brain pathology. These problems are often a result of lesions in the attentional networks.
9. Nonspatial cognitive problems, common in persons with CNS pathology, can include altered level of consciousness, change in mental status, and deficits in learning, memory, and attention. Behavioral problems are also and include apathy, aggression, low frustration tolerance, emotional lability, depression, and loss of behavioral inhibition that result in impulsivity.
10. Explicit and implicit learning and memory are differentially affected by CNS pathology because of their different anatomical substrates. In addition, the effect of providing explicit information on implicit learning of motor skills will also vary depending on the type and timing of instruction and the location of neural pathology.

CHAPTER 6

A Conceptual Framework for Clinical Practice

Learning Objectives

Following completion of this chapter, the reader will be able to:

1. Discuss the relationship between a conceptual framework and clinical practice.
2. Discuss each element in the American Physical Therapy Association's patient management process.
3. Describe components of the World Health Organization's International Classification of Functioning, Disability, and Health.
4. Define a hypothesis and describe how hypotheses are used in research versus clinical practice.
5. Define evidence-based practice and discuss the concept of levels of evidence.
6. Describe a task-oriented approach to examination and intervention.
7. Discuss factors that have an impact on the selection of tests and measures used to examine a patient with a movement disorder.
8. Describe the goal of treatment focused on recovery of function versus compensation; discuss factors that should be considered when choosing each approach.

INTRODUCTION

Clinicians responsible for retraining movement in a patient with neurologic impairments are faced with an overwhelming number of decisions. What is the most appropriate way to examine my patient? How much time should be spent on documenting functional ability and levels of participation versus evaluating underlying impairments leading to dysfunction? What criteria should I use in deciding what the priority problems are? How do I establish goals that are realistic and meaningful? What is the best approach to intervention and the most effective way to structure my therapy sessions? What are the most appropriate outcomes for evaluating the effects of intervention?

These questions reflect the critical need for a conceptual framework for clinical practice. A conceptual framework is a logical structure that helps the clinician organize clinical practices into a cohesive and comprehensive plan. It provides a context in which clinical information is gathered and interpreted (Campbell, 2006; Darrah et al., 2006; Schenkman et al., 2006; Trombly, 1995). A conceptual framework influences clinical practice in several ways. It influences decisions about what to measure during the examination of the patient, the selection of intervention strategies, and the conclusions drawn regarding the intervention process. It provides the clinician with guidelines for how to proceed through the clinical intervention process (Campbell, 2006; Darrah et al., 2006; Schenkman et al., 2006; Trombly, 1995). Finally, a conceptual framework also provides a structure that clinicians can use to organize the rapidly expanding body of research evidence that informs clinical practice. Finally, the development of conceptual frameworks within specialized clinical areas assists a clinician in organizing the most relevant rehabilitation outcomes as well as the aspect measured by such outcomes—impairment, function, or environmental aspects (Demers et al., 2004; Jesus & Hoening, 2015; King et al., 2018).

The growing recognition of the importance of conceptual frameworks to clinical practice is seen in the increasing number of publications related to this topic (Campbell, 2006; Darrah et al., 2006; Rothstein et al., 2003; Schenkman et al., 2006). As was true for theories of motor control, each conceptual framework represents an individual's perspective on the relative importance and usefulness of specific elements to their practice. There is no consensus on the best framework across all forms of practice.

The purposes of this chapter are to consider elements that contribute to a conceptual framework we find useful for organizing evidence-based research and guiding clinical practice and to describe a conceptual framework for retraining the patient with movement disorders, which we call a "task-oriented approach." A task-oriented approach is used in later chapters as the framework for retraining posture, mobility, and upper-extremity control in a patient with a neurologic deficit.

COMPONENTS OF A CONCEPTUAL FRAMEWORK FOR CLINICAL PRACTICE

While there are potentially many concepts that contribute to a conceptual framework for practice, we have identified five:

1. A model of practice, which outlines a method for gathering information and developing a plan of care consistent with the goals, problems, and needs of the patient
2. A model of function and disability, which describes a framework for examining the effects of a health condition on the individual and enables the clinician to identify the patient's strengths and limitations critical in developing a plan of care
3. Hypothesis-oriented clinical practice, which provides the means to test assumptions about the nature and cause of motor control problems systematically
4. Principles of motor control and motor learning, which help us to understand both the cause and the nature of normal and abnormal movement, as well as assumptions about how movement skills are learned or relearned
5. Evidence-based clinical practice, an approach to clinical practice that stresses the importance of integrating best research evidence with clinical expertise and patient values (Sackett et al., 1996)

The following sections describe each of these important components in detail.

Models of Practice

Remember in Chapter 1, we introduced you to a number of cases, including the case of Genise T., a 53-year-old woman who has had a stroke; Mike M., a 59-year-old man with Parkinson disease; John C., a 33-year-old with spinocerebellar degeneration; and Thomas L., a 7-year-old with spastic diplegia—a subtype of cerebral palsy. This diverse group of patients is typical of those referred to therapy for motor control problems affecting their ability to move and carry out activities of daily livings (ADLs). Can the same conceptual framework underlying the process for examining motor control in a man with Parkinson disease be appropriate for a 33-year-old man with cerebellar degeneration? Can the same conceptual framework underlying intervention strategies used with a 53-year-old woman with impaired balance following a stroke be used to habilitate mobility in a 7-year-old child with cerebral palsy?

As you will see, the answer to all of these questions is "yes." Despite the diversity of these patients, the conceptual framework underlying the process used to gather information and design an intervention program is similar for all patients. Thus, while each patient's motor control problems and therapeutic solutions may be different, the process used to identify those problems and solutions will be consistent across patients because the underlying conceptual framework is consistent.

American Physical Therapy Association Model of Practice

The American Physical Therapy Association (APTA) in its publication *Guide to Physical Therapist Practice 3.0* has described a process for managing patient and client care. The APTA's patient-oriented management process is composed of five elements: examination, evaluation, diagnosis, prognosis, and intervention. These elements are shown in Figure 6.1. The process is an iterative one, as you can see by the arrows connecting the various components of the process. Additionally, the "Guide to Physical Therapy Practice" has adopted a language that is consistent with the current version of the International Classification of Functioning, Disability and Health (ICF). The following section provides a brief overview,

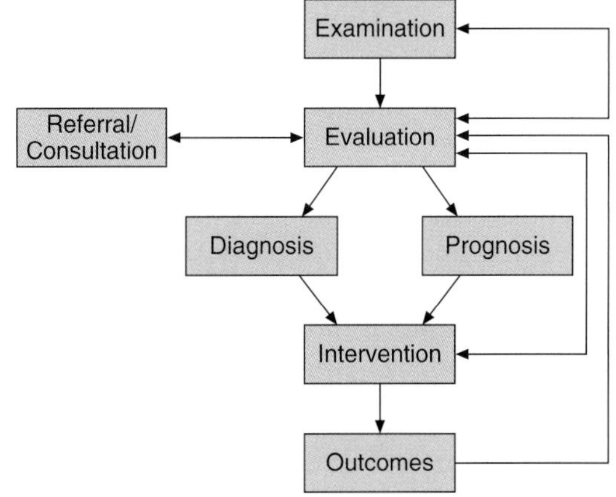

Figure 6.1 The patient and client treatment process suggested by the American Physical Therapy Association. (Adapted from American Physical Therapy Association. *Guide to physical therapist practice 3.0*. Alexandria, VA: American Physical Therapy Association, 2014, with permission.)

while a detailed explanation of this management process can be found on the APTA's website.

Examination. Examination is the process of obtaining data necessary to form a diagnosis, prognosis, and plan of care. There are three parts to the examination process: taking a history, reviewing relevant systems, and performing appropriate tests and measurements.

History. Information related to the patient's current and past health can be gathered directly from the patient, family, or caregiver; from medical records; and from other health care professionals. The types of data that might be generated from a patient history include general demographics (e.g., age, race, sex), current conditions and history of conditions (specific concerns expressed by patient/family/caregiver), living environment, growth and developmental history (if appropriate), family history, health status, social history (e.g., family and caregiver resources, cultural beliefs, social support), occupation or employment, functional status, and activity level (current and prior level of function with respect to self-care and home management [e.g., ADL and independent activities of daily living (IADL)]). Also included in the history is a list of medications and relevant lab and diagnostic tests from other medical specialties (APTA, 2014).

Interviewing the patient and/or the patient's family is a critical part of the examination process. The interview is the first step in establishing a good rapport between the patient and the therapist, a factor known to affect the outcome of therapeutic intervention. The interview is used to gather information on the patient's goals, expectations, and motivation, a central feature of a patient-oriented approach to clinical practice. The interview process also allows the therapist insight into the patient's level of understanding regarding their medical condition and the therapeutic process. Information on previous and current health behaviors, including exercise habits, is also critical information when planning intervention.

Systems review. The examination also includes a brief review of the relevant systems in order to help direct the selection of specific tests and measurements and to assist in determining diagnosis and prognosis. A review of the systems includes a brief determination of the anatomical and/or physiological status of the cardiopulmonary, integumentary, musculoskeletal, and neuromuscular systems. It also includes a brief examination of the patient's communication ability, cognition, language, and learning style.

Tests and measurements. The last part of the examination process includes the performance of specific tests and measurements that provide the clinician with insights into specific impairments and functional limitations that restrict the patient's ability to participate in the roles and activities that are important to their life. The tests and measures used by physical therapists are organized into 26 categories:

- Aerobic capacity and endurance
- Anthropometric characteristics
- Assistive technology
- Balance
- Circulation (arterial, venous, lymphatic)
- Community, social, and civic life
- Cranial and peripheral nerve integrity
- Education life
- Environmental factors
- Gait
- Integumentary integrity
- Joint integrity and mobility
- Mental functions
- Mobility (including locomotion)
- Motor function
- Muscle performance (including strength, power, endurance, and length)
- Neuromotor development and sensory processing
- Pain
- Posture
- Range of motion
- Reflex integrity
- Self-care and domestic life
- Sensory integrity
- Skeletal integrity
- Ventilation and respiration
- Work life

Evaluation. The next step in APTA's patient and client management process is evaluation, defined as the process of making clinical judgments based on the data gathered during the examination. The process of evaluation enables a therapist to

- interpret the individual's response to tests and measures,
- integrate the test and measure data with other information collected during the history,
- determine a diagnosis or diagnoses amenable to physical therapist management,
- determine a prognosis, including goals for physical therapist management, and
- develop a plan of care.

Factors that have an impact on the evaluation include not just clinical findings related to tests and measurements but the extent of loss of function, social considerations, overall physical function, and health status. The evaluation reflects the severity and duration of the current problem, the presence of coexisting conditions or diseases, and the stability of the condition.

Diagnosis. The next step in the management process is determining a physical therapy diagnosis. A diagnosis is a label that identifies the impact of a condition on the function at both the level of a system (e.g., the movement system) and the level of the whole person (APTA, 2014). The physical therapy diagnosis encompasses the signs and symptoms, syndromes, and categories of problems that are used to guide the therapist in determining the most appropriate intervention. The term "diagnosis" as it relates to the profession of physical therapy is distinguished from a diagnosis made by physicians. Sahrmann (1988, p. 1705) proposed the following definition of a physical therapy diagnosis: "Diagnosis is a term that names the primary dysfunction toward which the physical therapist directs treatment. The dysfunction is identified by the physical therapist based on information obtained from the history, signs, symptoms, examination and tests the therapist performs or requests." The physical therapy diagnosis allows the clinician to name and classify clusters of signs and symptoms that will potentially benefit from physical therapy treatment (Rose, 1989). Thus, the purpose of a physical therapy diagnosis is to direct treatment. It allows the identification of specific problems that will likely respond successfully to a specific treatment.

Prognosis and Plan of Care. The fourth stage in APTA's management process includes determining a patient's prognosis and plan of care. A prognosis includes both the level of functional independence the patient is expected to achieve following intervention and the expected amount of time required to get to that level. In determining a prognosis, the therapist identifies both the highest level of function the patient is capable of achieving and the highest level of function that is likely to be habitual for that patient. In addition, a part of prognosis is determining intermediate levels of function that will be accomplished during the course of therapy.

At this point in the management process, the therapist establishes a plan of care that specifies the goals, predicted level of optimal improvement, specific interventions to be used, and proposed duration and frequency of the interventions that are required to reach the goals and outcomes. Goals are the *intended* impact of the plan of care on functioning (body functions and structures, activities, participation). Goals should be measurable, functionally driven, and time limited and can be classified as either short term or long term (APTA, 2014).

Outcomes are the actual results of implementing the plan of care that indicate the impact of treatment on functioning, including body structure and functions, activities, and participation. Anticipated outcomes also address risk reduction, prevention, impact on societal resources, and patient and client satisfaction. The anticipated outcomes in the plan should be measurable within a specified time limit (APTA, 2014).

Expected outcomes reflect the therapist's professional judgment about the likely level of function the patient will achieve, while goals may be used to measure progress toward expected outcomes (Quinn & Gordon, 2003). In a patient-oriented approach to clinical practice, goal setting is a collaborative process involving the therapist, the patient (and family as appropriate), and often other health care professionals. Patient-centered goals—that is, goals that are relevant to the patient's desires—are important in ensuring successful outcomes (Payton et al., 1990; Quinn & Gordon, 2003).

Therapists are frequently asked to establish both short- and long-term goals for therapy. Short-term goals are those expected to be achieved in a reasonably short time, with the amount of time varying depending on where the patient is receiving care. For example, short-term goals in a rehabilitation program may be defined weekly; alternatively, short-term goals in an outpatient program may be defined monthly.

Long-term goals define the patient's expected level of performance at the end of the intervention process. Long-term goals are often expressed relative to functional gains, such as (a) amount of independence; (b) supervision, or level of assistance required to carry out a task; or (c) in relationship to the equipment or environmental adaptation needed to perform the task. Quinn and Gordon (2003) have proposed an alternative approach to describing goals for intervention. They suggest writing goals and outcomes at three different levels: disability goals, functional goals, and impairment goals. Disability goals indicate outcomes related to recovery of participation in the specific roles and activities important to the patient. Functional goals reflect recovery of performance of important functional tasks and ADL. Finally, impairment goals express changes in underlying impairments contributing to functional limitations; thus, these goals should be linked to a relevant functional goal (Quinn & Gordon, 2003).

Writing effective goals is facilitated by the use of a structure that guides the therapist in generating objective, measurable, patient-centered goals. The "ABCDE" structure shown in Figure 6.2 is based on five essential components of an effective goal (Quinn & Gordon, 2003). The first component is the actor (a), the individual who will accomplish the goal; the second is the behavior (b) or action that will be performed; the third component is the condition (c) under which the behavior will be performed; the fourth is the degree (d), quantifying the level of performance; and the fifth is the expected time frame (e) in which the goal is to be achieved.

Intervention. The last step in APTA's management process is intervention. Intervention is the purposeful and skilled interaction of the therapist with the patient. Physical therapist interventions are organized into nine categories:

- Patient or client instruction (used with every patient and client)
- Airway clearance techniques
- Assistive technology

Essential Components of a Well-Written Functional Goal: ABCDE

Actor
- Who will carry out the activity
- Usually the patient, occasionally family member or other caregiver
- e.g., "Patient will . . ." or "Patient's wife will . . ."

Behavior
- Description of the activity (in understandable terminology)
- E.g., ". . . will walk . . ." or ". . . will transfer . . ." or ". . . will put on shirt . . ."

Condition
- Circumstances under which the behavior is carried out
- Must include all essential elements of performance (e.g., assistive devices, environmental context)
- E.g., ". . . in hospital corridor with quad cane . . ."

Degree
- Quantitative specification of performance
- Examples of quantification: rate of success or failure, degree or level of assistance, time required, distance, number of repetitions, heart rate at end of activity, etc.
- ". . . 8/10 times successfully . . ." or ". . . in 4 minutes . . ." or ". . . three blocks . . ." or ". . . 500 feet . . ." or ". . . with increase of heart rate to no more than 110 beats/min . . ."
- Qualitative aspects of performance: "with effective toe clearance" "while maintaining proper body mechanics"

Expected Time
- How long it will it take to reach goal
- Stated in days, weeks, months, or, alternatively, number of visits
- E.g., ". . . within 2 weeks . . ." or ". . . within 3 therapy sessions . . ."

Figure 6.2 Five components of effective clinical goals and outcomes. (Adapted from Quinn L, Gordon J. *Functional outcomes: documentation for rehabilitation*. Philadelphia, PA: Saunders, 2003:104, Fig. 9.1.)

- Biophysical agents
- Functional training in self-care and domestic, work, community, social, and civic life
- Integumentary repair and protection techniques
- Manual therapy techniques
- Motor function training
- Therapeutic exercise

Based on information gained through the entire patient management process (examination, evaluation, diagnosis, and prognosis), the therapist selects, prescribes, and implements interventions appropriate for the goals of a specific patient. During an episode of care, the specific interventions used may change depending on the patient's response (APTA, Guide to Practice 3.0, 2014).

While a model of practice gives you a broad framework for proceeding through the therapeutic process, it does not provide details regarding how each step should be implemented. It does not provide answers to critical questions such as the following: How shall I measure the effect of disease or injury on my patient? Toward what goals should I direct my intervention? In what order should problems be tackled? A model of functioning and disablement can help to answer these questions.

Models of Functioning and Disability

Models of functioning and disability suggest a framework for structuring the effects of a health condition on aspects of function in an individual. The term "disablement" is a global one that refers to the impact of disease on human functioning at many different levels (Jette, 1994). As health care professionals, we deal with the consequences of disease, injury, and congenital abnormalities on the health and functioning of individuals (Rothstein, 1994). The goal of therapeutic intervention is to optimize function and thereby maximize participation; however, in order to accomplish these goals, we need to understand the effects of a health condition on the ability of individuals to function and participate in activities and roles that are important to them.

World Health Organization Model

The ICF is a framework proposed by the World Health Organization (WHO) for describing health and health-related states (WHO, 2001). It provides a standard language and framework to describe how people with a health condition function in their daily lives. The new ICF is a major revision of the original International

Classification of Impairments, Disabilities, and Handicaps (ICIDH) proposed in 1980 (WHO, 1980).

In 2001, the 191 Member States of the World Health Organization agreed to adopt the ICF as the basis for the scientific standardization of data on health and disability worldwide. The ICF for Children and Youth (ICF-CY) is a newly derived classification that shares the same common foundation of the ICF but addresses the learning and playing aspects while considering the developmental process across infancy, childhood, and adolescence. In June 2008, the APTA House of Delegates officially endorsed and adopted the WHO's ICF.

The ICF model, shown in Figure 6.3, classifies factors that have an impact on human functioning (and its restrictions) into two major parts, each of which has two components. Part 1, functioning and disability, includes the components of body functions/structures and activities and participation. Part 2, contextual factors, includes the components of environmental factors and personal factors. Each component can be expressed in either positive (functioning) or negative (disability) terms.

Within part 1, body functions include both physiological and psychological functions of the body, while body structures include anatomical parts of the body. The negative expression of these concepts is impairment, defined as a significant deviation or loss in body function or structure. Activity is defined as the execution of a task or action by an individual, and thus represents the individual perspective of function. Participation reflects involvement in a life situation and represents a societal perspective of functioning (WHO, 2001). Activity limitations and restricted participation are the negative aspects of these concepts.

The WHO lists nine domains of activities and participation: learning and applying knowledge, general tasks and demands, communication, mobility, self-care, domestic life, interpersonal interactions and relationships, major life areas, and community, social, and civic life, many of which can be considered as both an activity and a reflection of participation. For example, mobility is both an activity (a task the individual performs) and a component of participation (societal

	Part 1: Functioning and disability		**Part 2: Contextual factors**	
Components	Body functions and structures	Activities and participation	Environmental factors	Personal factors
Domains	Body functions Body structures	Life areas (tasks, actions)	External influences on functioning and disability	Internal influences on functioning and disability
Constructs	Change in body functions (physiologic) Change in body structures (anatomic)	Capacity Executing tasks in a standard environment Performance Executing tasks in the current environment	Facilitating or hindering impact of features of the physical, social, and attitudinal world	Impact of attributes of the person
Positive aspect	Functional and structural integrity	Activities Participation	Facilitators	Not applicable
	Functioning			
Negative aspect	Impairment	Activity limitation Participation restriction	Barriers/ hindrances	Not applicable
	Disability			

Figure 6.3 International Classification of Functioning and Disability. (Adapted from World Health Organization. *International Classification Functioning, Disability and Health [ICF]*. Geneva, Switzerland: World Health Organization, 2001:11, Table 1.)

perspective of moving around to different locations and using transportation).

The terms "performance" and "capacity" are used to describe behavior of the individual in the nine domains. The performance qualifier describes what the individual does in their current environment, that is, within the actual context in which one lives (WHO, 2001, p. 15). In contrast, the capacity qualifier describes the highest probable level of functioning a person could achieve in an environment adjusted to the ability of that person. Thus, "capacity" quantifies ability in a standard or uniform environment, in contrast to "performance," which quantifies ability in the person's actual environment.

Part 2 of the ICF model identifies contextual factors, both environmental and personal, that can modify and influence the effect of a health condition on functioning of the individual. Personal factors can include those such as age, education, socioeconomic status, and presence of other comorbidities. Other examples include lifestyle and health behaviors such as exercise and diet; psychosocial attributes such as positive affect, prayer, and self-efficacy; and the ability to adapt to and accommodate potential limitations (Verbrugge & Jette, 1994; WHO, 2001).

Environmental factors are external to the individual and include physical, social, and attitudinal factors. These factors can have an impact at the level of the individual, reflecting the immediate environment in which the person is living, or at the societal level, reflecting social agencies, services, laws, and regulations as well as attitudes and cultural values.

Environmental factors can have either a positive (enhancing function/participation) or a negative (limiting function/participation) effect. Environmental factors are critical because disability emerges from a complex relationship between factors in the individual and external factors reflecting the circumstances in which the person is living (WHO, 2001). Some environments facilitate functioning and reduce disability, while others restrict functioning and increase disability. Thus, determination of disability (restricted participation) cannot be made solely by factors intrinsic to the individual; demands of the environment must also be considered (Patla & Shumway-Cook, 1999). For example, a person who has limited walking ability due to a stroke may be less disabled in a flat geographical location such as Chicago than in a hilly location such as San Francisco. A person with limited visual acuity may be able to function independently in daylight hours but be restricted in their participation when light levels are low. Thus, the environment and characteristics of the individual conjointly determine the capacity to participate.

In summary, the ICF provides a framework for examining the components of functioning that are impacted by a health condition including personal, activity, and environmental. It is a tool that enables the collection of data as to how an individual with a health condition functions in their daily life, taking into consideration both environmental context and personal factors. It was developed and tested for cross-cultural applicability in over 40 countries, providing a common global framework for organizing and communicating information on human functioning (WHO, 2001).

Clinical Implications

Models of function and disability provide a conceptual framework for examining the effect of a health condition on the individual. They provide a common language for communicating information, and they improve our ability to be understood by both clinicians and nonclinicians. How do these models assist a clinician in formulating a clinical plan for intervention? Before continuing, complete Lab Activity 6.1.

Clinicians are involved in identifying and documenting the effects of a health condition on body structure and function (impairments), as well as activities and participation (functional limitations and restricted participation) (Campbell, 2006; Jette, 1994; Schenkman et al., 2006). During the examination, clinicians identify

LAB ACTIVITY 6.1

Objective: To apply the ICF framework to one of our case studies with neurologic pathology.

Procedure: Select one or more of the case studies presented in Chapter 1. View the video case study associated with your choice. Use the ICF framework to describe the effect of pathology on this individual.

Assignment

1. Define the health condition of the disease or injury.
2. Make a list of the probable impairments (limitations in body structure and function) associated with this disease.
3. How will limitations in body structure and function change as the patient moves from an acute to a chronic condition?
4. What functional activities are likely to be affected given the range of impairments? What may be spared?
5. What will this patient's level of participation be?
6. Will this person be restricted (disabled) in the roles and activities in which the person is able to participate?
7. Consider how contextual factors impact this case. What are the personal factors that influence the effect of this health condition on function in this patient? What environmental factors are likely to influence the patient's functioning?

and document the sensory, motor, and cognitive impairments that potentially constrain functional abilities and limit participation. These impairments can be the direct result of the neurologic lesion (e.g., paresis) or the indirect effect of another impairment (such as the development of contractures in the paretic and immobile patient). Examination also includes the identification and documentation of limitations in functional activities (tasks performed by the individual), for example, the ability to walk, transfer, reach for, and manipulate objects. The clinician also examines the effect of a health condition on the individual's ability to participate in the necessary activities and roles of their daily life. Finally, a comprehensive examination includes a description of the contextual factors (personal and environmental) that also influence functioning and disability in the individual.

The process of identifying functional problems and their underlying cause(s) is not always easy. Most CNS pathology affects multiple systems, resulting in a diverse set of impairments. This means that functional problems in a patient with a neurologic deficit are often associated with many possible causes. How does a therapist establish a link between impairments and functional limitations and restricted participation? Which impairments are critical to loss of function and which to reduced participation? Which impairments should be treated, and in what order? What is the most efficacious approach to intervention? Hypothesis-driven clinical practice can assist the clinician in answering some of these questions (Rothstein & Echternach, 1986; Rothstein et al., 2003).

Hypothesis-Oriented Clinical Practice

What is a hypothesis, and how do we use it in the clinic? A hypothesis can be defined as a proposal to explain certain facts. In clinical practice, a hypothesis can be considered one possible explanation of the cause or causes of a patient's problem (Platt, 1964; Rothstein & Echternach, 1986; Rothstein et al., 2003). To a great extent, the hypotheses generated reflect the theories a clinician has about the cause and nature of function and dysfunction in patients with neurologic disease. As noted in Chapter 1, there are many theories of motor control that present varying views on the nature and cause of movement. As a result, there can be many different hypotheses about the underlying cause(s) of motor control problems in patients with neurologic dysfunction.

Clarifying the cause(s) of functional movement problems requires the clinician to (a) generate several alternative hypotheses about the potential cause(s), (b) determine the crucial test(s) and their expected outcomes that would rule out one or more of the hypotheses, (c) carry out the tests, and (d) continue the process of generating and testing hypotheses, refining one's understanding of the cause(s) of the problem (Platt, 1964). Hypothesis testing can be used to explain factors associated with functional limitations and restricted participation.

For example, Genise, our patient with a right hemiplegia secondary to a CVA, is referred for balance retraining because of recurrent falls. During the course of your evaluation, you observe that she is unable to stand safely while performing functional tasks and has a tendency to fall primarily backward (a functional-level problem). Your knowledge of normal postural control suggests the importance of the ankle muscles during the recovery of stance balance. You generate three hypotheses regarding possible impairments that could explain why she is falling backward: (a) weak anterior tibialis muscle, (b) shortened gastrocnemius, and (c) a problem coordinating the anterior tibialis muscle within a postural response synergy. What clinical tests can be used to distinguish among these hypotheses? Strength testing indicates Genise has some ability to voluntarily generate force, thus weakening support for the first hypothesis. ROM tests suggest normal passive range of motion at the ankle, weakening support for the second hypothesis. In response to the nudge test (a brief displacement in the backward direction), Genise does not perform dorsiflexion of the foot of the hemiplegic leg. The inability to achieve dorsiflexion of the foot, even though the capacity to generate force voluntarily is present, suggests support for the third hypothesis. If it were available, surface electromyography could be used to investigate further whether the anterior tibialis muscle is activated as part of a postural synergy responding to backward instability.

The generation and testing of hypotheses are an important part of clinical practice. However, there is a difference between hypothesis testing in a research laboratory and that in a clinic. In the laboratory, it is often possible to set up a carefully controlled experiment that will test the hypothesis. The outcome is a "clean result," that is, a result that accepts one hypothesis and rejects the alternative hypothesis. In contrast, in the clinic, we are often unable to achieve this clean result. Clinical tests are often not sufficiently sensitive and specific to differentiate clearly between two hypotheses. Rather, they indicate the likelihood for the origin of the problem. For example, in the case presented previously, passive ROM tests may not be a valid way of predicting the active range of a muscle during dynamic activities. In addition, manual muscle testing may not be a valid way to predict the patient's ability to recruit that muscle automatically for tasks such as balance recovery or walking.

Despite the limitations of clinical tests in providing clean results, the generation, testing, and revision of alternative hypotheses is an important part of clinical care. Hypothesis generation assists the clinician in determining the relationship between functional limitations and underlying impairments. We treat the impairments that relate directly to functional limitations and are within the scope of treatments available to us (Rothstein & Echternach, 1986; Rothstein et al., 2003).

Theories of Motor Control and Learning

The fourth element that contributes to a comprehensive conceptual framework for clinical practice is our understanding of the neural basis for movement control and learning underlying the (re)acquisition of skill. As discussed in Chapters 1 and 2, theories of motor control and learning have led to the development of clinical practices that apply assumptions from these theories to improving the control of movement. Thus, the approach a clinician chooses when examining and treating a patient with movement disorders is based in part on both implicit and explicit assumptions associated with an underlying theory of motor control and motor learning (Gordon, 1987; Horak, 1991; Woollacott & Shumway-Cook, 1990). In this book, we use the term "systems theory" of motor control as part of our framework for clinical practice. In this theory, movement results from the dynamic interplay between multiple systems that are organized around a behavioral goal and constrained by the environment.

Clinical practices related to retraining patients with motor control problems are constantly changing, in part to reflect new views on the physiological basis of motor control and motor learning. As new models evolve, clinical practices are modified to reflect emerging concepts related to how the brain controls movement, factors affecting neural reorganization, plasticity, and motor learning underlying the (re)acquisition of skilled movement following injury. Thus, a conceptual framework for structuring clinical practice must be dynamic, changing in response to new scientific theories about motor control and learning.

Evidence-Based Clinical Practice

Evidence-based practice (EBP) is a philosophical approach to clinical practice that integrates the best available research, clinician expertise, and client characteristics (Jette et al., 2003; Sackett et al., 1996). As defined by Sackett et al. (1996, p. 71), evidence-based medicine is "the conscientious, explicit, and judicious use of current best evidence in making decisions about the care of individual patients. The practice of evidence-based medicine means integrating individual clinical expertise with the best available external clinical evidence from systematic research." Sackett et al. (1996) define "best available research" as clinically relevant research from both basic and clinical sciences that increases the accuracy and precision of diagnostic tests, prognostic markers, and the efficacy and safety of therapeutic, rehabilitation, and preventive interventions. EBP reflects a shift from clinical practices based on the opinions of authorities or anecdotal evidence to an emphasis on data-based, clinically relevant studies and research (Jette et al., 2003). In EBP, a comprehensive review of relevant research from *both* the basic and the clinical sciences contributes to the foundation of evidence for clinical practice.

Research can provide the underlying evidence critical to the clinical decision-making process. Basic research on the physiology and pathophysiology of motor control can provide the evidence base for clinical hypotheses about the underlying cause(s) of impairments, functional limitations, and restricted participation in a patient with a specific diagnosis. This research can also assist in the generation of hypotheses regarding the prognosis for the patient. Research on the psychometric properties of tests and measures, including validity, reliability, sensitivity, and responsiveness in different patient populations, can provide the clinician guidance when choosing appropriate tests and measures to evaluate a patient with a specific diagnosis. Finally, research on the relative effects of different therapeutic interventions provides the evidence base for choosing an intervention and determining both the appropriate dose and expected response of an intervention in a specific patient. Thus, evidence-based medicine is the integration of relevant research, clinician expertise, and patient preference into the decision-making process and is critical in ensuring that clinical practice is consistent with the evolving research basis for the field.

Applying a Conceptual Framework to Clinical Practice

How do these elements work together to provide a comprehensive framework for clinical practice? Theories of motor control and learning provide a framework of assumptions regarding the nature and cause of normal and abnormal movements, as well as factors affecting motor learning and recovery of function. A model of practice identifies the steps to follow during the course of clinical intervention, including examination, identification of goals and outcomes, and establishment of a plan for intervention to achieve them. A model of health-related function and disability provides a systematic way to examine the diverse effects of a health condition on the individual. It provides a common way of thinking and communicating information regarding underlying components of health and function in patients with motor control problems. Hypothesis-oriented practice helps us to explore the association between a health condition and components of functioning, including impairments of body structure and function and limitations and restrictions in domains of activities and participation. This allows us to develop an intervention program that takes into consideration both the resources and the constraints on health and functioning of the individual. Evidence-based clinical practice reinforces the importance of integrating the best research evidence from both basic and applied clinical sciences with clinical expertise and the goals and values of each individual patient.

Developing a Personal Conceptual Framework for Clinical Practice

This chapter presents the elements of a clinical framework that we, the authors, find useful and relevant to our own clinical practice. However, as we found in the discussion of motor control theories (see Chapter 1), there is no one clinical framework that is universally accepted by all clinicians. Whether clinicians are aware of it or not, an underlying conceptual framework is a driving factor to determine their clinical actions. Thus, we suggest that all clinicians try to become conscious of an underlying conceptual framework that would help in both rationalizing their therapeutic practice and justifying as many modifications as the clinical situation requires. In addition, as was true for motor control theories, the information that a conceptual framework brings to practice will change over time; and accordingly, the framework adopted by the clinician will also need to be changed in order to remain current with evidence-based information. We strongly believe that examining, and regularly updating, your own conceptual framework is critical to your clinical practice.

The remaining section of this chapter discusses how these concepts are integrated into a "task-oriented" approach to patient treatment. In later chapters, we will show the specific application of this approach to retraining posture, mobility, and upper-extremity function in the patient with neurologic dysfunction.

TASK-ORIENTED APPROACH TO EXAMINATION

A task-oriented approach to clinical practice uses a multifaceted approach to clinical management of motor control problems in patients with CNS pathology. A task-oriented approach, integrated within the ICF framework, examines behavior at a number of different levels, including (1) evaluation of functional activities and participation, (2) a description of the strategies used to accomplish functional skills, and (3) quantification of the underlying sensory, motor, and cognitive impairments (limitations in underlying body structure and function) that constrain performance of functional activities and restrict participation. In addition, a task-oriented approach recognizes the importance of contextual factors, including personal and environmental features that affect how an individual functions in a social and physical context. Since there is no single test or measure that allows one to collect information on all these components, clinicians are required to assemble a battery of tests and measures, enabling them to document problems at all levels of analysis.

Examination of Functional Activities and Participation

Examination of activities and participation looks at the ability of the individual to perform essential tasks and activities in a standard (clinical) environment (referred to in the ICF as "measurement of capacity") and the person's actual environment (referred to in the ICF as "measurement of performance"). Evaluation of functional activities and participation can involve self-report (or proxy report) and/or observation of the individual performing the test, also referred to as "performance-based measures."

Performance-based measures examine the patient's ability to perform functional tasks, while interview measures rely on the patient's (or a proxy's) report of their ability to perform functional activities and engage in all aspects of participation. Researchers have found a high correlation between self-report and performance-based measures, suggesting that self-report can be a valid way to examine functional activities and participation. Self-reported measures can be used when a patient is temporarily unable to perform certain activities (such as asking a patient who has had a recent hip fracture to report on their previous independence in ADLs).

Measuring Participation: Function in a Social and Physical Context

An important aspect of examination of patients with motor control problems is examining the effect of a health condition within the context of the person's life, referred to as participation in the ICF framework. Limitations in functional activities are defined by the individual's capacity to do specific tasks and activities in a standardized environment, while participation is defined with reference to behavior in a social and physical context (WHO, 2001). Measuring participation and its inverse, disability, is often difficult because of a lack of both a clear operational definition and valid methods of measurement. In addition, the concept of participation includes complex tasks, often performed with others and strongly influenced by environmental factors (Jette, 2003; Yorkston et al., 2008).

Participation has both objective and subjective dimensions. Traditional measures of participation and disability often focus on the objective dimension, quantifying frequency of participation or level of independence in performing ADL (either basic or instrumental). For example, the Late-Life Function and Disability Instrument (Haley et al., 2002; Jette et al., 2002) is an example of a measure designed to quantify activities (functional limitations) and participation (disability) as distinct dimensions. An example of a measure of disability that could be used with children is the Pediatric Evaluation of Disability

Inventory (Haley et al., 1992). In addition, many instruments that measure participation may only cover certain domains. For instance, in stroke rehabilitation, frequently used participation-related instruments include the Stroke Impact Scale (SIS), London Handicap Scale, Assessment of Life Habits (LIFE-H), Frenchay Activities Index, and Activity Card Sort (ACS). Each of these instruments covers different domains within the ICF framework for participation, for example: community, social and civic life, domestic life, and mobility. Currently, there is a paucity of instruments that examine other relevant participation domains such as learning and applying knowledge, general tasks, and demands or communication (Tse et al., 2013).

A second approach to measuring participation focuses on the subjective dimension in which individuals themselves report their opinions and feelings about their actual level of participation relative to their desired level of participation. For example, the Children's Assessment of Participation and Enjoyment (CAPE) and its companion measure, Preferences for Activities of Children (PAC), measures participation in children ages 6 to 21 years (King et al., 2004; Law et al., 2006). The CAPE is a 55-item measure of six dimensions of participation (diversity, intensity, where, with whom, enjoyment, and preference), with three levels of scoring: (a) overall participation scores; (b) domain scores reflecting participation in formal (i.e., organized or structured activities) and informal activities; and (c) scores in five types of activities (recreational, active physical, social, skill based, and self-improvement). The CAPE has been shown to have good reliability (King et al., 2004; Law et al., 2006) and construct validity (King et al., 2006).

Several researchers have found a low association between objective and subjective measures of participation, which implies that objective measures and subjective perceptions of participation are independent of each other (Brown et al., 2004; Johnston et al., 2002, 2005; Robinson, 2010; Yorkston et al., 2008). Researchers have found that frequency of participation in functional activities has only a slight relationship with perceived satisfaction and significance of these activities, suggesting that significance and satisfaction cannot be inferred from objective measures of frequency of participation. Thus, objective measures of participation must be supplemented by subjective measures that reflect an insider perspective.

Clinical Measures of Function

When measuring the ability to perform functional activities, clinicians have a wide variety of measures from which to choose, with more measures emerging in the clinical literature. Tests and measures can be task-, age-, or diagnosis-specific.

Task-Specific Tests and Measures. Some tests limit their focus to specific tasks such as balance, mobility, or upper-extremity control. Examples of these types of tools include the Berg Balance Scale (BBS) (Berg, 1993), the Performance-Oriented Mobility Assessment (Tinetti, 1986), and the Erhardt Test of Manipulatory Skills (Erhardt, 1982). These tests have been developed to provide clinicians with a clearer picture of the patient's functional skills related to a limited set of tasks the clinician will be directly involved in retraining. These task-specific tests will be covered in later chapters, which discuss retraining posture and balance, mobility, and upper-extremity functions.

Age-Specific Tests and Measures. Age-specific tests and measures have also been created. There are a number of tests available for examining pediatric patients, including the Gross Motor Function Measure (Russell et al., 1993), the Test of Infant Motor Performance (Campbell et al., 1995; Kolobe et al., 2004), the Peabody Developmental Motor Scales, the Bayley Scales of Infant Development, and the Pediatric Evaluation of Disability Index (Feldman et al., 1990). The Bruininks–Oseretsky test is often used for examining motor function in older school-aged children (Bruininks, 1978). At the other end of the age range are tests designed specifically for a geriatric population. Examples of these tests include the Performance-Oriented Mobility Assessment (Tinetti, 1986), the Functional Reach Test (Duncan et al., 1990), and the Physical Performance and Mobility Examination (Lemsky et al., 1991).

Pediatric versions of many tests developed for adults are now available, for example, the Functional Reach Test (Bartlett & Birmingham, 2003; Gan et al., 2008), the BBS (Gan et al., 2008; Kembhavi et al., 2002), the Clinical Test for Sensory Interaction in Balance (Gagnon et al., 2006; Richardson et al., 1992), and the Timed Up and Go (Gan et al., 2008; Williams et al., 2005).

Diagnosis-Specific Tests and Measures. A number of tools have been developed to examine functional limitations and underlying impairments in specific patient populations. The most prevalent of this type of tool relates to examining function following stroke. Examples of these include the Motor Assessment Scale for Stroke Patients (Carr et al.,1985), the Fugl-Meyer test (Fugl-Meyer et al., 1975), the Motor Assessment in Hemiplegia (Brunnstrom, 1966), and the Stroke Rehabilitation Assessment of Movement (STREAM) (Ahmed et al., 2003; Daley et al., 1999). Scales have been developed to evaluate the severity of symptoms associated with Parkinson disease, including the Unified Parkinson's Disease Rating Scale (Hoehn & Yahr, 1967) and the Schwab Classification of Parkinson Progression (Schwab, 1960) and—for persons with multiple sclerosis—the Expanded Disability Status Scale (Kurtzke, 1983).

Choosing Appropriate Tests and Measures. As you can see, a large number of tests and measures are available from which to choose. How does a clinician decide what tool to use? A number of factors can be considered when choosing an instrument. Patient-related factors such as age and diagnosis should be considered. Level of function must also be considered in order to avoid a measure with either floor or ceiling effects. Floor effects result when a test is chosen that is too difficult for the patient's level of function; thus, scores are all uniformly too low. Alternatively, a test that is too easy will result in scores that are all uniformly too high, thus creating a ceiling effect.

Test-related factors should also be considered when choosing a clinical test or measure. The purpose of the examination and the ability of a test to accomplish that purpose are important factors to consider when choosing a test or measure. An examination can serve different purposes; it can be used to discriminate, evaluate, or predict (Campbell, 1991; Ketelaar et al., 1998). Discriminative measures are used to distinguish individuals who have a particular problem from those who do not. For example, the Up and Go Test (Podsiadlo & Richardson, 1991) determines the relative risk for functional dependence in older adults. Based on results from this test, an older adult could be classified as being in a low-risk or a high-risk group. Another example is the BBS, which has been found useful in discriminating older adults who are prone to falling from those who are not (Muir et al., 2008; Shumway-Cook et al., 1997a, 1997b).

An evaluative measure is used to measure change over time or after treatment. The Gross Motor Function Measure is a standardized observational instrument developed to measure change in gross motor function over time in children with cerebral palsy (Russell et al., 1993). A predictive measure classifies people based on future status. The Bleck scale predicts ambulation in 7-year-olds using postural and reflex activity evaluated at a preschool age (Bleck, 1975). Results from the Walk and Talk test are predictive of future falls in a population of institutionalized elders (Lundin-Olsson et al., 1997).

Often, therapists choose a test or measure based on personal preference rather than for theoretical reasons, which can result in a number of problems. For example, your intent as a therapist may be to measure change following your intervention. If you select a measure designed primarily to discriminate among people, you may find no significant difference in preintervention and postintervention scores, not because your patient has not responded to your treatment but because you have chosen a test that may not be sensitive to change.

Psychometric properties such as reliability, validity, sensitivity, and specificity will vary from test to test. Reliability reflects the dependability or consistency of a test, that is, its ability to measure accurately and predictably without variation when no true change has occurred (Dobkin, 1996). Consistency is reflected through both intrarater and interrater reliability. Intrarater reliability indicates a high degree of correlation when performance is measured by the same therapist over repeated applications of the test; interrater reliability indicates a high degree of agreement among multiple raters. If more than one therapist is to examine a patient over time, interrater reliability is critical to accurate data collection (Guccione, 1991).

Validity of a test is a complex concept that reflects the degree to which an instrument measures what it purports to measure (Dobkin, 1996). There are many aspects to validity. Content validity, often determined by a panel of experts, is linked to the definition of the construct being examined. It objectively examines the extent to which a group of items represents the domain examined by the instrument or test. Similar to content validity, face validity indicates the subjective degree to which an instrument measures what it is supposed to measure. Construct validity determines whether the test construct (i.e., the theoretical or conceptualized idea under examination) measures what it has been hypothetically designed for in comparison with well-established measures that examines other constructs. Concurrent validity is the degree to which the performance of two instruments that measure the same factors and are carried out simultaneously agree with each other (Dobkin, 1996; DeVellis, 2017). Finally, both sensitivity and specificity are important attributes of an instrument to quantify its diagnostic ability. Sensitivity is the degree to which a diagnostic test detects a disorder or dysfunction when it is present (true positives). In contrast, specificity reflects the ability of a test to rule out a disorder or dysfunction when it is not present (or true negatives) (Altman & Bland, 1994).

New research examining the measurement properties of tests and measures commonly used in the rehabilitation process is continually emerging. This type of research enables both researchers and clinicians to judge the quality and value of a specific instrument. It is only through this type of research that clinicians can ensure the validity, reliability, and accuracy of the data collected on any patient and establish a strong evidence-based foundation on which to build a clinical-decision making process.

Finally, *resource-related* factors may be considered when choosing a test. Consideration must be given to the skill and level of training of the therapists giving the test. Many standardized tests require that therapists be trained to give the test with an established level of proficiency. This requires time and resources that a facility may not be willing to provide. The amount of time available for examination as well as available space and equipment also need to be considered.

Limitations of Functional Tests and Measures. There are a number of limitations inherent in clinical measures of function. While functional measures will allow a therapist to document functional status (e.g., level of independence associated with performing specific functional tasks and activities), they do not provide information as to why the patient is dependent in performing functional skills. Thus, functional tests will not allow the therapist to test hypotheses about the cause of motor dysfunction.

Therapists retraining patients with movement disorders are concerned about not just the degree to which patients can carry out a task but also about how they perform the task. Functional measures in general are limited to providing information on the former but rarely the latter. Finally, clinical measures of function are limited to evaluating performance at one instant in time, under a fairly limited, and often relatively ideal, set of circumstances. Results from a functional-based examination do not always predict participation, that is, performance in the home or community environment. For example, because a patient can walk safely and independently with a cane in the clinic does not necessarily mean the patient can (or will) walk safely and independently in a cluttered, poorly lit home environment.

Despite these limitations, clinical measures of function enable the clinician to document a patient's functional status and are an important part of justifying therapy to the patient, the patient's family, and third-party insurers.

Examination at the Strategy Level

Examination at the strategy level is a *qualitative* approach to measuring function activities, since it examines the strategies used to perform functional tasks. The term "strategy" is not limited to the evaluation of the movement pattern used to accomplish a task but includes how the person organizes sensory information necessary to performing a task in various environments as well as how attentional resources are allocated.

Why is it important for clinicians to examine the strategies a patient uses when performing a functional task? One answer is that the strategies used to perform a task largely determine the level of performance. According to Welford (1982), a psychologist from England, performance depends on four factors. The first relates to the demands of the task and the person's desire for particular standards of achievement. The second relates to the capacities, both mental and physical, that a person brings to the task. The third relates to the strategies that the person uses to meet the demands of the task, while the fourth relates to the ability to choose the most efficient strategy for a given task given the constraints.

Note that two of the four factors relate to strategies, emphasizing their importance in determining our level of performance. Thus, the strategies we use relate the demands of the task to our capacity to perform it. If we choose poor strategies, and the task is difficult, we may reach the limits of our capacities well before we have met the demands of the task. In contrast, inefficient strategies may still be effective in carrying out simple, less demanding tasks. As the capacity to perform a task declines because of either age or disease, we may be unable to meet its demands unless we use alternative strategies to maintain performance levels.

For example, as a young adult, you rise quickly out of a chair without the need to use your arms. You rely on the ability to generate momentum, using movements of your trunk, and the strength in your legs, to rise from the sitting position. As you age, strength may slowly decline without affecting your ability to use this strategy for getting up. But at some threshold, the loss of strength in your legs means that you are no longer able to get up using your once-effective momentum strategy. Instead, you begin to use your arms to get up, thereby maintaining the functional ability to rise from a chair, albeit with a new strategy. Thus, in an individual with a neurologic deficit, maintaining functional independence depends on the capacity of that individual to meet the demands of the task in a particular environment. When impairments limit the capacity to use well-learned strategies, the patient must learn new ways to accomplish functional tasks despite these limitations. An excellent example of this may be seen in the video case study of Genise as she recovers from an acute stroke. Prior to her stroke, Genise was able to stand up quickly and efficiently without the use of her arms. At 4 days poststroke, Genise is unable to stand up without significant physical assistance from her therapist, due to her profound hemiparesis. At 1 month poststroke, her paresis remains a significant impairment, but she has learned a new strategy for arising and is now able to stand up independently using primarily her nonparetic arm and leg. By 6 months poststroke, she is able to stand up from a chair again without the use of her arms.

Limitations to a Strategy Examination of Function

Clinicians are hampered in their ability to examine sensory, motor, and cognitive strategies used to perform daily tasks because methods for examining these strategies are just being developed. Only limited information exists defining sensory, motor, and cognitive strategies in neurologically intact subjects. In addition, we know very little about how compensatory strategies develop as a result of neurologic impairments.

Researchers have begun to quantify movement strategies used in functional tasks such as gait, stance postural control, and other mobility skills such as moving from sitting to standing, from a supine to a prone position, and from a supine to a standing position. Clinical tools to examine movement strategies have grown out of these analyses. An example is the use of observational gait analysis to define the movement strategies used during ambulation.

Examining Impairments of Body Structure and Function

Finally, examination at the third level focuses on identifying the impairments that potentially constrain functional movement skills. This requires examination of impairments within individual sensory, motor, and cognitive systems contributing to movement control, as well as multisystem impairments of posture, balance, and gait. Examination of the motor system includes both the neuromuscular and the musculoskeletal systems. Since perception is essential to action, examination of sensory and perceptual abilities in the control of movement is necessary. And since task-specific movement is performed within the context of intent and motivation, cognitive aspects of motor control, including mental status, attention, motivation, and emotional considerations, must be examined.

In summary, a task-oriented approach to examination is directed at answering the following questions:

1. What is the functional *capacity* of a patient during standardized testing? And to what degree can the patient *perform* functional tasks in less ideal more complex environments?
2. How do functional limitations restrict the patient's ability to participate in appropriate social roles and ADL (disablement)?
3. What strategies are used to perform functional tasks, and are those strategies adapted to changing task and environmental conditions?
4. What is the constellation of impairments that constrain how the patient performs the task, and can these impairments be changed through intervention?
5. Is the patient functioning at an optimal level given the current set of impairments, or can therapy improve either the strategies being used to accomplish functional tasks or the underlying impairments?

Once the examination is completed, the clinician can translate information gained through examination into a list of patient problems that reflect functional limitations and associated areas of disablement and underlying impairments constraining function. From this comprehensive list, the therapist and patient identify the most critical problems, which will become the focus for initial intervention strategies. Thus, a list of short- and long-term treatment goals is established and a specific treatment plan is formulated for each of the problems identified.

TASK-ORIENTED APPROACH TO INTERVENTION

A task-oriented approach to establishing a comprehensive plan of care includes intervention strategies designed to achieve the following goals derived from the examination:

1. Resolve, reduce, or prevent impairments in body structure and function.
2. Develop effective and efficient task-specific strategies for accomplishing functional task goals.
3. Adapt functional goal-oriented strategies to changing task and environmental conditions in order to maximize participation and minimize disablement.

These goals are not approached sequentially but, rather, concurrently. Thus, a clinician may use intervention strategies designed to focus on one or more of the aforementioned goals within the same therapy session. For example, when retraining mobility in Genise, our patient who has had a stroke, the clinician uses therapeutic techniques to (a) improve recruitment of muscles in the paretic limbs and decrease the effect of spasticity and abnormal synergies (impairments in body structure and function); (b) improve weight bearing on the involved leg during the stance phase of gait, to produce a more symmetrical gait pattern (strategy-level intervention); (c) practice walking a distance of 100 ft on a level surface in the clinic (improved performance of a functional activity); and (d) practice walking from the clinic to the car, crossing uneven surfaces while engaged in a conversation (participation-oriented intervention).

Recovery Versus Compensation

A question that frequently arises during the course of rehabilitating the patient with a CNS lesion regards how much emphasis should be placed on promoting recovery of "normal" strategies, that is, those strategies the patient used prior to the injury, versus teaching compensatory strategies for performing a task in light of current impairments. Recovery of pre-injury strategies (i.e., restorative interventions) for function is defined as the returning capability of the individual to perform a task using mechanisms used prior to the injury. Compensatory strategies can be defined as atypical approaches that take advantage of the patient's residual abilities. These strategies are designed to meet the requirements of the task using alternative mechanisms not typically used, for example, standing with the weight shifted to the nonparetic leg following a stroke. Compensatory strategies can also reflect modifications to the environment that simplify the demands of the task itself. For example, as shown in Figure 6.4, a

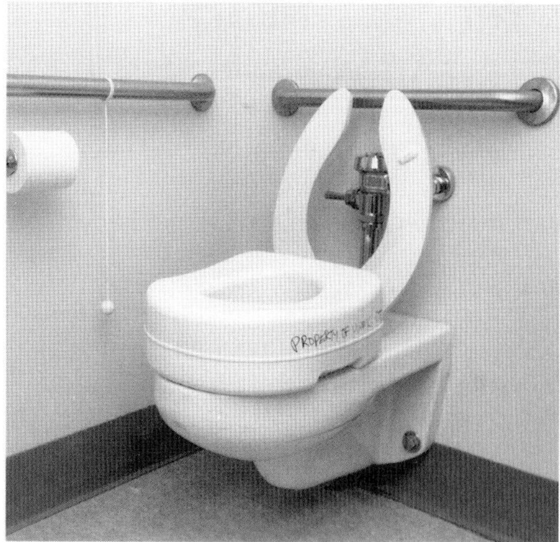

Figure 6.4 Changing the environment to accommodate functional limitations—raised toilet seat and bars around a toilet to facilitate transfers.

raised toilet seat and grab bars may be installed to assist a patient in transferring on to and off of the toilet.

When to facilitate pre-injury ("normal") strategies versus compensatory strategies is not easy to determine and will vary from patient to patient. Often, the criterion used to determine when compensatory strategies should be taught is time. That is, in the patient with an acute injury, emphasis is on recovery of pre-injury functional strategies, while in the patient with a chronic condition, the emphasis shifts to maximizing function through compensatory strategies.

We have found it helpful in the decision-making process to consider the nature of the impairments themselves in determining whether pre-injury versus compensatory strategies should be taught. Compensatory strategies will be needed in the case of permanent, unchanging impairments, regardless of whether the patient has an acute or a chronic condition. An example would be teaching a patient with a permanent loss of vestibular function to rely on alternative vision and somatosensory cues for maintaining balance during functional tasks or teaching a patient with a complete spinal cord lesion to become independent in ADLs using compensatory strategies. Alternatively, if impairments are temporary and changeable (either through natural recovery or in response to therapy), the emphasis would be on remediating impairments and recovery of pre-injury functional strategies for action.

A problem arises when it is not known whether impairments will resolve. For example, in Genise, our patient with an acute CVA with profound hemiparesis, it is not always possible to predict whether paresis will persist or whether she will regain control over one or both affected extremities. In this case, the clinician may revert to a time-based decision-making process, working toward recovery of normal strategies in the acute stage and switching to a compensatory focus in the chronic stage.

SUMMARY

1. The conceptual framework for clinical practice presented in this chapter is built on five key elements: (a) a model of practice that establishes the steps for intervention; (b) hypothesis-oriented practice, which provides a process for testing assumptions regarding the nature and cause of motor control problems; (c) a model of functioning and disability that examines the constituents of health and the effects of disease on the individual; (d) theories of motor control and learning that suggest essential elements to examine and treat; and (e) EBP, which emphasizes the integration of research evidence, clinical expertise, and patient characteristics in clinical practice.
2. The APTA model of practice is a five-step process including (a) examination, (b) evaluation, (c) diagnosis, (d) prognosis, and (e) intervention.
3. A model of functioning and disability provides a system for examining the effects of a health condition on functioning in the individual. Functioning and its inverse, disablement, can be used as a framework for organizing and interpreting examination data.
4. During the course of clinical intervention, the clinician will be required to generate multiple hypotheses, proposing possible explanations regarding the problem and its cause(s), and must investigate these hypotheses through observation, tests, and measurement.
5. A theory of motor control contributes assumptions regarding the nature and control of movement, movement disorders, and treatment, while theories of motor learning identify factors critical to the (re)acquisition of functional movement skills.
6. A task-oriented approach examines the effect of a health condition at many levels, including the ability and strategies used to perform functional tasks and activities, the extent to which limitations in performance of functional activities restrict participation in social and environmental contexts, and the underlying impairments in body structure and function, including sensory, motor, and cognitive impairments.
7. A task-oriented approach to intervention focuses on (a) resolving or preventing impairments, (b) developing effective task-specific strategies, and (c) adapting functional goal-oriented tasks to changing environmental conditions, thus maximizing participation and minimizing disablement.

ANSWERS TO LAB ACTIVITY ASSIGNMENTS

Lab Activity 6.1

If you selected Genise, our patient with an acute stroke, the following answers to this lab activity apply.

1. Health condition: Cerebrovascular accident
2. At 4 days poststroke, Genise's limitations in body structure and function (impairments) include problems in the neural control of force (paresis), abnormal muscle tone, decreased coordination, sensory loss, and impaired balance and gait; however, she has no problems with cognition including impaired memory, judgment, and attention.
3. At 1 month poststroke, Genise has improved her ability to generate and control muscle forces in her lower extremity, though recovery in her hemiparetic arm is limited. Abnormal muscle tone has actually become worse (increased spasticity). Persisting inactivity and increased tone are contributing to the development of secondary musculoskeletal problems, including tightness both at the ankle joint and in the wrist and hand flexors.
4. At 1 month, Genise is developing independence in all her functional tasks, including bed mobility, sitting, standing, and walking. She is independent in her personal ADLs but only because she has learned to use her nonparetic arm. She is unable to perform bimanual activities.
5. During her initial phase of recovery, Genise was severely restricted in participating in most activities and roles important to her. Over the 6 months of her recovery, participation has increased.

PART II

Postural Control

"The ability to control our body's position in space is fundamental to everything we do."

CHAPTER 7

Normal Postural Control

Learning Objectives

Following completion of this chapter, the reader will be able to:

1. Define postural control, distinguish between postural orientation and stability, and describe a dynamic definition of limits of stability.
2. Define steady-state, reactive, and proactive (anticipatory) postural control, and describe how each contributes to the control of functional movement.
3. Describe the action (motor) components of postural control, being able to define strategies and synergies and how they change according to the balance task (steady-state, reactive, and proactive) and environmental demands.
4. Describe sensory systems in postural control, including the role of individual senses, current theories for sensory organization, and how sensory organization is adapted to changing task and environmental demands.
5. Describe the cognitive demands of postural control and the implications of this for maintaining stability in multitask situations.
6. Describe the neural subsystems controlling postural orientation and stability.

INTRODUCTION

Why do we have an entire section of this book devoted to understanding postural control? Postural control is critical to independence in functional tasks, such as sitting, standing, and walking. Clinicians understand that impaired postural control is a common problem in both musculoskeletal and neurologic populations, and the consequences of impaired balance are significant. Impaired postural control contributes not only to loss of functional independence but also to reduced participation in daily life activities, increased risk for falls, and even increased risk for mortality and morbidity.

While there is universal agreement that postural control is critical to functional independence, clinicians do not necessarily agree on the best way to assess and treat impaired postural control in their patients. Multiple factors contribute to this lack of agreement, including a lack of consensus on the definitions of postural control and balance and on the neural mechanisms underlying the control of these functions. A clinician's approach to assessing and treating impaired postural control is dependent on both knowledge and skills, knowledge related to the research explaining the musculoskeletal and neural basis for normal and impaired balance control, and the skillful use of evidence-based clinical strategies for assessment and treatment.

Research and clinical practice have a profound influence on one another. As shown in Figure 7.1, research regarding the neural basis for normal and impaired postural control helps a clinician to identify the possible factors that are likely to contribute to imbalance in their patient. Research also helps a clinician to identify valid and reliable clinical measures used to assess and verify the specific factors that are actually contributing to imbalance. Finally, research helps a clinician to identify effective treatment strategies for improving impaired posture and balance control. So how can clinical practice influence research? Through their practice, clinicians identify an unmet need, which can serve as a catalyst for research. For example, many clinical measures were initially developed by clinicians in response to a need to assess a specific aspect of function not addressed in other measures. This initial development is then followed by a variety of research studies examining the reliability and validity of that clinical measure.

This chapter focuses on research explaining the neural basis for normal postural control. We begin our discussion with definitions of commonly used terms. We then go on to discuss a systems framework for normal

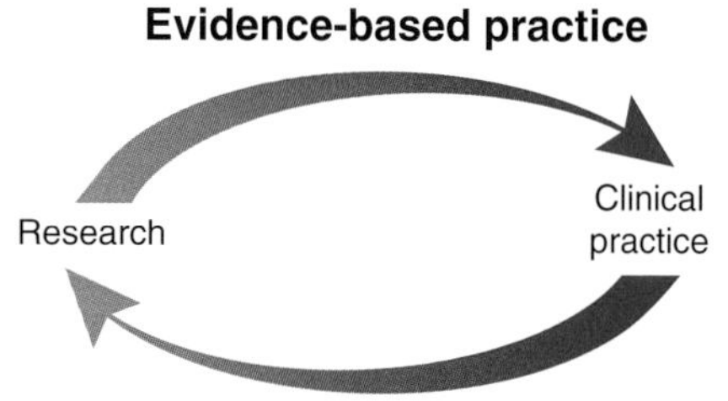

Evidence-based practice

Research → Clinical practice → Research

Neural basis for normal and impaired balance	What factors are likely contributing to imbalance in my patient?
Clinical methods (tests and measures) for examining balance	What strategies can I use to assess balance in my patient?
Evidence-based treatment of impaired balance	What strategies can I use to treat balance in my patient?

Figure 7.1 The interaction between research and clinical practice.

postural control including the motor, sensory, and cognitive contributions to the tasks of balance and consider how aspects of the environment constrain the organization of processes important to postural control.

Defining Postural Control

Postural control involves controlling the body's position in space for the dual purposes of stability and orientation. What is stability? Is it the same or different from orientation? **Postural orientation** is defined as the ability to maintain an appropriate relationship between the body segments and between the body and the environment for a task (Horak & Macpherson, 1996). The term "posture" is often used to describe both the biomechanical alignment of the body and the orientation of the body to the environment. We use the term "postural orientation" to include both of these concepts. For most functional tasks, we maintain a vertical orientation of the body. **Postural stability** is the ability to control the center of mass (COM) in relationship to the base of support (BOS). The **COM** is defined as a point that is at the center of the total body mass, which is determined by finding the weighted average of the COM of each body segment. The vertical projection of the COM is defined as the **center of gravity (COG)**. The **BOS** is defined as the area of the body that is in contact with the support surface. While researchers often talk about stability as controlling the COM relative to the BOS, they often mean controlling the vertical projection of the COM, the COG, relative to the BOS. In this book, we often use the terms "COM" and "COG" interchangeably. The term "postural control" is often used interchangeably with the terms "balance" and "equilibrium." In this text, we use the terms "posture," "balance," and "equilibrium" synonymously with the term "postural control."

What evidence do we have that the COM is the key variable being controlled by the nervous system during postural control? Research examining this question can be found in the Extended Knowledge 7.1.

What is the center of pressure (COP), and what role does it play in stability? As will be discussed in more detail in later sections of this chapter, to ensure stability, the nervous system generates forces to control motion of the COM. The COP is the center of the distribution of the total force applied to the supporting surface. The COP moves continuously around the COM to keep the COM within the support base (Benda et al., 1994; Winter, 1990). However, when the COM is outside the support base, it does not necessarily mean that a fall will occur. For instance, the COM of professional ice skaters (see Fig. 7.2A) is occasionally beyond the support base, yet the skater would still have full control of the body. As we will describe later in more detail, this example shows why we cannot fully define postural control without considering the task and the environment.

All tasks require postural control. That is, every task has an orientation component and a stability component. However, the stability and orientation requirements will vary with the task and the environment. Some tasks place importance on maintaining an appropriate orientation at the expense of stability. The successful blocking of a goal in soccer requires that the player always remain oriented with respect to the ball (see Fig. 7.2B), sometimes falling to the ground in an effort to block a goal. In contrast, the tightrope walker

Extended Knowledge 7.1

What does the postural control system actually control?

While most researchers hypothesize that it is the COM that is controlled during postural control, it is hard to experimentally verify this, as the COM is not a physical entity but is a virtual point in space that depends on the position of all body segments. Alternatively, the key variable controlled during balance could be joint positions or activation of specific muscles. If the nervous system controls the COM, it must be able to estimate the position of the COM using information from the various sensory receptors (Scholz et al., 2007). In order to determine whether the COM was the primary variable controlled by the nervous system during postural control, Scholz et al. (2007) used a new analysis tool, the uncontrolled manifold (UCM) approach. Using this approach, these researchers showed that when recovering from a loss of balance, subjects tend to reestablish the preperturbation COM position rather than the preperturbation joint configuration. This finding supports the hypothesis that the key variable controlled by the CNS during postural control is the COM (Scholz et al., 2007).

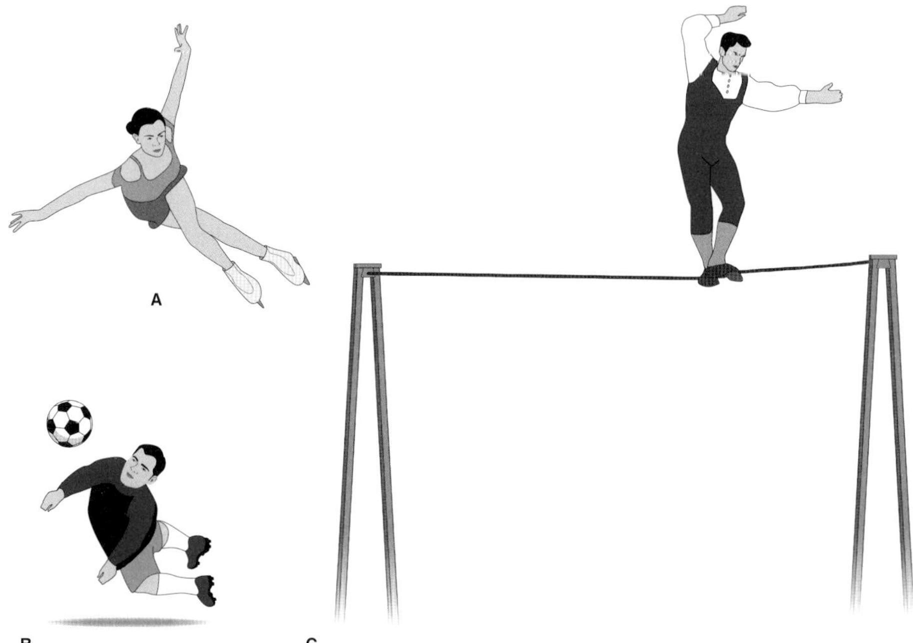

Figure 7.2 Stability and orientation requirements vary with the task. **(A)** The professional ice skater can maintain the center of mass beyond the base of support without falling. **(B)** Stability is sacrificed in order to maintain an appropriate orientation to the soccer ball. **(C)** In contrast, walking a tightrope requires careful control of stability.

in Figure 7.2C must maintain stability (i.e., keep the COM within the BOS) at all costs to prevent a fall and life-threatening injuries. Thus, while postural control is a requirement that most tasks have in common, stability and orientation demands change with each task (Horak & Macpherson, 1996; Shumway-Cook & McCollum, 1990).

Both the task and the environment influence the orientation and stability demands of a task. For example, the task of sitting on a bench and reading has a postural orientation requirement of keeping the head and gaze stable and fixed on the reading material (Fig. 7.3A). The stability requirements of this task are lenient. Since the contact of the body with the bench, back, and seat provides a fairly large BOS, the primary postural control requirement is controlling the unsupported mass of the head with respect to the mass of the trunk. In contrast, the task of standing and reading a book has roughly the same postural orientation requirement with respect to the head, eyes, arms, and book, but the stability requirement is considerably more stringent (Fig. 7.3B), as it involves

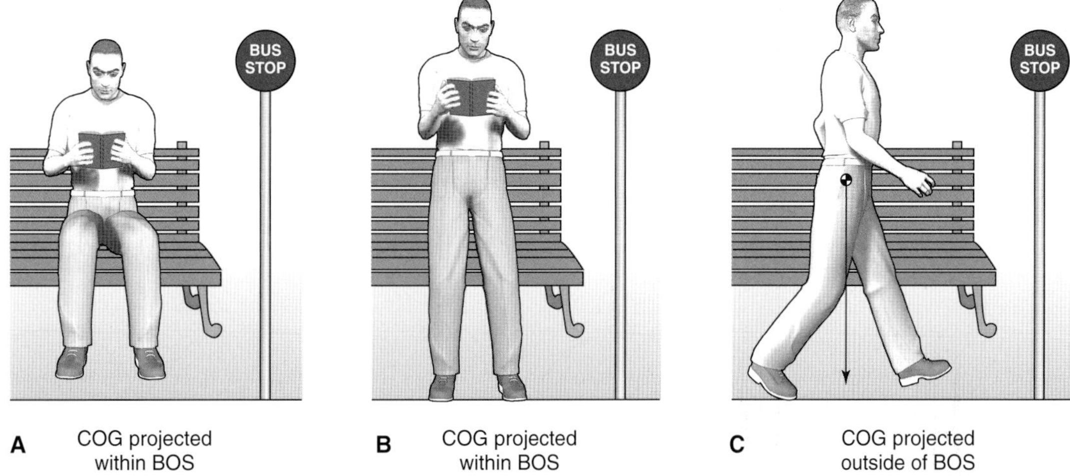

Figure 7.3 **(A)** Both the task and the environment influence the orientation and stability demands of a task. For example, the task of sitting on a bench and reading has a postural orientation requirement of keeping the head and gaze stable and fixed on the reading material. **(B)** The stability requirements of this task are lenient, since the contact of the body with the bench back and seat provides a fairly large base of support. The task of standing and reading a book has the same postural orientation requirement, but the stability requirement is more stringent. **(C)** The task of controlling stability during walking is very different from the task of balance during stance since when walking, the center of gravity often falls outside the base of support.

controlling the COM relative to a much smaller BOS defined by the two feet. Finally, the task of controlling stability during walking (Fig. 7.3C) is very different from the task of balance during stance (Winter et al., 1991). In walking, the COM does not stay within the support base of the feet, and thus, the body is in a continuous state of imbalance. To prevent a fall, the swinging foot is placed ahead of and lateral to the COG as it moves forward, thus ensuring control of the COM relative to a moving BOS. Thus, you can see that while these tasks demand postural control, the specific orientation and stability requirements vary according to the task and the environment.

A Systems Framework for Postural Control

As noted in Chapter 1, a systems framework suggests that postural control, like all aspects of motor control, emerges from an interaction of the individual with the task and the environment (Fig. 7.4).

Individual Systems for Postural Control

The ability to control our body's position in space emerges from a complex interaction of musculoskeletal and neural systems, collectively referred to as the "postural control system," as shown in Figure 7.5. Musculoskeletal components include such things as joint range of motion, spinal flexibility, muscle properties, and biomechanical relationships among linked body segments. Neural components essential to postural control include (a) motor processes, which include organizing muscles throughout the body into muscle synergies; (b) sensory processes that include detection of individual sensory signals (visual, vestibular, and somatosensory), and their integration and organization to produce limb and body orientation and motion in space or with respect to the environment; and (c) higher-level cognitive processes, including both cognitive resources and strategies essential for mapping sensation to action and ensuring anticipatory and adaptive aspects of postural control (Peterka, 2018).

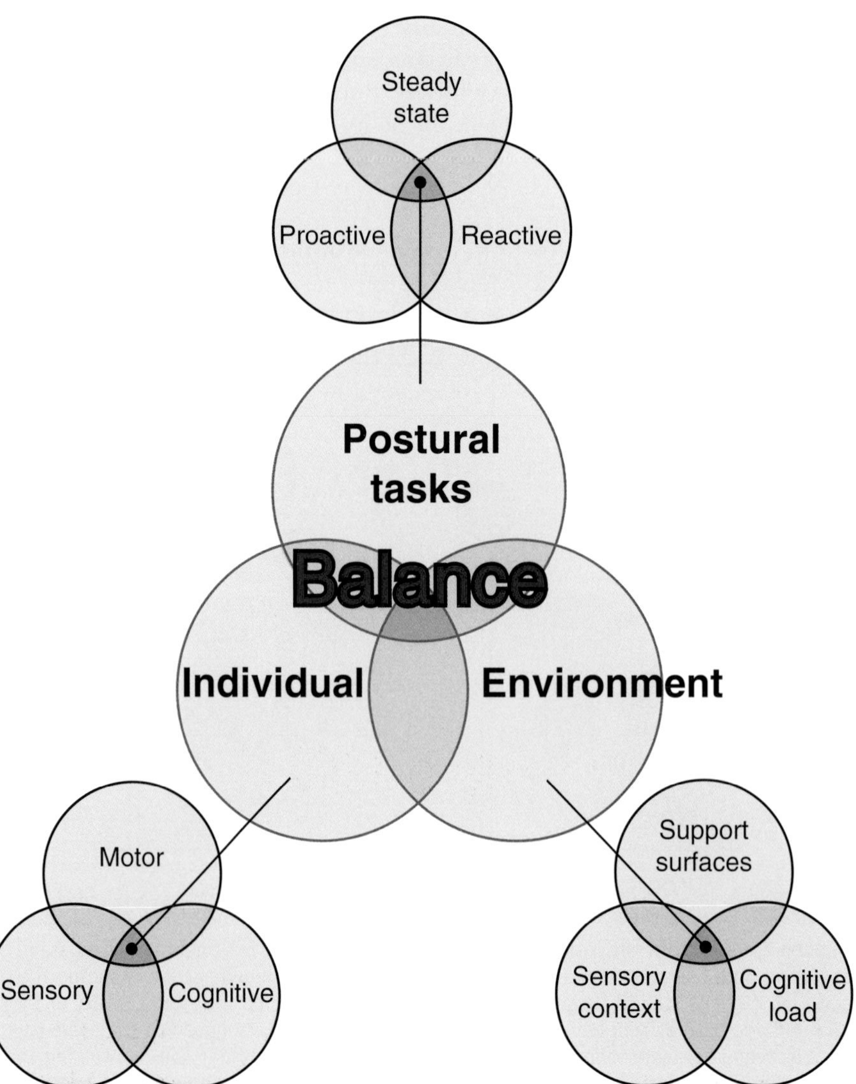

Figure 7.4 Balance emerges from the interaction of the individual, the task, and the environment, as represented by the central three circles in the figure. Functional tasks require three types of balance control: steady-state, reactive, and proactive. Environmental constraints such as type of support surface, sensory cues, and cognitive demands also impact the control of balance.

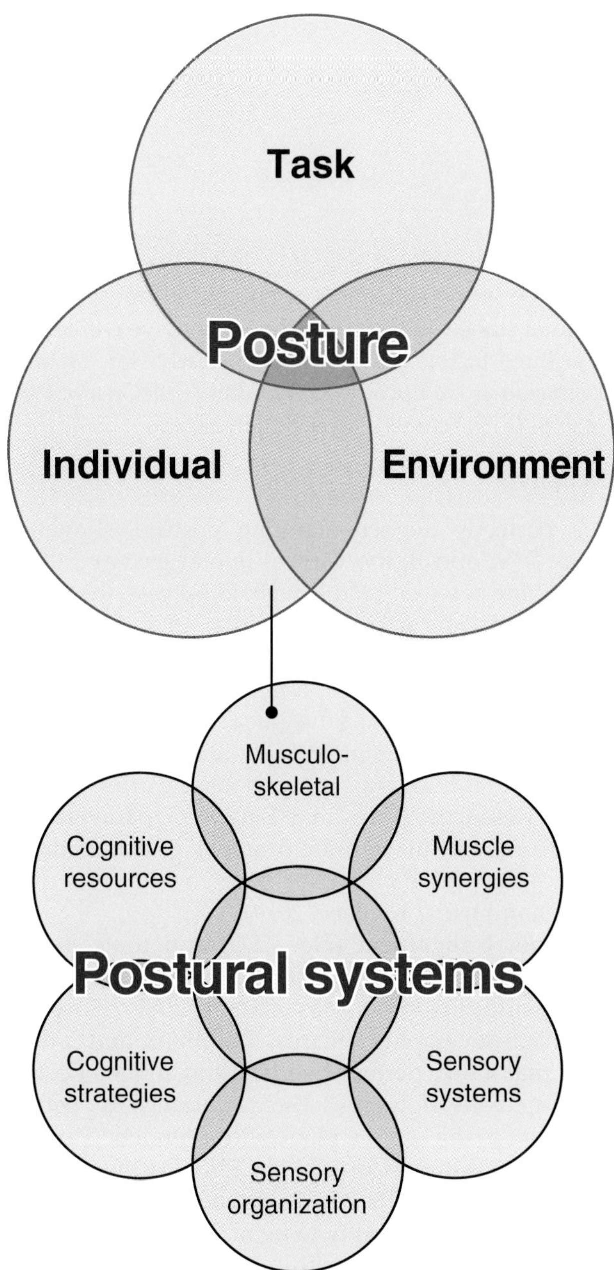

Figure 7.5 Conceptual model representing the many components of postural control that have been studied by researchers. Postural control is not regulated by a single system but emerges from the interaction of many systems.

In this text, we refer to higher-level neural processes as cognitive influences on postural control. It is very important to understand, however, that the term "cognitive" as it is used here does not necessarily mean conscious control. Higher-level cognitive aspects of postural control are the basis for learning and retention of adaptive and anticipatory aspects of postural control. Adaptive postural control involves modifying sensory and motor systems in response to changing task and environmental demands. Anticipatory aspects of postural control pretune sensory and motor systems for postural demands based on previous motor experience and learning. Other aspects of cognition that affect postural control include processes such as attention, motivation, and intent.

Thus, in a systems approach, postural control results from a complex interaction among many bodily systems that work cooperatively to control both orientation and stability of the body. The specific organization of postural systems is determined both by the functional task and the environment in which it is being performed.

Task Constraints

Daily life is characterized by the performance of a wide variety of functional tasks and activities requiring three types of balance control: steady-state, reactive, and proactive balance (refer back to Fig. 7.4). Steady-state balance is defined as the ability to control the COM relative to the BOS in fairly predictable and nonchanging conditions. Sitting, standing quietly, and walking at a constant velocity are examples of tasks that require steady-state balance control. Reactive balance control is the ability to recover a stable position following an unexpected perturbation. For example, walking and tripping over an obstacle or being bumped in a crowd requires the activation of multiple muscles in the legs and trunk to recover a stable position of the COM relative to the BOS. An inability to rapidly generate and apply appropriate corrective muscle forces to recover balance can result in a fall. Proactive or anticipatory balance is the ability to activate muscles in the legs and trunk for balance control in advance of potentially destabilizing voluntary movements. Lifting a heavy object, such as a bag of groceries, or stepping up onto a curb are two examples of tasks that require anticipatory balance. When anticipatory muscle activity is delayed or absent, performance of these tasks can lead to loss of balance and falls.

Reactive balance control relies on feedback mechanisms; in contrast, proactive balance utilizes primarily feedforward mechanisms. *Feedback control* refers to corrective postural control strategies that occur in response to detected sensory errors (visual, vestibular, or somatosensory) after an external perturbation. *Feedforward control* refers to anticipatory postural adjustments (APAs) that are executed in anticipation of a voluntary movement that is potentially destabilizing in order to maintain stability during the movement. These concepts are shown in Figure 7.6.

Most functional tasks require all three aspects of balance control at some point or another. For example, reaching for a heavy object while standing requires steady-state balance to maintain a stable position prior to the reach, anticipatory balance control to prevent loss of stability during the reach and lift, reactive balance control if the object is heavier than expected and lifting it causes us to lose balance, and then finally steady-state balance again after the task is completed.

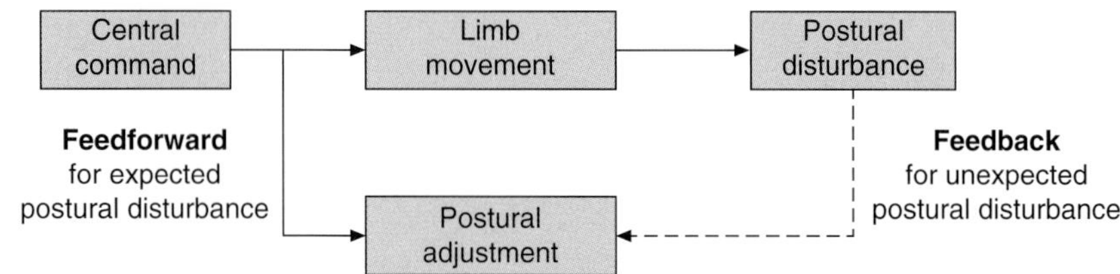

Figure 7.6 Feedforward versus feedback aspects of postural control.

Environmental Constraints

A systems framework also recognizes that environmental conditions (refer back to Fig. 7.4) impact the way sensory, motor, and cognitive systems are organized to control balance. Changes in support surfaces affect the organization of muscles and forces needed for balance. Differences in visual and surface conditions affect the way sensory information is used for balance control. Finally, daily life often requires that we perform multiple tasks, affecting the way cognitive systems like attention are used for balance.

The remainder this chapter discusses the motor contributions to steady-state, reactive, and proactive balance in sitting and standing, followed by the sensory and cognitive contributions to these aspects of balance control. Issues related to balance control during walking will be handled in Part III, "Mobility Functions."

MOTOR SYSTEMS IN POSTURAL CONTROL

Motor systems ensure the generation of sufficient coordinated forces in appropriate muscles to control the body's position and movement in space to ensure orientation and stability. Motor systems include systems involved in higher-level planning (frontal cortex and motor cortex), postural learning (basal ganglia and cerebellum), coordination (brainstem and spinal networks coordinating postural muscle synergies), and generation of forces (motor neurons and muscles) that produce movements effective in controlling the body's position in space.

Steady-State Balance

Stability underlying sitting and/or standing quietly has often been called "static balance," because the BOS is not changing. However, this term is misleading. Sitting or standing quietly is characterized by varying amounts of postural sway as the body moves continuously within its BOS. Thus, steady-state balance control is really quite dynamic.

A number of factors contribute to our ability to maintain steady-state stability, ensuring that we keep our postural sway within the BOS. First, body alignment can minimize the effect of gravitational forces, which tend to pull us off center. Second, muscle tone keeps the body from collapsing in response to the pull of gravity because of (a) the intrinsic stiffness of the muscles themselves and (b) the background muscle tone, which exists normally in all muscles because of neural contributions. Third, postural tone is the activation of antigravity muscles during quiet stance. In the following section, we will look at these three factors contributing to steady-state stability (Basmajian & De Luca, 1985; Kendall & McCreary, 1983; Roberts, 1979; Schenkman & Butler, 1992).

Alignment

In a perfectly aligned standing posture, shown in Figure 7.7A and B, the vertical line of gravity falls in the midline between (a) the mastoid process, (b) a point just in front of the shoulder joints, (c) the hip joints (or just behind), (d) a point just in front of the center of the knee joints, and (e) a point just in front of the ankle joints (Basmajian & De Luca, 1985). Activation of spinal muscles to maintain body alignment is a critical factor in minimizing postural sway during upright stance. Research shows that fatigue of paravertebral muscles may result in more dramatic postural control changes than fatigue of ankle, knee, or shoulder muscles (Ghamkhar & Kahlaee, 2019).

Skeletal alignment (Fig. 7.7C) and tonic muscle activity are also a critical aspect of maintaining steady-state balance in sitting (Masani et al., 2009). However, typically, developing infants, children, and adults rarely maintain a perfectly vertical and aligned posture in sitting; instead, there is a wide variance in postural alignment in the sagittal plane with a tendency toward a kyphotic posture (Curtis et al., 2015; Rachwani et al., 2017). Nonetheless, the ideal alignment when standing or sitting allows the body to be maintained in equilibrium with the least expenditure of internal energy.

Before we continue reviewing the research concerning postural control, be sure to review the information contained in Technology Tools 7.1, 7.2, and 7.3, which include a discussion of techniques for movement analysis at different levels of control, including electromyography (EMG) (Technology Tool 7.1), kinematics (Technology Tool 7.2), and kinetics (Technology Tool 7.3).

Muscle Tone

What is muscle tone, and how does it help us to keep our balance? "Muscle tone" refers to the force with which a muscle resists being lengthened, that is, its stiffness (Basmajian & De Luca, 1985). Muscle tone is often tested clinically by passively extending and flexing a relaxed patient's limbs and feeling the resistance offered by the muscles. Both nonneural and neural mechanisms contribute to muscle tone or stiffness.

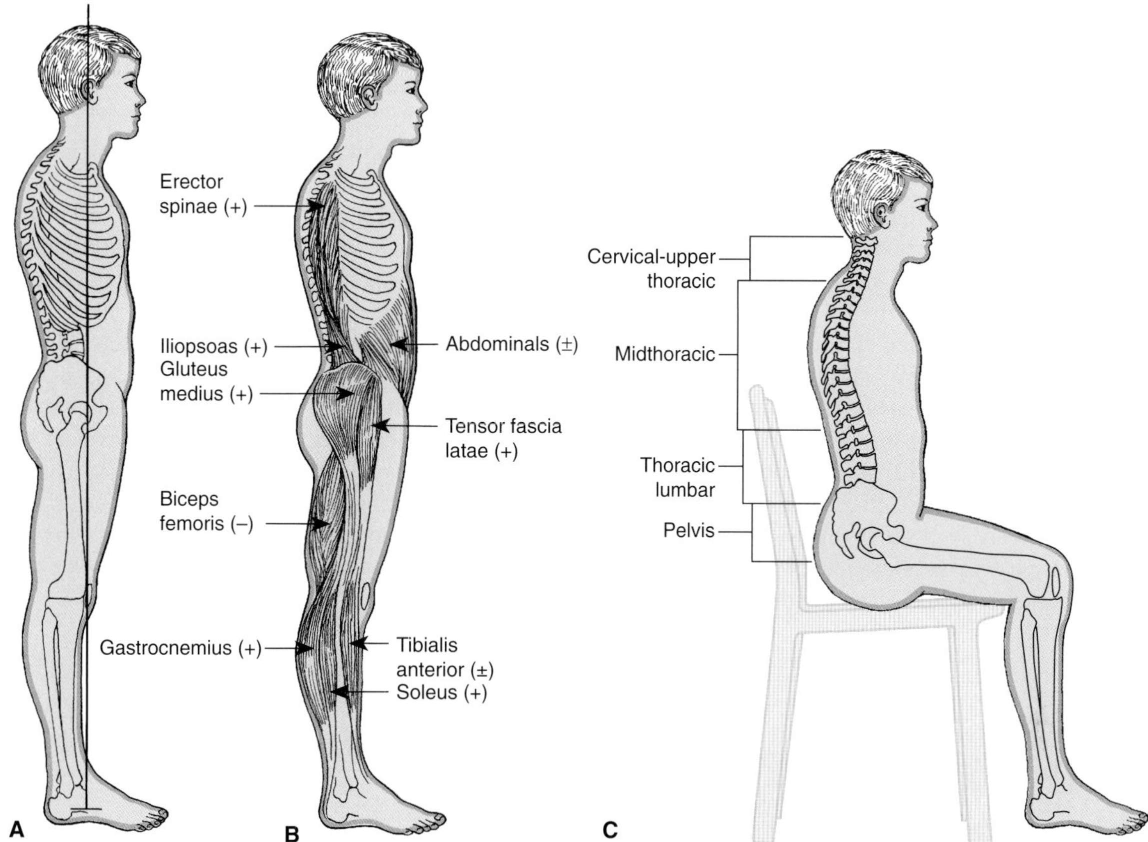

Figure 7.7 (A) The ideal alignment in stance, requiring minimal muscular effort to sustain the vertical position. **(B)** The muscles that are tonically active during the control of quiet stance. **(C)** Alignment in sitting, showing the proposed segments of trunk control including cervical–upper thoracic, midthoracic, thoracic–lumbar, pelvis. (Parts **A** and **B** adapted from Kendall FP, McCreary EK. *Muscles: testing and function*, 3rd ed. Baltimore, MD: Williams & Wilkins, 1983:280.)

TECHNOLOGY TOOL 7.1 Electromyography

Surface EMG is a technique used for measuring the activity of muscles through electrodes placed on the surface of the skin, over the muscle to be recorded, or in the muscle itself. The output signal from the electrode (the electromyogram, or EMG) describes the output to the muscular system from the motor neuron pool. It provides the clinician with information about (a) the identity of the muscles that are active during a movement, (b) the timing and relative intensity of muscle contraction, and (c) whether antagonistic or synergistic muscle activity is occurring. Surface electrodes are most often used; however, the ability of these electrodes to differentiate between the activity of neighboring muscles is not very effective.

The amplitude of the EMG signal is often interpreted as a rough measure of tension generated in the muscle. However, caution must be used when interpreting EMG amplitude measurements. There are many variables that can affect the amplitude of EMG signals, including how rapidly the muscle is changing length, resistance associated with cutaneous tissue and subcutaneous fat, and location of the electrode. Thus, generally, it is not accurate to compare absolute amplitudes of EMG activity of a muscle across subjects or within the same subject across different days. Researchers who use EMG amplitude data to compare temporal and spatial patterns of muscle activity across subjects or within a subject on different days generally convert absolute amplitude measures to relative measures. For example, one can determine the ratio between the response amplitude (the area under the curve of EMG activity for a specified time period, called "integrated EMG," or IEMG) and the amplitude of a maximum voluntary contraction of that muscle. Alternatively, the ratio of IEMG for agonist and antagonist muscles at a joint can be determined. Likewise, the ratio of IEMG for synergistic muscles can be found. One can then examine how this ratio changes as a function of changing task or environmental conditions (Gronley & Perry, 1984; Winter, 1990).

TECHNOLOGY TOOL 7.2 Kinematic Analysis

Kinematic analysis is the description of the characteristics of an object's movement, including linear and angular displacements, velocities, and accelerations. Displacement data are usually gathered from the measurement of the position of markers placed over anatomic landmarks and reported relative either to an anatomic coordinate system (i.e., relative joint angle) or to an external spatial reference system. There are various ways to measure the kinematics of body movement. Goniometers, or electrical potentiometers, can be attached to a joint to measure a joint angle (a change in joint angle produces a proportional change in voltage). Accelerometers are usually force transducers that measure the reaction forces associated with acceleration of a body segment. The mass of the body is accelerated against a force transducer, producing a signal voltage proportional to the acceleration. Finally, imaging measurement techniques, including cinematography, videography, or optoelectronic systems, can be used to measure body movement. Optoelectronic systems require the subject to wear special infrared lights or reflective markers on each anatomic landmark; one or more cameras record these lights. The location of the light, or marker, is expressed in terms of *x*- and *y*-coordinates in a two-dimensional system or *x*-, *y*-, and *z*-coordinates in a three-dimensional system. Output from these systems is expressed as changes in segment displacements, joint angles, velocities, or accelerations, and the data can be used to reconstruct the body's movement in space (Gronley & Perry, 1984; Winter, 1990).

TECHNOLOGY TOOL 7.3 Kinetic Analysis

Kinetic analysis refers to the analysis of the forces that cause movement, including both internal and external forces. Internal forces come from muscle activity, ligaments, or friction in the muscles and joints; external forces come from the ground or external loads. Kinetic analysis gives us insight into the forces contributing to movement. Force-measuring devices or force transducers are used to measure force, with output signals that are proportional to the applied force. Force plates measure ground-reaction forces, which are the forces under the area of the foot, from which COP data are calculated. The term "COG of the body" is not the same as the "COP." The COG of the body is the net location of the COM in the vertical direction. COP is the location of the vertical ground-reaction force on the force plate and is equal and opposite of all the downward-acting forces (Gronley & Perry, 1984; Winter, 1990).

A certain level of muscle tone is present in a normal, conscious, and relaxed person. However, in the relaxed state, no electrical activity is recorded in normal human skeletal muscle using EMG. This has led researchers to inferthat nonneural contributions to muscle tone are the result of small amounts of free calcium in the muscle fiber, which cause a low level of continuous recycling of cross-bridges (Hoyle, 1983).

The review of Lakie and Campbell (2019) shows that the viscoelastic characteristic of muscles contributes to the muscle property called thixotropy. Thixotropy is a passive, intrinsic, and nonlinear muscle property in which muscle resistance is greater during small movements and lower in larger movements. Interestingly, this muscle resistance during small movements goes away with movement repetition but rebuilds when there is no movement. Passive muscle properties, such as thixotropy, are of particular relevance to maintain muscle stiffness during quiet standing. In healthy conditions, long-lasting upright stance has low energy cost, and it is controlled through the activation of fatigue-resistant slow-twitch muscle fibers (Herbison et al., 1981; Ivanenko & Gurfinkel, 2018). However, quiet postural standing just requires low force generation through a partial number of motor units at submaximal activation to overcome the effect of gravity and the resistance offered by inactive muscle fibers. Research has shown that relaxed muscles make a large contribution to muscle stiffness. Lakie and Campbell (2019) propose that relaxed calf muscles may contribute up to 5% to 20% of the total stiffness of each ankle (300 N*m/rad). There are also important neural contributions to muscle tone or stiffness. Muscle tone is defined as long-lasting and fatigue-resistant muscle activity that is sensitive to head positions (tonic neck and vestibular reflexes). The control of muscle tone in the axial musculature (trunk and proximal limb segments) sustains posture during both static and dynamic conditions. The somatic descending brain stem pathways, monoaminergic descending systems (serotonergic, noradrenergic, and dopaminergic tracts), and even the limbic system modulate muscle tone (Gurfinkel et al., 2006). Within the motor cortex, there exist neurons that are specific to either load-related activity or movements, in such a way that load-related neurons only depolarize while maintaining posture but not during movement, and vice versa (Ivanenko & Gurfinkel, 2018). Another aspect of the modulation of muscle tone is that it may be regulated by *shortening* and *lengthening* reactions that increase and decrease muscle activity, respectively. Interestingly, this muscle effect is the opposite of the one observed in stretch reflexes (Gurfinkel et al., 2006). It is often assumed that stretch reflexes play a feedback role during the maintenance of stance posture. In other words, as we sway back and forth at the ankle while standing, the ankle muscles are stretched, activating the stretch reflex. This results in a reflex shortening of the muscle and subsequent control of forward and backward sway. However, researchers have shown that the gain of the spinal stretch reflex in the ankle muscles is quite low during stance, leading to doubts about the relevance of stretch reflexes in the control of stance (Gurfinkel et al., 1974).

Postural sway may play an important role in maintaining a flow of dynamic sensory inputs to the central nervous system (CNS; Carpenter et al., 2010). New evidence shows that the control of certain postural states in standing may be regulated by other peripheral neural mechanisms. Horslen and colleagues (2013, 2018) investigated the spinal stretch reflex of the soleus muscle at the tendon (T-reflex) and spinal (H-reflex) levels during tasks associated with balance threats (e.g., standing on elevated platforms causing a risk of falls). They found an amplification of tendon-mediated stretch reflexes without significant increases in H-reflex amplitudes or background muscle activity. Thus, the authors suggest that a critical increase in muscle spindle sensitivity is an adaptive strategy enabling an increase in sensory-related postural information to the CNS), which is essential when postural movement is restricted.

Postural Tone

When we stand upright, activity increases in antigravity postural muscles to counteract the force of gravity; this is referred to as *postural tone*. Sensory inputs from multiple systems are critical to postural tone. Lesions of the dorsal (sensory) roots of the spinal cord reduce postural tone, indicating the importance of somatosensory inputs to postural tone. Activation of cutaneous inputs on the soles of the feet causes a placing reaction, which results in an automatic extension of the foot toward the support surface, thus increasing postural tone in extensor muscles. Somatosensory inputs from the neck activated by changes in head orientation can also influence the distribution of postural tone in the trunk and limbs. These have been referred to as the "tonic neck reflexes" (Ghez, 1991; Roberts, 1979). Inputs from the visual and vestibular systems also influence postural tone. Vestibular inputs, activated by a change in head orientation, alter the distribution of postural tone in the neck and limbs and have been referred to as the "vestibulocollic" and "vestibulospinal" reflexes (Massion & Woollacott, 2004).

In the clinical literature, considerable emphasis has been placed on the concept of postural tone in trunk muscles as a major mechanism in supporting the body against gravity (Schenkman & Butler, 1989). In a study examining muscle activity before a seated reaching task in young adults with external trunk support, there was significant baseline tonic EMG activity in the lumbar, thoracic, and cervical paraspinal muscles during steady-state balance (Santamaria et al., 2018). Thus, it appears that trunk muscle activity is critical to the maintenance of steady-state balance in the seated position. What have EMG studies reported about the muscles active in quiet stance?

Researchers have found that many muscles in the body are tonically active during quiet stance (Basmajian & De Luca, 1985). Some of these muscles are shown in Figure 7.6B and include (a) the soleus and gastrocnemius, because the line of gravity falls slightly in front of the knee and ankle; (b) the tibialis anterior, when the body sways in the backward direction; (c) the gluteus medius and tensor fasciae latae but not the gluteus maximus; (d) the iliopsoas, which prevents hyperextension of the hips, but not the hamstrings (HAM) and quadriceps; and (e) the thoracic erector spinae in the trunk (along with intermittent activation of the abdominals), because the line of gravity falls in front of the spinal column. Research has suggested that appropriate activation of abdominal and other trunk muscles often discussed in relation to "core stability" is important for efficient postural control, including postural compensation for respiration-induced movement of the body (Hodges et al., 2002; Mok et al., 2004).

These studies suggest that muscles throughout the body are tonically active to maintain the body in a narrowly confined vertical position during quiet stance. Although *"static" postural control* may traditionally be used to describe postural control during quiet stance or sitting, you can see that control is actually dynamic. In fact, research suggests that postural control involves active sensory processing, with a constant mapping of perception to action, so that the postural system is able to calculate where the body is in space and can predict where it is going and what actions will be necessary to control this movement.

Movement Strategies

Is quiet stance really quiet? In addition, how do postural sway and the movements used to control postural sway vary depending on your BOS? To answer these questions for yourself, do Lab Activity 7.1. As you can see, "quiet" stance is not quiet from the perspective

LAB ACTIVITY 7.1

Objective: To explore the motor strategies used for steady-state and reactive postural control

Procedure: With a partner, observe body movement in the following conditions:

1. Stand with your feet shoulder distance apart for 1 minute. Observe the alignment of your partner and amount of body sway.
2. Try leaning forward and backward a little and then as far as you can without taking a step. Now lean so far forward or backward that you have to take a step.
3. Come up on your toes and do the same thing.
4. Put on a pair of ski boots (constraining ankle movement) and try swaying backward and forward.
5. Now have your partner place three fingers on your sternum and nudge you backward, first gently and then with more force.

Assignment

Write answers to the following questions, based on your observations of your and your partner's balance under the different conditions:

1. During quiet stance, did you stand perfectly still, or did you move very slightly? In which direction did you feel yourself swaying most? What type of balance control underlies the ability to stand safely and independently?
2. During active sway, describe the movement strategies you used to control body sway.
3. Describe the movement strategies used when reacting to nudges from your partner. What type of balance control underlies the ability to recover a stable position following an unexpected displacement to the COM?
4. Discuss how those strategies change as a function of (a) size of BOS, (b) speed of movement, (c) where the COM was relative to the BOS (well inside, near edge, outside), and (d) when movement was constrained at the ankle (wearing ski boots).
5. List the muscles you think were active to control sway in these conditions. (a) What muscles did you feel working to keep you balanced when you swayed a little? (b) What muscles worked when you swayed further? (c) What happened when you leaned so far forward that your COM moved outside the BOS of your feet?

of the neural control processes, since many mechanisms are active when we are trying to maintain the COM within stability limits. Previously, stability limits during stance were conceptualized rather statically, defined solely by the physical characteristics of the BOS, the feet. More recent research has suggested that stability limits are not fixed boundaries but change according to the task; characteristics of the individual, including such things as strength; range of motion; characteristics of the COM; and various aspects of the environment. While early research on stance postural control tended to emphasize the importance of the position of the COM relative to stability limits, more recent research has suggested that any understanding of stability must consider both the position and the velocity of the COM at any given moment (Pai et al., 2000). It is the interaction between these two variables, rather than just the position of the COM alone, that determines whether a person will be able to remain stable within their current BOS or be required to take a step or reach for support in order to regain stability. For further information on how position and velocity of COM interact in steady-state balance, refer to Extended Knowledge 7.2.

Extended Knowledge 7.2

Interactions Between COM Displacement and Velocity

Many factors have an impact on how the COM is controlled relative to the stability limits of the body in stance, including both the velocity and the position of the COM. Figure 7.8 illustrates this point. In this figure, three possible trajectories of the COM (combining velocity and displacement) in response to an external perturbation in standing are plotted. The shaded area indicates the region of the COM state space where stepping is predicted to be necessary. The initial position of the COM is indicated by the arrow head and is about midfoot prior to the perturbation. In trajectory 1, the combined change of COM position and velocity remains small enough so that stability is recovered without a change in the BOS. In contrast, in trajectory 2, displacement and velocity are sufficient to move the COM beyond the stability boundary, necessitating a step to recover stability. Trajectory 3 also requires a step, not because the amplitude of displacement of the COM is great but because the velocity is high, resulting in the need for a step to recover stability. For both trajectories 2 and 3, the final position of the COM is in front of the toe, indicating that a step has occurred (Pai et al., 2000).

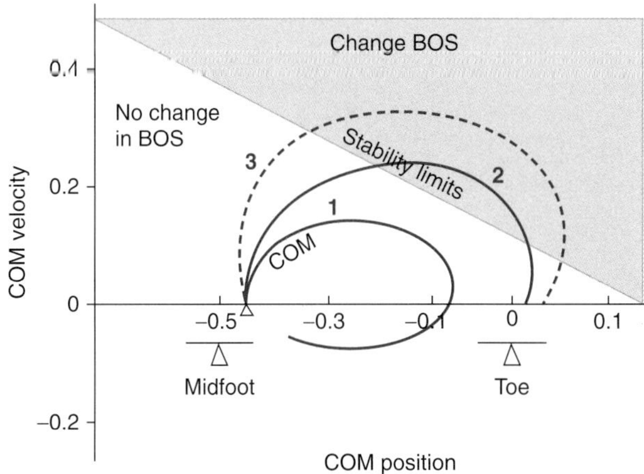

Figure 7.8 Interaction between center of mass motion (characterized by velocity on the *y*-axis and displacement on the *x*-axis) and type of response used to recover stability following an external perturbation. The shaded area indicates the region of the center of mass state space where stepping is predicted to be necessary. Three possible trajectories of the center of mass in response to a perturbation are shown. In trajectory 1, the combined change of center of mass position and velocity remains small enough so the center of mass does not cross the stability boundary; thus, stability is recovered without a step. In contrast, in trajectory 2, center of mass displacement and velocity are sufficient to move the center of mass beyond the stability boundary, necessitating a step to recover stability. The step is reflected by a trajectory that stabilized at a point beyond the toe of the original base of support. Trajectory 3 also requires a step, but this is because the initial center of mass velocity is high, though the displacement was initially small. The model illustrates the importance of center of mass velocity, not just position, in determining strategies for recovery of stability. (Adapted with permission from Pai YC, Maki BE, Iqbal K, et al. Thresholds for step initiation induced by support surface translation: a dynamic center of mass model provides much better prediction than a static model. *J Biomech*. 2000;33:390, Figure 3.)

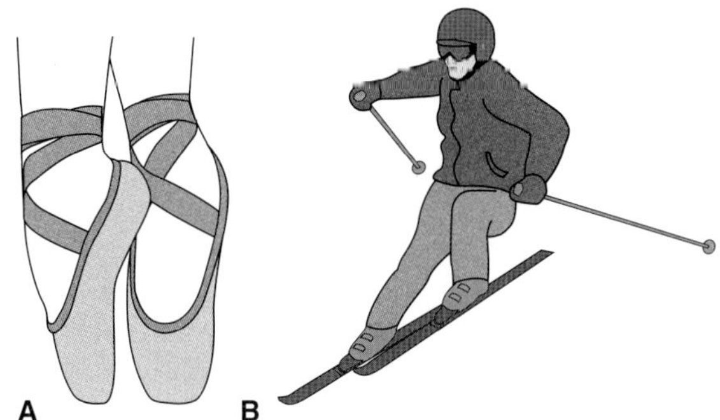

Figure 7.9 Stability limits vary as a function of the task. Stability limits in a dancer standing on point **(A)** are quite small. In comparison, stability limits are much larger in the person wearing skis **(B)**.

Stability limits (the point at which a person will change the configuration of their BOS to achieve stability) are also affected by other perceptual and cognitive factors, such as fear of falling and perception of safety (Pai et al., 2000). Thus, stability limits are not just defined by the biomechanics of the system, but perceptual and cognitive factors also contribute to the internal model we form related to our stability limits.

Because both quiet stance and sitting are characterized by body sway, passive skeletal alignment, in conjunction with muscle and postural tone, is not enough; rather, movement strategies are needed to maintain stability even when standing or sitting quietly. In addition, the movement strategies needed to control sway will also depend on the nature of the stability limits. For example, as shown in Figure 7.9A, stability limits for this dancer on point are quite small, necessitating minimal sway and movement control at the hip. In contrast, the person wearing skis has extended his BOS (Fig. 7.9B), has much larger stability limits, and thus is able to lean much further and still maintain stability.

Traditionally, researchers studying stance and seated postural control in humans have modeled the body as a single segment. In stance, sway occurs around the ankles, approximating an inverted pendulum, with the head, trunk, and legs moving as a single segment. In sitting, sway occurs around the hips, with the head, trunk, and arms considered a single body segment. In this model, sway is controlled mainly by movement about the ankle joint in standing or hips in the seated position.

More recently, research has shown that control is more complex than this. During quiet stance, the body behaves more like a multilink pendulum (legs and trunk) with two coexisting modes of control (Creath et al., 2005). These modes of control could be described as an ankle strategy (in which both leg and trunk segments move in phase) when sway frequencies are low (<1 Hz) or a hip strategy (in which the leg and trunk segments move out of phase) when sway frequencies are higher (>1 Hz). Depending on conditions, the CNS can move back and forth between these control modes. Both are always present, but one may predominate depending on sensory information and task conditions.

Goodworth and Peterka (2012) assumed a segmented model divided into upper and lower body to investigate how individuals maintain steady-state standing posture while standing with feet together on a tilting surface that was rotated at different amplitudes. Visual and vestibular information sources were manipulated. The findings of this experiment showed that lower-body control relied on reweighting sensory feedback, whereas upper-body control was mainly dependent on musculoskeletal mechanisms. The proper control of these intersegmental interactions assured effective maintenance of postural stance. Thus, new research is challenging the traditional inverted pendulum model as an explanation for the control of upright stance. This research concludes that quiet standing is multidimensional and may involve the coordination of many other joints along the longitudinal axis of the body aside from hips and ankles. Because there are many joints producing motion variability, the CNS needs to coordinate them to effectively maintain the body COM within the boundaries of the BOS (Hsu et al., 2007).

Research has shown that seated postural control is also more complex than previously thought. For example, recent studies have demonstrated that there is considerable intra- and intersubject variability in seated postural alignment, predominantly in the sagittal plane. During unsupported quiet sitting, typically developing individuals often assume a kyphotic posture. This same kyphotic posture if observed in a person with neurologic dysfunction would often be interpreted as a symptom of poor seated postural control (Curtis et al., 2015).

In addition, research has demonstrated that while the trunk can be controlled as a single segment, control also occurs in segmental zones (Saavedra et al., 2012; Santamaria et al., 2018). In typically developing infants and young adults, muscle activity underlying trunk postural control varies with the location and degree of external support provided, supporting the concept of segmental zones of control (Saavedra et al., 2012; Santamaria et al., 2018). As shown in Figure 7.7C, four segmental zones have been proposed: cervical–upper thoracic, midthoracic, thoracic–lumbar, and pelvis (Saavedra et al., 2012). This research supports the concept that the trunk is not controlled as a single segment in an inverted pendulum fashion but requires a complex coordination of muscle activity across specific segments of the trunk.

Clinical Applications of Research on Steady-State Balance

Clearly, steady-state balance is an important component of function since it enables us to maintain our body's position and movement in space under predictable and nonperturbed conditions, such as when sitting or standing quietly. Based on this research, how might you assess steady-state balance in a clinical setting? What are the tasks you would ask a patient to do in order to assess steady-state balance? Clinical tests and measures that examine a patient's ability to sit or stand independently, such as the Berg Balance Scale (BBS), are examining steady-state balance. Based on the research reviewed, what behaviors would you observe when the patient is sitting or standing quietly? Steady-state balance includes orientation, so observing the alignment of body segments, including different segments of the trunk, to one another and to gravity and the surface will be important. This includes examining anteroposterior (AP) as well as mediolateral (ML) alignment. Stability, which is the ability of the patients to maintain their COM within their BOS, is also important to observe. How much the COM moves relative to the BOS (postural sway) is also important to notice. Further information on tests of steady-state balance is found in Chapter 10.

Reactive Balance Control

Many research labs have studied reactive balance control, specifically the organization of movement strategies used to recover stability in response to brief displacements of the supporting surface, using a variety of moving platforms such as the one shown in Figure 7.10 (Allum & Pfaltz, 1985; Diener et al., 1982; Nashner, 1976). In addition, characteristic patterns of muscle activity, called "muscle synergies," which are associated with postural movement strategies used to recover stability in the sagittal plane, have been described (Horak & Nashner, 1986; Nashner, 1977; Nashner & Woollacott, 1979).

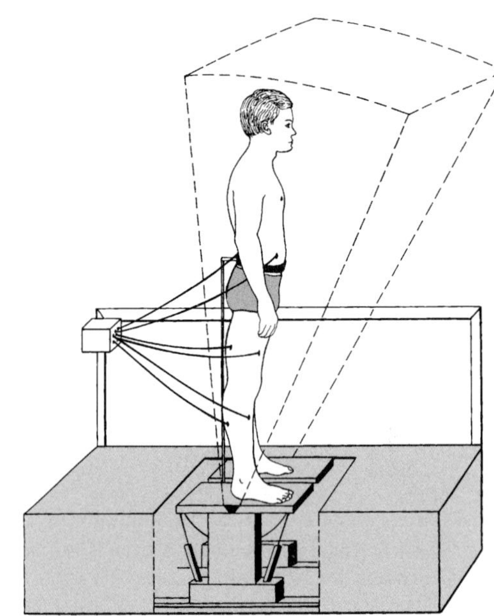

Figure 7.10 Moving platform posturography used to study postural control. (Adapted from Woollacott MH, Shumway-Cook A, Nashner LM. Aging and posture control: changes in sensory organization and muscular coordination. *Int J Aging Hum Dev.* 1986;23:108.)

What motor strategies do we use to respond to threats to balance? To answer this question, complete Lab Activity 7.2. As the lab exercise shows, the specific movement patterns used to recover stability following displacement of the COM are selected by the CNS based on a number of factors, including characteristics of the perturbation (e.g., direction and magnitude); biomechanical constraints, including musculoskeletal geometry and intersegmental dynamics of the individual's body (Kuo & Zajac, 1993); and environmental conditions. The motor patterns used for reactive balance control have been described as ankle, hip, step, and reach-to-grasp strategies (illustrated in Fig. 7.11). Alternatively, strategies have been characterized as fixed-support (ankle and hip) versus change-in-support (step or reach-to-grasp) strategies, depending on the research laboratory (Maki et al., 2003). Some researchers prefer the term "fixed-support" strategy rather than terms such as "ankle" or "hip" because discrete strategies are usually not observed during balance recovery following a slip or trip. Rather, subjects show a continuum of movements ranging from ankle through hip motion. In addition, as shown previously for quiet stance, these two modes

LAB ACTIVITY 7.2

Objective: To examine central organization and adaptation of sensory inputs to stance postural control.

Procedures: This lab *requires* a partner (for safety). Equipment needed is a stopwatch, an 18-by-18-by-3-inch piece of medium-density foam and a meter stick mounted horizontally on the wall at shoulder height, next to your partner. You will be measuring maximum sway in a forward or a backward direction during a 20-sec period of quiet stance in four conditions. In condition 1, your partner should stand on a firm surface (e.g., linoleum or wood) with feet together, hands on hips, and eyes open. Record the maximum shoulder displacement in the forward and backward directions. In condition 2, stand as previously mentioned, but with eyes closed. Record displacement. In condition 3, the subject should stand with feet together on the foam, with eyes open. Record displacement. In condition 4, stand on the foam with eyes closed. There is an increased risk for loss of balance in this condition, so be sure to stand close and guard your partner well. Record displacement.

Assignment

1. For each condition, make a list of the sensory cues that are available for postural control. Compare sway using your displacement measures across all conditions.
2. How does sway vary as a function of available sensory cues?
3. How do your results compare with Woollacott et al.'s (1986) results (conditions 1, 2, 4, and 5), found in Figure 7.16?

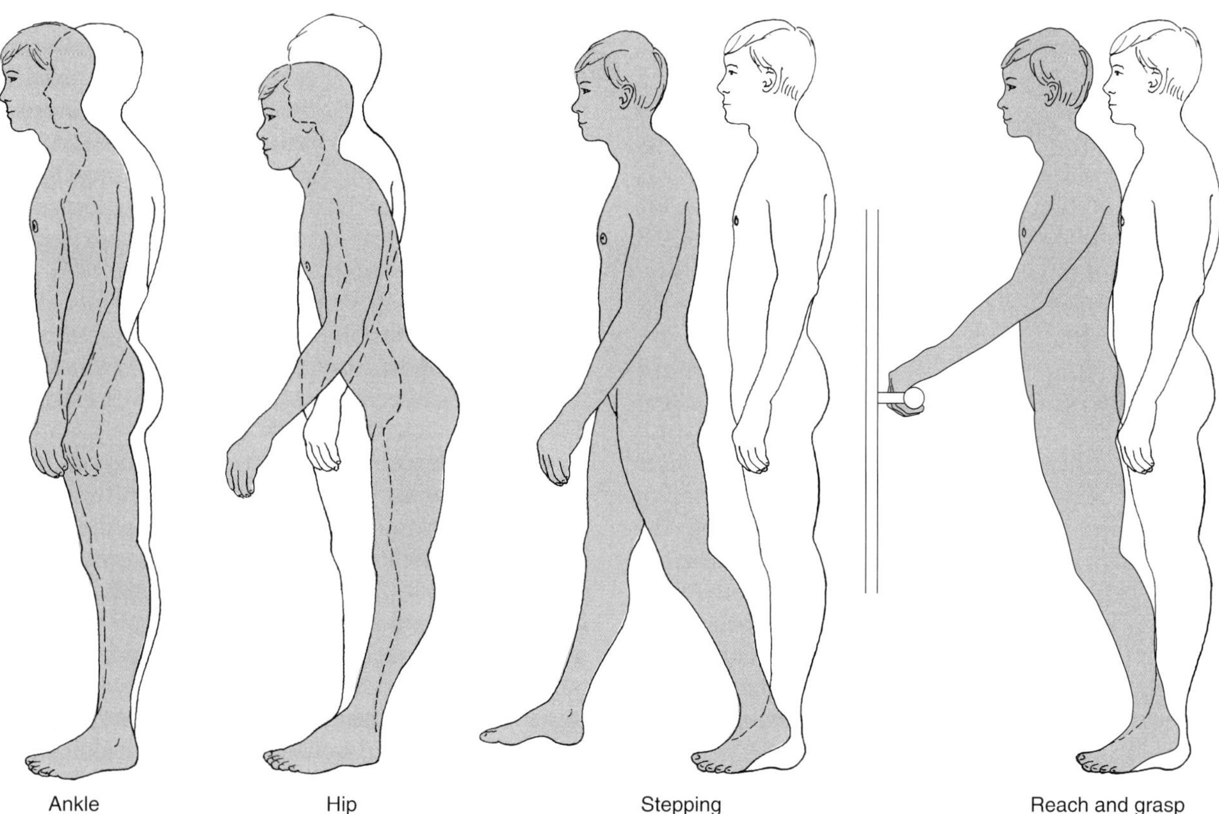

Figure 7.11 Four postural movement strategies used by normal adults when recovering stability following a threat to balance: ankle, hip, step, and reach. (Adapted from Shumway-Cook A, Horak F. Vestibular rehabilitation: an exercise approach to managing symptoms of vestibular dysfunction. *Semin Hearing*. 1989;10:199.)

may both be present in postural control, with one dominating, depending on the sensory and task conditions. Some authors also propose that upper extremity and trunk movements are also essential to the maintenance of balance during challenging dynamic balance tasks (Kim et al., 2018). Since the use of upper body movements to maintain or recover postural balance is more prevalent in challenging gait tasks such as walking on narrow beams, these upper body strategies will be further explained in Chapter 13.

Early postural control research by Nashner and colleagues (Horak & Nashner, 1986; Nashner, 1977; Nashner & Woollacott, 1979; Nashner et al., 1979) explored muscle patterns that underlie movement strategies for balance. Results from postural control research in neurologically intact young adults suggests that the nervous system combines independent, though related, muscles into units called "muscle synergies." A *synergy* is defined as the functional coupling of groups of muscles that are constrained to act together as a unit; this simplifies the control demands on the CNS.

What are some of the muscle synergies underlying movement strategies critical for reactive balance control? How do scientists know whether these neuromuscular responses are due to neural programs (i.e., synergies) or whether they are the result of independent stretch of the individual muscles at mechanically coupled joints? Are there different types of strategies and underlying muscle response synergies for AP stability versus ML stability? In the following sections, we examine strategies used for stabilization in multiple directions, including AP, ML, and also multidirectional planes of motion. We examine the research on motor strategies used to recover stability in standing as well as in sitting.

Anteroposterior Stability

As you discovered in Lab Activity 7.1, in both standing and sitting, among healthy adults, most sway occurs in the AP direction. This is the reason why researchers have studied movement strategies for postural recovery and muscle activity patterns to control AP stability.

Ankle Strategy. The ankle strategy and its related muscle synergy were among the first patterns for controlling upright sway to be identified. The ankle strategy restores the COM to a position of stability through body movement centered primarily about the ankle joints. Figure 7.12A shows the typical synergistic muscle activity and body movements associated with corrections for loss of balance in the forward direction during a translation of the platform in the backward direction. Muscle activity begins at about 90 to 100 ms after perturbation onset in the gastrocnemius, followed by activation of the hamstrings 20 to 30 ms later, and finally by the activation of the paraspinal muscles (Nashner, 1977, 1989).

Activation of the gastrocnemius produces a plantarflexion torque that slows, and then reverses, the body's forward motion. Activation of the hamstrings and paraspinal muscles maintains the hip and knees in an extended position. Without the synergistic activation of the hamstrings and paraspinal muscles, the indirect effect of the gastrocnemius ankle torque on proximal body segments would result in forward motion of the trunk mass relative to the lower extremities.

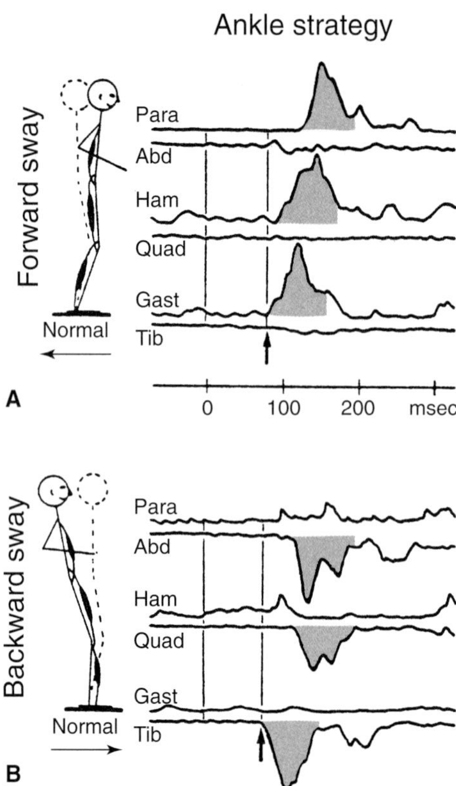

Figure 7.12 Muscle synergy and body motions associated with the ankle strategy for controlling forward sway **(A)** and backward sway **(B)**. (Reprinted with permission from Horak F, Nashner L. Central programming of postural movements: adaptation to altered support surface configurations. *J Neurophysiol.* 1986;55:1372.)

Figure 7.12B shows the synergistic muscle activity and body motions used when reestablishing stability in response to backward instability. Muscle activity begins in the distal muscle, the anterior tibialis, followed by activation of the quadriceps and abdominal muscles. How do scientists know that the ankle, knee, and hip muscles are part of a neuromuscular synergy, instead of being activated in response to stretching of each individual joint? The answer to this question is found in Extended Knowledge 7.3.

The ankle movement strategy described previously appears to be used most commonly in situations in which the perturbation to equilibrium is small and the support surface is firm. Use of the ankle strategy requires intact range of motion and strength in the ankles. What happens if the perturbation to balance is large or if we are in a situation in which we are unable to generate force using ankle joint muscles?

Hip Strategy. Scientists have identified another in-place strategy for controlling body sway, the hip movement strategy (Horak & Nashner, 1986). This strategy controls motion of the COM by producing large and rapid motion at the hip joints with antiphase rotations of the ankles.

Extended Knowledge 7.3

Neuromuscular synergy versus individual joint control: what is the evidence?

How do scientists know that the ankle, knee, and hip muscles are part of a neuromuscular synergy, instead of being activated in response to stretching of each individual joint? Some of the first experiments in postural control (Nashner, 1977; Nashner & Woollacott, 1979) provide some evidence for synergistic organization of muscles.

In these early experiments, the platform was rotated in a toes-up or toes-down direction. In a toes-up rotation, the platform motion provides stretch to the gastrocnemius muscle and dorsiflexion of the ankle, but these inputs are not associated with movements at the mechanically coupled knee and hip. The neuromuscular response that occurs in response to toes-up platform rotation includes activation of muscles at the ankle, knee, and hip joints, despite the fact that motion has occurred only at the ankle joint. Evidence from these experiments supports the hypothesis of a neurally programmed muscle synergy (Nashner, 1976, 1977; Nashner & Woollacott, 1979), including knee and hip muscles on the same side of the body as the stretched ankle muscle.

Since these responses to rotation are destabilizing, in order to regain balance, muscles on the opposite side of the body are activated. These responses have been hypothesized to be activated in response to visual and vestibular inputs (Allum & Pfalz, 1985) and are sometimes referred to as M3 responses, as opposed to an M1 response, that is, a monosynaptic stretch reflex, and the longer-latency stretch responses, which have been called M2 responses (Diener et al., 1982).

Figure 7.13A shows the typical synergistic muscle activity associated with a hip strategy. Motion of the platform in the backward direction again causes the subject to sway forward. As shown in Figure 7.13A, the muscles that typically respond to forward sway when a subject is standing on a narrow beam are different from the muscles that become active in response to forward sway while standing on a flat surface. Muscle activity begins at about 90 to 100 ms after perturbation onset in the abdominal muscles, followed by activation of the quadriceps. Figure 7.13B shows the muscle pattern and body motions associated with the hip strategy, correcting for backward sway.

Horak and Nashner (1986) suggest that the hip strategy is used to restore equilibrium in response to larger, faster perturbations or when the support surface is compliant or smaller than the feet—for example, when standing on a beam. As mentioned previously, researchers have noted that there is a continuum of movement strategies ranging from pure ankle to ankle plus hip when individuals respond to perturbations of increasing amplitudes and velocities. The CNS may also select a different control strategy depending on the conditions under which people are standing. For example, when healthy individuals stand holding onto a handrail, there is a predominant control at the wrist level compared to an ankle control strategy (Blenkinsop et al., 2017).

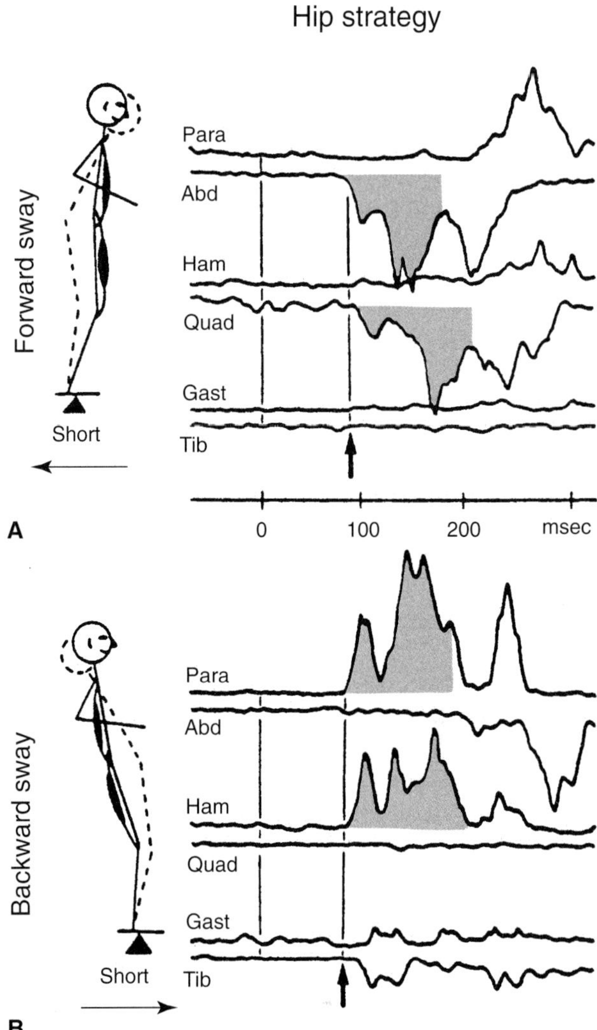

Figure 7.13 Muscle synergy and body motions associated with the hip strategy for controlling forward sway **(A)** and backward sway **(B)**. (Reprinted with permission from Horak F, Nashner L. Central programming of postural movements: adaptation to altered support surface configurations. *J Neurophysiol.* 1986;55:1372.)

Change-in-Support Strategies. In addition to fixed-support strategies (ankle and hip), the recovery of balance is also accomplished using "change-in-support" strategies. These involve rapidly moving the limbs to change the BOS, either by taking a step or by reaching and grasping an object for support. A step strategy realigns the BOS under the falling COM, while the reach-to-grasp strategy relies on extending the BOS by using the arms (see Fig. 7.11). Initially, researchers believed that "change-in-support" strategies were used when fixed-support strategies were inadequate to recover stability, such as in response to large perturbations that moved the COM outside the BOS (Horak, 1991; Nashner, 1989; Shumway-Cook & Horak, 1989). More recent research has found that in many conditions, stepping and reach-to-grasp occur even when the COM is well within the BOS (Brown et al., 1999; Maki et al., 2003; McIlroy & Maki, 1993). The control of change-in-support strategies is considered more complex than that of fixed-support strategies because complex limb movements are required that must be appropriate to both the characteristics of the balance disturbance and the constraints of the surrounding environment (e.g., presence of unobstructed space to allow stepping and handholds to support reach-to-grasp) (Maki et al., 2003).

Are change-in-support balance reactions the same or different from similar voluntary limb movements (e.g., voluntary stepping or reaching)? Research suggests that timing is a key difference between voluntary movements and balance reactions. Change-in-support balance reactions, including both stepping and reach-to-grasp, are initiated and completed in half the time it takes to perform a similar voluntary movement. Another key difference is that voluntary limb movements can be preplanned; in contrast, the direction, amplitude, and speed of compensatory change-in-support strategies must be programmed in response to unpredictable body movements (Gage et al., 2007; Maki et al., 2003).

Finally, voluntary stepping is always preceded by an ML APA that shifts the COM toward the stance limb prior to lifting the swing limb, thus avoiding a loss of balance toward the unsupported side. Does an APA also precede compensatory stepping? There is conflicting evidence related to the presence of APAs prior to a compensatory stepping response, with some researchers reporting the presence of APAs (Brauer et al., 2002); others report that the presence of APAs depends on task conditions. For example, following a novel perturbation, APAs are either missing or severely truncated, resulting in an increased frequency of lateral instability that must be countered after the swing limb makes contact with the floor (Maki et al., 2003; McIlroy & Maki, 1999).

Mediolateral and Multidirectional Stability

Early research on postural response strategies explored stability only in the AP direction. More recent research has revealed that alternative strategies are used to recover stability in the ML and other directions. This is because the alignment of body segments and muscles requires the activation of forces at different joints and in different directions to recover stability. For example, in the lower limb, very little ML movement is possible at the ankle and knee joints. Thus, the hip is the primary joint involved when recovering stability in the ML direction.

A number of researchers (Day et al., 1993; Kapteyn, 1973; Rozendal, 1986; Winter et al., 1996) have proposed that in contrast to AP postural control, ML control of balance occurs primarily at the hip and trunk, rather than at the ankle. They have noted that the primary ML motion of the body is lateral movement at the pelvis, which requires adduction of one leg and abduction of the other. With narrow stance widths, there is also motion at the ankle joint; however, this is minimal with stance widths wider than 8 cm (Day et al., 1993).

Researchers have begun to explore muscle activity patterns in response to instability in multiple directions, not just AP or ML. Henry et al. (1998) examined responses to platform perturbations in 12 different directions in standing humans (see Fig. 7.14A). EMGs were recorded from leg and trunk muscles; the timing and amplitude of muscle responses were then related to the direction of platform motion. As shown in Figure 7.14B and C, muscles tended to respond to movement in one of three directions. Two muscles (rectus femoris and tensor fasciae latae) tended to be most active in response to lateral perturbations (see Fig. 7.14B). The remaining muscles in both the leg and the trunk tended to be maximally active in response to diagonal perturbations (see Fig. 7.14C). While this finding is not surprising for muscles such as the anterior tibialis, which has an optimal line of pull for torque production on a 30 to 60 degree diagonal, it is surprising that both the flexors and extensors of the trunk and leg

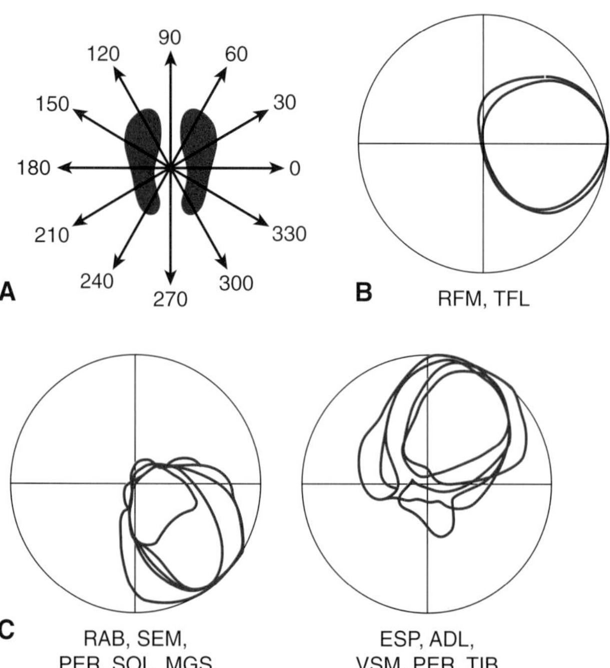

Figure 7.14 Muscle activation patterns in response to multidirectional perturbations. **(A)** Twelve directions of platform motion used to examine multidirectional instability. **(B)** Two muscles (rectus femoris and tensor fasciae latae) are activated (shown as *circles*) in response to lateral perturbations (indicated by the placement of the two circles) representing the muscle activation relative to the different directions of perturbation. **(C)** Remaining muscles in the leg and trunk (represented as *circles*) were activated in response to diagonal perturbations. The right side of the figure represents muscles activated in response to a backward diagonal perturbation; the left side of figure represents the muscles activated in response to a forward diagonal perturbation. *RAB*, right abdominal; *SEM*, semimembranosus; *PER*, peroneus longus; *SOL*, soleus; *MGS*, medial gastrocnemius; *ESP*, erector spinae; *TIB*, anterior tibialis; *VEM*, vastus medialis; *ADL*, adductor longus. (Adapted from Henry SM, Fung J, Horak FB. EMG responses to maintain stance during multidirectional surface translations. *J Neurophysiol.* 1998;80:1943–1944, Figures 3 and 4.)

would show this pattern, as they are largely responsible for sagittal plane movements (Henry et al., 1998).

In summary, this research examining multidirectional postural control modifies our understanding of the characteristics of fixed-support synergies used to recover from instability in the AP or ML directions. Early research suggested that specific muscle groups were combined into discrete synergies primarily responsive to instability in a single plane (e.g., either the AP or ML). Research by Henry et al. (1998) suggests that leg and trunk muscles appear to be grouped into three primary synergies that are dominantly active in the diagonal direction or the ML direction. This could be the result of both neural control and biomechanical reasons. For more information about how muscle synergy concepts are evolving, see Extended Knowledge 7.4.

Refining and Tuning Muscle Synergies

As the research discussed previously shows, postural synergies are not fixed, stereotypical reactions but are refined and tuned in response to changing demands in the task and environment. This process of refining and tuning movements in response to task demands is often called adaptation. Several studies have examined how individuals adapt movement strategies to changing task and environmental conditions. These studies suggest that subjects without neural pathology can shift and blend postural movement strategies as needed. We saw this in the research examining muscle responses to increasing velocities of platform perturbations. At small velocities, the ankle strategy response dominated. As platform velocities increased, the hip strategy was added and integrated with the ankle strategy. At some point, depending on the individual, there will be a shift from these fixed-support strategies to a change-in-support strategy.

Research has also shown that even when task demands do not change, we refine our responses, for example, reducing the amplitude of muscle activity in response to repeated perturbations of the same velocity, making them more efficient (Woollacott et al., 1988).

Finally, we also use anticipation when scaling the amplitude of postural adjustments to perturbations to balance. The amplitude of the muscle response is related to our expectations regarding the size or amplitude of the upcoming perturbation. For example, subjects overresponded when they expected a larger perturbation than they received and under-responded when they expected a smaller one. Practice also caused a reduction in postural response magnitude and in the amplitude of antagonist muscle responses (Horak et al., 1989a). This research has clinical implications. First, the specific instructions given to a patient during postural control training may have a substantial impact on how patients respond to postural disturbances. Instructions that allow a patient to predict the size (large or small) of the perturbation before experiencing it have a significant impact on their response. Thus, practice should include both predictable and unpredictable perturbations of varying size. Second, practice should involve perturbations in variable directions to avoid habituating postural responses with repeated trials in the same direction.

Extended Knowledge 7.4

Emerging Concepts in the Neural Control of Synergies

Recent research has begun to challenge early views (Horak & Nashner, 1986) that muscle synergies used to control posture were discrete entities. Runge and colleagues examined muscle activity in response to gradually increasing velocities of platform perturbations. Results showed that ankle and hip strategies were not distinctly and separately controlled but tended to blend in a more continuous manner. Subjects did not simply shift from using forces primarily at the ankles at low velocities to forces primarily at the hip for higher velocities. Instead, they continued to increase forces applied at the ankle and then began to add in forces at the hip. The specific point at which a person began to add hip forces varied from subject to subject, with some subjects using primarily forces at the ankle for most perturbation velocities. Pure hip strategies, previously identified using EMG patterns when subjects responded to postural perturbations while standing on a narrow support surface (Horak & Nashner, 1986), were never observed in subjects perturbed while standing on a flat surface, regardless of the size or speed of the perturbation (Jensen et al., 1996; Runge et al., 1999).

Latash et al. (2005) modified the concept of discrete and fixed synergies in his research, which showed that variability in muscle activity within the synergies is necessary for accurate control of the COM. A number of studies (Ting & Macpherson; 2005; Torres-Oviedo & Ting, 2007; Torres-Oviedo et al., 2006) have shown in both humans and cats that a limited number of synergies (five to six) are sufficient to explain muscle activity across all perturbation directions.

As shown in Figure 7.15, the COM controller specifies the twin goals of weight support and balance, which have associated synergies. In the figure, S1 is the synergy associated with weight support, while S2 through S5 are activated in varying amounts in order to control balance in response to instability in different directions. Each synergy activates a specific set of muscles in a fixed amount. In the figure, this is illustrated by the lines connecting each synergy to a different set of muscles (represented as circles). Activation of these muscles causes torques at the hip, knee, and ankle joints (circles labeled H [hip], K [knee], and A [ankle]). The combined torques from the three joints then create an end point force between the foot and the floor, which serves to control balance (position and motion of the COM). Thus, the end point force is the sum of the forces generated by several synergies.

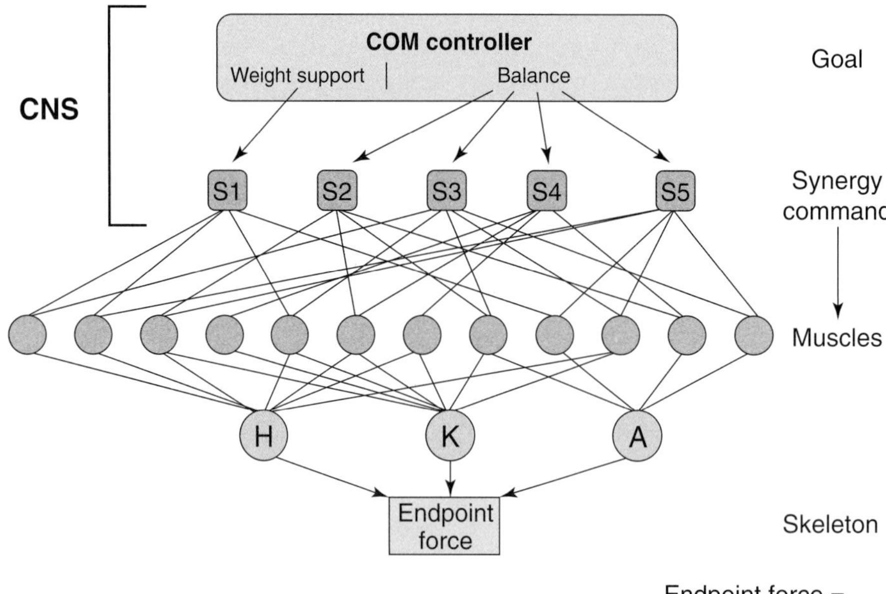

Figure 7.15 Synergy control structure. At the top of the schematic is the center of mass controller, which specifies the twin goals of postural control, weight support, and balance, which have associated synergies. One synergy (S1) is activated for weight support during quiet stance. The other four synergies (S2–S5) are activated in varying amounts in order to control balance in response to instability in different directions. Each synergy activates a specific set of muscles in a fixed amount. In the figure, this is illustrated by the lines connecting each synergy to a different set of muscles (represented as *circles*). Activation of these muscles causes torques at the hip (*H*), knee (*K*), and ankle (*A*) joints. The combined torques from the three joints then create an end point force between the foot and the floor, which serves to control balance (position and motion of the center of mass). Thus, the end point force is the sum of the forces generated by the activation of multiple synergies.

Reactive Balance Control in Sitting

Recovery of stability in the seated position is controlled similarly to that in stance. Which muscles are important in the recovery of balance following a seated perturbation? It depends. It depends on the specific task and environmental conditions. For example, in response to an AP platform perturbation to balance, a person seated unsupported on a stool, with the feet dangling, recovers stability using muscle activity in the trunk (Horak & Nashner, 1986). In contrast, the same platform perturbations will elicit activity in the legs when the person is seated with legs extended forward (Forssberg & Hirshfeld, 1994). Multidirectional perturbations in the seated position result in compensatory muscle responses that have many of the same characteristics of those seen in stance. Tonic muscle activity (in this case in the trunk) serves to support and stabilize the head and trunk during quiet sitting (steady-state balance). Phasic muscle responses to loss of balance are tuned to the direction of instability. In addition, muscle responses in sitting are initiated rapidly (faster than voluntary movements); they also involve the temporal and spatial coordination of muscle synergists, with relatively little activity in muscle antagonists. One approach to examining reactive balance in the seated position is shown in Figure 7.16A. A seated subject received perturbations directly to the trunk in multiple directions. Figure 7.16B illustrates the range of muscle activity in the abdominals and back muscles in response to perturbations in eight different directions. As in stance, individual muscles change their relative activation depending on the direction of instability. For example, as shown in Figure 7.16B, the abdominal muscles are most active in response to instability in the backward direction. In contrast, the back extensor muscles are most active in response to instability in the forward direction (Masani et al., 2009).

In addition to trunk muscle activity (responding with a fixed-support strategy), perturbations to balance in sitting can elicit a compensatory reach-to-grasp response (responding with a change-in-support strategy) (Gage et al., 2007). Compensatory reach-to-grasp responses occur faster than do voluntary reach-to-grasp movements (137 vs. 239 ms for voluntary reaches); however, the sequence of muscle activity and the kinematics of joint motion are similar (Gage et al., 2007).

Clinical Applications of Research on Reactive Balance

Reactive balance is clearly an important aspect of postural control underlying functional independence. Knowing this, how could you assess reactive balance control in sitting and standing in your patient? Remember that reactive balance is a response to an unexpected perturbation to stability. In the clinic, we could use gentle pushes to displace the COM in a standing or seated patient and observe the response. The nudge test, as

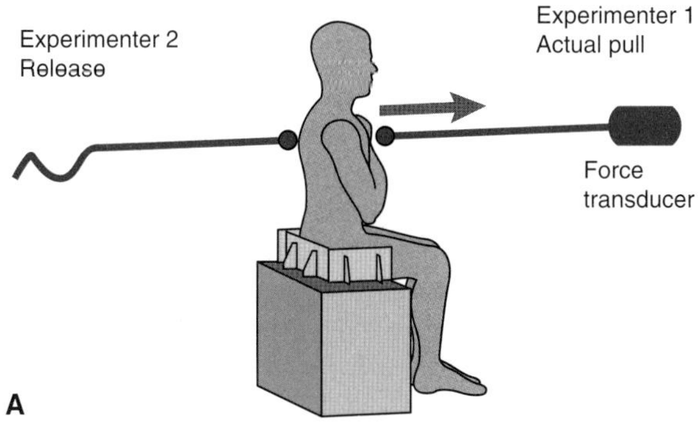

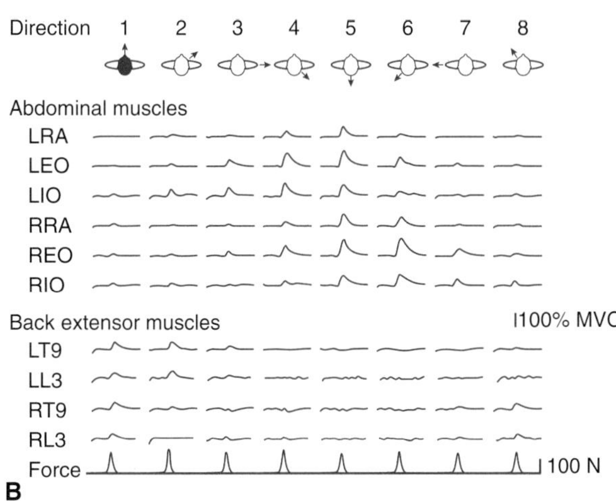

Figure 7.16 Muscle activity in response to center of mass perturbations in the seated position. **(A)** Seated subject is pulled off balance in one of eight directions. **(B)** Amplitude of muscle activity in the front (abdominals) and back (extensors) varies depending on the direction of instability. The eight directions of instability are shown in the row titled "Direction." (Adapted with permission from Masani K, Sin VW, Vette AH, et al. Postural reactions of the trunk muscles to multidirectional perturbations in sitting. *Clin Biomech*. 2009;24:176–182.)

part of the Performance-Oriented Mobility Assessment (POMA) or the Segmental Assessment of Trunk Control (SATCo), is an example of a clinical test of reactive balance that uses small nudges in the standing position to elicit a fixed-support response. A more recent test, the Seated Postural and Reaching Control (SP&R-co) test, uses a *hold-and-release* technique to examine reactive balance control. In this test, the patient is aware of the direction of the perturbation (just like in the nudge test) but remains unaware of the timing of the perturbation. More details about these tests are included in Chapter 11. Additional tests have been designed to examine change-in-support reactions, which are also essential in preventing falls (Okubo et al., 2017).

Research has demonstrated that during recovery of stability, we continuously modulate and add multiple synergies, depending on contextual factors. This suggests that when retraining balance, it will be important not to limit training to the activation of a single synergy (e.g., ankle vs. hip vs. step vs. reach) but to create conditions in which strategies are continuously modulated. For example, Creath et al. (2005) report that use of an ankle strategy (legs and trunk moving in phase) is predominant when standing on a firm surface; however, there is a shift to using a hip strategy (legs and trunk out of phase) when standing on a foam surface. Further ideas for assessing and training reactive balance are found in Chapter 10.

Proactive (Anticipatory) Balance Control

Did you ever pick up a box expecting it to be heavy and find it to be light? The fact that you lifted the box higher than you expected shows that your CNS preprogrammed force based on anticipation of what the task required. Based on previous experience with lifting other boxes of similar and different shapes and weights, the CNS forms a representation of what perception or action subsystems are needed to accomplish this task. It pretunes these systems for the task. Our mistakes are evidence that the CNS uses anticipatory processes in controlling action.

Perform Lab Activity 7.3. What you may notice through this lab experience is that you are able to use APAs when you are lifting the book out of your own

LAB ACTIVITY 7.3

Objective: To explore the use of APAs in a lifting task.

Procedure: Work with a partner. Tape a ruler vertically to the wall near where you are standing. Stand with your arm outstretched, at about waist height, palm up. Place a heavy book on your outstretched palm and have your partner note the vertical position of your hand on the ruler. Now, have your partner lift the book off that hand. Have your partner note the movement of your hand when they lift the book. Reposition the book. Now, lift the book off your own hand with your opposite hand. Have your partner note the movement of your hand in this condition.

Assignment

Answer the following questions.

1. What did the hand holding the book do when your partner lifted the book?
2. Was it steady? Or did it move upward as the book was lifted off? How much did it move?
3. What happened when you lifted the book yourself? Was it steady? How much did it move?
4. In which of these two conditions is there evidence for APAs?
5. What was necessary for the APA to occur?
6. Explain the differences between the two conditions.

hand, so that your hand does not involuntarily move upward, while you cannot use these adjustments when someone else is lifting the same book from your hand. In this case, you have to rely on sensory feedback regarding the change in arm position to counter the upward movement of the arm.

Anticipatory postural activity is also critical to lower-extremity activities such as standing on one leg or stepping up onto a curb. You can experience this yourself by trying the activity of lifting your right leg, described in the following experiment. As you can see, prior to lifting your right leg, you had to activate muscles in the left leg, shifting your weight toward the left leg, before you could lift the right. Man'kovskii and colleagues (1980) showed this when they asked young adults to lift their right leg in response to a light turning on (see Fig. 7.17A). EMGs were recorded, from both the right leg (prime mover) and the left leg. As shown in Figure 7.17B, for all subjects (each subject is represented by a line), muscle activity in the rectus femoris of the left leg occurred well before activation of the biceps femoris in the right leg. This demonstrates that postural activity anticipates the voluntary movement, ensuring stability of the body during the performance of this task.

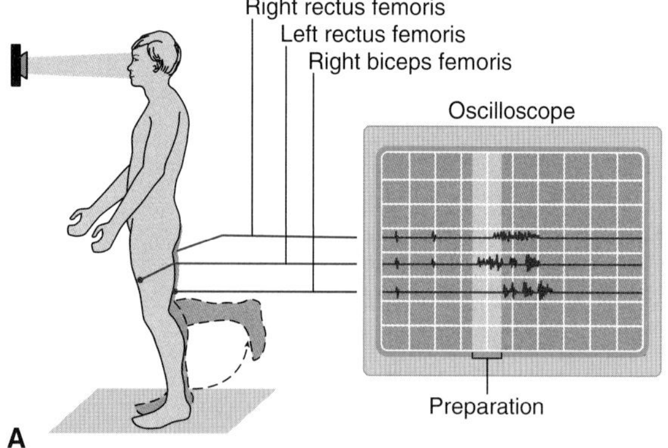

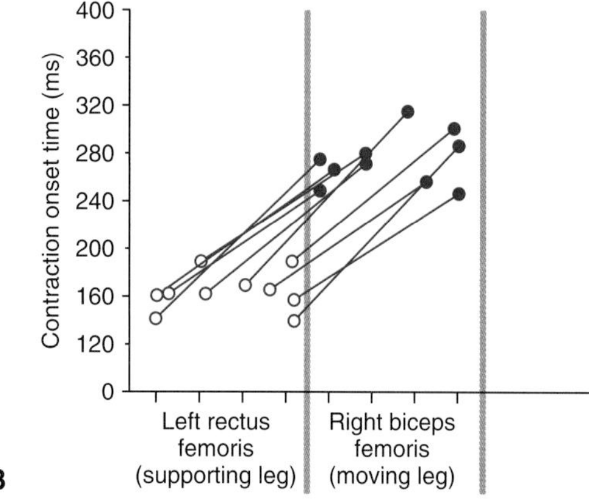

Figure 7.17 Research examining the presence of anticipatory postural activity prior to a voluntary leg task. **(A)** Young adults lift their right leg in response to a light. EMGs are from both the right leg (prime mover) and the left (stance) leg. **(B)** For all subjects, muscle activity in the left rectus femoris (the postural muscle) preceded activation of the right biceps femoris (voluntary prime mover) (the relationship between the postural and the voluntary muscles for each subject is represented by a line). (Part **A** adapted from Spirduso W, Physical dimensions of aging. Champaign, IL: Human Kinetics, 1995; Figure 6.7, page 166; Part **B** adapted from Man'kovskii NB, Mints AY, Lysenyuk VP. Regulation of the preparatory period for complex voluntary movement in old and extreme old age. *Hum Physiol Moscow*. 1980;6:46–50.)

Anticipatory postural muscle activity in the leg and trunk is also present prior to a voluntary arm movement (Belen'kii et al., 1967). Postural muscle activity accompanying a rapid arm movement occurs in two parts. The first is a preparatory phase, in which postural muscles are activated more than 50 ms in advance of the prime mover muscles (muscles that displace the body structure during the action), to compensate in advance for the destabilizing effects of the arm movement. The second phase is a compensatory phase, in which the postural muscles are again activated after the prime movers, in a feedback manner, to stabilize the body further. As mentioned, the sequence of postural muscles activated is specific to the nature of the task and context. APAs, like compensatory postural adjustments, are adapted to changing tasks and environmental contexts. For example, when external support to stabilize the body is provided prior to a potentially destabilizing arm movement, anticipatory postural muscle activity in the legs does not occur (Cordo & Nashner, 1982). In a study conducted by Hall and colleagues (2010), healthy adults performed random leg-lifting movements under four different conditions: unsupported standing, while holding a bilateral handgrip, while biting a plate, or a combination with the handgrip and bite plate. The data showed that anticipatory responses were modulated and appropriately adapted to the context—even during the most unfamiliar condition (biting a plate). Furthermore, the authors showed that APAs were further refined with practice.

Proactive Balance in Sitting

The organization of anticipatory postural muscle activity preceding voluntary movement appears to depend on characteristics of the demands of both the postural and the voluntary movement tasks (Moore et al., 1992; Shepherd et al., 1993; van der Fits et al., 1998). Van der Fits et al. (1998) examined changes in anticipatory postural muscle activity associated with unilateral and bilateral arm raises under different postural conditions (e.g., sitting and standing) (shown in Fig. 7.18). For all subjects, the organization of anticipatory postural muscle activity was dependent on the position of the person and thus the postural demands. For example, during stance (shown in Fig. 7.18 on the left), dorsal postural muscles in the leg, trunk, and neck were activated in a caudal-to-cranial order, prior to prime mover muscle activation. This ensured that the COM was maintained within the BOS during the arm movement. In contrast, when reaching was performed in sitting (shown on the right side of the figure), anticipatory

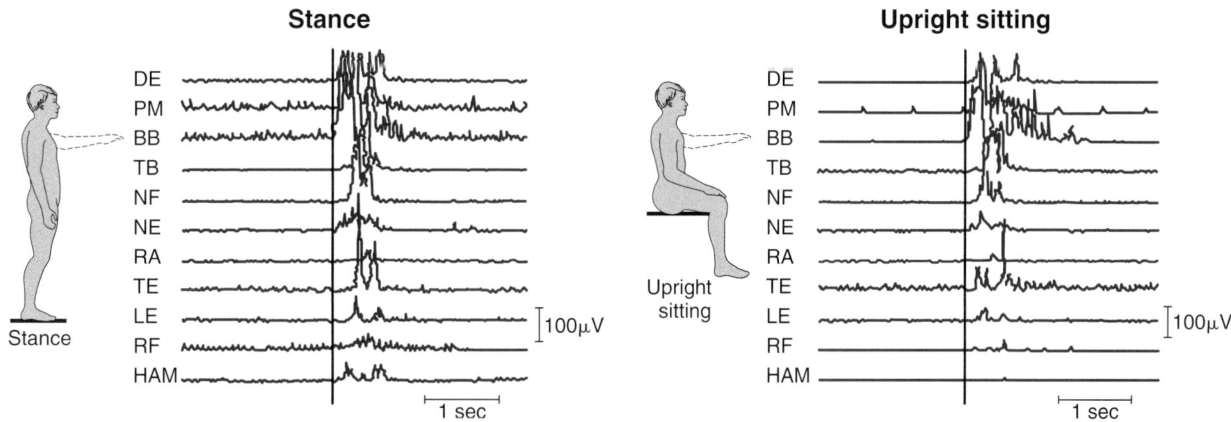

Figure 7.18 Position-dependent changes in anticipatory muscle activity. A rapid arm raise is performed in standing **(left)** or sitting **(right)**. In standing, postural muscle activity in the neck, trunk, and legs preceded that of the prime movers. In sitting, anticipatory muscle activity in the legs was absent. *DE*, deltoid; *PM*, pectoralis major; *BB*, biceps brachii; *TB*, triceps brachii; *NF*, neck flexor; *NE*, neck extensor; *TA*, rectus abdominis; *TE*, thoracic extensor; *LE*, lumbar extensor; *RF*, rectus femoris; *HAM*, hamstrings. (Adapted from van der Fits IBM, Klip AWJ, vanEykern LA, et al. Postural adjustments accompanying fast pointing movements in standing, sitting and lying adults. *Exp Brain Res*. 1998;120:202–216, Figures 1 and 2.)

muscle activity was absent in the hamstrings and delayed in the lumbar extensors (LE), causing a reversal in the order of recruitment (cranial to caudal). Thus, anticipatory postural muscle activity decreased as support to the body increased. In addition, anticipatory postural muscle activity increased when task load increased (during bilateral arm movements or unilateral arm movement with a load; data not shown) (van der Fits et al., 1998). An early phase to prepare the "postural set" before APAs may be present in some motor tasks. For instance, healthy adults show greater EMG activity of distal muscles in the leg (gastrocnemius) to prepare the postural configuration in sitting before performing a pushing task with hands. These distal muscles are not typically a part of anticipatory muscle adjustments. However, in this study, these early muscle adjustments were predominant when the person sat on an unstable surface during the pushing act (Tsai et al., 2018).

This research demonstrates that the organization of APAs in sitting, as in standing, varies as a function of both task demands and environmental characteristics.

Clinical Applications of Research on Proactive Balance

Proactive balance is an essential part of voluntary movements that are potentially destabilizing to the body. How could you assess proactive balance in the clinic? Asking a patient to stand on one leg requires anticipatory postural activity to stabilize the body prior to lifting the leg. Without this APA, the patient will either be unable to lift the limb or will lose balance while doing so. In addition, asking a patient to lift a heavy object also requires anticipatory postural activity. Clinical tests that include these types of tasks (such as the BBS) are examining proactive balance control. Further information on other tests can be found in Chapter 10.

SENSORY AND PERCEPTUAL SYSTEMS IN POSTURAL CONTROL

Effective postural control requires more than the ability to generate and apply forces for controlling the body's position in space. In order to know *when* and *how* to apply restoring forces, the CNS must have an accurate picture of *where* the body is in space and whether it is stationary or in motion. To do this, the CNS must organize information from sensory receptors throughout the body, including visual, somatosensory (proprioceptive, cutaneous, and joint receptors), and vestibular systems. Each sense provides the CNS with specific information about position and motion of the body; thus, each sense provides a different *frame of reference* for postural control (Gurfinkel & Levick, 1991; Hirschfeld, 1992).

Which sense is most important for postural control? The answer we shall see is "it depends!" The specific combination of sensory inputs most important for postural control depends on a number of factors, including characteristics of the individual (such as age), the environmental conditions, which influence the availability of sensory cues for balance, and finally the postural task being performed. Research suggests that how the CNS organizes and selects sensory information for postural control may be different during steady-state, reactive, and proactive postural control.

Sensory Inputs for Steady-State Balance

A wide range of research has shown that the CNS utilizes sensory information from visual, somatosensory, and vestibular systems for steady-state balance.

Visual Contributions

Visual inputs provide information regarding the position and motion of the head with respect to surrounding objects as well as a reference for verticality, since many things that surround us, like windows and doors, are aligned vertically. In addition, the visual system reports motion of the head, since as your head moves forward, surrounding objects move in the opposite direction. Visual inputs include both peripheral visual information and foveal information, although there is some evidence to suggest that a peripheral (or a large visual field) stimulus is more important for controlling posture (Paillard, 1987).

Visual inputs are an important source of information for steady-state postural control, but are they absolutely necessary? No, since most of us can keep our balance while standing even when we close our eyes or when we are in a dark room. In addition, visual inputs are not always an accurate source of orientation information about *self-motion*. If you are sitting in your car at a stoplight and the car next to you moves, what do you do? You quickly put your foot on the brake. In this situation, visual inputs signal *motion*, which the brain initially interprets as self-motion; in other words, *my car is rolling*. The brain therefore sends out signals to the motor neurons of the leg and foot, so you step on the brake to *stop* the motion. Thus, the brain may misinterpret visual information. The visual system has difficulty distinguishing between object motion, referred to as "exocentric motion," and self-motion, referred to as "egocentric motion."

A systematic review shows that people with congenital blindness may initially show deficits in postural control (static and dynamic); however, these deficits are compensated by the other functioning sensory systems—proprioceptive and vestibular—and through neuroplastic changes in the cerebral cortex (Parreira et al., 2017). Thus, vision is not absolutely necessary to the control of steady-state balance; however, when vision is present, it actively contributes to steady-state balance control during quiet stance (Edwards, 1946; Lee & Lishman, 1975; Paulus et al., 1984). For example, sway amplitude increases with eyes closed versus eyes open. The ratio of body sway during eyes-open and eyes-closed conditions has been referred to as the "Romberg quotient" and is frequently used as a measure of stability in the clinic (Romberg, 1853). In addition, research examining sway in response to continuous or transient visual motion cues also supports the importance of visual inputs to steady-state postural control (Brandt et al., 1976; Butterworth & Hicks, 1977; Butterworth & Pope, 1983; Lee & Lishman, 1975; Sundermier et al., 1996). The first experiments of this type were performed by David Lee and his colleagues from Edinburgh, Scotland, using a novel paradigm in which subjects stood in a room that had a fixed floor but with walls and a ceiling that could be moved forward or backward, creating the illusion of sway in the opposite direction (Lee & Lishman, 1975). The moving room was used to create either slow oscillations, simulating visual cues during quiet stance sway, or abrupt perturbations to the visual field, simulating an unexpected loss of balance. In response to small continuous room oscillations, neurologically intact adults sway with the room's oscillations, thus showing that visual inputs have an influence on steady-state balance of adults during quiet stance.

Somatosensory Contributions

The somatosensory system provides the CNS with position and motion information about the body with reference to supporting surfaces. In addition, somatosensory inputs throughout the body report information about the relationship of body segments to one another. Under normal circumstances, when standing on a firm, flat surface, somatosensory receptors provide information about the position and movement of your body with respect to a horizontal surface. However, if you are standing on a surface that is moving relative to you (e.g., a boat) or on a surface that is not horizontal (such as a ramp), it is not appropriate to establish a vertical orientation with reference to the surface, as under these conditions it is not a stable reference. In these situations, somatosensory inputs reporting the position of the body relative to the support surface are not helpful.

The importance of somatosensory cues in steady-state postural control is also demonstrated by studies showing that reducing afferent input from the lower limb due to vascular ischemia (anesthesia, or cooling) causes an increase in COP motion during quiet stance (Asai et al., 1994; Diener et al., 1984a,1984b; Magnusson et al., 1990). But it appears that somatosensory inputs from all parts of the body contribute to steady-state balance during quiet stance (Andersson & Magnusson, 2002; Kavounoudias et al., 1999; Roll & Roll, 1988). Studies using minivibrators to stimulate eye, neck, and ankle muscles produced directionally specific body sway in standing subjects (Kavounoudias et al., 1999, 2001; Roll & Roll, 1988). For example, vibrating the anterior tibialis (TA) muscle stretched and excited the muscle spindle afferents, as would happen with backward body sway. The CNS responded to the perceived backward body sway by contracting the TA, which produced a compensatory forward sway. When eye, neck, and ankle muscles were vibrated simultaneously, the effects were additive (Andersson & Magnusson, 2002).

Jeka (1997) showed that lightly touching a fingertip to a stable surface (see Fig. 7.19A) reduces postural sway in subjects standing with a reduced BOS. As shown in Figure 7.19B, sway was highest in the no-contact condition, especially with eyes closed. Sway was reduced equally in the light contact and force-contact conditions, suggesting that it was the somatosensory orientation cue rather than the available support that

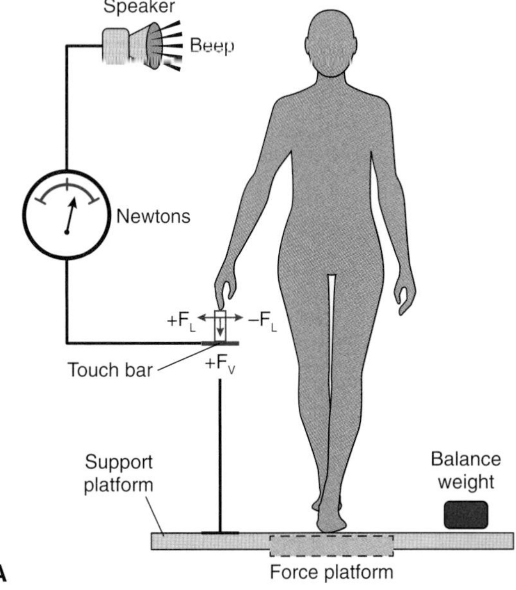

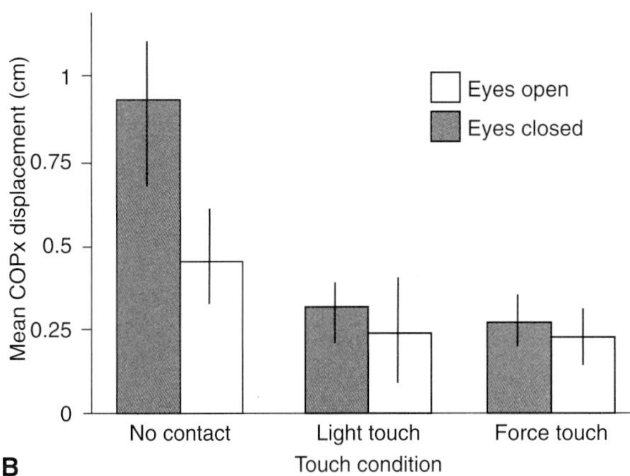

Figure 7.19 Effect of somatosensory inputs on steady-state stance balance. **(A)** Participant stands with a reduced base of support and lightly touches a solid surface. **(B)** Body sway is largest for the no-contact condition (especially with eyes closed) but is reduced equally in the light-touch and force-contact conditions. (Adapted from Jeka JJ. Light touch contact as a balance aid. *Phys Ther.* 1997;77:477–487, Figures 1 and 2.)

reduced sway. Results from all of these studies demonstrate that somatosensory information from all parts of the body plays an important role in the maintenance of steady-state postural control. This paradigm has been shown to have clinical applicability for older adultsand also for people with bilateral vestibular dysfunction, Down syndrome, or injured musculoskeletal components (anterior cruciate ligament). Research suggests that even minimal additional somatosensory information can reduce postural sway in these patients (Baldan et al., 2014).

Vestibular Contributions

Information from the vestibular system is also a powerful source of information for steady-state postural control. The vestibular system provides the CNS with information about the position and movement of the head with respect to gravity and inertial forces, providing a *gravitoinertial* frame of reference for postural control. Vestibular signals alone cannot provide the CNS with a true picture of how the body is moving in space. For example, the CNS cannot distinguish between a simple head nod (movement of the head relative to a stable trunk) and a forward bend (movement of the head in conjunction with a moving trunk) using vestibular inputs alone (Horak & Shupert, 1994).

Sensory Integration

Daily life requires that we maintain our balance in a wide variety of sensory environments, for example, dark rooms, moving surface, and visual environments. How does the CNS organize and select sensory information for postural control under these varied conditions? Nashner and colleagues examined how the CNS organizes the three sensory inputs for steady-state balance. They used a moving platform and visual surround to control the availability and accuracy of sensory inputs to steady-state standing balance (Nashner, 1976, 1982). In Nashner's protocol, body sway is measured while the subject stands quietly under six different conditions that alter the availability and accuracy of visual and somatosensory inputs for postural orientation. These conditions are shown in Figure 7.20, which also describes the accurate and inaccurate sensory inputs available within each condition. In conditions 1 to 3, the subject stands on a firm, flat surface with eyes open (1), with eyes closed (2), or within a boxlike enclosure that moves in the same direction and speed as the person sways, giving the visual illusion that the person is not moving. Conditions 4 to 6 are identical to 1 to 3 except that the support surface now rotates with body sway as well. Differences in the amount of body sway in the different conditions are used to determine a subject's ability to maintain balance when there is a change in sensory inputs.

Average differences in body sway across the six sensory conditions within a large group of neurologically intact adults are shown in Figure 7.21. Adults sway the least when the surface is firm and flat; in this condition, support-surface orientation inputs are accurately reporting the body's position in space relative to the surface regardless of the availability and accuracy of visual inputs (conditions 1, 2, and 3). When support-surface information is no longer available as an accurate source of orientation information (e.g., in conditions 4, 5, and 6, when the surface is rotated in conjunction with the subject's AP sway), adults begin to sway more. The greatest amount of sway is seen in conditions 5 and 6, in which only one accurate set of inputs, the vestibular inputs, is available to mediate postural control (Peterka & Black, 1990). The application of this concept can be found in Lab Activity 7.2.

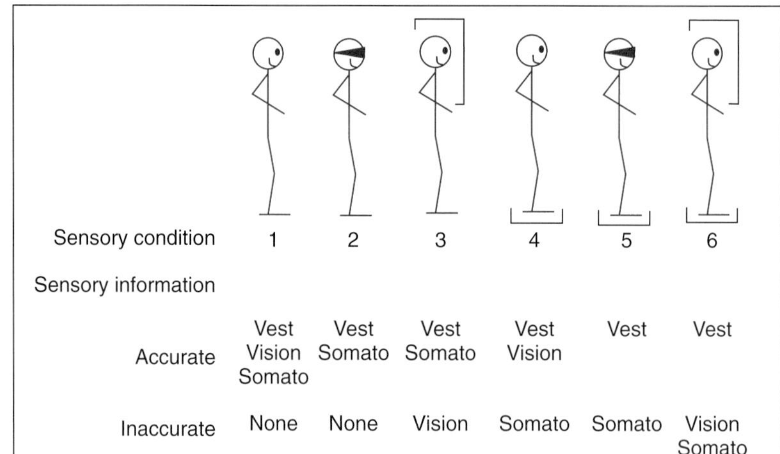

Figure 7.20 The six sensory conditions used to test how people adapt the senses to changing sensory conditions during the maintenance of stance. (Adapted from Horak F, Shumway-Cook A, Black FO. Are vestibular deficits responsible for developmental disorders in children? *Insights Otolaryngol.* 1988;3:2.)

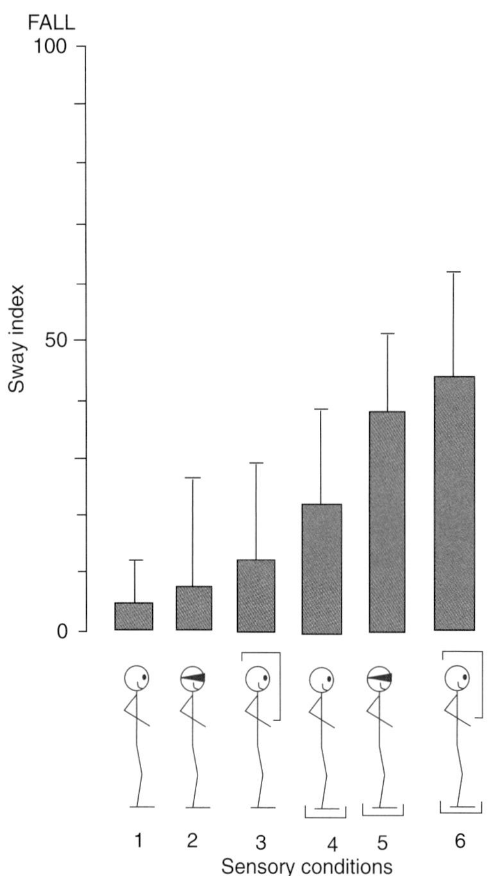

Figure 7.21 Body sway in healthy young adults in the six sensory conditions used to test sensory adaptation during stance postural control. *RMS*, root mean square. (Adapted from Woollacott MH, Shumway-Cook A, Nashner L. Aging and posture control: changes in sensory organization and muscular coordination. *Int J Aging Hum Dev.* 1986;23:108.)

This and other studies have shown that adults and children over the age of 7 maintain balance (i.e., keep their COM well within their stability limits) under all six sensory conditions (Jeka et al., 2000; Nashner, 1982; Peterka, 2002; Peterka & Black, 1990; Peterka & Loughlin, 2004; Woollacott et al., 1986).

What can we conclude from these studies? They suggest that in healthy young adults, when all three senses are present, they each contribute to postural control during steady-state balance. However, in environments in which a sense is not providing optimal or accurate information regarding the body's position, the CNS is able to modify how it uses sensory information for balance. This is called sensory reweighting. Sensory reweighting occurs when reliance on one sensory system for postural control increases while, at the same time, reliance of another sensory system decreases (Peterka, 2002). For example, in environments in which vision is inaccurate (such as when the environment is in motion relative to the individual), the CNS reduces its use of vision and relies on the alternative accurate sensory inputs (e.g., somatosensory and vestibular). Because the CNS is able to modify the relative importance of any one sense for postural control, individuals are able to maintain stability in a variety of environments. Failure to properly make use of sensory reweighting can lead to impaired balance and falls (Nashner, 1982; Peterka, 2002). For further information on how the CNS accomplished the integration of sensory information for steady-state postural control, see Extended Knowledge 7.5.

Task-Dependent Sensory Reweighting

We have seen how sensory reweighting is critical to being able to maintain steady-state balance in changing "sensory" environments. Research suggests that the CNS reweights sensory information for postural control under changing task conditions as well. For example, the sensory inputs used to control steady-state balance depend on the characteristics of the BOS during stance. When healthy adults assume a narrow BOS (such as standing feet together), sensory reweighting is used to shift reliance from proprioceptive cues to vestibular and/or visual cues that orient the body to upright. This is shown by the increase in postural sway

Extended Knowledge 7.5

Theories Explaining the Process of Sensory Integration

Adapting how we use the senses for postural control is a critical aspect of maintaining stability in a wide variety of environments and has been studied by several researchers. There are two hypotheses describing the process by which the CNS organizes sensory information for postural orientation. In the intermodal theory of sensory orientation, all three senses contribute equally to postural orientation at all times. It is only through the interaction of all three senses that the CNS is able to maintain appropriate postural orientation. In contrast to this theory is the sensory weighting model, which suggests that the CNS modifies the weight, or importance, of a sensory input depending on its relative accuracy as a sensory input for orientation. In this model, the CNS has to resolve sensory conflicts (situations in which there is disagreement among sensory inputs) by changing the relative weight of a sensory input to postural control.

Intermodal Theory of Sensory Organization

Stoffregen and Riccio (1988) used an ecological approach to describe how sensory information is used for orientation. They suggest that information critical for postural orientation is gained through the interaction of the different sensory systems. The organization of sensory information for postural orientation is based on lawful relationships between patterns of sensory stimulation and properties of the environment, and these lawful relationships are called "invariants." Invariants describe intermodal relationships across perceptual systems. In this view, there is never sensory conflict; rather, all the senses provide information that increases specificity in control and perception. There is no relative weighting of sensory information; rather, orientation emerges from an interaction of all three senses. They use a triangle to illustrate this concept of intermodal organization. It is the relationship among three lines that makes a triangle; you understand a triangle only by understanding the relationship of the three lines to one another. Similarly, it is the relationship of the three senses to one another that provides the CNS with the essential information for postural orientation.

Sensory Weighting Hypothesis

In contrast to the intermodal theory is the sensory weighting theory, which suggests that the postural control system is able to reweight sensory inputs in order to optimize stance in altered sensory environments (Oie et al., 2002). The sensory weighting hypothesis predicts that each sense provides a unique contribution to postural control. In addition, the sensory weighting hypothesis predicts that changes in postural responses in different sensory conditions are due to changes in sensory weights. Sensory weighting implies that the "gain" of a sensory input will depend on its accuracy as a reference for body motion. For example, as vision becomes less reliable as an indicator of self-motion, the visual input will be weighted less heavily and somatosensory cues will be weighted more heavily. In contexts in which touch becomes a less reliable indicator of self-motion, the visual inputs are weighted more heavily. The sensory weighting hypothesis is supported by a number of researchers (Jeka & Lackner, 1994, 1995; Kuo et al., 1998; Nashner, 1976, 1982). This research suggests that sensory strategies, that is, the relative weight given to a sense, vary as a function of age, task, and environment.

Research by Peterka (2002) provided evidence for the sensory reweighting hypothesis. His experiments examined the relative contribution of somatosensory and vestibular inputs to the control of balance and orientation by measuring body sway while blindfolded subjects stood quietly on a surface that rotated continuously up and down by varying amounts, up to 8 degrees in magnitude. They tested both healthy young adults and people with loss of vestibular function. Figure 7.22 summarizes their findings; the graph on the left compares body sway measures relative to vertical, which are expressed as root mean square (RMS) sway in degrees. The dashed line plots the situation in which body sway and platform sway are exactly comparable. In the healthy participant (red trace), body sway and platform sway were equal for low-amplitude stimuli of less than 2 degrees, suggesting that this participant oriented the body axis relative to the support surface using somatosensory information. At larger amplitudes of surface rotation, the healthy participant maintained a more vertical posture, minimizing body sway, suggesting that they were relying more on vestibular and less on somatosensory inputs for postural control. In contrast to the healthy participant, when the blindfolded participant with loss of vestibular function (gray trace) stood on the rotating platform, the participant oriented the body axis to the surface and maintained balance during small-amplitude platform rotations (relying on somatosensory inputs for postural control) but could not maintain balance on the large-amplitude tilts. Lacking visual (blindfold) and vestibular inputs, the participant persisted in orienting the body axis to the surface (relying on somatosensory inputs for balance), but this was not effective in the face of large-amplitude platform tilts, resulting in imbalance and falls. The graph on the right illustrates this shift in the dominance of a specific sense with a shift in conditions. During the control of balance, the influence of somatosensory information decreases while the influence of vestibular information increases with increasing platform tilt; thus, body sway is minimized as participants shift and orient to gravitational vertical rather than the support surface.

This research suggests a number of things about how the CNS organizes and adapts sensory information for postural control. It supports the concept of hierarchical weighting of sensory inputs for postural control based on their relative accuracy in reporting the body's position and movements in space. In environments in which a sense is not providing optimal or accurate information regarding the body's position, the weight given to that sense as a source of orientation is reduced, while the weight of other more accurate senses is increased. Because of the redundancy of senses available for orientation and the ability of the CNS to modify the relative importance of any one sense for postural control, individuals are able to maintain stability in a variety of environments.

---

when healthy young adults stand with a narrow BOS and with their eyes closed in comparison to standing with eyes open. In contrast, wider-than-normal BOS stance does not appear to require sensory reweighting, since postural sway is identical in adults in eyes-open and eyes-closed conditions. These results suggest that visual orientation cues have little influence on balance control during wide stance (Goodworth et al., 2014).

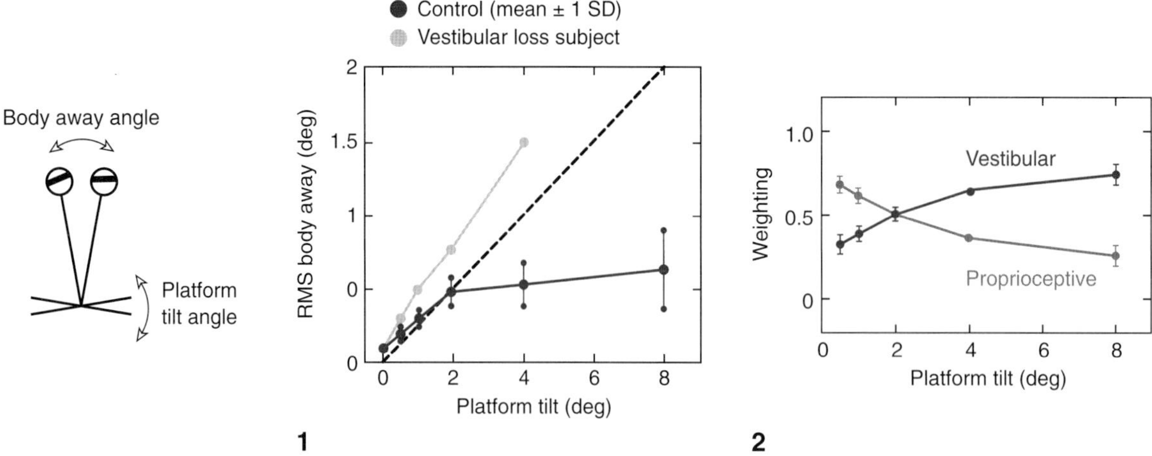

Figure 7.22 An experiment to illustrate the dynamic use of sensory information under varying conditions. See text for detailed explanation. (Adapted from Peterka RJ. Sensorimotor integration in human postural control. *J Neurophysiol.* 2002;88:1102, Figure 4.)

Similarly, sensory reweighting appears to occur during the process of learning new motor skills. Lee and Lishman (1975) found increased weighting of visual inputs when adults were just learning a task. As the task became more automatic, there was a decrease in the relative importance of visual inputs for postural control and increased weighting given to somatosensory inputs. Van Dieën and colleagues (2015) investigated how healthy adults learn to balance the body during a novel task—one-leg stance on a board that fully rotates in the frontal plane. They manipulated the visual and vestibular systems and trained individuals during 30-minute sessions. Results showed that adults relied more on visual inputs during the initial learning of the task, whereas later changes in postural sway were due to an increase in the use of proprioceptive feedback.

The reweighting of visual information for postural control when learning a new task may also apply to adults recovering from a neurologic lesion. Early on in recovery, postural control relies primarily on visual inputs. As motor skills are regained, patients appear to become less reliant on vision and are better able to use somatosensory inputs for postural control (Mulder et al., 1993).

Sensory Inputs for Reactive Balance

How do visual, vestibular, and somatosensory inputs contribute to reactive postural control? Let us look at some of the research examining this question.

Visual Contributions

Moving rooms have also been used to examine the contribution of visual inputs to recovery from transient perturbations. When abrupt room movements are made, young children (1-year-olds) compensate for this illusory loss of balance with motor responses designed to restore the vertical position (Lee & Aronson, 1974; Lee & Lishman, 1975). Older children and adults typically do not show large sway responses to these movements, indicating that in adults, vision does not play an important role in compensating for transient visual perturbations. Visual cues are very important contributions when change-in-support strategies are used to recover stability. In this case, visual information regarding the environment (e.g., unobstructed space to step or the availability of handholds for support) is a critical determinant of whether these strategies can be used. Visual information is gathered as soon as a person enters an environment to form a map of environmental affordances; it is not obtained after the perturbation to balance has occurred (Maki et al., 2003).

Somatosensory Contributions

Somatosensory inputs appear to be very important in reactive postural control, especially in response to surface perturbations. In addition, muscle response latencies to somatosensory cues signaling perturbations to balance are activated at 80 to 100 ms; in contrast, response latencies to visual cues are quite slow, on the order of 200 ms (Dietz et al., 1991; Nashner & Woollacott, 1979). In healthy subjects, when somatosensory inputs are reduced using a blood pressure cuff to cause partial anesthesia of the feet and ankles, the onset latency of compensatory muscle activity responses did not change; subjects instead shifted from an ankle to a hip strategy when recovering balance (Horak et al., 1990). However, in a second study in which somatosensory inputs of the foot were reduced by foot cooling, the onset latency of the soleus was delayed and the amplitude of the soleus and gastrocnemius increased (Ferguson et al., 2017). In addition, compensatory muscle responses in persons with peripheral neuropathy are significantly slower (Inglis et al., 1994).

Because somatosensory responses to support-surface translations appear to be much faster than those triggered by visual or vestibular systems, researchers have suggested that the nervous system preferentially relies on somatosensory inputs for controlling body sway when imbalance is caused by rapid displacements of the support surface.

Vestibular Contributions

What is the relative contribution of the vestibular system to postural responses to support surface perturbations? Experiments by Dietz et al. (1991, 1994) and Horak et al. (1994) indicate that the contribution of the vestibular system is much smaller than that of somatosensory inputs. In these experiments, the onset latency and amplitude of muscle responses were compared for two different types of perturbations of stance: (a) the support surface was moved forward or backward, stimulating somatosensory inputs, and (b) a forward or backward displacement of a load (2 kg) attached to the head was applied, stimulating the vestibular system (the response was absent in patients with vestibular deficits). For comparable accelerations, muscle responses to vestibular signals were about 10 times smaller than the somatosensory-evoked responses induced by the displacement of the feet. This suggests that vestibular inputs may play only a minor role in recovery of postural control when the support surface is displaced horizontally.

However, under certain conditions, vestibular and visual inputs are important in controlling responses to transient perturbations. For example, when the support surface is rotated toesupward, stretching and activating the gastrocnemius muscle, this response is destabilizing, pulling the body backward. Allum's research shows that the subsequent compensatory response in the tibialis anterior muscle, used to restore balance, is activated by the visual and vestibular systems when the eyes are open. When the eyes are closed, it is primarily (80%) activated by the vestibular semicircular canals (Allum & Pfaltz, 1985). The velocity at which the surface tilts can also be a significant factor in the control of postural stance. Horak and colleagues (2016) have shown that people with bilateral vestibular deficits consistently lose balance (90% of the trials) when the tilting board rotates at 4 deg/s (the approximate rate of physiological postural sway). Interestingly, when the board rotates at slower (0.25–1 deg/s) or faster (16–32 deg/s) velocities, people with bilateral vestibular loss rarely fall. According to the authors, people with bilateral vestibular loss without vision might use "very-low-threshold receptors"—gravitational information from alimentary pressure sensors and Golgi tendon organs (torque-related information), feet pressure sensors, and otoliths (if available)—to control balance. During fast tilts, however, they could be relying on "high-threshold-receptors" like muscle spindles. Moreover, the CNS of persons with vestibular loss may be unable to distinguish different sensory stimuli within natural sway frequencies without creating a reference between the body, surface, and space.

These studies suggest that all three sensory inputs play a role in the recovery of stability following an unexpected perturbation. The relative contribution of individual senses appears to depend on many factors, including the processing speed within each sensory system. For example, early postural responses to transient horizontal perturbations to stance may rely heavily on somatosensory inputs, because of their fast processing speed. However, vision and vestibular inputs, which have slower processing speeds, do contribute to early responses, albeit to a much lesser degree. Vision and vestibular inputs may be more important, however, in later aspects of the postural response. Altogether, these studies justify the use of equipment (e.g., tilting boards) in the clinic to examine and/or challenge sensory-related balance deficits in people with neuromotor disorders.

Clinical Applications of Research on Sensory and Perceptual Aspects of Postural Control

As you can see from this review of the research on sensory aspects of postural control, the ability to organize and select appropriate sensory inputs is an important aspect of maintaining stability under changing task and environmental contexts. As discussed in Chapter 10, instability can result from not only the loss of an individual sensory input important to postural control (e.g., loss of vision or somatosensory inputs) but also an inability to effectively organize and select sensory inputs appropriate to the task and environmental context. Balance rehabilitation must include clinical strategies for assessing both the integrity of individual sensory systems and the ability to organize sensory inputs for balance control.

Clinical strategies for improving balance should include not only activities to improve the organization of muscle activity but also the way in which sensory information is used for balance control. In the case when a specific sensory input is permanently lost (e.g., loss of vestibular inputs following head injury or some types of medications), activities that promote the reliance on alternative senses such as vision and somatosensory inputs can be used.

COGNITIVE SYSTEMS IN POSTURAL CONTROL

Many daily life tasks involve doing more than one task at a time (e.g., maintaining standing balance while talking on the phone to a friend). Since normal postural control occurs automatically, without conscious effort, it was traditionally assumed that few attentional resources were needed when controlling balance. Attentional resources are defined as the information-processing resources that are required to complete a task. When two tasks are performed simultaneously, the competition for available attentional resources may cause a decrease in performance on one or more tasks. This is called dual-task interference. One of the ways we examine attentional demands of postural control is to perform a postural task alone and then simultaneously with another task and measure change in performance from single- to dual-task conditions. This dual-task research has shown that there are significant attentional requirements for postural control. In addition, attentional requirements are not constant but vary depending on the postural task, on the age of the individual and on the individual's balance abilities (Woollacott & Shumway-Cook, 2002).

Kerr et al. (1985) performed the first research to demonstrate the attentional demands of stance postural control. They hypothesized that a difficult balance task would interfere with a spatial (visual) memory but not a verbal memory task, because postural control is assumed to involve visual and spatial processing. The visual and spatial cognitive task was the Brooks spatial memory task, which involved placing numbers in imagined matrices and then remembering the position of these numbers. The nonspatial verbal memory task involved remembering similar sentences. They found that performing the memory task with the concurrent balance task caused an increase in the number of errors in the spatial but not in the nonspatial memory task and that there was no significant difference in postural sway during the performance of either cognitive task. They concluded that postural control in young adults is attentionally demanding.

A study by Lajoie et al. (1993) determined that attentional demands vary as a function of the type of postural task being performed. They asked young adults to perform an auditory reaction time (RT) task while sitting, standing with a normal versus a reduced BOS, and during walking (single- vs. double-support phase). They found that RTs were fastest for sitting and slowed for the standing (slower in narrow stance than normal stance) and walking (slower for single-support phase compared with double-support) tasks. They concluded that as the demand for stability increases, there is a concomitant increase in attentional resources used by the postural control system.

Attentional demands also vary as a function of sensory context. As sensory inputs for postural control are reduced (such as standing eyes closed or on foam), attentional demands associated with maintaining stability increase (Lajoie et al., 1993; Redfern et al., 2001; Shumway-Cook & Woollacott, 2000). This can be seen in Figure 7.23, which compares visual and auditory

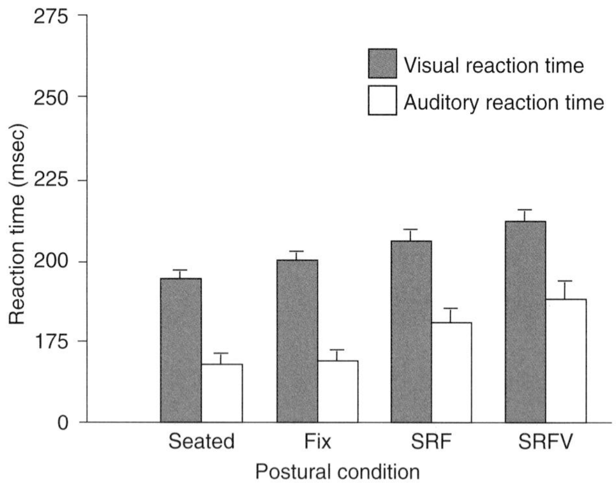

Figure 7.23 Attentional demands increase with the demands of the postural task. Visual (*colored bars*) and auditory (*white bars*) reaction times are compared in young adults under four postural conditions: seated, standing on a fixed surface (fix), standing on a sway-referenced floor (which changes the availability of accurate somatosensory inputs), and sway-referencing of both floor and vision (SRFV), which change the availability of accurate somatosensory and visual inputs. Reaction times increase significantly as the postural tasks get more difficult, with the highest reaction times found in the hardest sensory condition SRFV. (Adapted from Redfern MS, Jennings JR, Martin C, et al. Attention influences sensory integration for postural control in older adults. *Gait Posture*. 2001;14:211–216, Figure 2b.)

reactions under four postural conditions, including seated, standing on a fixed surface (fix), standing on a sway-referenced floor (SRF) (which changes the availability of accurate somatosensory inputs), and sway-referenced floor and vision (SRFV), which changes the availability of accurate somatosensory and visual inputs. RTs increased significantly as the postural tasks became more difficult, with the highest RTs found in the hardest sensory condition SRFV (Redfern et al., 2001).

The performance of a secondary task does not always have a detrimental effect on postural control. Stoffregen et al. (2000) showed that when individuals were asked to fixate on a visual target and perform a visual task (counting the frequency of letters in a block of text), they showed less sway than when inspecting a blank target. In addition, focusing on a near target caused sway to be reduced relative to focusing on a distant target. In this case, postural control is enhanced, not reduced, during the performance of a secondary task. The authors conclude that postural control is organized as part of an integrated perception and action system and can be modified to facilitate the performance of other tasks.

Similar to the results of Stoffregen and colleagues, other researchers have shown that adding a variety of secondary tasks can reduce both stance sway and sway variability in young adults and offer other possible explanations for these findings (Huxhold et al., 2006; Riley et al., 2005; Vuillerme & Nafati, 2007). For example, Huxhold et al. (2006) showed that when young adults were asked to perform a secondary task (working memory task, in which they had to remember numbers presented 1, 2, or 3 items back in an auditory recording) while standing with feet shoulder width apart, they showed reduced postural sway in the dual-task condition. The authors proposed that improvements in postural control under these dual-task conditions were due to the possibility that directing subjects' attention to a highly automatic process like postural control may actually reduce the efficacy of postural mechanisms and that directing attention toward a secondary task may actually improve the automaticity and efficacy of the postural control processes. Other researchers have proposed that reduced sway in a dual-task setting may be due to heightened arousal when performing a secondary task, causing improved performance (Andersson et al., 2002). It is interesting that though these effects are typically present in young adults, they are only present in older or balance-impaired individuals when performing a very simple cognitive task; with increased cognitive task difficulty, postural sway and variability increase in older and balance-impaired populations (Huxhold et al., 2006).

Under dual-task conditions, does maintaining balance take precedence over other tasks? The answer appears to be "it depends." Whether the control of balance is a priority depends on how great the threat to stability is. When threats to stability are great, healthy young adults prioritize postural control over other tasks, and this is referred to as "postural prioritization" or the "posture first" strategy. Müller et al. (2007) demonstrated a posture-first control strategy by examining RT to either a visual or auditory RT task prior to, during, and following a platform perturbation in healthy young adults. They reported that RTs were slowest just prior to a platform perturbation; as postperturbation time increased (once an appropriate postural response was initiated), RT became gradually faster. Differences in RT suggest evidence for postural prioritization; RT task processing on a secondary task is delayed in anticipation of postural events still to occur; once the nature of the postural stimulus has been determined and the appropriate postural responses have been initiated, RT processing becomes faster. As we will discuss in later chapters, postural prioritization does not occur in many balance-impaired older adults and in patients with neurologic pathology.

In summary, dual-task research suggests that postural control is attentionally demanding in young adults and that when threats to stability are great, postural control becomes a priority. In healthy young adults, attentional effects are small unless you increase the difficulty of the postural control task or, alternatively, ask subjects to perform more complex secondary tasks. In addition, some secondary tasks can increase postural sway (often interpreted as interference with postural control), but others decrease sway (often interpreted as improved postural control). As will be discussed in later chapters, the attentional demands associated with postural control appear to be different in older adults with balance impairments and individuals with neurologic impairment.

Clinical Applications of Research on Cognitive Aspects of Postural Control

Daily life requires that we maintain balance while doing a range of attentionally demanding tasks. Since research has demonstrated that performing an additional task can have a detrimental effect on postural stability, which may not be evident when the postural task is performed alone, it is very important to assess balance under both single- and dual-task conditions. In addition, treatment designed to improve postural stability under both single- and dual-task conditions is essential.

NEURAL SUBSYSTEMS CONTROLLING POSTURAL ORIENTATION AND STABILITY

What are the different neural subsystems that contribute to the control of postural orientation and stability? A systematic review found that the control of balance is a whole-brain phenomenon. However, among the 71 brain structures most studied and involved in the control of balance, the cerebellum, the basal ganglia, the thalamus, the hippocampus, the inferior parietal cortex, and the frontal lobe are of particular relevance (Surgenta et al., 2019). Figure 7.24 summarizes the hypothesized contributions of the brain and spinal cord systems to different aspects of postural control.

Spinal Contributions

To determine spinal contributions to postural control, research has examined animals with intact versus transected spinal cords (spinal preparation). It was found that the spinal cord contributions to the orientation component of postural control included tonic activation of extensor muscles for weight support. In addition, directionally specific responses to perturbations were also present at the spinal cord level. However, evidence suggests that while reactive postural control is present in spinal preparations in animals, responses are dramatically reduced without supraspinal drive, so that they are not functional (Deliagina et al., 2012).

What somatosensory inputs contribute to posture control? It has been shown that both group I and group II muscle spindle afferents are very sensitive to postural sway and postural disturbances and both contribute to directionally specific postural responses

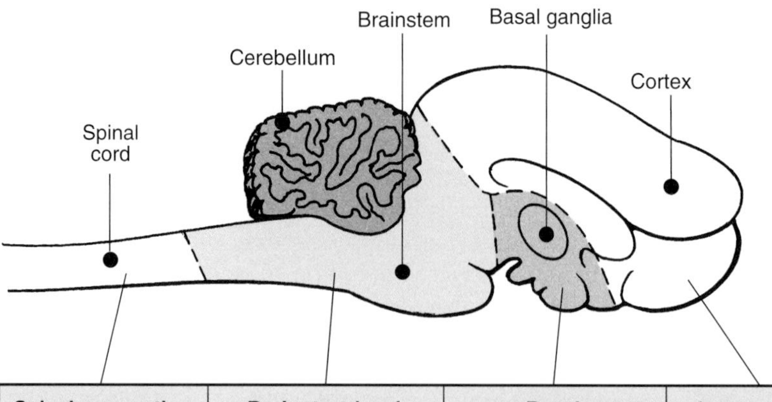

Spinal preparation	Brainstem level	Basal ganglia/cerebellum	Intact system
Ground reaction forces for orientation present though diminished Tonically active extensor muscle for antigravity support for postural orientation No lateral stability Somatosensory contributions to postural control	Controls level of postural tone in combination with cerebellum Circuits for automatic postural synergies (hypothesized) Vestibular contributions to postural control	*Cerebellum* Control of adaptation — abilities to modify postural muscle amplitude in response to changing task and environmental conditions *Basal ganglia* Control of postural set—ability to quickly change muscle patterns in response to changing task and environmental conditions	Adaptable postural control system to meet the goals of stability and orientation in any environment Visual contribution to postural control

Figure 7.24 Proposed contributions of brain and spinal circuitry in postural control.

(Deliagina et al., 2012; Honeycutt et al., 2012). In addition, cutaneous afferents contribute to the amplitude of postural responses, though not to directional specificity (Honeycutt & Nichols, 2010). Finally, Golgi tendon organs (GTOs) also contribute to postural control (Dietz et al., 1992). What allows these somatosensory inputs to create functional circuitry for postural control? It is the descending drive from both brainstem and higher brain centers.

Brainstem Contributions

Research on brainstem nuclei has shown that these centers are active in the regulation of postural tone and automatic postural synergies and include important nuclei for processing vestibular inputs to postural control. For example, the brainstem has important centers for controlling the facilitation (through raphespinal and cerulospinal tracts) and inhibition of muscle tone (the pedunculopontine tegmental nucleus in the mesopontine tegmentum and the reticulospinal tract) important for the control of posture.

Stapley and Drew (2009) have shown that pontomedullary reticular formation neurons in the brainstem of the cat discharge strongly in response to support surface perturbations, suggesting that nuclei in the brainstem contribute to the restoration of equilibrium following a balance threat.

The brainstem is also important in the regulation of anticipatory postural control. Massion (1979) trained animals to perform a leg-lifting task that required the activation of postural muscles simultaneously in the other three legs when it lifted the prime mover leg. They found that they could also directly stimulate the motor cortex or the red nucleus in the area of the forelimb flexors and produce the leg-lifting movement. When they did this, the movement was always accompanied by a postural adjustment in the other limbs, initiated in a feedforward manner. They suggest that APAs are organized at the brainstem level and that the pyramidal tract (from the motor cortex) activates brainstem pathways for anticipatory postural muscle activity as it sends descending commands to activate the prime mover muscles.

Finally, when the brainstem reticular formation is inactivated by pharmacologic means, APAs that would normally be activated to stabilize a voluntary movement initiated through activation of the motor cortex are no longer activated, supporting the importance of brainstem nuclei in anticipatory postural control (Takakusaki et al., 2004).

Basal Ganglia and Cerebellar Contributions

Research on postural control in patients with pathology in the basal ganglia and cerebellum, discussed in detail in Chapter 10, is increasing our understanding of the contributions of these neural structures to postural control. The cerebellum is known to control adaptation of postural responses—that is, the ability to modify postural muscle response amplitudes in response to changing environmental and task conditions. For example, patients with cerebellar disorders cannot adapt responses to changing perturbation amplitudes (Horak & Diener, 1994). The basal ganglia are involved in the control of postural set—that is, the ability to quickly change reactive balance muscle patterns in response to changing task and environmental conditions (e.g., sitting vs. fixed-support or change-in-support strategies). Patients with Parkinson disease cannot shift movement strategies appropriately for changes in task and environmental demands (Horak et al., 1992) (see Chapter 10 for research details).

Finally, when all systems are intact, the individual shows adaptable postural control and is able to meet the goals of stability and orientation in any environment.

SUMMARY

1. The task of postural control involves controlling the body's position in space for (a) stability, defined as controlling the center of body mass relative to the BOS, and (b) orientation, defined as the ability to maintain an appropriate relationship between the body segments and between the body and the environment for a task.
2. A number of factors contribute to postural control during steady-state balance in sitting and standing, including (a) body alignment, which minimizes the effect of gravitational forces; (b) muscle tone; and (c) postural tone, which keeps the body from collapsing in response to the pull of gravity.
3. Reactive balance, defined as the recovery of stability following an unexpected displacement of the COM, requires movement strategies that are effective in bringing the COM back within stability limits determined primarily by the BOS.
4. Movement patterns used to recover balance are categorized into fixed-support (ankle and hip) and change-in-support (stepping and reach-to-grasp) strategies. Healthy young adults can adapt to changing task and environmental constraints by shifting relatively quickly from one postural movement strategy to another.
5. The CNS activates synergistic muscles at mechanically related joints, possibly to ensure that forces generated at one joint for balance control do not produce instability elsewhere in the body.
6. Postural muscles are also activated before voluntary movements to minimize potential disturbances to balance that the movement may cause. This is called *anticipatory postural control*.
7. Inputs from visual, somatosensory (proprioceptive, cutaneous, and joint receptors), and vestibular systems are important sources of information about the body's position and movement in space with respect to gravity and the environment. Each sense provides the CNS with a different kind of information about position and motion of the body; thus, each sense provides a different frame of reference for postural control.
8. Because of the redundancy of senses available for orientation and the ability of the CNS to modify the importance of any one sense for postural control, individuals are able to maintain stability in a variety of environments.
9. Postural tasks require attentional processing and thus can reduce the performance of a second task performed simultaneously. In addition, complex secondary tasks can, in some cases, reduce the performance of a concurrently performed postural task. However, attention to some secondary tasks improves postural control, through improving the automaticity of postural control, through increased arousal, or through the use of reduced postural sway to support the efficiency of performance of the suprapostural task.
10. The neural control of posture is widely distributed among spinal and brain systems.

ANSWERS TO LAB ACTIVITY ASSIGNMENTS

Lab Activity 7.1

1. You probably moved slightly, since it is rare to stand perfectly still. You also would typically move most in the AP direction, but there would also be a certain amount of ML sway. We call the type of balance used to control quiet stance and sitting "steady-state" balance control.
2. Movement would be at the ankle for small amounts of AP sway; movements would be about the hip when swaying close to your stability limits.
3. The toes came up when responding to the light nudge, indicating that the tibialis anterior muscle was activated; you probably took a step backward in response to a harder nudge. The type of balance

used to recover stability following an unexpected displacement in stance or sitting is called *reactive balance control*.

4. (a) It would be easier to balance using an ankle strategy with a larger BOS; (b) harder to recover from a faster movement; (c) hardest to respond with an ankle movement when the COM was already close to the edge of the BOS; a person tends to use a hip or stepping strategy; and (d) could not use an ankle strategy, so would shift to movement about the hips. If there were a handhold available, the person might reach for support.
5. (a) One would use predominantly ankle muscles for AP sway and hip muscles for ML sway. (b) Hip muscles. (c) Took a step.

Lab Activity 7.2

1. **Condition 1**: Firm surface (e.g., linoleum or wood) with feet together, hands on hips, and eyes open. Sensory cues available: vision, vestibular, and somatosensory. Shoulder displacement amplitude: low levels.

   Condition 2: Eyes closed, firm surface: Sensory cues available: somatosensory and vestibular.

   Shoulder displacement amplitude: slightly higher.

   Condition 3: Feet together on the foam, with eyes open. Sensory cues available: vision, vestibular, and distorted somatosensory.

   Shoulder displacement amplitude: higher than in conditions 1 and 2.

   Condition 4: Feet together on foam with eyes closed. Sensory cues available: vestibular and distorted somatosensory.

   Shoulder displacement amplitude: highest of the four conditions.
2. It becomes larger as sensory cues are removed or made less accurate.
3. They should be similar in relative amplitude for the same four conditions.

Lab Activity 7.3

1. It moved upward.
2. This will vary depending on the person: if a person is very relaxed, the hand may move more; if the person is very stiff, it may move less.
3. It was nearly steady, moving very little, if at all.
4. The second.
5. The lifting of the book must be internally generated rather than externally generated.
6. When the subject lifts the weight, the arm does not move, due to anticipatory inhibition of the biceps muscle, but when someone else lifts the weight, the arm moves up, as there is no anticipatory inhibition of biceps.

CHAPTER 8

Development of Postural Control

Learning Objectives

Following completion of this chapter, the reader will be able to:

1. Describe the development of postural control using a systems framework. Contrast the systems framework to the reflex/hierarchical framework of postural development.
2. Outline the milestones that characterize postural development, and the ages at which the milestones typically appear.
3. Discuss the contributions of sensory and motor systems to the emergence of steady-state, reactive, and anticipatory postural control underlying development of head control, trunk control (sitting balance), and independent stance.
4. Describe the development of adaptive capacity in postural control; discuss how learning and practice affects the development of postural control.

INTRODUCTION

During the early years of life, children develop an incredible repertoire of skills, including crawling, independent walking and running, climbing, eye–hand coordination, and the manipulation of objects in a variety of ways. The emergence of all these skills requires the development of postural activity to support the primary movement.

To understand the emergence of mobility and manipulatory skills in children, therapists need to understand the postural substrate for these skills. Similarly, understanding the best therapeutic approach for a child with difficulties in walking or reaching skills requires the knowledge of any limitations in their postural abilities. Understanding the basis for normal postural development, then, is a necessary first step in understanding impaired postural development, both of which are necessary to determining the best therapeutic approach for improving functional postural skills.

This chapter discusses the research on the development of postural control and how it contributes to the emergence of stability and mobility skills. Later chapters consider the implications of this research when assessing and treating postural control in populations with atypical development.

Postural Control and Development

Let's first look at some of the evidence showing that postural control is a critical part of motor development. Research on early development has shown that the simultaneous development of the postural, locomotor, and manipulative systems is essential to the emergence and refinement of skills in all these areas. In a neonate, when the chaotic movements of the head that regularly disturb the infant's seated balance are stabilized, movements and behaviors normally seen in more mature infants emerge (Amiel-Tison & Grenier, 1980). For example, as shown in Figure 8.1, when the clinician stabilizes the head of a newborn, they begin to attend to the clinician, reach for objects, and maintain their arms at the side, with the fingers open, suggesting inhibition of the grasp and Moro reflexes.

These results support the concept that an immature postural system is a limiting factor or a constraint on the emergence of other behaviors, such as coordinated arm and hand movements, as well as the inhibition of reflexes. It has also been suggested that delayed or abnormal development of the postural system may also constrain a child's ability to develop independence in mobility and manipulatory skills.

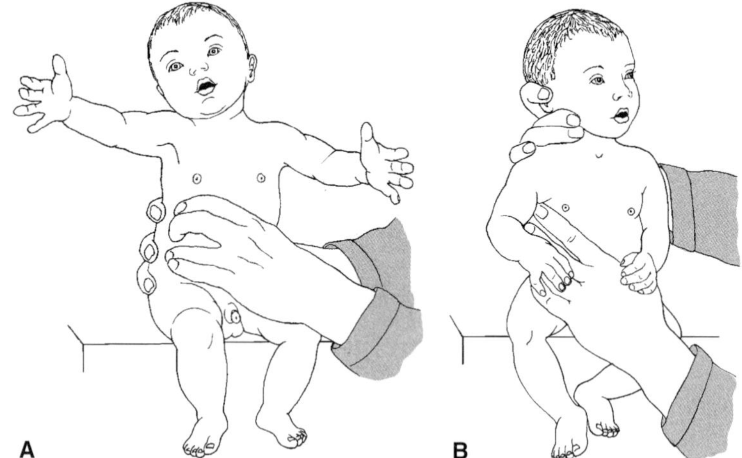

Figure 8.1 Stabilizing the head in a neonate can produce dramatic changes in behavior. **(A)** Uncontrolled movements of the head produce a Moro response. **(B)** External support to the child's head and trunk results in more mature behaviors, including attending to people and objects, and even reaching. (Adapted from Amiel-Tison C, Grenier A. *Evaluation neurologique du nouveau-né et du nourrisson*. [Neurological evaluation of the newborn and the infant.] Paris, France: Masson, 1980:82.)

Motor Milestones and Emerging Postural Control

The development of postural control has traditionally been associated with a predictable sequence of motor behaviors, referred to as "motor milestones." Some of the major motor milestones in development are typically displayed in a chart with the average onset age and/or percentiles, as shown in Figure 8.2. They include head control, rolling, sitting, pull to stand, creeping/crawling, cruising, independent stance, and walking. The sequence and timing of the emergence of these motor milestones have been well described by the early pioneers in developmental researcher.

In 1946, Arnold Gesell, a pediatrician, described the emergence of general patterns of behavior in the first few years of life. He noted the general direction of behavioral development as moving from head to pelvis, and proximally to distally within segments. Thus, he formulated the law of developmental direction

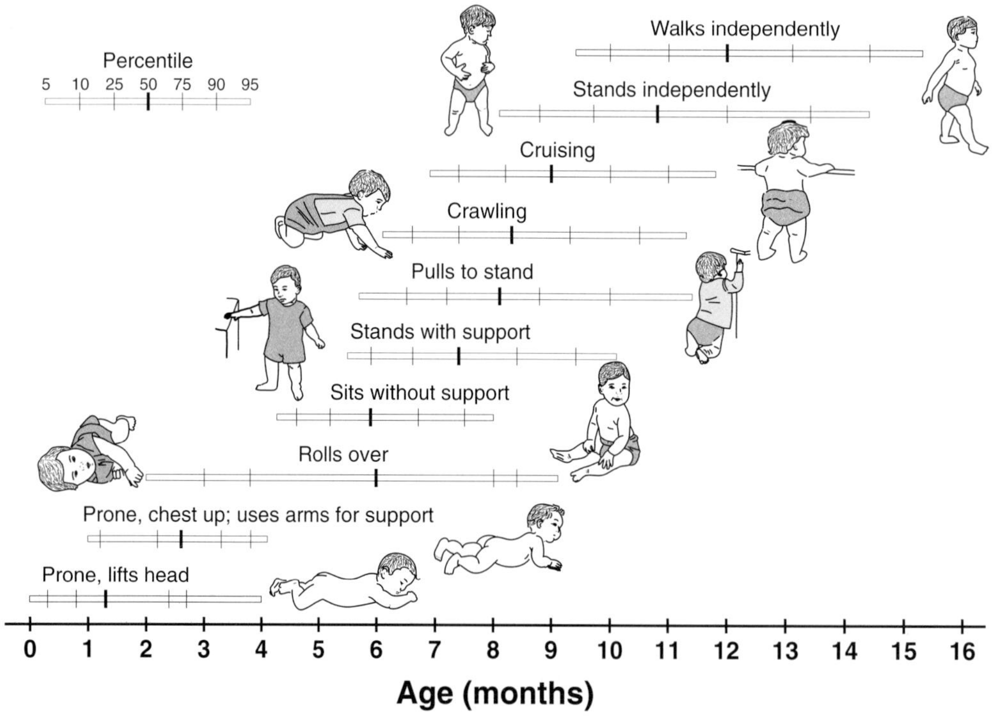

Figure 8.2 Major motor milestones that emerge with the development of postural control. The length of the horizontal bars represents the 5th to 95th percentiles, and ticks denote the 10th, 25th, 50th, 75th, and 90th percentiles. Normative data for lifting the head, propping the chest up while prone, rolling, and pulling to stand are from the Alberta Infant Motor Scale (AIMS). Data for sitting with support, crawling, cruising, independent stance, and walking are from the World Health Organization (WHO) standards. (Adapted from Rachwani J, Hoch JE, Adolph KE. Action in development: Variability, flexibility, and plasticity. In C.S. Tamis-LeMonda & J.J. Lockman (Eds.). *Handbook of infant development*. Cambridge University Press. 2020; Figure 17.1.)

(Gesell, 1946). In addition, Gesell portrayed development as a spiraling hierarchy. He suggested that the development of skilled behavior does not follow a strict linear sequence, always advancing, constantly improving with time and maturity. Instead, Gesell believed that development is much more dynamic in nature and seems to be characterized by alternating advancement and regression in the ability to perform skills.

Gesell gave the example of children learning to crawl and then creep. Initially, in learning to crawl, the child uses a primarily symmetrical arm pattern, eventually switching to a more complex alternating arm pattern as the skill of crawling is perfected. When the child first begins to creep, there is a return to the symmetrical arm pattern. Eventually, as creeping becomes perfected, the emergence of an alternating arm pattern occurs. Thus, as children progress to each new stage in the development of a skill, they may appear to regress to an earlier form of the behavior as new, more mature and adaptive, versions of these skills emerge.

The dynamic nature of motor development has also been described by modern developmental researchers. They noted that infants can acquire skills in various orders, skip stages, and revert to earlier forms (Adolph et al., 2011; Atun-Einy et al., 2012). For example, most infants learn to crawl before cruising, but some infants learn to cruise before crawling, and some infants never learn to crawl at all (Adolph et al., 2011). Although crawling and cruising skills eventually disappear from infants' repertoires as walking emerges, infants exhibit both skills simultaneously for prolonged periods before they begin walking, suggesting that there is a temporal overlap in practicing skills rather than a stage-like advancement of skills, as implied by the depictions of typical milestone charts.

What are the causes for these individual differences in motor development? Of course, individual motor abilities are a primary reason for seeing individual developmental trajectories. However, the type of skills infants acquire, the ages they appear, and the subsequent trajectories of skills are also highly responsive to cultural and historical differences in childrearing practice, infants' everyday experiences, and infants' motivation to move (Adolph & Hoch, 2019).

Most of the traditional assessment scales created to evaluate the emergence of motor behaviors use developmental norms established by McGraw (1932) and Gesell (1946). Using these scales, the therapist evaluates the age and performance of the infant or child on functional skills that require postural control. These skills include sitting, standing, walking unsupported, reaching forward, and moving from a sitting to a standing position. Examples of developmental tests and measures include the Gross Motor Function Measure (GMFM) (Russell et al., 1993), the Peabody Developmental Motor Scales (Folio & Fewell, 2000), the Bayley Scales of Infant and Toddler Development (Bayley, 2006), and the Alberta Infant Motor Scale (AIMS) (Piper et al., 1994). These and other tests follow normal development and are used to differentiate typical from atypical development. However, because of the dynamic nature of motor skill acquisition, children's performance on these tests should be used as a guidance and in conjunction with other factors (e.g., childrearing practice) that may be contributing to atypical development.

THEORIES OF DEVELOPING POSTURAL CONTROL

What is the basis for the development of postural control underlying this predictable sequence of motor behaviors? Several theories of child development try to relate neural structure and behavior in developing infants.

Reflex/Hierarchical Theory

Classic theories of child development place great importance on a reflex substrate for the emergence of mature human behavior patterns. This means that in the normal child, the emergence of posture and movement control is dependent on the appearance and subsequent integration of reflexes. According to these theories, the appearance and disappearance of these reflexes reflect the increasing maturity of cortical structures that inhibit and integrate reflexes controlled at lower levels within the central nervous system (CNS) into more functional postural and voluntary motor responses (refer back to Fig. 1.5). This classic theory has been referred to as a reflex/hierarchical theory (Horak & Shumway-Cook, 1990; Woollacott & Shumway-Cook, 1990). For a detailed explanation of the reflex/hierarchical theory of postural development, see Extended Knowledge Box 8.1.

Systems Theory

More recent theories of motor control, such as the systems theory, suggest that development involves much more than the maturation of reflexes within the CNS. Development is a complex process, with new behaviors and skills emerging from an interaction of the child (and the maturing nervous and musculoskeletal system) with the environment. In the systems theory, the emergence of postural control results from a complex interaction between neural and musculoskeletal systems including the development of the following:

1. Muscle strength and changes in relative mass of the different body segments
2. Motor coordination strategies for the control of steady-state, reactive, and anticipatory balance
3. Individual sensory systems, including somatosensory, visual, and vestibular systems

Extended Knowledge 8.1

Reflex/Hierarchical Theory of Postural Control

Postural reflexes were studied in the early part of the 20th century by investigators such as Magnus (1926), DeKleijn (1923), Rademaker (1924), and Schaltenbrand (1928). In this early work, researchers selectively produced lesions in different parts of the CNS and examined an animal's capacity to orient. Magnus and associates took the animal down to what they referred to as the "zero condition," a condition in which no postural reflex activity could be elicited. Subsequent animals received selective lesions, leaving systematically greater and greater amounts of the CNS intact. In this way, Magnus identified individually and collectively all the reflexes that worked cooperatively to maintain postural orientation in various types of animals.

Postural reflexes in animals were classified by Magnus as local static reactions, segmental static reactions, general static reactions, and righting reactions. Local static reactions stiffen the animal's limb for support of body weight against gravity. Segmental static reactions involve more than one body segment and include the flexor withdrawal reflex and the crossed extensor reflex. General static reactions, called "attitudinal reflexes," involve changes in position of the whole body in response to changes in head position. Finally, Magnus described a series of five righting reactions, which allowed the animal to assume or resume a species-specific orientation of the body with respect to its environment.

Many researchers have tried to document accurately the time frame for the appearance and disappearance of postural reflexes in normal children, with widely varying results. There is little agreement on the presence and time course of these reflexes, or on the significance of these reflexes to normal and abnormal development (Claverie et al., 1973).

Attitudinal Reflexes

According to the reflex theory of postural control, tonic attitudinal reflexes produce persisting changes in body posture that result from a change in head position and include (a) the asymmetric tonic neck reflex (ATNR), (b) the symmetric tonic neck reflex (STNR) (shown in Fig. 8.3A), and (c) the tonic labyrinthine reflex (TLR) (Milani-Comparetti & Gidoni, 1967). The ATNR produces extension in the face arm and flexion in the skull arm when the head is turned. The STNR results in flexion in the upper extremities and extension in the lower extremities when the head is flexed; however, when the head is extended, the upper extremities extend while the lower extremities flex.

Righting Reactions

According to a reflex/hierarchical model, the interaction of five righting reactions produces orientation of the head in space and orientation of the body in relationship to the head and ground. Righting reactions are considered automatic reactions that enable a person to assume the normal standing position and maintain stability when changing positions (Barnes et al., 1978). Three righting reactions (Fig. 8.3B) orient the head in space and include (a) the optical righting reaction, which contributes to the reflex orientation of the head using visual inputs; (b) the labyrinthine righting reaction, which orients the head to an upright vertical position in response to vestibular signals (Ornitz, 1983; Peiper, 1963); and (c) the body-on-head righting reaction, which orients the head in response to proprioceptive and tactile signals from the body in contact with a supporting surface. The Landau reaction combines the effects of all three head-righting reactions (Cupps et al., 1976). Two reflexes interact to keep the body oriented with respect to the head and the surface. The neck-on-body righting reaction (Fig. 8.3C) orients the body in response to cervical afferents, which report changes in the position of the head and neck. The body-on-body righting reaction, shown in Figure 8.3C, right, keeps the body oriented with respect to the ground, regardless of the position of the head.

Balance and Protective Reactions

According to the reflex/hierarchical theory, balance emerges in association with a sequentially organized series of equilibrium reactions, including the tilting reactions (Fig. 8.3D), used for controlling the center of gravity in response to a tilting surface; the parachute, or protective, responses (Fig. 8.3E), which protect the body from injury during a fall; and the staggering reactions (sideways stepping), a response to instability in the lateral direction.

Much debate has occurred in recent years over the relative merits of the reflex/hierarchical versus the systems models in explaining postural development. In many respects, the two models are consistent. Their differences include the following: (a) The reflex/hierarchical model views balance control from a reactive perspective, while the systems model stresses the importance of proactive, reactive, and adaptive aspects of the system, and (b) the reflex/hierarchical model tends to weight the role of CNS maturation more heavily than experience, while the systems model does not emphasize the role of one over the other.

4. Sensory strategies for organizing these multiple inputs in the control of steady-state, reactive, and anticipatory postural control
5. Cognitive resources and strategies critical to controlling posture under multitask conditions

An important part of interpreting sensory information and coordinating actions for postural control is the presence of an internal representation of the body, or body schema. In this body schema, multisensory inputs are integrated to establish a postural frame of reference that the brain can use to generate motion. The CNS can correct the body's motion based on the error between the body schema and received sensory signals (Chiba et al., 2016). It has been hypothesized that this body schema is not only used as a comparison for incoming sensory inputs but is also an essential part of interpreting self-motion and is used to calibrate motor actions (Gurfinkel & Levik, 1978).

Development of sensory, motor, and cognitive aspects of postural control has been hypothesized to involve the capacity to build up appropriate internal representations related to posture that reflect the rules for organizing sensory inputs and coordinating them with motor actions. For example, as the child gains experience moving in a gravity environment, sensory/motor

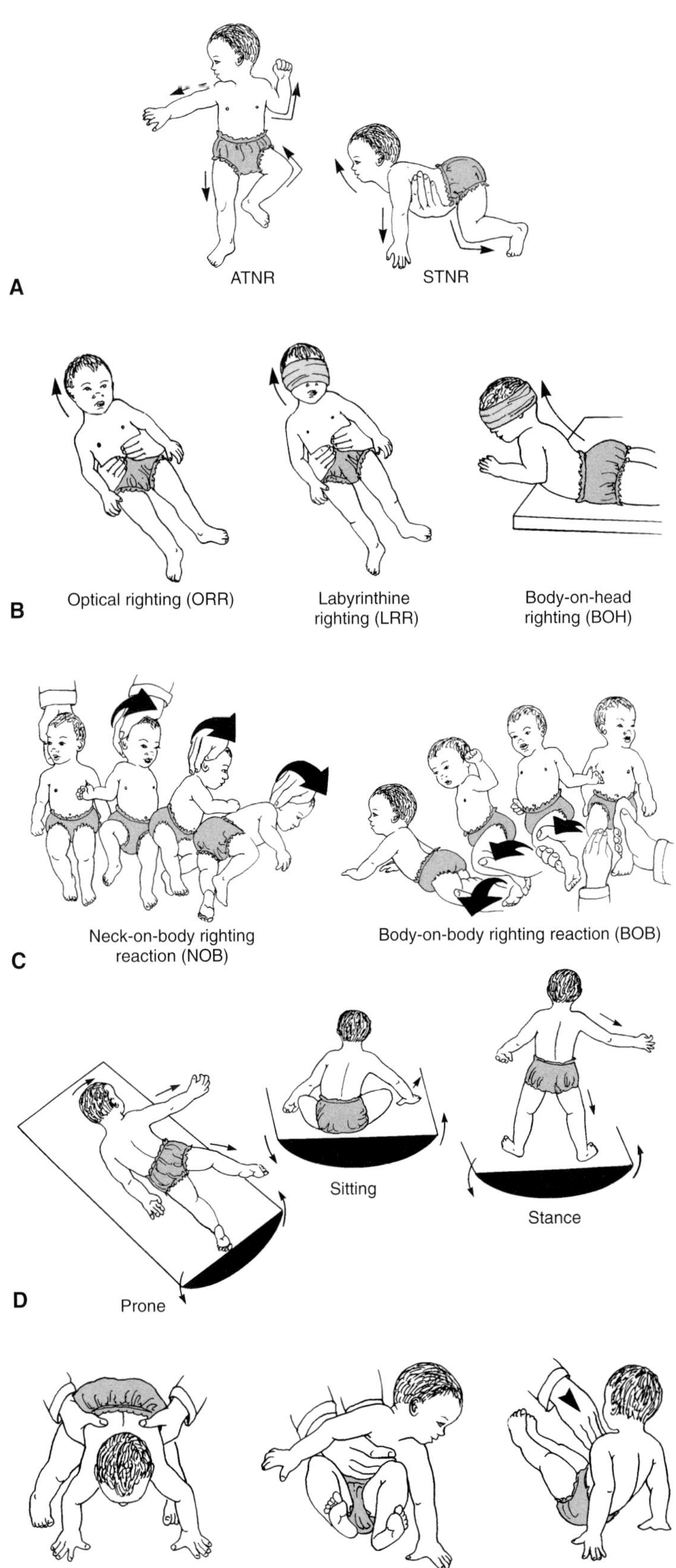

Figure 8.3 (A) Attitudinal reflexes. **Left:** The ATNR reflex: extension in the face arm, and flexion in the skull arm when the head is turned. **Right:** The STNR reflex: head flexion causes flexion of the upper extremities and extension of the lower extremities; head extension causes extension in the upper extremities and flexion in the lower extremities. **(B)** Righting reactions that orient the head. **Left:** The optical righting reaction orients the head to visual vertical. **Center:** The labyrinthine righting reaction orients the head in response to vestibular signals signaling vertical. **Right:** The body-on-head righting reaction uses tactile and neck proprioceptive information to orient the head to vertical. **(C)** Righting reactions of the body. Shown are the mature form of (L), the neck-on-body righting reaction **(left)** and the body-on-body righting reaction **(right)**. **(D)** Tilting reactions. Tilting responses are purported to emerge first in prone **(left)**, then supine (not shown), then sitting **(center)**, then emerge in all fours (not shown), and finally standing **(right)**. **(E)** Protective reactions. These reactions protect the body from injury resulting from a fall and develop first in the forward direction **(left)**, then sideways **(center)**, and then backward **(right)**. (Adapted from Barnes MR, Crutchfield CA, Heriza CB. *The neurophysiological basis of patient treatment*. Morgantown, WV: Stokesville, 1978:222.)

maps would develop. These maps would relate actions to incoming sensory inputs from visual, somatosensory, and vestibular systems. In this way, rules for moving would develop and be reflected in altered synaptic relationships. Thus, researchers argue that the path from sensation to motor actions proceeds via an internal representational structure or body schema (Gurfinkel & Levik, 1978; Hirschfeld, 1992).

Since different systems affecting postural control develop at different rates, it is important to understand which components are rate limiting at each developmental stage or, conversely, which ones push the system to a new level of function when they have matured. According to newer models of development, finding the connection between critical postural components and development ultimately guides the clinician in determining which systems should be examined and how the contribution of these systems changes at various developmental stages. It also allows the clinician to determine appropriate interventions specific to the system that is dysfunctional.

DEVELOPMENT OF POSTURAL CONTROL: A SYSTEMS PERSPECTIVE

Since Gesell's original studies in 1946 describing the cephalocaudal nature of development, many researchers have found exceptions to some of his general developmental rules. For example, studies have found that when infants are strapped to a reclined board to stabilize balance, infants as young as 8 weeks of age were able to successfully reach for toys with their feet—a month earlier than when the same infants were able to reach with their hands (Galloway & Thelen, 2004). Thus, infants show control of the legs well before they can control their arms in space. However, in the area of balance and postural control, it does appear as if development follows a cephalocaudal sequence.

General Movements in Infants

Heinz Prechtl (1986), a researcher and physician from the Netherlands, has studied the general movements that are part of the spontaneous repertoire of infants from fetal development through the end of the first 6 months of life, when intentional and antigravity movements become more predominant. He has noted that early in development, there is an appearance of complex writhing movements, involving the whole body (arm, leg, neck, and trunk movements in variable sequences), which occur often from early fetal life until the end of the second month post-term. These movements appear to have a gradual beginning and ending and vary in intensity and velocity, showing coordination and fluidity. At 6 to 9 weeks post-term, writhing movements gradually disappear whereas fidgety movements—small movements of the neck, trunk, and limbs performed at medium speed—gradually emerge. Fidgety movements are predominant in awake typically developing 3- to 5-month-olds. His research also indicates that when the nervous system is impaired, movements become monotonous and poorly differentiated. In fact, two specific changes in the movement patterns have been reliably shown to predict a later diagnosis of cerebral palsy. These include (a) cramped synchronized general movements (lacking a normal fluid character) and (b) absence of general movements of a fidgety character (Einspieler & Prechtl, 2005). This research has led to the development of the General Movements Assessment, a measure of spontaneous movement patterns from the preterm period to 15 weeks post-term. This measure has been shown to be a valid and reliable prognostic tool to identify infants with neurodevelopmental disabilities (Darsaklis et al., 2011).

Emerging Head Control

Motor Coordination

Steady-state postural control, which involves antigravity control of the head in space, is not present at birth. Is this due to lack of muscle strength (a musculoskeletal constraint) or, alternatively, a lack of coordinated muscle activity for controlling the head relative to gravity? Prechtl and colleagues examined spontaneous head movements using both electromyographic (EMG) and video recordings to determine whether coordinated muscle activity was present. They found no organized patterns of muscle activity that appeared to counteract the force of gravity on any consistent basis, suggesting that the lack of head control in newborns is not solely the result of a lack of strength but also results from a lack of organized muscle activity (Schloon et al., 1976).

When does reactive balance control of the head develop? Experiments examining infants' development of reactive balance control have been performed in many labs (Harbourne et al., 1993; Hedberg et al., 2005; Hirschfeld & Forssberg, 1994; Woollacott et al., 1987). Figure 8.4 compares the experimental paradigm used for examining reactive balance in infants at varying developmental levels. To test reactive balance in the control of head posture, infants are placed in an infant seat on a moveable postural platform (a) or seated supported by experimenters' hands and then released as the platform moves (b); to test reactive balance in sitting, infants sit unsupported on the platform, which is then moved (c). Finally, reactive balance during the emergence of stance postural control is tested with children standing on the moveable platform (d). Using the experimental paradigm shown in Figure 8.4A, Hedberg and colleagues found that the emergence of directionally specific postural responses in neck muscles underlying reactive balance control begins in

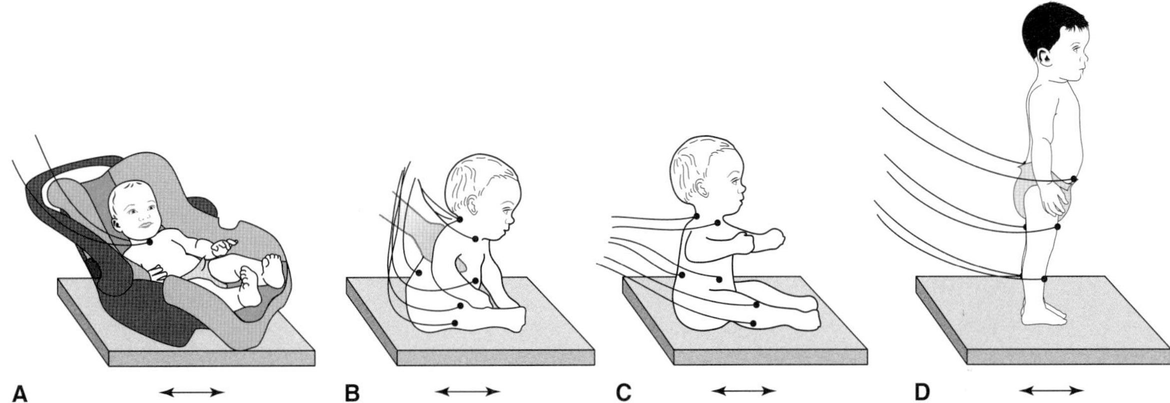

Figure 8.4 Moving platform posturography and electromyography used to study postural response patterns in infants in response to a moving surface in various stages of sitting. **(A)** Stage 1, holding up head, with trunk support supplied by an infant seat; muscle responses are recorded from neck muscles. **(B)** Stage 2, propping on arms during sitting or sitting independently for brief periods. Experimenter releases their manual trunk support of the infant just before the perturbation; muscle responses are recorded from neck, trunk, and leg. **(C)** Stage 3, sitting independently without falling. **(D)** Standing. Perturbation is given without external support for both **(C** and **D)**, and muscle activity recorded from the legs and trunk. (Adapted from Harbourne RT, Stergiou N. Nonlinear analysis of the development of sitting postural control. *Dev Psychobiol*. 2003;42:368.)

infants as young as 1 month of age, although responses are present in only 28% to 30% of trials across infants for neck flexors (Hedberg et al., 2004, 2005).

Sensory Contributions

As discussed in Chapter 7, all three sensory inputs are important to the control of steady-state balance in adults. Which combination of senses contributes most according to the task and the environmental context? To what extent do the individual sensory systems contribute to the development of steady-state postural control underlying the emergence of head control?

Visual Contributions. Studies on infants with early blindness suggest that vision contributes to the development of head orientation in complex ways. It appears to be important in the calibration of both the vestibular and proprioceptive systems, which contribute to the development of internal models of posture, essential to the emergence of postural control and functional skills. Interestingly, the effect of loss of vision on the emergence of head control is not readily evident until approximately 2 to 3 months post-term, when infants normally demonstrate antigravity control of the head using visual inputs to orient the head in space. Blind infants are unable to use their normal vestibular inputs to orient the head to vertical when tilted, suggesting the importance of visual inputs to calibration of the labyrinthine function. Finally, blind infants demonstrate impairments in fine manipulation of objects compared to sighted infants, even when sighted infants are not looking at their hands, suggesting the importance of peripheral visual inputs in calibrating proprioceptive function (Prechtl et al., 2001).

Babies with intact vision as young as 60 hours old are able to orient themselves toward a source of visual stimulation, and they can follow a moving object by correctly orienting the head (Bullinger, 1981; Bullinger & Jouen, 1983). It appears that the neural programs underlying visual orientation are present at birth; however, they appear to require experience and learning in order to be maintained and refined. Blind infants reorient their head in the direction of an object placed in their hand (as if to "look" at it) at the age of 6 months. However, this behavior disappears at the age of about 10 months, suggesting that the orienting response is built in but maintenance is normally provided by the visual system. Thus, in the absence of vision (such as in blind infants), head orientation disappears (Prechtl et al., 2001).

As discussed earlier, one approach to studying the role of vision in the emergence of postural control is comparing development of head control in sighted and blind infants. Alternatively, researchers have used moving visual stimuli to examine the role of vision in postural control. Jouen and colleagues (Jouen, 1993; Jouen et al., 2000) examined the postural reactions of the head and neck of neonates in response to moving visual stimuli, which create the illusion of a movement of the head in space. This paradigm and results are shown in Figure 8.5. Video monitors on either side of the head provided optic flow stimuli (pseudo-random dot patterns moving horizontally) to 3-day-old infants while they reclined 25° in an infant seat. The head rested on a pressure-sensitive pillow, which was used to measure changes in pressure associated with postural adjustments of the head (Fig. 8.5A). The infant and monitors were inside a dark chamber. Researchers found that as angular velocity of the optic flow increased, there was a corresponding increase in head pressure (Fig. 8.5B); for example, when the visual patterns moved toward the infants, the infants moved their head backward into the pillow, as though to compensate for perceived forward sway of the head. These results support Prechtl's

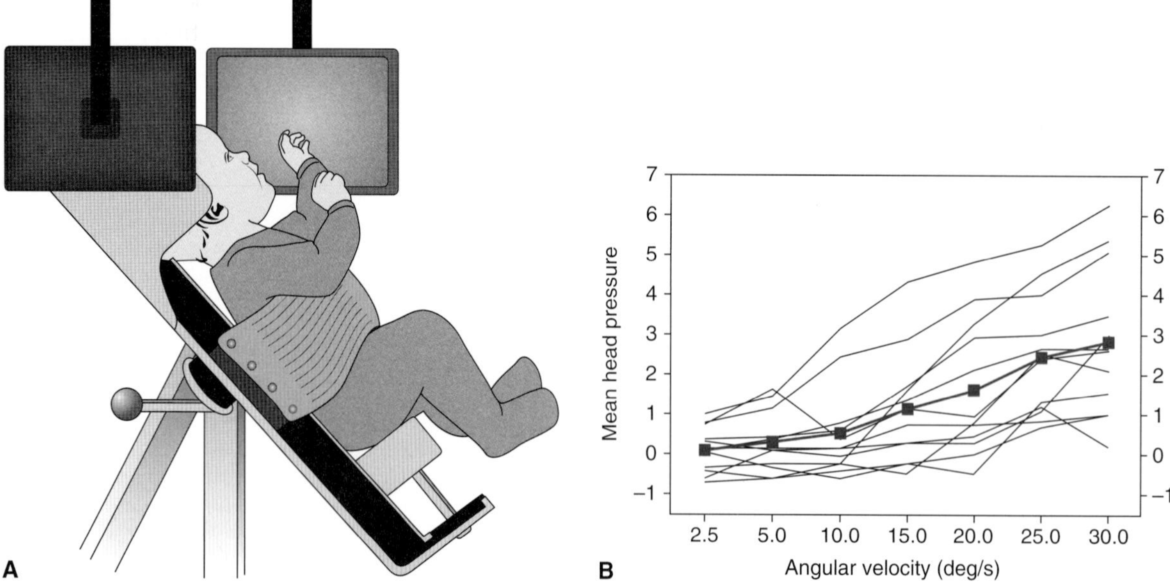

Figure 8.5 Examining the effect of optic flow on postural control of the head in neonates. **(A)** Infant lies supported in an infant seat with head on a pressure-sensitive pillow; monitors provide the optic flow stimuli. **(B)** For all infants (shown as individual lines), head pressure increases with an increase in angular velocity of optic flow. *Red line* and *red squares* represent the mean of the group of infants. (Part **B** data from Jouen F, Lepecq JC, Gapenne O, et al. Optic flow sensitivity in neonates. *Infant Behav Dev.* 2000;23:271–284.)

findings of early optic flow sensitivity in infants and suggest that (a) the subcortical neural networks that contribute to visual proprioceptive control of posture are present at birth and (b) while learning is not required for the initial emergence of optic flow sensitivity, experience and visual feedback are important for the maintenance and refinement of visual–postural coupling (Jouen et al., 2000; Prechtl et al., 2001).

Vestibular Contributions. Maturation of the vestibular system is genetically programmed but also depends on the exposure to vestibular inputs. Vestibular development is essential for functions such as postural control (head and trunk with respect to space and head in relation to the trunk), gaze stabilization, homeostatic regulation, and spatial memory (Jamon, 2014). Children with vestibular deficits, mainly bilateral deficits, may show problems in developing brain representations of body parts relative to one another or body orientation and position within the environment (Wiener-Vacher et al., 2013). For example, children born deaf who have abnormal vestibular function show significantly delayed acquisition of head control and independent walking compared to children who are deaf but have normal vestibular function (Inoue et al., 2013). But as we have seen, visual information appears to be critical in calibrating vestibular information for postural control.

Somatosensory Contributions. By the age of 3 months post-term, the primary somatosensory cortical circuits are being developed together with the primary motor and visual cortexes (Hadders-Algra, 2018a). At this age, there is an important transition of sensorimotor behaviors. For example, goal-oriented movements (i.e., reaching) replace spontaneous movements, and infants develop the ability to maintain the head with respect to the trunk while held in a sitting position (Hadders-Algra, 2018b). Thus, somatosensory inputs also contribute to the emergence of head control in normal infants, but like the contributions of vestibular inputs, visual information appears to be critical in calibrating somatosensory inputs for control of head posture.

Modifiability of Head Control

What is the effect of practice on the emergence of head control? Lee and Galloway (2012) examined the effect of training on the development of head control. Infants received postural and movement activities provided by their caregiver for 20 minutes daily for 4 weeks when they were 1 month of age. The activities targeted the neck, shoulder girdle, and trunk muscles, and the use of arm movements for reaching. Trained infants had increased head control during the training period and after the training compared to the nontrained infants. Moreover, trained infants maintained their heads in a vertical and midline position longer compared with nontrained infants. These results provide a basis for treatment. Therapists might consider using similar activities when targeting children lacking head control.

Emergence of Independent Sitting

As infants begin to sit independently, and thus develop trunk control, they must learn to master the control of spontaneous background sway of both the head and the trunk and to respond to perturbations of balance. This requires the coordination of sensory/motor information relating two body segments (the head and the trunk) together in the control of posture. Are the rules that newborns use regarding sensory/motor relationships for head postural control already available for controlling trunk musculature, or do they need to be learned with experience in sitting? As you will see in the research discussed in the following section, it appears as though there may be both innate components of control, available in the newborn, and emergent aspects of control, resulting from the infant interacting with the environment in a dynamic way.

Motor Coordination

The emergence of independent sitting requires the coordination of multiple muscles to control the position of the head and trunk during steady-state, reactive, and anticipatory balance control.

Steady-State Balance. The emergence of independent sitting is characterized by the infant's ability to control spontaneous sway sufficiently to remain upright. This occurs at approximately 6 to 8 months of age (Butterworth & Cicchetti, 1978). Research on the emergence of steady-state balance control during sitting (sometimes called "static balance") supports the hypothesis that postural development of the head and trunk is an emergent dynamic skill.

In studies on the development of control of steady-state balance in sitting, Harbourne and Stergiou (2003) used methods from nonlinear dynamics to analyze the complexity (level of predictability) and dimensionality (degrees of freedom) of center of pressure (COP) data across three stages of sitting development: Stage 1 (defined as the time when infants were able to hold up the head and upper trunk, but not sit independently; age range, 4 to 5.5 months), stage 2 (infants able to sit independently briefly, i.e., 10 to 30 seconds, or prop themselves on their arms; age range, 5 to 6.5 months), and stage 3 (independent sitting, but not yet crawling; age range, 6 to 8 months). They found that there was a high complexity and dimensionality in stage 1 sitting that decreased as infants reached stage 2 sitting, indicating a reduction in the degrees of freedom of movement and possibly homing in on a strategy for trunk control. This is often found when individuals are learning a new skill. They then found that dimensionality increased from stage 2 to stage 3, indicating a subsequent increase in degrees of freedom of trunk/head movement, as infants mastered sitting skills and increased their adaptability and flexibility in postural control. This research suggests that the development of sitting postural control is a dynamic process in which the infant gradually learns to control the degrees of freedom involved in head/trunk control through three stages of the development of sitting balance.

Though the trunk has traditionally been modeled as a single segment when postural development has been studied in infants, the trunk is clearly made up of multiple segments, controlled by a combination of muscles. Saavedra et al. (2012) studied how infants solve the problem of learning to sit upright and whether a specific sequence of changes in the control of trunk segments underlies the process of learning to sit independently. In a longitudinal study of infants from 3 to 9 months of age, they examined steady-state postural control at four levels of support (under the arms, midribs, waist, and hips) and found that control of the trunk in sitting develops in a top–down manner, between 3 (no control) and 9 (functional control) months of age. They found that control of independent sitting developed gradually, with four different stages present in most infants (no control, attempts to initiate upright sitting, partial control with large range of body sway, and functional control with minimal sway). This is shown in Figure 8.6. The figure illustrates the longitudinal development of sitting balance in a single child over time and also includes an adult subject. The infant is supported by the researcher at the hips only, as shown by the placement of the researcher's hands. Shown is the sway of the trunk at each of the stages of control, with the circle showing the base of support circumference at the level of the hips. Note that at stage 1, the child simply collapses forward and cannot recover sitting balance. At stage 2, the infant attempts to initiate balance but continually loses balance either forward or backward. At stage 3, he can stay upright but is "wobbly" and leans forward, while in stage 4, he shows controlled sitting balance. Histograms showing the amount of time spent at various positions in the anteroposterior plane (vertical bar is midline) also show this shift from no control through functional control, across time. Data from an adult are shown at the right of the figure, for comparison.

In addition, this study found that stability and control of the head in sitting improved with the development of control over sequential trunk segments. This finding has contributed to the development of a clinical strategy for assessing and treating the impaired trunk segment for sitting balance in children with neurologic pathology. Targeted training systematically uses external support at different trunk segments to progressively train sitting balance in children and adults with impaired trunk control. This treatment approach and the associated assessment tools are discussed in detail in Chapter 11.

Reactive Balance Control. Does reactive balance control for sitting develop at the same time as steady-state balance control, or is it available earlier? Results of experiments (Harbourne et al., 1993; Hedberg et al., 2005;

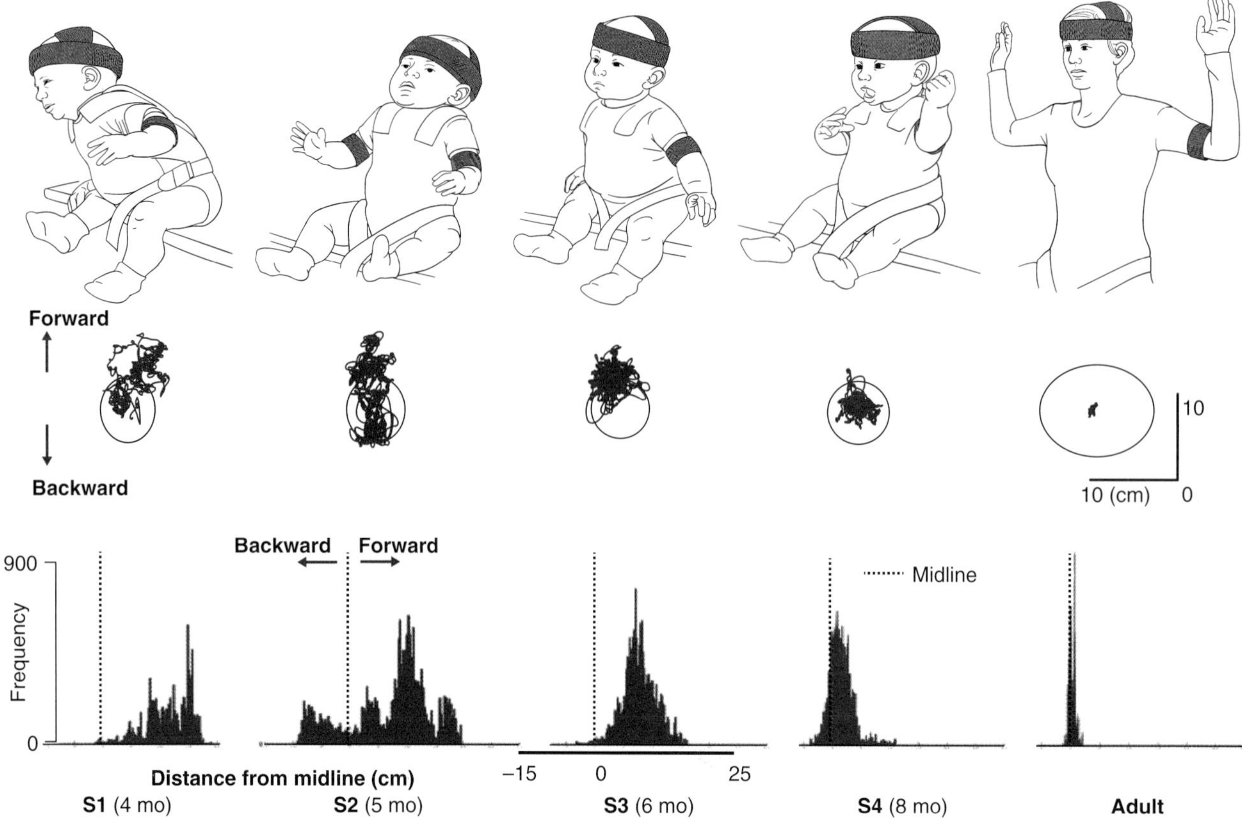

Figure 8.6 Illustrations of a child showing the four stages involved in mastering trunk control, along with an adult with full control. The circles immediately following the illustrations indicate the base of support circumference at the level of the hips and the sway of the trunk in relation to this base of support circumference during the period of data collection. Note that at stage 1 **(far left)**, the child simply collapses forward and cannot recover sitting balance. At stage 2, the infant attempts to initiate balance but continually loses balance either forward or backward. At stage 3, he can stay upright but is "wobbly" and leans forward, while in stage 4, he shows controlled sitting balance. However, sway is still higher than for the adult **(far right)**. At the bottom of the figure are shown histograms indicating the amount of time spent at various positions in the anteroposterior plane (vertical bar is midline) for each stage of hip control development. Data for the adult are shown on the right. (Data from Saavedra S, Woollacott MH. Contributions of spinal segments to trunk postural control during typical development. *Dev Med Child Neurol.* 2009;51(Suppl. 5):82.)

Hirschfeld & Forssberg, 1994; Woollacott et al., 1987) suggest that reactive balance control in the trunk appears to be available to a limited extent in infants well before sitting develops (as early as 1 month of age) and continues to develop through the onset of independent sitting. Thus, there may be innate components available at birth, which are refined with practice.

The study by Hedberg et al. (2005) discussed earlier for reactive balance control of the head also examined the development of reactive sitting balance, including measurements of trunk and leg muscle responses during recovery from balance threats while sitting. Figure 8.7 shows the probability of seeing complete response patterns (all three flexor or extensor muscles) to forward and backward translations in children from 1 to 10 months of age. Note that complete responses are present at low probabilities at 1 month, then diminish further in probability through 3 months, and finally begin to increase again at 4 to 5 months of age.

Hirschfeld and Forssberg (1994) showed that platform movements causing backward sway give much stronger and less variable postural muscle-response synergies than those causing forward sway. This may be caused by the larger base of postural support in the forward direction in seated infants (Hirschfeld & Forssberg, 1994). In this study, infants too young to sit independently (5 to 7 months) responded with only one to two muscles for most forward perturbations, with all three anterior muscles (neck flexors, rectus abdominis, and rectus femoris) being activated in 25% of the trials. By the time infants were independent sitters (7 to 8 months), all three muscles were activated in 100% of the trials. These results also suggest that response synergies are being shaped during the months prior to the emergence of independent sitting and are organized appropriately in all trials by the time infants are able to sit independently.

By 1 month of age, postural response synergies are present; however, they are highly variable and present in only a small percentage of trials. Paradoxically, they appear less frequently in infants at 3 to 4 months of age (Hedberg et al., 2005; Woollacott et al., 1987) and then reappear with greater frequency and refinement as the child learns to sit independently. Thus, these early more variable synergies present in young infants may

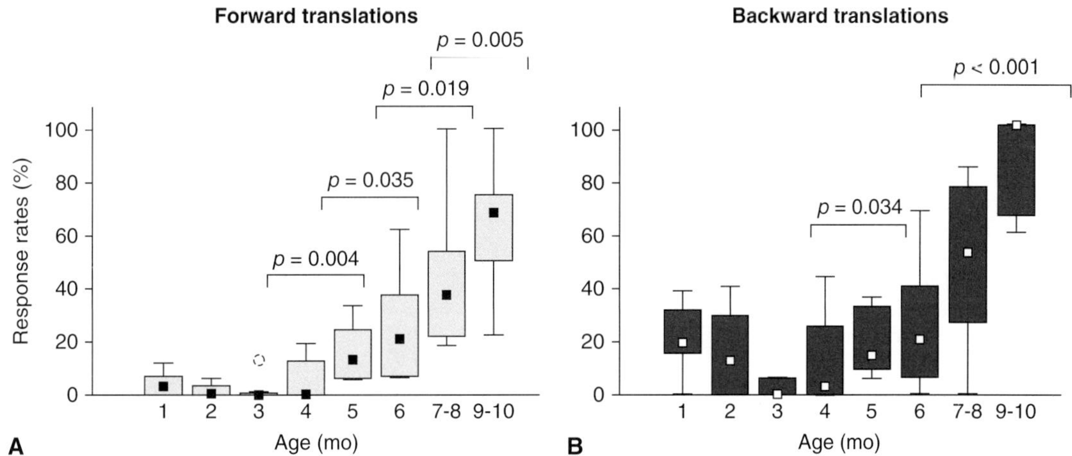

Figure 8.7 Response rates of complete EMG patterns (from neck, trunk, and leg muscles) during seated perturbations for children from 1 through 10 months of age. **(A)** Responses to forward translations. **(B)** Responses to backward translations. Vertical bars show ranges, rectangular boxes show interquartile ranges, and small squares show median values for each group. Light-colored boxes indicate responses of the three flexor muscles (neck, trunk, and hip), while dark orange boxes indicate extensor muscles (neck, trunk, and hip). The *p* values show significantly different distributions of response rates across age groups. (Reprinted with permission from Hedberg, A, Carlberg EB, Forssberg H, et al. Development of postural adjustments in sitting position during the first half year of life. *Dev Med Child Neurol.* 2005;47:318.)

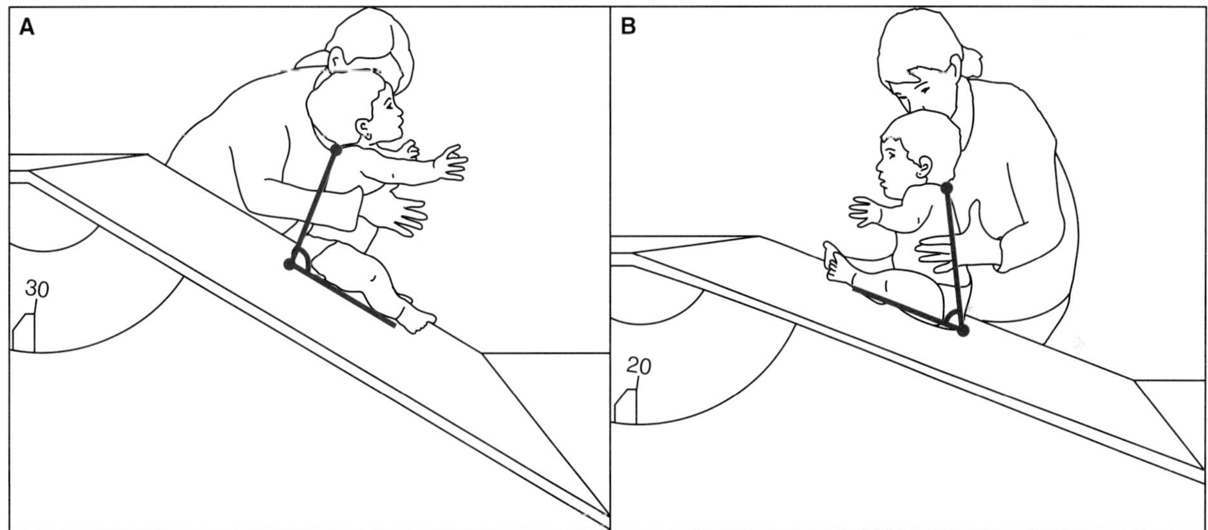

Figure 8.8 Example of an infant in the forward **(A)** and backward **(B)** directions, at the average steepest slopes, infants were able to sit without falling. Orange lines represent trunk–thigh angles. In the forward direction, the trunk–thigh angle increases to 98°, so the infant is leaning backward. In the backward direction, the trunk–thigh angle decreases to 63°, so the infant is leaning forward. (Adapted from Rachwani J, Soska KC, Adolph KE. Behavioral flexibility in learning to sit. *Dev Psychobio.* 2017;59:8, Figure 3.)

be considered precursors to later more refined postural synergies underlying the development of seated postural control.

With greater refinement of postural synergies, infants can react under varying sitting conditions—not only to a horizontal platform. For example, Rachwani et al. (2017) showed that by the time infants can sit independently, they quickly adjust their sitting posture by increasing their trunk–thigh angle on steep forward slopes or decreasing their trunk–thigh angle on steep backward slopes to maintain stability (example shown in Fig. 8.8). Most impressive are infants' systematic adjustments to each incremental change in slant. Moreover, similar to a horizontal platform, postural adjustments on slopes are also direction specific—infants are more successful at keeping balance on steeper forward than backward slopes, most likely due the larger base of support in the forward direction.

Anticipatory Balance Control. Research has examined the development of anticipatory postural control and its relationship to reaching in seated infants, as well as the effects of providing external trunk support on reaching behavior (Rachwani et al., 2015). Ten infants were studied every 2 weeks from age 2.5 to 8 months of age. As shown in Figure 8.9, infants were seated and

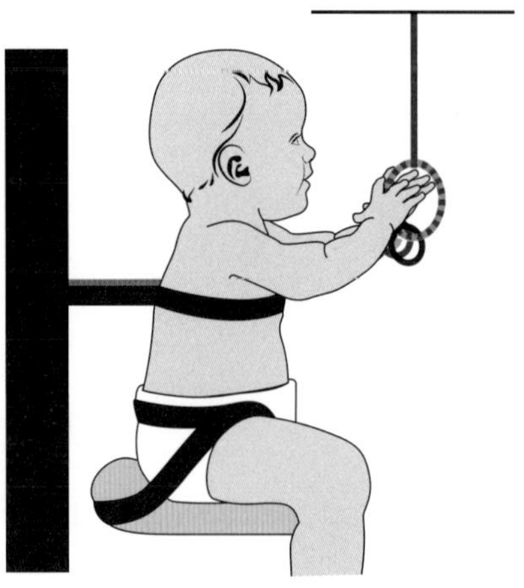
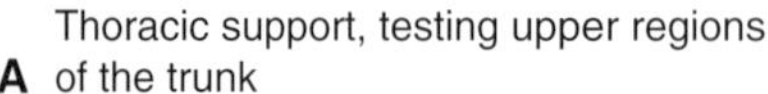

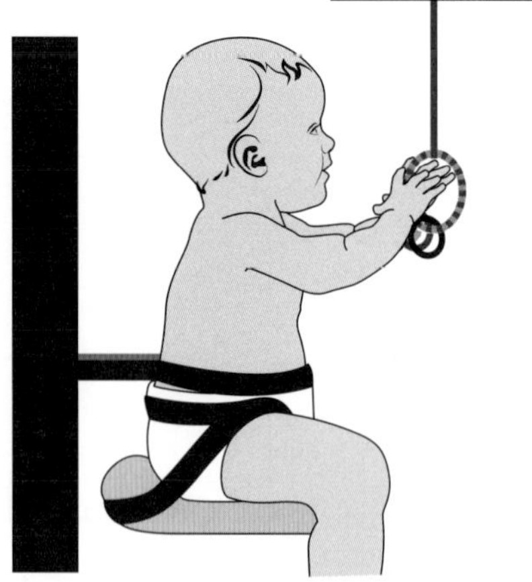

Figure 8.9 Research paradigm for studying anticipatory seated postural control. Infants are seated and provided either thoracic support **(A)** or pelvic support **(B)**, and a toy is dropped in front of the child at arm's length. Kinematics of trunk motion and arm reaches are recorded as is EMG in the trunk and arm. (Adapted from Rachwani J, Santamaria V, Saavedra SL, et al. The development of trunk control and its relation to reaching in infancy: a longitudinal study. *Front Hum Neurosci*. 2015;9:94, Figure 1.)

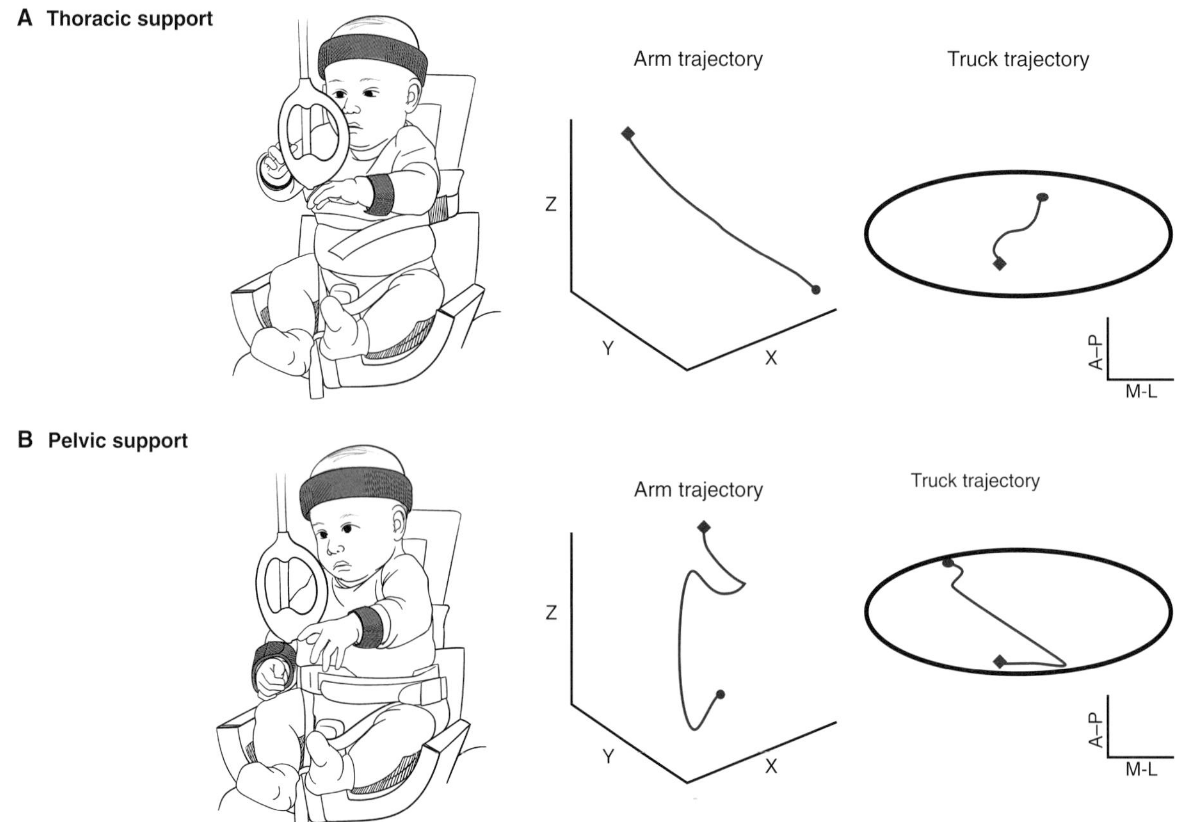

Figure 8.10 The effect of external support on trunk control and reaching in a 4-month-old nonindependent sitter. With only pelvic support (shown on the **bottom**), the infant sways forward (as indicated by the trunk trajectory) and the arm trajectory associated with the reach is jerky and much longer. In contrast, when thoracic support is provided (shown on the **top**), trunk sway is much less and the reach trajectory is smoother and faster. A-P, anterior-posterior; M-L, medio-lateral; X, Y, Z represents the three dimensional Cartesian coordinate system. (Data obtained from Rachwani J, Santamaria V, Saavedra SL, et al. The development of trunk control and its relation to reaching in infancy: a longitudinal study. *Front Hum Neurosci*. 2015;9:94.)

were provided with either thoracic or pelvic support, and a toy was dropped in front of the child at arm's length. Kinematics of trunk motion and arm reaches were recorded, as was EMG in the trunk and arm. Let's first explore the effect of trunk support on reaching in a 4-month-old nonindependent sitter (shown in Fig. 8.10). With only pelvic support (shown on the bottom), the infant sways forward (as indicated by the trunk trajectory) and the arm trajectory associated with the reach is jerky and much longer. In contrast, when thoracic support is provided, trunk sway is much less and the reach trajectory is smoother and faster. This supports earlier research that postural control, specifically control of the trunk, is the rate-limiting factor in reaching in young infants.

As shown in Figure 8.11, as infants develop, trunk control improves (note change in trunk trajectory over time), and this is associated with improved reach trajectories. EMG analysis of muscles in the trunk (data not shown) demonstrated that anticipatory postural activity, beginning about 300 ms prior to the reach, was present in 40% of the trials as early as 3 months of age. As infants developed, the probability for anticipatory activity in the trunk increased to 60% (Rachwani et al., 2015). It is interesting to note that in the youngest infants, while anticipatory postural activity occurred in only 40% of the trials, compensatory postural activity was present in almost 80% of the trials. This suggests that reactive balance control emerges prior to anticipatory control.

Data from these studies of segmental control of posture during development refute the concept that the trunk develops as a single unit; rather development of trunk control underlying sitting balance involves the sequential development of control over successive segments of the trunk in a top–down order (Rachwani et al., 2015; Saavedra et al., 2012).

Sensory Contributions. Early research investigated the role of vision in seated postural control by examining the response of infants at different stages in the development of independent sitting to visual stimuli, giving the illusion of a postural perturbation (the moving room paradigm) (Butterworth & Hicks, 1977; Butterworth & Pope, 1983). Infants with relatively little experience in sitting independently showed a complete loss of balance in response to the visual stimulation (a single ramp stimulus); with increasing experience in sitting, the response amplitude declined. This implies that newly sitting infants rely heavily on visual inputs when controlling sway, and that this dependence decreases with increasing experience in independent sitting, as infants rely more on somatosensory inputs.

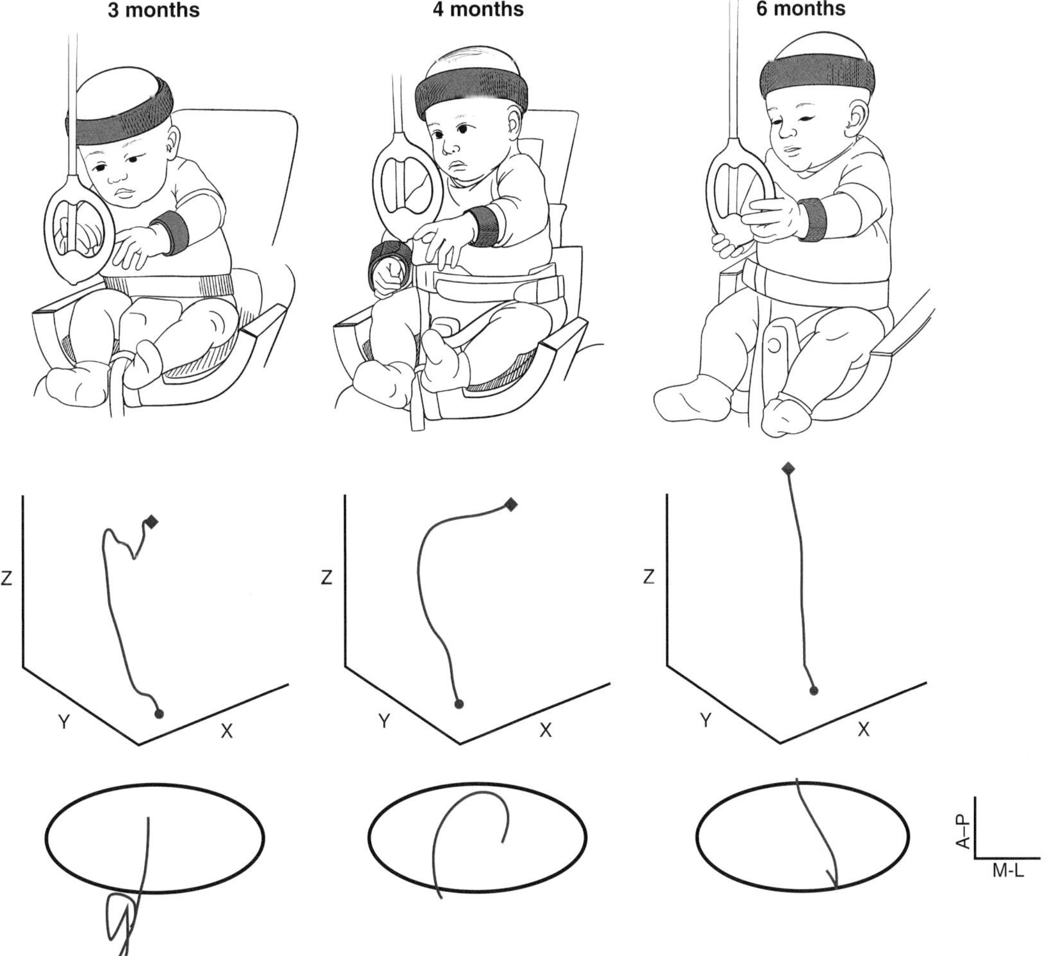

Figure 8.11 Data from an infant at 3, 4, and 6 months of age, showing the longitudinal development of anticipatory postural control supporting reaching. As the infant develops, trunk control improves (note change in trunk trajectory over time, shown in the *circle*, which is the boundary of the base of support), and this is associated with improved reach trajectories (shown in the **middle** row). A-P, anterior-posterior; M-L, medio-lateral; X, Y, Z represents the three dimensional Cartesian coordinate system. (Data obtained from Rachwani J, Santamaria V, Saavedra SL, et al. The development of trunk control and its relation to reaching in infancy: a longitudinal study. *Front Hum Neurosci*. 2015;9:94.)

Experiments by Bertenthal et al. (1997) have also examined the responses of infants to visual cues using continuous oscillations, as they mastered independent sitting. In this study, infants 5 to 13 months old sat on a child's bicycle seat (with a back) in a room that continuously oscillated at a variety of speeds and amplitudes. The postural responses were measured with a force plate under the bicycle seat. They noted that even 5-month-old infants who were not yet sitting independently showed some entrainment to the moving visual stimuli; however, this response became more consistent with age and experience. They concluded that during the process of learning to sit independently, infants are learning to scale or map visual sensory information to their postural activity.

Other studies have examined sensory contributions to the emergence of independent sitting balance using support-surface perturbations that activate all three senses, rather than just vision alone. Woollacott et al. (1987) studied muscle patterns in the head and trunk in response to platform perturbations in seated infants with and without vision. They found that taking away visual stimuli did not change the muscle activation patterns in response to a moving platform. They concluded that somatosensory and vestibular systems are capable of eliciting postural actions in isolation from vision in infants first learning to sit.

In an effort to understand the relationship among vestibular and visual inputs reporting head motion, and proprioceptive inputs from the trunk, Hirschfeld and Forssberg (1994) performed experiments in which head orientation was systematically varied in seated infants undergoing platform perturbations. Coordinated muscle activity stabilizing the trunk did not change regardless of how the head was oriented. This suggests that in the seated position, postural responses to perturbations are largely controlled by somatosensory inputs at the hip joints, not by vestibular or visual stimulation alone.

Recent studies have shown infants' capability of adapting to changes in somatosensory input. For example, Kokkoni et al. (2017) examined infants—all independent sitters—sitting on a force plate. Somatosensory information was altered at the base of support of sitting using foam of different densities. Results showed that after allowing infants to settle in the support condition, infants' body sway was not affected by the alteration in the support surface, suggesting that independent sitters are able to quickly detect and adapt to the distortion of the support surface. Kyvelidou & Stergiou (2018) then compared the effects of altered somatosensory (sitting on a foam pad) and visual (sitting while the lights were turned off) stimuli on infants' sitting postural control and found that infants' body sway increased in the lights off conditions, regardless of whether or not there was a foam pad underneath.

All these studies suggest that as infants learn to sit, they acquire a coherent and consistent relationship between the sensory and motor systems. At first, control of infant's sitting posture is highly reliant on the visual system and thus it is disrupted by conflicting visual information (e.g., a moving room). However, with increasing sitting experience, infants are capable of scaling their postural responses to changes in visual, somatosensory, or vestibular input with adult-like precision. Altogether, the data suggest that it is important for therapists to target all three sensory systems when training infants and children with neuromotor deficits to sit independently.

Modifiability of Postural Responses

What is the effect of practice on the emergence of seated postural responses? Hadders-Algra et al. (1996) examined the effect of training on the development of postural adjustments in infants who were not yet sitting independently (they used parents to train the infants at home [5 minutes, three times a day for 3 months]). The training consisted of toy presentation to the side or semibackward at the infant's limits of stability. When comparing EMG responses to platform perturbations pretraining versus post-training, they found that the trained infants (as compared with nontrained infants) showed a higher probability of complete responses to perturbations and increased response modulation at higher perturbation velocities, along with decreased pelvic displacement. There were no changes in muscle-response onsets.

These results provide a rationale for similar types of postural training programs in children with motor delays. As discussed in more detail in Chapter 11, training seated postural control in children with cerebral palsy was effective in decreasing postural sway in sitting (Curtis et al., 2018).

Transition to Independent Stance

Motor Coordination

Development of Steady-State Balance. The postural demands of steady-state sitting and stance balance are very different. During the process of learning to stand independently, infants must learn to (a) balance within significantly reduced stability limits compared to those used during sitting; (b) control many additional degrees of freedom, as they add the coordination of the leg and thigh segments to those of the trunk and head; and (c) recalibrate sensorimotor representations for postural control to include the thigh, shank, and foot for balance to create an improved internal model for postural control of independent stance. Research suggests that an important part of transitions in development of new behaviors is the recalibration of the sensorimotor systems.

Chen et al. (2007) examined whether infants' sitting postural control changed during the transition to independent walking. They longitudinally assessed infants' postural sway monthly from the onset of sitting through the 9th month of independent walking while they sat on a saddle-shaped chair positioned on a force plate, as shown in Figure 8.12. It was hypothesized that the transition to bipedal locomotion would be associated with decreases in the stability of sitting posture, suggesting a recalibration or tuning of a generalized internal representation for the sensorimotor control of sway. When sitting data across the 11 months were compared, sway amplitude, variability, area, and velocity of COP trajectory showed a peak just before or at the onset of walking, as shown in Figure 8.13, and at this point, peak sway was greater than at any other stage. The authors concluded that this transient disruption in sitting posture results from a process involving recalibration of the infants' internal model for the sensorimotor control of posture as they practice the newly emerging bipedal behavior of independent walking.

Research suggests that the process of recalibration in the sensorimotor system does not seem to affect relatively simple, well-mastered skills. Boxum et al. (2019) tested infants' muscle activity during reaching in two conditions: while sitting in an infant chair providing trunk support and during unsupported "long-leg" sitting on the floor. They found no changes in muscle activity across time—not before, during, or after the development of independent walking—and postural activity was similar between the two sitting positions. Thus, the transient disruption in sitting posture during the emergence of independent walking is dependent on the testing situation or the challenge to balance during testing.

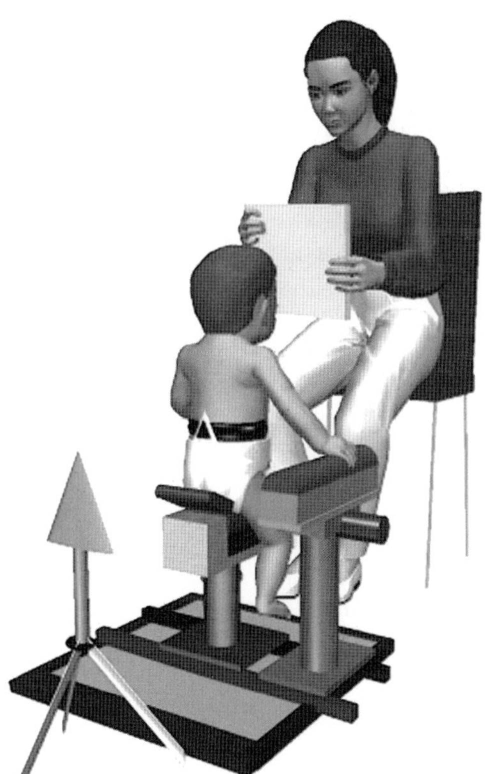

Figure 8.12 The infant sits independently on a saddle-shaped chair attached to the force platform in either the no-touch condition or in the touch condition (pictured), in which they place the hand on the touchpad. The experimenter sits in front of the infant to keep attention on the task. (Reprinted with permission from Chen LC, Metcalfe JS, Jeka JJ, et al. Two steps forward and one back: learning to walk affects infants' sitting posture. *Infant Behav Dev*. 2007;30:19.)

Why do infants just learning to stand and walk appear to sway so much? Is it a lack of control? Newell and others have proposed that infants first learning to stand and walk combine two mechanisms or strategies to control postural sway: The first is exploratory and the second is performatory (Newell, 1991; Reed, 1982; Riley et al., 1997). Exploratory postural sway is used to investigate and explore the sensorimotor workspace for posture control; increased exploratory sway creates sensory information essential to refining sensorimotor relationships underlying postural control. Performatory postural sway, on the other hand, uses sensory information to control posture. Thus, it is possible that exploratory sway behavior of infants learning to stand and walk may mask improvements in the ability to control sway.

Role of Strength. Several researchers have suggested that a primary rate-limiting factor for the emergence of independent stance and gait is the development of sufficient muscle strength to support the body during standing and walking (Thelen & Fisher, 1982). Can leg muscle strength be tested in the infant to determine whether this is the case?

Researchers have shown that by 6 months of age, infants are capable of producing forces well beyond their own body weight (Roncesvalles & Jensen, 1993). These experiments suggest that the ability to support weight against the force of gravity in the standing position occurs well before the emergence of independent stance, so it is probably not the major constraint to emerging stance postural control in infants.

Reactive Balance: Development of Muscle Synergies. How do postural response synergies compensating for threats to balance begin to emerge in the newly standing infant? Longitudinal studies have explored the emergence of postural response synergies in infants from ages 2 to 18 months, during the transition to independent stance (Sveistrup & Woollacott, 1996; Woollacott & Sveistrup, 1992). Infants stood with varying degrees of support, on the moving platform while EMGs were used to record muscle activity in the leg and trunk in response to loss of balance.

Figure 8.14 shows EMG responses from one child during the emergence of coordinated muscle activity in the leg and trunk muscles in response to a fall backward. Infants tested at 2 to 6 months of age did not show coordinated muscle responses (Fig. 8.14A). As pull-to-stand behavior progressed (7 to 9 months), the infants began to

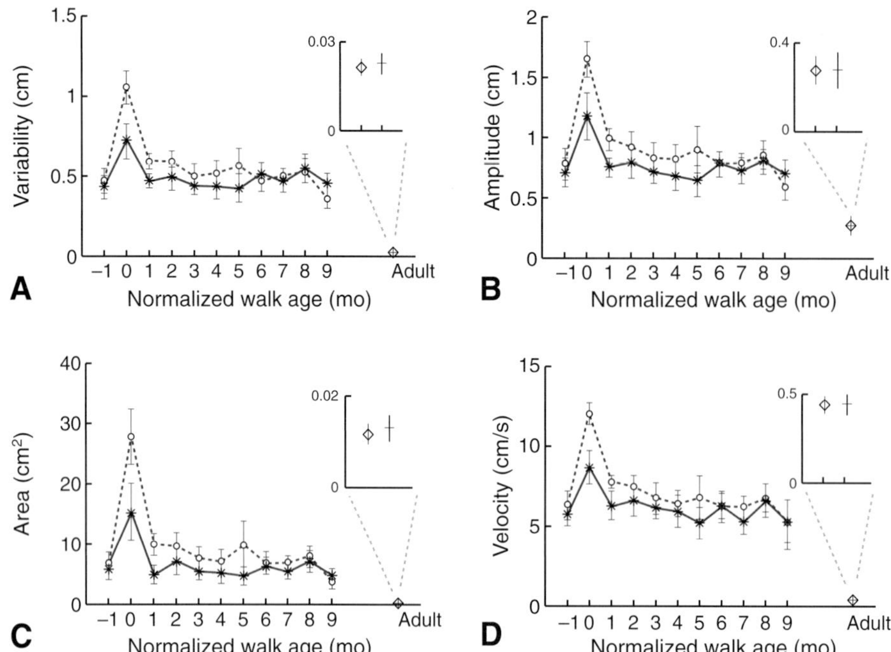

Figure 8.13 Force platform data from the experimental paradigm shown in Figure 8.12. Resultant COP sway was derived from mediolateral and anteroposterior COP. Resultant COP sway: **(A)** variability (cm), **(B)** amplitude (cm), **(C)** area of 90% ellipse (cm2), and **(D)** velocity (cm/sec) across normalized walk ages and touch conditions. Infants' postural sway was presented as means ±SE. Note that the peak in all COP variables in the seated position occurs at the age of walking onset. Adults' averaged postural sway was presented for comparison (•) infant no-touch; (*) infant touch; (♦) adult no-touch; (+) adult touch. Note the difference in scale between infants and adults. (Reprinted with permission from Chen LC, Metcalfe JS, Jeka JJ, et al. Two steps forward and one back: learning to walk affects infants' sitting posture. *Infant Behav Dev.* 2007;30:22.)

show directionally appropriate responses in their ankle muscles (Fig. 8.14B). As pull-to-stand skills improved, muscles in the thigh segment were added, and a consistent distal-to-proximal sequence began to emerge during late pull-to-stand and independent stance and walking (9 to 11 months) (Fig. 8.14C–E); at this point, trunk muscles were consistently activated, resulting in a complete synergy. Figure 8.15 shows that there is a gradual reduction in one-muscle responses (shown in deep orange) during this transition; at the same time, there is a gradual increase in the two- and three-muscle response patterns (shown in light orange and beige).

Sensory Contributions

Once an infant learns how to organize synergistic muscles for controlling stance in association with one sense, will this automatically transfer to other senses reporting sway? This may not always be the case. It appears that vision maps to muscles controlling stance posture by at least 5 to 6 months, prior to somatosensory system mapping, and long before the infant has much experience in the standing position (Foster et al., 1996). This suggests that the infant has to reassemble the synergies when somatosensory inputs are mapped for stance postural control.

EMG responses and sway patterns in response to visual flow created by a moving room were examined in infants and children of varying ages and abilities and compared with those of young adults (Foster et al., 1996). Figure 8.16 shows an example of an infant positioned in a moving room. The child's sway was recorded through one-way glass with a video camera mounted outside the room, and muscle responses were recorded from the legs and hips. Infants who were unable to stand independently were supported about the hip by their parents.

Children as young as 5 months of age swayed in response to room movements; sway amplitudes increased in the pull-to-stand stage, peaked in the independent walkers, and dropped to low levels of sway in experienced walkers (Foster et al., 1996). Sway responses were associated with clear patterns of muscle responses that pulled the child in the direction of the visual stimulus.

These experiments demonstrate that the visual system elicits organized postural responses in standing infants at an earlier age than does the somatosensory system.

Modifiability of Postural Responses

Development of Adaptation. To determine when adaptive processes are available to infants, researchers examined the attenuation of postural responses to visual flow (the moving room) (Foster et al., 1996). Infants at all stages of development (pull-to-stand, stance, and

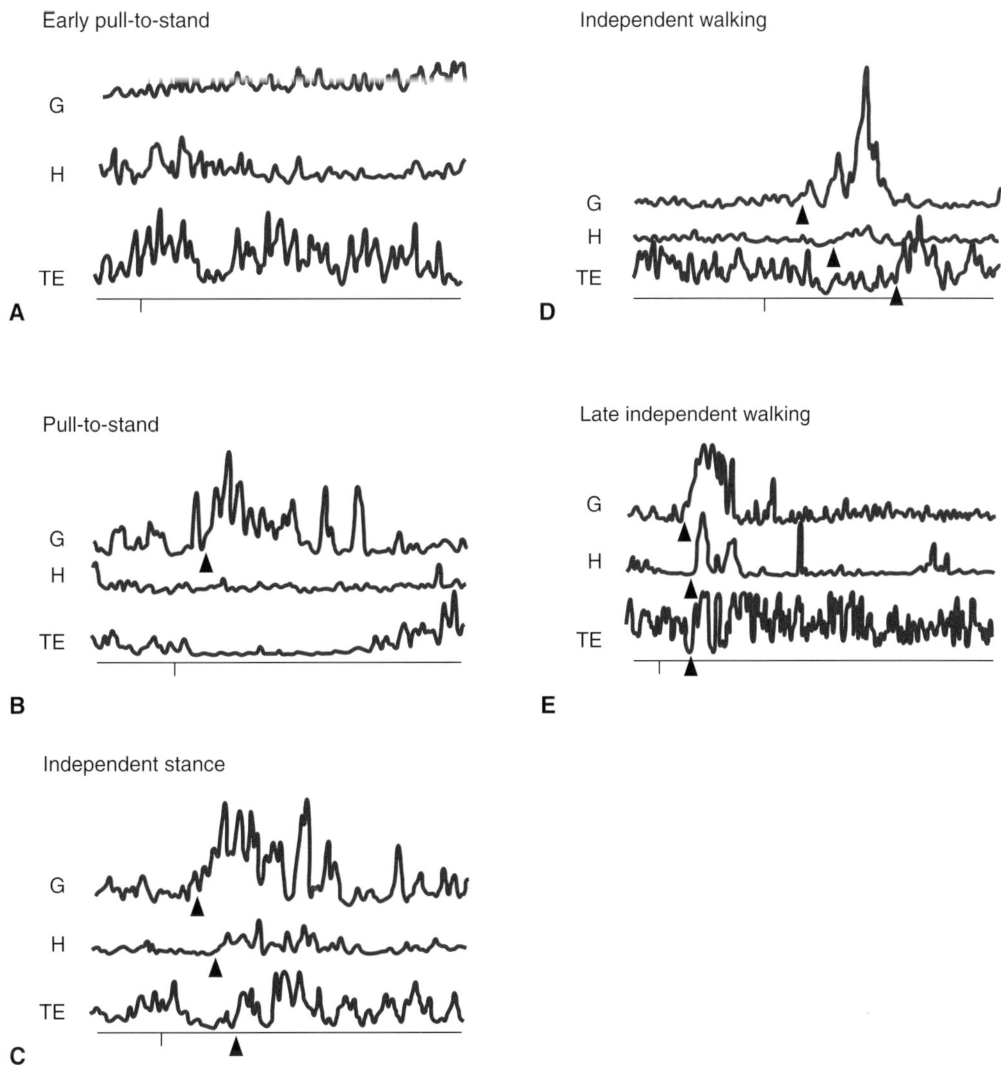

Figure 8.14 Responses from one child during the emergence of coordinated muscle activity in the leg and trunk muscles in response to platform perturbations in the following: **(A)** early pull-to-stand, **(B)** pull-to-stand, **(C)** independent stance, and **(D and E)** independent walking and late independent walking. Note that there was no response in early pull-to-stand and responses gradually developed at subsequent behavioral levels. *G*, gastrocnemius; *H*, hamstrings; *TE*, trunk extensors. The vertical line under the TE muscle indicates the onset of platform movement. Arrows indicate the onset of muscle responses. Each trace corresponds to a 1-second recording. (Adapted with permission from Sveistrup H, Woollacott MH. Longitudinal development of the automatic postural response in infants. *J Motor Behav.* 1996;28:63.)

walking) had inappropriately large muscle responses to the first visual perturbation (causing loss of balance) and were unable to adapt the magnitude of these postural responses over the next five trials. The researchers concluded that higher-level adaptive processes related to postural control have not yet matured by the time of emergence of independent walking.

When does the ability to adapt responses to changes in support-surface characteristics emerge? A study examined the ability of 13- to 14-month-old infants to adapt to altered support-surface conditions, including high-friction (high-friction plastic), low-friction (Formica coated with baby oil), and foam surfaces, as well as standing crosswise on a narrow beam (Stoffregen et al., 1997). The infants had two poles available to hold to help with balance. The greatest amount of time spent in free standing was on the high-friction surface, with minimal hand support used. As the surfaces became more compliant (foam) or lower friction (baby oil), pole holding increased substantially, with a concomitant drop in free standing. Finally, it was impossible for the infants to stand crosswise on the beam while standing independently. Since standing crosswise on a beam requires active control of the hips, rather than purely control of ankle movements, this suggests that this adaptive ability to use the hips in balance is not mastered in infants during the emergence of walking.

Previous research on adults has shown that increasing the size of a balance threat will often elicit a hip strategy (activated by abdominal muscle activity), rather than an ankle strategy, as the center of mass (COM) nears the edges of the base of support. In order to determine

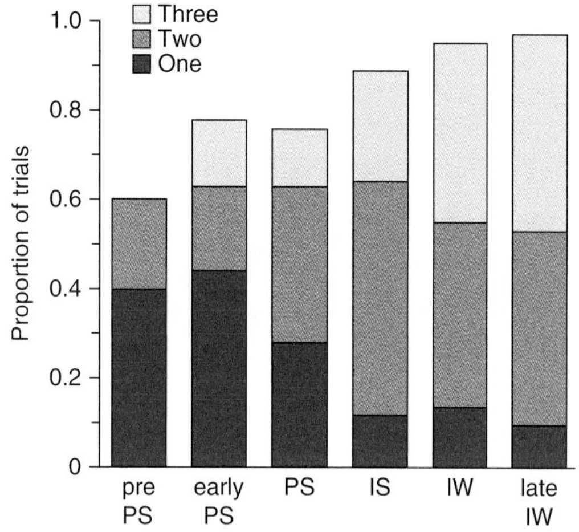

Figure 8.15 Proportion of trials with responses recorded in one, two, or three muscles following the platform perturbation, in each of the stages of stance development. *PS*, pull-to-stand; *IS*, independent stance; *IW*, independent walking. (Adapted with permission from Sveistrup H, Woollacott MH. Longitudinal development of the automatic postural response in infants. *J Motor Behav.* 1996;28:67.)

when the ability to control the hips during balance recovery emerges, researchers (Roncesvalles et al., 2003; Woollacott et al., 1998) gave children from new walkers (10 to 17 months) through hoppers (2 to 3 years), gallopers (4 to 6 years), and skippers (7 to 10 years) increasing magnitudes of balance threats in order to elicit a hip strategy, if it was available in these children. They found that hip-dominated responses were present in the walkers with only 3 to 6 months of walking experience. However, these responses were passively activated, with minimal abdominal activity used. It was not until the children reached 7 to 10 years of age (skippers) that they began to show consistent active control of the strategy with high levels of abdominal muscle activity.

Effect of Practice. To determine whether experience is important in the development of postural response characteristics in infants learning to stand, postural responses were compared in two groups of infants in the pull-to-stand stage of balance development (Sveistrup & Woollacott, 1997). One group of infants was given extensive experience with platform perturbations, receiving 300 perturbations over 3 days. The second (control) group of infants did not receive this training.

Infants who had extensive experience on the platform were more likely to activate postural muscle responses, and these responses were better organized. Figure 8.17 shows the probability of seeing a response in tibialis anterior, quadriceps, and abdominal muscles in response to platform movements causing backward sway, both before and after training. Note that the probability of seeing a response in all three muscles was significantly increased. However, onset of activation of postural responses did not change.

These results suggest that experience may influence the strength of the connections between the sensory and motor pathways controlling balance, thus increasing the probability of producing postural responses. However, the lack of a training effect on muscle response onset suggests that neural maturation may be a rate-limiting factor in reducing muscle onsets with development. It is probable that the myelination of nervous system pathways responsible for reducing onset of postural responses during development is not affected by training.

Refinement of Postural Control

Up until now, we have examined changes within the postural control system in the first 12 months of life that contribute to the emergence of sitting and stance. Researchers have found that postural control is essentially mature by 10 to 12 years of age. What are the key changes that contribute to this refinement of postural control? It appears that the emergence of adult levels of control occurs at different times for different aspects of postural control.

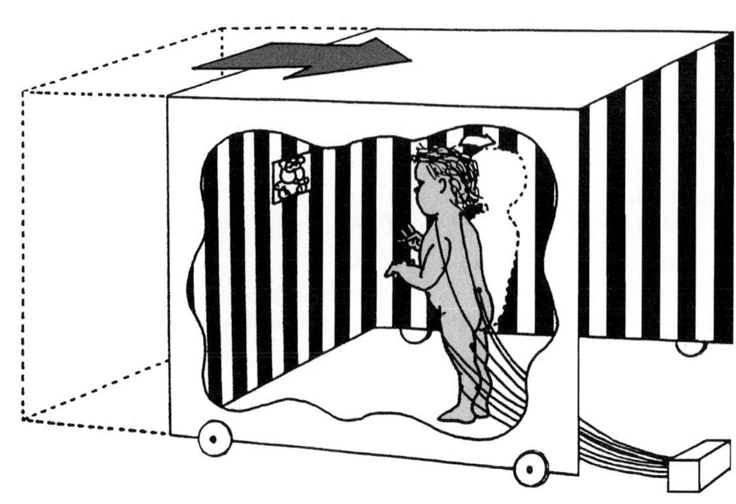

Figure 8.16 Diagram showing the moving room paradigm used to examine the development of visual contributions to postural control. When the room moves toward the child, they perceive forward sway and respond by swaying backward. (Reprinted with permission from Sveistrup H, Woollacott MH. Systems contributing to the emergence and maturation of stability in postnatal development. In: Savelsbergh GJP, ed. *The development of coordination in infancy*. Amsterdam, Netherlands: Elsevier, 1993:324.)

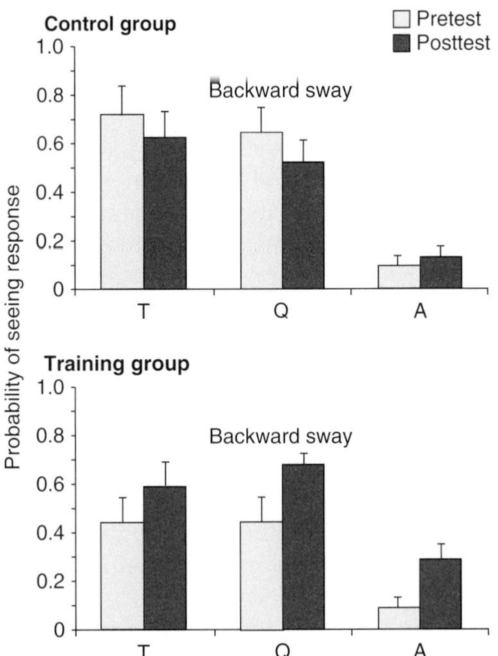

Figure 8.17 Probability of seeing a response in tibialis anterior (*T*), quadriceps (*Q*), and abdominal (*A*) muscles in response to platform movements causing backward sway, both before and after 3 days of balance training. Note that the probability of seeing a response in all three muscles was significantly increased. (Adapted with permission from Sveistrup H, Woollacott M. Can practice modify the developing automatic postural response? *Exp Brain Res.* 1997;114:41.)

Musculoskeletal System: Changes in Body Morphology

Are children inherently more stable than adults? Children are shorter and therefore closer to the ground. Does their height make balancing an easier task? Anyone who has watched a fearless young child ski down a steep slope with relative ease, falling and bouncing back up, might assume that their task is easier. They don't have as far to fall! It turns out that while children are shorter than adults, they are proportioned differently. Children are top-heavy. The relative size of the head, in comparison to the lower extremities, places the COM at about T12 in the child, as compared with L5 to S1 in the adult. Because of their shorter height, and the difference in the location of their COM, children sway at a faster rate than adults. Thus, the task of balance is slightly more difficult, since the body is moving at a faster rate during imbalance. However, after 7 years of age, there is no correlation between structural growth of the human body (body height, body mass, and age) and sway during normal quiet stance (Lebiedowska & Syczewska, 2000; Zeller, 1964).

Motor Coordination

Refinement of Steady-State Stance. How is the control of spontaneous sway during steady-state stance refined as children develop beyond early independent stance? A number of studies have examined refinement in spontaneous sway with development (e.g., from 2 to 14 years of age) and have shown that both the amplitude and the frequency of postural sway decreased during this period (Hayes & Riach, 1989; Kirshenbaum et al., 2001; Taguchi & Tada, 1988). Young children used a high-velocity balance strategy, making large, fast corrections of the COP as they attempted to maintain their COM within their base of support, while at around 8 to 9 years of age, they show shorter excursions and more accurate control (Riach & Starkes, 1994).

Research also shows considerable variability in sway amplitude in the young children. This variance became systematically lower with age and with the children's improved balance. Effects of eye closure were represented by the Romberg quotient (eyes-closed sway expressed as a percentage of eyes-open sway), giving an indication of the contributions of vision to balance during quiet stance. Very low Romberg quotients were recorded for the youngest children who completed the task (4-year-olds), with values of less than 100%. This indicates that these children were swaying more with eyes open than with eyes closed (Hayes & Riach, 1989). Spontaneous sway in children reached adult levels by 9 to 12 years of age for eyes-open conditions and at 12 to 15 years of age for eyes-closed conditions. Sway velocity also decreased with age, reaching adult levels at 12 to 15 years of age (Taguchi & Tada, 1988).

Research using nonlinear analysis techniques (correlation dimension and complexity, described earlier) to examine changes in balance control during quiet stance has shown that 3-year-old children show a decreased COP dimensionality and complexity, indicating that they are using restricted degrees of freedom in balance during quiet stance. Five-year-olds showed significantly increased dimensionality and complexity of their COP path, similar to that of adults, indicating that they have more control and adaptability in their balance abilities during quiet stance (Newell, 1997).

Refinement of Reactive Postural Control. Refinement of compensatory balance adjustments in children 15 months to 10 years of age has been studied by several researchers using a movable platform to examine changes in postural control (Berger et al., 1985; Forssberg & Nashner, 1982; Hass et al., 1986; Shumway-Cook & Woollacott, 1985a). Research has shown that compensatory postural responses of young children (15 months of age) are more variable and slower than those of adults (Forssberg & Nashner, 1982). These slower muscle responses and the more rapid rates of sway acceleration observed in young children cause sway amplitudes (in response to balance threats) that are bigger and often more oscillatory than those of older children and adults.

Even children of 1.5 to 3 years of age generally produce well-organized muscle responses to postural perturbations while standing (Shumway-Cook & Woollacott, 1985a; Forssberg & Nashner, 1982). However, the amplitudes of these responses are larger, and the onsets and durations of these responses are longer than those of adults. Other studies have also found a longer duration of postural responses in young children and have also noted the activation of monosynaptic stretch reflexes in young children in response to platform perturbations. These responses disappear as the children mature (Berger et al., 1985; Hass et al., 1986).

Surprisingly, postural responses in children 4 to 6 years of age are, in general, slower and more variable than those found in children 15 months to 3 years old, those 7 to 10 years old, or adults, suggesting an apparent regression in the postural response organization. Figure 8.18 compares EMG responses in the four age groups.

In these studies, by 7 to 10 years of age, postural responses were basically like those in adults. There were no significant differences in onset of activation, variability, or temporal coordination between muscles within the leg synergy between this age group and adults (Shumway-Cook & Woollacott, 1985a).

Why are postural actions so much more variable in 4- to 6-year-old children? It may be significant that the variability in response parameters of 4- to 6-year-old children occurs during a period of disproportionate growth with respect to critical changes in body form. It has been suggested that discontinuous changes seen in the development of many skills, including postural control may be the result of critical dimension changes in the body of the growing child (Kugler et al., 1982). The system would remain stable until dimensional changes reached a point at which previous motor programs were no longer highly effective. At that point, the system would undergo a period of transition marked by instability and variability and then a new plateau of stability.

Research analyzing the movements of different segments of the body, in response to platform perturbations in both children and adults (Woollacott et al., 1988), has shown that the kinematics of passive body movements caused by platform translations are very similar in the 4- to 6-year-olds, 7- to 9-year-olds, and adults. Thus, it is more probable that changes in response onsets and variability seen in 4- to 6-year-olds represent developmental changes in the nervous system itself.

In addition to looking at the development of reactive balance control from a neurophysiological perspective, one can look at it from a biomechanical perspective, examining the development of forces used to recover from balance threats. Studies have used kinetics to examine the refinement in the development of force capabilities in children from 9 months to 10 years of age, as they recover from balance threats (Roncesvalles et al., 2001). In examining COP trajectories used to recover from balance threats, it was noted that children just learning to stand and walk were the slowest to recover stability (about 2 seconds) with COP trajectories more than twice as large as those of the older children (7- to 10-year-olds, 1.1 seconds). Why was this the case? Examination of the torque profiles

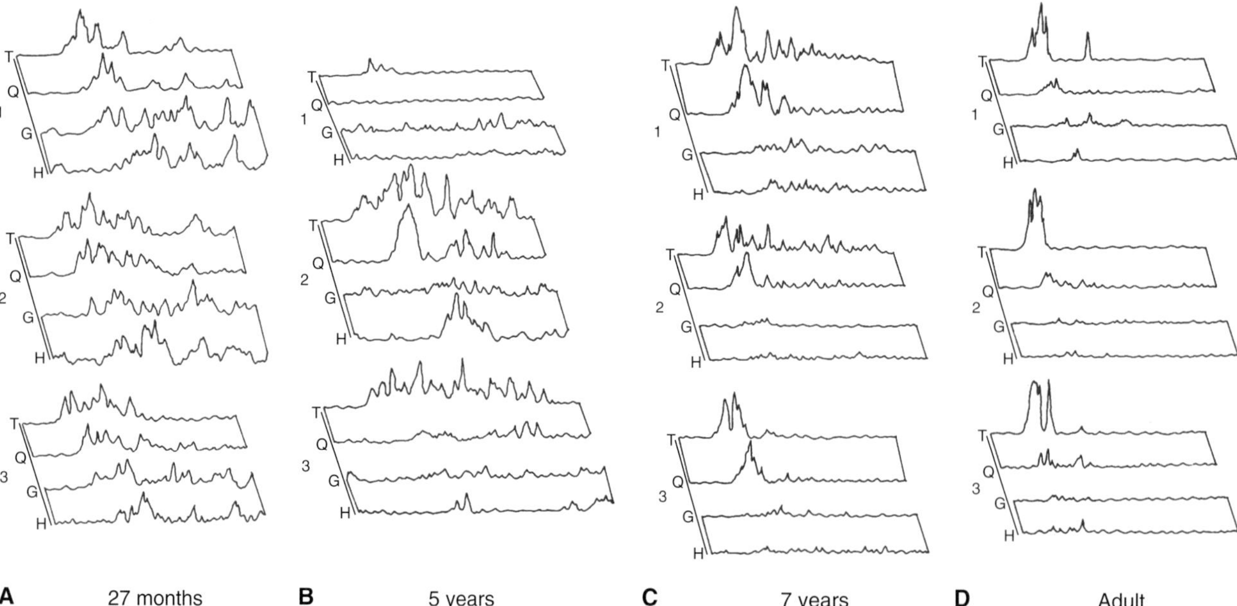

Figure 8.18 A comparison of muscle activation patterns in leg and trunk muscles in response to forward platform perturbations causing backward sway in children from four age groups: **(A)** 27 months, **(B)** 5 years, **(C)** 7 years, and **(D)** adult. Three successive responses to platform perturbations are shown for each child. Platform perturbation started at the onset of the EMG recording. Recording is 600 ms. *T*, tibialis anterior; *Q*, quadriceps; *G*, gastrocnemius; *H*, hamstrings. (Reprinted with permission from Shumway-Cook A, Woollacott M. The growth of stability: postural control from a developmental perspective. *J Mot Behav*. 1985;17:136.)

at the ankle, knee, and hip showed that in contrast to older children and adults, who rapidly generated large torques, the younger children (standers and walkers, 9 to 23 months of age) used multiple torque adjustments before regaining control. Figure 8.19 shows torque profiles of children from 9 to 13 months (new standers), 14 to 23 months (advanced walkers), 2 to 3 years (runners/jumpers), 4 to 6 years (gallopers), and 7 to 10 years (skippers). Note that there are at least three bursts of torque production at the ankle, knee, and hip in the stander and walker, while this is reduced to two bursts and then one burst in the older age groups. The youngest age groups tended to overshoot and undershoot torque requirements, with many torque reversals.

These data support the previous work found on refinement of balance strategies using neurophysiological and kinematic measures (Forssberg & Nashner, 1982; Shumway-Cook & Woollacott, 1985a) that showed that children 1 to 3 years of age exhibited large and oscillatory sway excursions, while response patterns were gradually refined and became similar to those of adults by 7 to 10 years of age.

Is the refinement of reactive postural control direction specific? By 7 years of age, children show

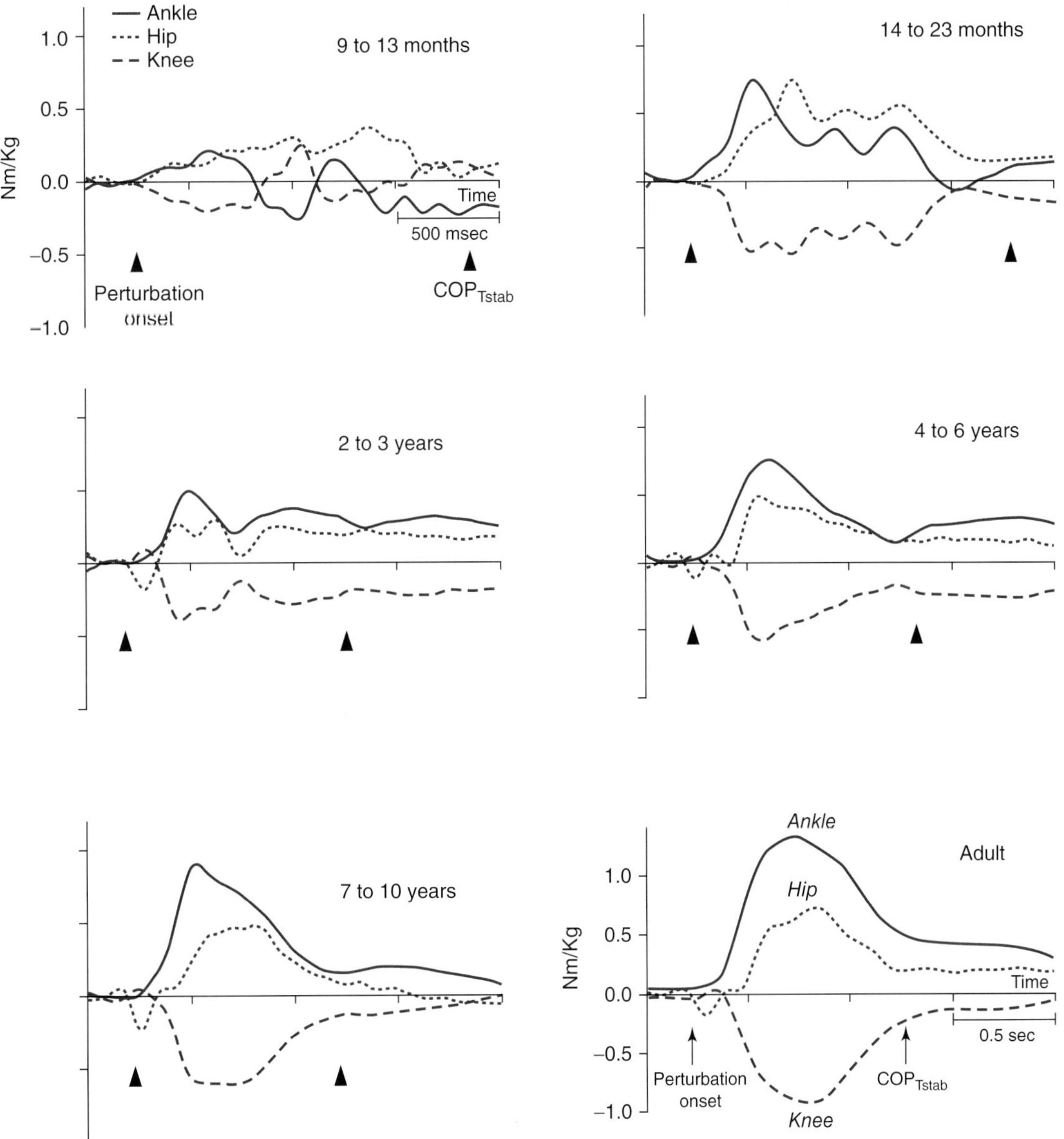

Figure 8.19 Torque profiles of children from 9 to 13 months (new standers), 14 to 23 months (advanced walkers), 2 to 3 years (runners/jumpers), 4 to 6 years (gallopers), and 7 to 10 years (skippers) in response to backward platform movements causing forward sway. Note that there are at least three bursts of torque production at the ankle, knee, and hip in the stander and walker, while this is reduced to two bursts and then one burst in the older age groups. The onset of perturbation and recovery of balance are marked by arrowheads. The ankle and hip torques are extensor (positive) and responsible for returning the COM to its resting range. Knee torque was flexor, counterbalancing the extensor torques generated at ankle and hip. Muscle torques were normalized to body mass, and all graphs were plotted on the same scale. The time scale is 500 ms. Nm/kg, Newton meters/kilogram; COP$_{Tstab}$ time to stabilization of COP.

consistent activity of the ankle and hip strategy; however, recent research has shown that performance to anterior–posterior and mediolateral balance threats do not mature at the same rate. Walchli et al. (2018) found that 6- to 7-year-olds have more sway in response to balance threats in the anterior-posterior plane than 11- to 13-year-old children; in contrast, the authors found no age differences in the ability to counteract perturbations in the medio-lateral plane. In response to this finding, the authors propose that the control of responses to balance threats in the medio-lateral direction is either matured by the age of 6 years or that the main adaptation in this direction occurs after the age of 13 years.

Refinement of Anticipatory Postural Control. Skilled movements, such as reaching, have both postural and voluntary components; the postural component establishes a stabilizing framework that supports the second component and that of the primary movement (Gahery & Massion, 1981). Without this supporting postural framework, skilled action deteriorates, as seen in patients with a variety of motor problems. As discussed in earlier sections, the development of anticipatory postural control in sitting infants underlies the emergence of efficient reaching.

In standing, children as young as 10 months old are able to activate postural muscles in advance of arm movements (Forssberg & Nashner, 1982; Witherington et al., 2002). In a cross-sectional study examining the development of preparatory postural control during standing in infants from 10 to 17 months of age, standing infants were asked to open a cabinet drawer to retrieve a toy while a force resisting the pull was applied to the drawer. Results showed that both timing and the proportion of trials involving anticipatory postural activity in the gastrocnemius before the biceps was activated (to pull the drawer open) progressively improved from 10 to 17 months. At 10 to 11 months (infants were just beginning to stand independently), anticipatory activity was present, but highly inconsistent. By 13 months, as they gained experience walking, infants began to show consistent anticipatory postural activity. After the onset of independent walking, over half of the infants' pulls involved anticipatory adjustment in the gastrocnemius muscle within 240 ms of pull onset. However, the ability of the infants to deal with different external resistances during the drawer pull (adaptational abilities) did not occur until about 15 months of age (Witherington et al., 2002).

By 4 to 6 years of age, anticipatory postural adjustments preceding arm movements while standing are essentially mature (Nashner et al., 1983; Woollacott & Shumway-Cook, 1986).

Refinement of Sensory Organization

Postural control is characterized by the ability to adapt how we use sensory information about the position and movement of the body in space to changing task and environmental conditions. How does the CNS learn to interpret information from vision, vestibular, and somatosensory receptors and relate it to postural actions? One theory is that children and adults learn to reweight sensory inputs under changing sensory conditions in order to primarily rely on inputs that are giving accurate information within the environmental context. For example, if visual information from the environment gives the illusion of sway when the individual is actually remaining steady, then the CNS would reduce the reliance on vision and rely primarily on somatosensory and vestibular inputs.

We have already described evidence from moving room experiments suggesting that the visual system plays a predominant role in the development of postural actions. That is, visual inputs reporting the body's position in space appear to be mapped to muscular actions earlier than inputs from other sensory systems. In young children, the invariant use of visual inputs for postural control can sometimes mask the capability of other senses to activate postural actions. Results from the experiments in which children balanced without visual inputs suggest that in certain age groups, postural actions activated by other sensory inputs can be better organized than those associated with vision.

Moving platform posturography in conjunction with a moving visual surround has also been used to examine the development of intersensory integration and the ability to reweight sensory inputs for postural control. The platform protocols used to study the organization and selection of senses for postural control were described in detail in Chapter 7.

The development of sensory adaptation in children ages 2 to 14 years of age has been studied by a number of investigators using this protocol (Ferber-Viart et al., 2007; Forssberg & Nashner, 1982; Foudriat et al., 1993; Shumway-Cook & Woollacott, 1985a). The results of the combined studies suggest that 1.5- to 3-year-olds sway more than older children and adults, even when all three sensory inputs are present (condition 1). Performance continues to improve slightly across all age groups through 14 years of age. With eyes closed (condition 2), children's stability did not significantly decrease further, in the youngest age groups (Forssberg & Nashner, 1982); however, studies testing children 4 years and older have shown slight decreases in stability in most age groups either with eyes closed or the visual surround stabilized (conditions 2 and 3). Stability in these conditions improves through 14 years of age, as shown in Figure 8.20.

Reducing the accuracy of somatosensory information for postural control by rotating the platform surface in correlation with the infant's sway, reducing reliable ankle–joint inputs (condition 4), further reduced the stability of all age groups substantially.

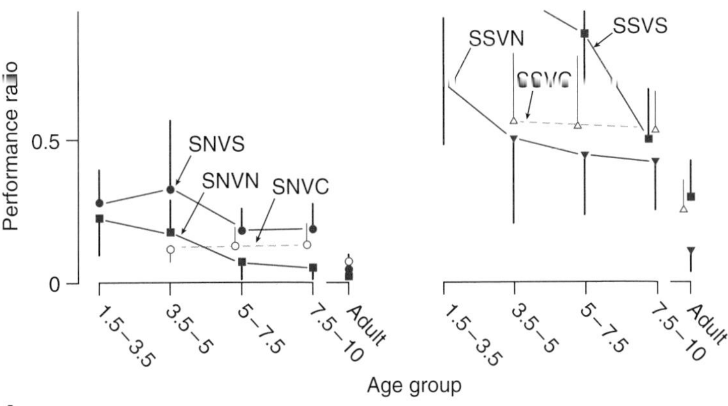

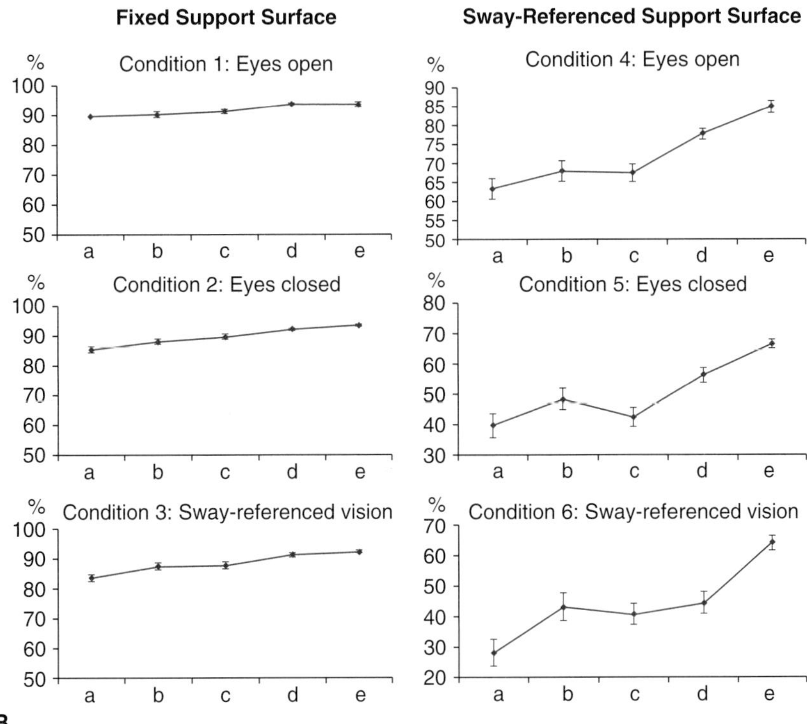

Figure 8.20 **(A)** Average (±SD) performance ratios of different age groups of children standing under the six different conditions of the Sensory Orientation Test (*SOT*): on the left side with fixed support surface and eyes open (*SNVN*), eyes closed (*SNVC*), and the visual surface stabilized (SNVS); on the right side with support surface stabilized and eyes open (*SSVN*), eyes closed (*SSVC*), and the visual surface also stabilized (*SSVS*) (on the *x*-axis, 1 is equal to a fall and 0 is equal to perfect stability with no sway). (Data from Forssberg H, Nashner L. Ontogenetic development of postural control in man: adaptation to altered support and visual conditions during stance. *J Neurosci*. 1982;2:549.) **(B)** SOT Equilibrium scores for each group (a, 6–8; b, 8–10; c, 10–12; d, 12–14; and e, 20-year-olds) in both normal (fixed support) surface (left) and sway-referenced support surface (right) platform trials (on the *x*-axis, 100% is equal to perfect stability and 0 is equal to a fall). (Part **A** data from Forssberg H, Nashner L. Ontogenetic development of postural control in man: adaptation to altered support and visual conditions during stance. *J Neurosci*. 1982;2:549. Part **B** reprinted with permission from Ferber-Viart C, Ionescu E, Morlet T, et al. Balance in healthy individuals assessed with Equitest: maturation and normative data for children and young adults. *Int J Pediatr Otorhinolaryngol*. 2007;71:1043–1044.)

Finally, when children closed their eyes (condition 5) or balanced in the support surface and visual surround sway-referenced conditions (condition 6), stability continued to decrease, especially in the youngest age groups (Fig. 8.20).

These results suggest that children under 7 to 8 years of age are unable to balance efficiently when both somatosensory and visual cues are inaccurate or removed, leaving only vestibular cues to control stability. In addition, children younger than 7 to 8 years of age show a reduced ability to adapt senses for postural control appropriately when one (or more) of these senses is inaccurately reporting body orientation information.

Another way of examining the development of the ability to adapt to changing sensory inputs is to put children into a context in which they perceive simultaneous small-amplitude somatosensory movement (of a movable bar they touch with a finger) and visual environmental movement (of a visual scene in front of them), as shown in Figure 8.21. In the experimental protocol, the amplitude of these movements is varied independently across different conditions. The experimenters then measure body sway amplitude relative to each stimulus amplitude in order to determine touch gain and vision gain. The gain of sensory systems is defined as the amount that the system amplifies a signal between its input and output; thus, it indicates the manner in which children reweight these sensory inputs as they attempt to balance under the different conditions (Bair et al., 2007).

Bair et al. (2007) asked children 4 to 10 years of age to perform this task. They observed that children could reweight responses to multisensory inputs as early as 4 years of age. They define *intramodal reweighting* as, for example, the dependence of visual system gain on visual movement amplitude, and they define *intermodal reweighting* as the dependence of visual system gain on

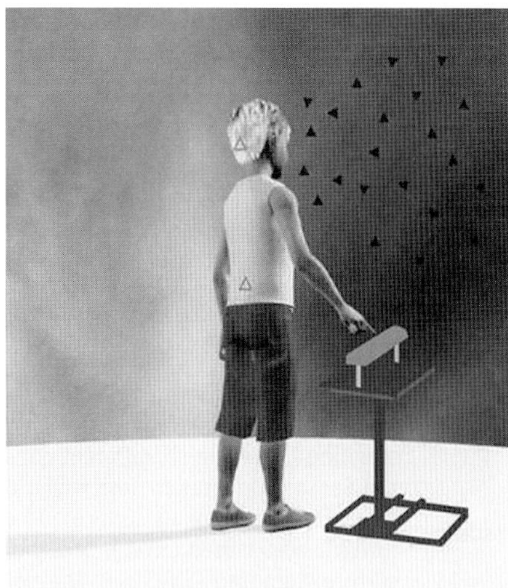

Figure 8.21 Experimental setup in which a child is performing the multisensory posture task (room illumination not dimmed for illustrative purposes; fewer dots are plotted for a clear view of child's posture). (Reprinted with permission from Bair WN, Kiemel T, Jeka JJ, et al. Development of multisensory reweighting for posture control in children. *Exp Brain Res.* 2007;183:437.)

touch bar movement amplitude. They found that intramodal reweighting was present in 4-year-old children; however, intermodal reweighting was observed only in the older children (10 years). With older age, children showed an increase in the amount of reweighting, suggesting better adaptation to changing sensory conditions. Thus, these results add elegantly to the previous results of others using the Sensory Organization Test, to show that the development of multisensory reweighting is present at 4 years of age and contributes to more stable and flexible control of upright stance.

Cognitive Systems in Postural Development

As we mentioned in Chapter 7, postural control requires attentional resources, and additional resources are required with increasing postural task complexity. Since many activities that children perform have both a postural and a cognitive component, it is possible that performance on the postural task, the cognitive task, or both will deteriorate if the attentional capacity of the child is exceeded while performing the two tasks. For example, in the academic setting, when children are performing a postural task (standing, walking, or reaching for an object) while also performing a cognitive task, the attentional requirements of the motor task may compete for processing resources within the limited attentional capacity of the child.

In order to determine whether there are changing attentional demands of postural control during development, researchers asked children of two different age levels (4 to 6 years and 7 to 13 years) and adults to perform postural tasks both alone and in combination with a cognitive task (a visual memory task, in which they had to hold in memory a set of colored squares and then determine whether a new set of squares was the same as the set they had seen 5 seconds earlier). They then examined the extent to which performance on either the postural or cognitive task decreased during simultaneous dual-task performance. Although the cognitive task was calibrated so that all groups showed the same accuracy on the task when they performed it alone (the different groups had to remember different numbers of squares), the adults and older children were 2.5 and 1.7 times more likely to have greater accuracy on the cognitive task than the younger children when performing a demanding postural task (the modified Romberg task) at the same time. In addition, the younger children showed greater increases in postural instability (greater COP velocity) than the older children and adults when they were asked to balance in the tandem Romberg task simultaneously with the cognitive task (Reilly et al., 2008a). This suggests that the postural demands of younger children tax their attentional resources more than for older children, and this may affect both their postural and cognitive performance in dual-task situations.

Olivier et al. (2007) have also shown decreased abilities of children (7 years of age) to perform cognitive tasks (modified Stroop task) while simultaneously performing postural tasks of varying levels of complexity (quiet stance vs. standing with an ankle vibrator attached to the Achilles tendon to activate muscle spindle reflexes and thus cause a perturbation to postural sway). They found that in the ankle vibration perturbation condition, the sway was significantly higher for the children while performing the cognitive task. In adults, there was no effect of cognitive task on mean velocity of COP. Interestingly, as the cognitive task difficulty increased, sway decreased slightly in the 7-year-old group and the adults. The authors interpret this to mean that the children adopted a different postural strategy, which gave more stability, under more complex cognitive task conditions.

At first, this type of behavior may seem counterintuitive, as the children are showing more stability under more complex cognitive task conditions. However, this type of behavior has also been seen in some other experiments under certain dual-task conditions. This increased performance has been hypothesized to be due to a number of possible factors, including the possibility of increased arousal, anchoring vision more consistently to the visual task, or shifting attention from the task of postural control to another task, thus allowing the task to be more automatic. These authors showed in a second study that children from 4 to 11 years of age were more stable when looking at a video (without instruction about posture) as compared with looking at a cross at the center of the TV screen with the instruction to remain as stable as possible. Similarly,

7-month-old sitting infants sway less when visually attending to a toy someone else is holding compared to when infants hold the toy (Arnold et al., 2020). All this research lends support to the automaticity hypothesis as one important contributor to improved postural sway under certain dual-task conditions.

This research has described some of the critical refinements in the components of the postural control system that occur between 10 months and 13 years of age. Changes in the motor components involve changes in body morphology as well as refinement of the muscular response synergies, including (a) a decrease in onset latencies, (b) improvement in the timing and amplitude of muscle responses, and (c) a decrease in the variability of muscle responses. Refinements in postural motor behavior are associated with a decrease in sway velocity and a reduction of oscillatory sway behavior.

Refinements in the sensory aspects of postural control include a shift from predominance of visual control of balance to a somatosensory control of balance by 3 years of age. With increasing age, the automaticity of postural control is increased, thus requiring less attentional resources. Both (a) the ability to adapt senses for postural control appropriately when one or more of these senses are inaccurately reporting body orientation information and (b) the ability to perform both postural and cognitive tasks in dual-task situations are significantly improved in children over the age of 7 years.

SUMMARY

1. The development of postural control is an essential aspect of the development of skilled actions, like locomotion and manipulation.
2. Consistent with Gesell's developmental principles, postural development appears to be characterized by a cephalocaudal progression of control.
3. The emergence of postural control can be characterized by both the presence of limited innate components of reactive control and the subsequent development of more refined rules that relate sensory inputs reporting the body's position with respect to the environment, to motor actions that control the body's position.
   a. Control begins in the head segment. The first sense that is mapped to head control appears to be vision.
   b. As infants begin to sit independently, they learn to coordinate sensory/motor information relating the head and trunk segments, extending the sensorimotor rules for head postural control to trunk muscles.
   c. The mapping of individual senses to action may precede the mapping of multiple senses to action, thus creating internal neural representations necessary for coordinated postural abilities.
4. Anticipatory, or proactive, postural control, which provides a supportive framework for skilled movements, develops in parallel with reactive postural control, though in reaching, reactive or compensatory control is present before anticipatory control.
5. Adaptive capabilities that allow a child to modify sensory and motor strategies to changing task and environmental conditions develop later. Experience in using sensory and motor strategies for posture may play a role in the development of adaptive capacities.
6. The development of postural control is best characterized as the continuous development of multiple sensory and motor systems, which manifests behaviorally in a discontinuous steplike progression of motor milestones. New strategies for sensing and moving can be associated with seeming regression in behavior as children incorporate new strategies into their repertoire for postural control.
7. Not all systems contributing to the emergence of postural control develop at the same rate. Rate-limiting components limit the pace at which an independent behavior emerges. Thus, the emergence of postural control must await the development of the slowest critical component.

CHAPTER 9

Aging and Postural Control

Learning Objectives

Following completion of this chapter, the reader will be able to:

1. Describe factors contributing to aging and discuss their implications for the rehabilitation of older adults.
2. Describe Spirduso's continuum of physical function and discuss factors contributing to the heterogeneity of aging.
3. Discuss the prevalence of falls in older adults and review intrinsic and extrinsic risk factors for falls among community-dwelling versus hospitalized older adults.
4. Describe age-related changes in the systems important to postural control, including both the musculoskeletal and the neural systems.

INTRODUCTION

Why is it that George M, at the age of 90, is able to run marathons, while Lew N, at the age of 78, is in a nursing home, confined to a wheelchair, and unable to walk to the bathroom without assistance? Clearly, the answer to this question is complex. Many factors affect how we age with respect to health and functional abilities. These factors contribute to the tremendous differences found among older adults.

This chapter does not describe all aspects of aging. Rather, the focus is on age-related changes that occur in systems critical to postural control. We review the research examining age-related changes in systems whose dysfunction may contribute to instability among older adults. Some introductory comments about research examining changes in older adults are important.

Factors Contributing to Aging

Although a variety of studies have examined the process of aging and have shown a decline in a number of sensory and motor processes in many older adults, a surprising feature of most studies is the great heterogeneity in the aging process, with older adults of the same chronologic age showing physical function that ranges from the physically elite to the physically dependent and disabled (Aniansson et al., 1978; Duncan et al., 1993; Kosnik et al., 1988; Lewis & Bottomly, 1990; Sloane et al., 1989; Spirduso et al., 2005; Tinetti & Ginter, 1988). This has led to the understanding that there are many factors that contribute to health and longevity, including internal factors, such as genetics, and external factors, such as a person's lifestyle and the environment in which they live (Birren & Cunningham, 1985; Davies, 1987; Woollacott, 1989).

One set of theories on aging says that an important factor contributing to aging is DNA damage. For example, research has shown that the cells of our bodies undergo about 800 DNA lesions per hour, or 19,200 per cell per day (Lu et al., 2004; Vilenchik & Knudson, 2000). Though most of these lesions are repaired, there are some errors. Nonreplicating cells in the brain, muscle, and liver accumulate the most damage. Interestingly, the principal source of DNA damage leading to normal aging is reactive oxygen, from normal metabolism, and this is something that can be affected by diet and exercise. Specific genetically associated diseases, in which symptoms of aging occur early in life (Werner's syndrome, with a mean life span of 47 years, and progeria, with a mean life span of 13 years), are due to inherited defects in the enzyme that causes DNA repair and thus offer support for this theory (Ly et al., 2000; Spirduso, et al., 2005). They suggest that the efficiency of DNA repair is a factor contributing to longevity, and in fact, DNA repair capacity is highly correlated with longevity in both humans and other animals (Bürkle et al., 2005).

The second category includes factors contributing to longevity that are external to the organism and includes insults and damage caused by environmental factors such as radiation (causing genetic mutation), pollutants, bacteria/viruses, foods/toxins, and catastrophic insults that cause damage to the system and positive influences on longevity such as exercise. Interestingly, research indicates that genetic factors contribute about 20% to longevity, while health-related behaviors, including lifestyle, diet, and levels of exercise, stress, and self-efficacy (a person's perception of their ability to succeed), contribute 80% (Bortz & Bortz, 1996).

However, a focus on genetic components alone as the primary determinant of nervous system function with age creates a rather pessimistic view of aging, since it suggests that functional loss is an invariant part of growing old. This type of reasoning can lead to self-limiting perceptions on the part of older individuals regarding what they can do (Tinetti et al., 1990). Self-limiting perceptions are often inadvertently reinforced by the medical professionals, who may hold a limited view regarding what older adults can accomplish. For example, when assessing an older adult, a therapist may perceive that the patient's strength is good, considering the patient's age. As a result, a strength grade of 3 out of 5, which would never be accepted in a 30-year-old, is often accepted as normal in a 70-year-old.

In contrast, a focus on secondary factors that contribute to longevity leads to a more optimistic view (Woollacott, 1989). In this model, in the presence of optimal experiential factors, one expects high levels of function in the central nervous system (CNS) unless unexpected pathology occurs. Experiential factors involve leading a healthy and active life. Thus, when therapists with this perspective on aging evaluate an older person, they anticipate that function will be optimal. If a decline is detected in any area of the nervous system, this perspective will allow the therapist to work on rehabilitation strategies aimed at returning function toward that of a healthy young adult.

Interactions between Primary and Secondary Factors

Research supports the profound role of secondary or experiential factors on aging (Colman et al., 2009; van Praag, 2009; Wang et al., 2002). Secondary, or experiential, factors are more or less under our control, and include nutrition, stress, exercise, and pathologies that affect our mind and body.

Scientists have shown that proper nutrition results in prolonged and healthier lives (Lee et al., 1993). Further, animal studies have shown that dietary restriction extends the life span (Colman et al., 2009). In addition, exercise programs have been shown to improve cardiovascular health, control obesity, and increase physical and mental function (Kramer et al., 2006). The resultant gains in aerobic power, muscle strength, and flexibility can improve biologic age by 10 to 20 years. This can result in delaying the age of dependency and increasing the quality of the remaining years of life (Fries, 2002; Wang et al., 2002). Psychosocial factors—social relationships, feelings of loneliness, and satisfaction with life and aging—are known to be associated with longevity (Ailshire & Crimmins, 2011). This knowledge that how we age is largely determined by how we live leads to an emphasis on preventive health care measures. It also has implications for rehabilitation. Therapists work to assist older patients who have experienced pathology to return to optimal lifestyles (Tinetti, 1986).

Thus, the factors that determine the health and mobility of George M versus Lew N are a combination of primary aging factors, mainly genetics, over which they have limited control, and secondary (experiential) aging factors, over which they have considerable control.

It also appears that aging, whether it is due to genetic or lifestyle factors, may not necessarily be characterized by an overall decline in function. Rather, decline may be limited to specific neural structures and functions. This is consistent with a major theme in this book, in which function and dysfunction are not generalized but emerge through the interaction of the capacities of the individual carrying out particular tasks within specific environmental contexts.

Heterogeneity of Aging

A review of the literature on aging shows that some studies report no change in function of the neural subsystems controlling posture and locomotion with age (Gabell & Nayak, 1984), while others show a severe decline in function in older adults (Imms & Edholm, 1981). How can there be such a discrepancy in studies reporting age-related changes in systems for posture and gait? This may be due to fundamental differences in the definition that researchers use in classifying an individual as an older adult.

For example, some researchers have classified the older adult as anyone over 60 years of age. When no exclusionary criteria are used in the study of older adults, results can be very different from when researchers use restrictive criteria for including subjects for study. For example, a study on the effects of aging on walking ability selected a group of 71 subjects ranging in age from 60 to 99 years, using no exclusion criteria for possible pathology (Imms & Edholm, 1981). These researchers noted that the mean walking velocities for their older adults were slower than were those reported in any previous studies.

In contrast, another study examined walking in healthy older adults. In this study, 1,187 individuals 65 years of age and older were screened to find 32 who were free of pathology, that is, who had no disorders of the musculoskeletal, neurologic, or cardiovascular systems or any previous history of falls (Gabell & Nayak, 1984). Interestingly, this study found no significant differences between their younger and older adult groups when comparing four parameters measuring the variability of gait. They thus concluded that an increase in variability in the gait cycle among older adults was not normal, but was always due to some pathology.

These types of results suggest that there is much heterogeneity among older adults. This amazing variability reminds us that it is important not to assume that physical capabilities decline in all older adults and that studies should also consider categorizing older adults based on variability of skill performance rather than age alone.

This continuum of function among older adults has been nicely described by Spirduso et al. (2005), who have illustrated the continuum of function found among older adults. This continuum is illustrated in Figure 9.1. At the high end of the continuum are older adults who are physically elite, who engage in competitive sports, and who are considered to undergo optimal aging. Moving down the continuum are older adults who are physically fit, that is, who engage in sports, games, and hobbies, and who are capable of moderate physical work. Physically independent adults are also active, but engage in less physically demanding activities, such as golf or social dancing. Independence in all basic activities of daily living (BADLs) and instrumental activities of daily living (IADLs) is characteristic of this group. Adults in the physically frail group are usually independent in BADLs but are dependent in many IADLs. They are capable of light housekeeping, but often require assistance to continue living independently. Physically dependent adults are disabled; they are dependent in both BADLs and IADLs. They require full-time assistance or institutional care. Using this continuum, you can see that George M would fall at the upper end of the continuum, in the physically elite group, while Lew N would fall at the lower end.

BEHAVIORAL INDICATORS OF INSTABILITY

Defining Falls

Before we can discuss falls and their causes in more detail, it is important to have a clear understanding of the definition of a fall and the different categories of falls that can be experienced. This knowledge allows the therapist to question patients more effectively regarding the frequency and nature of their falls; it also offers a better understanding of the types of rehabilitative strategies appropriate for situations with a variety of types of balance risk. Falls are often defined differently in the clinic versus in the research environment. For example, in the clinic, a fall is often defined as a situation in which the older adult falls to the ground

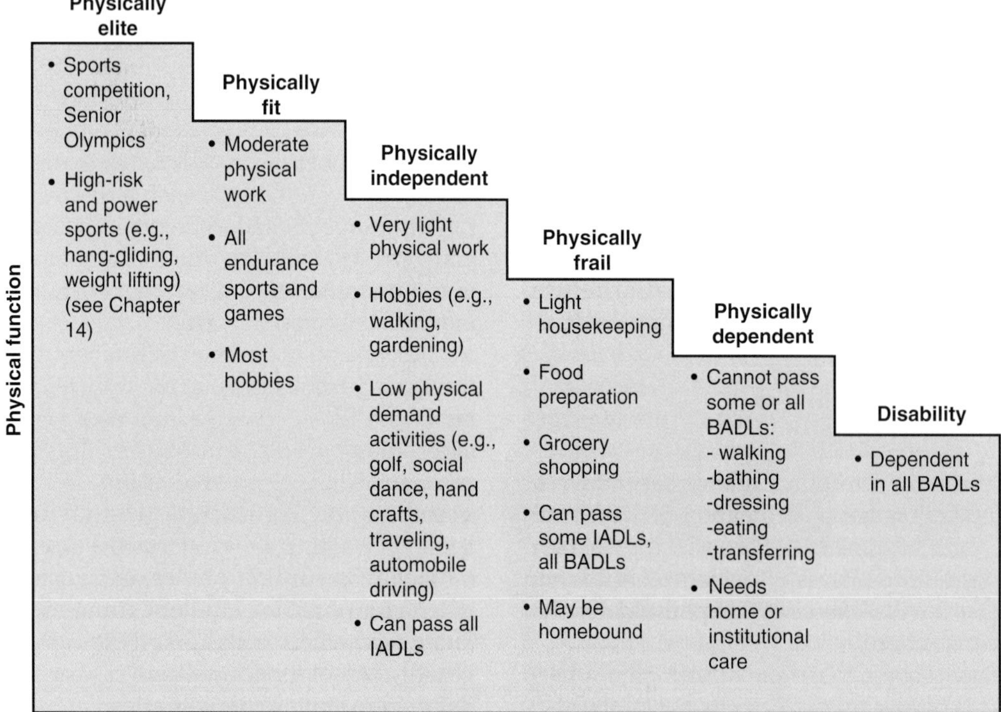

Figure 9.1 Continuum of physical function among older adults. (Adapted from Spirduso W, Francis K, MacRae PG. *Physical dimensions of aging*. Champaign IL: Human Kinetics, 2005:264, Figure 11.1.)

or is found lying on the ground. In addition, it is often defined as any unintended contact with a supporting surface, such as a chair, counter, or wall.

In the research environment, the safety of older adults is considered of utmost importance, and thus, balance testing is typically done with a safety harness protecting the older adult from actual falls. In the laboratory, balance threats are often simulated by moving the support surface varying distances underneath the older adult or moving (pushing or pulling) the center of mass of the person varying distances away from the center of their base of support. A fall is defined as the inability to recover stability independently, thus requiring assistance (either by another person or by a harness) to prevent a fall.

Since the term "fall" is used in a variety of contexts, it is important for clinicians to define their own meaning of the term when talking to patients about falls. One clinical definition used to define a fall is an event that results in a person coming to rest inadvertently on the ground or other lower level and other than as a consequence of the following: sustaining a violent blow; loss of consciousness; sudden onset of paralysis, as in a stroke; or an epileptic seizure (Hauer et al., 2006). In this definition, a supporting surface is not defined solely by the floor, but could be a chair (as when a person begins to rise and falls back unexpectedly into the chair) or a wall (as when a person loses their balance and staggers into a wall with the hip or shoulder).

LAB ACTIVITY 9.1

Objective: To explore issues related to determining fall risk.

Procedure: Ask yourself how many times you have fallen in the past 12 months. Think about and list the activities you were performing at the time you fell. What were the environmental conditions like when you fell? What were the consequences of your falls? Were you injured? Since the fall, have you been afraid or reluctant to return to those activities? Now, find an older adult living within the community or within a residential facility like an assisted living retirement center or skilled nursing facility. Ask this older adult the same set of questions. What is their fall rate? What activities were they performing at the time of the fall? What was the environment like? Was the older adult injured, and what was the psychological consequence of the fall? Was the older adult more fearful and reluctant to return to prior levels of activity?

Assignment

1. Write answers to the above questions, and compare your responses to those of the older adult. What is the difference between your falls and those you would expect to see in 70- to-80 year-olds? What were the consequences?

Risk Factors for Falls

Statistics show that unintentional injuries are the seventh leading cause of death among older adults (after cardiovascular disease, cancer, pulmonary disorders, stroke, Alzheimer's disease, and diabetes), and falls account for the largest percentage of those deaths (CDC, 2016). Approximately one in four U.S. residents aged ≥65 years report falling each year (Bergen et al., 2016). Of significance, about three-fourths of the deaths from falls occur in people over 65 years (Ochs et al., 1985; Rubenstein, 2006). In addition, fall rates in persons 65 years of age or older are at least 33% per year in community-dwelling older adults, with women being found to fall more frequently than do men (Campbell et al., 1981; Nevitt et al., 1989; Shumway-Cook et al., 2009). What factors contribute to these losses of balance? Many early studies on balance loss among older adults expected to isolate a single cause of falls for a given older adult, such as vertigo, sensory neuropathy, or postural hypotension. In contrast, more current research indicates that many falls among older adults have multiple contributing factors, including extrinsic environmental factors and intrinsic factors such as physiological, musculoskeletal, and psychosocial factors (Campbell et al., 1989; Lipsitz et al., 1991; Tinetti et al., 1986).

Perform Lab Activity 9.1 to explore issues related to determining fall risk. You may have discovered that when attempting to determine fall risk, it is critical to know both the activity level and the risk of falls for the activity in which the person is engaged. Falls are not determined solely by factors within the individual (e.g., poor balance); falls emerge from an interaction of the individual performing specific tasks in certain environments. In fact, research shows that older adults (>75 years) tend to fall at home, while younger old adults (70 to 75 years) fall more frequently away from home (and suffer more serious injuries) (Shumway-Cook et al., 2009; Speechley & Tinetti, 1991; Tinetti et al., 1988).

According to the "Guidelines for Prevention of Falls in Older Persons," published by the American and British Geriatrics Societies and the American Academy of Orthopedic Surgeons (Kenny et al., 2011), there are a number of risk factors associated with falls among community-living older adults, including muscle weakness, history of falls, gait deficits, balance deficits, use of an assistive device, visual deficits, arthritis, impaired activities of daily living (ADLs), depression, cognitive impairment, and age greater than 80 years. Environmental factors that increase fall risk include the presence of stairs, throw rugs, slippery surfaces, and poor lighting (Kenny et al., 2011; Rubenstein et al., 1988; Sheldon, 1960). Based on this research, Rubenstein et al. (2011) developed and validated a self-rated fall questionnaire to identify

Assessment Tool 9.1

Fall Risk Questionnaire

1. I have fallen in the last 6 months. Yes = 2 points
2. I am worried about falling. Yes = 1 point
3. Sometimes, I feel unsteady when I am walking. Yes = 1 point
4. I steady myself by holding onto furniture when walking at home. Yes = 1 point
5. I use or have been advised to use a cane or walker to get around safely. Yes = 2 points
6. I need to push with my hands to stand up from a chair. Yes = 1 point
7. I have some trouble stepping up onto a curb. Yes = 1 point
8. I often have to rush to the toilet. Yes = 1 point
9. I have lost some feeling in my feet. Yes = 1 point
10. I take medicine that sometimes makes me feel light-headed or more tired than usual. Yes = 1 point
11. I take medicine to help me sleep or improve my mood. Yes = 1 point
12. I often feel sad or depressed. Yes = 1 point

Total __________/14

Increased risk for falls ≥4

Reprinted from Rubenstein LZ, Vivrette R, Harker JO, Stevens JA, et al. Validating an evidence-based, self-rated fall risk questionnaire (FRQ) for older adults. *J Safety Res.* 2011;42:493–499, with permission.

older adults at risk for falls. The questionnaire, shown in Assessment Tool 9.1, was strongly correlated with clinical findings related to fall risk. A cut point of greater than 4 points indicates an increased risk for future falls. Indeed, older adults who have an increased risk for falls often show great difficulties when performing the items described on the questionnaire. For example, Ko and colleagues (2020) showed that older adults who failed an obstacle crossing task (stepping over a curb) reported a greater likelihood of falling the previous year, had more balance problems, lower walking ability, and needed longer time to complete five chair stands compared to older adults who successfully completed the obstacle crossing task. Moreover, older adults who failed the obstacle crossing task walked slower with smaller knee range of motion than those who passed the task. The authors conclude that an obstacle crossing task may be useful for identifying older adults who appear to be functionally intact but none the less are at increased risk for falls.

Falls are a great problem among hospitalized older adults and those living in residential facilities as well (Oliver et al., 2004). Falls by inpatients are associated with an increased duration of hospitalization and a greater chance of unplanned readmission or of discharge to residential or nursing home care (Bates et al., 1995). Are risk factors the same for older adults in hospital and residential facilities as for those living in the community? Many factors predictive of falls among older adults in the community may not apply to hospital inpatients, for whom recovery from acute illness that is associated with changing mobility is more common. Since the occurrence of falls depends on patient characteristics and institutional characteristics, such as clinical and nursing practice, risk factors may be specific to particular hospital units (e.g., acute medical versus inpatient rehabilitation) (Oliver et al., 1997). Many studies have examined risk factors for falls among hospitalized older adults, and they have consistently identified the following factors: gait instability, lower-extremity weakness, urinary incontinence or frequency or need for assistance in toileting, impaired cognition (agitation, confusion, or impaired judgment), history of falls, and the use of certain medications, in particular centrally acting sedatives (Oliver et al., 2004).

The identification of factors predictive of falls in hospitalized older adults has led to the development of a number of risk factor assessment tools for use in hospitals and residential settings (see Oliver et al., 2004; Perell et al., 2001, for reviews of risk assessment tools). Assessment Tool 9.2 is an example of one such tool, STRATIFY (St. Thomas's risk assessment tool in falling older adult inpatients), developed and validated by British researchers to predict falls in hospitalized older adults. Among hospitalized older adults, a risk score of 2 or more had a sensitivity of 93% and a specificity of 88% for predicting inpatient falls (Oliver et al., 1997).

Among older adults, fall risk is also high 1 to 6 months after discharge from the hospital. Several studies have examined post-discharge fall rates among older adults hospitalized for hip fracture. McKee et al. (2002) followed 57 patients for 2 months and reported that 17.5% of those with a hip fracture went on to fall again. Colon-Emeric et al. (2000) reported that 19% of community-dwelling men and male veterans sustained a second hip or pelvic fracture within 1 year after the initial hip fracture. Shumway-Cook et al. (2005a) followed 90 older adults for 6 months after discharge for a fall-related hip fracture and reported that 53.3% of patients (48 of 90) reported one or more falls in the 6 months after hospitalization. Older adults who fell after discharge had significantly greater declines in independence in ADLs and lower performance on balance and mobility measures. These authors found that two factors—premorbid history of falls and use of a gait-assistive device (indicating impaired mobility)—predicted falls in the 6 months after discharge. The authors suggest that identification of older adults at risk for poor outcomes early in their hip fracture care could

Assessment Tool 9.2

Stratify

1. Did the patient present to hospital with a fall, or has the patient fallen on the ward since admission?
(Yes = 1, No = 0)

(Questions 2–5) Do you think the patient:

2. Is agitated?
(Yes = 1, No = 0)
3. Is visually impaired to the extent that everyday function is affected?
(Yes = 1, No = 0)
4. Is in need of especially frequent toileting?
(Yes = 1, No = 0)
5. Has a transfer and mobility score of 3 or 4*?
(Yes = 1, No = 0)

Total score (range, 0–5)

Score ≥2 indicates an increased risk for falls

*Transfer score: 0 = unable, 1 = major help needed (one or two people, physical aids), 2 = minor help (verbal or physical), 3 = independent; mobility score: 0 = immobile, 1 = independent with aid of wheelchair, 2 = walks with help of one person, 3 = independent.

Reprinted from Oliver D, Britton M, Seed P, et al. Development and evaluation of evidence based risk assessment tool (STRATIFY) to predict which elderly inpatients will fall: case–control and cohort studies. *BMJ* 1997;315:1049–1053, with permission.

result in improved discharge planning. Specifically, older adults determined to be at risk for additional falls could be referred for further physical therapy after fracture healing for exercises specifically designed to improve balance and mobility function in order to reduce the risk for falls (Shumway-Cook et al., 2005a).

Many studies have examined the physiological factors that contribute to a risk of falls (Campbell et al., 1989; Lipsitz et al., 1991; Lord et al., 1993; Maki et al., 1994; Nevitt et al., 1989; Tinetti et al., 1988). The conclusions of these studies were that most falls in older adults involve multiple risk factors and that many of these factors may be remediated. The risk of falling increases with the number of risk factors. In a cohort of older adults living in the community, the risk for falling increased from 8% among those with no risk factors to 78% among those with four or more risk factors (Tinetti et al., 1988). Thus, it has been suggested that the clinician who is working with an older adult should determine both intrinsic and extrinsic factors associated with a particular fall and reduce or correct as many of these as possible (Lipsitz et al., 1991).

Studies examining intrinsic factors leading to falls have included examining the role of balance control. Several researchers, including Tinetti et al. from the United States, Berg et al. from Canada, and Mathias et al. from England, have measured functional skills related to balance in order to identify people at high risk for falls (Berg et al., 1989; Mathias et al., 1986; Speechley & Tinetti, 1990; Tinetti et al., 1986). Functional skills include sitting, standing, and walking unsupported; standing and reaching forward; performing a 360-degree turn; and moving from a sitting to a standing position. A more recent approach to understanding the balance function in older adults examines specific variables relating to normal postural control and determines the extent to which deterioration in their function contributes to loss of stability and mobility in older adults.

In the remaining sections of this chapter, we examine the intrinsic factors related to balance problems in older adults from a systems perspective. We discuss changes in the motor system, the sensory systems, and higher-level adaptive and cognitive systems as well as the use of anticipatory postural responses before making a voluntary movement. Studies on the ability of older adults to integrate balance adjustments into the step cycle are covered in the mobility section of this book.

AGE-RELATED CHANGES IN THE SYSTEMS OF POSTURAL CONTROL

Bonnie B is a 90-year-old woman with impaired balance resulting in multiple falls, two of which required hospitalization. Bonnie has a number of underlying sensory, motor, and cognitive impairments that contribute to her impaired balance. What have researchers learned about how age-related changes in these systems contribute to an increased likelihood for falls in older persons like Bonnie?

Motor Systems

Problems in the motor systems contributing to age-related changes in postural control include impairments in both neuromuscular and musculoskeletal systems. Many of these changes, such as kyphosis, are similar to those found in patients with neurological pathology, but are found in milder forms in many older adults.

Musculoskeletal System

Muscle Strength. Several researchers have reported changes in the musculoskeletal system in many older adults (Aniansson et al., 1986; Buchner & deLateur, 1991; Frontera et al., 2000; Narici et al., 2008). Strength, or the amount of force a muscle produces, declines with age. Lower-extremity muscle strength (defined as the amount of force produced during a single maximum contraction of a muscle) can be reduced by as much as 40% between the ages of 30 and 80 years (Aniansson et al., 1986). Longitudinal studies following muscle strength changes across 10 years in older adults (mean age at the start of the study, 60 years) showed a 12% to 17% loss of knee flexor and extensor strength over the two types of muscles. Plantar flexion, dorsal flexion, hip flexion, hip abduction, and hip adduction strength also play an important role in balance recovery and are also reduced with age (Afschrift et al., 2019; Inacio et al., 2019; Koushyar et al., 2019; Porto et al., 2019). However, strength gains were also seen in some individuals, showing the heterogeneity of the aging process (Hughes et al., 2001). Muscle strength reduction is more severe in older nursing home residents with a history of falls (Whipple et al., 1987). In these subjects, the mean knee and ankle muscle strength was reduced twofold and fourfold, respectively, as compared with those with no history of falls.

Endurance, which is the capacity of the muscle to contract continuously at submaximal levels, also decreases with age. However, endurance is better preserved with age than is strength. As muscles age, they become smaller; this reduction in muscle mass is greater in the lower extremities than in the upper extremities (Medina, 1996). As muscle cells die, they are replaced with connective tissue and fat. A number of studies have examined the preferential loss of muscle fiber types with aging, with mixed results. There appears to be an age-related loss of both type I (slow oxidative, used in activities such as postural control and long-distance running) and II (fast twitch, used for sprinting, etc.) muscle fiber types. It used to be thought that with aging, type II fast-twitch fibers may be lost at a faster rate than type I fibers (Timiras, 1994), but new evidence suggests that an increasing number of muscle fibers simply become more of a blend of type I and type II, with characteristics of both (Anderson et al., 1999; Spirduso et al., 2005). Researchers have also shown that the number of motor units declines with age; there is a reduction in both large and small myelinated fibers. In addition, there are age-related changes at the neuromuscular junction (Medina, 1996).

Changes in skeletal muscle affect the functional capacity of the muscles. Maximum isometric force decreases, the muscles fatigue more rapidly, and the rate of tension development is slower. It appears that concentric contractions are more affected by age-related changes in the neuromuscular system than are eccentric contractions. Rapid-velocity contractions are more affected than are slow-velocity contractions.

Researchers have shown that the association between strength and physical function is large, with over 20% of the variance in functional status explained by relative strength (Buchner & deLateur, 1991). In addition, lower-extremity lean muscle mass and reduced strength were strong independent predictors of severe functional impairment in older adults (Reid et al., 2008). Interestingly, muscle power has been found to be even more highly correlated with physical function than muscle strength, with power training being more effective than strength training for improving physical function in older adults with muscle weakness (Bean et al., 2003; Miszko et al., 2003).

However, the amount of strength or power needed for physical function is dependent on the task. For example, it has been suggested that the typical healthy 80-year-old woman is very near, if not at, the threshold value for quadriceps strength necessary to rise from a chair (Young, 1986). When strength falls below the threshold needed for a task, functional disability occurs.

Range of Motion. Decreased range of motion and loss of spinal flexibility in many older adults can lead to a characteristic flexed or stooped posture (Fig. 9.2) (Balzini et al., 2003; Katzman et al., 2007). Spinal flexibility, particularly spinal extensibility, shows the greatest decline with age (Einkauf et al., 1987; Katzman et al., 2007). This may be primarily a cause of the types of daily activities most often performed by older adults, with few activities requiring a backward extension (Spirduso et al., 2005). Loss of spinal flexibility can be associated with other changes in postural alignment,

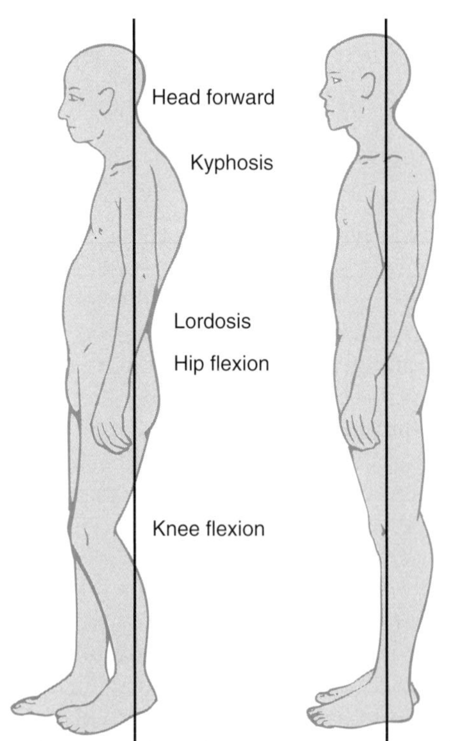

Figure 9.2 Comparison of postural alignment in a young versus an older adult. Changes in spinal flexibility can lead to a stooped or flexed posture in many older adults. (Adapted from Lewis C, Bottomley J. Musculoskeletal changes with age. In: Lewis C, ed. *Aging: health care's challenge*, 2nd ed. Philadelphia, PA: FA Davis, 1990:146.)

including a compensatory shift in the vertical displacement of the center of body mass backward toward the heels. Starting at around 50 years of age, adults have increased cervical lordosis, thoracic kyphosis, and knee flexion, and these changes are more marked among women (Gong et al., 2019). Ankle-joint flexibility, critical for postural control, also declines by 50% in women and 35% in men between the ages of 55 and 85 (Vandervoort et al., 1992). Other conditions, such as arthritis, can lead to decreased range of motion in many joints throughout the body. In addition, pain may limit the functional range of motion of a particular joint (Horak et al., 1989). Increased kyphosis is associated with a decrease in spinal extensor muscle strength as well as impaired balance, slower walking and stair climbing, a shorter functional reach, and decreased ADL performance (Balzini et al., 2003; Katzman et al., 2007).

In addition to the musculoskeletal systems, aging results in changes to the neuromuscular system, specifically the coordination of forces controlling steady-state, reactive, and proactive balance control.

Clinical Implications

When evaluating balance in older adults, such as Bonnie, the clinician should be sure to include evaluation of both primary neuromuscular and secondary musculoskeletal contributions to instability, as deficits have been found in these systems in many older adults with balance impairments.

Changes to Steady-State Balance

Traditional methods for assessing steady-state balance function in older adults have used global indicators of balance control, such as determination of spontaneous sway during quiet stance. One of the earliest studies examined the extent to which subjects in age groups from 6 years through 80 years swayed during quiet stance. Subjects at both ends of the age spectrum (ages 6 to 14 and 50 to 80) had greater difficulty in minimizing spontaneous sway during quiet stance than did the other age groups tested (Sheldon, 1963). This study tested a great variety of older adults and did not try to limit subjects in the older groups to those who were free of pathology.

A number of studies have measured spontaneous sway in different age groups using stabilometry, or static force plates. Several have documented increased sway with increasing age, particularly among adults with a history of falls (Fernie et al., 1982; Shumway-Cook et al., 1997c; Toupet et al., 1992), while others have found few differences in sway between young and older adults (Peterka & Black, 1991; Wolfson et al., 1992).

Several researchers have expressed caution about using measures of sway during quiet stance to infer balance abilities. Patla et al. (1990) note that while large excursions of center of pressure (COP) are generally interpreted as a reflection of a poor balance control system, some older adults use larger and higher-frequency excursions of COP to enhance sensory information about their posture while remaining well within their limits of stability (Patla et al., 1990). They suggest that static balance be assessed under challenging conditions such as tandem stance with eyes open versus closed. Horak et al. (1992) also remind us that there are a variety of patients with neurologic disorders, such as Parkinson's disease, who have normal, or even reduced, sway in quiet stance. This may be due to the fact that they show increased stiffness or rigidity and this limits sway to a smaller area during quiet stance. This is one reason that measurement of sway with eyes open during normal quiet stance may not be the best way to evaluate balance dysfunction in older adults.

Age-Related Changes in Functional Stability Limits

Researchers have examined changes in functional stability limits by measuring the COP trajectory (COP movement during anteroposterior, lateral, and diagonal maximum sway efforts) in relation to estimated geometric stability boundaries (borders of the feet). In a study examining subjects from 60 to 96 years of age, it was shown that the ratio of the area of motion of the COP to the area of both geometric and functional stability boundaries increased with age. Functional stability boundaries were much smaller than were geometric boundaries and became smaller with increasing age, suggesting that measures of stability limits using only foot boundaries may be inappropriate in older adults. A measure of virtual time to contact with the postural stability boundary also decreased with age, suggesting that older adults are at higher risk of instability that would necessitate taking a step or risking a fall (Slobounov et al., 1998). Other researchers examined functional stability limits as the percentage of the base of support that individuals are willing to use when extending their COP (Holbein-Jenny et al., 2007). They found that functional stability limits significantly decreased with age.

Functional stability limits are often inferred by examining how far an individual can lean or reach in multiple directions. Using this approach, researchers have reported that functional stability limits are reduced with age (Horak et al., 1989). Thompson and Medley (2007) measured forward and lateral reach in sitting across four age groups. Results are shown in Figure 9.3 and demonstrate that distance reached in both directions significantly declines with age, supporting the concept that functional stability limits ("dynamic sitting balance" is their term) decline with age. Unlike standing, changes in distance reached in sitting were unrelated to anthropometric measurements.

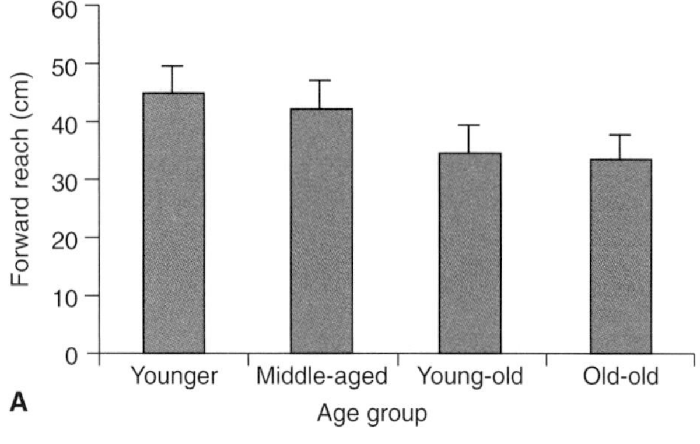

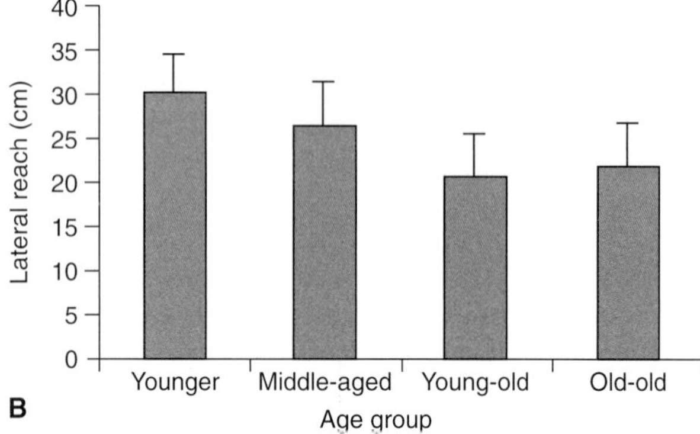

Figure 9.3 Bar graph illustrating the mean and standard deviation of sitting forward reach **(A)** and lateral reach **(B)** for four different age groups (Young: 21–39; Middle-aged: 40–59; Young-old: 60–79; Old-Old: 80–97 years). The younger and middle-aged participants reached further than did the older participants (Reprinted from Thompson M, Medley A. Forward and lateral functional reach in sitting in younger, middle aged, and older adults. *J Ger Phys Ther*. 2007;30:46, Figures 2, 3, with permission.)

Clinical Implications of Age-Related Changes to Steady-State Balance

As there are a variety of patients with neurologic disorders, and older adults with balance impairments, who have normal, or even reduced, sway in quiet stance, measurement of sway with eyes open during normal quiet stance may not be the best way to evaluate balance dysfunction in these populations. Thus, more challenging quiet stance conditions, such as tandem Romberg, with eyes closed, will allow the clinician to determine the true capacity of the older adult to balance under changing steady-state balance conditions.

Changes in Reactive Balance Control

Extensive research has been performed on age-related changes in the coordination of postural muscle synergies (both in-place and change-in-support strategies) that affect the ability to recover stability following an unexpected threat to balance. Problems affecting the coordination of muscle response synergies are classified into (a) sequencing problems, (b) problems with the timely activation of postural responses, and (c) problems adapting postural activity to changing task and environmental demands.

In-Place Strategies

Is the older adult capable of activating muscle response synergies with appropriate timing, force, and muscle response organization when balance is threatened? Most research addresses this question by using a moving platform to provide an external threat to balance. In the following pages, we summarize the studies that have examined changes in electromyography (EMG), kinematic, and kinetic variables that are correlated with aging and with falls.

Woollacott et al. (1986) performed one of the first studies to examine age-related changes in postural muscle response characteristics elicited when balance was threatened. They found that the muscle response organization of older adults (61 to 78 years) and younger adults (19 to 38 years) was generally similar, with responses being activated first in the stretched ankle muscle and radiating upward to the muscles of the thigh.

However, there were also differences between the two groups in certain response characteristics. The older adults showed significantly slower onset latencies in the ankle dorsiflexors in response to anterior platform movements, causing backward sway. This has been observed in other laboratories as well (Studenski et al., 1991). In addition, in some older adults, the muscle response organization was disrupted, with proximal muscles being activated before distal muscles (a sequencing problem). This response organization has also been seen in patients with CNS dysfunction (Nashner et al., 1983).

The older adult group also tended to coactivate the antagonist muscles along with the agonist muscles at a given joint significantly more often than did the younger adults. Thus, many of the older adults studied tended to stiffen the joints to a greater degree than did young adults when compensating for sway perturbations.

Several labs have found that many older adults used a strategy involving hip movements rather than ankle movements significantly more often than did young adults (Horak et al., 1989; Manchester et al., 1989). Hip movements are typically used by young adults when balancing on a short support surface that does not allow them to use ankle torque in compensating for sway. It has been hypothesized that this shift toward use of a hip strategy for balance control in older adults may be related to pathologic conditions such as ankle-muscle weakness or loss of peripheral sensory function. Horak et al. (1989) have suggested that in older adults, some falls, particularly those associated with slipping, may be the result of using a hip strategy in slippery conditions in which the surface cannot resist the sheer forces associated with the use of this strategy, for example, when on ice.

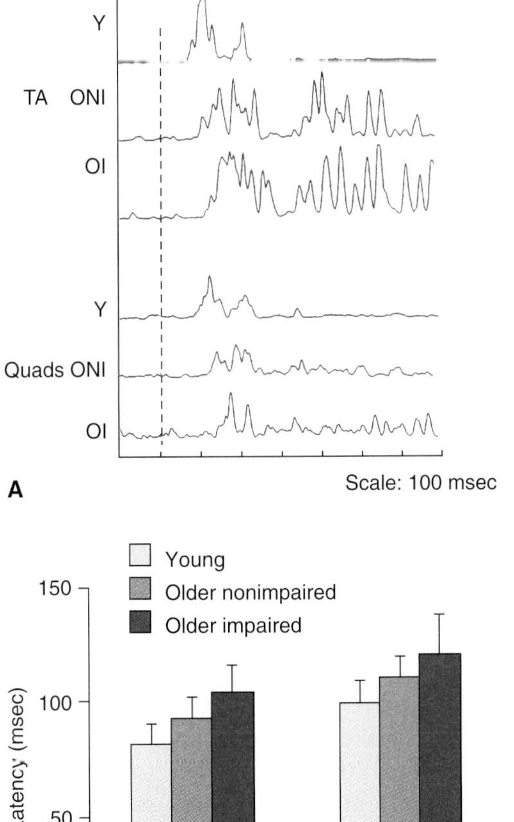

Figure 9.4 Changes in timing of muscle response synergies in older adults. **(A)** Examples of muscle responses to an anterior platform movement causing posterior sway in a young adult (*Y*), a healthy older adult (older nonimpaired, *ONI*), and an older adult who had problems with balance and falls (older impaired, *OI*). Note that the onset latencies for the tibialis anterior (*TA*) and quadriceps (*Quads*) postural muscles become progressively later for the stable (*ONI*) and then the unstable older adults (*OI*). **(B)** Graphs showing mean response onset latencies for *TA* and *Quads* in each subject group.

More recent studies have extended this research and have compared young adults with stable older adults and with older adults with balance problems (Chandler et al., 1990; Lin & Woollacott, 2002). Figure 9.4 summarizes some of the effects found in these studies. Figure 9.4A shows examples of responses (from individual trials) to anterior platform movements causing posterior sway in a young adult, a healthy older adult, and an older adult who had problems with balance and falls. Note that the contraction onset for the tibialis anterior (TA) and quadriceps postural muscles becomes progressively later for the stable and then the unstable older adults. Figure 9.4B shows the mean muscle contraction onset for all individuals in each group.

Maintaining balance control while turning is difficult for older adults and may even lead to falls. Mileti and colleagues (2019) observed that abnormal reactive postural responses may be a contributing factor to this difficulty. Young and older adults underwent external continuous yaw perturbations provided by a movable platform. Older adults had significant reduction in horizontal rotations of body segments and joints compared to young adults, as well as reduced center of mass displacement. The authors note that this more conservative and less destabilizing motion may be a more cautious postural strategy used by older adults to compensate for reduced physical capabilities.

Furthermore, older adults had a greater variability in reactive postural responses than young adults.

Changes in Adaptation: Modifying Movements to Changing Tasks and Environments

These early research studies provided information on age-related changes in responses to balance threats of a single size. It is possible that these changes in postural response characteristics in older adults are simply indications of deterioration in postural muscle response efficiency, as implied in the earlier literature. However, it is also possible that some of these changes may be due to the older adults using a different response strategy than that seen in young adults, as a way of adapting to certain constraints associated with aging, such as muscle weakness, reduced ankle-joint sensation, or joint stiffness. For example, it is possible that a shift toward the use of hip movements in balance control may be due to ankle-muscle weakness and the inability to generate large amounts of force at the ankle joint (Horak et al., 1989; Manchester et al., 1989). This might be seen more clearly as an older adult is subjected to larger balance threats that exceed their muscle response capacity at the ankle. In addition, older adults with balance problems may show more severe constraints within their neural and musculoskeletal systems and therefore show more limited response capacity.

In order to explore this question further, studies have examined the response characteristics of both well-balanced and less-stable older adults during balance threats of increasing magnitude and velocity, in order to simulate environmental situations with changing balance conditions (Lin & Woollacott, 2002; Lin et al., 2004). Young (mean [±SD] age, 25±4 years) and older adults were recruited from the community for the study. Older adults (mean age, 75±4 years) were divided into stable and unstable groups according to their scores on three clinical balance tests (Berg [Berg et al., 1992], Dynamic Gait Index [Shumway-Cook et al., 2013], and self-perceived balance ability).

In response to small or slow perturbations, the onset of postural muscle activity was delayed in both groups of older adults compared with the young adults, but for the large or fast perturbations, only the unstable older adults showed muscle onset delays. This suggests that the stable older adults had difficulty in sensing the onset of small or slow perturbations but were able to compensate adequately for larger scaling factors.

In response to large perturbations, both groups of older adults showed smaller amplitude muscle responses compared to young adults. In response to small perturbations, only the unstable older adults showed smaller amplitude muscle responses, suggesting that both older stable and unstable adults show a limited response capacity as compared with young adults, but this is not apparent in stable older adults until balance threats are large.

Were older adults using a higher percentage of maximal voluntary capacity in responding to balance threats? Lin and Woollacott (2002) compared postural response amplitudes during perturbations to amplitudes of a maximum voluntary gastrocnemius contraction. Figure 9.5 shows that for small perturbations, the young and stable older adults used similar amounts of maximum capacity (about 20%), but the unstable older adults used significantly more (almost 40%). As perturbation velocity increased to 40 cm/s, the stable older adults also showed significantly larger amounts of maximum capacity utilization than did the young adults.

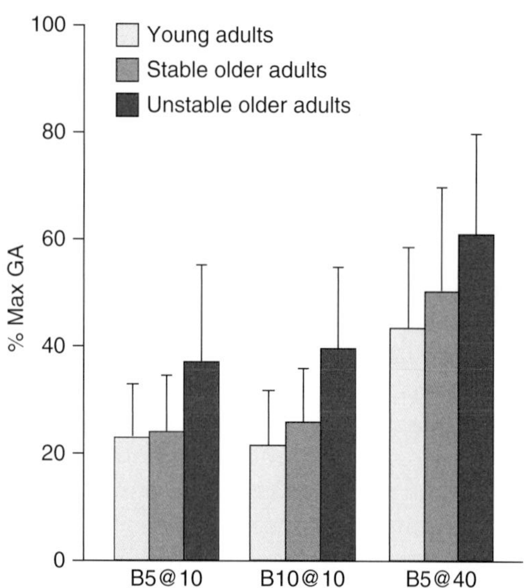

Figure 9.5 Comparison of postural response amplitudes (IEMG) of young stable adults, stable older adults, and unstable older adults for similar intervals when standing maximally on toes (maximum gastrocnemius capacity) versus when responding to balance threats of different sizes and velocities. Note that for small perturbations, the young and stable older adults used similar amounts of maximum capacity (about 20%), but the unstable older adults used significantly more (almost 40%). As perturbation velocity increased to 40 cm/s, the stable older adults also showed significantly larger amounts of maximum capacity utilization than did the young adults. *GA*, gastrocnemius; *B5@10*, backward perturbation of 5 cm at 10 cm/s; *B10@10*, backward perturbation of 10 cm at 10 cm/s; *B5@40*, backward perturbation of 5 cm at 40 cm/s. (Adapted from Lin S-I, Woollacott MH. Differentiating postural responses following dynamically changing balance threats in young adults, healthy older adults and unstable older adults: electromyography. *J Mot Behav*. 2002;34:42, Figure 5.)

How were these age-related changes in neuromuscular responses correlated with behavioral changes during balance recovery? For even very small or slow perturbation conditions that did not require a step, there were clear differences in strategies used by the groups. Both stable and unstable older adults used significantly less ankle-dominated responses and more hip-dominated responses than did young adults. In addition, unstable older adults use alternative strategies such as bending at the knee and using the arms to balance. These differences were increased for faster perturbations, with older adults showing a significant percentage of stepping responses when young adults were still using in-place (ankle or hip) responses.

These differences can also be seen in the quantitative data showing COP changes in response to platform perturbations for young stable and unstable older adults. Figure 9.6 shows that when young adults were given a platform perturbation, they efficiently returned the COP to a stable position, whereas the stable and unstable older adults each showed more COP oscillation before coming to a stable position, with the unstable group showing the largest excursion of the COP. This was accompanied by an increased time for the COP to come to stabilization. It is interesting that, in spite of the increases in these variables, there were no differences in peak center of mass (COM) displacements between the groups (Lin et al., 2004). This suggests that each group aimed at keeping a fairly low COM displacement, and when it went beyond this point, the older adults simply shifted strategies and took a step.

What might be the causes of these age-related changes in postural response characteristics to perturbations? Clinical tests showed that muscle strength was significantly lower for the unstable older adults than for the young and stable older adults for most muscles tested. In addition, the strength of the muscles tested was found to be significantly correlated with the scores of the three functional balance tests for almost all muscles tested. Other studies that have examined correlations between balance performance and sensory or motor system function have shown significant correlations between visual acuity, low vibrotactile thresholds, isometric muscle strength, and high psychomotor speed (reaction time [RT] and movement time) (Era et al., 1996; Kristinsdottir et al., 2001). For example, Craig and Doumas (2019) investigated whether postural aftereffects witnessed during transitions from a moving to a stable support are accompanied by a delayed perception of platform stabilization in older adults. They found that older adults took 5 times longer than young adults to perceive platform stabilization,

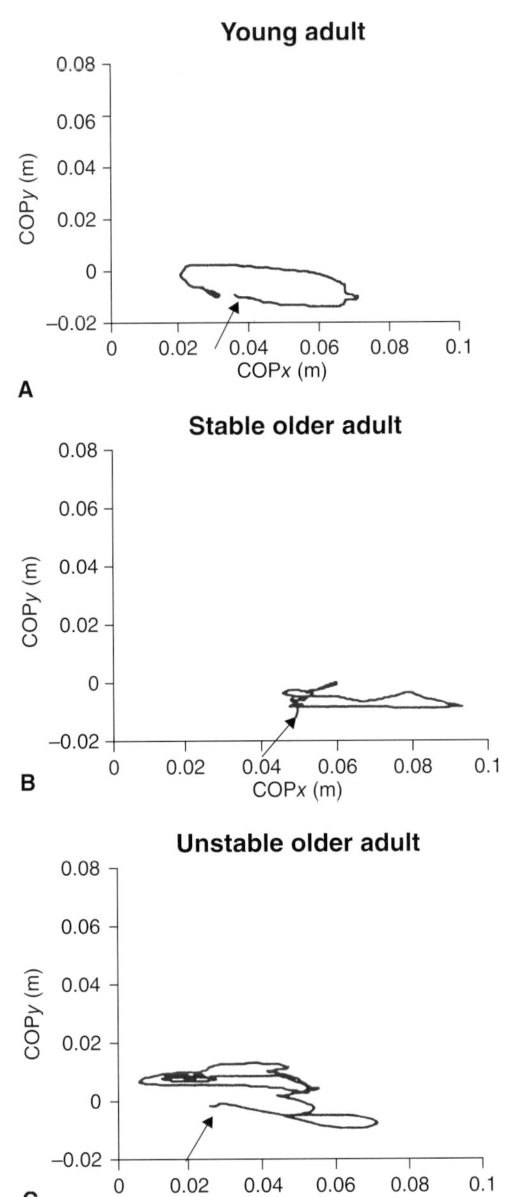

Figure 9.6 Graphs showing COP trajectory (in *x*- and *y*-coordinates) from perturbation onset to 2 seconds after the perturbations for young **(A)**, stable **(B)**, and unstable **(C)** older adults. The *arrow* indicates perturbation onset. Note that the COP trajectory shows much more movement within the 2-second period for unstable older adults. (Reprinted from Lin S-I, Woollacott MH, Jensen J. Differentiating postural responses following dynamically changing balance threats in young adults, healthy older adults and unstable older adults: kinematics and kinetics. *Aging Clin Exp Res*. 2004;16:373, Figure 4, with permission.)

and this was more pronounced in fall-prone older adults. These results further support studies indicating that older adults (especially fallers) have a less efficient sensory reintegration capacity, which can further disrupt balance control.

Changes in steady-state balance, as indicated by increased postural sway and the need for close guarding, can be seen in the postural control segment of Bonnie's case study video.

Change in Base-of-Support Strategies: Stepping and Reaching

When do compensatory steps during balance recovery cause falls? Table 9.1 shows features of compensatory stepping and reaching reactions related to aging and increased fall risk (Maki & McIlroy, 2006). Note that taking one or more additional steps after the initial stepping response during recovery is associated with both aging and fall risk. Moreover, older adults have a deficiency in the execution of these reactive steps, which may be associated with an elevated risk of falls (Shulman et al., 2019). Using a side-step sequence (SSS) more frequently results in balance recovery compared to a crossover step (COS) (Borrelli et al., 2019a). Thus, a SSS during recovery is associated with aging, but sustaining limb collisions during lateral stepping is associated with both aging and falls. Finally, slowed initiation and execution of reach-and-grasp movements is associated with both aging and falls. The presence of multiple steps during recovery was also reported by Mille et al. (2013), who noted that among older adult fallers, interlimb collisions during recovery from lateral instability were increased compared to nonfallers and younger adults.

The need for multiple steps and assistance to prevent a fall may be seen in the postural control segment of Bonnie's video. In response to both small and large perturbations, Bonnie is unable to recover stability without the physical assistance of another person. She does step, but her steps are insufficient to recover her stability.

What are the potential mechanisms that underlie the need for multiple steps among balance-impaired older adults? Ochi et al. (2014) used EMGs to investigate the characteristics of stepping responses in older women (mean age 81) with and without a history of falls. Older adults with a history of falls had a shorter step length and slower step velocity compared to nonfallers. EMG time to peak in the gastrocnemius (which provides the push-off force prior to foot-off) was slower in fallers, and there was increased coactivation of agonist and antagonist muscles during stepping. The authors suggest that impairments in muscle activation patterns among older adults who fall contribute to an inability to recover stability using a single step.

With repeated exposure to perturbations requiring a step, some older adults, who initially used multiple steps to recover, adapt their responses such that they are able to use a single step by the 4th trial (Barrett et al., 2012). However, the degree to which this type of adaptation is retained is unclear; thus, its relevance to preventing falls in the real world (which occur on the first, not the fourth, trial) is uncertain. For example, in another study by König and colleagues (2019), older adults had the ability to adapt to repeated trip-like perturbations during gait (by maintaining a stable stance after a single recovery step) but needed more recovery steps during the first trial compared with young adults.

TABLE 9.1 Features of Compensatory Stepping and Reaching Reactions Related to Aging and Increased Falling Risk

Feature of the reaction	Example	Significant association with	
		Aging	Falling risk
Stepping reactions			
Takes one or more additional steps after the initial stepping reaction	NOTE: arrow indicates direction of falling motion	Yes	Yes (AP falls)
Follows a forward or backward stepping reaction with one or more lateral steps		Yes	Yes (ML falls)
Tends to use a side-step sequence (SSS), rather than a crossover step (COS), during lateral stepping reactions	SSS; COS	Yes	No
Sustains limb collisions during lateral stepping reactions (during stance but particularly when walking in place)		Yes	Yes (AP falls)
Reaching reactions			
Initiates arm movements despite instructions not to move the arms		Yes	Yes (AP falls)
Slowed initiation and execution of reach-to-grasp movements		Yes	Yes (all falls)

AP, anteroposterior; *ML*, mediolateral.

Adapted from Maki BE, McIlroy WE. Control of rapid limb movements for balance recovery: age-related changes and implications for fall prevention. *Age Ageing*. 2006;35–S2:ii14.

Nevertheless, older adults were not able to retain the initially acquired recovery response adaptations 14 weeks after experiencing the repeated trials and just like in the first trial of the training, they required more than one recovery step. Moreover, for all adults, the perturbation-training did not generalize to an untrained lean-and-release task, despite both tasks' similarities in reactive gait stability. The authors put forth the hypothesis that reactive balance control is rapid, task specific, and independent of age, but retention of these learning effects is age dependent and there is limited inter-task transfer (this is illustrated in Fig. 9.7).

Similar to the stepping response, adults may display an arm reaction induced by a sudden loss of balance. When a handrail is present, these arm reactions often (71% of times) involve a reach-to-grasp reaction. But in the absence of a handrail, the induced arm movement occurs in effort to either counterbalance the falling motion (27% of times) or to protect against impact (13% of times). Thus, these arm reactions are dependent on task conditions and protective reactions are relatively infrequent (Borrelli et al., 2019b). Older adults display a delay in these arm reactions. Komisar and colleagues (2019) tested the time and speed of a reach-to-grasp balance reaction while adults walked along an 8° slope mounted to a robotic platform. They saw that aging was associated with slower EMG latency, reduced hand acceleration time, and increased hand deceleration time.

It is also important to note that holding a cane interferes with grasping a handrail during balance recovery

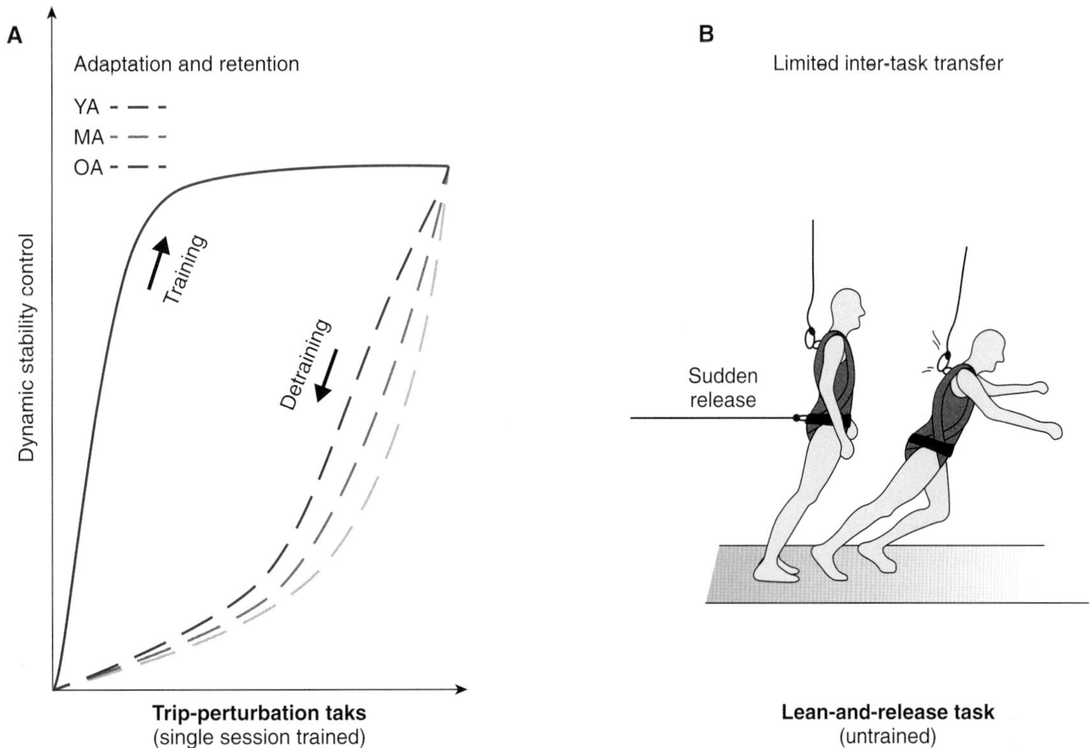

Figure 9.7 A schematic illustration of adaptability of reactive balance control. **(A)** The acquisition of reactive stability is independent of age, as indicated by the observed similar rates and magnitudes of balance recovery-response adaptations due to trip-perturbations training in young (*YA*), middle-aged (*MA*), and older adults (*OA*) (Training). Retention of learning diminishes with increasing age (Detraining). **(B)** Adaptations to gait-trip perturbation training does not transfer to an untrained balance task (lean-and-release task), despite the similarity of the reactive stability control mechanisms. (Adapted from König M, Epro G, Seeley J, et al., Retention and generalizability of balance recovery response adaptations from trip perturbations across the adult life span. *J Neurophysiol.* 2019;122:1890, Figure 6.)

(Bateni et al., 2004a, 2004b). When subjects had either a cane or just a cane top, they seldom reached for a handrail, and when the rail was not contacted, balance was lost. This suggests that when we have something in our hands, the nervous system gives priority to that object rather than reaching to aid in balance.

In summary, these data suggest that older adults with and without balance problems show changes in the motor systems affecting postural control and that these can contribute significantly to an inability to maintain balance. Some of these motor system changes include (a) muscle weakness; (b) impaired timing and organization among synergistic muscles activated in response to instability; and (c) limitations in the ability to adapt movements for balance in response to changing task and environmental demands.

Clinical Implications of Reactive Balance

Research suggests that it is important to evaluate the following aspects of reactive balance control in older adults: (a) the type of motor strategy used for balance recovery (e.g., the use of in-place versus stepping [including use of single versus multiple steps] or reaching strategies); (b) the timing and speed of response (e.g., does the patient sway a prolonged period of time when given a nudge to the sternum, before recovering?); (c) the sequence of muscle activation (this can be seen by examining interjoint coordination problems, such as buckling at the knees during recovery); and (d) adaptation (e.g., the ability to modify the response to changing sizes of a manual perturbation).

Changes in Anticipatory Postural Control

Postural adjustments are often used in a proactive manner, to stabilize the body before making a voluntary movement. Adults in their 70s and 80s may begin to have more difficulty maneuvering in the world because they have lost some of their ability to integrate balance adjustments into ongoing voluntary movements such as lifting or carrying objects. Thus, it is important to study the effects of age on the ability to use postural responses proactively within the context of voluntary movements. It is under these dynamic conditions, including walking, lifting, and carrying objects, that most falls occur.

One of the first researchers to study age-related changes in anticipatory postural adjustments was Man'kovskii, from Russia (1980). He compared the characteristics of anticipatory postural responses and prime mover (voluntary) responses for young (19 to 29 years of age), medium old (60 to 69), and very old (90 to 99) adults who were asked to do the simple task of flexing one leg at the knee (prime mover response) while using the other leg for support (postural response), both at a comfortable and at a fast speed. Both the medium old adults and very old adults showed a slowing in both the postural (contralateral rectus femoris) and prime mover (ipsilateral biceps femoris) muscle response onsets for the movements at a comfortable speed, but this slowing did not result in an increased probability of losing balance. However, as shown in Figure 9.8, at the fast speeds, for both medium and very old adults: (a) the correlation between the postural and prime mover muscles decreased, and (b) there was a decrease in the time between the response onsets for postural and prime mover muscles. In the very old, postural and prime mover muscles were activated almost simultaneously. This inability to activate postural muscles far enough before the prime mover caused a loss of balance in many trials (Man'kovskii et al., 1980).

Impaired anticipatory postural control is evident in Bonnie, our balance-impaired older adult. In the postural control segment of her video, impaired anticipatory postural control is evident in her inability to reach forward, lean over and pick up an object, or step up onto a curb or box without loss of balance.

In Chapter 7, we mentioned that in the healthy young adult, the same postural response synergies that are activated during stance balance control are activated in an anticipatory manner before making a voluntary movement while standing. Thus, when a young adult is asked to pull on a handle, first the gastrocnemius is activated, followed by the hamstrings, trunk extensors, and then the prime mover muscle, the biceps of the arm. A slowing in onset of contraction or a disruption of the sequence of activation of these postural synergies could affect the ability of an older adult to make movements such as lifting objects.

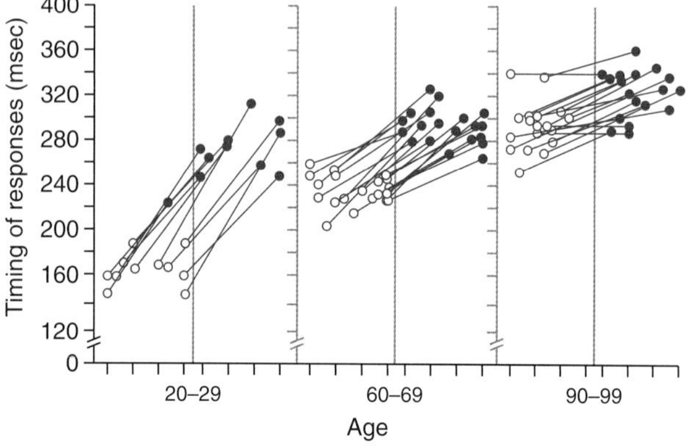

Figure 9.8 Timing of anticipatory postural responses (*open circles*) and prime mover (voluntary) responses (*filled circles*) for individuals in three age categories: 20 to 29 years, 60 to 69 years, and 90 to 99 years. (Adapted from Man'kovskii NB, Mints AY, Lysenyuk VP. Regulation of the preparatory period for complex voluntary movement in old and extreme old age. *Hum Physiol.* 1980;6:49, Figure 2.)

Experiments were performed to explore age-related changes in the ability of older adults to activate postural muscle response synergies in an anticipatory manner (Frank et al., 1987; Inglin & Woollacott, 1988). In one study, standing young (mean age, 26 years) and older (mean age, 71 years) adults pushed or pulled on a handle that was adjusted to shoulder level, in response to a visual stimulus. Results of the study showed that the contraction onsets of the postural muscles were significantly longer in the older adults than in the younger adults when they were activated in a complex RT task. There was also a large age-related slowing in onset time for voluntary muscles. According to a systems perspective, this slowing in voluntary RT in older adults could be caused either by the need for advanced stabilization by the already delayed and weaker postural muscles or to slowing in the voluntary control system itself. Since the absolute differences in onset times between the young and the older adults were larger for the voluntary muscles than for the postural muscles, there may be slowing in both systems in the older adult (Woollacott et al., 1988).

In a study of interactions between anticipatory and reactive postural control in a sit-to-stand task in older adults (Pai et al., 2003), older adults were given unexpected forward slips as they stood up from a chair. It was found that with repeated trials, the older adults made adaptive adjustments in advance (anticipatory control) to improve their stability. When exposed to both slip and nonslip trials, the older adults began to select optimal movements that improved stability under both conditions. The authors suggest that these results can be explained if it assumed that an internal representation of COM stability limits guides the improvements in the anticipatory control of stability.

Another study looked at the interactions between anticipatory and steady state postural control in older adults (Kasahara & Saito, 2019). The authors tested participants standing on a force plate while performing a forward movement of the center of pressure as fast as possible when they were given a visual cue; then participants were required to stop rapidly to match the center of pressure position with the target position on the monitor as accurately as possible. The reaction and movement times of the older-adult group were significantly longer than those of the younger-adult group. Moreover, the sequence of propulsion and braking was longer in the older-adult group.

The results of these studies suggest that many older adults have problems making anticipatory postural adjustments quickly and efficiently, especially without prior practice. This inability to stabilize the body in association with voluntary movement tasks such as lifting or carrying may be a major contributor to falls in many older adults.

Clinical Implications of Anticipatory Balance

The prevalence of impaired anticipatory postural activity and its detrimental effect on performance of voluntary functional tasks suggests it is a critical aspect of balance control to evaluate in aging adults. Clinical tests for evaluating anticipatory postural control, such as the Functional Reach test, are discussed in Chapter 11.

AGING IN THE SENSORY OR PERCEPTUAL SYSTEMS

How do changes in the sensory systems, which are important for posture and balance control, contribute to declining stability as people age? The following sections review changes within individual sensory systems and then examine how these changes affect stability in quiet stance as well as our ability to recover from loss of balance.

Changes in Individual Sensory Systems

Somatosensory

Studies have shown that *vibratory* sensation threshold at the great toe increases threefold by the age of 90 (Kenshalo, 1979). Vibratory thresholds in general increase more in the lower extremities than in the upper extremities. In fact, in some cases, researchers reported an inability to record vibratory responses from the ankle, because many of the older subjects were not able to perceive sensation there (Whanger & Wang, 1974).

Many studies have shown that *tactile* sensitivity decreases with age, as measured by threshold to touch stimuli (Bruce, 1980; Kalisch et al., 2009) or passive motion (Barela et al., 2018). Researchers have documented a decline in fine touch and pressure or vibration sensation mediated by Meissner end organs and Pacinian corpuscles. Aging affects both the quantity and the quality of the Meissner and Pacinian corpuscles; however, it is thought that functional effects are determined primarily by the number of receptors lost. In addition to receptor loss, there is a decline of up to 30% of the sensory fibers innervating the peripheral receptors, causing peripheral neuropathy. The deficient somatosensation contributes to functional and subjective balance problems and increased fall risk in older adults (Hafström, 2018). Nevertheless, adding haptic input helps prevent falls in older adults. For example, a study by Oates and colleagues (2020) examined the effects of added haptic input—via light touch on a railing while walking—in older adults. They found that adding haptic input resulted in a more cautious gait pattern, improved balance and gait pattern, and increased muscle activity.

This peripheral neuropathy will cause increased reliance on other sensory systems, such as the visual and vestibular systems. Studies examining postural responses in patients with somatosensory deficits caused by peripheral neuropathy have shown significant delays in muscle response onset latencies in response to platform perturbations and an inability to modulate response amplitudes in relation to stimulus size. Figure 9.9A shows EMGs from a patient with peripheral neuropathy and a healthy subject in response to a platform perturbation. Figure 9.9B compares the

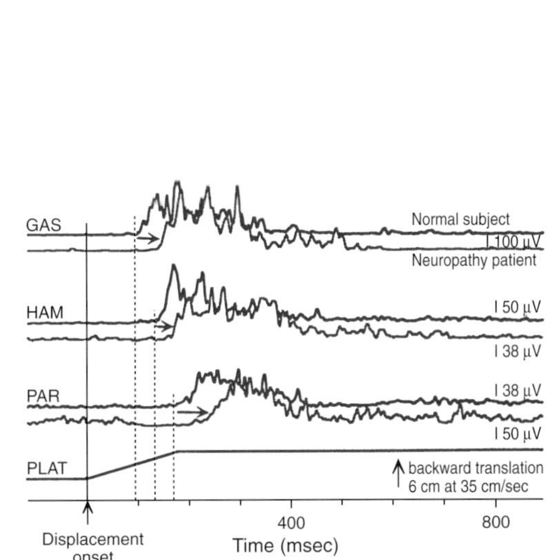

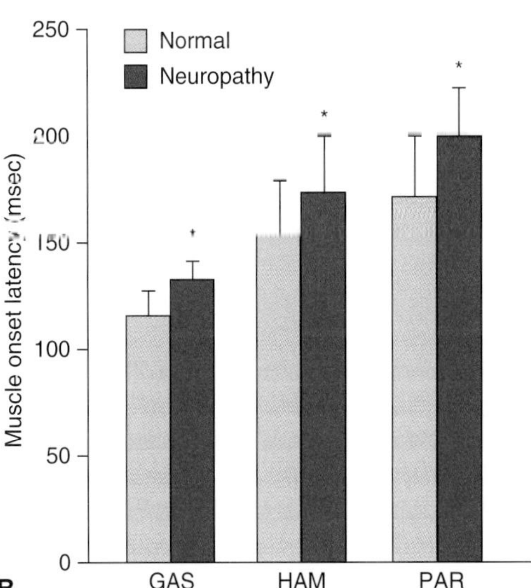

Figure 9.9 (A) EMGs from the leg and trunk muscles of a patient with peripheral neuropathy and a healthy subject in response to a platform perturbation. Note that EMGs from all recorded muscles slow equally. *GAS*, gastrocnemius; *HAM*, hamstrings; *PAR*, paraspinal muscles; *PLAT*, platform displacement. **(B)** Mean onset latencies for GAS, HAM, and PAR muscles in control subjects (normal) versus patients with peripheral neuropathy. (Reprinted from Inglis JT, Horak FB, Shupert CL, et al. The importance of somatosensory information in triggering and scaling automatic postural responses in humans. *Exp Brain Res*. 1994;101:161, with permission.)

onset latencies of muscles in the healthy subjects with those of the subjects with neuropathy. Note that EMGs from all recorded muscles slow equally (Inglis et al., 1994). Patients with multiple sclerosis show problems similar to those in patients with peripheral neuropathy (Jackson et al., 1995; Nelson et al., 1995).

In addition, osteoarthritis and accompanying reduced joint position sensitivity cause increased sway during quiet stance balance with either eyes open or closed in older adults. However, it does not affect reactive balance (McChesney & Woollacott, 2000).

Vision

Studies on the visual system show similar declines in function. Because of multiple changes within the structure of the eye itself, less light is transmitted to the retina; thus, the visual threshold (the minimum light needed to see an object) increases with age. In addition, there is typically a loss of visual field, a decline in visual acuity, and visual contrast sensitivity, which causes problems in contour and depth perception (Sturnieks et al., 2008). Loss of visual acuity can result from cataracts and macular degeneration, and loss of peripheral vision can be due to ischemic retinal or brain disease. These age-related changes in the visual system affect a broad range of functional skills, including postural control (Pastalan et al., 1973; Pitts, 1982). For example, a number of studies have indicated that age-related increases in sway during quiet stance become larger when visual cues are removed (eyes-closed condition) (Patla et al., 1990; Schultz et al., 1993; Sheldon, 1963; Wolfson et al., 1992).

As mentioned in Chapter 8, one can test the influence of vision on balance control by creating the illusion of postural sway through visual flow generated by an experimental moving room. Normally, young adults show small amounts of sway in response to visual flow giving the illusion of sway. A study by Wade et al. (1995) comparing the effects of visual flow on postural responses (COP measurements) in older adults indicated that healthy older adults show increased sway as compared with young adults under these conditions. The authors suggest that this may be due to decreased somatosensory information available to older as compared with younger subjects.

A second study, by Sundermeier et al. (1996), compared the effects of visual flow on postural responses of young, stable older, and unstable older adults. Figure 9.10A shows the paradigm used. As the room moves forward (a), the subjects perceive that they are swaying backward (b) and sway forward (c) to compensate. Figure 9.10B shows the COP responses of individuals in each group. As you can see, the unstable older adults showed significantly more reliance on the visual flow than did the young or stable adults as measured by COP. In addition, they showed continuing COP oscillations after the room movements had stopped. The investigators also noted that the unstable older adults used higher levels of sheer forces when compensating for the simulated postural sway, thus suggesting greater use of hip strategies even in response to visual perturbations to posture. When analyzing muscle response characteristics to these room movements, they found that when the room moved away from the

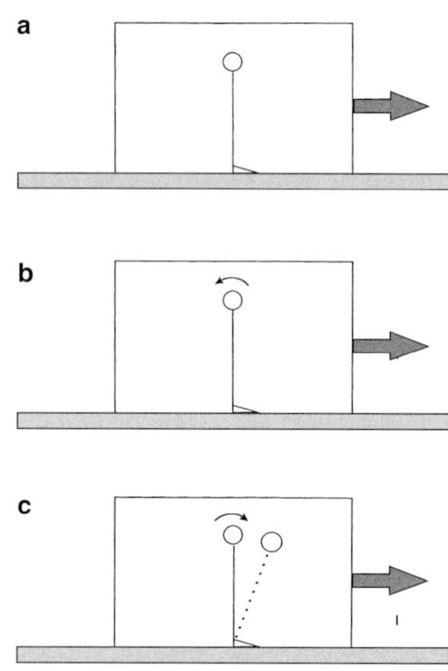

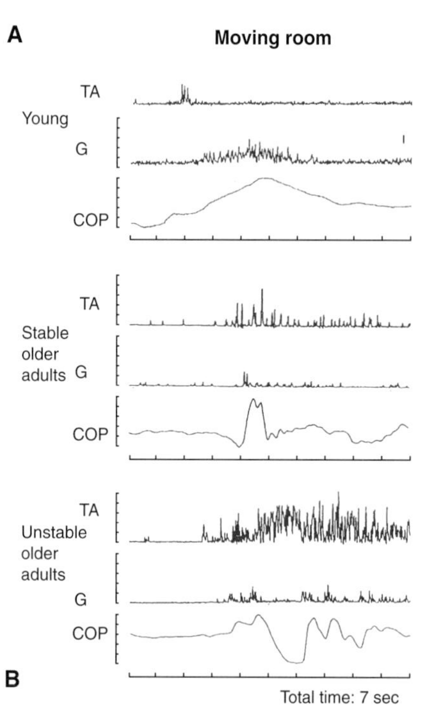

Figure 9.10 Effect of moving room on subject's sway. **(A)** Room moves forward (*a*) causing perception of backward sway (*b*) and active forward sway (*c*). **(B)** EMGs from tibialis anterior (*TA*), gastrocnemius (*G*), and COP movement versus time for young, stable, and unstable older adults in response to room movements. (Adapted from Sundermeier L, Woollacott M, Jensen J, Moore S. Postural sensitivity to visual flow in aging adults with and without balance problems. *J Gerontol.* 1996;51:M49, with permission.)

subjects, the unstable older adults used larger ankle dorsiflexor (TA) responses, which caused high amounts of sway in the forward direction (Fig. 9.10B).

In a similar study, Ring et al. (1988) used a visual image on a screen in front of subjects to create the illusion of movement toward the subject. In these "visual push" experiments, he noted that subjects who had recently fallen (within 2 weeks) and those who had fallen within the past year swayed significantly more than older adults (65 to 86 years of age) who had not fallen. He thus concluded that the visual push test might be capable of identifying older adults who are at risk for falls.

Another study looked at how adults quickly adjust their goal-directed hand movements to an unexpected visual perturbation (Zhang et al., 2018). They found that even though young and older adults tapped equally accurately to both visual stimuli (a target jump or background motion), the older adults took longer to respond in comparison to the younger adults, and were more sensitive to the motion of the background than the target jump, most likely because older adults relied more on visual information for maintaining balance.

Vestibular

The vestibular system also shows a reduction in function, with a loss of 40% of the vestibular hair and nerve cells by 70 years of age and a 3% loss per decade of vestibular nucleus cells from 40 to 90 years (Rosenhall & Rubin, 1975).

One of the functions of the vestibular system is that of an absolute reference system with which the other systems (visual and somatosensory) may be compared and calibrated (Black & Nashner, 1985). The vestibular system would be especially important for balance control in situations of visual and somatosensory system conflict. A decline in vestibular function with age would cause this absolute reference system to be less reliable, and thus the nervous system would have difficulty dealing with conflicting information coming from the visual and somatosensory systems. This may be the reason that older adults with vestibular deficits have problems with dizziness and unsteadiness when they are in environments with conflicting visual and somatosensory inputs.

In addition to the vestibular system's function as an absolute reference system, vestibular inputs contribute to the amplitude of automatic postural adjustments to balance threats. Thus, older adults with vestibular deficits would show postural responses that were inappropriately small (Allum et al., 1994).

Multisensory Deficit

"Multisensory deficit" is a term used to describe the loss of more than one sense important for balance and mobility functions (Brandt & Daroff, 1979). In many older people with multisensory deficits, the ability to compensate for the loss of one sense with alternative senses is not possible because of numerous impairments in all the sensory systems important for postural control. Indeed, the magnitude of multisensory integration is a strong predictor of balance performance and incidence of falls. A study by Mahoney and colleagues (2019) showed that older adults with decreased visual-somatosensory integration had decreased performance in a balance task (unipedal stance) and increased incident of falls.

Adapting Senses for Postural Control

In addition to showing declines in function within specific sensory systems, research from many labs has indicated that some older adults have more difficulty than do younger adults in maintaining steadiness under conditions in which sensory information for postural control is severely reduced (Brandt & Daroff, 1979; Horak et al., 1989; Peterka & Black, 1990–1991; Raffalt et al., 2019; Speers et al., 2002; Teasdale et al., 1991; Toupet et al., 1992; Wolfson et al., 1985; Woollacott et al., 1986).

To understand the contribution of vision to the control of sway during quiet stance in older adults, researchers examined sway under altered visual conditions. When young people closed their eyes, they showed a slight increase in body sway, and this was also true for healthy older adults (Teasdale et al., 1991; Woollacott et al., 1986).

In addition, when their eyes were open, healthy older adults were often as steady as young adults when standing on a compliant surface, such as foam, a condition that reduces the effectiveness of somatosensory inputs reporting body sway. However, when healthy older adults were asked to stand on a compliant surface with their eyes closed, thus using vestibular inputs alone for controlling posture, sway significantly increased as compared with young adults (Teasdale et al., 1991).

Several studies have examined the ability of healthy older adults to adapt senses to changing conditions during quiet stance using posturography testing (Horak et al., 1989; Peterka & Black, 1990; Speers et al., 2002; Wolfson et al., 1985; Woollacott et al., 1986). Most studies found that healthy active older adults did not show significant differences from young adults in the amount of body sway (Fig. 9.11), except under conditions in which both ankle-joint inputs and visual inputs were distorted or absent (conditions 5 and 6). In one study, increased variability of shank and hip angles was found for older adults in conditions 2 (eyes closed), 4 (somatosensory inaccurate, eyes open), 5 (somatosensory inaccurate eyes closed), and 6 (somatosensory and vision inaccurate). The authors suggested that the increased sway in the older adults was due to their decreased ability to detect small movements of the platform (Speers et al., 2002).

When both visual and somatosensory inputs for postural control were reduced (conditions 5 and

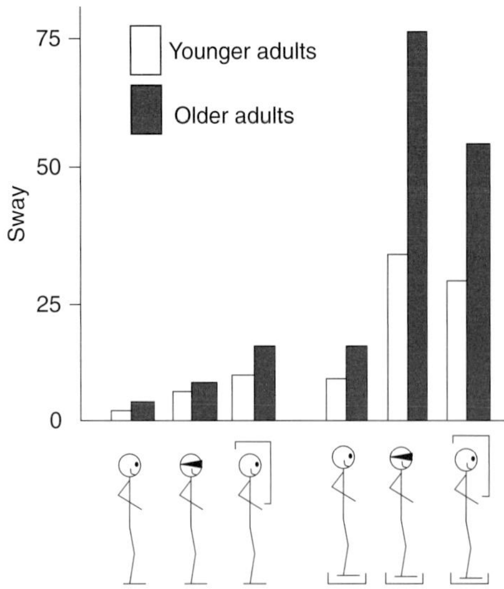

Figure 9.11 Comparison of body sway in the six sensory conditions in young versus active older adults. (Adapted from Woollacott MH, Shumway-Cook A, Nashner LM. Aging and posture control: changes in sensory organization and muscular coordination. *Int J Aging Hum Dev.* 1986;23:340.)

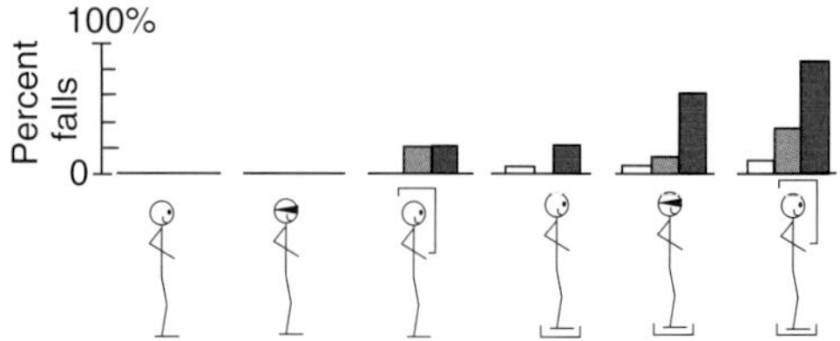

Figure 9.12 Comparison of number of falls in the six sensory conditions in young adults, older adults with no history of falling, and older adults with a history of falling. Open bar = adults 20 to 39 years old; lightly shaded bar = adults >70 years old who had no history of falling; darkly shaded bar = adults >70 years old who had a history of falling. (Reprinted from Horak F, Shupert C, Mirka A. Components of postural dyscontrol in the elderly: a review. *Neurobiol Aging*. 1989;10:732, with permission.)

6), half of the older adults lost their balance on the first trial for these conditions and needed assistance. However, most of the older adults were able to maintain balance on the second trial within these two conditions. Thus, they were able to adapt senses for postural control, but only with practice in the condition (Woollacott et al., 1986).

These results suggest that healthy older adults do not sway significantly more than young people when there is a reduction in the availability or accuracy of a single sense for postural control. However, in contrast to young adults, reducing the availability of two senses appears to have a significant effect on postural steadiness in even apparently healthy older adults.

Are the changes summarized above the result of an inevitable decline in nervous system function, or are they the result of borderline pathology in specific subsystems contributing to postural function?

To determine whether evidence of borderline pathology existed in subjects who participated in a postural study and who considered themselves fit, active older adults, researchers gave each subject a neurologic exam and then correlated the existence of borderline pathology with performance on the balance tasks. Although all the older adults considered themselves to be healthy, a neurologist participating in the study found neural impairment, such as diminished deep tendon reflexes, mild peripheral nerve deficits, distal weakness in the TA and gastrocnemius muscles, and abnormal nystagmus in many adults in the population. Loss of balance in two subjects accounted for 58% of total losses of balance (Manchester et al., 1989).

These subjects had no history of neurologic impairment, but the neurologist diagnosed them as having borderline pathology of CNS origin. These results again suggest the importance of pathologies within specific subsystems contributing to imbalance in older adults, rather than a generalized decline in performance.

Other researchers have also studied the adaptation to changing sensory information during quiet stance in older adults (Horak et al., 1989). One group of older adults was active and healthy and had no history of falls (labeled "asymptomatic"). The second group was symptomatic for falling. Figure 9.12 illustrates some of the results of their study, showing that over 20% of the older adults (both symptomatic and asymptomatic) lost their balance when visual information was inaccurate for balance (condition 3), as compared with none of the young subjects, ages 20 to 39. Forty percent of the asymptomatic older adult patients lost their balance under condition 6, when both visual and somatosensory information were inaccurately reporting body sway. By contrast, less than 10% of the healthy young adults fell under this condition. The symptomatic older adult had a larger percentage of falls in any condition that was sway referenced, that is, with misleading somatosensory cues (conditions 4, 5, and 6).

This led researchers to conclude that the inability to select and weight alternative orientation references adaptively is a crucial factor contributing to postural dyscontrol in many older adults. This is especially true for those who are symptomatic for balance problems (Horak et al., 1989).

Another approach to studying adaptation of sensory systems involves the use of rotational movements of a platform. These experiments were described in more detail in earlier chapters. Results from platform rotation studies with older adults found that 50% of the healthy older subjects lost their balance on the first trial. However, all but one of the subjects was able to maintain their balance on subsequent trials (Woollacott et al., 1986). This finding could suggest a slower ability to adapt postural control in this population.

A propensity for falls in the first trial of a new condition is a recurring finding in many studies examining postural control in older adults (Horak et al., 1989; Peterka &

Black, 1990, 1991; Teasdale et al., 1991; Woollacott et al., 1986). Perhaps this means that slowing occurs, rather than a total lack of adaptability, in many older adults. A propensity to fall in new or novel situations could also be the result of impaired anticipatory mechanisms. Anticipatory processes related to postural control enable the selection of appropriate sensory and motor strategies needed for a particular task or environment.

Zettel et al. (2008) have explored whether there are age-related changes in the ability of older adults to use vision for clearing an obstacle during balance recovery. They found that older adults, like young adults, rarely looked downward for obstacle clearance when they were also performing a second visual task, though they usually cleared the obstacle effectively. This suggests that both young and older adults use stored visuospatial information, gained when they first enter a new environment, for stepping over obstacles. Kunimune and Okada (2019) further corroborated this by testing the role of the visual field in maintaining postural stability during obstacle crossing in young and older adults. Participants wore an accelerometer and liquid crystal shutter goggles while crossing an obstacle under three conditions: (a) full vision, (b) total visual field occlusion at two steps before the obstacle, and (c) lower visual field occlusion at two steps before the obstacle. The authors found no effect of visual condition. However, postural lateral instability was higher for older compared to younger adults. Thus, peripheral visual information appears to contribute minimally to the maintenance of stability during obstacle crossing, at least when participants have the chance to perceive the surrounding environment and the size of the obstacle well before approaching it.

Clinical Implications of Age-Related Change to the Sensory or Perceptual Systems

Research on age-related changes in the sensory systems important to postural control suggests that in addition to evaluating the integrity of individual sensory systems, it is important to examine sensory organization and adaptation during postural control. Evaluating the individual's ability to maintain stability under changing sensory conditions is critical to understanding the capacity to maintain stability under complex and changing environmental conditions.

COGNITIVE ISSUES AND POSTURE CONTROL

Mrs. Eulalia H, who is 80 years old, normally has no problems with falls. She is walking down a busy sidewalk in the city, talking to a friend, while carrying a fragile piece of crystal she just bought at the department store. Suddenly, a dog runs in front of her. Will she be able to balance in this situation as well as she does when she is walking down a quiet street by herself?

Eulalia's friend Mr. Shelby L has within the past 6 months recovered from a series of serious falls. These falls have led to a loss of confidence and fear of falling, which have resulted in a reduction in his overall activity level and an unwillingness to leave the safety of his own home. Can fear of falling significantly affect how we perceive and move in relation to balance control?

Determining the answer to these and other questions related to the complex role of cognitive issues in postural control may be a key to understanding loss of balance in some older adults.

As we mentioned in the first part of this chapter, the capacity of an individual, the demands of a task, and the strategies the person uses to accomplish a task are important factors that contribute to the ability of a person to function in different environments. As individuals get older, their capacities to perform certain tasks such as balance control may be reduced as compared with their abilities at age 20, but they will still be able to function in normal situations, in which they can focus on the task. However, when they are faced with situations in which they are required to perform multiple tasks at once, such as the one just described, they may not have the attentional capacity to perform both tasks, as attentional or information-processing capacity and processing robustness is reduced with aging (Gilchrist et al., 2008; Li et al., 2004). Among frail older adults, an inability to walk while talking (a dual task involving gait and a secondary cognitive task) is a predictor of future falls (Lundin-Olsson et al., 1997). In addition, performing a postural task (such as recovery of balance) in conjunction with another motor task (such as carrying a glass of water, or a tray loaded with items) can result in instability in many older adults (Papegaaij et al., 2012). Researchers are beginning to explore the question of how our attentional capacities affect our balance abilities in different environments (see Woollacott & Shumway-Cook, 2002 for a review).

We know from Chapter 7 that, as stability demands increase, attentional resources needed to maintain stability also increase. The question is, are attentional demands needed to maintain stability greater in older adults compared to young adults? Lajoie et al. (1996) compared attentional demands (using an auditory RT task) between young and older adults under increasingly difficult balance conditions. Results, summarized in Figure 9.13, demonstrate that even in the simplest condition (sitting), RTs were slower in older adults compared to younger adults. RTs became even slower in the older adults in the most difficult balance task (standing with a narrow support), suggesting that attentional demands increase in older adults compared to young adults when stability is challenged. It is not clear whether this is because attentional resources were

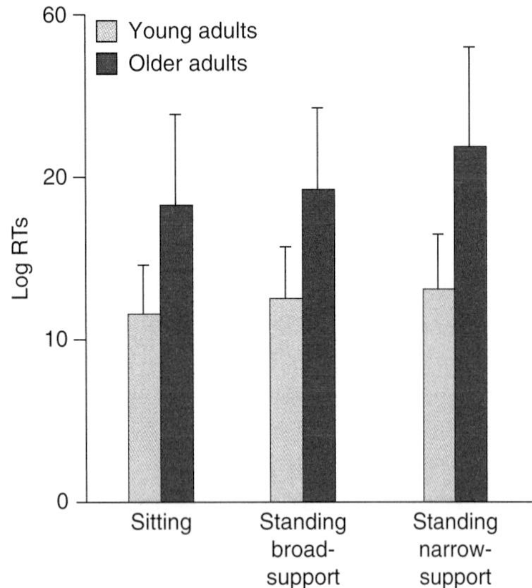

Figure 9.13 A comparison of RTs in older adults versus young adults under three postural conditions, sitting, standing with a broad base of support, and standing with a narrow base of support. (Adapted from Woollacott M, Shumway-Cook A. Attention and the control of posture and gait: a review of an emerging area of research. *Gait Posture*. 2002;16:6, Figure 5.)

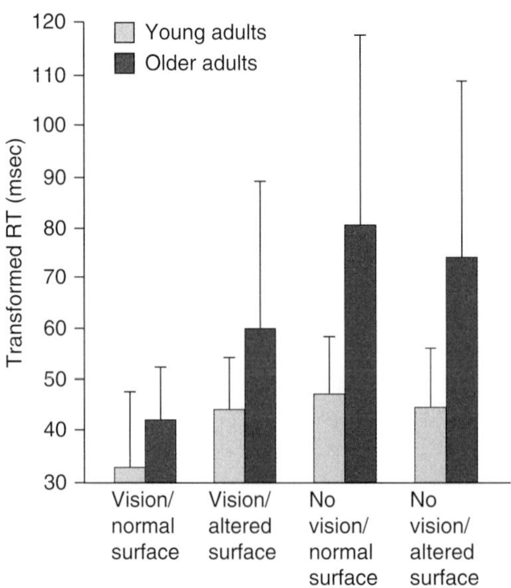

Figure 9.14 Transformed reaction time (RT) scores of young adults versus older adults for a dual-task paradigm consisting of an RT cognitive task and a postural task that was performed under four sensory conditions. Note that as sensory information decreased, RTs on the cognitive task became significantly longer for older adults as compared with young adults. This implies that the amount of attention used for postural control is dependent on the degree of instability inherent in the task. (Adapted from Teasdale N, Bard C, LaRue J, et al. On the cognitive penetrability of postural control. *Exp Aging Res*. 1993;19:8.)

limited in the older adults in this study compared to younger adults or if, in fact, postural control required more attentional resources.

If increasing the difficulty of the postural task requires more attentional processing in older adults than young adults, one might ask whether decreasing sensory information would also demand more attention and whether older adults would have more difficulty than young adults under these circumstances.

Teasdale et al. (1993) studied the balance (COP measurements) of young and older adults while sitting (control condition) versus standing with eyes open versus closed on a normal surface versus a foam surface. The foam surface was used to decrease sway-related somatosensory information available for balance control. They also measured RT on a secondary task, in which the subject pressed a button at the sound of an auditory cue. Figure 9.14 shows the RTs for the young versus older adults under the four conditions. Note that as sensory information decreased, RTs became significantly longer for both younger and older adults, but the effect was exaggerated in the older adults. This implies that the amount of attention is dependent on the degree of sensory input available during the task and that older adults require more attention than do young adults to perform tasks with reduced sensory input.

More recently, Doumas et al. (2008) asked how older adults share dual-task costs when balancing under the six sensory conditions of the Sensory Organization Test (described above), especially when sensory information from the different senses was in conflict or reduced. In this case, the cognitive task was the N-back task, in which participants continuously monitor a stream of numbers on a screen and must say the digit seen two or three cycles before (level of difficulty was chosen based on responses being 80% correct). They found that older adults on the stable surface had a 40% increase in sway in the dual-task condition, while the young adults did not. However, in the sway-referenced condition, the postural performances in the single- and dual-task conditions were the same, with a 15% increase in costs for the cognitive task in the dual-task condition. Why was this the case? On the stable surface, the older adults had the flexibility to increase their sway in the dual-task condition, as they diverted attention to the secondary task, as they were well within their stability limits. However, on the sway-referenced surface, they had high levels of sway, even in the single-task condition, and thus could not afford to divert attentional resources to the dual-task condition and increase sway, so instead, they diverted attention from the cognitive task and reduced the cognitive task performance. This shows the flexible nature of attentional resource allocation in healthy older adults.

How do older adults deploy sensory information under dual-tasks conditions? Dominquez-Zamora and colleagues (2020) looked at the different gaze patterns between young and older adults when navigating around a series of obstacles under dual-task conditions (walking while counting or looking for relevant landmarks). They found that older adults transferred gaze away from obstacles earlier and contacted obstacles more frequently than young adults. In addition, older adults had to allocate gaze to landmarks to a greater extend in the landmark-search condition to maintain a similar search performance during the dual-task condition compared to the single-task condition. Thus, older adults use different gaze strategies while navigating around a series of obstacles compared to young adults and have greater difficulty under dual-tasking conditions.

How does performing an attentionally demanding task affect postural sway in healthy older adults versus those with a history of falling? A number of laboratories have examined this question (Redfern et al., 2001; Shumway-Cook et al., 1997c; Shumway-Cook & Woollacott, 2000). Shumway-Cook et al. (1997c) examined the ability of young adults, healthy older adults, and older adults with a history of, or recent recurrent episodes of, falling to perform postural tasks of varying difficulty (standing on a normal surface versus foam) while performing cognitively demanding secondary tasks. They found that during the simultaneous performance of a postural and a cognitive task, there were decrements in performance in the postural stability measures rather than the cognitive measures for young adults, healthy older adults, and balance-impaired older adults. It is interesting that differences between the young and healthy older adults became apparent only when task complexity was increased—either by adding the secondary task or by adding the more challenging postural condition. However, balance-impaired older adults showed problems even in less-complex-task conditions.

The effect of a secondary task on postural sway in stance in older adults with and without a history of falls can be seen in Figure 9.15. Sway was larger in the older faller compared to the nonfaller, when each was standing quietly with no secondary task (boxes on the left). When a secondary task was added (a sentence-completion task), sway increased significantly in the faller (bottom right box) compared to the nonfaller (top right box).

Interestingly, the task of reintegrating sensory information after it has been removed causes increased attentional demands in older adults. In a study in which visual and ankle proprioceptive inputs were removed or perturbed and suddenly reinserted, older adults showed a faster COP velocity than did young adults when required to reintegrate proprioceptive inputs. This increased COP velocity in spite of the fact that there was increased availability of sensory information suggests that for older adults, sensory reweighting requires additional attentional resources as compared with young adults (Teasdale & Simoneau, 2001).

These experiments examined attentional constraints on older adults in quiet-stance situations, but it would also be important to know whether recovery from

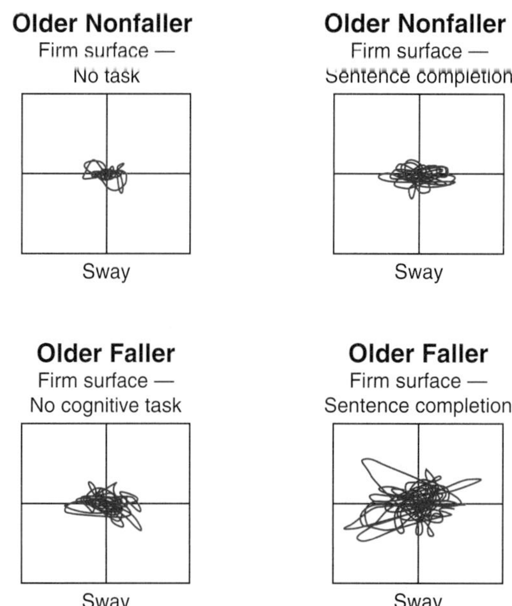

Figure 9.15 A comparison of displacement of the COP when standing on a firm surface with no secondary task (no task) versus standing and performing the sentence completion task (dual-task condition) in an older adult with no history of falls and an older adult with a history of falls. (Adapted from Shumway-Cook A, Woollacott, M. Baldwin M, et al. The Effects of Two Types of Cognitive Tasks on Postural Stability in Older Adults With and Without a History of Falls. *J Gerontol A Biol Sci Med Sci.* 1997;52A:M237, Figure 4.)

perturbations to stance requires more attention for older than for young adults, thus contributing to an increased likelihood of falls in these situations. To explore this, Brown et al. (1999) asked older and younger subjects to respond to unexpected platform displacements either with no secondary task or while performing a math task (count backward by threes). They found that attentional requirements for the recovery of balance are higher for older adults than for young adults. Performing a secondary task caused subjects to step earlier when using a stepping strategy. It is interesting to note that the postural muscle responses of the older adults were smaller when performing the secondary cognitive task. This may have been the reason the subjects were required to step earlier; their muscle responses were too small to use an in-place strategy (Rankin et al., 2000).

In a second study exploring the temporal dynamics of attention during postural perturbations in young versus older adults, Redfern et al. (2002) asked participants to perform a simple visual or auditory RT task at different delays from the onset of a platform perturbation. They found that RT was slowed (more for auditory than for visual cues) both before and during the platform movement, particularly for the older adults; however, by 250 msec after the perturbation, the effects had disappeared.

This type of study was extended to compare the effects of a secondary task on balance recovery

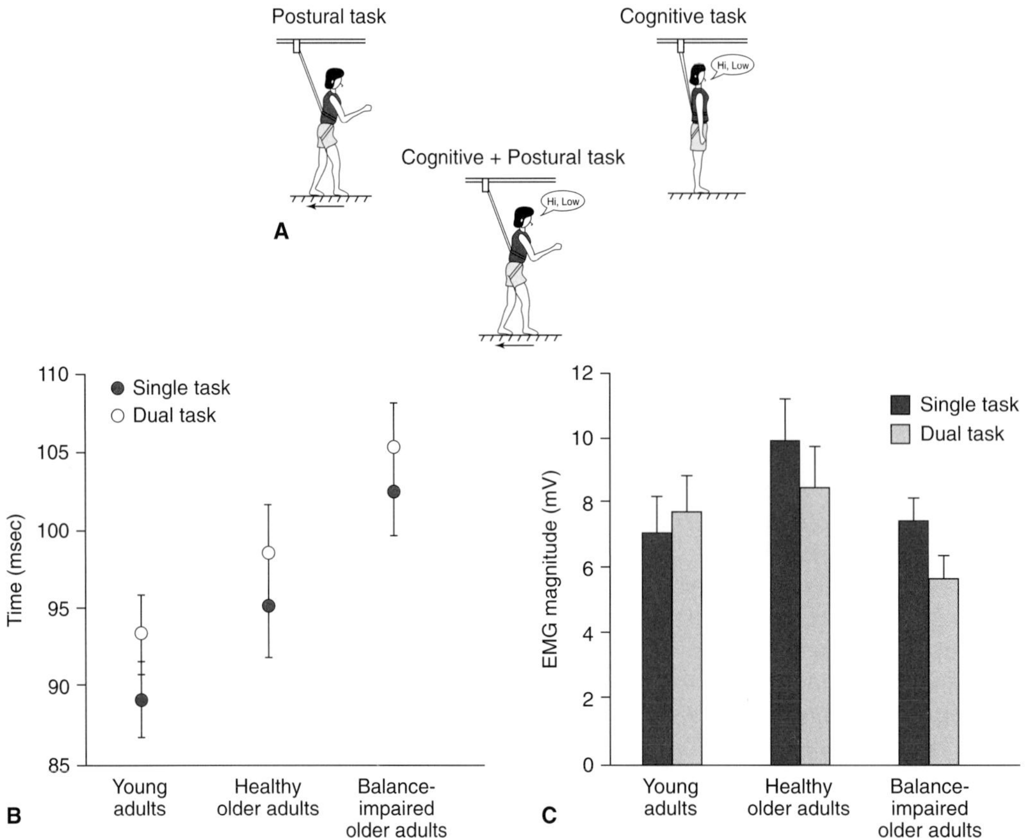

Figure 9.16 Single- and dual-task paradigms. **(A)** Postural and cognitive task performance is measured in isolation ("postural task" and "cognitive task") and when performed simultaneously ("cognitive + postural task"), and differences are compared between single- and dual-task conditions. **(B)** Time of contraction onset for the gastrocnemius muscle for young, healthy older adults and balance-impaired older adults in the single- versus dual-task conditions. Note that all three groups show delays in the dual-task as compared with the single-task conditions, in addition to the delays in responses associated with age and balance impairment. **(C)** Changes in muscle response (EMG) magnitude of the gastrocnemius muscle for the three subject groups in the single- and dual-task conditions. Note that the healthy older and balance-impaired older adults show a reduction of response amplitude in the dual-task condition. (Reprinted from Brauer SG, Woollacott M, Shumway-Cook A. The influence of a concurrent cognitive task on the compensatory stepping response to perturbations in balance-impaired and healthy elders. *Gait Posture*. 2002;15:91, Figure 4, with permission.)

from a perturbation in balance-impaired older adults (Brauer et al., 2001, 2002). Results showed that balance-impaired older adults took a longer time to regain a stable posture in the dual-task condition than when responding to the postural task alone. When a compensatory step was required to regain balance, RTs were longer in all subjects than when recovering balance with an in-place strategy and longer in balance-impaired older adults than in young adults (see Fig. 9.16A for a picture of the dual-task paradigm). The authors noted that this difference between young and balance-impaired older adults may have been related to prioritization of the two tasks, rather than to attentional demands, because the older adults completed the step before the RT task, while the young adults performed both concurrently.

Healthy older adults and balance-impaired adults also showed a delayed muscle response onset and reduced response amplitude when taking a compensatory step in the dual-task paradigm as compared with young adults. This is shown in panels B and C of Figure 9.16. Note that the time of onset of the gastrocnemius muscle response is delayed for young, healthy, and balance-impaired older adults (B) and muscle response magnitude is reduced for both healthy and balance-impaired older adults (C) in the dual-task condition.

Although many studies have explored differences in postural performance between those with a history and those with no history of falling, very few have explored the effect of fear of falling on the control of balance. There is now experimental evidence that anxiety and fear of falling affect the performance of older adults on tests of balance control (Maki et al., 1991; Tinetti et al., 1990). As a result, older adults probably modulate strategies for postural control based on their perception of the level of postural threat. Thus, older adults who have a great deal of anxiety about falling related to poor perceptions regarding their level of balance skills will move in ways that reflect these perceptions. More work is needed to fully understand the relationship between fear of falling and postural control. Lab Activity 9.2 applies many concepts discussed in this chapter.

LAB ACTIVITY 9.2

Objective: Through the interview process, to explore the balance abilities of a healthy versus a balance-impaired older adult, and to define possible events that led up to their current functional status.

Procedure: Find two older adults in your community who you can interview, one who is very active and has good balance and the other with balance problems and a history of falling. In your interview, ask the following questions:

1. What is your age?
2. Do you exercise regularly? If so, how much?
3. Have you had any medical problems that have affected your balance abilities?
4. Ask them to try standing in a tandem Romberg position (one foot in front of the other) for 20 seconds. Time their attempt.
5. Ask them to get up out of a chair, walk 10 feet, turn around, and walk back, sitting down again in the chair. Using a watch with a second hand, determine the time taken for the task (Timed Up and Go [TUG] test).

Assignment: Write up an evaluation of each of the older adults, based on the following information:

1. Where do you think each of the people you interviewed would fit on Spirduso's (2005) scale: Physically Elite, Physically Fit, Physically Independent, Physically Frail, and Physically Dependent.
2. What do you think are their physiological ages as compared with their chronological ages?
3. Compare their performance on the static balance task and on the TUG test. How did each of them do when getting up out of the chair during the TUG test?
4. What do you think are factors contributing to their current balance status?

A CASE STUDY APPROACH TO UNDERSTANDING AGE-RELATED POSTURAL DISORDERS

Bonnie B is a 90-year-old woman with impaired balance resulting in multiple falls, two of which required hospitalization. Bonnie lives alone in an apartment; she has a home health aide who comes in 3 times a week for 4 hours to assist her with shopping, cooking, cleaning, and laundry. Bonnie's main concerns relate to her declining balance. She is increasingly fearful because of her multiple falls.

Bonnie has a number of underlying sensory, motor, and cognitive impairments that are illustrated in the impairment section of her case study video. She has reduced spinal flexibility that constrains her ability to rotate her trunk. She has reduced strength in her arms and legs and is able to move against gravity but cannot take any additional resistance. She has age-related changes in vision and reduced somatosensory sensitivity. In addition, she has bilateral sensorineural hearing loss and a previous history of vertigo, due to partial loss of vestibular function. Bonnie has mild cognitive deficits affecting her memory and executive function.

These sensory, motor, and cognitive impairments all contribute to her significantly impaired postural control, which can be seen in the postural control segment of her case study video. Bonnie is able to sit unsupported with her feet on the floor. She is able to stand unassisted, but requires close supervision when not holding on to her walker, suggesting impaired steady-state balance in stance.

Bonnie has impaired reactive balance control and uses her arms to recover stability in response to both small and large perturbations. However, as can be seen in her video, she requires assistance to prevent a fall. Researchers have shown that impaired reactive postural activity in older adults like Bonnie affects both in-place and stepping strategies. Impaired strategies (both in-place and stepping) are due to slower muscle responses, inappropriate temporal coordination among proximal and distal muscles, smaller amplitude, and increased coactivation of agonist and antagonist muscle groups. In the case of stepping responses, multiple steps are often required, and there is frequent interlimb collision, particularly during lateral stepping.

Bonnie has impaired sensory organization that contributes to her instability in certain environments. Though she requires close guarding, she is able to stand on a firm surface with her eyes open, a condition in which all three senses are available for balance control. When standing on a firm surface with her eyes closed, she shows increased sway and requires assistance. She is unable to stand on the foam surface with her eyes open or closed. This pattern suggests Bonnie has difficulty maintaining her balance when any sensory input for postural control is reduced. This is consistent with her complaints of loss of balance when walking on carpeted surfaces or in areas with low lighting levels. When taking a shower, she must use a shower stool since she cannot maintain balance and close her eyes to wash her hair.

Bonnie has significantly impaired proactive balance control, which reduces her ability to perform tasks such as leaning and reaching forward, or leaning over to pick up an object from the floor. She has had several falls in her apartment trying to pick up objects from the floor and now uses an assistive device (extended reacher) to assist her in picking up objects from the floor. She is unable to step up or down without assistance even with her walker. Researchers have found delayed onset of anticipatory postural adjustments associated with voluntary movements in many older adults.

Finally, Bonnie has significant problems maintaining balance under dual-task conditions. This is due to several causes, including decreased attentional capacity and the increased attentional demands associated with maintaining stability under even the simplest postural conditions.

As you can see, many factors contribute to Bonnie's impaired balance control. Some of these factors reflect age-related changes in the systems important to balance control. Others are less related to aging and more related to her sedentary lifestyle. Balance impairments significantly affect Bonnie's life. They reduce her independence and significantly increase her likelihood for future falls. Because she has had several fall-related injuries, she is very fearful of falling again and is restricting her activity level because of this.

SUMMARY

1. Many scientists believe that factors contributing to aging can be considered either primary or secondary. Primary factors, such as genetics, contribute to the inevitable decline of neuronal function in a system. Secondary factors are experiential, and include nutrition, exercise, insults, and pathologies.
2. Researchers in all areas find much heterogeneity in function among older adults, suggesting that assumptions about declining physical capabilities cannot be generalized to all older adults.
3. Unintentional injuries are the seventh leading cause of death in older adults, and falls make up two-thirds of these deaths. Falls in older adults have multiple contributing factors, including intrinsic physiological and musculoskeletal fac tors and extrinsic environmental factors. Understanding the role of declining postural and balance abilities is a critical concern in helping to prevent falls among older adults.
4. Older adults typically show impaired reactive control with delays in the onsets of muscle responses and smaller response magnitudes, resulting in a longer time required to restabilize balance. Activation of postural responses during anticipatory or proactive balance control is often delayed, causing instability in performing tasks such as leg lifting or opening a door. In addition, when sensory inputs for balance control are reduced or distorted, older adults have difficulty maintaining balance and sway excessively or lose balance. Finally, many falls occur due to impaired postural responses under dual-task conditions.
5. Many factors can contribute to declining balance control in older adults who are symptomatic for imbalance and falls. Researchers have documented impairments in all of the systems contributing to balance control; however, there is no one predictable pattern that is characteristic of all older adults with a history of falling.
6. On a positive note, there are many older adults who have balance function that is equivalent to that of young people, suggesting that balance decline is not necessarily an inevitable result of aging. Experiential factors such as exercise can aid in the maintenance of good balance and decrease the likelihood for falls as people age.

ANSWERS TO LAB ACTIVITY ASSIGNMENTS

Lab Activity 9.1

Question 1. Responses will differ, depending on the person interviewed.

Lab Activity 9.2

Questions 1, 2, 3, 4. Results will differ, depending on the people interviewed.

CHAPTER 10

Abnormal Postural Control

Learning Objectives

Following completion of this chapter, the reader will be able to:

1. Discuss changes to steady-state balance in persons with neurologic pathology and describe some of the factors contributing to impaired steady-state balance.
2. Discuss the effects of neural pathology on postural movement strategies used to recover stability following an unexpected perturbation during quiet stance and sitting. Give examples of sequencing and timing problems that affect the coordination of postural motor responses; discuss the neural pathology likely to result in these types of problems.
3. Discuss the effect of impaired segmental trunk control on steady-state, reactive, and anticipatory balance control in sitting.
4. Discuss the influence of impaired anticipatory postural control on voluntary movement; discuss the neural pathology likely to result in these types of problems.
5. Describe the effect of different types of sensory problems on steady-state, reactive, and anticipatory postural control; describe impaired perceptions important to the control of posture.
6. Discuss the effect of different types of cognitive problems on steady-state, reactive, and anticipatory postural control.
7. Compare and contrast postural control deficits found in persons with stroke, Parkinson's disease, cerebral palsy, cerebellar ataxia, and multiple sclerosis.

INTRODUCTION

Balance is critical to independence in activities of daily living (ADLs). Impairments in postural control producing loss of stability have a profound impact on the daily life of individuals with neurologic pathology. The consequences of impaired stability include loss of functional independence, reduced or restricted participation in ADLs, reduced confidence in the ability to perform ADLs safely, and increased risk for falls.

Falls in Persons with Neurologic Pathology

Falls are a major problem among persons with neurologic pathology, with prevalence varying by diagnosis and setting. The rate of falls among survivors of stroke ranges from 25% to 46% and appears to be a problem at all stages in the recovery process (Ashburn et al., 2008; Divani et al., 2009; Nyberg & Gustafson, 1997; Teasell et al., 2002; Ugur et al., 2000). Falls following stroke vary by setting and acuity, from 36% among acute stroke survivors to 46% in chronic survivors of stroke living in the community (Divani et al., 2009; Kerse et al., 2008; Lamb et al., 2003; Nyberg & Gustafson, 1997). Many falls occur while performing complex walking tasks; inability to safely walk over obstacles is a predictor of falls among persons with stroke (Said et al., 2013).

Approximately 15% of falls require medical attention (Divani et al., 2009), with a reported fourfold increase in the risk for hip fracture (Smith et al., 2001), due to an increased incidence of osteoporosis in both paretic and nonparetic limbs (Jørgensen et al., 2000; Poole et al., 2009; Ramnemark et al., 1999).

Falls are also a significant problem in Parkinson's disease (PD), with fall rates ranging from 40% to 68% (Ashburn et al., 2001; Bliem et al., 2001; Gray & Hildebrand, 2000; Wielinski et al., 2005; Wood et al., 2002; Woodford & Walker, 2005). In addition, fall rates are high among persons with multiple sclerosis (MS) (Cattaneo et al., 2002; Finlayson et al., 2006; Matsuda et al., 2009; Nilsagård et al., 2009a, 2009b; Peterson et al., 2007, 2008). As was true for older adults, the majority of falls in persons with neurologic pathology are associated with mobility, occurring during walking, transfers, and stair climbing (Forster & Young, 1995; Lamb et al., 2003; Matsuda et al., 2009; Nilsagård et al., 2009a, 2009b; Teasell et al., 2002).

Impaired balance has been found to be a major risk factor for falls among all persons with neurologic pathology, underscoring the importance of recovery of balance control in these populations (Ashburn et al., 2001; Bloem et al., 2000; Finlayson et al., 2006; Harris et al., 2005; Hyndman & Ashburn, 2003; Marchese et al., 2003; Matsuda et al., 2009; Nilsagård et al., 2009a, 2009b).

In the therapeutic environment, the ability to retrain postural control to improve balance requires a conceptual framework that incorporates information on the physiological basis for normal postural control as well as knowledge regarding the basis for instability. Our understanding of the physiological basis for instability comes from research examining postural control in different categories of neurologic pathology, such as post-cerebrovascular accident hemiparesis, traumatic brain injury, PD, MS, cerebellar disorders, and developmental disorders such as Down syndrome and cerebral palsy (CP). This has led to an understanding of the different types of sensory, motor, and cognitive problems that underlie impaired steady-state, reactive, and anticipatory postural control. As we shall see, often the same type of postural control problem (e.g., delayed onset of postural responses) can manifest in a wide variety of neurologic disorders.

We begin by exploring studies that have examined problems in the motor systems of postural control affecting the ability to (a) maintain a stable position (steady-state balance), (b) recover stability following a perturbation (reactive balance), and (c) prevent instability by activating postural muscles in advance of a potentially destabilizing voluntary movement (anticipatory balance) in persons with neurologic deficits. We will also review studies exploring the effect of sensory/perceptual problems on these three aspects of postural control. Finally, research examining the effects of cognitive problems on postural control will be reviewed. The chapter will conclude with a summary of postural control problems in our case studies in order to provide an understanding of the types of problems found in people with different types of neurologic diagnoses.

PROBLEMS IN THE MOTOR SYSTEMS

Problems in the motor systems contributing to abnormal postural control include impairments in both neuromuscular and musculoskeletal systems. Many of the most common neuromuscular and musculoskeletal problems resulting from neurologic pathology were discussed in detail in Chapter 5 and thus will not be repeated here. The focus instead will be on problems affecting the ability to activate and coordinate muscle activity in order to maintain, recover, or prevent loss of stability when standing or sitting.

Impaired Steady-State Balance

Impaired steady-state balance leading to an inability to maintain a stable standing or seated position has enormous functional consequences for persons with neurologic pathology. Inability to assume and maintain a stable position from which to move often necessitates using the arms for support and balance, thus limiting the availability of the arms for functional tasks of daily living. In addition, impaired steady-state balance increases the risk for falls and injury. As discussed in Chapter 7, a number of factors contribute to steady-state stability, including body alignment, muscle and postural tone, and movement strategies that control spontaneous sway.

Alignment

Alignment of the body refers to the relationship of body segments to one another as well as to the position of the body with reference to the surroundings, gravity, and the base of support. Alignment of body segments over the base of support determines to a great extent the effort required to support the body against gravity. In addition, alignment determines the constellation of movement strategies that will be effective in controlling posture. Changes in initial position or alignment are often characteristic of a person with a neurologic deficit. Abnormalities in alignment can reflect changes in the alignment of one body part to another or in alignment of the center of mass relative to the base of support.

The characteristically stooped posture of persons with PD is an example of changes in the alignment of body segments with respect to vertical. Stooped posture results from a forward trunk inclination and increased flexion at the hips and knees. This typical stooped posture may be seen in the postural control segment of the video case study on Mike, our patient with PD. Stooped posture in persons with PD may result from both neuromuscular impairments, such as flexor rigidity, and secondary musculoskeletal limitations, such as reduced trunk motion and spinal flexibility (Schenkman, 1990).

Children with CP frequently show restricted range of motion in many joints, including the ankle, knee, and hip. Contractures of the hip, knee, and ankle muscles result in atypical postural alignment in sitting (Fig. 10.1A) and standing (Fig. 10.1B and C) that cause postural control deficits (Domagalska-Szopa & Szopa, 2017; Abd El-Nabie & Saleh, 2019). Atypical posture in both sitting and standing may also be seen in the postural segment of the video case study on Thomas, our child with spastic diplegia CP. Postural alignment influences how muscles are recruited and coordinated for recovery of stability. For example, in their study on postural control in children with spastic diplegia, Burtner and colleagues (1999) found that the children with spastic diplegia who maintained a crouched (flexed knees and hips) stance posture showed significant coactivation of

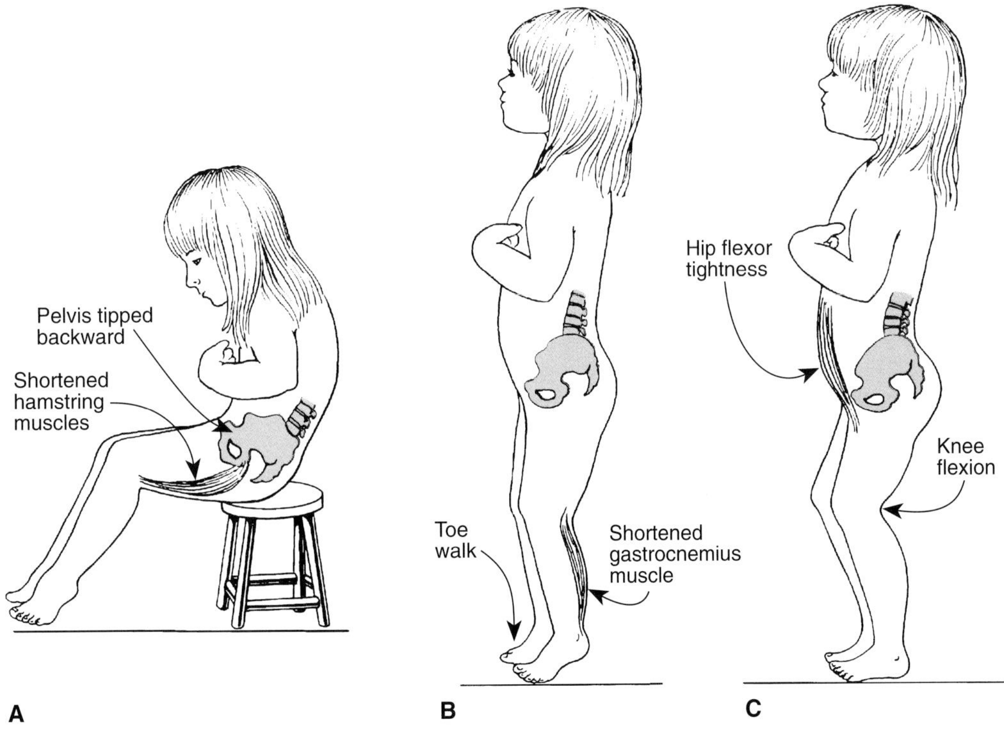

Figure 10.1 Atypical postures due to musculoskeletal impairments. **(A)** Excessive posterior tilt of the pelvis in sitting accommodates shortened hamstrings. **(B)** Shortening of the gastrocnemius muscle results in toe walk. **(C)** Hip flexor tightness can result in tilting of the pelvis and flexion of the knee. (Adapted from Reimers J. Static and dynamic problems in spastic cerebral palsy. *J Bone Joint Surg.* 1973;55:822-827.)

leg and trunk muscles during recovery of balance following a perturbation. Interestingly, healthy children standing in a crouched position, mimicking the posture of the children with diplegia, used antagonistic muscles more often in response to platform perturbations, suggesting that the musculoskeletal constraints associated with standing in a crouched posture may play a significant role in the atypical postural muscle response patterns seen in children with spastic diplegia, described in more detail in the section on impaired movement strategies during perturbed stance (Burtner et al., 1999; Woollacott et al., 1998).

Abnormal alignment can also be expressed as a change in the position of the body with reference to the environment, gravity, and the base of support. For example, upright stance among individuals who have had a stroke is characterized by weight-bearing asymmetry (WBA), with more weight on the nonparetic leg (Duncan & Badke, 1987; Shumway-Cook et al., 1988).

Asymmetric alignment following stroke may also develop as part of a compensatory strategy. As shown in Figure 10.2A, the lateral shift in body alignment and asymmetric weight-bearing seen in a person with hemiplegia compared to a healthy control (see Fig. 10.2B) may be due to perceptual impairments related to body scheme. Stroke patients may lack the ability to make use of the afferent information pertaining to standing postural sway, which in turn relates to their postural asymmetry. For example, Pollock and colleagues (2019) found that the ankle plantarflexion muscle activation in patients with stroke was not attuned to changes in anterior–posterior sway in the

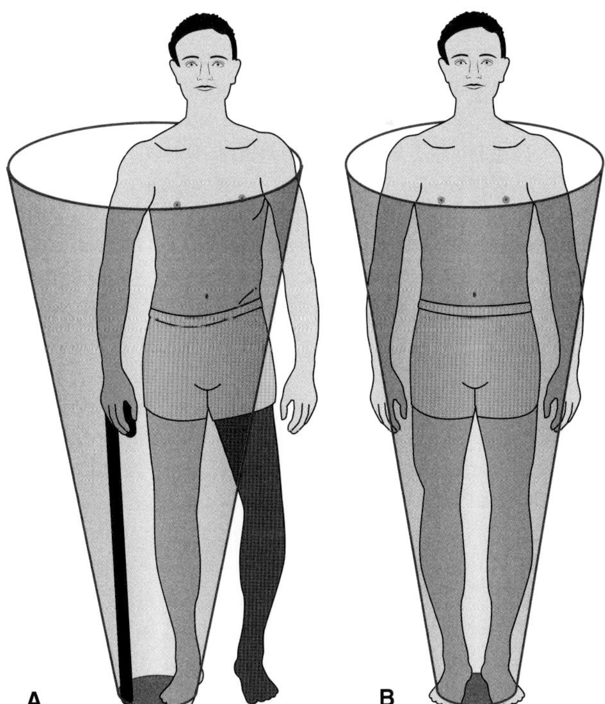

Figure 10.2 Asymmetrical alignment and stability limits in a person with stroke **(A)** compared to a healthy control **(B)**.

paretic leg compared to the nonparetic leg. Alternatively, persons with hemiplegia may develop a strategy to compensate for motor impairments, such as paresis in the hemiparetic leg, which is no longer capable of supporting the body's weight. Both Genise and Jean, our patients with hemiparesis secondary to a cerebral vascular accident, stand with an asymmetric posture. (See postural control segments of both video case studies.) Understanding these differences is important, since achieving a symmetrically aligned position may not be a reasonable goal for the person with hemiplegia until underlying impairments have resolved sufficiently to ensure that the hemiparetic leg will not collapse under the weight of the body.

Many persons with neurologic deficits stand with the center of mass displaced either forward or backward. For example, it has been reported that older adults with a fear of falling tend to stand in a forward-lean posture, with the center of mass displaced anteriorly (Maki et al., 1991). However, persons with other types of postural deficits stand with the center of mass displaced posteriorly (Shumway-Cook & Horak, 1992). Changes in body alignment influence many aspects of postural control, including the characteristics of body sway in quiet stance and the way muscles are activated during recovery of stability following a perturbation.

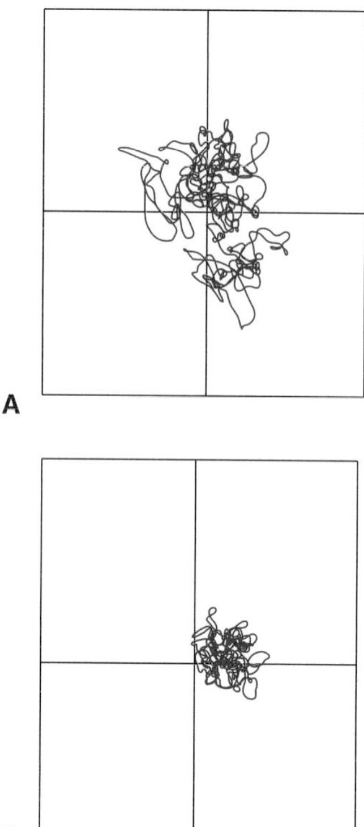

Figure 10.3 Changes in COP during quiet stance in a person in the early stages of PD off levodopa medication **(A)** and on medication **(B)**. (Adapted from Beuter A, Hernández R, Rigal R, et al. Postural sway and effect of levodopa in early Parkinson's disease. *Can J Neurol Sci*. 2008;35:67.)

Postural Sway

One of the most common approaches to assessing stability during quiet stance is the use of single or dual force plates to quantify characteristics of the center of pressure (COP) excursion. While most studies use COP trajectories as an indicator of sway and thus a sign of postural stability, Patla and colleagues (2002) demonstrated that the changes in the COP may also be related to joint moments needed to maintain body alignment and prevent collapse of the body with respect to gravity.

Individuals with PD have abnormal postural sway in stance, including increased sway area and velocity (Rocchi et al., 2004). Increased mediolateral sway has been reported in several studies (Beuter et al., 2008; Viitasalo et al., 2002), while anteroposterior sway has been reported as comparable to normal in one study (Viitasalo et al., 2002) but increased in another (Rocchi et al., 2002). Rocchi and colleagues reported that treatment with levodopa increased postural sway abnormalities, while treatment with deep brain stimulation improved postural sway (Rocchi et al., 2004, 2006). In contrast, in a study on people in the early stages of PD, levodopa significantly reduced postural sway in quiet stance. Figure 10.3 illustrates changes in COP displacement in a person with PD off medication (A) and on medication (B). Differences in postural sway on and off medication may also be seen in the postural control segment of Mike's case study video.

Pathology in different parts of the cerebellum may result in directionally specific increased postural sway (Dichgans & Fetter, 1993; Diener et al., 1984a, 1984b; Mauritz et al., 1979; Sullivan et al., 2006). Several studies have reported that pathology in the spinocerebellar (upper vermal and intermediate) part of the anterior lobe results in predominantly anteroposterior body sway, with a frequency of about 3 Hz (Dichgans & Fetter, 1993; Diener et al., 1984a, 1984b; Mauritz et al., 1979; Sullivan et al., 2006). Lesions of the lower (vestibulocerebellar) vermis are associated with increased omnidirectional postural sway, while lesions of spinocerebellar afferents (Friedreich's ataxia) are associated with a low-frequency, large-amplitude lateral sway pattern (Dichgans & Fetter, 1993; Diener et al., 1984a, 1984b; Mauritz et al., 1979). Finally, among patients with anterior-lobe cerebellar pathology, postural sway was significantly increased in the absence of visual inputs but reduced with additional orientation inputs from the somatosensory system (light fingertip touch) (Sullivan et al., 2006). In the postural control segment of the case study on John, our patient with spinocerebellar degeneration, he stands with a wide base of support, and when asked to stand with feet shoulder width apart, postural sway is significantly increased.

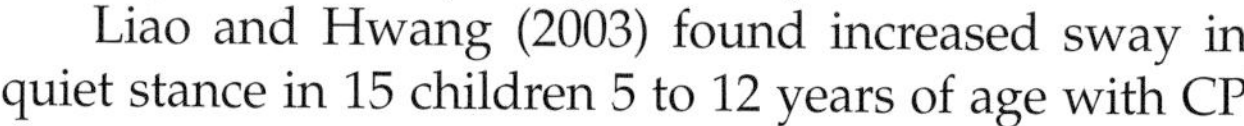
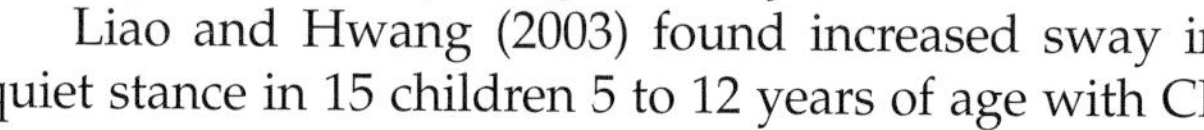

Liao and Hwang (2003) found increased sway in quiet stance in 15 children 5 to 12 years of age with CP (type not specified) and reported that postural stability in the eyes-closed condition was the best predictor of gross motor function. Rojas and colleagues (2013) showed that children with diplegic CP have increased sway with either eyes open or closed compared with children with hemiplegia. However, not all children with diplegic CP demonstrate abnormal postural sway in quiet stance. In a study of 23 ambulatory children and adolescents with spastic diplegia CP (518 years of age), the majority (14) had normal standing balance values (Rose et al., 2002).

Donker and colleagues (2007) used a dynamical analysis to examine the structure of COP trajectories in 10 children with CP and 9 typically developing (TD) children in quiet stance with eyes open, eyes closed, and while performing a concurrent visual feedback task, which created a more external focus of attention. They reported that sway amplitude was larger and more regular in children with CP as compared with TD children (Donker et al., 2007; Roerdink et al., 2006). In addition, providing concurrent visual feedback, which created a more external focus of attention, decreased both the amount and the regularity of sway. Similarly, when TD infants, premature infants, and infants with CP were tested in a seated motor task that was associated with focused attention (visual-manual exploration of a toy), TD infants and infants with CP made fewer trunk/pelvic movements in comparison to when they were not exploring the toy (Berger et al., 2019). This is consistent with the proposal by Wulf and colleagues (2001) that adopting an external focus of attention—focusing on the action outcome instead of the movement *per se*—is beneficial when performing or learning a motor skill. In contrast, an internal focus of attention (e.g., directing attention to one's own body) is detrimental because it disrupts the automatic control of posture and movement (for a review, see Wulf & Prinz, 2001; see also, McNevin & Wulf, 2002; McNevin et al., 2003; Wulf et al., 2001).

Several researchers have quantified COP trajectories following stroke, reporting both asymmetrical and increased sway area in quiet stance (DiFabio & Badke, 1991; Genthon et al., 2008; Shumway-Cook et al., 1988). These studies have shown that many factors contribute to WBA following stroke, including motor weakness (Bohannon, 1990; Genthon et al., 2008), asymmetric muscular tone (Pérennou, 2005), somatosensory deficits (DiFabio & Badke, 1991; Genthon et al., 2008), and neglect syndrome and distorted body scheme (Pérennou, 2006). In addition, spatial cognitive disorders, such as impaired perceptions related to visual vertical and postural vertical, may also be involved (Barra et al., 2009; Bonan et al., 2006; Genthon et al., 2008).

Does asymmetrical stance alignment improve over time? A number of researchers have examined the recovery of stance postural control following stroke (de Haart et al., 2004; Geurts et al., 2005; Roerdink et al., 2009). de Haart et al. (2004) did a longitudinal follow-up of 30 patients after stroke to examine the contribution of paretic and nonparetic limbs to stance postural control. This study used two force plates to study COP under each limb separately at baseline (when patients were first able to stand for 30 s unsupported) then at 2, 4, 8, and 12 weeks later. Patients stood under three conditions, eyes open, eyes closed, and while performing a math task (dual-task condition). Early in recovery, there was significant asymmetry in stance, with increased area and velocity in the nonparetic as compared with the paretic limb. Sway area and WBA both improved significantly with follow-up assessments; however, the nonparetic limb continued to provide the majority of dynamic stabilization. Changes in sway under the three conditions over time are shown in Figure 10.4. The authors suggest that increased WBA and lateralized control (active control by the nonparetic limb) are effective compensatory strategies for maintaining a stable stance position, particularly in patients with significant motor impairments. In addition, they suggest that rehabilitation strategies to reduce WBA in patients with severe motor impairments of the paretic limb may not be advisable, since this may be a reasonable compensatory strategy in the face of significant motor, sensory, and cognitive impairments.

Functional Stability Limits

As discussed in Chapter 7, a main goal of the postural control system is to ensure stability by controlling the center of mass relative to functional stability limits. Stability limits are determined in part by the biomechanics of the body but are also influenced by other factors, including subjective perceptions, postural control abilities, and environmental factors (Holbein & Redfern, 1997; Mancini et al., 2008). Functional limits of stability are often quantified by asking an individual to lean as far forward or backward as possible and recording the maximum COP

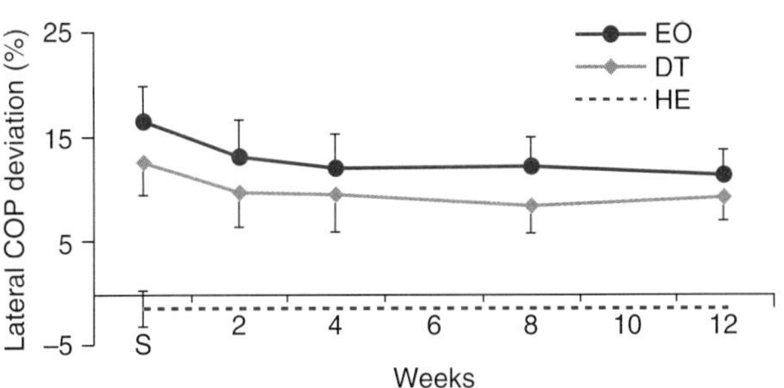

Figure 10.4 Changes in postural sway over a 12-week period in patients with stroke standing with eyes open (*EO*) and while performing a dual task (*DT*). Also shown is postural sway in healthy older adults (*HE* shown as a *dotted line*) over the same 12-week period. (Adapted from de Haart M, Geurts AC, Huidekoper SC, et al. Recovery of standing balance in postacute stroke patients: a rehabilitation cohort study. *Arch Phys Med Rehabil.* 2004;85:886–895.)

excursion (Adkin et al., 2005; Bartolic et al., 2005; Mancini et al., 2008; Schieppati et al., 1994; van Wegen et al., 2001). Figure 10.5 compares the response of two older adults who have been asked to lean as far forward as they safely can in order to explore functional stability limits. The older adult man (A) is able to sway forward, while the older adult woman (B) flexes at the hips in order to avoid moving the COM forward relative to her base of support (BOS). When asked to lean back, she steps (C).

Reduced limits of stability as indicated by reduced COP excursion during voluntary leaning have been reported among children with developmental coordination disorder (DCD) (Fong et al., 2016), adults with MS (Karst et al., 2005), and persons with PD (Adkin et al., 2005; Bartolic et al., 2005; Mancini et al., 2008; Schieppati et al., 1994; van Wegen et al., 2001). The use of levodopa improves functional limits of stability in subjects with PD (Mancini et al., 2008). Several factors may contribute to reduced forward functional limits of stability in PD, including stooped posture (Bloem et al., 1999; Mancini et al., 2008), increased rigidity, and impaired postural preparation for the voluntary leans (Mancini et al., 2008).

Steady-State Balance in Sitting

In a prospective study on steady-state sitting balance involving 93 patients with stroke, 48% were unable to sit independently at the onset of rehabilitation, while 27% were still unable to sit at the end of rehabilitation (Mayo et al., 1991). Moreover, patients with acute stroke were more unsteady (greater sway) than were healthy controls during unsupported sitting tasks (Genthon et al., 2008; Harley et al., 2006). Along this line, people with spinal cord injury (SCI), regardless of whether their spinal lesion is low thoracic (T_7–T_{12}) or high thoracic (T_1–T_6), demonstrate increased postural sway during a 30-s unsupported static sitting (Chen et al., 2003b). In a 30-s seated task, with and without vision, individuals with SCI shows impaired steady-state balance control in the anteroposterior and mediolateral directions compared to healthy controls. This lack of static sitting control was characterized by increased COP range and postural sway variability (Serra-Añó et al., 2013).

Sitting balance has also been shown to be a good prognostic indicator of functional outcomes following stroke (Feigin et al., 1996; Kwakkel et al., 1996; Loewen & Anderson, 1990; Morgan, 1994; Sandin & Smith, 1990) and traumatic brain injury. Impaired sitting balance on admission to rehabilitation was associated with dependence in locomotion and transfers at discharge and at 1 year after traumatic brain injury (Duong et al., 2004). Black et al. (2000) followed 237 patients with traumatic brain injury who were admitted to a rehabilitation unit and found that, next to age, the ability to sit independently at admission was the best predictor of scores at discharge on the functional independence measure (FIM).

Studies have also confirmed the importance of age of sitting onset as a predictor of walking in children with neurologic pathology; studies report that sitting by 18 to 24 months predicts walking outcomes in children with spastic diplegia forms of CP (Badell-Ribera, 1985; Wu et al., 2004b).

An important component of steady-state sitting balance is control of the trunk. Clinicians and researchers have often modeled the trunk as a single segment. However, more recent research has questioned this model, suggesting that a segmental control of the trunk may be critical to achieve or fully recover seated postural control. As we saw in Chapter 8, development of trunk control underlying steady-state sitting balance in TD

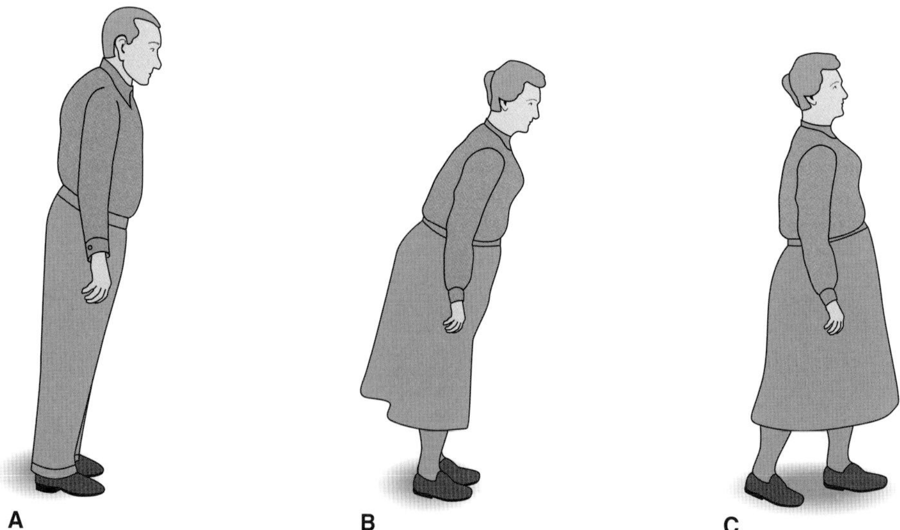

Figure 10.5 Functional stability limits in two older adults. When asked to sway forward to his limits of stability, the older adult man **(A)** is able to sway forward, bringing his COM forward over his BOS. In contrast, the older adult woman **(B)** bends at the hip, avoiding forward movement of her COM, and, when asked to lean back **(C)**, steps. (Adapted from Horak FB, Shupert CL, Mirka A. Components of postural dyscontrol in the elderly: a review. *Neurobiol Aging*. 1989;10:727–738.)

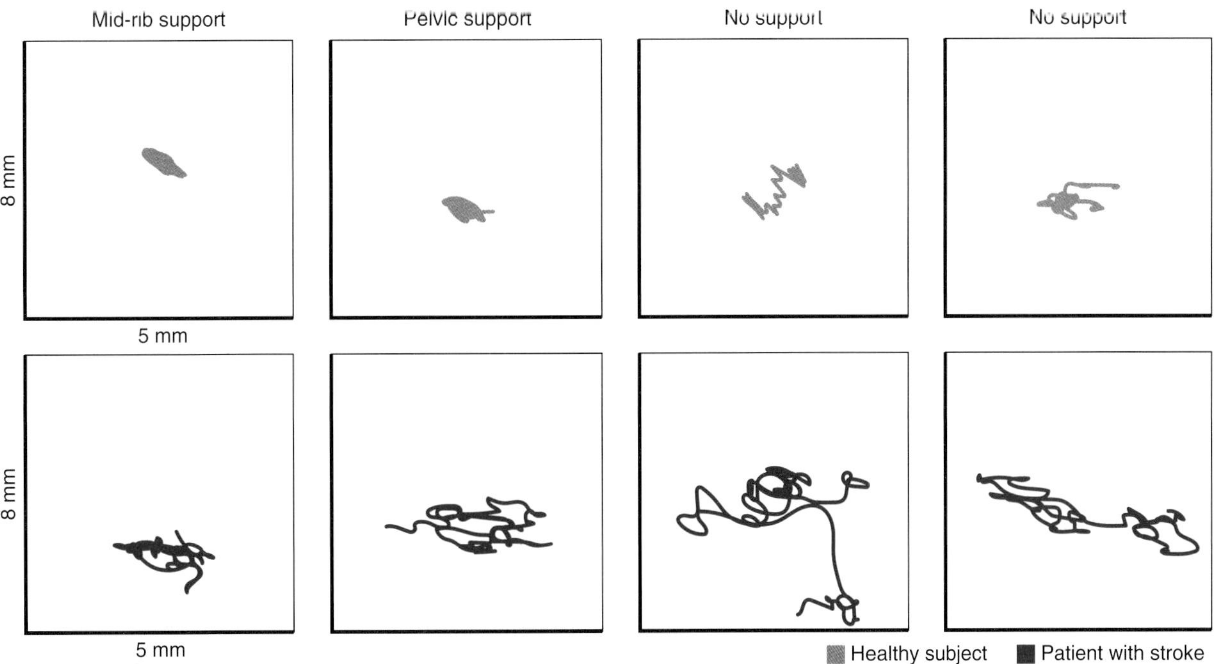

Figure 10.6 A comparison of external trunk support on steady-state postural sway in sitting. In a patient with stroke who has poor segmental trunk control, postural sway in the seated position decreases in direct proportion to the amount of external support that is provided to the trunk (lower trace). In contrast, a healthy age-matched control shows relatively little sway across all levels of support because he has intact segmental trunk control (upper trace) (Woollacott M, unpublished data).

children involved sequential development of control over successive segments of the trunk in a top–down order (Rachwani et al., 2015; Saavedra et al., 2012). Researchers have begun to demonstrate that among patients with neurologic pathology, development or recovery of sitting balance follows a similar pattern. As shown in Figure 10.6, in a patient with stroke who has poor segmental trunk control, postural sway in the seated position decreases in direct proportion to the amount of external support that is provided to the trunk (lower trace). In contrast, a healthy age-matched control shows relatively little sway across all levels of support because he has intact segmental trunk control (upper trace).

Impaired sitting balance is a characteristic of children with moderate-to-severe CP (Saavedra & Woollacott, 2015). In order to understand the contribution of segmental trunk control to seated balance control, researchers have quantified head and trunk kinematics under four levels of external support (axillae, midrib, waist, and hip) in children with moderate and severe CP (Gross Motor Function Classification Systems [GMFCS] levels IV and V). The apparatus used to provide the four levels of support is shown in Figure 10.7 (left column). Postural orientation and stability of the trunk were measured by evaluating angular displacement of estimated center of mass of the head in relation to a vertical line located at the center of the base of support. Results are shown in Figure 10.7 middle and right columns. With hip support alone, trunk stability (as indicated by head movement) in the children with CP is significantly impaired. This can be seen in the lowest part of Figure 10.7, which traces head movement relative to the base of support (showing both alignment and stability) in two children with CP (GMFCS IV on the left and GMFCS V on the right). As the level of trunk support increased from hips up through axillae, trunk stability significantly improved in both children, as can be seen by the decreased motion of the head. When no or minimal support was provided to the severely involved child (GMFCS level 5), he showed no capability for controlling the head or any portion of the trunk (lowest trace). However, when provided with support at a high level (upper thoracic), control of the head and trunk segments above the level of support emerged (upper two traces). Similarly, when a moderately involved child (GMFCS IV) was provided support at the low-to-midthoracic level, the ability to control the head and trunk segments above this level of support emerged (compare top two traces to the lowest trace). While stability improved in both children with external support, there were differences in alignment of the head relative to the base of support; the less involved child (GMFCS IV) maintained the head over the support, while the more involved child (GMFCS V) maintained the head forward and lateral to the base of support.

This research suggests that a critical part of understanding a child's capability for head and trunk control, and thus steady-state balance in sitting, is finding the optimal level of trunk support at which this behavior emerges (Saavedra & Woollacott, 2015). The effect

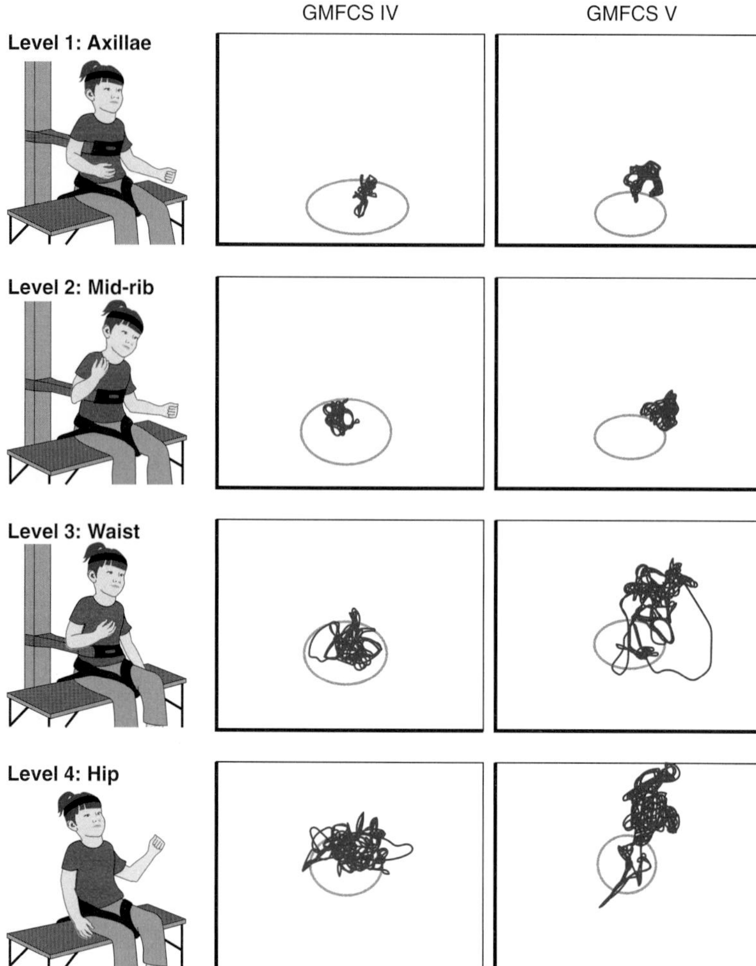

Figure 10.7 The apparatus used to provide four levels of trunk support in the seated position **(left)** and traces of head COM movement (*lines*) in relation to the base of support (*circle*) of a child classified as GMFCS level IV **(middle)** and V **(right)** during steady-state sitting at each level of support. As you see, in children with severe CP, trunk stability was inversely related to level of trunk support. (Adapted from Saavedra SL, Woollacott MH. Segmental contributions to trunk control in children with moderate-to-severe cerebral palsy. *Arch Phys Med Rehabil.* 2015;96(6):1088–1097.)

of external support on control of the head and trunk in space is also illustrated in the postural control segment of our case study of Malachi, our child with athetoid/spastic CP, and in the video on assessment and treatment of segmental trunk control.

Clinical Implications of Research on Steady-State Balance

As you can see from the research, assessment of steady-state balance in sitting or standing involves the examination of multiple factors, including alignment, postural sway, and stability limits. In addition, as we begin to appreciate the importance of segmental trunk control, particularly in seated postural control, the assessment of the ability to control different segments of the trunk will be important. New clinical tools such as the Segmental Assessment of Trunk Control (SATCo) and the Seated Postural and Reaching Control (SP&R-co) have been developed to examine segmental trunk control in steady-state, reactive, and proactive sitting balance. These measures will be discussed in more detail in Chapter 11.

Impaired Reactive Balance

A number of researchers have begun to explore how neurologic deficits influence the coordination of postural muscle synergies (both in-place and change-in-support strategies) that affect the ability to recover stability following an unexpected perturbation. Problems affecting the coordination of muscle response synergies are classified into (a) sequencing problems, (b) problems with the timely activation of postural responses, and (c) problems adapting postural activity to changing task and environmental demands.

Impaired In-Place Strategies

As discussed in Chapter 7, in-place strategies are defined by the ability to recover stability without changing the base of support. In stance, they are categorized as either an ankle or a hip strategy.

Sequencing Problems. One of the earliest studies reporting information on motor coordination problems affecting reactive balance was by Nashner and

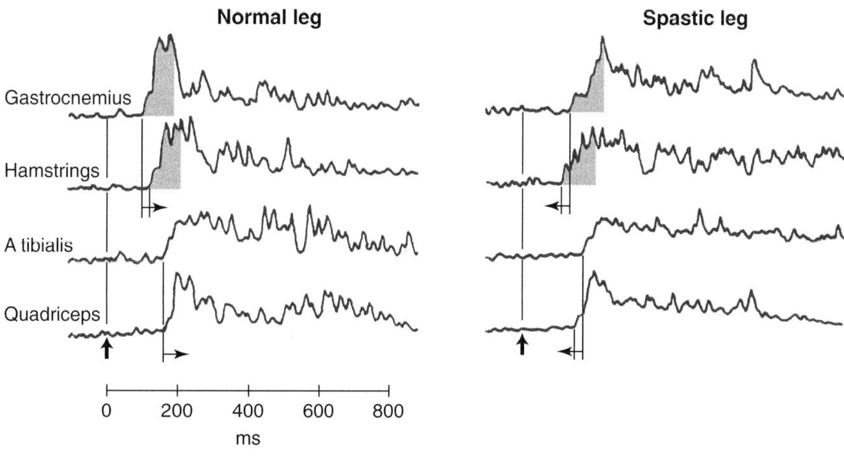

Figure 10.8 Abnormal sequencing of muscles in a child with hemiplegia responding to a backward translation of a moving platform. EMG recordings show an inappropriate activation of muscles responding to forward sway, with proximal muscles (hamstrings) activated in advance of the so-called spastic distal muscles (gastrocnemius). The upward arrow indicates the onset of platform movement. The horizontal arrows indicate the onset of muscle activity. (Reprinted from Nashner LM, Shumway-Cook A, Marin D. Stance posture control in select groups of children with cerebral palsy: deficits in sensory organization and muscular coordination. *Exp Brain Res*. 1983;49: 393–409, with permission.)

colleagues (1983), who studied reactive postural control in children with different types of CP. Ambulatory children (7 to 10 years of age) with different types of CP stood on a platform that perturbed stance balance in the forward or backward direction. Electromyograms (EMGs) and ground reaction forces were used to examine the coordination of leg muscles responding to this induced sway. Figure 10.8 is an example of the EMG records from one of the children with spastic hemiplegia. Shown is muscle activity (gastrocnemius, hamstrings, anterior tibialis, and quadriceps) in both the spastic hemiplegic and nonhemiplegic legs in response to a backward platform perturbation producing forward sway. The sequencing of muscle activity in the nonhemiplegic leg (labeled normal) began in the gastrocnemius muscle at approximately 100 ms, followed 30 ms later by activation of the hamstrings muscle. In contrast, muscle activity in the spastic leg began first in the hamstrings, followed 30 to 50 ms later by delayed activation of the gastrocnemius.

Burtner and colleagues (2007) also investigated reactive balance control in children with spastic diplegia CP as well as both age-matched and developmentally matched children. Children with CP stepped more frequently (or lost balance, being caught by the support harness they were wearing) at lower platform velocities than did either of the control groups. In addition, children with CP showed significant problems in scaling the muscle activity to changes in perturbations (Mills et al., 2018; Roncesvalles et al., 2002). Inability to recover stability following a gentle perturbation to stance balance may be seen in the postural control segment of Thomas, one of our children with spastic diplegia. Thomas was unable to recover from a small perturbation in any direction and had to be caught to prevent a fall.

What is the consequence of impairments in the timing and scaling of postural muscles responding to a loss of balance? This can be seen in Figure 10.9, which plots the COP trajectory in a TD child and one with CP. The recovery trajectory path in the typical child is much shorter, reflecting the normal timing and sequencing of muscle activity. In contrast, the COP recovery trajectory in the child with CP is much longer and has multiple reversal postural directions, reflecting impairments in the organization of muscle responses for recovering balance after the perturbation.

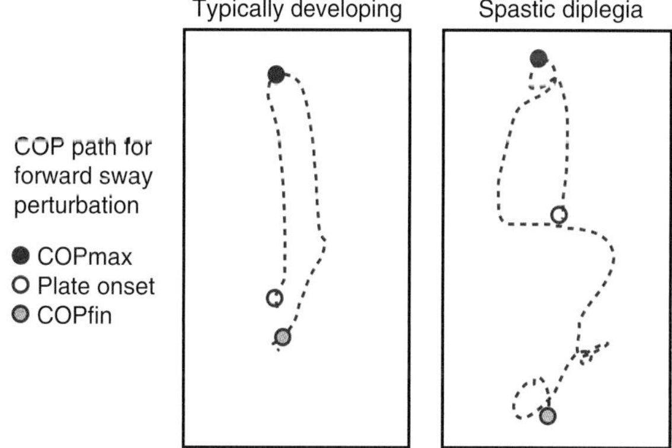

Figure 10.9 Sample COP profiles from a typical child and a child with CP, spastic diplegia in response to a platform perturbation. The open circle represents the initial starting position prior to platform motion. The filled circle represents the maximum forward movement of the COP as a result of the platform movement in the backward direction. The path between the COPmax (*filled circle*) and COPfin (*light colored filled circle*) is the recovery trajectory of the COP. (Adapted from Burtner PA, Woollacott MH, Craft GL, et al. The capacity to adapt to changing balance threats: a comparison of children with cerebral palsy and typically developing children. *Dev Neurorehabil*. 2007;10:249–260.)

Extended Knowledge 10.1

Ankle–Foot Orthoses

What is the effect of constraining movement at a joint on the organization of muscle activity used to recover balance? AFOs are often used by clinicians to control spasticity and prevent excessive plantar flexion. A variety of orthoses are used, including both solid AFOs, which do not allow movement at the ankle joint, and spiral or hinged AFOs, which allow a degree of dynamic ankle–joint movement. Burtner and colleagues (1999) examined the effects of solid versus dynamic AFOs on the coordination of muscles for postural control in both children with spastic diplegia and TD children. For both TD children and children with spastic diplegia, the percent of trials in which the ankle strategy was used was significantly reduced when balancing with the solid AFO compared to the no-AFO and dynamic-AFO conditions. Use of a solid AFO was associated with significantly delayed response onset in the gastrocnemius muscle and a reduction in the frequency of the normal distal-to-proximal muscle response sequence. These results are shown in Figure 10.10A and B and suggest that the types of devices used to control position and motion at the ankles can have a significant impact on the sequencing and timing of muscle responses used for recovery of balance. AFOs that restrict motion at the ankle will reduce the participation of ankle–joint muscles in the control of stability, resulting in an increased use of hip and trunk muscles for balance control.

The delay, noted earlier, in the activation of the gastrocnemius in the spastic leg was surprising for a number of reasons. Given the presence of gastrocnemius spasticity in these children, one might predict a hyperactive stretch response in the gastrocnemius when it is stretched by a rapid platform motion. However, in response to platform-induced stretch, the gastrocnemius muscle was slow to become active, and the amplitude of the muscle activity was low as compared with the uninvolved side. The finding of delayed activation of a stretched "spastic" muscle is consistent with the findings of other investigators, who have reported an inability to recruit and regulate the firing frequency of motor neurons in people with hypertonia (Badke & DiFabio, 1990; Sahrmann & Norton, 1977).

What is the effect of restricting movement at one or more joints through the use of braces on sequencing of muscle activity? Research into this question may be found in Extended Knowledge Box 10.1.

Sequencing problems can also manifest as abnormally long delays in the recruitment of proximal muscle synergists. This type of timing problem has been reported in children with Down syndrome (Shumway-Cook & Woollacott, 1985b) and in adults with traumatic brain injuries with focal cortical contusions (Shumway-Cook & Olmscheid, 1990). Delayed activation of proximal muscles following platform perturbations can be seen in Figure 10.11, which compares EMG responses in a child with Down syndrome to an age-matched normal child. In the normal child, proximal muscle delays were on the order of 36 ms, as compared with 60 to 80 ms in the child with Down syndrome (Shumway-Cook & Woollacott, 1985b). The biomechanical consequences of the delayed activation

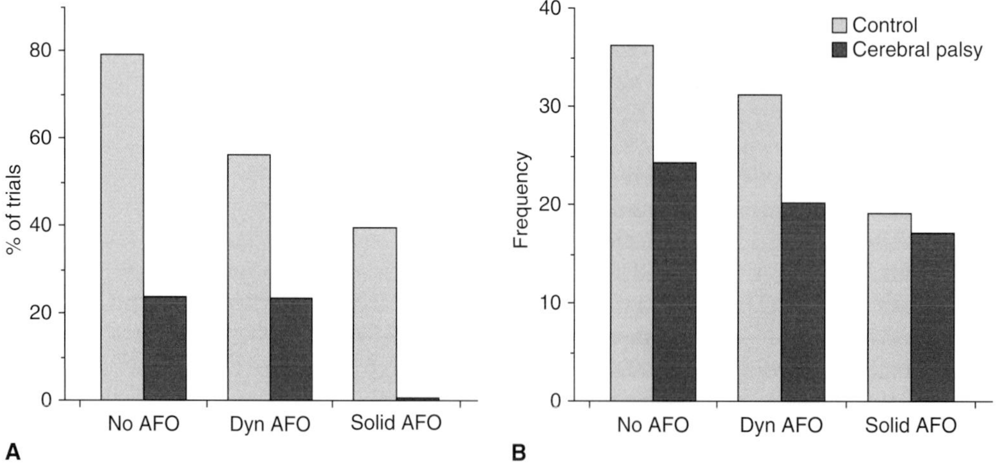

Figure 10.10 (A) Percent of trials in which the ankle strategy was used in both control children and in children with cerebral palsy when wearing no AFO, a dynamic AFO, or a solid AFO. **(B)** Frequency of observing the normal distal-to-proximal muscle response in both control children and those with cerebral palsy, in the no-AFO condition compared with the dynamic and solid AFO conditions. Note that solid AFOs caused a reduction in both use of the ankle strategy and in distal-to-proximal response sequencing. (Adapted from Burtner PA, Woollacott MH, Qualls C. Stance balance control with orthoses in a group of children with spastic cerebral palsy. *Dev Med Child Neurol.* 1999;41:748–757.)

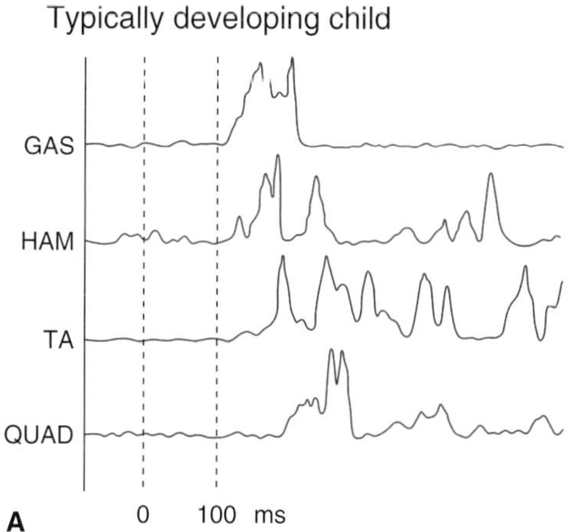

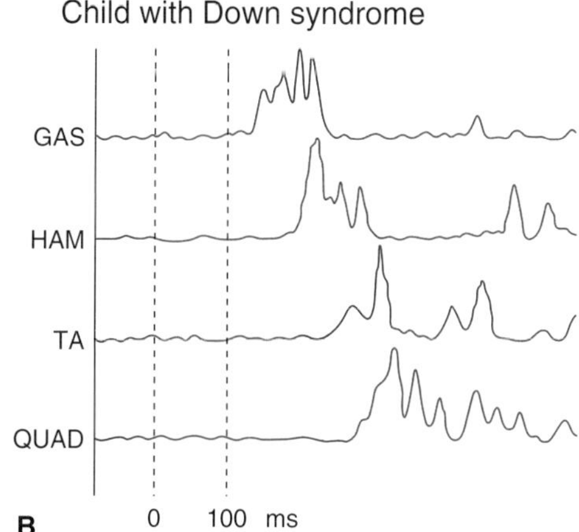

Figure 10.11 Comparison of EMG responses in a child with Down syndrome **(B)** with an age-matched TD child **(A)**, illustrating the delay in proximal muscle activation during recovery of balance. In the TD child, proximal muscle delays were about 35 ms, as compared with 60 to 80 ms in the child with Down syndrome. *GAS*, gastrocnemius; *HAM*, hamstrings; *QUAD*, quadriceps; *TA*, tibialis anterior. (Adapted from Shumway-Cook A, Woollacott M. Postural control in the Down's syndrome child. *Phys Ther.* 1985;9:1317, with permission.)

of the proximal muscles compared with the distal muscles include excessive motion at the knee and hip. This is because the timing of synergistic muscles is not efficient in controlling the indirect effects of forces generated at the ankle on more proximal joints.

Coactivation. Muscle coactivations are usually defined as the simultaneous activation of paired agonist–antagonist muscles during movements. However, muscle coactivations may extend to other muscles and even large groups of muscles. A main mechanical effect of muscle coactivations is the reduction of movement. Muscle coactivations used to maintain balance are task specific and can be observed among individuals with no neurologic pathology (non-impaired individuals) upon unexpected perturbations (Latash, 2018).

The presence of coactivation is a common postural coordination strategy reported in both very young healthy children and a wide variety of people with neurologic deficits, including CP (Crenna & Inverno, 1994; Nashner et al., 1983; Woollacott et al., 1998), CVA (Duncan & Badke, 1987), traumatic brain injury (Shumway-Cook & Olmscheid, 1990), Down syndrome (Shumway-Cook & Woollacott, 1985b), and PD (Dimitrova et al., 2004a; Horak et al., 1992b. A study by Chalard and colleagues (2019) found that, more than spasticity, co-contraction is highly associated with an impairment in the production of active movements. Furthermore, abnormal muscle coactivations may also be present after musculoskeletal surgery (e.g., ligament knee reconstruction) and impair stepping up tasks (Song et al., 2018)

Coactivation in an individual with PD can be seen in Figure 10.12, which compares EMG responses in a person without PD and an older adult person with PD. This activation of muscles on both sides of the joint results in a stiffening of the body and is a very inefficient strategy for the recovery of balance (Horak et al., 1992b). Carpenter et al. (2004) reported increased coactivation in people with PD in response to multidirectional support surface rotations, and Colebatch and Govender (2019) reported increased trunk and thigh muscle tonic activation in response to forward and backward perturbations in people with severe PD. These results are not consistent with the classic work on PD by Purdue Martin (1967), who reported an absence of equilibrium and righting reactions in people with PD. The rigidity and loss of balance found during tilt tests suggested that equilibrium reactions were absent. However, placing EMG electrodes on the muscles of people with PD has allowed researchers to see that individuals with PD do indeed respond to disequilibrium, but the pattern of muscular activity used is ineffective in recovering balance.

Delayed Onset of Postural Responses. Researchers have also found that significant delays in the onset of postural responses can contribute to instability in persons with neurologic deficits. Muscle activity in response to platform perturbations (both horizontal translations and rotations) has been studied in persons with hemiplegia resulting from a CVA (Diener et al., 1984a, 1984b; DiFabio et al., 1986; Ikai et al., 2003; Slijper et al., 2002). Researchers have reported deficits in the sequencing, timing, and amplitude of postural muscle activity in the paretic limb. Figure 10.13 shows the EMG responses in the paretic and nonparetic legs of a person with hemiplegia in response to a forward sway perturbation (DiFabio et al., 1986). Onset latencies in the paretic distal muscles were significantly longer and smaller in amplitude than on the nonparetic side. Delays in the activation of distal muscles in the paretic limb were compensated for by early activation of proximal muscles in the nonparetic limb.

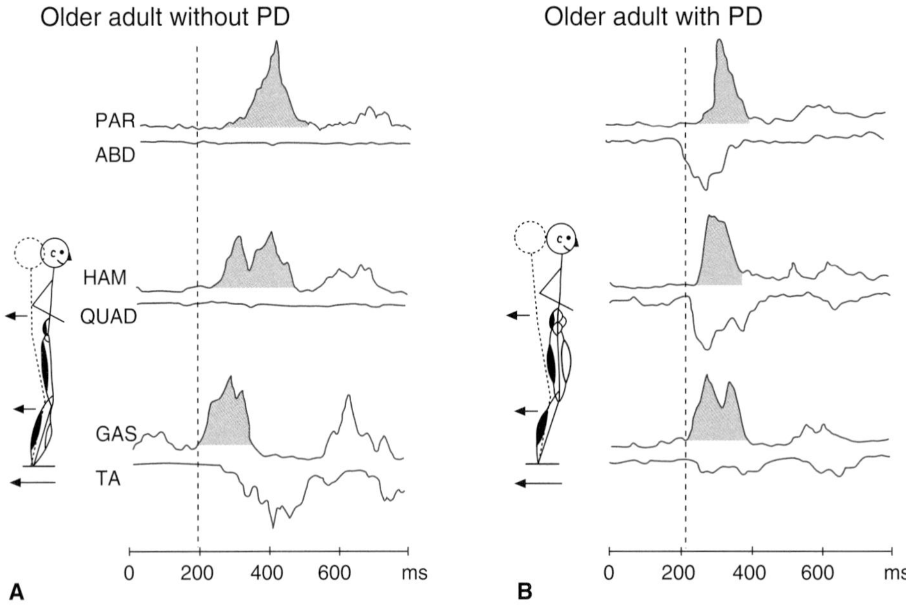

Figure 10.12 Comparison of muscle activation patterns in an older adult without PD **(A)** and an older adult with PD **(B)**, illustrating muscle activation patterns in response to forward sway. The person with PD coactivates antagonistic muscles around the hip and knee, while the subject without PD does not. Shown are the EMG response and a schematic representation of the responses. *ABD*, abdominals; *GAS*, gastrocnemius; *HAM*, hamstrings; *PAR*, paraspinals; *QUAD*, quadriceps; *TA*, tibialis anterior. (Adapted from Horak FB, Nutt JG, Nashner LM. Postural inflexibility in Parkinsonian subjects. *J Neurol Sci*. 1992;111:49, Figure 1, parts B and C.)

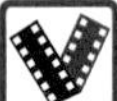

Following stroke, problems in the timing and organization of muscle activity during recovery from a perturbation can contribute to increased risk for falls. Marigold and Eng (2006) examined differences in body kinematics and postural muscle activity (surface EMGs) in 44 persons after they had had a stroke (11 fallers and 33 nonfallers) in response to forward and backward perturbations to stance. EMG analysis, shown in Figure 10.14, demonstrated that in the faller group, postural responses in the paretic, but not the nonparetic limb, were slower and smaller in amplitude as compared with the nonfaller group (131 and 119 ms, respectively). In addition, in the faller group, the activation of the proximal synergist (the right rectus femoris) was significantly delayed in both the paretic and nonparetic limbs as compared with the nonfallers, suggesting impaired intralimb coupling among muscle synergists. In the video segments on postural control for both Genise and Jean, our patients with stroke, both demonstrate an inability to recover balance independently and require physical assistance to prevent a fall. In response to a small perturbation in any direction, Jean reaches for support with her nonparetic limb. Both Jean and Genise have significantly impaired reactive balance responses in the paretic leg, which is a major factor in recurrent falls.

Significant delays in the onset of postural activity have been reported in developmental abnormalities, including Down syndrome (Shumway-Cook & Woollacott, 1985b) and some forms of CP (Nashner et al., 1983). Children with CP spastic hemiplegia and diplegia (GMFCS I-III) show large COP excursions, take longer time to recover balance, and frequently use stepping rather than in-place reactions after moving platform-induced perturbations compared to TD children (Pavão et al., 2013). This can be seen in Figure 10.15, which compares muscle response onset to forward sway in healthy control children, children with Down syndrome, and children with CP (spastic hemiplegia and ataxia).

Postural response onsets were significantly longer in persons with MS (average, 161 ± 31 ms) as compared with control subjects (102 ± 21 ms), with considerable asymmetry between the two legs, both of which were correlated with somatosensory conduction delays. The authors suggest that demyelination of the posterior columns of the spinal cord is the direct cause of the somatosensory conduction delays and that this causes delayed postural responses and imbalance in most people with MS (Cameron et al., 2008). These results also support the hypothesis that postural responses to surface translations are likely triggered by primary and/or secondary afferents from muscle spindles (Stapley et al., 2002). In the video case study of Sue, our patient with relapsing remitting MS, she is unable to recover stability following even a small perturbation to balance and requires assistance to prevent a fall.

Problems Modifying Postural Strategies. Normal postural control requires the ability to modify postural strategies in response to changing tasks and environmental demands. This includes the ability to modify postural activity with practice, referred to as "postural

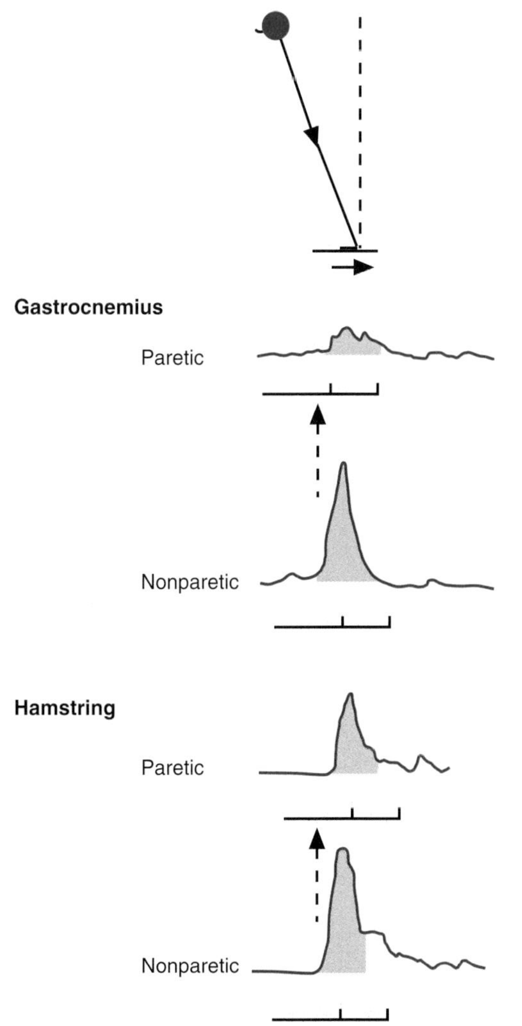

Figure 10.13 EMG responses in the gastrocnemius and hamstrings muscles in paretic and nonparetic limbs of a person with hemiplegia following a CVA in response to a forward sway perturbation. Muscle responses in the paretic limb are slow and reduced in amplitude. (Adapted from DiFabio RP, Badke MB, Duncan PW. Adapting human postural reflexes localized cerebrovascular lesion: analysis of bilateral long latency responses. *Brain Res*. 1986;363:259.)

adaptation," and the ability to change the pattern of postural muscle activity quickly in response to changing task conditions, referred to as shifting central set (Chong et al., 2000; Hall et al., 2010; Horak, 1996). The inability to modify postural responses to changing task demands is a characteristic of many people with neurologic pathology.

Maintaining balance requires that forces generated to control the body's position in space are appropriately scaled to the degree of instability. This means that a small perturbation to stability is met with an appropriately sized muscle response. Thus, force output must be appropriate to the amplitude of instability. Neurologically intact people use a combination of feedforward, or anticipatory, and feedback control mechanisms to scale forces needed for postural stability. These control mechanisms engage different neural substrates—anticipatory control via cortico-ponto-cerebellar pathways and real-time sensory feedback via spinocerebellar connections. Constraints on adaptation can be due to a variety of problems, including limitations in ability to increase the recruitment of agonist muscles in response to increasing perturbation size (strength problems) or problems in the ability to scale, or modulate, the amplitude of postural responses either up or down in response to different-sized perturbations to balance.

Researchers have found that children with CP have significant problems in adapting the amplitude of postural responses to perturbations of increasing distance and velocity (Roncesvalles et al., 2002). This reduced ability to adaptively increase the amplitude of the agonist muscle can be seen in Figure 10.16, which gives an example of muscle activity in a TD child and a child with CP in response to three levels of perturbation difficulty. While the TD child increased the amplitude of the gastrocnemius muscle in response to increasing perturbation size and velocity, the child with CP did not. Similarly, Mills and colleagues (2018) found that in comparison to TD children, mildly impaired children with CP struggled to maintain their balance as the frequency of platform-induced perturbations increased. This was evidenced by a higher number of steps, inefficient joint control, and low percentage of postural muscle bursting activity in the posterior muscles of the lower extremity. These findings were consistent with research showing that maximum voluntary contraction levels for muscles in the lower extremities, and especially distal ankle joint muscles, are significantly lower in children with CP (Wiley & Damiano, 1998). This suggests that constraints on the ability to modulate the amplitude of muscle activity found in children with CP affect both the voluntary control system and the automatic postural response system.

Inability to grade or scale force output to perturbations of varying sizes has been reported in individuals with anterior cerebellar lesions (Horak & Diener, 1994; Horak et al., 1989a, 1990). Individuals with unilateral cerebellar pathology affecting the anterior lobe show hypermetric postural responses on the involved side of the body. Hypermetric postural responses are too large and are associated with excessive compensatory body sway in the direction opposite the initial direction of instability. Hypermetric balance responses can be seen in the video case study of John, who has spinocerebellar degeneration.  An example of hypermetric postural responses found in people with anterior-lobe cerebellar damage is shown in Figure 10.17. EMG responses in people with cerebellar disease are larger in amplitude and longer in duration than are those found in controls. An examination of the sway and torque records shown in Figure 10.17 shows that hypermetric muscle activity resulted in both excess torque and an overcorrection in

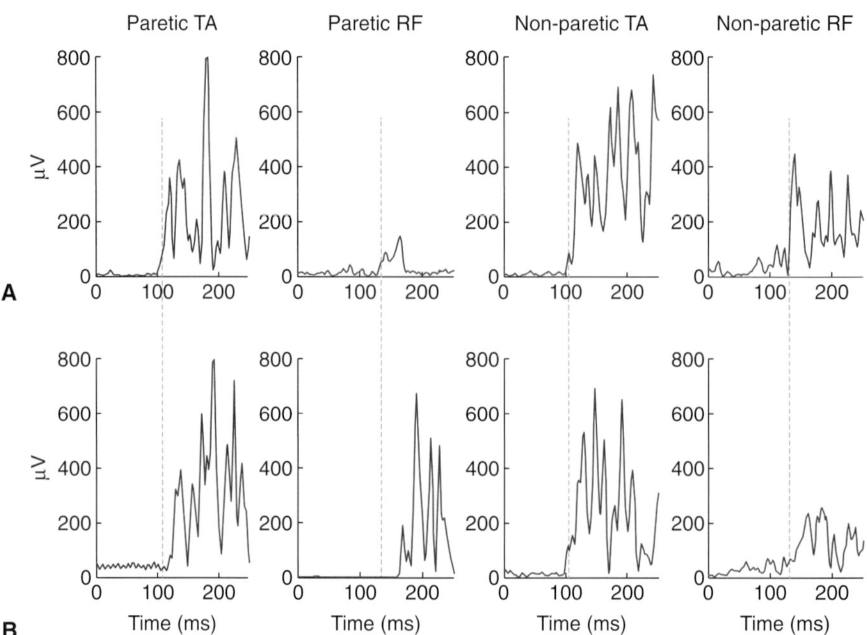

Figure 10.14 Differences in muscle activity in the paretic and nonparetic tibialis anterior (*TA*) and rectus femoris (*RF*) in response to a forward platform translation inducing backward sway in two subjects with stroke. In comparison to the nonfaller **(A)**, the subject who fell **(B)** had slower onset latencies in the paretic TA and slower responses in both the paretic and nonparetic RF, suggesting poor intralimb coupling. (Adapted from Marigold DS, Eng JJ. Altered timing of postural reflexes contributes to falling in persons with chronic stroke. *Exp Brain Res*. 2006;171:454, Figure 3, with permission.)

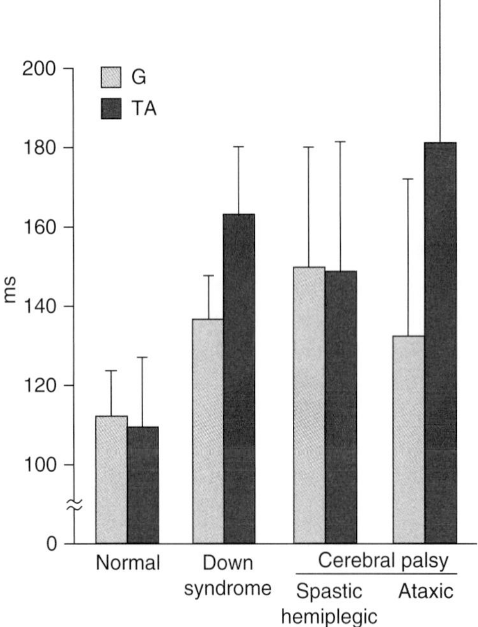

Figure 10.15 Onset of contraction of postural muscles to platform perturbations in TD children, children with Down syndrome, and children with cerebral palsy (spastic hemiplegic and ataxic). Onset of muscle contraction in the children with neurologic deficits is significantly slower than in the TD children. *G*, gastrocnemius; *TA*, tibialis anterior.

sway (seen as full body oscillations) during the recovery of stability (Horak & Diener, 1994). Hypermetric postural responses resulting in full body oscillations can be seen in the postural control segment of John's video case study. In response to small perturbations to balance, John is able to recover independently; however, his body oscillates prior to reestablishing a stable position. Hypermetric postural activity in persons with cerebellar pathology has also been reported in response to multidirectional perturbations (Kung et al., 2009). Finally, postural responses also appear to be larger than normal in persons with MS, possibly to compensate for their delayed onset of contraction. The larger postural responses seen in subjects with MS were similar to, but not as large as, the hypermetric postural responses seen in subjects with cerebellar ataxia (Cameron et al., 2008). There is evidence indicating that children with CP also show greater number of muscle torque bursts to regain postural stability and less efficient temporal–spatial organization of torque activation patterns in response to support-surface perturbations of various magnitudes (Chen & Woollacott, 2007).

Impaired Central Set. Inability to change movement strategies quickly to adapt to changes in support surface characteristics has been found in people with PD (Horak et al., 1992b). In this study, normal controls and a group of individuals with PD were asked to maintain stance balance in a variety of situations, including standing on a flat surface, standing with both feet on a narrow beam, and sitting on a stool with the feet unsupported. People in the control group were able to modify postural muscle responses quickly in response to changing task demands (Fig. 10.18A). In contrast, individuals with PD were unable to modify the complex movement strategy used in recovering balance while standing on a flat surface, for use while standing on the beam or while seated, showing an inability to modify how they moved in response to changes in environmental and task demands (Fig. 10.18B). Researchers believe that these results suggest that the basal ganglia functions to prime or set the nervous system to achieve its goal (Chong et al., 2000). Individuals with PD have difficulty changing from one

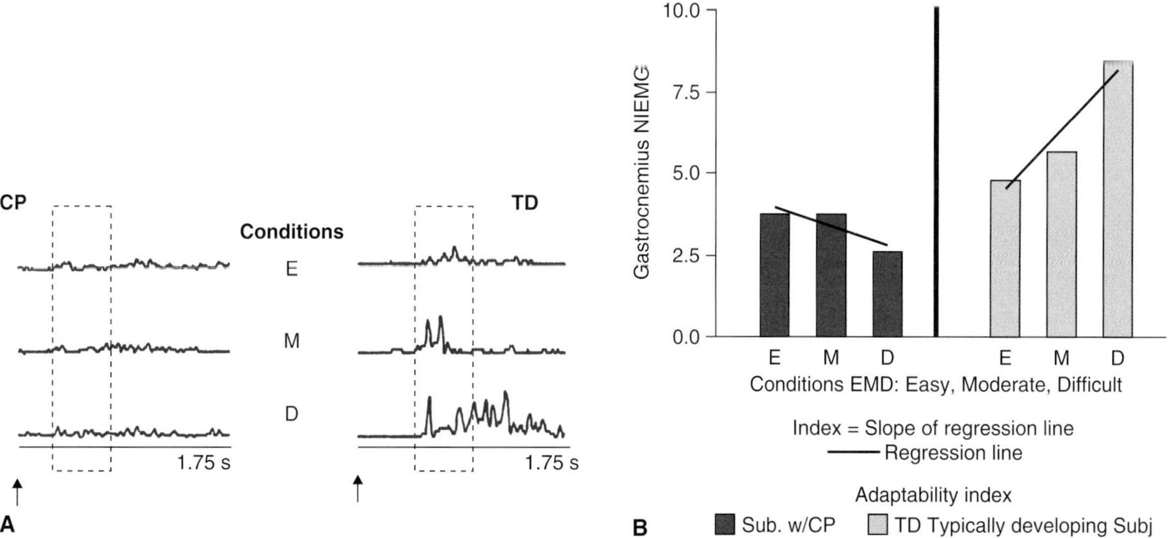

Figure 10.16 (A) Surface gastrocnemius EMG from one child with cerebral palsy (*CP*) and one typically developing (TD) child, illustrating difficulty in adaptively increasing muscle activity to easy (*E*), moderate (*M*), and difficult (*D*) platform perturbations. Notice that the size of the muscle responses increases as the difficulty of the perturbation increases. In contrast, there is no change in the level of muscle activity in the different platform conditions in the child with CP. The *arrow* indicates the time of platform movement onset. The window marked by dotted lines indicates the EMG data used to compare responses across groups of children. **(B)** Adaptability index showing the change in average gastrocnemius amplitude in each condition in the children with CP (on the **left**) and the TD children (on the **right**). (Adapted from Roncesvalles MN, Woollacott MW, Burtner PA. Neural factors underlying reduced postural adaptability in children with cerebral palsy. *NeuroReport*. 2002;13:2409, Figure 1, with permission.)

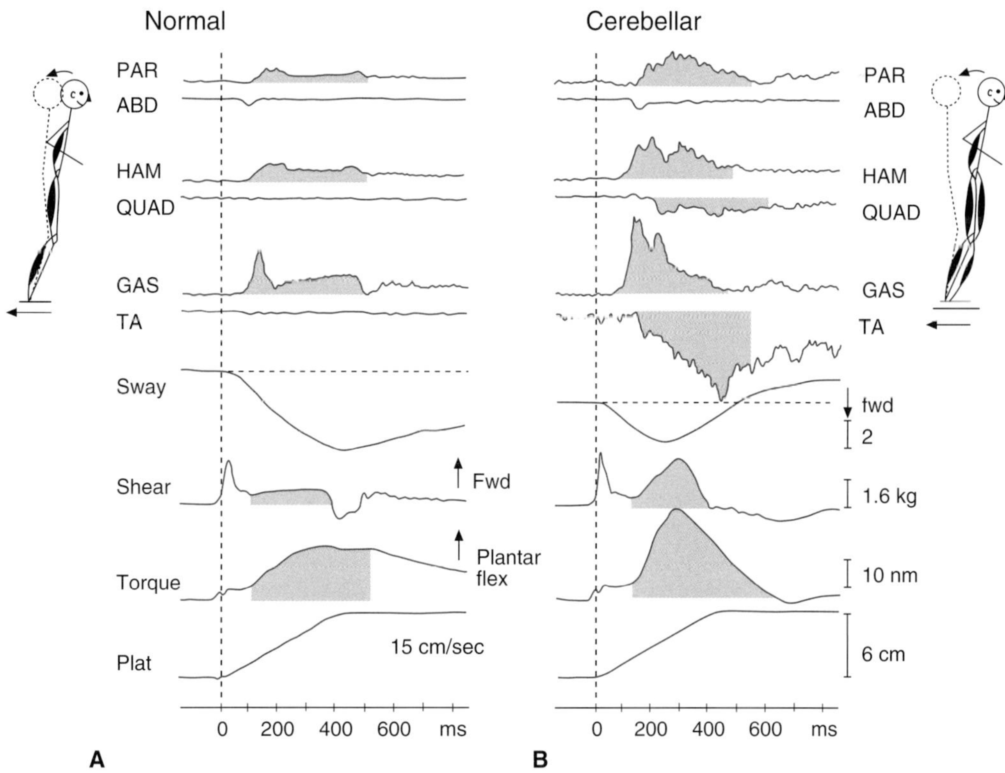

Figure 10.17 EMG activity in controls **(A)** versus persons with anterior-lobe cerebellar degeneration **(B)**. Muscle responses of the person with cerebellar degeneration are hypermetric, that is, significantly larger in amplitude and longer in duration than in controls. *ABD*, abdominals; *GAS*, gastrocnemius; *HAM*, hamstrings; *PAR*, paraspinals; *QUAD*, quadriceps; *TA*, tibialis anterior. (Adapted from Horak FB, Diener HC. Cerebellar control of postural scaling and central set in stance. *J Neurophysiol*. 1994;72:483, with permission.)

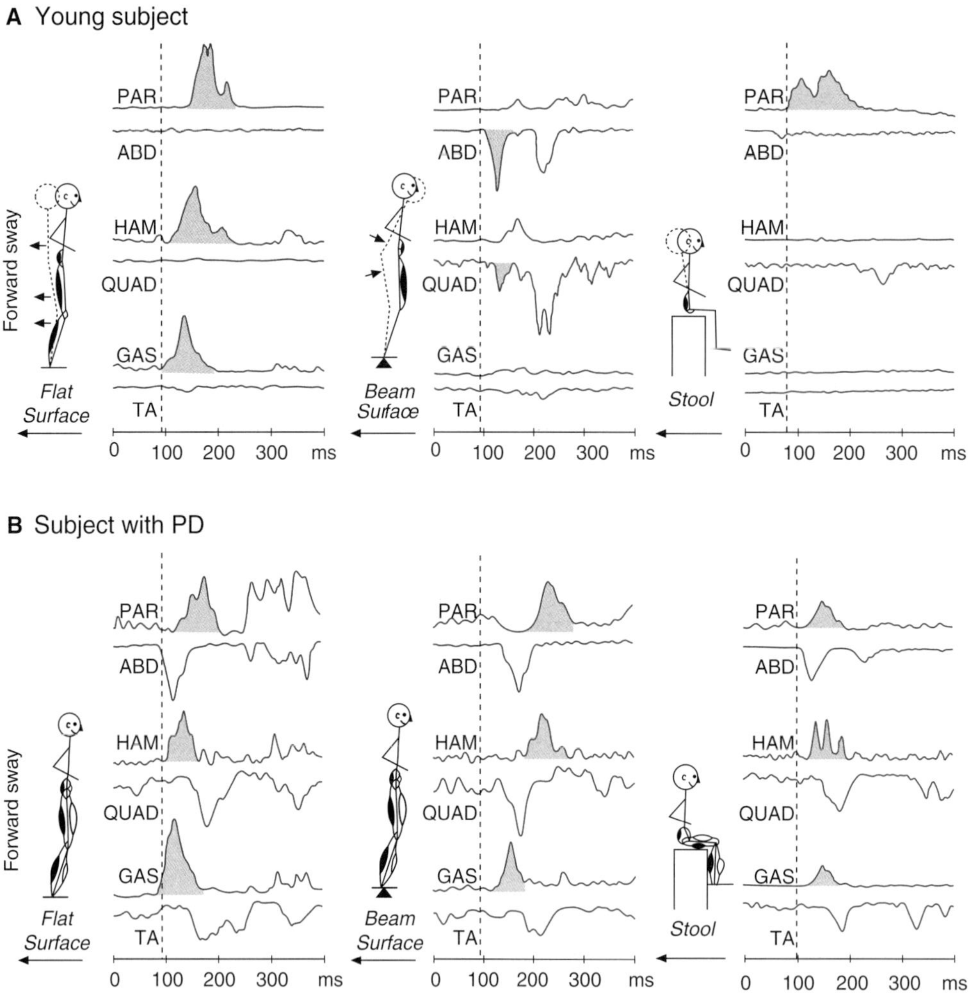

Figure 10.18 Normal and abnormal postural set changes. **(A)** Normal modulation of muscle activity in response to perturbations producing forward sway under three different task conditions: standing on a flat surface, standing on a beam surface, and sitting on a stool. **(B)** In contrast to a young subject in the control group **(A)**, EMG patterns in a person with PD revealed a complex strategy of muscle activity that did not change in response to task demands. *ABD*, abdominals; *GAS*, gastrocnemius; *HAM*, hamstrings; *PAR*, paraspinals; *QUAD*, quadriceps; *TA*, tibialis anterior. (Adapted from Horak FB, Nutt JG, Nashner LM. Postural inflexibility in Parkinsonian subjects. *J Neurol Sci*. 1992;111:52.)

movement set to another. A reduced ability to modify postural strategies in people with PD has also been shown in response to multidirectional surface perturbations and in response to changing stance width (Dimitrova et al., 2004a, 2004b; Horak et al., 2005).

The inability to modify postural activity in response to changing task and environmental conditions is found in people with varying types of neural pathology, suggesting that mechanisms underlying postural flexibility are distributed among many neural structures.

Impaired Change in Support Strategies

Very few researchers have studied the effect of neural pathology on the organization and timing of automatic stepping or reach-for-support strategies used to recover from an unexpected perturbation. Much of the research related to stepping in persons with neurologic pathology has been done in the context of voluntary stepping and is covered in the section on gait initiation in Chapter 14, on abnormal mobility.

King and Horak (2008) examined lateral stepping strategies in persons with PD on and off medication. A movable force plate was used to elicit lateral steps in participants with PD and healthy controls. Participants with PD used a similar lateral stepping strategy to that of controls in response to lateral translations; however, a lack of an anticipatory lateral weight shift and delayed onset reduced the effectiveness of the lateral stepping strategy, resulting in a significant number of losses of balance (requiring assistance) among the group with PD. In addition, while the healthy controls tended to recover with a single lateral step, participants with PD took several small steps to recover. Though less frequent than the lateral step, both groups also used a crossover strategy—one leg crosses the midline of the body—to recover from the lateral perturbations; however, this crossover strategy was frequently associated with falls in the PD group.

Reactive Balance in Sitting

Several studies have examined reactive balance control in sitting in children with CP and other types of developmental motor disorders. These studies used surface EMGs to study muscle activation patterns underlying the recovery of stability in sitting in children with various types of CP (Brogren et al., 1996, 1998; van der Heide et al., 2004). They have consistently reported the presence of directionally specific postural responses (muscles opposed to the direction of body sway are activated); however, the recruitment order was not that used in typical children. Rather than a bottom-up recruitment pattern seen in TD children over 8 to 10 months, children with CP showed a top–down recruitment order to prioritize head control and had difficulty modulating muscle activity in response to changing task context (Carlberg & Hadders-Algra, 2005). In addition, there was a high level of coactivation in the antagonist muscles. Changes reported by Brogren et al. (1996) in muscle recruitment in response to a perturbation to sitting balance can be seen in Figure 10.19.

Similar findings were reported by Washington et al. (2004), who compared muscle activation patterns in response to seated perturbations in TD infants at 8 months of age and in high-risk infants with developmental delays. In general, muscle activity in high-risk infants was characterized by increased tonic rather than phasic muscle activity. In addition, when high-risk infants did recruit muscles phasically, the patterns were direction specific, but recruited in a top–down rather than a bottom–up order, and there was considerable coactivation.

The effect of external support on reactive balance in sitting was tested in children with CP using the clinical measure SATCo (described in detail in Chapter 11). As was true for steady-state balance in sitting, in children with moderate-to-severe CP, optimizing trunk support enabled the emergence of reactive balance control in the head and trunk as indicated by the ability to recover a stable position following nudges in all directions, above the level of support (Saavedra & Woollacott, 2015).

Is impaired postural control in children with CP due to biomechanical reasons (children seated in a flexed posture) or to a neural deficit? To answer this question, Brogren et al. (2001) examined reactive postural adjustments during sitting in an erect and a flexed position in 20 children 3 to 7 years of age with mild-to-severe forms of spastic diplegia and 10 age- and sex-matched TD children. Children with severe spastic diplegia had significantly impaired muscle activation patterns during recovery from platform translations. This included loss of direction-specific activation of muscles during recovery from backward sway, which was more pronounced in the erect sitting posture as compared with the flexed position. The authors suggest that the flexed sitting pattern adopted by many children with CP may in part be a compensatory solution to the instability experienced in the erect position.

The effect of segmental trunk control on the ability to recover from an unexpected perturbation to seated posture is being examined in adults following stroke. As shown in Figure 10.20, in response to a small

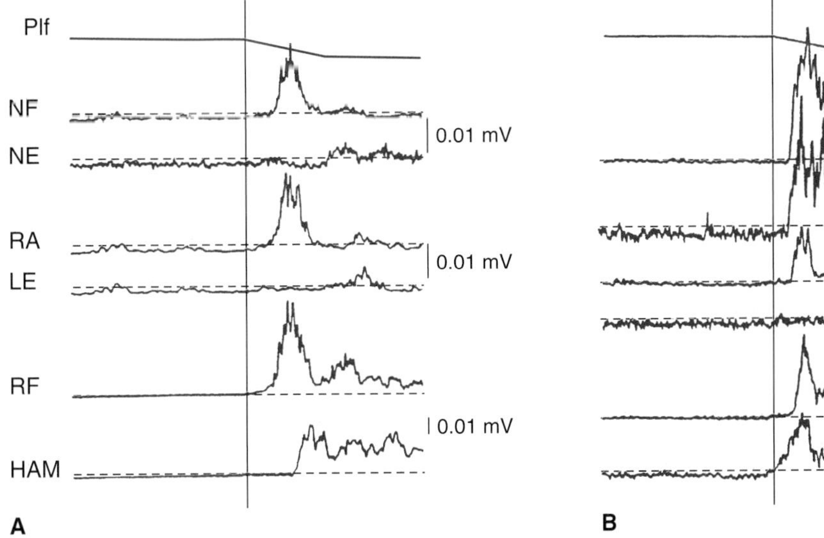

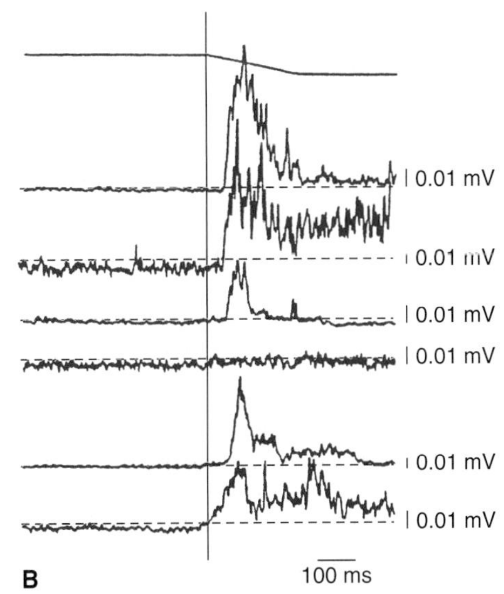

Figure 10.19 Comparison of EMG records from a control child **(A)** and a child with spastic diplegia **(B)**. The sequencing of muscles in a child with spastic diplegia responding to a backward translation of a moving platform (*Plf*) while in the seated position is abnormal as compared with the muscles of the control child. EMG records show an inappropriate activation of muscles responding to forward sway, with proximal neck flexors and extensors (*NF* and *NE*) firing simultaneously with distal trunk (*RA* and *LE*) and leg (*RF* and *HAM*) muscles. (Reprinted from Brogren E, Hadders-Algra M, Forssberg H. Postural control in children with spastic diplegia: muscle activity during perturbations in sitting. *Dev Med Child Neurol.* 1998;38:381, with permission.)

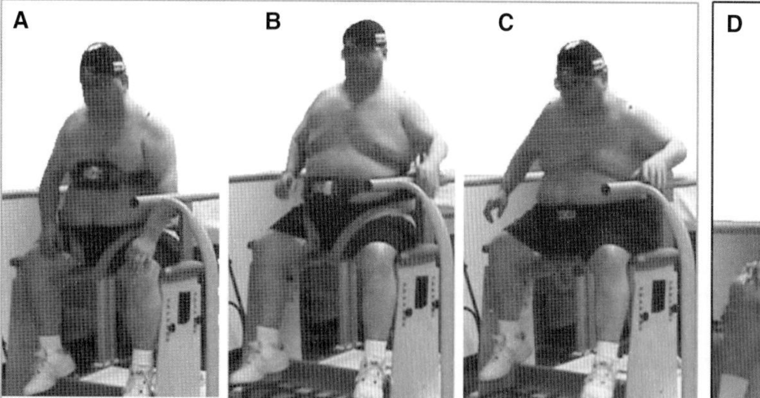

Figure 10.20 Images showing the effect of external support on the recovery strategy used in response to platform perturbations while seated. With no support **(C)**, the patient with stroke uses a reach-for-support strategy in response to a small platform perturbation, unlike the healthy age-matched control who recovers with an in-place strategy **(D)**. With pelvic support **(B)**, the trajectory associated with the compensatory reach-for-support strategy is straighter and more efficient; at midrib support **(A)**, an in-place strategy emerges. (Woollacott, unpublished data; images courtesy of Jaya Rachwani and Victor Santamaria.)

platform perturbation, a healthy age-matched control is able to recover stability using an in-place (trunk alone) recovery strategy (D). In contrast, in response to the same perturbation, the patient with stroke in an unsupported position (C) must reach for support to recovery stability. With the addition of pelvic support, the patient still requires a reach for support (B); however, with additional external support at the midrib level, an in-place strategy emerges (A).

Clinical Implications of Research on Impaired Reactive Balance

The previously mentioned research suggests that impairments in reactive balance control significantly impact functional independence in adults and children with neurologic pathology. Factors contributing to impaired reactive balance are complex, including problems with timing, sequencing, and adapting muscle responses to external threats to balance. A comprehensive approach to balance rehabilitation must include assessment of reactive balance as well as treatment programs designed to improve recovery strategies. These are discussed in detail in the next chapter.

Impaired Anticipatory Postural Control

Another source of postural dyscontrol is the loss of anticipatory processes that activate postural adjustments in advance of potentially destabilizing voluntary movements. Anticipatory postural activity is heavily dependent on previous experience and learning.

Inability to activate postural muscles in anticipation of voluntary arm movements has been described in both adults and children with neurological pathology, including individuals who have had a stroke (Horak et al., 1984; Slijper et al., 2002), traumatic brain injury (Arce et al., 2004), children with CP (Nashner et al., 1983; Santamaria, 2015; van der Heide et al., 2004), children with Down syndrome (Shumway-Cook & Woollacott, 1985b), and people with PD (Aruin and Almeida, 1996; Latash et al., 1995; Rogers, 1990, 1991).

Problems in initiating postural muscle activity prior to a voluntary arm movement in a child with spastic hemiplegia are shown in Figure 10.21. There is a lack of preparatory postural activity in leg muscles of the hemiparetic side, as compared with the normal side when the child was asked to push or pull on a handle while standing (Nashner et al., 1983). Similarly, when compared to TD children, children with spastic diplegia show a delay and decreased activity of the gastrocnemius muscle prior to lifting a load, which is unlikely attributable to their differences in initial standing posture before lifting (Tomita et al., 2011). When TD children were tested in an upright versus a crouched standing posture (to mimic those in the CP group), no significant changes were found in the timing of gastrocnemius anticipatory postural adjustments (APAs). This suggests that impaired anticipatory postural control found in children with CP are unlikely to be the result of biomechanical factors associated with impaired initial alignment.

Impaired anticipatory postural adjustments associated with a rapid upper-extremity movement in individuals who have had a stroke have been reported in several studies (Garland et al., 2003; Horak et al., 1984; Slijper et al., 2002). Garland et al. (2003) recorded EMG activity from the legs and trunk during a rapid arm flexion movement immediately after stroke and 1 month after rehabilitation. Immediately after the stroke, there was a significant delay in the activation of the paretic hamstrings muscle during the arm raise task, indicating impaired anticipatory postural control. After a month of rehabilitation, improvements in

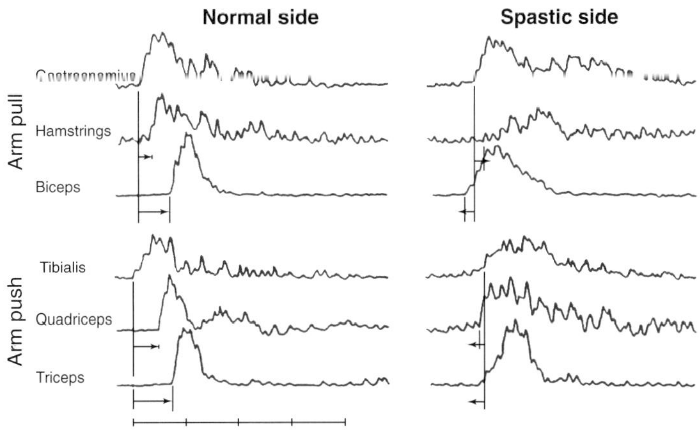

Figure 10.21 Normal and abnormal anticipatory postural control. EMG responses in arm (biceps/triceps) and leg (gastrocnemius/hamstrings and tibialis/quadriceps) muscles during a push or pull task on the normal versus the spastic side of a child with spastic hemiplegia. Muscle responses on the normal side show the activation of postural muscles in the leg in advance of the prime mover in the arm. In contrast, on the spastic side, muscle activity in the arm precedes postural activity in the legs, resulting in instability. (Adapted from Nashner LM, Shumway-Cook A, Marin O. Stance posture control in select groups of children with cerebral palsy: deficits in sensory organization and muscular coordination. *Exp Brain Res*. 1983;49:401.)

anticipatory postural activity varied among participants. Figure 10.22 illustrates the three patterns of change that emerged over the 1 month of rehabilitation. In the first group (A in the figure), there was significant improvement in the recruitment of both paretic and nonparetic hamstrings, but no appreciable change in arm acceleration. In the second group (B), there was significant improvement in the paretic hamstrings only, without any notable change in arm acceleration. Finally, in the third group (C), there was a significant improvement in the nonparetic hamstrings that was associated with improved arm acceleration, which the authors called a compensatory recovery.

What type of rehabilitation techniques can improve APAs in stroke patients? Curuk and colleagues (2020) tested the effects of a single session of practice consisting of pushing and catching a medicine ball with the unaffected arm to target both the anticipatory and reactive postural mechanisms. Figure 10.23 illustrates the exercise and also shows the pre- and posttest involving a pendulum impacting their raised arm. With a single session of 120 repetitions of pushing and catching with a 2 minute rest after each 40 repetitions, stroke patients showed improved APAs during arm lifts and reactive muscle response latencies after the pendulum impact on both sides of the body (the affected and non-affected sides).

Why do lesions in so many areas of the nervous system produce problems in anticipatory postural control? The circuitry underlying anticipatory postural control involves many neural structures, including supplementary motor cortex, basal ganglia, and the cerebellum. Thus, lesions in any one of these areas can disrupt critical pathways contributing to learning and executing anticipatory postural strategies.

Anticipatory Balance in Sitting

Dickstein and colleagues (2004) examined muscle activity in persons with stroke and controls during voluntary trunk flexion and extension and while performing voluntary arm and leg movements. They found that trunk velocity during voluntary flexion and extension was slower in persons with stroke as compared with controls, and muscle activity on the paretic side was both reduced in magnitude and delayed relative to the unaffected side. Muscle activity in the trunk was also delayed and reduced during anticipatory postural adjustments associated with voluntary arm or leg movements performed in sitting.

Providing external trunk support can reduce the effect of impaired anticipatory postural adjustments in the trunk on voluntary reaches in stroke. This is shown in Figure 10.24, which compares voluntary reaches in a person with stroke under different levels of external support. With no external trunk support (no support condition), the reach trajectory is long and uncoordinated, and AP trunk movement is large (in ovals, bottom). With higher levels of trunk support (pelvic support and midrib support), arm trajectory improves and AP trunk movements decrease. Finally, with the highest level of support (axillae support), arm trajectory and AP trunk motion in the patient are closer to that of the unsupported age matched control (B).

Improvement in voluntary reaching with external support to the trunk has also been shown in children with CP. This can be seen in Figure 10.25, which shows a child with CP reaching for an object placed at midline under three levels of support. With only pelvic support (figure on far right), trunk stability is severely impaired (trunk motion is shown on the bottom right trace) and reach trajectory is irregular (shown in the three-dimensional trajectory plot on the middle row). In contrast, as support increases from pelvis to midrib and to axillae, both trunk stability and reach trajectory improve (Santamaria et al., 2016).

EMG analysis indicated that in contrast to the children with CP who have more severe trunk control impairments (axillae and thoracic subregions), children with mild trunk control impairments (low-thoracic and lumbar subregions) demonstrated anticipatory postural adjustments that were closer to the onset of

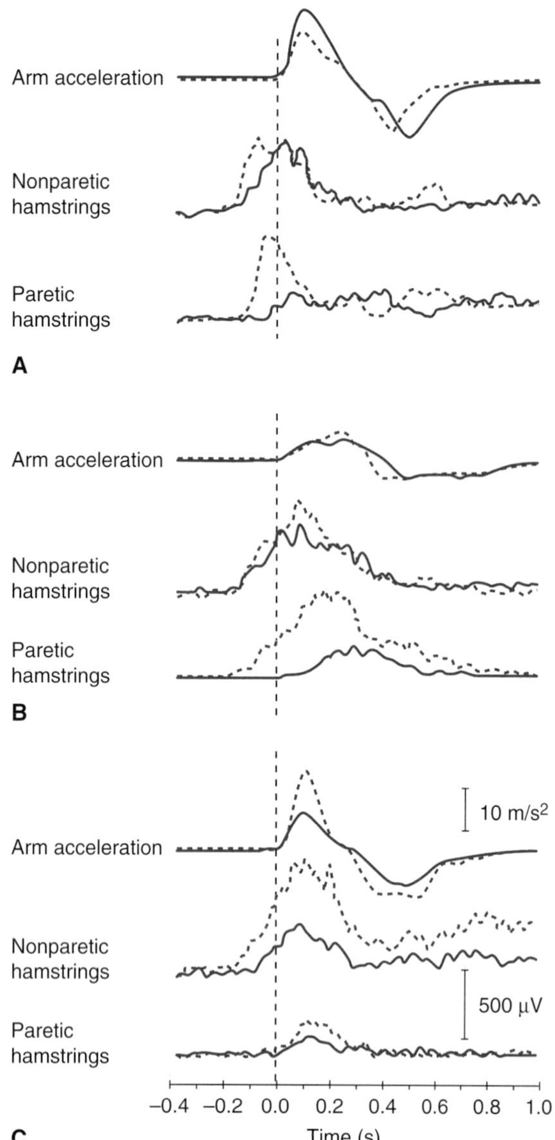

Figure 10.22 Three patterns of change in anticipatory postural activity in the paretic and nonparetic hamstrings muscles associated with a rapid arm movement prior to (*solid line*) and following (*dotted line*) 1 month of rehabilitation for stroke. In the first group **(A)**, there was significant improvement in the recruitment of both paretic and nonparetic hamstrings (compare *dotted* to solid lines), but no appreciable change in arm acceleration. In the second group **(B)**, there was significant improvement in the paretic hamstrings only, without any notable change in arm acceleration. Finally, in the third group **(C)**, there was a significant improvement in the nonparetic hamstrings that was associated with improved arm acceleration, which the authors called compensatory recovery. (Adapted from Garland SJ, Willems DA, Ivanova TD, et al. Recovery of standing balance and functional mobility after stroke. *Arch Phys Med Rehabil.* 2003;84:1753–1759, Figure 3.)

reaches. In addition, as trunk deficits increased, the ability to produce anticipatory postural adjustments in the trunk decreased (Santamaria, 2015).

This effect of external trunk support on anticipatory postural control and upper-extremity function can be seen quite dramatically in Malachi, our video case study of sitting balance in a child with severe athetoid/spastic CP.

Clinical Implications of Research on Impaired Anticipatory Postural Control

Anticipatory postural control is a critical component of the efficient and safe performance of many activities of daily life. Activities such as reaching for and lifting objects that are potentially destabilizing (such as a heavy grocery bag), opening a heavy door, or stepping up onto a curb all require activation of postural muscles, which stabilize the COM prior to the voluntary movement. Impaired anticipatory postural control significantly impacts these activities and is therefore a critical aspect of balance control that needs to be assessed in children and adults with neurologic pathology. In addition, treatment strategies that improve anticipatory postural control, such as providing segmental trunk support, will significantly improve functional skills. Clinical strategies for assessing and treating anticipatory postural control are discussed in Chapter 11.

PROBLEMS IN THE SENSORY/PERCEPTUAL SYSTEMS

Normal postural control requires the organization of sensory information from visual, somatosensory, and vestibular systems that provide information about the body's position and movement with respect to the environment and the coordination of sensory information with motor actions.

Sensory problems can disrupt postural control by affecting a person's ability to adapt sensory inputs to changes in task and environmental demands, disrupting the control of steady-state, reactive, and anticipatory balance. In addition, sensory problems disrupt the development of accurate internal models and perceptions of the body critical for postural control.

Sensory Problems Affecting Steady-State Balance

Researchers examining the effect of neurologic injury on a person's ability to organize and select appropriate sensory inputs for postural control have focused primarily on the use of computerized force platforms in conjunction with moving visual surrounds, first developed by Nashner and colleagues (Black et al., 1988; Horak et al., 1990; Shumway-Cook et al., 1988). This approach, described in detail in the chapter on normal postural control, measures changes in body sway during stance in situations in which sensory information is reduced or made inaccurate for postural control. Alternatively, therapists have used compliant foam surfaces in conjunction with a visual dome to examine sensory

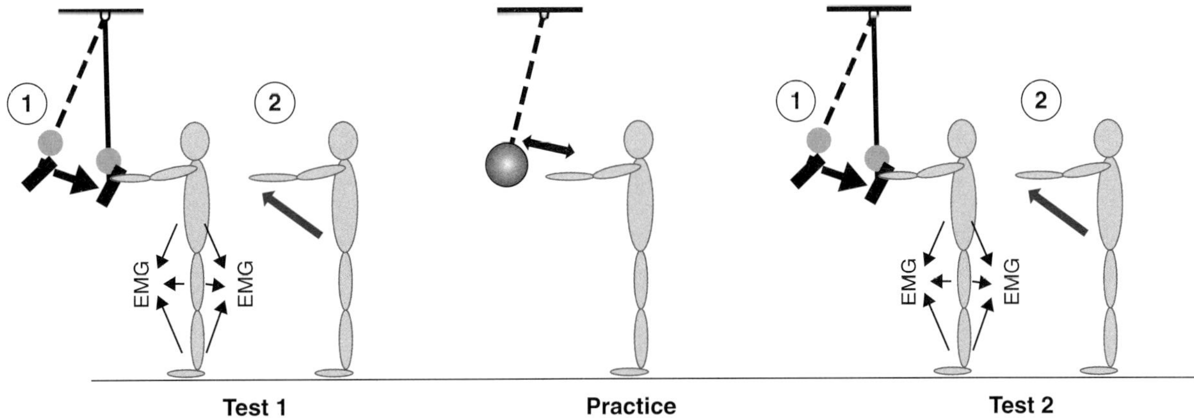

Figure 10.23 Schematic representation of a practice session consisting of pushing and catching a medicine ball with the unaffected arm, as well as pre- and posttests involving anticipatory (arm lift) and reactive postural mechanisms (in response to a pendulum impact). (Adapted from Curuk E, Lee Y, Aruin AS. Individuals with stroke improve anticipatory postural adjustments after a single session of targeted exercises. *Hum Mov Sci*. 2020;69:3.)

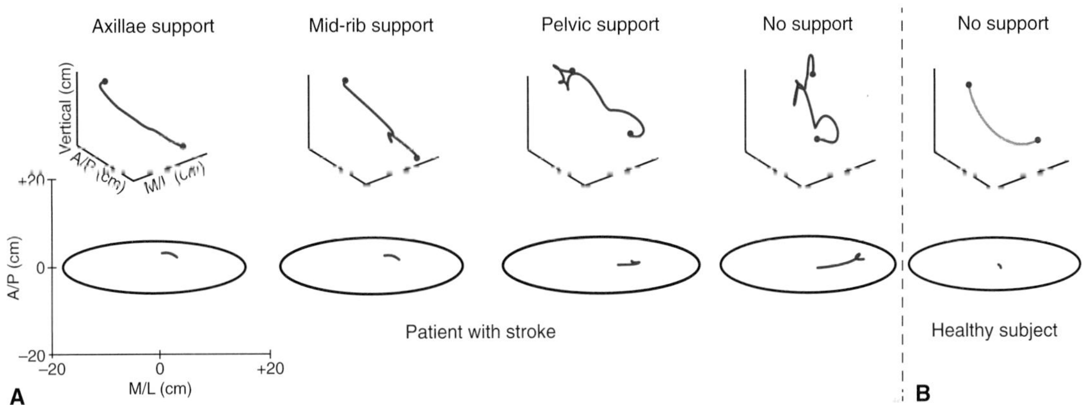

Figure 10.24 Comparison of voluntary reach trajectories in a patient with stroke with varying levels of trunk support **(A)** compared to a healthy control **(B)**. With no external trunk support (no support condition), trajectory of reach in the patient was longer and uncoordinated (**top** trace). In addition, AP trunk movement (**bottom** figure) was large (shown in the ovals, which signify the boundary of the base of support). With the next higher level of trunk support (pelvic support), arm trajectory improved and AP trunk movements decreased. Finally, with the highest levels of support (axillae support and midrib support), arm trajectory and AP trunk motion in the patient were closer to that of the unsupported age-matched control **(B)** (Woollacott, unpublished data).

adaptation in the clinic. This test, referred to as the Clinical Test of Sensory Interaction in Balance (CTSIB), measures the number of seconds (30 s maximum) a person can stand under six different sensory conditions (Horak, 1987; Shumway-Cook & Horak, 1986).

What is the effect of loss of a sensory input on postural control? It depends! Some important factors include (a) the availability of other senses to detect the position of the body in space, (b) the availability of accurate orientation cues in the environment, and (c) the ability to correctly interpret and select sensory information for orientation. Researchers are beginning to examine the extent to which persons with a loss of one sense can compensate by increasing the sensitivity of the remaining senses.

As shown in Figure 10.26, persons with loss of vestibular information for postural control may be stable under most conditions as long as alternative sensory information from vision or the somatosensory systems is available for orientation. In situations in which vision and somatosensory inputs are reduced, leaving mainly vestibular inputs (the last two conditions in Fig. 10.26) for postural control, the person may experience sudden falls, indicated by the score of 100 on the sway index (Horak et al., 1990).

Functionally, persons with this type of postural dyscontrol might perform normally on most tests of balance as long as they are carried out in a well-lit environment and on a firm, flat surface. However, performance on balance tasks under ideal sensory conditions will not necessarily predict the person's likelihood for falls in more complex conditions, such as when getting up to go to the bathroom at night and negotiating a carpeted surface in the dark.

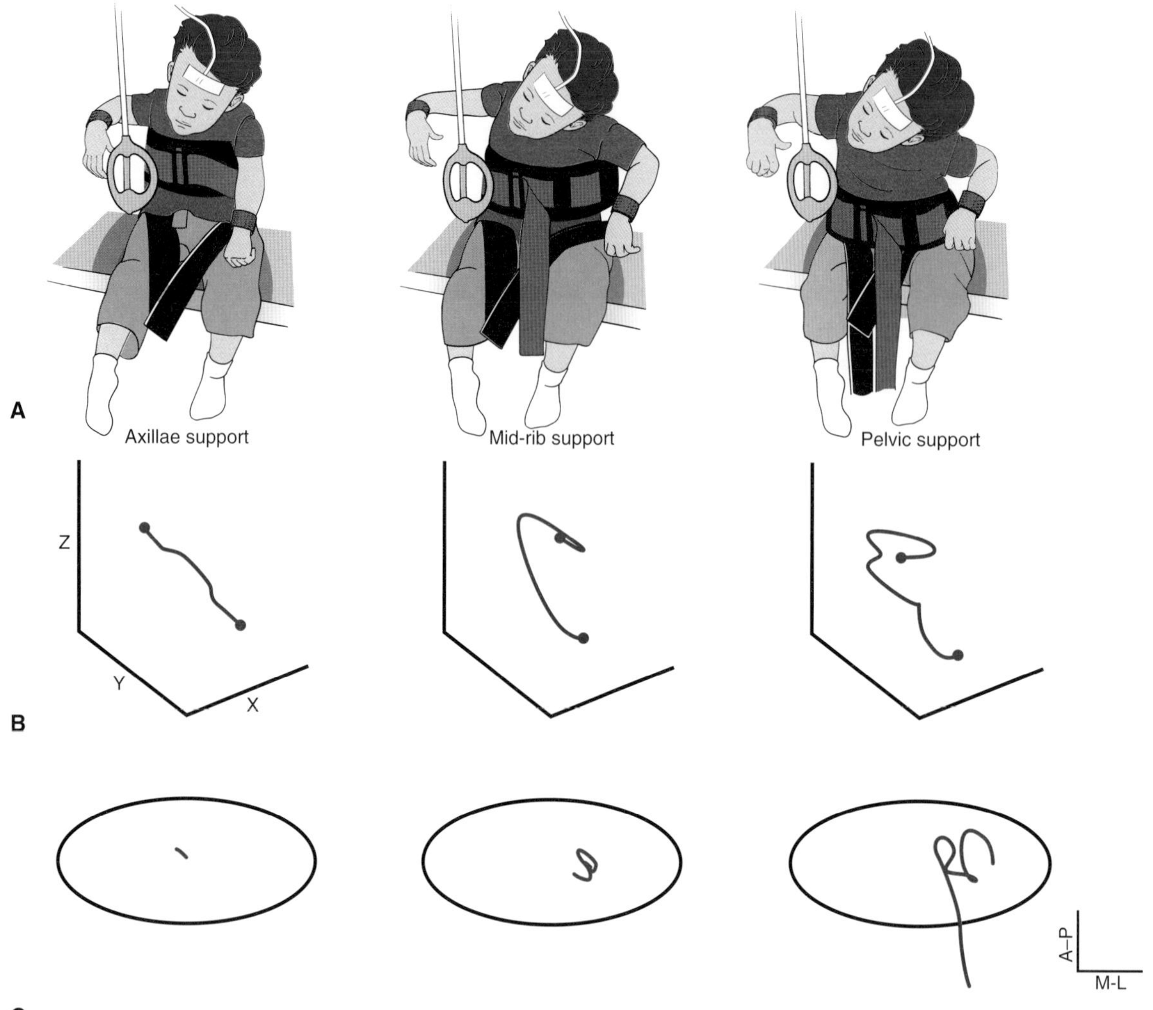

Figure 10.25 Improvement in voluntary reaching with external support to the trunk in a child with CP (classified as GMFCS level IV) shown in **(A)**. With only pelvic support (figure on far **right**), trunk stability (trunk data shown in row **C** of this figure) is severely impaired (trunk motion during the reach is shown within an oval showing the boundary of the base of support); reach trajectory (reach data shown in row **B** of this figure) is less direct (shown in the three-dimensional trajectory plot). In contrast, as support increases from midrib to axillae, both trunk stability and reach trajectory improve. *A-P*, anterior-posterior plane of motion; *M-L*, medio-lateral plane of motion. (Reprinted, with permission of author, from Santamaria V. The effect of different levels of external trunk support on postural and reaching control in children with cerebral palsy. Ph.D. Dissertation, University of Oregon, 2015; Figure 19.)

How does disruption of somatosensory information affect steady-state postural control? One might expect that a person with a sudden loss of somatosensory information could maintain stability as long as alternative information from vision and vestibular senses was available. Horak and colleagues (1990) examined this question by applying pressure cuffs to the ankles of normal adults and inflating them until cutaneous sensation in the feet and ankles was temporarily lost. As shown in Figure 10.27, neurologically intact persons were able to maintain balance on all sensory conditions, despite the loss of somatosensory cues from the feet and ankles, as they always had an alternative sense (either vision or vestibular) available for orientation.

What happens in neurologically affected individuals? Jayakaran and colleagues (2018) explored postural control in children with strabismus (demonstrating visual suppression from the deviating eye) and in children with normal vision (without strabismus) on the Sensory Organization Test (SOT). The authors found that in comparison to children with normal vision, the postural control in children with strabismus was worse when all sensory systems were available and children with strabismus were highly dependent on the somatosensory system for maintaining balance.

Jeka and colleagues (1996) studied the use of sensory cues for steady-state postural control in sighted and blind individuals. They were interested in understanding whether increasing haptic cues could improve postural orientation in blind individuals. Haptic perceptual cues involve both cutaneous receptors that provide information about surface properties (such as friction)

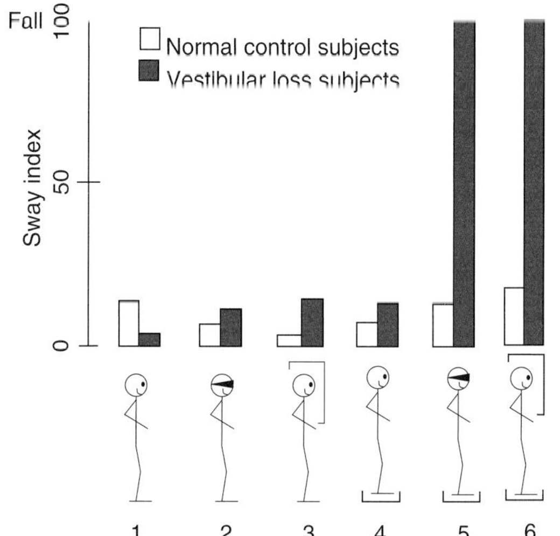

Figure 10.26 Comparison of body sway in the six sensory conditions of the Sensory Organization Test (SOT) in neurologically intact adults versus persons with loss of vestibular function. Results show that instability in persons with loss of vestibular function occurs only in conditions in which vision and somatosensory inputs are not available for postural control (conditions 5 and 6). (Adapted from Horak F, Nashner LM, Diener HC. Postural strategies associated with somatosensory and vestibular loss. *Exp Brain Res*. 1990;82:418.)

and kinesthetic receptors that provide information about body movement and position. In sighted and blind individuals maintaining a tandem Romberg position, haptic cues were provided by contact with a cane. Touch contact with a slanted cane reduced postural sway more than did physically supportive forces with a perpendicular cane.

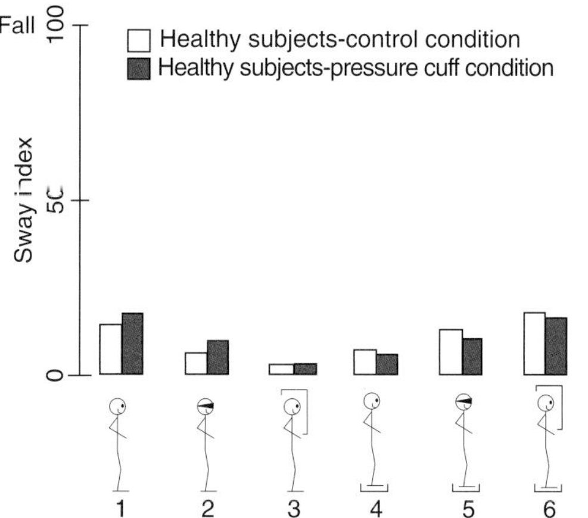

Figure 10.27 Body sway in the six sensory conditions of the Sensory Organization Test (SOT) in normal persons before use of pressure cuffs at the ankle (*white bars*) and after subsequent temporary loss of cutaneous sensation with the use of pressure cuffs (*orange bars*). Loss of somatosensory inputs below the pressure cuffs did not affect the ability of these neurologically intact persons to maintain balance because of the availability of alternative senses and the capacity to adapt remaining senses to the changing demands. (Adapted from Horak F, Nashner LM, Diener HC. Postural strategies associated with somatosensory and vestibular loss. *Exp Brain Res*. 1990;82:418.)

This suggests that a handheld cane provides haptic sensory cues with sufficient precision to improve postural stability substantially in blind individuals.

Providing additional sensory information for steady-state postural control through the use of haptic cues (fingertip touch to a supporting surface) has been found to improve postural stability in a number of persons with neurologic pathology, including those with cerebellar pathology (Sullivan et al., 2006); in adults with Down syndrome (Gomes & Berela, 2007); in adults with stroke (Martinelli et al., 2018); and in persons with peripheral neuropathy due to long-standing diabetes (Dickstein et al., 2001, 2003). Researchers have also shown that somatosensory loss in persons with diabetic peripheral neuropathy was associated with an increased sensitivity to vestibular stimulation (Horak & Hlavacka, 2001). This type of sensory substitution mechanism is consistent with research showing an adaptive increase in somatosensory system input gain in persons with chronic loss of vestibular cues (Strupp et al., 1999).

In this line of research, new technology has been developed to apply mechanical or electrical sub-sensory stochastic resonance stimulation, which is a continuous low-level noise that forces weak signals to cross the receptor's sensory threshold and then be detected, to improve sensory sensitivity. Stochastic resonance stimulation enhances balance during upright standing in people with diabetic neuropathy and stroke. In one study, the stimulating electrodes were placed on the lateral side of the leg and ankle ligaments while children with CP and TD controls stood on a force plate with and without vision. The stimulation reduced COP sway in children with CP and it had a greater rate of balance improvement in the CP group compared to the TD group (Zarkou et al., 2018). The findings of this study highlight how the enhancement of somatosensory inputs, reducing sensory deficits, can improve steady-state balance control.

In some cases, instability results from an inability to effectively organize and select appropriate sensory inputs for postural control. Sensory organization problems can manifest as an inflexible weighting of sensory information for orientation. This means that a person may depend heavily on one particular sense for postural control; for example, they may be either vision dependent or somatosensory system dependent. When presented with a situation in which that sense is either not available or not accurately reporting self-motion, persons will continue to rely on the preferred sense, even though instability may be a consequence. For example, several studies have reported that following a stroke, there is an increased reliance on visual inputs for stance postural control in the early stages of recovery (Bonan et al., 2004; Geurts et al., 2005). Some have reported that over time, with recovery, there is a decreased reliance on visual inputs for stance postural control (de Haart et al., 2004), while others have reported that an increased reliance on vision persists (Laufer et al., 2005).

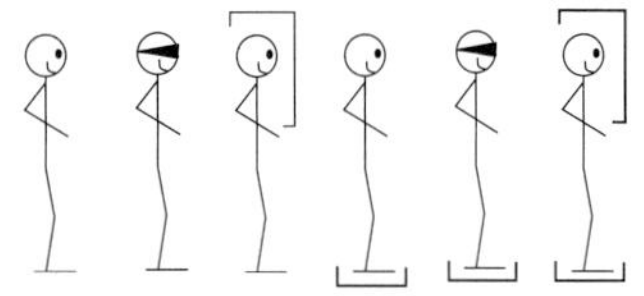

	1	2	3	4	5	6
Normal						
Adults (7–60)	N	N	N	N	N	N
Children (1–7)	N	N	A	A	A	A
Abnormal						
Visually dependent	N	N/A	A	N	N/A	A
Surface dependent	N	N	N	A	A	A
Vestibular loss	N	N	N	N	A	A
Sensory selection problems	N	N	A	A	A	A

Figure 10.28 Classification scheme for identifying different problems related to organizing sensory information for stance postural control based on patterns of normal and abnormal sway in six sensory conditions of the Sensory Organization Test (SOT) used during dynamic posturography testing. *A*, abnormal sway; *N*, normal sway.

Patterns of sway associated with this type of sensory inflexibility are summarized in Figure 10.28. Persons who are dependent on visual information for postural control (referred to as "visually dependent" in Fig. 10.28) tend to show abnormally increased sway in any condition in which visual cues are reduced (such as standing with eyes closed) or made inaccurate (such as standing in the presence of visual motion in the environment) (Black & Nashner, 1984a, 1984b).

Persons who demonstrate an inflexible use of somatosensory inputs for postural control (surface dependent) become unstable in conditions in which surface inputs do not allow them to establish and maintain a vertical orientation (Horak & Shupert, 1994). This can be seen as excessive amounts of body sway in conditions 4–6 (Fig. 10.28). Thus, when standing on a compliant surface, like sand or thick carpet; on a tilted surface, like a ramp; or on a moving surface, like a boat, the position of the ankle joint and other somatosensory and proprioceptive information from the feet and legs does not correlate well with the orientation of the rest of the body (Horak & Shupert, 1994). An overreliance on somatosensory inputs for postural control in these environments will result in instability.

Inability to appropriately select a sense for postural control in environments in which one or more orientation cues inaccurately report the body's position in space has been referred to as a "sensory selection problem" (Horak et al., 1988; Shumway-Cook et al., 1988). Persons with a sensory selection problem are often able to maintain balance in environments where sensory information for postural control is consistent; however, they are unable to maintain stability when there is incongruence among the senses. Persons with a sensory selection problem do not necessarily show a pattern of overreliance on any one sense but rather appear to be unable to correctly select an accurate orientation reference; therefore, they are unstable in any environment in which a sensory orientation reference is not accurate. This is shown in Figure 10.28, where abnormal sway is seen in conditions 3–6.

Sensory selection problems have been reported in persons with stroke (Bensoussan et al., 2007; DiFabio & Badke, 1990; Laufer et al., 2005; Marigold et al., 2004). Using the CTSIB test, Laufer et al. (2005) examined sensory organization ability in 20 patients currently receiving stroke rehabilitation. Sway was measured while patients stood on a force plate under the six sensory conditions; testing was done twice, at 1 and 2 months poststroke. A group of age-matched controls was also tested. Results are shown in Table 10.1. In the group with stroke, compared to the eyes-open condition, changing visual cues for balance (eyes-closed or dome conditions) resulted in significantly increased sway on both the firm and foam surfaces at 30 days poststroke (T1) and continued to be significant even 60 days poststroke (T2). Interestingly, with eyes open, the shift from firm surface to foam surface did not increase sway in persons with stroke, but did in the healthy controls. These results suggest that following stroke, patients show a greater dependency on visual inputs for postural control than do age-matched controls. Inability to maintain balance under altered sensory condition following a stroke can be seen in Jean's video (postural

TABLE 10.1 Sway Index of the Control Group of the Patients at First (T1) and Second (T2) Examination in Each Stance Position (mean ± SD)

	Firm surface			Foam surface		
Stance position	***Eyes open***	***Eyes closed***	***Dome***	***Eyes open***	***Eyes closed***	***Dome***
Control	15.6 ± 5.7	18.7 ± 5.7	19.5 ± 6.4	19.7 ± 7.9	30.3 ± 8.8	27.1 ± 4.7
Patients at T1	32.5 ± 16.3	43.2 ± 23.8	40.7 ± 21.6	33.9 ± 14.5	45.8 ± 15.2	42.0 ± 16.6
Patients at T2	28.3 ± 14.1	43.8 ± 22.5	36.6 ± 20.9	28.8 ± 12.6	49.8 ± 21.6	44.2 ± 15.8

control segment). Though she requires close guarding, Jean is able to maintain stance balance when all sensory inputs are present; however, when asked to close her eyes (removing visual inputs for postural control), she loses balance and requires assistance to prevent a fall. This suggests that Jean is visually dependent, that is, she relies on visual inputs for postural control.

Sensory organization problems have also been reported following traumatic brain injury (Shumway-Cook & Olmscheid, 1990) and in children with developmental disorders, including CP (Cherng et al., 1999; da Costa et al., 2019; Nashner et al., 1983), Down syndrome (Shumway-Cook & Woollacott, 1985b), and learning disabilities (Shumway-Cook et al., 1988). Thomas, our child with CP, also demonstrates problems with maintaining stability under altered sensory conditions. This can be seen in the postural control segment of his video. While he is able to maintain a stable position with eyes open and closed, he loses balance when wearing the visual dome (inaccurate visual inputs for balance).

Gatev et al. (1996) reported that participants with cerebellar pathology swayed more than did control participants under all six sensory conditions, and most fell in conditions 5 and 6, when both visual and somatosensory inputs were reduced. The authors note that testing standing balance under altered sensory conditions had better sensitivity than did normal stance testing (e.g., standing with eyes open or closed). Consistent with this research, John, our patient with cerebellar dysfunction, demonstrated a reduced ability to maintain balance under altered sensory conditions, as indicated by his performance on the CTSIB test. (See postural control segment on his video.)

Cherng et al. (1999) reported that sway was not significantly different between children with spastic diplegia as compared with TD children when somatosensory information was reliable (fixed foot support), regardless of the visual conditions. (See Fig. 10.29, conditions 1–3 on the SOT test.) In contrast, when somatosensory information was unreliable (compliant foot support), the difference in stance stability between the children with spastic diplegic CP and their matched controls was significantly greater when the visual input was deprived (occluded) or unreliable (sway referenced) than when it was reliable, suggesting the presence of sensory selection problems.

Not all children with CP demonstrate the same pattern of sensory organization problems. For example, sway in children with hemiplegia was not significantly different from age-matched controls in sensory conditions 1–5; however, they were less steady in condition 6. This is likely because children with hemiplegia have one normal leg to help regulate sway. Children with significant ataxia demonstrated significant increases in sway, compared to age-matched controls, in all six sensory conditions. Among all the children with CP, there was enormous variability in performance in the six sensory conditions; while some children had a lot of difficulty regulating sway, others did not (Nashner et al., 1983).

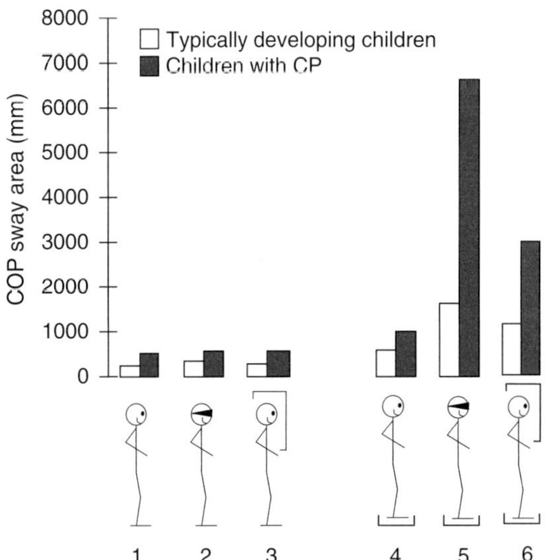

Figure 10.29 A comparison of COP area in the six sensory conditions of the Sensory Organization Test (SOT) in two groups of standing children, nondisabled healthy controls versus children with spastic diplegia cerebral palsy. (Adapted from Cherng RJ, Su FC, Chen JJ, et al. Performance of static standing balance in children with spastic diplegic cerebral palsy under altered sensory environments. *Am J Phys Med Rehabil.* 1999;78:336–343.)

Finally, sensory organization problems were reported in adults with MS (Cattaneo & Jonsdottir, 2009). Among persons with MS, there was no correlation between performance on the instrumented sensory organization tests and clinical measures of balance, including the Berg Balance Scale, Dynamic Gait Index, and the Activities-Specific Balance Confidence scale, leading the authors to conclude that the tests assessed different aspects of balance control (Cattaneo & Jonsdottir, 2009). Consistent with this research, Sue, our patient with MS, has difficulty maintaining balance under altered sensory conditions, as indicated by her poor performance on the CTSIB test. (See accompanying video.)

Sensory Problems Affecting Reactive Balance

As discussed in Chapter 7 on normal postural control, somatosensory inputs from the lower extremities play an important role in reactive balance, specifically in triggering muscle responses to support surface perturbations. To investigate the effect of impaired somatosensory inputs on stance reactive balance control, Inglis et al. (1994) examined muscle responses in patients with diabetic neuropathy and healthy controls in response to platform perturbations. While patients with neuropathy showed the same distal-to-proximal muscle

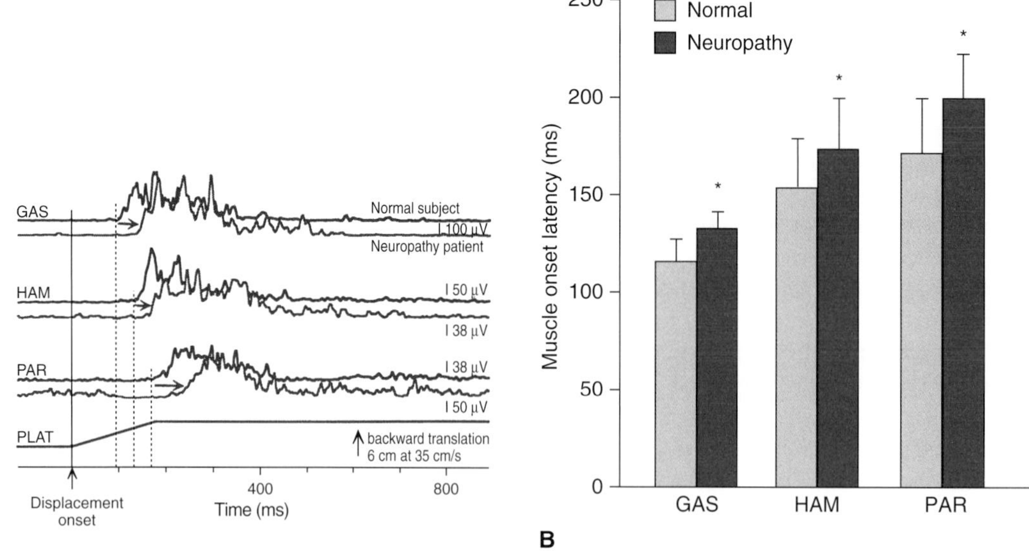

Figure 10.30 (A) EMG activity in lower extremity muscles in response to a backward platform translation from a patient with peripheral neuropathy and a healthy control participant. **(B)** Onset of muscle activity in all three lower extremity muscles is delayed in the patients with peripheral neuropathy compared to the healthy controls. *GAS*, gastrocnemius; *HAM*, hamstrings; *PAR*, paraspinals; *PLAT*, platform movement. (Reprinted from Inglis JT, Horak FB, Shupert CL, et al. The importance of somatosensory information in triggering and scaling automatic postural responses in humans. *Exp Brain Res*. 1994;101:159–164, with permission.)

activation pattern as the healthy controls, the onset of muscle responses was delayed by 20 to 30 ms in all muscles. This is shown in Figure 10.30A, which compares the EMG responses in the lower extremities from one healthy control and one patient with neuropathy in response to a backward platform translation. Onset of muscle activity in all three lower extremity muscles (Fig. 10.30B) is delayed. In addition, patients showed an impaired ability to scale muscle response amplitudes to change in both the velocity and amplitude of surface translations. Results suggest that somatosensory information from the lower limb impacts reactive balance control in two ways: (a) Triggering centrally organized postural synergies and (b) providing direct sensory feedback, which combined with prior experience, are essential in scaling the magnitude of automatic postural responses.

Sensory Problems Affecting Anticipatory Balance

Most of the studies examining the effect of sensory problems on anticipatory balance have been done in the context of locomotion and consequently are covered in detail in that chapter. However, this research has provided some interesting insights. For example, in locomotion, patients with stroke use visual information (through a fixed-point gaze or downward gaze) as a compensatory strategy to help maintain balance (Aoki et al., 2017). Similarly, a loss of somatosensory inputs in individuals with peripheral neuropathy results in profound changes in motor adaptation and an earlier activation of anticipatory postural adjustments as a compensatory strategy (Bunday & Bronstein, 2009). It is likely that impaired sensation may result in earlier activation of anticipatory postural activity in stance and sitting as well, but this awaits further research.

Perceptual Problems Affecting Postural Control

We have discussed how sensory problems affecting the selection and organization of sensory information can significantly impact steady-state, reactive, and anticipatory postural control. The following sections discuss the impact of perceptual problems on postural control.

Perceptions of Verticality

Many studies have shown that the perception of vertical in humans is extremely precise, particularly in the upright position. The brain integrates sensory inputs from visual, vestibular, and somatosensory systems to create perceptions related to verticality (Barra et al., 2010). Perceptions of vertical can be subdivided into several components. The subjective visual vertical (SVV) is determined by having subjects adjust a visible luminous line in complete darkness to what they consider to be upright, earth vertical; haptic vertical (HV) is determined by manipulation of a rod to the earth vertical position while the subject's eyes are closed. The subjective postural vertical (SPV) is the perception of the position of the head or body with respect to true vertical, usually tested with eyes closed.

Impaired perceptions related to verticality are found in many patients with neurologic impairment and are strongly associated with impaired balance control. Clinicians involved in balance rehabilitation need to be aware of the effect of impaired perceptions on the control of balance. Subjective VV is impaired in many patients with acute stroke and is significantly correlated with impaired balance (Bonan et al., 2006) and WBA (Barra et al., 2009). Impaired perceptions of visual vertical are worse among patients with somatosensory loss (Barra et al., 2010).

SPV (the perceived sense of "uprightness" of one's own body) is also significantly impaired in many patients with neurologic pathology. Pérennou and colleagues (1998) reported that even with visual cues present, the majority of patients with stroke studied (19/22) had impaired SPV. Impaired SPV was not correlated with age, severity of weakness, or spasticity; however, it was dependent on both the severity of spatial neglect and degree of sensory loss on the hemiparetic side (Pérennou, 2006). Finally, there is some evidence that contraversive pushing ("pusher syndrome"), in which a person uses the nonparetic limbs to actively push the body toward the paretic limbs, may result from impaired perceptions of postural vertical. Interestingly, these patients often demonstrate normal visual vertical (Karnath & Broetz, 2003; Karnath et al., 2000).

Clinical Implications of Research on Impaired Sensation/Perceptions and Postural Control

These studies demonstrate that impaired sensation has a significant effect on all aspects of postural control and suggest a number of important clinical implications. First, pathology in widely distributed areas of the brain can disrupt the ability to organize and select sensory information essential to steady-state, reactive, and proactive postural control. The research on impaired sensory organization and selection problems reminds us that instability in patients with neurologic pathology can be "context specific." This means that instability can be present in some environments but not in others. For example, a person with stroke or traumatic brain injury may be able to maintain balance in an environment in which sensory information is optimal (e.g., standing on a firm surface in a well-lit environment) but may lose balance in an environment in which sensory conditions are less than optimal (e.g., standing on an incline or carpeted surface in low-light conditions). This research also suggests that therapists must carefully consider the conditions under which balance is tested in persons with neurologic pathology. Since postural instability may not be readily apparent when a patient is tested in ideal or optimal sensory conditions (e.g., on a firm flat surface with eyes open), balance may need to be tested and treated under more complex sensory conditions, such as when surface and/or visual inputs for postural control are disrupted. Sensory organization capability may not be readily identified using common clinical measures of balance that do not examine balance under altered sensory conditions. As discussed in more detail in the next chapter, different tests of balance measure different aspects of postural control. Finally, it is clear that problems in organizing sensory information related to the body's position and movement in space also affect the development of perceptions relevant to balance control. It is important to understand the relative role of impaired perceptions to functional balance control. Thus, balance rehabilitation programs must include the assessment and treatment of misperceptions affecting the control of balance.

PROBLEMS IN COGNITIVE SYSTEMS

There is increasing evidence demonstrating the interacting effects of impaired cognition and postural control in persons with neurologic pathology. Research in this area is expanding rapidly. In the following section, we review studies in three areas: (a) impaired balance self-efficacy and its relationship to participation in daily life activities, (b) the impact of cognitive load on postural stability in persons with neurologic pathology, and (c) studies examining postural deficits in individuals with different forms of dementia, including Alzheimer's disease.

Balance and Falls Self-Efficacy

The consequences of impaired balance are significant, leading to increased risk for falls as well as loss of functional independence. In addition, balance abilities influence balance and falls self-efficacy, which reflect how confident persons are in their ability to perform daily activities without losing their balance (balance self-efficacy) or falling (falls self-efficacy). Poor balance and falls self-efficacy are reported in many persons with neurologic pathology including those with stroke (Robinson et al., 2011; Salbach et al., 2006), MS (Matsuda et al., 2011), and PD (Rahman et al., 2011) and can be present even among persons who have no history of falls (Matsuda et al., 2011). Impaired balance and falls self-efficacy are associated with avoidance of physical activity and restrictions in daily life activities (Bertera & Bertera, 2008; Peterson et al., 2007). In addition, balance self-efficacy is a major factor predicting participation in community mobility following stroke (Robinson et al., 2011; Schmid et al., 2012). It is clear that willingness to engage in daily life activities is influenced not only by a person's actual balance abilities but also by their perceived balance abilities. Clinical measures of balance and falls self-efficacy are discussed in Chapter 11.

Impaired Postural Stability and Dual-Task Interference

We saw in Chapter 7 that even among healthy young adults, normal postural control requires attentional resources; the amount of attention required depends on the difficulty of the postural task being performed. Does impaired postural control found in patients with neurologic pathology increase the attentional demands of balance? The answer is yes. This can be seen in Figure 10.31, which summarizes the results of an experiment that examined how different postural tasks affect performance (reaction times) on a secondary task in persons with hemiplegia and healthy controls. Remember from Chapter 7 that researchers use changes in performance on a secondary task (in this case, reaction time) to infer attentional requirements of the primary task. In healthy controls, reaction times were not different in sitting, standing feet apart, or standing feet together (StandTo), suggesting all three tasks had comparable attentional demands for this group. In contrast, participants with stroke showed increasingly slowed reaction times as postural tasks became more difficult, suggesting that attentional demands for this group increased with increased demands of the postural task (Brown et al., 2002).

This research suggests that impaired postural control impacts the attentional demands associated with maintaining balance, with more difficult balance tasks requiring more attention. Do increased attentional demands associated with impaired postural control affect the performance of tasks performed in daily life, such as recognizing familiar faces?

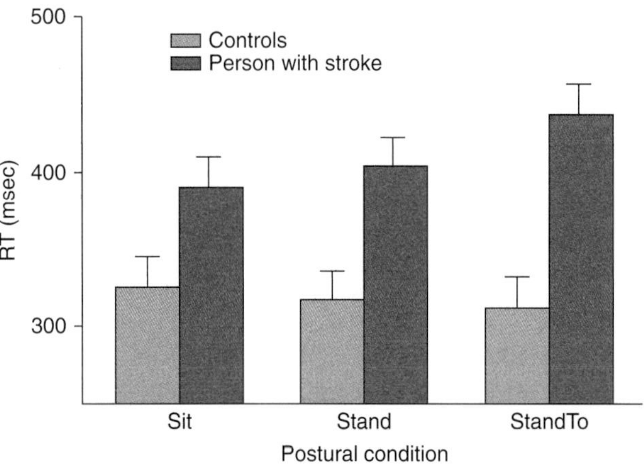

Figure 10.31 Attentional demands associated with three different postural tasks (sitting, standing, and standing with feet together [StandTo]) in persons with stroke and age- and gender-matched controls. Reaction times (RTs) to a secondary verbal RT task are slower in subjects with stroke as compared with controls in all three conditions. In addition, RT is significantly faster in sitting as compared with standing tasks in patients with stroke but not in controls, suggesting that postural control is more demanding after stroke. (Reprinted from Brown LA, Sleik RJ, Winder TR. Attentional demands for static postural control after stroke. *Arch Phys Med Rehabil.* 2002;83:1732–1735, Figure 1, with permission.)

In order to answer this question, Suzuki et al. (1997) used dual-task methods to examine the effects of increasing postural demands on facial recognition in patients with right hemisphere versus left hemisphere stroke who had unilateral spatial neglect (USN). They examined the patient's ability to perceive faces presented to the right or left of midline while sitting, standing, or stepping in place. Performance on the test for each patient is summarized in Table 10.2. Some patients (e.g., subjects 8 and 12) were able to recognize all faces when they were presented on the ipsilesional side but were unable to recognize any faces when they were presented on the contralesional side, and this was true across all postural tasks. However, some patients (e.g., subjects 1, 5, and 6) were able to observe all 15 faces presented on the contralesional side when sitting or standing; however, they were unable to perceive any faces (score of 0) while stepping in place. These findings indicate that USN is context specific; that is, it may only interfere with a spatial task when postural demands are great but may not be apparent when postural demands are less. Interestingly, two of the individuals with USN (subjects 9 and 10) who performed normally on the video face test in stepping (score of 15) required more assistance to step during the test, suggesting that they allocated attention to the video task rather than to the stepping task. Other subjects were able to keep stepping with minimal or no assistance (Suzuki et al., 1997).

The research reviewed so far demonstrates that impaired postural control impacts the amount of attention required to maintain balance, and this can interfere with the performance of other tasks, such as recognizing the faces of familiar people. How does performance of a secondary task impact postural stability in patients with neurologic pathology?

Researchers have shown that a reduced ability to maintain balance while performing multiple tasks is common among persons with various types of neurologic pathology. Dual-task interference with steady-state stance balance has been shown in some, but not all, people with PD. Marchese et al. (2003) examined the effect of a secondary task on COP area (steady-state stance balance) in patients with PD and healthy controls. As shown in Figure 10.32A, compared to healthy controls (NC), sway area was not greater in the baseline condition (quiet stance alone) but was significantly increased in PD (orange) on both the subtraction (Calc) and thumb/fingers opposition (Seq) tasks. However, not all patients showed the problem. As shown in Figure 10.32B, dual-task interference was greatest among persons with PD with instability (shown in orange) compared to more stable individuals with PD (shown in black) (Marchese et al., 2003). Similarly, postural stability is more compromised

TABLE 10.2 Scores on the Video Face Test in Patients With Unilateral Spatial Neglect: Number of Correct Identifications of Faces Presented on the Right or Left Side in Sitting, Standing, and Walking

		Sitting		Standing		Stepping	
Subject no.	**Hemisphere lesion side**	**RT**	**LT**	**RT**	**LT**	**RT**	**LT**
1	Right	15	15	15	15	14	0
2	Right	15	15	15	15	15	7
3	Right	14	15	15	15	13	7
4	Right	14	13	15	15	15	0
5	Right	15	15	15	15	15	0
6	Right	15	15	15	15	15	0
7	Right	15	15	15	15	15	9
8	Right	15	0	15	0	15	0
9	Right	15	15	15	15	15	15
10	Right	14	15	15	15	15	15
11	Left	14	15	15	15	10	15
12	Left	0	15	0	15	0	15

Total possible, 15. *RT*, right; *LT*, left.

Reprinted from Suzuki E, Chen W, Kondo T. Measuring unilateral spatial neglect during stepping. *Arch Phys Med Rehabil.* 1997;78:176, with permission.

during dual tasking in individuals with PD with freezing of gait than nonfreezers (Bekkers et al., 2018). Bloem et al. (2006) also reported impaired stability under dual-task conditions in persons with PD and suggested that individuals with PD use a "posture second" strategy, in which cognitive rather than balance tasks are prioritized under dual-task conditions.

Impaired dual-task performance has also been shown following traumatic brain injury (Brauer et al., 2004) and stroke (Bensoussan et al., 2007,

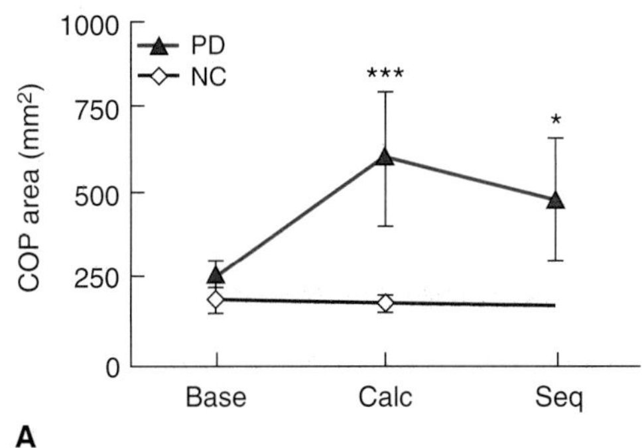

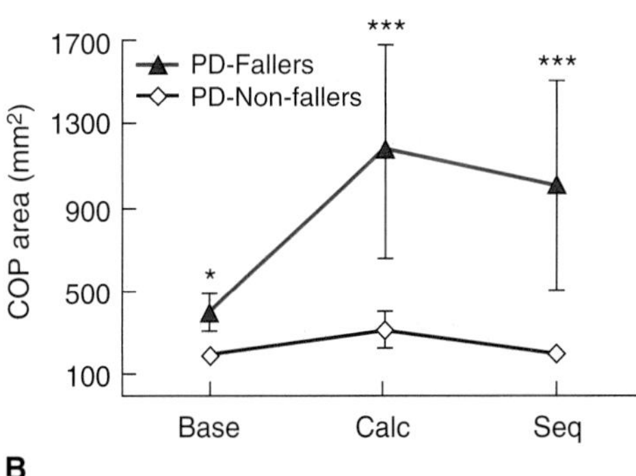

Figure 10.32 Examining the effect of a secondary task on COP area (during steady-state stance balance) in patients with PD and healthy controls (NC). **(A)** Sway area was not greater in the single baseline stance condition but was significantly increased in PD (*orange*) on both the subtraction (Calc) and thumb/fingers opposition (Seq) tasks. **(B)** Dual-task interference was greatest among persons with PD with more instability (prev. falls, orange) compared to individuals with PD with good balance. (Adapted from Marchese R, Bove M, Abbruzzese G. Effect of cognitive and motor tasks on postural stability in Parkinson's disease: a posturographic study. *Mov Disord.* 2003;18:652–658.)

Cockburn et al., 2003; Hyndman & Ashburn, 2003; Hyndman et al., 2009). Bensoussan et al. (2007) reported increased sway under dual-task conditions, especially among stroke survivors with a history of falls, whereas Hyndman and colleagues (2009) reported decreased sway during the dual-task condition following stroke, even for those with a history of falls. Hyndman et al. suggest that reduced sway under dual-task conditions was a strategy to preserve balance; participants prioritized the balance task over the secondary task (what others have termed a "posture-first strategy"). However, the authors did not report changes in the secondary task under any of the conditions; thus, it is difficult to determine whether preserving balance (the posture-first hypothesis) was done at the expense of performance on the secondary task.

Impaired dual-task performance has also been reported in children with neurologic pathology. Children (mean age, 5 years) with DCD demonstrated increased sway under dual-task conditions (naming objects) as compared with TD children. Cognitive performance was affected by the dual tasks in the TD children but not in those with DCD. Thus, under dual-task conditions, children with DCD had increased sway but no change in cognitive task performance, suggesting that they were prioritizing the cognitive task (Laufer et al., 2008). Finally, Reilly et al. (2008b) investigated the effects of a secondary task on balance in children with spastic versus ataxic CP and TD children. A dual-task paradigm was used in which the children stood in either a wide or a narrow stance position while simultaneously performing a visual working memory task. For both stance positions, the children with CP were more unstable than were comparably aged TD children, but only in the dual-task condition (i.e., showed greater dual-task interference). In addition, the children with ataxic CP showed greater dual-task interference affecting postural control compared to those with spastic diplegia. Figure 10.33 compares COP under single- and dual-task conditions in a TD child and one with ataxic CP. In addition, for the children with ataxia, increasing postural demands (standing with feet together) resulted in reduced performance on the secondary memory task. This was not found in the children with spastic diplegia CP. Likewise, it has been shown that the constraints on performance during dual-tasks are less in children with mild CP (Palluel et al., 2019).

It is clear from this brief review that dual-task interference is a significant contribution to instability in many types of neurologic pathology. Instability under dual-task conditions may arise for a number of reasons. Neurologic pathology may affect attentional capacity; under dual-task conditions, limited attentional capacity is exceeded and stability is compromised. Neurologic pathology may produce deficits in executive attention, which influences the allocation of attention under dual-task conditions, also impairing balance. Finally, researchers have shown that maintaining stability requires more attentional resources in persons with neurologic pathology as compared with individuals without disability, and this may contribute to instability under dual-task conditions. Regardless of the underlying cause, examining the effect of performing a second task on balance control is critical to understanding stability problems in persons with neurologic pathology.

Impaired postural control leading to reduced function and increased likelihood for falls is common among persons with dementia. A review of the research on postural control in persons with dementia may be found in Extended Knowledge Box 10.2.

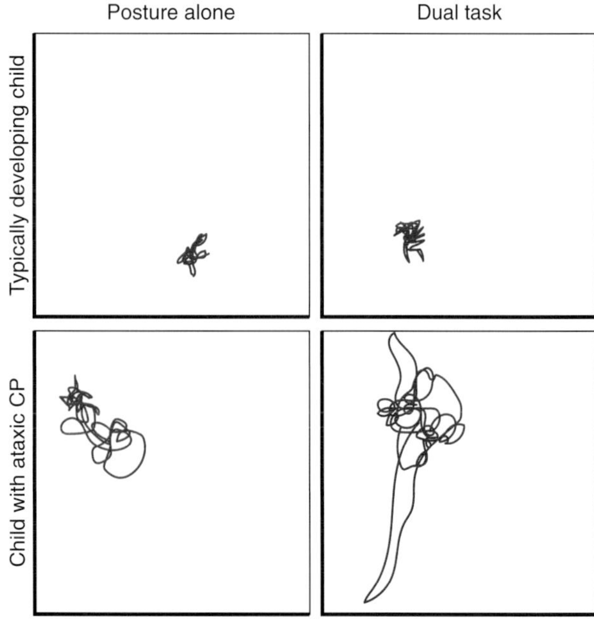

Figure 10.33 A comparison of COP excursion under single- (posture alone) and dual-task conditions in a TD child and one with ataxic cerebral palsy. (Adapted with permission from Reilly DS, Woollacott MH, van Donkelaar P, et al. The interaction between executive attention and postural control in dual-task conditions: children with cerebral palsy. *Arch Phys Med Rehabil.* 2008b;89:834–842.)

Extended Knowledge 10.2

Postural Control in Persons with Dementia

The relationship between impairments in cognitive function and postural control is being studied by many researchers, in part because of the high rates of falls reported in persons with various types of dementia, including Alzheimer's disease (Ballard et al., 1999; Camicioli & Licis, 2004; Kallin et al., 2005). Cognitive impairment is a known predictor of falls in older adults (Buchner & Larson, 1987; Morris et al., 1987; Tinetti et al., 1995). The incidence of mortality and morbidity following falls is much higher among persons with cognitive impairments as compared with those with no cognitive impairments (Buchner & Larson, 1987; Lord et al., 2001). Risk factors for falls in persons with dementia include impairments of motor function, balance, and gait (Alexander et al., 1995; Camicioli & Licis, 2004; Kallin et al., 2005; Visser, 1983). Poor performance under dual-task conditions has been reported as a risk factor for falls in some studies (Hauer et al., 2003; Pettersson et al., 2005) but not in others (Camicioli & Licis, 2004; Camicioli et al., 1997).

Researchers have begun to study the effects of impaired cognition on different components of postural control in order to better understand the neural mechanisms underlying the increased risk of falls in persons with dementia.

Motor Coordination

Moving-platform methods have been used to study postural motor activity in individuals with Alzheimer's disease. Problems in central set underlying the ability to change postural motor strategies with changing task conditions were examined in individuals with Alzheimer's disease (Chong et al., 1999). Leg-muscle activity during backward platform translations was examined in people with and without Alzheimer's disease when they stood freely, held on to a supporting frame, or sat. Surprisingly, individuals with Alzheimer's disease were able to quickly suppress leg-muscle activity when in the supported condition, suggesting that central set was not impaired.

Anticipatory postural activity preceding a voluntary movement of the arms also appears to be intact in individuals with Alzheimer's disease (Elble & Leffler, 2000). Individuals with Alzheimer's disease were asked to push or pull on a rigid horizontal bar in order to quickly move a cursor into a target window on a computer screen placed in front of them while they were standing unsupported. Although individuals with Alzheimer's disease had slower reaction times and were significantly less accurate in the task than were controls, anticipatory postural activity in the legs was the same in the two groups.

In summary, results from studies involving individuals with Alzheimer's-type dementia have shown relatively few deficits in the motor component of postural control, although research is just beginning in this area, and the number of studies available is relatively limited.

Sensory Organization

The ability to organize sensory information for postural control was examined in individuals with mild versus moderate Alzheimer's dementia using the moving-platform and visual-surround methods described earlier (Chong et al., 1999; Dicken & Rose, 2004). Individuals with Alzheimer's disease had more difficulty than did age-matched controls in maintaining stability when only vestibular information was available for postural control (condition 6 on the SOT test), despite normal vestibular function. In addition, individuals with mild Alzheimer's disease had more difficulty than did those with moderate disease when visual information was disrupted. The authors interpret these findings to suggest that with increasing severity of dementia, there is a reduced dependence on visual information for postural control. As a result, disrupting visual information has less effect in individuals with moderate-to-severe Alzheimer's disease as compared with those with mild dementia. Research exploring deficits in postural control in persons with dementia are improving our ability to reduce fall rates in this vulnerable population.

A CASE STUDY APPROACH TO UNDERSTANDING POSTURAL DYSCONTROL

Until now, our discussion of postural dyscontrol following neurologic pathology has focused on presenting a wide variety of sensory, motor, and cognitive problems leading to instability. You can see that the range of problems is great, and this reflects the complexity of problems that affect the central nervous system. In the last section of this chapter, we use our case studies to summarize postural control problems by diagnosis. Several warnings must be given prior to beginning this section. Remember that even persons with the same diagnosis can present with very different postural problems. Differences in postural control problems can result from variability in type, location, and extent of neural lesions. Other factors, such as age, premorbid status, and degree of compensation, also have a profound impact on the behavior seen. Before reading the case studies, complete Lab Activity 10.1. The answers to this lab activity may be found in the case studies. Remember that each case study has an accompanying video; in the postural control, segment of each patient video is an example of the types of postural problems described in this chapter. Also shown are many of the clinical tests used to examine postural control problems in patients with neurologic diagnoses.

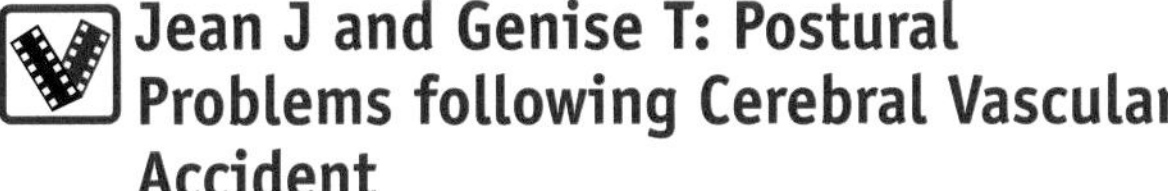

Jean J and Genise T: Postural Problems following Cerebral Vascular Accident

Jean J, our 82-year-old woman who has a right hemiparesis following a stroke 4 years ago, and Genise, our 53-year-old woman who had a stroke 1 month ago, both have significant postural control problems affecting the ability to function independently. Postural responses are delayed and reduced in amplitude in the paretic right limb.

Both Jean and Genise demonstrate asymmetric weight-bearing when sitting or standing quietly.

LAB ACTIVITY 10.1

Objective: To translate research on the physiological basis for abnormal postural control into hypotheses about the potential underlying cause(s) of instability in a patient with a specific neurologic diagnosis.

Assignment

1. For each patient case study listed at the end of this chapter, generate a list of hypotheses regarding the potential sensory, motor, and cognitive factors contributing to instability in each patient. How would you expect these impairments to impact steady-state, reactive, and proactive balance in sitting and standing?
2. Based on the information presented in this chapter, what research supports your hypotheses?

In addition, postural sway is increased, suggesting impairments in steady-state balance. In response to manual perturbations, Jean relies on reaching with her nonhemiparetic arm to recover balance or, in most cases, has to be caught to prevent a fall. Genise is unable to generate force with her paretic limb and is unable to recover from even a small perturbation to balance.

If we were to look at the synergistic organization of muscles in the paretic limbs of these two patients, we would find significant disruption of the temporal and spatial sequencing of muscle activity in the nonhemiparetic limb as well as a reduced ability to recruit muscles in the paretic limb.

Loss of anticipatory activation of postural muscles during voluntary movements is also present. This results in unsteadiness when carrying out functional activities such as lifting, reaching, or carrying physical loads. Difficulty modifying and adapting postural movements to changing task demands is also present in persons with stroke. This makes it difficult to maintain stability in response to a change in the base of support or in appropriately responding to challenges to balance that vary in speed and amplitude.

Neuromuscular problems resulting from stroke have also produced secondary musculoskeletal problems that affect postural control in both Genise and Jean. Weakness has developed in both the hemiparetic and the nonparetic limb. Limitations in range of motion in the arm and leg have also developed.

In addition to motor changes, both Genise and Jean have a number of sensory problems that are contributing to impaired postural control. Though neither Jean nor Genise does, many persons with stroke have reduced sensory information from the visual system (hemianopsia). Genise has significantly reduced somatosensation in the hemiparetic limbs. In addition, both women have difficulty in adapting sensory information to changing environmental demands. This affects the ability to maintain stability in certain environments, such as under low-light levels or when the surface is soft or unsteady. Inability to maintain balance in conditions in which there is a loss of sensory redundancy is a critical factor in understanding Jean's balance problems. You can see this in her inability to stand when any sensory input is reduced (such as when standing with eyes closed or on a foam surface). Jean has difficulty maintaining balance while performing other attentionally demanding tasks, though this is not shown in the video. Finally, because of sensory/motor impairments, both Jean and Genise have had several falls and are at increased risk for falls in the future.

 Mike M: Postural Problems in Parkinson's Disease

Mike is our 67-year-old man with PD. He is having increasing difficulty with mobility skills, including bed mobility, transfers, and gait. Postural problems affecting orientation and stability are a significant factor in his declining independence, particularly when he is off his medication. As you can see on the video, steady-state balance (orientation, alignment, and sway) when on medication is fairly good, though he stands with a typically flexed posture. When he is off medication, his flexed posture worsens. Though he is able to correct this posture with verbal cueing, when distracted, he reverts back to a kyphotic stance. His reactive balance on medication is good; he is able to use an in-place recovery strategy in response to small perturbations. In response to larger perturbations, when a change-in-support (step) is required, you see the effect of medication. On medication, he is able to recover using a single step. Off medication, multiple steps (retropulsion) occur. If we were using EMGs to record his muscle activity, we would find that despite the fact that he has significant bradykinesia, or slowed voluntary movement, which is common in PD, the onset latencies of his automatic postural responses are likely to be normal. However, we would likely find that he uses a complex pattern of muscle activity involving coactivating muscles on both sides of the body when responding to instability. This coactivation of muscles on both sides of his body results in a rigid body and an inability to recover stability adequately. In addition, he would be unable to modify movement patterns quickly in response to changing task demands. This problem with central set causes him to use the same pattern of muscle activity when responding to perturbations to balance while sitting or standing.

Because of impaired anticipatory postural control, he is unsteady when carrying out functional tasks that are potentially destabilizing, such as lifting or reaching for objects. You see that off medication, he is slower in performing tasks such as the stool touch that require anticipatory postural adjustments. In addition to primary neuromuscular impairments such as rigidity and bradykinesia, secondary musculoskeletal problems have developed, further limiting movements for postural control.

Mike, like many others with PD, has sensory organization problems. He has difficulty organizing and selecting sensory information for postural control indicated by his increased sway under the four sensory conditions shown on the video, particularly off medication. In addition, he has difficulty maintaining balance under dual-task conditions.

John C: Postural Problems in Cerebellar Disorders

John is our 33-year-old man with spinocerebellar degeneration, type 2, resulting in severe ataxia. Much of the research on postural control in persons with cerebellar disorders has been with persons who have anterior-lobe cerebellar degeneration. Thus, findings from these studies may not necessarily completely apply to John, who has more generalized damage to the cerebellum, or to other persons with specific lateral hemisphere lesions or vestibulocerebellar lesions. Certainly, however, impaired postural control is a hallmark of cerebellar disorders.

You can see from the video that steady-state balance control is disrupted in John. He stands with a wide base of support, and when asked to narrow his base, sway increases dramatically and he has to be closely guarded to prevent a fall. In response to a small perturbation to balance, John is able to recover using an in-place strategy, but you can see that during recovery, he oscillates before coming to a stable position. If we were recording EMGs, we would likely find that onset of contraction of postural muscles in John is likely to be normal, although in children with ataxic forms of CP, contraction onsets are often delayed. John has difficulty scaling postural activity, resulting in hypermetric postural responses. This means that in response to a small backward perturbation to balance, John overcorrects, and this results in significant oscillation of his body. Research suggests that this overcorrection results from hypermetric muscle responses, that is, responses that are too large compared to the size of the challenge. Thus, he overshoots when trying to return to a stable position. In response to larger perturbations, he takes multiple steps initially but is able to adapt and scale responses appropriately with practice. John has significant problems with anticipatory postural control, as indicated by his instability when performing tasks such as the stool touch, in which the therapist has to catch him to prevent a fall.

John also has problems with adapting how sensory information is used for postural control in response to changing environmental demands. He has difficulty when trying to maintain balance in conditions in which he must adapt sensory information for postural control. He is unable to maintain balance when standing on a firm surface with his eyes closed but is able to maintain stability but with increased sway on the foam surface with eyes open. He loses balance on the foam surface with eyes closed. This pattern suggests that John is dependent on vision for balance control, and this may partly explain why he loses balance and falls at night.

Thomas L: Postural Problems in Spastic Diplegic CP

Thomas is a 7 year-old boy with spastic diplegia form of CP. He is moderately involved, scoring a 3 on the Gross Motor Function Classification Scale. He has both neuromuscular and musculoskeletal problems affecting postural control, and this results in multiple falls on a weekly basis. Thomas has significantly impaired steady-state balance in both sitting and standing. As you can see on the video, he is able to sit on the floor independently, but with a posterior tilt of his pelvis, a kyphotic trunk and forward head position. He is internally rotated and flexed at the hips, knees, and ankles and has difficulty maintaining a stable position. He is able to stand independently, but with significant hip flexion and an anterior tilt of the pelvis. He uses excessive lordosis to get his head and trunk vertical. His knees are hyperextended, and ankles are plantarflexed. Without support, his sway increases significantly.

Reactive balance is impaired as well. In standing, Thomas is unable to recover from a small perturbation in either the forward or backward direction; he uses his arms to stabilize and requires assistance to prevent a fall. In response to a larger perturbation, he uses a step response but requires assistance to prevent a fall. He is unable to step in response to a larger backward perturbation. If we were recording EMGs on Thomas during recovery from a perturbation, we would likely find that the onset of contraction of his postural muscles is quite delayed and reduced in amplitude, despite the presence of hyperactive stretch reflexes in spastic muscles. In addition to delayed onset of spastic muscles, he is likely to show a disruption of the normal sequencing of muscle activation patterns. Other factors contributing to muscle sequencing problems are changes in postural alignment (specifically, his crouched stance posture) and the use of Ankle–foot orthoses (AFOs). He has anticipatory postural control problems that also affect his stability during performance of voluntary motor acts. Musculoskeletal problems, including weakness, reduced range of motion, and changes to the structure and function of skeletal muscles, will also contribute to balance problems. Thomas also shows problems in anticipatory postural control as indicated by his reduced ability to reach forward, or kick a ball, without losing his balance.

Problems in sensory adaptation do not appear to be present consistently in all children with spastic hemiplegia forms of CP; however, they do appear to be a problem in spastic diplegia and ataxic forms of CP. This can be seen in Thomas's reduced ability to maintain stance stability when standing under altered sensory conditions. While he is able to stand independently on a firm surface, with eyes open or closed or when wearing the visual conflict dome, he is only able to stand 15 s on the foam surface with eyes open or closed and falls immediately with the visual conflict dome.

Malachi: Postural Problems in Severe Athetoid/Spastic CP

Malachi is a 4-year-old boy with a severe, mixed form of CP. While predominantly athetoid with a dystonic component, he has spasticity in the lower extremities and has had surgery to release contractures in the hamstrings, adductors, and Achilles tendons. He is classified as a level IV on the Gross Motor Function Classification System. Functionally, Malachi requires assistance to move into the seated position; once he is there, he can prop for short periods before collapsing. He cannot stand or walk independently.

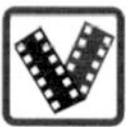

Sue: Postural Problems in Multiple Sclerosis

Sue is our patient with relapsing remitting MS. As can be seen in her video case study, Sue has significant postural dyscontrol that affects primarily her ability to stand and walk independently. Postural control in sitting, including steady-state, reactive, and proactive balance, is good. However, all three aspects of balance control are significantly impaired in standing. She is able to stand without support but shows significantly increased postural sway, suggesting impaired steady-state balance in stance. She is unable to recover from small or large perturbations when standing, suggesting significantly impaired reactive balance. Research on reactive balance in persons with MS suggests that significantly delayed postural muscle responses are one of the factors contributing to impaired reactive balance in Sue. In addition, Sue has difficulty performing tasks that require anticipatory postural adjustments, such as reaching forward or leaning over to pick up an object from the floor. Research suggests that delay in the activation of postural muscles prior to a voluntary movement contributes to impaired anticipatory postural control in MS.

On the modified CTSIB test, Sue has difficulty maintaining balance when any sensory input for balance is reduced (standing with eyes closed or on the foam surface). This is consistent with research suggesting that persons with MS have difficulty organizing and selecting sensory inputs for postural control.

Sue is able to complete the Timed Up and Go test in 22 s in both the single- and dual-task conditions; however, she makes numerous errors on the secondary task, suggesting that dual-task interference is present during walking.

SUMMARY

1. An enormous range of problems can contribute to postural dyscontrol in individuals with a neurologic deficit. In the therapeutic environment, the ability to retrain postural control requires a conceptual framework that incorporates information on the physiological basis for normal postural control, as well as knowledge regarding the basis for instability.
2. Neurologic pathology can affect many aspects of balance control, including the ability to maintain stability when sitting or standing. Several behaviors are used to evaluate steady-state balance including alignment and sway. Sway during quiet stance and sitting (as indicated by COP or COM excursion) is often, but not always, increased. Many factors contribute to atypical sway patterns, including problems in alignment, changes in muscle tone, impairments in the sensory/perceptual system, and secondary musculoskeletal problems.
3. Reactive balance in stance and sitting is also impaired in neurologic patients; the extent of impairment will depend on the extent and location of pathology. Neuromuscular problems that disrupt the coordination of postural movement strategies affect the ability to recover from an external perturbation. Coordination problems include (a) sequencing problems, (b) problems with the timely activation of muscle response synergies, (c) disorders related to the scaling of postural muscle activity, and (d) problems adapting motor responses to changing task conditions.
4. Anticipatory postural problems also contribute to loss of functional independence in many patients with neurologic pathology. Inability to activate postural muscles prior to a voluntary movement of the arm or leg results in instability and increased risk for falls. External support to the trunk can reduce the effects of impaired anticipatory postural control and improve upper-extremity function.
5. Sensory problems can disrupt postural control by (a) affecting a person's ability to adapt sensory inputs to changes in task and environmental demands and (b) preventing the development of accurate internal models of the body essential to accurate perceptions related to postural control.
6. Cognitive problems also significantly affect postural stability, including inability to maintain stability when engaged in multiple tasks.
7. Differences in postural control problems can result from variability in type, location, and extent of the neural lesion. Other factors, such as age, premorbid status, and degree of compensation, also have a profound impact on postural behavior.

CHAPTER 11

Clinical Management of the Patient with a Postural Control Disorder

Learning Objectives

Following completion of this chapter, the reader will be able to:

1. Understand the relationship between research on normal and abnormal postural control and clinical methods for assessing and treating impaired postural control in patients with movement disorders.
2. Discuss the clinical implications of both the ICF (International Classification of Functioning, Disability and Health) and systems framework on the assessment and treatment of balance disorders.
3. Discuss clinical tests and measures for assessing balance and consider the evidence regarding the reliability, validity, sensitivity, and specificity of these tests in pediatric, geriatric, and neurologic populations.
4. Develop a clinical decision-making process for selecting appropriate tests and measures when assessing postural control in patients with varying levels of functional ability.
5. Describe a task-oriented approach to improving postural control in sitting and standing, providing a rationale for intervention practices based on a systems theory of normal and abnormal postural control.
6. Discuss the evidence for best practices related to balance retraining in geriatric and neurologic populations.

INTRODUCTION

This chapter focuses on clinical methods for assessing and treating persons with postural control disorders. We will examine research evidence that supports the effectiveness of specific therapeutic methods used to assess and treat postural disorders, including those related to orientation and balance (control of the center of mass [COM] relative to the base of support). Although there is a growing body of research related to the effectiveness of balance training, it is often difficult to apply this research to the clinical treatment of persons with balance problems. In many cases, researchers have demonstrated the efficacy of training on a variety of balance outcomes but have provided limited information on what specific strategies were used to improve balance.

Consequently, researchers are now emphasizing the need to design interventions characterized by a high level of therapeutic fidelity. In rehabilitation, intervention fidelity addresses a systematic and correct implementation of the key features upon which the intervention is built, to avoid compromising the effectiveness of its outcomes (An et al., 2020). An and colleagues (2020) suggest a multidimensional approach to quantify therapeutic fidelity that includes adherence (adequate delivery of key intervention components), intervention quality (means by which the intervention is delivered following the defined therapeutic strategies of implementation), dosage (amount of intervention delivered), participant responsiveness (participants' engagement during the intervention), and program differentiation (difference in the therapeutic process and components between interventions). Intervention fidelity would be particularly important when therapists plan to implement two related interventions and need to evaluate the one most beneficial for a specific patient. Researchers can now improve intervention fidelity through the use of the Template for Intervention and Replication Purposes (TIDieR)—a 12-item checklist that describes interventions with sufficient details to ensure their replicability (Hoffmann et al., 2014).

While there is growing evidence examining the effect of improved balance on functional activities, there is limited evidence on the effects of improved balance on participation in social roles and complex daily life activities. This makes it difficult for clinicians to identify best practices related to balance rehabilitation. Questionnaires and self-perceived balance confidence scales, described in the Examination section of this chapter, may be good tools to help researchers and clinicians explore how balance is related to patient activity and participation. In older adults, Pua and colleagues (2017) used the Modified Falls Efficacy Scale (MFES) (a questionnaire to measure self-perceived confidence during the performance of indoor and outdoor activities) to measure the interaction between falls efficacy and postural balance (examined with computerized posturography), and its association with fall risk. They found that older adults with high MFES scores (more confidence and less fear of falling) but poor postural balance were at high risk for falls. Furthermore, the authors found that low MFES scores strongly predict poor gait performance.

Conceptual Framework for Balance Rehabilitation

How then shall we assess and treat postural control in our patients? What outcome measures are most appropriate for evaluating balance in our patients? As discussed in Chapter 6, there are a number of websites that present detailed information on clinical outcome measures; however, none provide a decision-making framework to help therapists select the most appropriate outcome measures for a specific patient. This is a significant limitation since clinicians report that one of the barriers to using standardized outcome measures is understanding how to select and apply the best measure for a specific patient (Huijbregts et al., 2002). This is true in the area of balance as well. A conceptual framework provides guidance when making decisions about the most appropriate outcome measures and treatment strategies to use with a specific patient. While several decision-making models have been presented, there is as yet no consensus regarding the most appropriate model clinicians should use in selecting outcome measures (Potter et al., 2011; Schenkman et al., 2006; Sibley et al., 2015).

Our task-oriented approach to balance rehabilitation is based on a conceptual framework that incorporates both the International Classification of Functioning, Disability and Health (ICF) and the systems model of postural control. Where does postural control or balance fit into the ICF framework? This is not an easy question to answer, since postural control does not easily fit into one of the three ICF domains (Body Structure and Function, Activities, or Participation). Balance is assessed within the context of functional activities, such as sitting, standing, or walking, which is why some believe that balance belongs in the ICF domain of activity. However, performance of a functional activity such as standing or walking requires many components (e.g., strength, coordination, and range of motion), not just balance; therefore, we do not consider balance an independent functional activity. As shown in Figure 11.1A, in our framework, postural control (balance) is a multisystem function of the body and thus is placed in the ICF domain of Body Structure and Function. A systems model of postural control (Fig. 11.1B) also contributes to our task-oriented framework. Sensory, motor, and cognitive systems within the individual are organized to meet postural demands (steady-state, reactive, and proactive balance) within the functional activity being performed (e.g., sitting and typing, standing while preparing coffee, or walking to do household chores) and are further constrained by contextual factors (both personal, such as motivation and general health, and environmental, such as accessibility to buildings or public transportation). Thus, a task-oriented framework examines the effect of impaired postural control on different aspects of participation. In addition, steady-state, reactive, and proactive balance control are examined within a continuum of functional activities (e.g., sitting, standing, and mobility) under varying sensory and cognitive contexts. Finally, underlying impairments in motor (musculoskeletal and neuromuscular), sensory, and cognitive systems that may be contributing to impaired balance control are identified.

Our clinical framework for assessing postural control is complex, with many dimensions. Since no single test examines all of these dimensions, assessment requires the use of multiple tests and measures. Unfortunately, there is rarely enough time during an initial assessment to examine all aspects of balance across all levels of function. In addition, in order to reduce the burden of testing on the patient, clinicians need to be selective and avoid using multiple measures that provide redundant information. Thus, each measure should provide

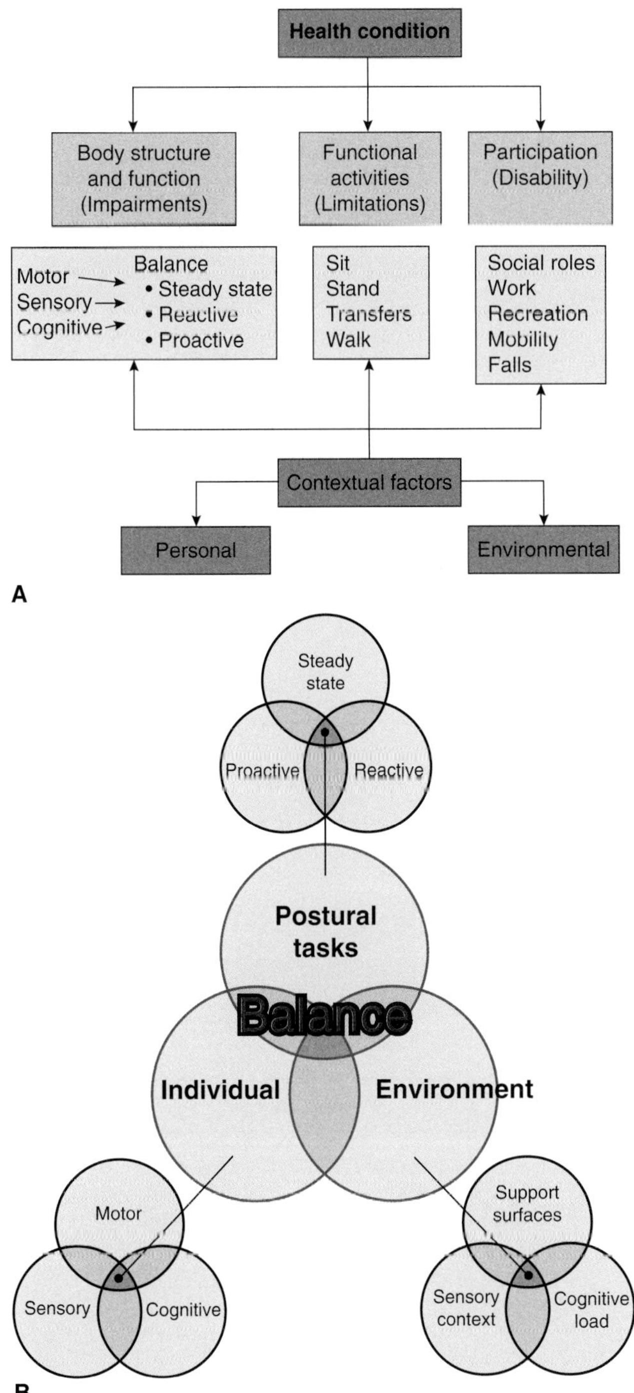

Figure 11.1 Two models underlying a task-oriented approach to balance rehabilitation. **(A)** Balance in the International Classification of Function, a multisystem function of the body. **(B)** Systems model of balance control.

insight into a unique aspect of balance control. When time and patient characteristics constrain the number of tests that can be used in an initial evaluation, a clinician must understand not only what aspects of balance are being assessed given the range of tests being used but also which aspects of balance are not being tested.

In this chapter, balance rehabilitation refers to the assessment and treatment of postural control problems within the context of sitting and standing; however, the framework presented serves as the basis for retraining balance within the context of mobility, which is discussed in detail in Chapter 15. For the most part, clinical tests of balance performed in sitting and standing are presented in this chapter, while clinical tests of mobility (even those designed to evaluate balance) are included in Chapter 15. Thus, a comprehensive approach to balance rehabilitation includes concepts in both this chapter and Chapter 15.

EXAMINATION

Safety—The First Concern

During the course of examining postural control, patients will be asked to perform a number of tasks that will likely cause instability. Safety is of paramount importance. All patients should wear an ambulation belt during testing and be closely guarded at all times. In determining which tasks and activities cause loss of balance, the patient must be allowed to experience instability. However, the therapist should protect the patient at all times to prevent a fall.

Examining the Effect of Balance on Participation

An important part of balance assessment is gathering self-report information on the effect of balance on participation in social roles and activities considered by the patient (or the patient's family) to be essential to daily life.

Falls

A critical aspect of evaluating the effect of balance on daily life function includes asking about the frequency of falls (defined as unintentionally coming to rest on a lower surface) and the circumstances leading to the fall(s). The Centers for Disease Control has developed the STEADI Algorithm for Fall Risk Screening, Assessment, and Intervention (Fig. 11.2). STEADI offers a step-by-step guide to screen people who may be at risk for falls, including the balance tests that should be applied if the person is categorized as a potential faller. The STEADI algorithm also identifies other factors related to postural imbalance such as medications that increase the likelihood of falls, home hazards, blood pressure, vision, feet status and footwear, vitamin D intake, and other medical comorbidities.

In addition, frequency of "near falls" or missteps (defined as trip, slip, or other loss of balance in which recovery prevented a fall) is important, since missteps often occur more frequently than do falls themselves (Srygley et al., 2009). Self-report information on conditions in which instability and/or falls are experienced can help the clinician to generate hypotheses about which aspects of postural control are impaired and to

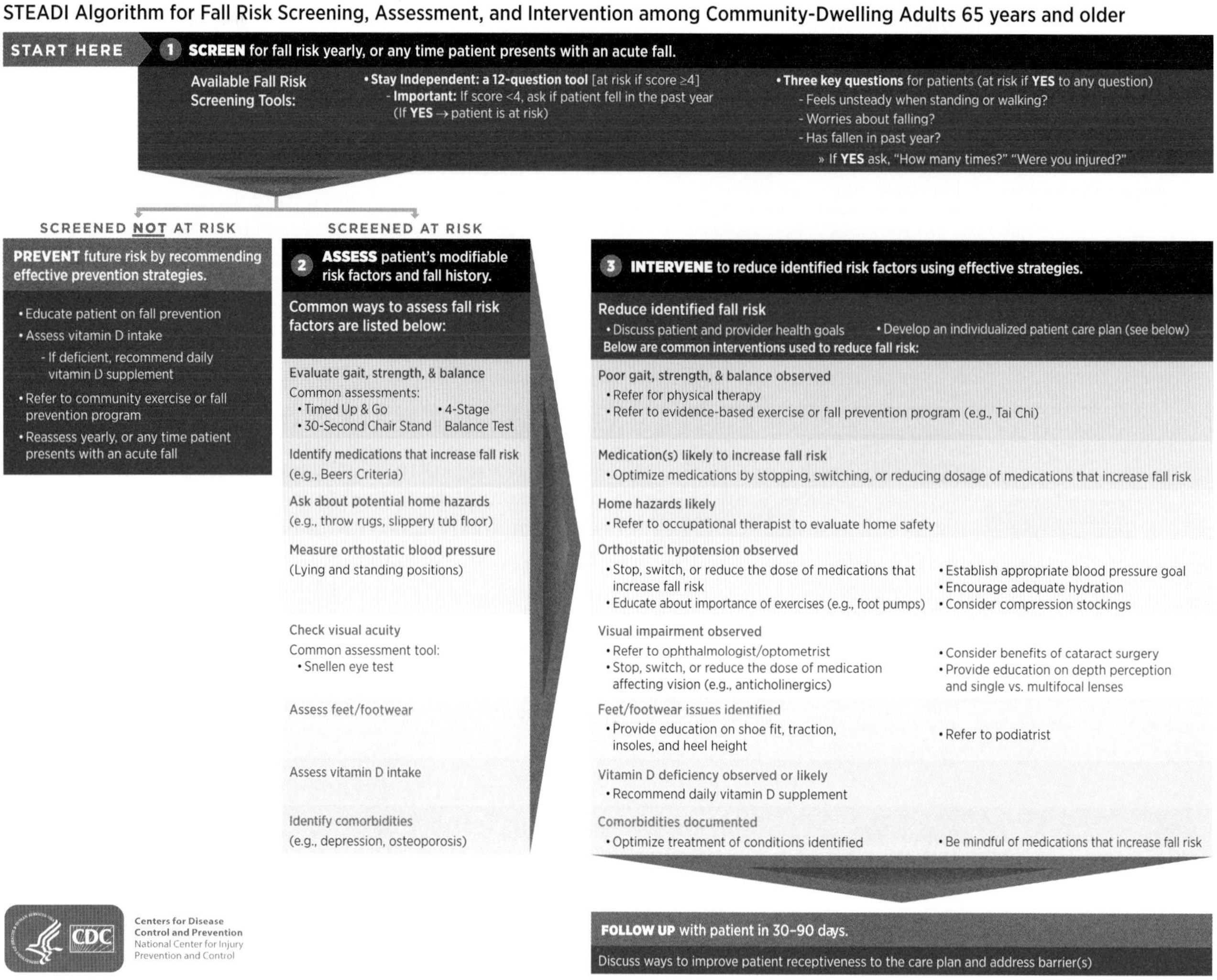

STEADI Algorithm for Fall Risk Screening, Assessment, and Intervention among Community-Dwelling Adults 65 years and older

START HERE → **1 SCREEN** for fall risk yearly, or any time patient presents with an acute fall.

Available Fall Risk Screening Tools:

- **Stay Independent: a 12-question tool** [at risk if score ≥4]
  - **Important:** If score <4, ask if patient fell in the past year (If **YES** → patient is at risk)
- **Three key questions** for patients (at risk if **YES** to any question)
  - Feels unsteady when standing or walking?
  - Worries about falling?
  - Has fallen in past year?
    - » If **YES** ask, "How many times?" "Were you injured?"

SCREENED NOT AT RISK

PREVENT future risk by recommending effective prevention strategies.

- Educate patient on fall prevention
- Assess vitamin D intake
  - If deficient, recommend daily vitamin D supplement
- Refer to community exercise or fall prevention program
- Reassess yearly, or any time patient presents with an acute fall

SCREENED AT RISK

2 ASSESS patient's modifiable risk factors and fall history.

Common ways to assess fall risk factors are listed below:

- Evaluate gait, strength, & balance
  Common assessments:
  - Timed Up & Go
  - 30-Second Chair Stand
  - 4-Stage Balance Test
- Identify medications that increase fall risk (e.g., Beers Criteria)
- Ask about potential home hazards (e.g., throw rugs, slippery tub floor)
- Measure orthostatic blood pressure (Lying and standing positions)
- Check visual acuity
  Common assessment tool:
  - Snellen eye test
- Assess feet/footwear
- Assess vitamin D intake
- Identify comorbidities (e.g., depression, osteoporosis)

3 INTERVENE to reduce identified risk factors using effective strategies.

Reduce identified fall risk

- Discuss patient and provider health goals
- Develop an individualized patient care plan (see below)

Below are common interventions used to reduce fall risk:

Poor gait, strength, & balance observed
- Refer for physical therapy
- Refer to evidence-based exercise or fall prevention program (e.g., Tai Chi)

Medication(s) likely to increase fall risk
- Optimize medications by stopping, switching, or reducing dosage of medications that increase fall risk

Home hazards likely
- Refer to occupational therapist to evaluate home safety

Orthostatic hypotension observed
- Stop, switch, or reduce the dose of medications that increase fall risk
- Educate about importance of exercises (e.g., foot pumps)
- Establish appropriate blood pressure goal
- Encourage adequate hydration
- Consider compression stockings

Visual impairment observed
- Refer to ophthalmologist/optometrist
- Stop, switch, or reduce the dose of medication affecting vision (e.g., anticholinergics)
- Consider benefits of cataract surgery
- Provide education on depth perception and single vs. multifocal lenses

Feet/footwear issues identified
- Provide education on shoe fit, traction, insoles, and heel height
- Refer to podiatrist

Vitamin D deficiency observed or likely
- Recommend daily vitamin D supplement

Comorbidities documented
- Optimize treatment of conditions identified
- Be mindful of medications that increase fall risk

FOLLOW UP with patient in 30–90 days.

Discuss ways to improve patient receptiveness to the care plan and address barrier(s)

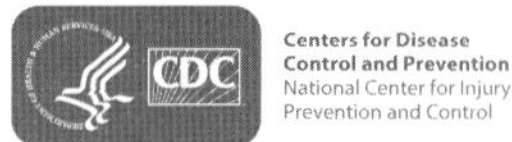

Check Your Risk for Falling

Circle "Yes" or "No" for each statement below			Why it matters
Yes (2)	No (0)	I have fallen in the past year.	People who have fallen once are likely to fall again.
Yes (2)	No (0)	I use or have been advised to use a cane or walker to get around safely.	People who have been advised to use a cane or walker may already be more likely to fall.
Yes (1)	No (0)	Sometimes I feel unsteady when I am walking.	Unsteadiness or needing support while walking are signs of poor balance.
Yes (1)	No (0)	I steady myself by holding onto furniture when walking at home.	This is also a sign of poor balance.
Yes (1)	No (0)	I am worried about falling.	People who are worried about falling are more likely to fall.
Yes (1)	No (0)	I need to push with my hands to stand up from a chair.	This is a sign of weak leg muscles, a major reason for falling.
Yes (1)	No (0)	I have some trouble stepping up onto a curb.	This is also a sign of weak leg muscles.
Yes (1)	No (0)	I often have to rush to the toilet.	Rushing to the bathroom, especially at night, increases your chance of falling.
Yes (1)	No (0)	I have lost some feeling in my feet.	Numbness in your feet can cause stumbles and lead to falls.

Figure 11.2 (A) STEADI Algorithm for Fall Risk Screening, Assessment, and Intervention among community-dwelling adults 65 years and older. (Adapted from Centers for Disease Control and Prevention. (2019). National Center for Injury Prevention and Control. Available at https://www.cdc.gov/steadi/pdf/STEADI-Algorithm-508.pdf.)

Yes (1)	No (0)	I take medicine that sometimes makes me feel light-headed or more tired than usual.	Side effects from medicines can sometimes increase your chance of falling.
Yes (1)	No (0)	I take medicine to help me sleep or improve my mood.	These medicines can sometimes increase your chance of falling.
Yes (1)	No (0)	I often feel sad or depressed.	Symptoms of depression, such as not feeling well or feeling slowed down, are linked to falls.
Total		Add up the number of points for each "yes" answer. If you scored 4 points or more, you may be at risk for falling. Discuss this brochure with your doctor.	

Figure 11.2 *(continued)* **(B)** Twelve-question tool for screening in step 1. (National Center for Injury Prevention and Control, and Centers for Disease Control and Prevention. [2017]. Stay Independent brochure [Data set]. Retrieved from https://www.cdc.gov/steadi/pdf/STEADI-Brochure-StayIndependent-508.pdf.)

determine the next steps in the examination process. For example, if a patient reports instability when leaning over to pick something up, the clinician may hypothesize that impaired anticipatory aspects of postural control may be a contributing factor and choose a test or measure that specifically examines anticipatory aspects of postural control in standing (e.g., stool touch or lean over and pick up a slipper from the floor, which are tasks on the Berg Balance Scale [BBS]). In contrast, a patient reporting loss of balance when washing her hair in the shower suggests a hypothesis related to sensory components of balance control, specifically difficulty in maintaining balance when visual cues are removed and standing on a reduced slippery surface. This could also be the case for a patient with long hair who reports balance loss and dizziness while drying the hair. This action typically involves several dynamic and static head movements with respect to a relatively stable standing position. These functional situations can then be tested specifically, for example, by observing whether the patient increases sway or requires assistance to prevent a fall during tests such as the 4-Stage Balance Step, the Clinical Test for Sensory Interaction on Balance (CTSIB), or the Balance Evaluation Systems Test (BEST) among others.

Balance or Falls Self-Efficacy

Because perceptions related to balance strongly influence participation in everyday life, assessing a patient's perceptions related to balance (balance self-efficacy or falls efficacy) is critical (Robinson et al., 2011a; Schmid et al., 2012). This can be done using a standardized self-report scale such as the Activities-Specific Balance Confidence (ABC) Scale (Powell & Myers, 1995) or the Falls Efficacy Scale (Tinetti et al., 1990), shown in Assessment Tool 11.1. Clinicians rarely use both tests as they measure similar constructs. Balance self-efficacy (as measured by the ABC scale) and not the Falls Efficacy Scale has been shown to predict levels of participation in persons with stroke, so this may be a better choice for this population (Robinson et al., 2011b; Schmid et al., 2012).

To save time, a self-report measure can be given to the patient to complete prior to the initial visit and then reviewed in person. Alternatively, if there is not enough time to complete a standardized scale such as the ABC, a limited set of questions can be used. For example, asking a patient to rate on a scale of 1 (not at all confident) to 5 (completely confident): (a) How confident are you that you can perform your daily activities without losing your balance (or falling), and (b) how often do you avoid doing an activity because of poor balance (or fear of falling)? Assessing balance confidence is critical in light of research demonstrating that balance confidence is one of the strongest predictors of participation following a stroke (Robinson et al., 2011b). A lack of confidence in one's ability to perform activities safely indicates not just a need for balance retraining but training strategies to enhance self-efficacy as balance improves. Understanding the impact of treatment on falls as well as balance perceptions requires repeating outcome measures following training.

Examining Balance in Functional Activities

Examination of balance from a functional perspective uses tests and measures that indicate how well a person can perform a variety of functional tasks that place different demands on the postural control system. Some functional tasks, for example, bed mobility tasks such as rolling or scooting, require more orientation and intersegmental coordination control (orienting parts of the body to each other and the task) and minimal stability control (control of the center of gravity), since the body is fully supported. However, most functional tasks such as sitting or standing reflect the need for some combination of (a) steady state (e.g., maintaining a stable position), (b) anticipatory (e.g., ability to maintain a stable position while performing tasks that are potentially destabilizing, such as reaching, leaning, or lifting a heavy object), and/or (c) reactive postural control (e.g., recovering a stable position following an unexpected perturbation).

Standardized measures of functional skills requiring balance provide the clinician with information on the patient's ability relative to established norms. Results can indicate the need for therapy, can serve as a baseline level of performance, and, when repeated at regular intervals, can provide both the therapist and the patient with objective documentation about a change in functional status. The following section reviews some of

Assessment Tool 11.1

Two Examples of Self-Report Measures of Balance Confidence

Activities-Specific Balance Confidence (ABC) Scale[a]

Rate confidence in ability to carry out the following activities (0 = no confidence, 100 = complete confidence). Total score is average of 16 individual scores.

1. Walk around house
2. Up and down stairs
3. Pick up slipper from floor
4. Reach at eye level
5. Reach up on tiptoes
6. Stand on chair to reach
7. Sweep floor
8. Walk outside to nearby car
9. Get in/out of car
10. Walk across parking lot
11. Walk up and down ramp
12. Walk in crowded mall
13. Walk in crowd/bumped
14. Ride escalator holding on
15. Ride escalator not holding rail
16. Walk on icy sidewalk

Falls Efficacy Scale[b]

Rate level of confidence in doing each of the activities without falling (0 = not at all, 10 = completely confident). Total score is sum of 10 individual scores (range: 0 [low self-efficacy] to 100 [high self-efficacy]).

1. Cleaning house
2. Getting dressed and undressed
3. Preparing simple meals
4. Taking a bath or shower
5. Simple shopping
6. Getting in and out of car
7. Going up and down stairs
8. Walking around neighborhood
9. Reaching into cabinets and closets
10. Hurrying to answer the phone

[a]Reprinted from Powell LE, Myers AM. The Activities-specific Balance Confidence (ABC) scale. *J Gerontol A Biol Sci Med Sci.* 1995;50A(1):M28–M34, with permission.

[b]Reprinted from Tinetti ME, Richman D, Powell L, Falls efficacy as a measure of fear of falling. *J Gerontol Psychol Sci.* 1990;45:P239–P243, with permission.

the available tests that measure functional skills related to postural control. Many of these tests have been used to determine the risk for falls as well.

As we review each test, the reader is encouraged to think about where the test (both individual items as well as the total test) fits into the framework presented in Table 11.1. What functional tasks are included in the measure (e.g., sitting, standing, mobility, including walking)? Which aspect of postural control is being examined (steady state, reactive, or anticipatory)? What aspects of functional task performance are used in scoring (e.g., time, level of assistance needed)? What behaviors related to balance are being observed and scored (e.g., alignment, sway, strategy used, or requirement for assistance)? Finally, consider whether motor, sensory, or cognitive aspects of balance control are being manipulated. For example, examining standing quietly with eyes open versus eyes closed measures steady-state balance during the manipulation of sensory conditions, while changing from a normal to narrow base of support is an example of a motor manipulation. Finally, comparing performance under single- versus dual-task conditions modifies cognitive demands.

Berg Balance Scale

The BBS was developed by Kathy Berg, a Canadian physical therapist (Berg, 1993). This test, shown in Assessment Tool 11.2, uses 14 different items, which are rated 0 to 4. The test is reported to have good test–retest and interrater reliability (intraclass correlation coefficient = 0.98) and good internal consistency (Cronbach's alpha = 0.96) (Berg et al., 1989). The Berg has good correlation with other tests of balance and mobility, including the Tinetti Performance-Oriented Mobility Assessment (POMA) ($r = 0.91$) and the TUG ($r = 0.76$) (Berg et al., 1992).

TABLE 11.1 Framework for Determining the Range-of-Balance Demands and Functional Tasks Included in Clinical Measures of Balance

	Sit	Stand	Walk
Steady-state			
Reactive			
Anticipatory			

Assessment Tool 11.2

Berg Balance Scale[c]

1. **Sitting to standing**
Instruction: Use a chair with arms. Ask the patient to stand up. If the patient stands up using the arms of the chair, ask him or her to stand up without using his or her hands, if possible.
Grading: Mark the lowest category that applies. ______
_____ (4) able to stand, no hands, and stabilize independently
_____ (3) able to stand independently using hands
_____ (2) able to stand using hands after several tries
_____ (1) needs minimal assistance to stand or to stabilize
_____ (0) needs moderate or maximal assistance to stand

2. **Standing unsupported**
Instruction: Stand for 2 minutes without holding on to any external support.
Grading: Mark the lowest category that applies. ______
_____ (4) able to stand safely for 2 minutes
_____ (3) able to stand for 2 minutes with supervision
_____ (2) able to stand for 30 seconds unsupported
_____ (1) needs several tries to stand for 30 seconds unsupported
_____ (0) unable to stand for 30 seconds unassisted
If subject is able to stand 2 minutes safely, score full marks for sitting unsupported. Proceed to position change from standing to sitting.

3. **Sitting unsupported feet on floor**
Instruction: Sit with arms folded for 2 minutes.
Grading: Mark the lowest category that applies. ______
_____ (4) able to sit safely and securely for 2 minutes
_____ (3) able to sit for 2 minutes under supervision
_____ (2) able to sit for 30 seconds
_____ (1) able to sit for 10 seconds
_____ (0) unable to sit without support for 10 seconds

4. **Standing to sitting**
Instruction: Sit down.
Grading: Mark the lowest category that applies. _____
_____ (4) sits safely with minimal use of hands
_____ (3) controls descent by using hands
_____ (2) uses backs of legs against chair to control descent
_____ (1) sits independently but has uncontrolled descent
_____ (0) needs assistance to sit

5. **Transfers**
Instruction: Move from this chair (chair with arm rests) to this chair (chair without arm rests) and back again.
Grading: Mark the lowest category that applies. ______
_____ (4) able to transfer safely with only minor use of hands
_____ (3) able to transfer safely with definite need for hands
_____ (2) able to transfer with verbal cueing and/or supervision
_____ (1) needs one person to assist
_____ (0) needs two people to assist or supervise to be safe

6. **Standing unsupported with eyes closed**
Instruction: Close your eyes and stand still for 10 seconds.
Grading: Mark the lowest category that applies. ______
_____ (4) able to stand for 10 seconds safely
_____ (3) able to stand for 10 seconds with supervision
_____ (2) able to stand for 3 seconds
_____ (1) unable to keep eyes closed for 3 seconds but stays steady
_____ (0) needs help to keep from falling

7. **Standing unsupported with feet together**
Instruction: Place your feet together and stand without holding on to any external support.
Grading: Mark the lowest category that applies. ______
_____ (4) able to place feet together independently and stand for 1 minute safely
_____ (3) able to place feet together independently and stand for 1 minute with supervision
_____ (2) able to place feet together independently but unable to hold for 30 seconds
_____ (1) needs help to attain position but able to stand for 15 seconds feet together
_____ (0) needs help to attain position and unable to hold for 15 seconds
The following items are to be performed while standing unsupported.

8. **Reaching forward with outstretched arm**
Instruction: Lift arm to 90 degrees. Stretch out your fingers and reach forward as far as you can. Examiner places a ruler at end of fingertips when arm is at 90 degrees. Fingers should not touch the ruler while reaching forward. The recorded measure is the distance forward that the fingers reach while the subject is in the most forward-leaning position.
Grading: Mark the lowest category that applies. ______
_____ (4) can reach forward confidently >10 inches
_____ (3) can reach forward >5 inches safely
_____ (2) can reach forward >2 inches safely
_____ (1) reaches forward but needs supervision
_____ (0) needs help to keep from falling

9. **Pick up object from the floor**
Instruction: Pick up the shoe/slipper that is placed in front of your feet.
Grading: Mark the lowest category that applies. ______
_____ (4) able to pick up slipper safely and easily
_____ (3) able to pick up slipper, but need supervision

(continued)

Assessment Tool 11.2

Berg Balance Scale (*continued*)

_____ (2) unable to pick up but reaches 1 to 2 inches from slipper and keeps balance independently
_____ (1) unable to pick up, and needs supervision while trying
_____ (0) unable to try, and needs assistance to keep from falling

10. **Turning to look behind over left and right shoulders**
Instruction: Turn to look behind you over your left shoulder. Repeat to the right.
Grading: Mark the lowest category which applies. _____
_____ (4) looks behind from both sides and shifts weight well
_____ (3) looks behind one side only, other side shows less weight shift
_____ (2) turns sideways only, but maintains balance
_____ (1) needs supervision when turning
_____ (0) needs assist to keep from falling

11. **Turn 360 degrees**
Instruction: Turn completely around in a full circle. Pause. Then, turn a full circle in the other direction.
Grading: Mark the lowest category that applies. _____
_____ (4) able to turn 360 degrees safely in <4 seconds each side
_____ (3) able to turn 360 degrees safely one side only in >4 seconds
_____ (2) able to turn 360 degrees safely but slowly
_____ (1) needs close supervision or verbal cueing
_____ (0) needs assistance while turning

12. **Count number of times step stool is touched**
Instruction: Place each foot alternately on the stool. Continue until each foot has touched the stool four times for a total of eight steps.
Grading: Mark the lowest category that applies. _____
_____ (4) able to stand independently and safely and complete eight steps in 20 seconds
_____ (3) able to stand independently and complete eight steps in >20 seconds
_____ (2) able to complete four steps without aid with supervision
_____ (1) able to complete less than 4 steps, needs minimal assistance
_____ (0) needs assistance to keep from falling/unable to try

13. **Standing unsupported, one foot in front**
Instruction: (Demonstrate to subject.) Place one foot directly in front of the other. If you feel that you cannot place your foot directly in front, try to step far enough ahead that the heel of your forward foot is ahead of the toes of the other foot.
Grading: Mark the lowest category that applies. _____
_____ (4) able to place foot tandem independently and hold for 30 seconds
_____ (3) able to place foot ahead of other independently and hold for 30 seconds
_____ (2) able to take small step independently and hold for 30 seconds
_____ (1) needs help to step but can hold for 15 seconds
_____ (0) loses balance while stepping or standing

14. **Standing on one leg**
Instruction: Stand on one leg as long as you can without holding on to an external support.
Grading: Mark the lowest category that applies. _____
_____ (4) able to lift leg independently and hold for >10 seconds
_____ (3) able to lift leg independently and hold for 5 to 10 seconds
_____ (2) able to lift leg independently and hold for 3 seconds or more
_____ (1) tries to lift leg, unable to hold for 3 seconds, but remains standing independently
_____ (0) unable to try or needs assistance to prevent fall

[c]Reprinted from Berg K. Measuring balance in the elderly: validation of an instrument. Dissertation. Montreal, QC: McGill University, 1993, with permission.

What aspects of postural control does the BBS assess? Take a moment and complete Lab Activity 11.1. Review each item in the BBS. Does it measure steady-state, reactive, or proactive balance? What functional activities are being tested (e.g., sitting, standing, walking)? Is the BBS a complete measure of balance control, that is, does it measure all aspects of balance within a systems framework? If a clinician chooses to use the BBS, what additional tests and measures will have to be selected to give a complete view of the patient's balance control according to a systems framework?

As you can see from the lab activity, the Berg examines a combination of steady-state balance (items 2, 3, and 6) and anticipatory aspects (items 1, 4, 5, 7, 8, 9, 10, 11, 12, 13, and 14) of balance control, primarily within the context of sitting and standing; it also includes some tasks related to mobility (change in base of support) (items 1, 4, 5, 11, and 12). It does not examine reactive balance control, and it does not examine balance in the context of gait.

Two versions of a shortened form of the Berg have been proposed (Chou et al., 2006; Hohtari-Kivimaki et al., 2012). The original Berg appears to be more sensitive for detecting change in balance abilities compared to the short form; hence, it is the preferred form for persons with stroke (Chen et al., 2015).

Shumway-Cook and colleagues (1997a) reported that the BBS was the best single predictor of fall status in community-dwelling older adults without neurologic pathology. Declining BBS scores were associated with increased fall risk, but as can be seen in Figure 11.3, this

LAB ACTIVITY 11.1

Objective: To examine the relationship between a clinical test of balance and specific aspects of the systems framework of postural control, specifically the range of tasks and environments examined

Procedures: Examine Assessment Tool 11.2, which outlines the BBS. By each test item, indicate whether the task requires steady-state, reactive, or proactive postural control. Examine the environmental condition for each item.

Assignment

1. How many items test steady-state balance control?
2. How many items test anticipatory balance control?
3. How many items test reactive postural control?

TABLE 11.2 Gradient of Fall Risk and Berg Balance Scale Scores in Community-Living Older Adults

BBS score	Likelihood for multiple falls
≥55	10%
50–54	11%
45–49	16%
40–44	31% (2.07 × more likely to fall)
<40	54% (5.19 × more likely to fall)

Source: Adapted from Muir SW, Berg K, Chesworth B, et al. Use of the BBS for predicting multiple falls in community-dwelling elderly people: a prospective study. *Phys Ther.* 2008;88:449–459.

relationship was nonlinear. In the score range of 56 to 54, each 1-point drop in the Berg score was associated with a 3% to 4% increase in fall risk. However, in the score range of 54 to 46, a 1-point change in the Berg score was associated with a 6% to 8% increase in fall risk. Below the score of 36, fall risk was close to 100%. Thus, a 1-point change in the Berg score can lead to a very different predicted probability for a fall, depending on where the baseline score is on the scale.

A study by Berg and colleagues (Muir et al., 2008) examined the predictive validity of the BBS in identifying single versus recurrent falls among 187 older adults followed prospectively for 1 year. Like Shumway-Cook et al. (1997a), they reported a nonlinear relationship between fall risk and BBS scores, showing an increasing gradient of risk associated with decreasing Berg scores, shown in Table 11.2. They reported that while 58% of those scoring lower than 45 (the commonly used cutoff point for fall risk) fell, 39% of older adults who scored greater than 45 also fell. The authors concluded that the BBS had good discriminative ability to predict multiple falls; however, the use of the BBS as a dichotomous scale, with a threshold of 45, was inadequate for the identification of the majority of people at risk for falling in the future. They therefore recommend discontinuing the use of 45 as a cutoff point for identifying fall-prone older adults. These data suggest that the Berg would be a good test to use with Bonnie, our balance-impaired older adult who has functional capability in sitting, standing, and walking, with a total score that is predictive of future recurrent falls.

The BBS may not necessarily be a good predictor of fall risk in individuals with neurologic impairment. Harris et al. (2005) examined the relationship between BBS and falls in 99 community-dwelling people with chronic stroke and found that performance on the BBS was not different between those with a high risk of falling and those with a low risk and therefore

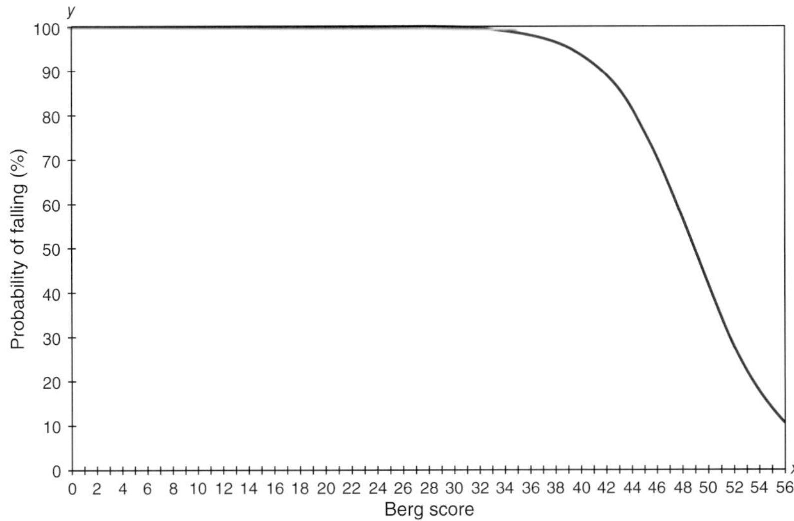

Figure 11.3 Relationship between scores on the BBS and risk for falls. On the *y*-axis is the predicted probability for being at risk for falling; scores from the BBS are on the *x*-axis. (Reprinted from Shumway-Cook A, Baldwin M, Pollisar N, et al. Predicting the probability of falls in community dwelling older adults. *Phys Ther.* 1997;77:817, with permission.)

suggested that clinicians use caution when using the BBS to predict fall risk in a patient with chronic stroke. These data suggest that while the BBS is a good test for examining steady-state and proactive balance in both Genise and Jean, our two persons with stroke, the total score may not be a good predictor of future falls.

The pediatric version of the Berg (the Pediatric Balance Scale, or PBS) has been shown to be a reliable and valid measure of balance in children with cerebral palsy (Franjoine et al., 2003; Gan et al., 2008; Kembhavi et al., 2002). The PBS was correlated with gross motor function measure (GMFM) total scores but did not distinguish between children with cerebral palsy with gross motor function classification system (GMFCS) levels I and II (Gan et al., 2008). The PBS would be an appropriate choice for examining components of balance in Thomas, our child with moderate cerebral palsy, but would be inappropriate for Malachi, who is unable to sit or stand independently.

Donoghue and Stokes (2009) reported that the minimal detectable change—defined as the smallest true change in the outcome that is not owed to measurement error—in the BBS varies as a function of the baseline score. The minimal detectable change is 4 points when the baseline Berg score is between 45 and 56, 5 points if the score is between 35 and 44, 7 points if the score is between 25 and 34, and 5 points if the score is within 0 to 24.

Reach Tests

Functional Reach Test. The Functional Reach Test is a single-item test developed as a quick screen for balance problems and falls risk in older adults (Duncan et al., 1990). As shown in Figure 11.4A, subjects stand with feet shoulder distance apart and with one arm (hand in a fist) raised to 90 degrees of flexion. Without moving their feet, subjects reach as far forward as they can while still maintaining their balance (Fig. 11.4B). The distance reached is measured and compared with that of age-related norms, shown in Table 11.3. The Functional Reach Test has good interrater reliability and has been shown to be predictive of falls among neurologically intact older adults (Duncan et al., 1990).

A modified version of the Functional Reach Test (modified Functional Reach Test [MFRT]) has been developed and tested in the acute (14 to 21 days) phase of stroke recovery. The test involves measuring unsupported reaching in the forward and lateral directions in the seated position. This test has high reliability and is responsive to improved motor performance on the paretic side (effect size, 0.80) (Katz-Leurer et al., 2009). In addition, Thompson and Medley (2007) have published reference age- and gender-related norms for the forward and lateral reach performed in sitting in three healthy age groups: 21 to 39 years, 40 to 59 years, and 60 to 97 years.

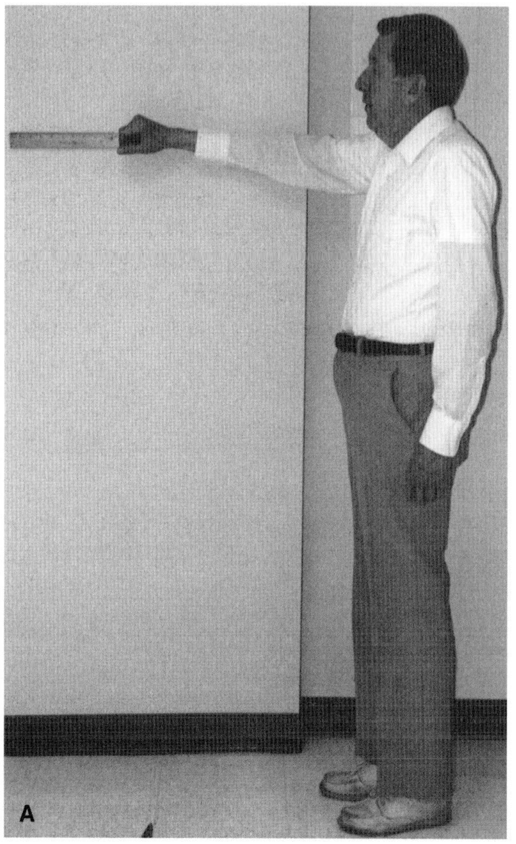

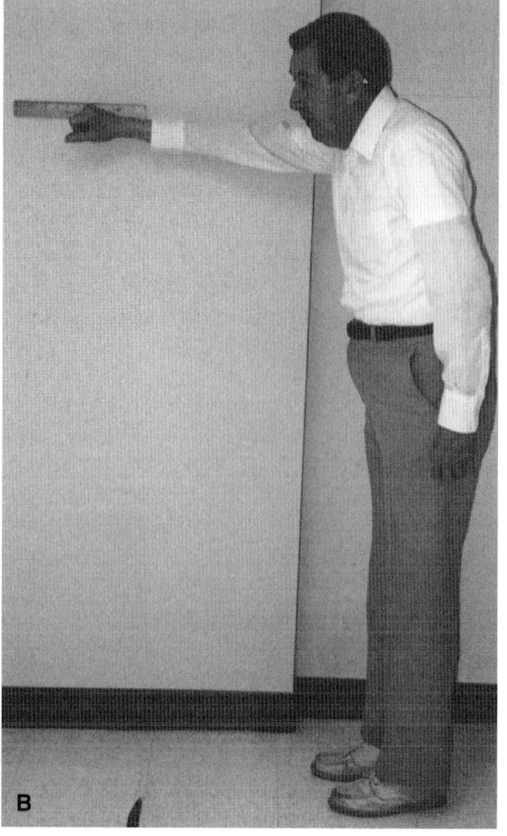

Figure 11.4 Functional Reach Test. **(A)** Subjects begin by standing with feet shoulder distance apart and arm raised to 90 degrees of flexion. **(B)** Subjects reach as far forward as they can while still maintaining their balance.

TABLE 11.3 Functional Reach Norms

Age (in years)	Men (means and SD in inches)	Women (means and SD in inches)
20–40	16.7 ± 1.9	14.6 ± 2.2
41–69	14.9 ± 2.2	13.8 ± 2.2
70–87	13.2 ± 1.6	10.5 ± 3.5

Source: Reprinted from Duncan PW, Weiner DK, Chandler J, et al. Functional reach: a new clinical measure of balance. *J Gerontol.* 1990;45:M195, with permission.

The Pediatric Reach Test (PRT) measures forward and lateral reach in both the seated and standing positions and has been shown to have good interrater and intrarater reliability in both typically developing children and those with cerebral palsy. Construct validity was established through a high correlation with the GMFCS (Bartlett & Birmingham, 2003). Forward reach tests are used to evaluate both anticipatory postural control and perceived functional stability limits. Given the availability of norms, it would be a good measure for Thomas, our child with moderate cerebral palsy.

Multidirectional Reach Test. The Multidirectional Reach Test (MDRT) was proposed to examine the limits of stability not only in the forward and backward directions but also in the medial and lateral directions. As shown in Figure 11.5, a yardstick is fixed to a telescoping tripod, allowing the vertical height of the yardstick to be adjusted so that it is at the level of the subject's acromion process. Instructions are "without moving your feet or taking a step, reach as far [direction given] as you can and try to keep your hand along the yardstick" (Newton, 2001, p. M249). Subjects are allowed to use their arm of choice for the forward and backward reaches, but both the right and the left arms are tested. Newton examined

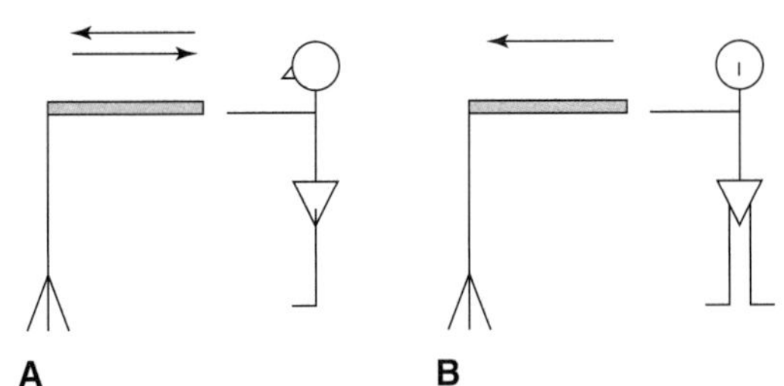

Figure 11.5 Positions for the Multidirectional Reach Test. **(A)** Position for the forward and backward reach. **(B)** Position for the right lateral lean (yardstick would be repositioned for left lateral lean). (Reprinted from Newton R. Validity of the Multi-Directional Reach Test: a practical measure for limits of stability in older adults. *J Gerontol Med Sci.* 2001;56A:M249, with permission.)

TABLE 11.4 Multidirectional Reach Test Scores in a Sample of 254 Community-Dwelling Older Adults (mean [±SD] age, 74.1 ± 7.9 y)

Test (In.)	Mean	SD	Minimum	Maximum
FR	8.89	3.4	0.5	16.8
BR	4.64	3.1	0.4	14.0
RR	6.86	3.0	0.7	18.2
LR	6.61	2.9	0.0	14.4

FR, arm stretched forward; BR, leaning backward; RR, arm stretched to the right; LR, arm stretched to the left.

Source: Adapted from Newton R. Validity of the multi-directional reach test: a practical measure for limits of stability in older adults. *J Gerontol Med Sci.* 2001;56A:M250, with permission.

the MDRT in 254 community-dwelling older persons; the mean distance reached (in inches) for this group is shown in Table 11.4. The MDRT was correlated with the BBS (r = 0.476 to 0.356) and inversely related to scores on the Timed Up and Go (TUG) (r = −0.26 to −0.442), with the strongest correlations shown for the forward direction.

The Functional Reach Test (whether performed in sitting or standing, in any direction) is often used as a measure of functional stability limits and anticipatory postural control, both important aspects of balance to assess. The standing Functional Reach (in the forward direction) is included in the BBS; however, to understand functional stability limits and anticipatory postural control in the lateral directions (or in the seated position), it would require adding additional tests.

There are many aspects to the reach tests that are not clearly defined; for example, should the fingers be extended or fisted? Should the feet be together or shoulder-width apart? Can patients change their base of support (go up on toes)? Can they rotate around the vertical axis of the body? In the absence of clear instructions, we suggest that clinicians establish guidelines for themselves and their clinic and be consistent. This is true for any standardized test.

Performance-Oriented Mobility Assessment

Mary Tinetti, a physician-researcher at Yale University, published a test called the Performance-Oriented Mobility Assessment (POMA) to screen balance and mobility skills in older adults and to determine the likelihood for falls (Tinetti, 1986; Tinetti & Ginter, 1988). Assessment Tool 11.3 presents Tinetti's balance and mobility scale, which rates performance on a three-point scale.

Assessment Tool 11.3

Performance-Oriented Mobility Assessment[d]

I Balance Tests

Initial instructions: Subject is seated in a hard, armless chair. The following maneuvers are tested.

1. Sitting balance _____
   Leans or slides in chair = 0
   Steady, safe = 1
2. Arises _____
   Unable without help = 0
   Able, uses arms to help = 1
   Able without using arms = 2
3. Attempts to arise _____
   Unable without help = 0
   Able, requires >1 attempt = 1
   Able to rise, 1 attempt = 2
4. Immediate standing balance (first 5 seconds) _____
   Unsteady (staggers, moves feet, trunk sways) = 0
   Steady, but uses walker or other support = 1
   Steady without walker or other support = 2
5. Standing balance _____
   Unsteady = 0
   Steady but wide stance (medial heels >4 inches apart) and uses cane or other support = 1
   Narrow stance without support = 2
6. Nudged (subject at maximum position with feet as close together as possible, examiner pushes lightly on subject's sternum with palm of hand three times) _____
   Begins to fall = 0
   Staggers, grabs, catches self = 1
   Steady = 2
7. Eyes closed (at maximum position no. 6) _____
   Unsteady = 0
   Steady = 1
8. Turning 360 degrees _____
   Continuous steps = 0
   Discontinuous steps = 1
   Unsteady steps (grabs, staggers) = 2
9. Sitting down _____
   Unsafe (misjudged distance, falls into chair) = 0
   Uses arms, or not a smooth motion = 1
   Safe, smooth motion = 2

Balance score:____/16

II Gait Tests

Initial instructions: Subject stands with the examiner and walks down hallway or across room, first at usual pace and then back at rapid, but safe pace (usual walking aids).

10. Initiation of gait (immediately after told to "go") _____
    Any hesitancy or multiple attempts to start = 0
    No hesitancy = 1
11. Step length and height _____
    a. Right swing foot
       Does not pass left stance foot with step = 0
       Passes left stance foot = 1
       Right foot does not clear floor completely with step = 0
       Right foot completely clears floor = 1
    b. Left swing foot
       Does not pass right stance foot with step = 0
       Passes right stance foot = 1
       Left foot does not clear floor completely with step = 0
       Left foot completely clears floor = 1
12. Step symmetry _____
    Right and left step length not equal (estimate) = 0
    Right and left step appear equal = 1
13. Step continuity _____
    Stopping or discontinuity between steps = 0
    Steps appear continuous = 1
14. Path (estimated in relation to floor tiles, 12-inch diameter; observe excursion of 1 foot over about 10 ft of the course) _____
    Marked deviation = 0
    Mild/moderate deviation or uses walking aid = 1
    Straight without walking aid = 2
15. Trunk _____
    Marked sway or uses walking aid = 0
    No sway, but flexion of knees or back pain or spreads arms out while walking = 1
    No sway, no flexion, no use of arms, and no use of walking aid = 2
16. Step width _____
    Heel apart = 0
    Heels almost touching while walking = 1

Gait score: ____/12

Balance and gait score:_____/28

[d]Reprinted from Tinetti, M. Performance-oriented assessment of mobility problems in elderly patients. *J Am Geriatr Soc.* 1986;34:119–126, with permission.

The maximum score is 28 points. An examination of the individual items in the balance portion of the POMA suggests that it evaluates steady-state balance in sitting and standing (items 1 and 5), proactive balance (items 2, 3, 6, and 9), and reactive balance (item 6) and includes a sensory component (item 7).

The POMA has been shown to be a good measure of fall risk in neurologically intact older adults living in the community. A score of less than 19 indicates a high risk for falls. Scores in the range of 19 to 24 indicate a moderate risk for falls. The test takes about 10 to 15 minutes to administer, and the interrater reliability of this test is good (Tinetti & Ginter, 1988). In a comparison of four tests of balance (TUG, One-Leg Stand, Functional Reach, and POMA), the POMA was found to have the best test–retest reliability and discriminant and predictive validities for fall risk in 1,200 people 65 years of age or older and was the most responsive to change in status with regard to activities of daily living (Lin et al., 2004).

The POMA is a good outcome measure for Bonnie, our balance-impaired community-dwelling older adult. It is not normed for children, or patients with ataxia; therefore, while the test could be used to examine balance in mobility in persons such as John, our patient with cerebellar dysfunction, the total score could not be used to predict falls.

Fullerton Advanced Balance Scale

The Fullerton Advanced Balance Scale (FAB) was developed for higher-functioning adults to avoid the ceiling effect sometimes found when using the BBS (Rose, 2003). The FAB includes 10 items (shown in Assessment Tool 11.4) scored from 0 to 4, with a score range of 0 (poor balance) to 40 (good balance).

Assessment Tool 11.4

Ten Test Items from the Fullerton Advanced Balance (FAB)[e] Scale

1. Stand with feet together, eyes closed
2. Reach forward to retrieve object
3. Turn in a full circle to the right and left
4. Step up and over bench
5. Tandem walk
6. Stand on one leg, eyes open
7. Stand on foam, eyes closed
8. Two-footed jump for distance
9. Walk with head turns
10. Unexpected backward release

[e]Reprinted from Rose D. Fall proof: a comprehensive balance and mobility program. Champaign, IL: Human Kinetics, 2003, with permission.

Balance Evaluation Systems Test

The BEST was developed by Horak and colleagues (2009) to examine multiple aspects of postural control. The BESTest consists of 36 items, grouped into six systems: Biomechanical Constraints, Stability Limits/Verticality, Anticipatory Postural Adjustments, Postural Responses, Sensory Orientation, and Stability in Gait. It has good reliability and is correlated with scores on the ABC Test (Horak et al., 2009). By systematically examining different components of balance, this test allows a clinician to determine the specific factors contributing to instability, increasing the specificity of treatment aimed to improve balance. Rasch analysis was used to develop a shorter version of the BESTest, called the mini-BESTest (Franchignoni et al., 2010). The mini-BESTest contains 14 items that group into four of the original six sections: Anticipatory Postural Adjustments (sit-to-stand, rise to toes, stand on one leg), Reactive Postural Responses (stepping in four different directions), Sensory Orientation (stance—eyes open; foam surface—eyes closed; incline—eyes closed), and Balance during Gait (gait during speed change, head turns, pivot turns, obstacles; TUG test with dual tasks). In addition, the mini-BESTest uses a three-level ordinal scoring system instead of the original four levels. Table 11.5 summarizes the categories and items for both the original and mini-BESTest. The mini-BESTest is an APTA-recommended outcome measure for many diagnoses. However, neither the BESTest nor the mini-BESTest provides information on balance in sitting, and thus they may not be appropriate for patients with a low level of function.

A number of clinical measures are available to assess patients with low functional capacity and are often used in acute care settings.

Boston University's Activity Measure for Postacute Care: Basic Mobility Short Form

The Boston University's Activity Measure for Post-acute Care (AM-PAC) is an activity limitation measure developed for use in post-acute care settings. The AM-PAC measures activity limitation in three functional domains: Basic Mobility, Daily Activities, and Applied Cognitive, with items in each domain scaled along a continuum of difficulty to create item banks. A subset of items is used to create eight short forms: two inpatient forms (Basic Mobility and Activities of Daily Living), three generic outpatient forms (Basic Mobility, Activities of Daily Living, Applied Cognitive Domains), and three forms for Medicare patients in outpatient settings (Basic Mobility, Activities of Daily Living, Applied Cognitive Domains).

The 6-Clicks basic mobility short form for use in acute care quantifies both level of difficulty and assistance required to complete 6 tasks related to basic mobility skills, such as turning over in bed, sit-to-stand,

TABLE 11.5 Summary of BESTest Items and Subsystem Categories

The 14 items forming the mini-BESTest for dynamic balance are in bold. Only the worst performance in items 11 (Stand on one leg) and 18 (Lateral stepping) have to be taken into account for the score. Moreover, the performance in item 27 (Cognitive Get up and Go) must be compared with that in the baseline item 26.

I. Biomechanical Constraints	II. Stability Limits	III. Anticipatory Transitions
1. Base of support	6 a. Lateral lean L	**9. Sit-to-stand**
2. Alignment	b. Lateral lean R	**10. Rise to toes**
3. Ankle strength	c. Sitting verticality L	**11. Stand on one leg (both right and left)**
4. Hip strength	d. Sitting verticality R	
5. Sit on floor and stand up	7. Reach forward	12. Alternate stair touch
	8 a. Reach L	13. Standing arm raise
	b. Reach R	
IV. Postural Responses	V. Sensory Orientation	VI. Dynamic Gait
14. In-place forward	**19 a. Stance EO (firm surface)**	21. Gait natural
15. In-place backward		**22. Change speed**
16. Stepping forward	b. Stance EC	**23. Head turns**
17. Stepping backward	(firm surface)	**24. Pivot turns**
18. Lateral stepping (both right and left)	c. Foam EO	**25. Obstacles**
	d. Foam EC	26. Get up and go
	20. Incline EC	**27. Cognitive get up and go**

EC, eyes closed; EO, eyes open; L, left; R, right.

Source: Reproduced from Franchignoni F, Horak F, Godi M, et al. Using psychometric techniques to improve the Balance Evaluation System's Test: The mini-BESTest. *J Rehabil Med.* 2010;42:323–331. doi: 10.2340/16501977-0537, with permission.

supine to sit, bed to chair transfers, walking, and climbing stairs. It has good interrater reliability (Jette et al., 2014). It would not be an appropriate test for Jean, our chronic stroke patient, but would be a good choice for Genise, our patient with acute stroke. Further information on AM-PAC short forms is available through the Mediware website.

Postural Assessment Scale for Stroke

The Postural Assessment Scale for Stroke patients (PASS) was developed to examine postural control when maintaining or changing a position in patients with stroke who have very limited postural control (Benaim et al., 1999). The scale is shown in Assessment Tool 11.5. It has had extensive psychometric testing, with good reliability, construct and predictive validity, and internal consistency (Benaim et al., 1999). It is among the highly recommended outcome measures from the APTA StrokEDGE task force and would be a good choice for Genise, our patient with acute stroke.

Segmental Assessment of Trunk Control

The Segmental Assessment of Trunk Control (SATCo) provides a systematic method for assessing balance function in sitting. The test specifically assesses discrete levels of trunk control in healthy infants born at term and preterm, and children with CP (Butler et al., 2010; Pin et al., 2018). It includes tests of (a) static or steady-state balance, examining the person's ability to maintain a steady posture without support; (b) anticipatory balance adjustments, examining the person's ability to balance while turning the head; and (c) reactive balance, examining the person's ability to regain balance following a brief perturbation, such as a nudge. The person sits on a bench with a strapping system to stabilize the pelvis and hold it in a neutral

Assessment Tool 11.5

PASS Scoring Form[f]

Maintaining a Posture

Give the subject instructions for each item as written below. When scoring the item, record the lowest response category that applies for each item.

1. **Sitting without Support**
   Examiner: Have the subject sit on a bench/mat without back support and with feet flat on the floor.
   _____ (3) Can sit for 5 minutes without support
   _____ (2) Can sit for more than 10 seconds without support
   _____ (1) Can sit with slight support (e.g., by 1 hand)
   _____ (0) Cannot sit

2. **Standing with Support**
   Examiner: Have the subject stand, providing support as needed. Evaluate only the ability to stand with or without support. Do not consider the quality of the stance.
   _____ (3) Can stand with support of only 1 hand
   _____ (2) Can stand with moderate support of 1 person
   _____ (1) Can stand with strong support of 2 people
   _____ (0) Cannot stand, even with support

3. **Standing without Support**
   Examiner: Have the subject stand without support. Evaluate only the ability to stand with or without support. Do not consider the quality of the stance.
   _____ (3) Can stand without support for more than 1 minute and simultaneously perform arm movements at about shoulder level
   _____ (2) Can stand without support for 1 minute or stands slightly asymmetrically
   _____ (1) Can stand without support for 10 seconds or leans heavily on 1 leg
   _____ (0) Cannot stand without support

4. **Standing on Nonparetic Leg**
   Examiner: Have the subject stand on the nonparetic leg. Evaluate only the ability to bear weight entirely on the nonparetic leg. Do not consider how the subject accomplishes the task.
   _____ (3) Can stand on nonparetic leg for more than 10 seconds
   _____ (2) Can stand on nonparetic leg for more than 5 seconds
   _____ (1) Can stand on nonparetic leg for a few seconds
   _____ (0) Cannot stand on nonparetic leg

5. **Standing on Paretic Leg**
   Examiner: Have the subject stand on the paretic leg. Evaluate only the ability to bear weight entirely on the paretic leg. Do not consider how the subject accomplishes the task.
   _____ (3) Can stand on paretic leg for more than 10 seconds
   _____ (2) Can stand on paretic leg for more than 5 seconds
   _____ (1) Can stand on paretic leg for a few seconds
   _____ (0) Cannot stand on paretic leg

Maintain Posture SUBTOTAL______

Changing a Posture

6. **Supine to Paretic Side Lateral**
   Examiner: Begin with the subject in supine on a treatment mat. Instruct the subject to roll to the paretic side (lateral movement). Assist as necessary. Evaluate the subject's performance on the amount of help required. Do not consider the quality of the performance.
   _____ (3) Can perform without help
   _____ (2) Can perform with little help
   _____ (1) Can perform with much help
   _____ (0) Cannot perform

7. **Supine to Nonparetic Side Lateral**
   Examiner: Begin with the subject in supine on a treatment mat. Instruct the subject to roll to the nonparetic side (lateral movement). Assist as necessary. Evaluate the subject's performance on the amount of help required. Do not consider the quality of the performance.
   _____ (3) Can perform without help
   _____ (2) Can perform with little help
   _____ (1) Can perform with much help
   _____ (0) Cannot perform

8. **Supine to Sitting Up on the Edge of the Mat**
   Examiner: Begin with the subject in supine on a treatment mat. Instruct the subject to come to sitting on the edge of the mat. Assist as necessary. Evaluate the subject's performance on the amount of help required. Do not consider the quality of the performance.
   _____ (3) Can perform without help
   _____ (2) Can perform with little help
   _____ (1) Can perform with much help
   _____ (0) Cannot perform

9. **Sitting on the Edge of the Mat to Supine**
   Examiner: Begin with the subject sitting on the edge of a treatment mat. Instruct the subject to return to supine. Assist as necessary. Evaluate the subject's performance on the amount of help required. Do not consider the quality of the performance.
   _____ (3) Can perform without help
   _____ (2) Can perform with little help
   _____ (1) Can perform with much help
   _____ (0) Cannot perform

10. **Sitting to Standing Up**
    Examiner: Begin with the subject sitting on the edge of a treatment mat. Instruct the subject to stand up without support. Assist as necessary. Evaluate the subject's performance on the amount of help required. Do not consider the quality of the performance.

(continued)

Assessment Tool 11.5

Changing a Posture (*continued*)

____ (3) Can perform without help
____ (2) Can perform with little help
____ (1) Can perform with much help
____ (0) Cannot perform

11. **Standing Up to Sitting Down**
Examiner: Begin with the subject standing by the edge of a treatment mat. Instruct the subject to sit on the edge of the mat without support. Assist as necessary. Evaluate the subject's performance on the amount of help required. Do not consider the quality of the performance.
____ (3) Can perform without help
____ (2) Can perform with little help
____ (1) Can perform with much help
____ (0) Cannot perform

12. **Standing, Picking Up a Pencil from the Floor**
Examiner: Begin with the subject standing. Instruct the subject to pick up a pencil from the floor without support. Assist as necessary. Evaluate the subject's performance on the amount of help required. Do not consider the quality of the performance.
____ (3) Can perform without help
____ (2) Can perform with little help
____ (1) Can perform with much help
____ (0) Cannot perform

Changing Posture SUBTOTAL____

TOTAL ____

[f]Reprinted from Benaim C, Pérennou DA, Villy J, Rousseaux M, et al. Validation of a standardized assessment of postural control in stroke patients: the Postural Assessment Scale for Stroke Patients (PASS). *Stroke.* 1999;30:1862–1868, with permission.

position. The evaluator progressively changes the level of trunk support, beginning with a high level of support at the shoulder girdle to assess cervical (head) control, through support at the axillae (upper thoracic control), inferior scapula (midthoracic control), lower ribs (lower thoracic control), below ribs (upper lumbar control), pelvis (lower lumbar control), and, finally, no support, in order to identify the level of functional trunk control (e.g., the level of support required to optimize steady-state, reactive, and anticipatory balance control in the seated position). The SATCo is shown in Assessment Tool 11.6. Details for completing the SATCo may be found in Butler et al. (2010). In addition, a demonstration of the SATCo being administered to a typically developing infant and a child with cerebral palsy may be found in the video case study entitled "Assessment and Treatment of Segmental Trunk Control." The SATCo has been recommended as an appropriate outcome measure for children and adults with cerebral palsy (Saether et al., 2013). The SATCo has good reliability and shows responsiveness in detecting trunk control changes across the first months of life (Butler et al., 2010). However, in infants, examiners should be careful during testing because 5- to 6-month-olds and independent sitters tend to use hands for support. Also, the SATCo can discriminate reactive trunk control between full-term and preterm infants at 8 months but not earlier (Pin et al., 2018).

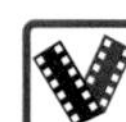

The Seated Postural and Reaching Control Test

The Seated Postural and Reaching Control (SP&R-co) test has been validated for children with CP. Like the SATCo, the SP&R-co test applies a segment-by-segment approach to evaluate and objectively score postural and reaching control in the sitting position across four postural dimensions: static, active, proactive (bimanual and unimanual), and reactive. The static dimension evaluates steady-state postural control for 20 seconds. The active dimension measures how the child can perform head rotations while maintaining the trunk steady. Proactive control is measured with fast goal-oriented bimanual and unimanual reaches (reaching for a basketball or pointing to a target). And reactive control is measured with a *hold-and-release* technique to determine the child's ability to execute direction-specific postural muscle contractions and counteract the amount of force voluntarily generated against the resistance exerted by the examiner. The SP&R-co test shows acceptable-good score consistency, good-excellent internal consistency, fair-excellent item-by-item reliability, good-excellent interrater and intrarater reliability, moderate-excellent correlations with CP-related measurements (GMFCS, GMFM, Manual Ability Classification System, Jebsen–Taylor Hand Function Test, and Box & Blocks) and excellent concurrent validity with the SATCo. Responsiveness, which is defined as the ability of the SP&R-co scores to change over time, has not yet been investigated (Santamaria et al., 2020).

Sitting Balance Scale

The Sitting Balance Scale is an 11-item test developed to examine balance in sitting in nonambulatory frail older adults who would demonstrate floor effects on most measures of balance (Medley & Thompson, 2011). This 11-item test focuses on steady state (sitting unsupported) and anticipatory (including items such as lateral reach, leaning over and lifting a leg) aspects of balance control in the seated position. It also varies the availability of sensory information during testing. It has good reliability

Assessment Tool 11.6

SATCo Assessment[a]

Client Name: Ref #: Tester Name: Date:	Level of Manual Support Pelvic/thigh strap used except as indicated	Functional Level Arms and hands in air except as indicated	Static	Active	Reactive	Comments
			Maintain vertical neutral position of head and trunk above manual support level.			
			Minimum of 5 seconds	While turning head with arms lifted	Maintain/ quickly regain following brisk nudge	
	Shoulder girdle Tester's hand position may vary from horizontal.	**Head control** Arms may be supported throughout.			NOT tested for head control	
	Axillae	**Upper thoracic control**				
	Inferior scapula	**Midthoracic control**				
	Over lower ribs	**Lower thoracic control**				
	Below ribs	**Upper lumbar control**				
	Pelvis	**Lower lumbar control**				

(continued)

Assessment Tool 11.6

SATCo Assessment[a] *(continued)*

Client Name: Ref #: Tester Name: Date:	Level of Manual Support Pelvic/thigh strap used except as indicated	Functional Level Arms and hands in air except as indicated	Static: Maintain vertical neutral position of head and trunk above manual support level. Minimum of 5 seconds	Active: While turning head with arms lifted	Reactive: Maintain/ quickly regain following brisk nudge	Comments
	No support given and pelvic/ thigh straps removed	**Full trunk control**				

Fixed spinal deformity? Yes ____ No___ Comments ____________

Limitation of cervical rotation Left ______ Right _____ Comments ____________

[a]Reprinted from Butler P, Saavedra S, Sofranac M, et al. Refinement, reliability and validity of the segmental assessment of trunk control (SATCo). *Ped Phys Ther*. 2010;22:257, Appendix 1, with permission.

and validity for use with older adults; however, its utility in other populations has not been examined.

There are many more measures examining balance developed for specific patient populations, with more emerging constantly. A complete review of all measures is not feasible. However, as shown in Table 11.6, there are a number of excellent websites that review outcome measures and summarize the research on their psychometric properties. We believe the framework presented in this chapter offers clinicians a way to understand which aspects of balance are included in any assessment, in order to understand how they contribute to an overall assessment of balance control in patients with different levels of function and diagnoses.

Limitations of Functional Tests and Measures

How well do functional tasks capture postural control from a systems perspective? Most functional measures have limitations. First, a patient's performance is examined under a limited set of environmental conditions; thus, it may not always predict actual performance in more complex environments. In addition, few tests examine all three aspects of postural control, including steady-state, reactive, and anticipatory postural control across a range of functional activities (e.g., sitting, standing, and walking). In addition, most functional tests provide little insight into the sensory, motor, and cognitive strategies used to achieve balance. Finally, most functional tests provide little insight into the specific subsystems within the body responsible for a decline in performance. To gain insight into the movement strategies used to accomplish balance and the underlying system impairments contributing to imbalance, additional tests are needed.

Assessing Strategies for Balance

Understanding balance impairments requires insight into the motor, sensory, and cognitive strategies used to maintain or regain stability.

Motor Strategies

Examination of motor strategies for postural control evaluates both the alignment of body segments during unperturbed sitting and standing (alignment in mobility tasks is discussed in Chapter 15) and the patient's ability to generate multijoint movements, or strategies that effectively control motion of the COM and/or changing the base of support to maintain stability (Shumway-Cook & Horak, 1990; Shumway-Cook & McCollum, 1990; Woollacott & Shumway-Cook, 1990).

Orientation (Alignment). Postural alignment is categorized within the "Body Functions and Structures" component of the ICF. Examination of postural control includes observation of the patient's orientation or alignment in sitting and standing. Is the patient vertical? Is weight symmetrically distributed right to left and forward and backward? A plumb line in conjunction with a grid can be used to quantify changes

TABLE 11.6 Websites with Information on Outcome Measure Psychometrics and Clinical Utility

Site name	Site creator
Hooked on Evidence	American Physical Therapy Association
Physiotherapy Evidence Database	Center for Evidence-Based Physiotherapy
Neurology Section Outcome Measures Recommendations	American Physical Therapy Association Neurology Section EDGE Task Force
Center for Outcome Measurement in Brain Injury	Rehabilitation Research Center at Santa Clara Valley Medical Center
Rehabilitation Assessment Measures in Multiple Sclerosis	MS Society
Clinical Practice Guidelines for Patients with Parkinson's Disease	Royal Dutch Society for Physiotherapy
Stroke Engine-Assess	Canadian Stroke Network & McGill University
Evidence-Based Review of Stroke Rehabilitation	Canadian Stroke Network
Rehabilitation Measures Database	Shirley Ryan Ability Lab

in orientation at the head, shoulders, trunk, pelvis, hips, knees, and ankles. In addition, the width of the patient's base of support upon standing can be measured and recorded using a tape to measure the distance between the medial malleoli (or, alternatively, the metatarsal heads). There are standardized tests that aim to address postural alignment and muscle status such as the Spinal Alignment and Range of Motion Measure (SAROMM). The SAROMM is designed to be used with people with CP and requires trained personnel in rehabilitation; it may take from 15 to 30 minutes, and two people might be required to administer the test if the patient cannot maintain independent sitting. The SAROMM has two sections: spinal alignment and range of motion and muscle extensibility. The examinee is required to actively correct spinal alignment and posture, and if this is successful the patient receives a

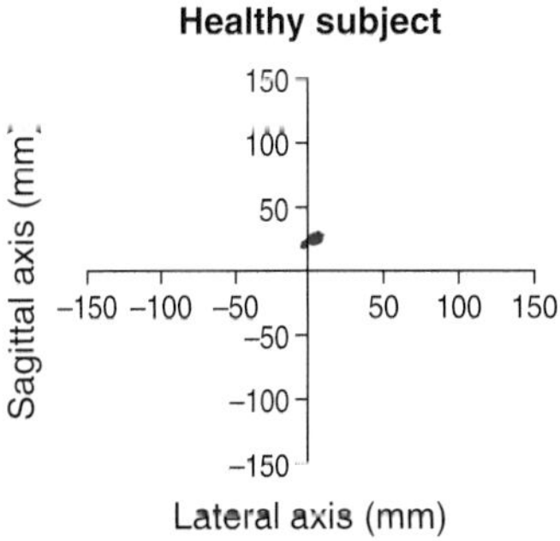

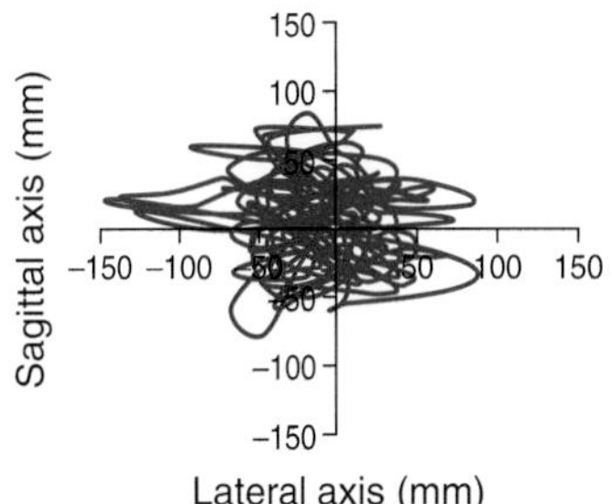

Figure 11.6 Dynamic posturography used to demonstrate the significant increase in COP displacement in a person with severe cerebellar ataxia (on **bottom**) compared to an age-matched healthy control (on **top**). (Adapted from Marquer A, Barbieri G, Pérennou D. The assessment and treatment of postural disorders in cerebellar ataxia: A systematic review. *Ann Phys Rehabil Med*. 2014;57:68.)

score of 0. If the person cannot achieve "normal" alignment after three trials, identified by alignment diagrams which are part of the test, passive corrections are conducted and the limitation is scored based on a specific set of criteria (Bartlett & Purdie, 2005).

Alternative ways to quantify displacement of the COM more objectively in the standing position include the use of static force plates (dynamic posturography) to measure displacement of the center of pressure (COP). For example, Figure 11.6 illustrates the use of dynamic posturography to compare COP displacement in a patient with degenerative cerebellar pathology to an age-matched control. This type of technology could be used to document increased sway in John, our patient with cerebellar degeneration. In the clinic, two standard scales can be used to determine whether there is weight discrepancy between the two sides (Fig. 11.7). During balance retraining, both of these methods can also be used to provide feedback to a person learning to control the position and displacement of the body.

Reactive Balance Movement Strategies. Both in-place and change-of-support strategies are necessary for postural stability. In addition, because instability is not confined to one plane, we must be able to control movements of the COM in all planes of movement in a variety of contexts. Movement strategies used to control the body in space are often examined during

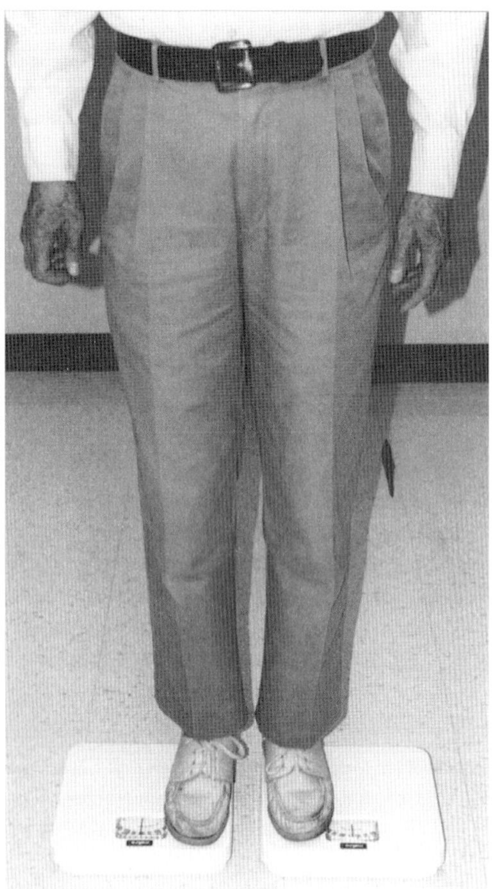

Figure 11.7 Two standard scales can be used to quantify static asymmetric standing alignment.

self-initiated sway, in response to externally induced sway, and anticipatory to a potentially destabilizing upper- or lower-extremity movement.

Movements used to control self-initiated body sway are observed while the patient voluntarily shifts the weight forward, then backward, and then side to side. The patient is tested in both the sitting and the standing positions. Figure 11.8 illustrates the range of movement patterns seen in a seated neurologically intact individual as she shifts the trunk further and further laterally while seated. As weight is transferred to one side of the body, the trunk begins to curve toward the unweighted side, resulting in elongation of the weight-bearing side and shortening of the trunk on the unweighted side (Fig. 11.8A). As weight continues to be shifted laterally, maintaining stability requires the subject to execute compensatory postural adjustments—by flexing and abducting the contralateral arm and leg in order to keep the trunk mass within the base of support (Fig. 11.8B). Finally, the arm is extended toward the surface, changing the base of support and preventing a fall (Fig. 11.8C).

Figure 11.9 illustrates two types of movement strategies being used to control forward voluntary sway in standing. Patient A (Fig. 11.9A) is using an ankle strategy to sway, while Patient B (Fig. 11.9B) is using a hip strategy to minimize forward motion of the COM.

The presence of coordinated movement strategies can also be examined during recovery from an external perturbation. Figure 11.10 illustrates one approach to assessing movement patterns used to recover stability in response to an external displacement at the hips (Carr & Shephard, 1998; Shumway-Cook & Horak,

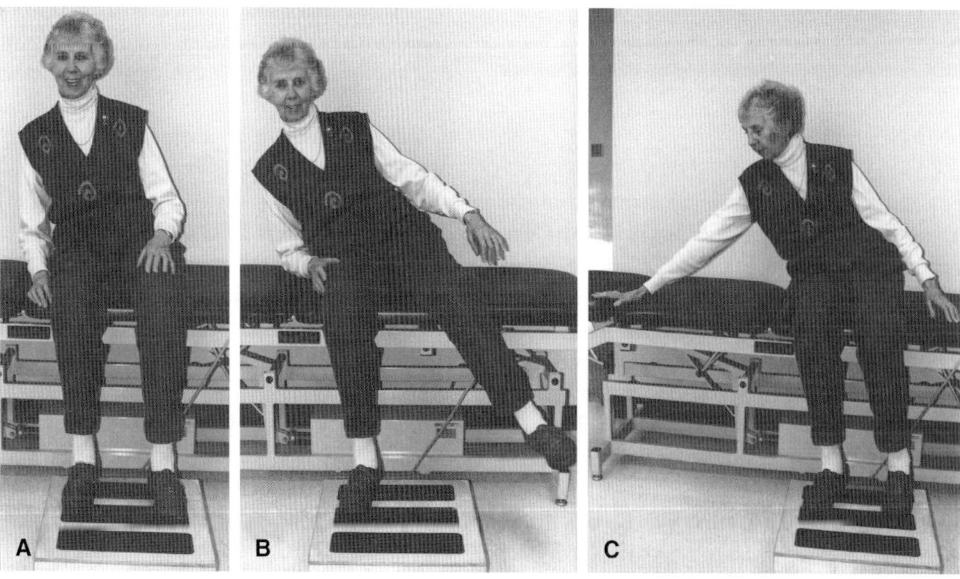

Figure 11.8 Maintaining stability during self-initiated weight shifts with trunk movements in sitting. **(A)** Small movements produce adjustments at the head and trunk. **(B)** Larger movements require counterbalancing with the arms and legs. **(C)** When movements of the head and trunk can no longer control stability with the current base of support, the arm reaches out to change the base of support and prevent a fall.

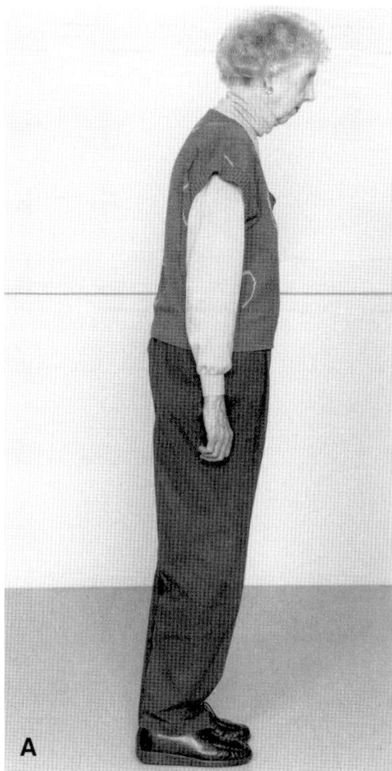

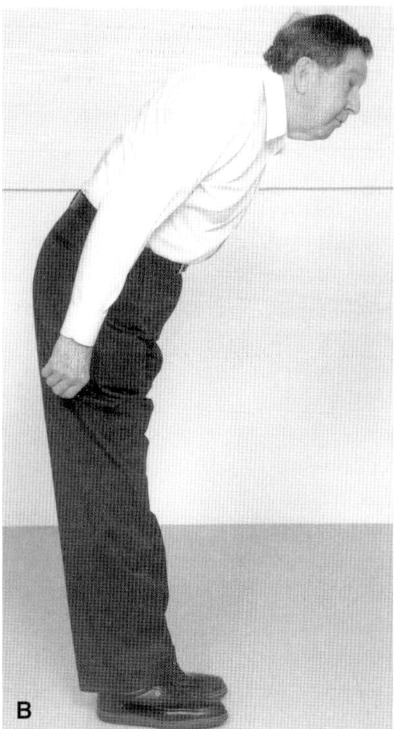

Figure 11.9 Voluntary sway in stance is a clinical strategy used to examine functional stability limits and movement strategies used to control stability. Shown are two types of movement strategies being used to control self-initiated voluntary sway in standing: the ankle strategy, which is associated with greater movement of the COM (and larger stability limits) **(A)**, and the hip strategy, which is associated with restricted functional stability limits **(B)**.

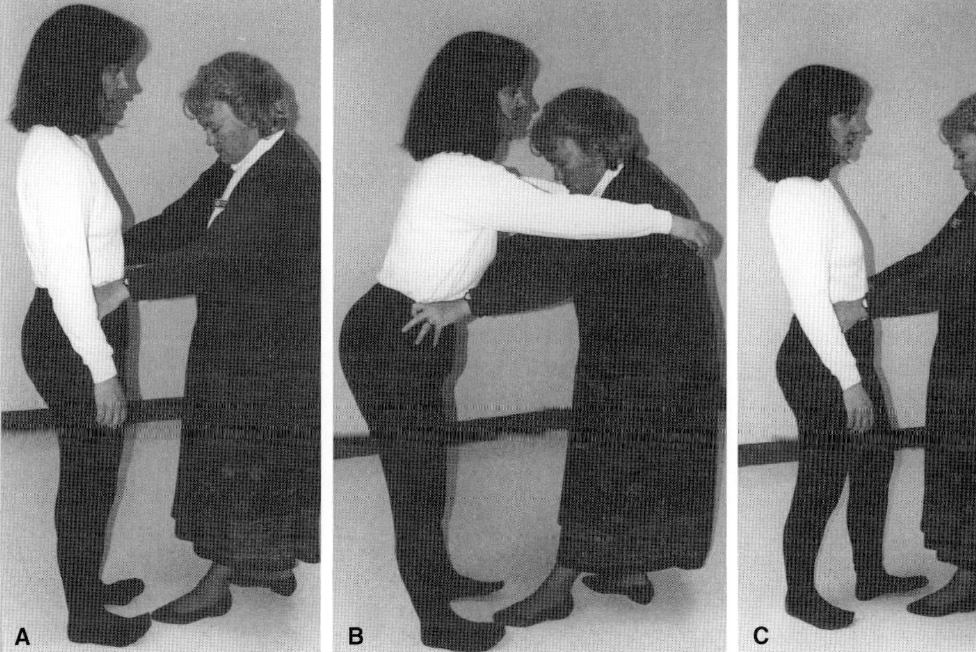

Figure 11.10 The technique to elicit movement strategies used to recover from an external perturbation to balance. **(A)** An ankle strategy is used to recover from a small displacement at the hips. **(B)** A larger displacement, with instructions not to step, produces a hip strategy. **(C)** When in-place strategies can no longer control the COM with respect to the existing base of support, a step is used to change the base of support and thus prevent a fall.

1992). Holding the patient about the hips, the therapist displaces the hips in multiple directions (forward, backward, side to side, and on diagonals). Strategies to recover stability in response to sagittal-plane perturbations are shown in Figure 11.10A and B; in-place strategies (ankle or hip) are used to recover from small displacements, while a step (Fig. 11.10C) may be used to recover stability when in-place strategies will not suffice.

An alternative approach to examining reactive balance is described in the BESTest and shown in the postural control segment of all the case study videos. To elicit an in-place strategy, a small amount of pressure is

applied at each shoulder and then released unexpectedly. Asking the patient to lean into the examiner's hands, bringing the COM to the limits of stability, and then releasing is used to elicit a stepping response (Horak et al., 2009; see also Jacobs et al., 2006). The BESTest examines the ability to recover from small versus large perturbations in all directions. Remember that many factors will determine how and when motor strategies are changed, including the amplitude and velocity of the destabilizing stimulus, as well as perceptions related to stability limits, perceived ability to recover balance, and fear of falling. As described before, the SP&R-co applies the *hold-and-release* technique to test reactive trunk control in seated children with CP. The *hold* phase tests whether the child has the ability to elicit direction-specific contractions in agonist muscles; whereas the "*release*" phase tests if the antagonist muscles can efficiently react to prevent sitting failure with "in-place" or "change-in-support" (e.g., reaching for support) strategies.

Movement strategies used to minimize instability in anticipation of potentially destabilizing movements can be assessed by asking a patient to lift a heavy object as rapidly as possible (Fig. 11.11) or by placing one foot on top of a stool. Both of these tasks require subtle shifts of the COM prior to the voluntary movement (of the arms in the lifting task or the leg in the stepping task) in order to maintain stability. Delayed or absent anticipatory adjustments are associated with reduced stability during performance of the task, and in some cases, the task may be performed more slowly. Finally, observing movements made to maintain stability in response to changing task demands can provide insight into the range of coordinated movement strategies available for postural control. Commonly used balance tasks such as standing on one foot (Fig. 11.12A) or in a tandem Romberg (heel/toe) position (Fig. 12.11B) reduce the

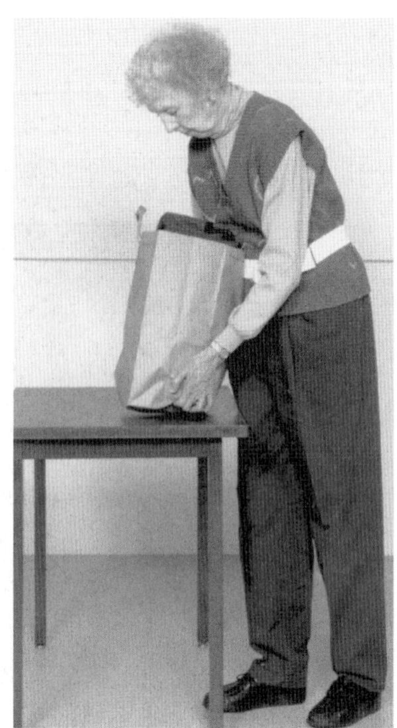

Figure 11.11 Anticipatory postural control can be examined by having patients perform tasks that are potentially destabilizing, such as lifting a heavy bag of groceries.

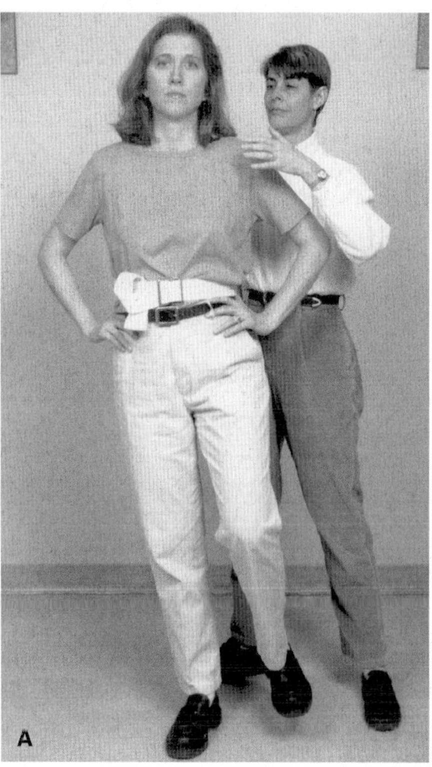

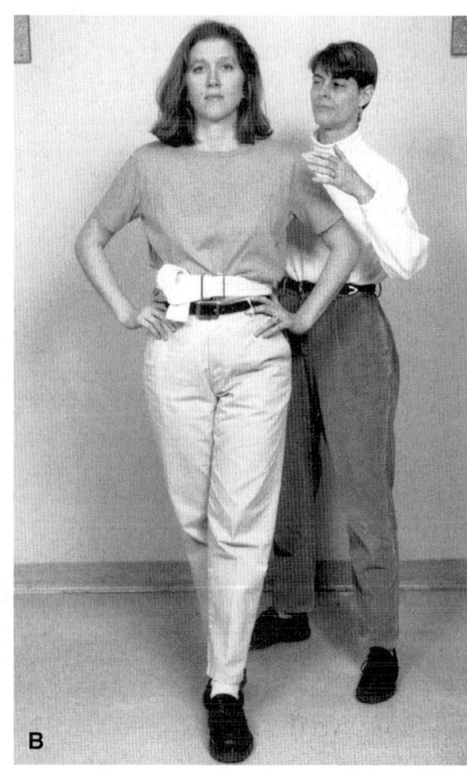

Figure 11.12 Adapting movement strategies to changes in the base of support either through the one-foot stance **(A)** or through the tandem Romberg **(B)** position.

base of support and increase the demands for frontal plane stability. They often result in the use of a hip or a stepping strategy to maintain stability and prevent a fall.

Research has shown that muscles in the leg and trunk are activated synergistically during recovery of stability, and this multijoint coordination is a hallmark of normal postural control. The most common clinical approach to evaluating multijoint dyscoordination within movement strategies used for postural control is through observation and description during tests such as the nudge test (Tinetti, 1986) or the reactive balance items from the BESTest (Horak et al., 2009). Following a small perturbation in the backward direction (Fig. 11.13A), the clinician may note that during recovery of stance balance, the patient demonstrates excessive flexion of the knees or excessive flexion or rotation of the trunk. Differences in onset of muscle responses on the two sides can often be noted by testing for symmetry when the toes come up in response to a backward perturbation (Fig. 11.13B and C). However, determining the underlying nature of the dyscoordination, that is, specific timing and or amplitude errors in synergistic muscles responding to instability, most often requires the use of technical tests such as electromyography (Shumway-Cook & McCollum, 1990).

Sensory Strategies

Stability must be maintained in a wide variety of environments (in well-lit environments, in the dark, in the presence of moving visual cues, and on surfaces with different geographic and physical features), necessitating a change in the way sensory information is used for postural control. An important part of assessing postural control is examining a person's ability to organize and select sensory information in response to changing sensory conditions. Instability when certain sensory cues are unavailable can provide insight into environmental conditions likely to produce instability.

Clinical Test for Sensory Interaction in Balance. Shumway-Cook and Horak suggested a method for assessing sensory organization components of stance postural control (Horak, 1987; Shumway-Cook & Horak, 1986). The CTSIB uses a 24- by 24-inch piece of medium-density temper foam in conjunction with a modified Japanese lantern. A large Japanese lantern's back is cut down and attached to a headband. Vertical stripes are placed inside the lantern, and the top and bottom of the lantern are covered with white paper (Fig. 11.14).

The method is based on concepts developed by Nashner (1982), and it requires the subject to maintain standing balance for 30 seconds under six different sensory conditions that either eliminate input or produce inaccurate visual and surface orientation inputs. These six conditions are shown in Figure 11.15. Patients are tested in the feet-together position, with hands placed on the hips. If unable to stand with feet together, patients are allowed to stand with a normal base of support, and this is noted in the evaluation.

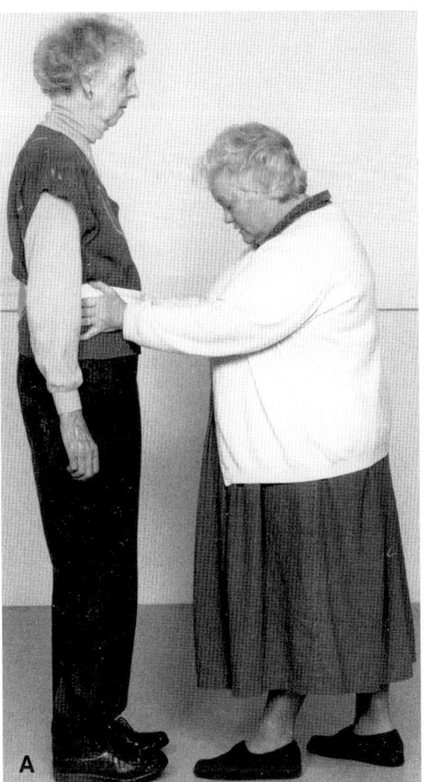

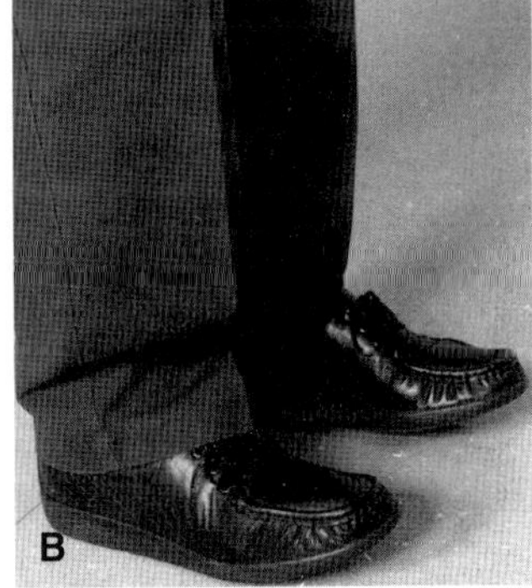

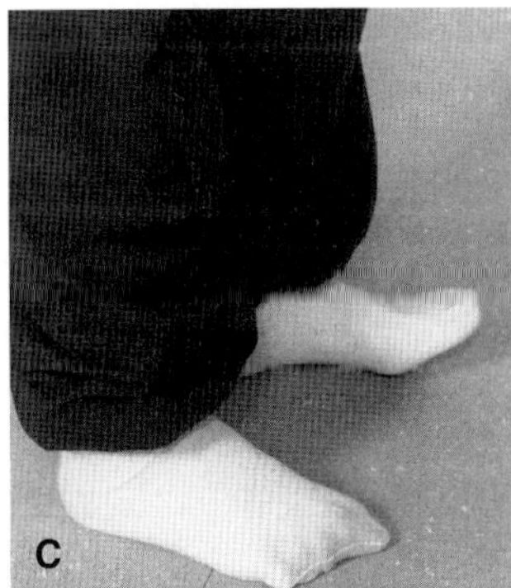

Figure 11.13 Symmetry of muscle responses at the ankle can be observed in response to displacement in the backward direction. **(A)** The patient is given a small displacement in the backward direction. **(B)** Normal response is dorsiflexion of both feet. **(C)** An abnormal response in a patient with hemiparesis is loss of the dorsiflexion response in the hemiparetic leg.

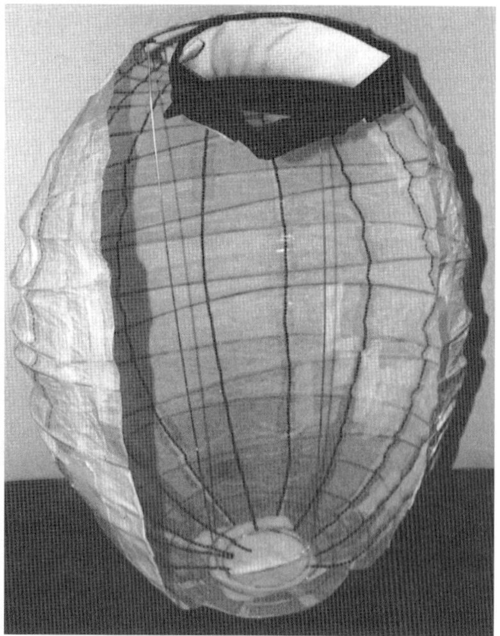

Figure 11.14 A modified Japanese lantern is used to change the accuracy of visual input for postural orientation.

Using condition 1 as a baseline reference, the therapist observes the patient for changes in the amount and direction of sway over the subsequent five conditions. If the patient is unable to stand for 30 seconds, a second trial is undertaken (Horak et al., 1992b).

Neurologically intact young adults are able to maintain balance for 30 seconds on all six conditions with minimal amounts of body sway. As was true for the computerized sensory organization testing, normal adults sway on average 40% more in conditions 5 and 6 than in condition 1 (Horak et al., 1992b). A modified version of the CTSIB has been proposed, eliminating the dome conditions and retaining four conditions—firm surface eyes open and closed and foam surface eyes open and closed (Allison, 1995; Whitney & Wrisley, 2004). One reason given for eliminating the dome condition was its lack of sensitivity in identifying patients who are sensitive (demonstrated by increased sway) to visual motion in the environment. Performance on the CTSIB may be seen in the postural control segments of the case study videos. 

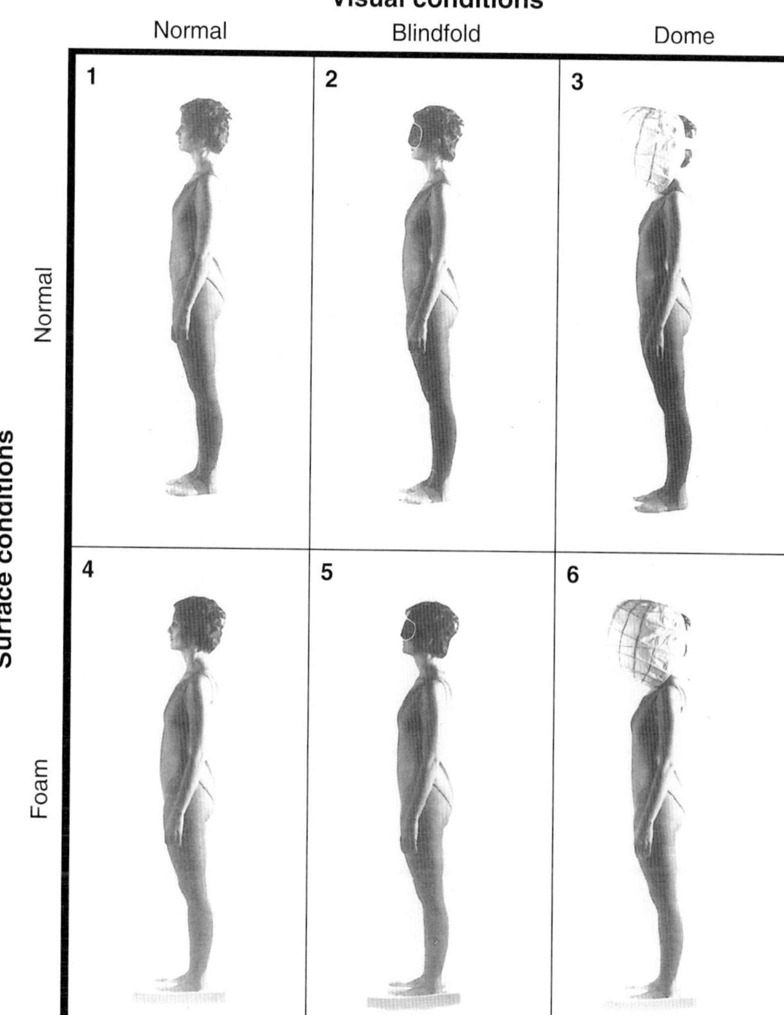

Figure 11.15 Six sensory conditions used to examine postural orientation under altered sensory contexts. The approach tests the ability to adapt how senses are used to maintain orientation. (Reprinted from Shumway Cook A, Horak F. Assessing the influence of sensory interaction on balance. *Phys Ther*. 1986;66:1549, with permission of the American Physical Therapy Association. This material is copyrighted, and any further reproduction or distribution requires written permission from APTA.)

Results from a number of research studies that have used either a moving platform or the CTSIB (Cohen et al., 1993; DeFablo & Badke, 1990, Horak et al., 1992b; Peterka & Black, 1990–1991) suggest the following scoring criteria. A single fall (i.e., requiring assistance from the therapist to recover stability), regardless of the condition, is not considered abnormal. However, two or more falls are indicative of difficulties adapting sensory information for postural control.

A proposed model for interpreting results is summarized in Figure 11.16. Patients who show increased amounts of sway or lose balance on conditions 2, 3, and 6 are thought to be visually dependent, that is, highly dependent on vision for postural control. Patients who have problems on conditions 4, 5, and 6 are thought to be surface dependent, that is, dependent primarily on somatosensory information from the feet in contact with the surface, for postural control (Shumway-Cook & Horak, 1990). Patients who sway more, or fall, on conditions 5 and 6 demonstrate a vestibular-loss pattern, suggesting an inability to select vestibular inputs for postural control in the absence of useful visual and somatosensory cues. Finally, patients who lose balance on conditions 3, 4, 5, and 6 are said to have a sensory selection problem. This is defined as an inability to effectively adapt sensory information for postural control (Shumway-Cook & Horak, 1992).

It is important to remember the following caution when interpreting results showing increased sway on a compliant surface. While we suppose that the primary effect of standing on a foam surface relates to altering the availability of incoming somatosensory information for postural orientation, additional factors can affect performance in this condition. Standing on foam changes the dynamics of force production with respect to the surface, and this may be a significant factor affecting performance in this condition. In a study with healthy adults, assessing anteroposterior and lateral torque variance with eyes open and eyes closed using three different types of foam block placed on a force platform, the authors found significant differences among conditions (Patel et al., 2008). Thus, clinicians should be careful in interpreting results when using the foam condition because the foam properties may influence the recorded body movements.

The six-item CTSIB test has been shown to have good test retest reliability in community-dwelling older adults and young adults (Cohen et al., 1993), is a valid way to evaluate and monitor change over time in patients with vestibular dysfunction (Allison, 1995; Cohen et al., 1993; Weber & Cass, 1993), and is used to determine fall risk in older adults (Anacker & DiFabio, 1992) and following stroke (DeFabio & Badke, 1990). Pediatric versions of both the CTSIB (Crowe et al., 1990; Gagnon et al., 2006; Richardson et al., 1992) and the modified CTSIB (Geldhof et al., 2006) have been used to examine sensory organization components of postural control in typically developing children and those with traumatic brain injury (Gagnon et al., 2004). Richardson and colleagues (1992) showed that the CTSIB, including heel-to-toe position, can discriminate age- and gender-related differences in children as young as preschoolers (4 to 5 years).

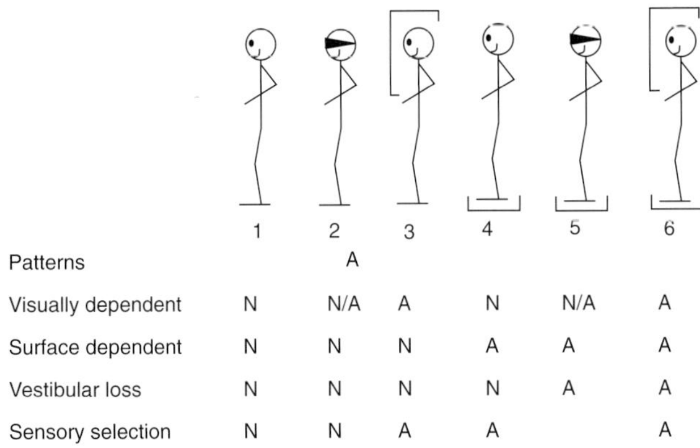

Patterns	1	2 A	3	4	5	6
Visually dependent	N	N/A	A	N	N/A	A
Surface dependent	N	N	N	A	A	A
Vestibular loss	N	N	N	N	A	A
Sensory selection	N	N	A	A		A

N = Body sway within normal limits
A = Body sway abnormal

Figure 11.16 Proposed model for interpreting the CTSIB test based on information gained through dynamic posturography testing.

Incline Test. Horak and colleagues (2009) in their BESTest have proposed another approach to examining the ability to maintain balance in the absence of useful vision and somatosensory inputs for postural control. In this test, orientation and sway are measured with eyes closed while standing on a firm surface as compared to a 10-degree-angle incline board (Fig. 11.17A and B). This test is based on research by Kluzik et al. (2005; 2007), who demonstrated that healthy subjects stood with trunk and legs aligned near gravity-vertical in both conditions. Patients with vestibular loss, however, have difficulty maintaining balance and orienting to vertical while standing on the inclined surface with eyes closed (Horak et al., 2009).

Cognitive Strategies

There is considerable research evidence to show that performing a secondary cognitive or motor task can have a detrimental effect on the ability to maintain balance in older adults and in people with neurological disorders. Dual tasks make automatic movements more attentionally demanding. Divided attention, or the attentional ability to perform two tasks simultaneously, is required in dual tasks (Fritz et al., 2015). Dual tasks can impair balance when performing dual motor tasks (i.e., standing on a firm or complaint surface while tapping or performing coordinative bimanual tasks or holding a trade or a glass with a liquid during walking at different speeds), dual cognitive-motor tasks (counting backward,

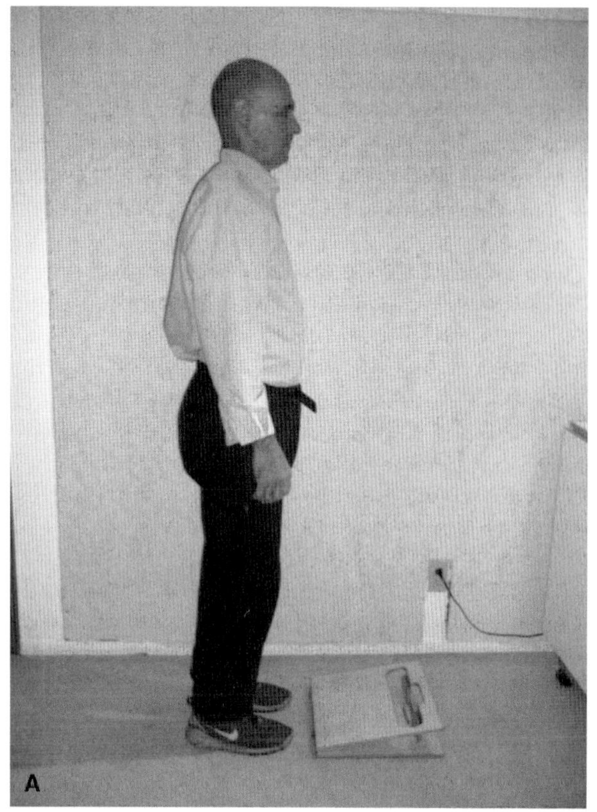
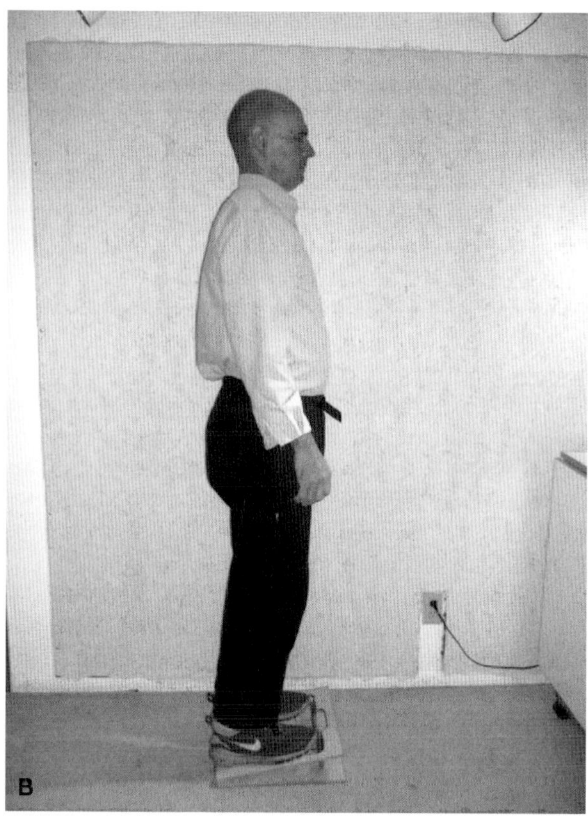

Figure 11.17 Incline Test. The Incline Test is part of the Balance Evaluation Systems Test (BESTest) and examines the individual's ability to maintain balance using vestibular inputs to orient to vertical in the absence of useful visual cues (eyes closed) and surface inputs (standing on an incline). Patients are tested with eyes closed standing on a firm flat surface **(A)** and then while standing with eyes closed on a 10-degree angle incline board **(B)**.

mental calculations, word spelling, verbal working memory tasks, or visual search activities), or complex actions (i.e., driving). The effect of the additional task on motor performance can be measured with the relative dual-task cost equation:

$$DTC = \frac{(DTmotor - STmotor)}{STmotor} * 100$$

Where
DTC = dual-task cost
DT = dual-task outcome (during simultaneous performance of the two tasks)
and ST = single task outcome

Specifically, balance impairments during dual tasks can be documented through validated clinical tests such as TUG or BBS (Fritz et al., 2015; Ghai et al., 2017; Leone et al., 2017; Matthews et al., 2006; Tajali et al., 2017; Rabaglietti et al., 2019; Sertel et al., 2017). However, the only standardized tests examining the effect of a secondary task on balance control have been done in the context of walking; hence, they are presented in Chapter 15. However, examining balance in sitting and standing under single- and dual-task conditions would provide insight into this important aspect of postural control. A major limitation to this is the lack of standardized protocols and normative data to guide clinicians as they assess cognitive strategies during balance.

Examination of Underlying Impairments

The final step in a task-oriented approach is examining the sensory, motor (neural and musculoskeletal), and cognitive subsystems that contribute to postural control. During this portion of the examination, the emphasis is on examining impairments that will have the most direct impact on postural control. Thus, examination of strength may focus on examining lower-extremity muscle strength, with particular attention to ankle muscles such as the anterior tibialis and gastrocnemius or soleus, because of the role of these muscles in the control of upright stance—ankle strategy. For that same reason, examining range of motion at the ankle is also considered critical. In a similar line of thinking, the assessment of muscle-force generation of abdominal, paravertebral, and neck muscles as well as potential vertebral column or chest deformities are of critical importance in the examination of seated postural control.

Understanding the integrity of sensory inputs critical to postural control, such as vision and somatosensation in the feet and ankles, is also an important part of examination at the impairment level. For a discussion of methods for examining impairments, refer to Chapter 5. Before moving on to treatment, the reader is encouraged to examine Figure 11.18 and complete Lab Activity 11.2, applying a task-oriented approach to examination.

Genise T. is a 53-year-old woman, admitted to the hospital with right-sided weakness. An MRI indicated an ischemic stroke affecting the left internal capsule with some extension in the external capsule. She is currently 1 month poststroke. To see a video of Genise, refer to her video case study which examines her underlying impairments and functional skills at 1 month poststroke.

Reason for referral: Outpatient therapy for continued impairments and functional limitations related to her stroke.

Medical history: She has a history of type II diabetes, hypertension, and hyperlipidemia, for which she takes medication. Following her 4-day stay in acute care, she spent 2 weeks in rehabilitation and was discharged to her home.

Social and work history: Genise lives with her husband in a single-level home. Prior to her stroke she was independent in all ADLs and IADLs. Prior to her stroke she worked as a worship leader in her church, composing and performing music.

ON EXAMINATION

I. Self-report participation and fall/balance history

Genise relies primarily on her wheelchair for mobility in her home and community. She reports walking in her own home with her cane and posterior stop AFO. She is independent in self-care activities (grooming, dressing, toileting, etc.), but requires assistance for all IADLs. Her primary social support is her husband, however, her mother and sister live nearby and are available to provide assistance as needed.

II. Impairments in Body Structure and Function

A. Motor System Impairments

1. Voluntary, isolated movement: When asked to move her right arm, she has partial flexion at the elbow and shoulder, performed within a flexor synergy. With her arm supported to minimize the effect of gravity, she has no active extension in her paretic arm. She has no active wrist or finger extension. When she tries to extend her hand and wrist, instead of recruiting the extensors, a flexor synergy is recruited resulting in flexion of the arm. When asked to flex her paretic leg, she flexes at the hip and knee and is beginning to recruit ankle dorsiflexors within a flexor synergy pattern. Similarly, when extending her leg, plantarflexors are recruited within an extensor synergy pattern. When asked to move only her ankle, she is not able to isolate ankle movement and instead recruits both the ankle dorsiflexors and plantarflexors within a total synergy pattern.

2. Range of motion: She has full range of motion at the shoulder and elbow but is beginning to develop tightness in her wrist and fingers flexors. She has limited range of motion in her right dorsiflexors.

3. Spasticity: Quick stretch of the biceps, wrist flexors and ankle plantarflexors indicates the presence of spasticity. Her Ashworth score is 3.

B. Sensation

Genise has impaired light touch, two point discrimination, and proprioception in both her paretic arm and leg; distal loss is greater than proximal loss. She has no visual problems.

C. Cognition

She has no cognitive impairments.

III. Postural Control

Impaired postural control is a significant factor contributing to Genise's limited functional abilities. She has had several falls since her return home; several while standing and leaning over to pick something up, or while walking.

A. Berg Balance Scale. At one month post stroke, Genise scores 19 out of 56 on the BBS; her scores on specific items are as follows:

1. Sit to Stand – 2: able to stand using hands after several tries
2. Stand – 1: needs several tries to stand for 30 seconds unsupported
3. Sitting Unsupported – 4: able to sit safely and securely for 2 minutes
4. Stand to Sit – 3: controls descent by using hands
5. Transfers – 3: able to transfer safely with definite need for hands
6. Standing Eyes Closed – 3: able to stand for 10 seconds with supervision
7. Standing Feet Together – 0: needs help to attain position, unable to hold for 15 seconds
8. Reaching Forward – 1: reaches forward but needs supervision
9. Leaning Over – 1: unable to pick up, and needs supervision while trying
10. Turn to look over shoulder – 1: needs supervision when turning
11. 360 degree turn – 0: needs assistance while turning
12. Stool touch – 0: needs assistance to keep from falling/unable to try
13. One leg stand – 0: loses balance while stepping or standing
14. Heel Toe stand – 0: unable to try or needs assistance to prevent fall

Figure 11.18 Case study of Genise T., a patient with acute stroke.

(continued)

B. Components of Postural Control

1. Sitting

Steady-state balance: Steady-state sitting balance is fairly good; her weight is slightly displaced to her left but she shows minimal sway. However, when her attention shifts to respond to questions, sway increases. She is able to maintain independent steady-state sitting balance with eyes closed. When displaced off vertical, with her eyes closed, she is not able to return to a symmetrical vertical position, suggesting verticality perceptions may be impaired.

Reactive balance: She is able to recover independently from small perturbations in all directions while sitting. However, in response to a large displacement to her paretic side, she is unable to reach for support with her paretic arm and has to be caught to prevent a fall.

Proactive balance: She has good proactive balance in sitting, and is able to reach forward > 10", pick things up from the floor, and turn her head and trunk without loss of balance.

2. Standing

Steady-state balance: At 1 month, her steady-state balance in standing is significantly impaired. She maintains stability but only for a few minutes, and stands asymmetrically with her weight shifted to the left. When distracted, she loses balance backwards and requires assistance to prevent a fall. Steady-state balance does not change when she closes her eyes, suggesting that she is not overly reliant on vision, and is able to use somatosensory and vestibular inputs for postural control.

Reactive balance: She is unable to recover from loss of balance in either the forward or backward direction using an inplace strategy, and requires assistance to prevent a fall. In response to the lean and release test, Genise does step with her nonparetic leg, but requires assistance with recovery. When she loads the paretic leg in order to step with the nonparetic leg, the knee snaps back into hyperextension to prevent collapse of the paretic leg. She is unable to step quickly enough with her paretic limb to prevent a fall.

Proactive balance: She has difficulty maintaining her balance during forward reach, and requires assistance to perform the task. She reports several falls when leaning over to pull up her pant legs when standing.

Figure 11.18 *(continued)*

LAB ACTIVITY 11.2

Objective: To apply a task-oriented approach to examining postural control to a patient with hemiplegia and to establish goals and a plan of care for improving posture and balance based on assessment information

Procedure: Read the case study of Genise T. in Figure 11.18.

Assignment: Based on the information you have, answer the following questions:

1. What are her functional limitations?
2. Based on her BBS score, what is her current fall risk (see Fig. 11.2)?
3. Does she have steady-state balance problems? Anticipatory control problems? Reactive control problems? Are these problems primarily in sitting or standing?
4. What movement strategies does she use for control of balance? What impairments are contributing to her choice of movement strategy?
5. How well is she able to organize sensory information for postural control? Based on the results from her CTSIB test, in what environments would you expect her to have difficulty maintaining balance?

EVALUATION: INTERPRETING THE RESULTS OF THE EXAMINATION

As was discussed in Chapter 1, movement emerges from the interaction among the individual, the task, and the environment. Specifically, when evaluating movement in a patient, clinicians should be familiarized with the terms: "capacity," "capability," and "performance." These three constructs are related but their operational definitions are distinct. *Capacity* is what a patient *can do* in a standardized and controlled environment. *Capability* refers to what a patient *can do* during ADLs. And *performance* describes what the patient *actually does* during ADLs (Holsbeeke et al., 2009).

Once the clinician is aware of a patient's performance during valid standardized postural tests, what they can achieve, and what patients truly do during ADLs, the clinician must interpret results, identify the problems, and establish short- and long-term goals and a plan of care for achieving those goals. An important part of establishing an appropriate plan of care is considering the evidence to support different therapeutic approaches to improving balance, restoring function, and maximizing participation.

TASK-ORIENTED BALANCE REHABILITATION

A task-oriented approach to treating the patient with postural control problems utilizes therapeutic strategies to (a) modify (or prevent) impairments in body structure and function impacting postural control and (b) improve the ability to meet the demands of balance during the performance of functional activities. Improving balance during the performance of functional activities requires facilitating the development of sensory, motor, and cognitive strategies that are effective in meeting stability (steady-state, anticipatory, and reactive) demands associated with a variety of functional tasks and teaching the patient to adapt these strategies to changing environmental contexts.

The ultimate goal of task-oriented balance rehabilitation is to improve participation outcomes, reflected in an improved ability to safely participate in the social roles, tasks, and activities that are important in the daily life of the patient. Improved participation can be demonstrated by increased frequency of participation or increased independence and safety (reduced falls and near falls) when performing daily tasks and activities. Improved participation may also be reflected in increased confidence, reduced fear, and increased satisfaction with one's level of participation. Tests that score balance control deficits and predict the probability of falls are of special interest for clinicians who apply therapeutic task-oriented approaches. Among older adults, for instance, Lusardi et al. (2017) proposed that a BBS score ≤50 points, a completion time in the TUG ≥12 s and in the 5 times sit-to-stand test ≥12 s accurately predict the risk of potential future falls.

The following sections discuss therapeutic strategies targeting motor, sensory, and cognitive systems for balance control. We begin with a review of treatment at the impairment level (targeting underlying body structure and function) and then discuss treatments designed to improve balance (steady-state, reactive, and proactive) during the performance of functional activities. Each section begins with a review of different types of treatment and then considers the evidence to support these treatments. We finish with a discussion of an integrated approach to balance rehabilitation and discuss the impact on measures of participation, specifically falls.

Motor System

Treating Underlying Motor Impairments

The priority for intervention at the impairment level is to reduce those impairments that have the greatest impact on postural control in functional tasks. For example, in our case study of Jean, underlying impairments related to paresis, weakness, and restricted range of motion in her hemiparetic leg limit her ability to effectively and efficiently meet the stability demands of functional tasks such as sitting, standing, and walking. Because of impairments in her legs, among other possible neuromotor factors, she must rely on reaching with her nonhemiparetic arm to maintain stability. When support is not available in her environment, a fall occurs. Chapter 5 summarized treatments used to impact underlying impairments resulting from pathology in the motor systems. What evidence do we have that treatments aimed at underlying motor impairments (in the absence of additional task training) will result in improved balance in functional tasks?

Effect of Strength Training on Balance. A number of studies have found that muscle-strength deficits are at least partially reversible in pediatric, geriatric, and neurologic populations. The evidence demonstrating the relationship between increased muscle strength and improved balance remains mixed, however.

Among older adults, many studies have shown that resistance strength training is effective in increasing strength; however, while in some studies this was associated with improved balance (Chandler & Hadley, 1996; Fiatarone et al., 1990; Fiatarone et al., 1994; Hess & Woollacott, 2005; Hess et al., 2006; Wolfson et al., 1996), in others it was not (Judge et al., 1994). Orr et al. (2008) conducted a systematic review of randomized controlled trials to examine the effect of progressive resistive strength training on balance in older adults. A total of 14 out of 29 studies met their inclusion criteria and reported balance improvements with strength training. However, they also suggest that resistance training alone may not be a robust enough intervention to improve balance control in older adults.

Similar to the research with older adults, the results of strength training on balance control in neurologic populations are mixed. Among persons with MS, DeBolt and McCubbin (2004) reported that resistance exercise resulted in a significant increase in lower-extremity power; however, there was no significant effect on postural-sway measures (anteroposterior and mediolateral sway and sway velocity) or on TUG performance. The authors conclude that resistance strength training is possible in persons with MS, with no adverse effects on the disease, but while this form of exercise improves power, it does not result in improved balance and mobility (as determined by their measures). Ada et al. (2006) reviewed data from 15 trials to determine whether strength training in participants who have had a stroke improves strength without increasing spasticity and whether increased strength resulted in improved function, though balance was not specifically identified. The meta-analysis found that strengthening interventions had a small positive effect on both strength and functional activities, with very little effect on spasticity. They concluded that strengthening programs should be a part of stroke rehabilitation. Results from these studies suggest that while there is considerable evidence demonstrating the effect of training on improved strength, the degree to which strength training alone will result in improved balance remains unclear. Thus, the task-oriented approach to balance rehabilitation presented in this book combines treatment of underlying impairments with clinical activities to improve balance within the context of functional task practice. Similar outcomes have been observed in CP. Strength training has been found to have benefits on ambulation in adults with CP (>18 years) but inconsistent positive modifications in activity and participation. In children diagnosed with ambulatory CP, the use of strength training seems to improve self-selected gait speed but does not improve overall gait velocity. With regards to the type of training, function and gait seem to improve more following isotonic rather than isokinetic training. Also, the benefit of strength training is more accentuated in younger compared to older individuals (Moreau et al., 2016; Ross et al., 2016)

Functional Electrical Stimulation. As discussed in Chapter 5, functional electrical stimulation (FES) is often used to improve recruitment and strengthen paretic muscles in persons with stroke. FES to the lower extremity, particularly the ankle dorsiflexors, is used to improve performance in functional tasks such as standing and walking. Does the position in which FES is delivered impact outcome? The answer appears to be "yes." A small study compared the effect of FES applied to the dorsiflexors of the paretic limb in 9 individuals with subacute stroke, 5 of whom received the treatment in standing and 4 in supine. FES was applied at the intensity of maximal contraction, for 30 minutes, 6 × a week for 8 weeks. Outcome measures including the TUG and the BBS, as well as FES intensity, were measured every 2 weeks for 8 weeks. Results demonstrated that FES applied in the standing position improved performance on the BBS and TUG greater than when it was applied in the supine position. Thus, treatment to improve an underlying impairment (recruitment of the ankle dorsiflexors), combined with task-specific training (in this case practice of steady-state balance in the stance position), was more effective than the same treatment provided in the absence of functional task practice (Kim et al., 2012b). This and other studies suggest that while treatments aimed at underlying impairments can impact balance, their effectiveness is increased significantly when combined with appropriate functional task training. For example, among children with cerebral palsy, task-specific practice of functional tasks was preceded by 30 minutes of stretching and active movement training using a robotic device attached to the ankle; this resulted in significant improvements in ankle joint range of motion, decreased plantarflexor spasticity, improved strength in both ankle dorsi- and plantarflexors, as well as showing significant improvements in both the TUG and the Pediatric Balance Scale (pediatric version of the BBS) (Sukal-Moulton et al., 2014). In line with these results, Moll and colleagues (2017) did a systematic review on FES applied to ankle dorsiflexors in adolescents with spastic CP, with reference to the ICF framework. They found evidence that FES has benefits in the body structure and function domain as justified by studies reporting improved ankle angle (dorsiflexion), strength, selective motor control, balance, and gait kinematics associated with decreased walking speed. Nonetheless, there is limited evidence showing that FES improves activity and participation.

Functional Balance Training: Improving Motor Strategies

Training balance within the context of function includes (a) improving underlying movement strategies used for steady-state, reactive, and anticipatory balance control and (b) adapting functional tasks to changing environmental conditions.

Steady-State Balance Control. Improving steady-state balance control most often focuses on retraining orientation and alignment to help the patient develop an initial position that (a) is appropriate for the task; (b) is efficient with respect to vertical alignment, that is, with minimal muscle activity requirements for maintaining the position; and (c) maximizes stability, that is, places the vertical line of gravity well within the patient's stability limits; this allows the greatest range of movements for postural control. Many tasks use a symmetrical vertical position, but this may not be a realistic goal for all patients (Shumway-Cook & McCollum, 1990).

Cohen and colleagues (2015) investigated if therapeutic programs that target postural alignment could have a positive impact on balance-related deficits. They investigated whether the Alexander Technique—which is used to reduce excessive muscle activity—could reduce axial rigidity, increase upright postural alignment, and be beneficial for postural sway and mobility in people diagnosed with Parkinson's disease and stooped posture. The authors compared the Alexander Technique (a muscle activity reduction technique) with another postural program to increase muscle activity and trunk stabilization and a control group with a relax condition. They showed that both postural alignment programs improve upright postural alignment compared to the control group. However, only the program based on postural instructions to decrease muscle activity (the Alexander Technique) reduced postural sway and axial muscle tone and consequently improved mobility—smooth COP trajectories during step initiation (Cohen et al., 2015).

A number of approaches can be used to help patients develop a symmetrically vertical posture. Commonly, verbal and manual cues are used by the clinician to assist a patient in finding and maintaining an appropriate vertical posture. Patients practice with eyes open and closed, learning to maintain a vertical position in the absence of visual cues. Mirrors can also be used to provide patients

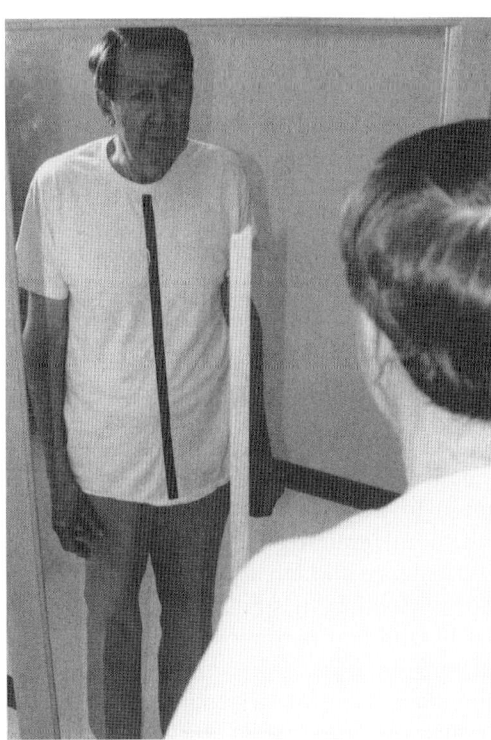

Figure 11.19 Using a mirror to provide visual feedback when retraining alignment. The patient is asked to line up the vertical stripe on his T-shirt with a vertical stripe on the mirror.

with visual feedback about their position in space. The effect of a mirror can be enhanced by having the patient wear a white T-shirt with a vertical stripe down the center and asking the patient to try to match the stripe on the T-shirt to a vertical stripe on the mirror (Fig. 11.19). The patient can use the mirror and T-shirt approach while performing a variety of tasks, such as reaching for an object, which require that the body be moved away from the vertical line and then returned to a vertical position. Given the results from motor learning research on the frequency of knowledge of results (KR) summarized in Chapter 2, learning might be better if visual feedback regarding midline alignment is given intermittently, rather than during every trial. For example, the therapist could turn or cover the mirror and ask the patient to repeat the task in the absence of visual feedback.

Another approach to retraining vertical symmetrical alignment, shown in Figure 11.20, uses flashlights attached to the patient's body in conjunction with targets on the wall (Shumway-Cook & Horak, 1992). In this task, the patient is asked to bring the light (or lights) in line with the target(s). Again, lights can be turned on and off during the task so that visual feedback is intermittent.

Another approach to retraining vertical posture involves having patients stand (or sit) with their back against the wall, which provides enhanced somatosensory feedback about their position in space. This feedback can be further increased by placing a yardstick or small roll vertically on the wall (Fig. 11.21) and having the patient lean against it. Somatosensory feedback can be made intermittent by having the patient lean away from the wall, only occasionally leaning back to get KR.

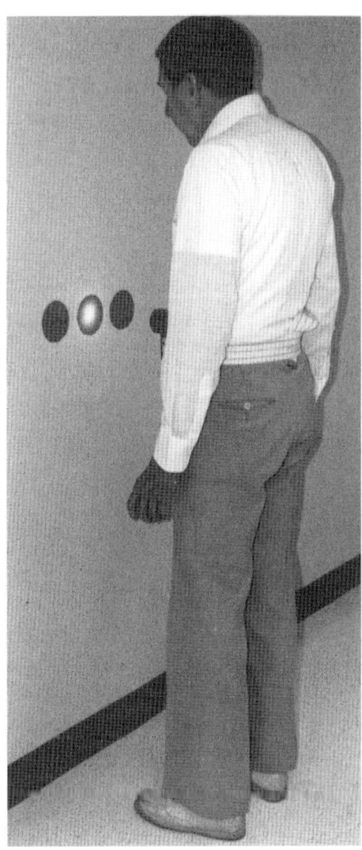

Figure 11.20 Using a flashlight in conjunction with targets on a wall to help a patient learn to control COM movements using continuous visual feedback.

Kinetic- or force-feedback devices are often used to provide patients with information about postural alignment and weight-bearing status (Herman, 1973; Shumway-Cook et al., 1988). Kinetic feedback can be provided with devices as simple as bathroom scales. Alternatively, kinetic feedback can be given through load-limb monitors (Herman, 1973), feedback canes (Baker et al., 1979), or force-plate biofeedback systems such as the one shown in Figure 11.22.

Research evidence. What evidence do we have that the use of force-plate biofeedback methods helps patients reestablish symmetrical postural alignment? In one of the earliest studies, Shumway-Cook and colleagues (1988) compared the effect of postural sway biofeedback to usual-care physical therapy in reestablishing symmetrical weight bearing during standing in patients with hemiparesis. Six months after a cerebrovascular accident (CVA), 16 patients were randomly assigned to feedback or usual-care groups. Prior to treatment, all patients carried about 70% of their total body weight on the noninvolved leg. The feedback group received 15 minutes of stance force-plate visual biofeedback twice a day for 2 weeks. The usual-care group received 15 minutes of balance retraining for the same amount of time.

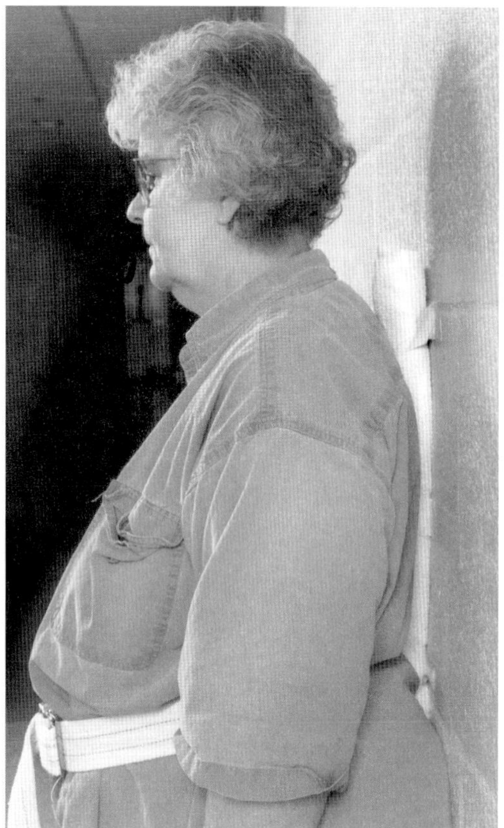

Figure 11.21 Enhancing somatosensation regarding verticality when retraining vertical posture by having the patient lean against a small roll placed vertically on the wall.

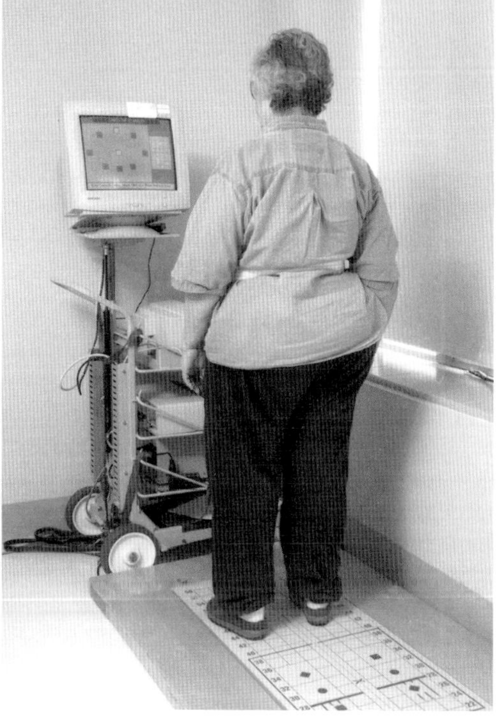

Figure 11.22 Use of a force-plate biofeedback system to provide visual feedback regarding alignment and weight-bearing status.

Following 2 weeks of training, the experimental group had significantly less lateral displacement than did the patients in the control group (six of whom were more asymmetric at the end of 2 weeks of therapy).

Winstein and colleagues (1989) also examined the effects of providing visual feedback about relative weight distribution over paretic and nonparetic limbs on standing balance and locomotor performance in patients with hemiplegia. They provided visual feedback through a standing feedback trainer to 21 patients randomly assigned to the experimental treatment; 21 patients served as controls and received conventional therapy. Consistent with the previous study, results showed that stance symmetry significantly improved with the visual-feedback therapy; however, there was no change in their asymmetrical locomotor pattern. These authors remind us that while control mechanisms for balance and locomotion may be highly interrelated, a reduction in standing asymmetry will not necessarily lead to a reduction in asymmetric locomotion patterns.

There have been two systematic reviews examining the effectiveness of force-plate biofeedback methods to improve standing balance after stroke. In their review, Barclay-Goddard et al. (2004) concluded that providing feedback from a force platform resulted in patients standing more symmetrically; however, this did not result in improved balance during functional activities, nor did it improve overall independence. The review by van Peppen et al. (2006) found a nonsignificant effect of visual-feedback therapy on weight distribution, postural sway, balance, and gait speed in persons with stroke. They concluded that visual-feedback therapy did not show an advantage over conventional therapy for improving weight-bearing asymmetry after stroke. Similar to the caution by Winstein et al. (1989), they suggest that many questions remain regarding the relationship between asymmetrical alignment and balance during stance and gait following stroke.

Clinicians routinely provide unsteady patients with assistive devices such as canes or walkers. What effect does providing external support such as a cane have on postural alignment and stability? An assistive device such as a cane increases the base of support. Since stability requires keeping the center of gravity within the base of support, increasing the base of support makes the task of stability easier. Milczarek and colleagues (1993) studied the effects of a cane on standing balance in patients with hemiparesis, using a force plate to record changes in COP under various conditions of support. As illustrated in Figure 11.23, they found that using a cane resulted in a significant shift in the position of the COP toward the cane side and a decrease in both anteroposterior and mediolateral postural sway. Thus, although using a cane reduced postural sway, it increased the asymmetric alignment of patients toward the side holding the cane (Milczarek et al., 1993). More recently, Bateni et al. (2004a) demonstrated that in

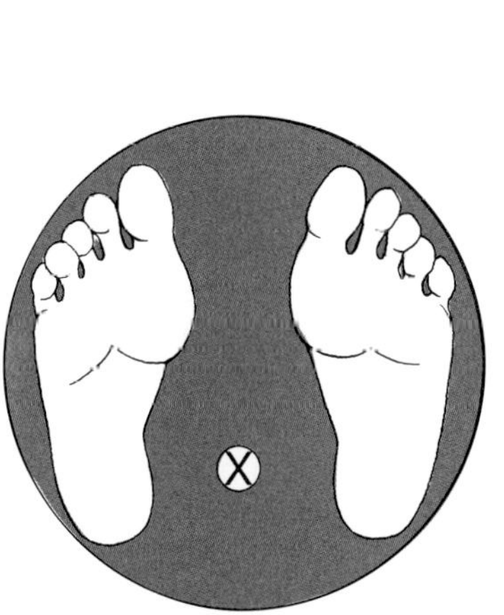

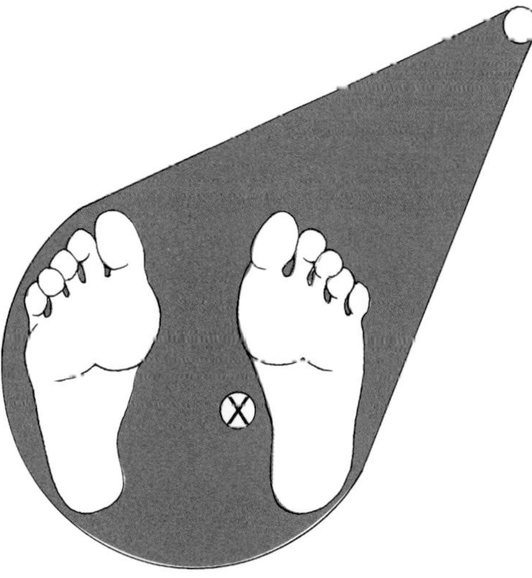

Figure 11.23 The effects of holding a cane while standing include widening the base of support and shifting the mean position of the COP laterally toward the cane side. (Adapted from Milczarek JJ, Kirby LM, Harrison ER, et al. Standard and four-footed canes: their effect on the standing balance of patients with hemiparesis. *Arch Phys Med Rehabil*. 1993;74:283.)

healthy subjects, the use of a cane or walker interfered with compensatory stepping responses. Use of an assistive device resulted in collisions between the swing foot and the assistive device and a significant reduction in lateral step length, pointing out the inherent limitations in assistive devices as an aid in recovery of postural stability in response to external perturbations.

Retraining Reactive Balance Control. The goal when retraining reactive balance control is to help the patient develop coordinated multijoint movements, including both in-place and change-in-support strategies, that are effective in recovery of stability following an unexpected loss of balance. Training involves exposing the patient to external perturbations that vary in direction, speed, and amplitude. External perturbations can include manual pulls and pushes applied to the hips or shoulders and the use of moving surfaces (such as rocker boards) or a variety of cable release systems. Small perturbations can facilitate the use of in-place strategies for balance control, while larger and faster perturbations encourage the use of a step or a reach.

Perturbation training programs to improve both stepping and reaching reactions have been developed (Maki & McIlroy, 2006; Mansfield et al., 2007, 2010). Environmental conditions are varied to encourage the use of stepping or reaching. For example, to improve reaching reactions, handholds in the environment are used to facilitate reaching, in combination with foam blocks placed around the person's legs, used to discourage stepping (shown in Fig. 11.24). Large perturbations in the standing position are combined with instructions to reach (or step) as quickly as possible.

Figure 11.25 illustrates a technique to facilitate a stepping response during reactive balance training. The therapist uses the gait belt to quickly and smoothly displace the patient first to the left (unloading the right limb and loading the left limb) then forward and to the right while providing manual assistance to step with the right limb.

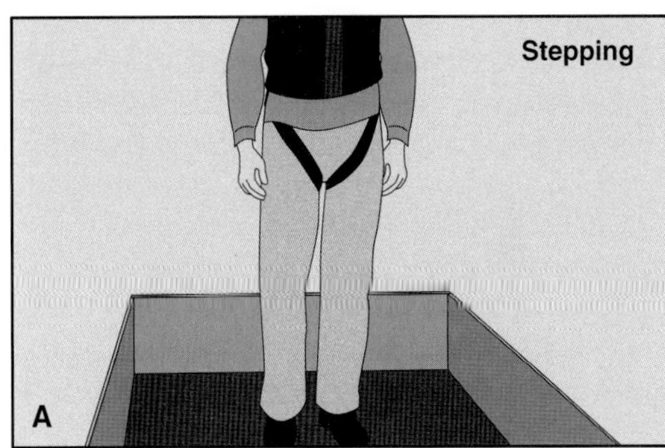

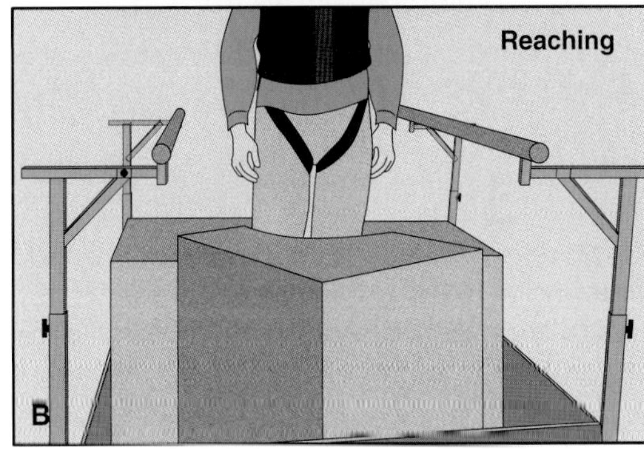

Figure 11.24 Environmental conditions used to facilitate change in support reactions. **(A)** Absence of handrails and a floor space large enough to accommodate steps are used to facilitate stepping. **(B)** Handrails in conjunction with foam blocks are used to facilitate reaching and discourage stepping. (Adapted from Mansfield A, Peters AL, Liu BA, et al. Effect of a perturbation-based balance training program on compensatory stepping and grasping reactions in older adults: a randomized controlled trial. *Phys Ther*. 2010;90:476, Figure 1 A, page 479.)

Responses to external perturbations are practiced in sitting or standing (depending on the patient's ability), in multiple directions, and under varying conditions in order to facilitate development of effective in-place and change-in-support (step and reaching) reactions. Examples of reactive balance training in a patient with stroke can be seen in the video case study on treatment of stroke. As patients improve, exercises

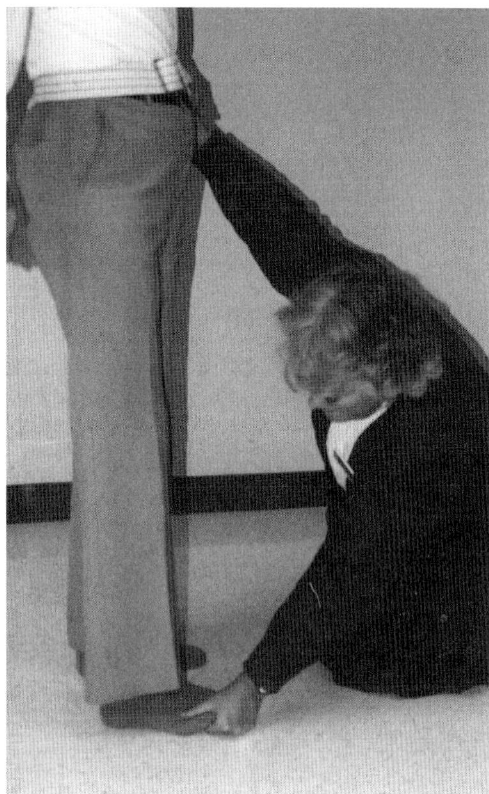

Figure 11.25 Facilitating automatic stepping by manually shifting the patient's COM laterally and forward of the base of support to trigger an automatic step while at the same time assisting the patient manually with the step.

are made progressively more difficult by changing the sensory conditions (e.g., with and without vision and on firm, foam, and inclined surfaces) and cognitive conditions (both alone and while practicing other tasks).

Research evidence. There is mounting evidence that training of reactive balance control does improve the organization and timing of postural responses in patients with neurologic deficits and can, in some cases, reduce the risk for falls (see Mansfield et al., 2015 for a review). Marigold et al. (2005) found improvements in the onset latency of paretic lower-extremity muscles in response to platform perturbations in people with chronic stroke after 10 weeks of balance training that incorporated reactive balance training. Improvements in the onset latency and organization of lower-extremity muscle responses to platform perturbations were also reported in children with spastic hemiplegic and diplegic forms of cerebral palsy following 5 days of intensive (100 perturbations of varying size and amplitude a day) reactive balance training on a movable platform (Shumway-Cook et al., 2003; Woollacott et al., 2005).

A randomized controlled trial was used to demonstrate improvements in the ability to step or reach following a training program in balance-impaired older adults (Mansfield et al., 2010). Thirty balance-impaired older adults were randomized to either the perturbation training program designed to improve stepping and reaching or a relaxation/flexibility program. Training was 30 minutes, 3 × a week for 6 weeks. Only the group receiving the perturbation training showed improvements in stepping reactions (indicated by fewer multiple steps and interlimb collisions) and reaching (faster handrail contact).

Other forms of training have also been shown to improve postural control at the impairment level—organization and timing of muscle responses—to recover balance following an unexpected perturbation. Gatts and Woollacott (2006; 2007) examined the effect of 3 weeks of intense (1½ hours, 5 days per week) Tai Chi training on the ability to recover from an unexpected perturbation while walking, in balance-impaired older adults. The authors found that Tai Chi training significantly enhanced balance responses by improving the organization and timing of stepping strategies of the swing leg. In addition, there was a significant reduction in co-contraction of antagonist muscles of the perturbed leg. These studies provide evidence that training can improve the organization and timing of muscle responses used to recover stability following an unexpected perturbation to stability. In some instances, perturbation training can significantly reduce the risk for falls (Mansfield et al., 2014). More research is needed to determine the types of interventions that are effective in improving reactive postural control in both neurologic and geriatric populations. Research examining the effectiveness of reactive balance training during gait is discussed in Chapter 16.

Retraining Anticipatory Balance Control. Movement strategies to control the COM can also be practiced during voluntary sway in all directions. With practice, patients learn to control COM movements over increasingly larger areas while varying speed. KR regarding how far the COM is moving during self-initiated sway can be facilitated using static force-plate retraining systems. Flashlights attached to the patient in conjunction with targets on the wall can also be used to encourage patients to move from side to side.

Patients who are very unsteady or extremely fearful of falling can practice movements while in the parallel bars or when standing close to a wall or in a corner with a chair or table in front of them (Fig. 11.26). Modifying the environment (either home or clinic) in this manner allows a patient to continue practicing movement strategies for balance control safely and without the continual supervision of a therapist.

When training anticipatory postural control, patients can be asked to carry out a variety of manipulation tasks, such as reaching, lifting, and throwing, thus helping patients to develop strategies for anticipatory postural control. A hierarchy of tasks reflecting increasing anticipatory postural demands can be helpful when retraining patients in this important area. The magnitude of anticipatory postural activity is directly related

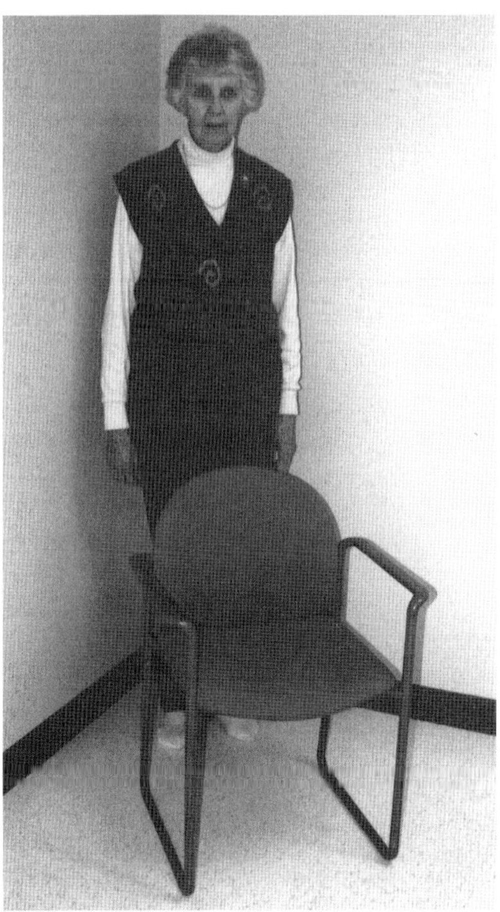

Figure 11.26 Placing a patient near a wall with a chair in front of her increases safety when retraining standing balance in a fearful or unstable patient.

to the potential for instability inherent in a task. Potential instability relates to speed, effort, degree of external support, and task complexity. Thus, asking a patient who is externally supported by the therapist to lift a light load slowly requires minimal anticipatory postural activity. Conversely, an unsupported patient who must lift a heavy load quickly must use a substantial amount of anticipatory postural activity to remain stable.

Research evidence. While many studies have documented that repetitive practice of functional tasks significantly improves performance on functional balance measures such as the BBS, the Functional Reach, and the TUG, few studies have examined the underlying muscle activity to determine whether improved task performance is associated with improved anticipatory aspects of postural control. Garland et al. (2003) used surface electromyography to examine the timing of muscle activity in the lower extremities (hamstrings and soleus) relative to the initiation of arm movement in an arm-raising task in persons with poststroke hemiparesis. Prior to rehabilitation, muscles in the paretic lower extremity were activated after the initiation of arm movement, rather than before, as was true in the nonparetic limb. Following 1 month of rehabilitation, arm movement was faster and recruitment of hamstring and soleus muscles was significantly faster in both limbs. While 10 of 27 patients showed activation of anticipatory muscle activity in the hemiparetic limb prior to arm movement (what the authors refer to as "true recovery"), 12 showed no change in the timing of muscle activity in the hemiparetic side, though they improved timing in the nonhemiparetic limb (a compensatory strategy). This research provides evidence that anticipatory aspects of postural control can be improved with training in some patients. More research is needed to verify and expand these findings to other patient populations.

Training Balance in Sitting

As discussed in Chapter 10, poor segmental trunk control is a major factor contributing to postural imbalance in many patients with severe neurologic pathology. For instance, segmental trunk control deficits have been shown to be associated with impaired gross motor function and mobility in children with CP (Curtis et al., 2015). Research in this area has led to the development of Targeted Training (Butler, 1998; Curtis et al., 2018). Targeted Training uses a rigid system to isolate specific trunk segments during postural training. Theoretically, targeted training gradually improves trunk control over an increased number of trunk segments when maintaining an upright sitting posture in individuals with moderate to severe disabilities. This approach is based on the system's theory, in which the number of degrees of freedom (trunk sub-regions in this case) is artificially constrained by following a top–down sequence with an external device until the individual acquires control over sequential trunk regions. The training system (which can be seen in the video entitled "Assessment and Treatment of Segmental Trunk Control") uses special equipment to establish and maintain an optimal vertical position. This equipment is used to provide an individual with support at the required segmental level of the trunk, that is, the level at which the subject displays lack of balance control of the upper body, and then challenges active and reactive control of trunk segments *above* that support level. The level of support needed is determined by using the SATCo test (described earlier). The clinical decision-making model for interpreting SATCo results and determining initial training conditions is shown in Figure 11.27. Progression in training is achieved by moving the support lower so the subject has to gain control over an increasing number of trunk segments and by increasing the postural control challenge (e.g., moving from a firm surface to a rocking surface). Recommended training is 30 minutes a day, 5 to 6 days a week (training is often provided in a home or school setting). A randomized clinical trial (Curtis et al., 2018) reported the effectiveness of Targeted Training on

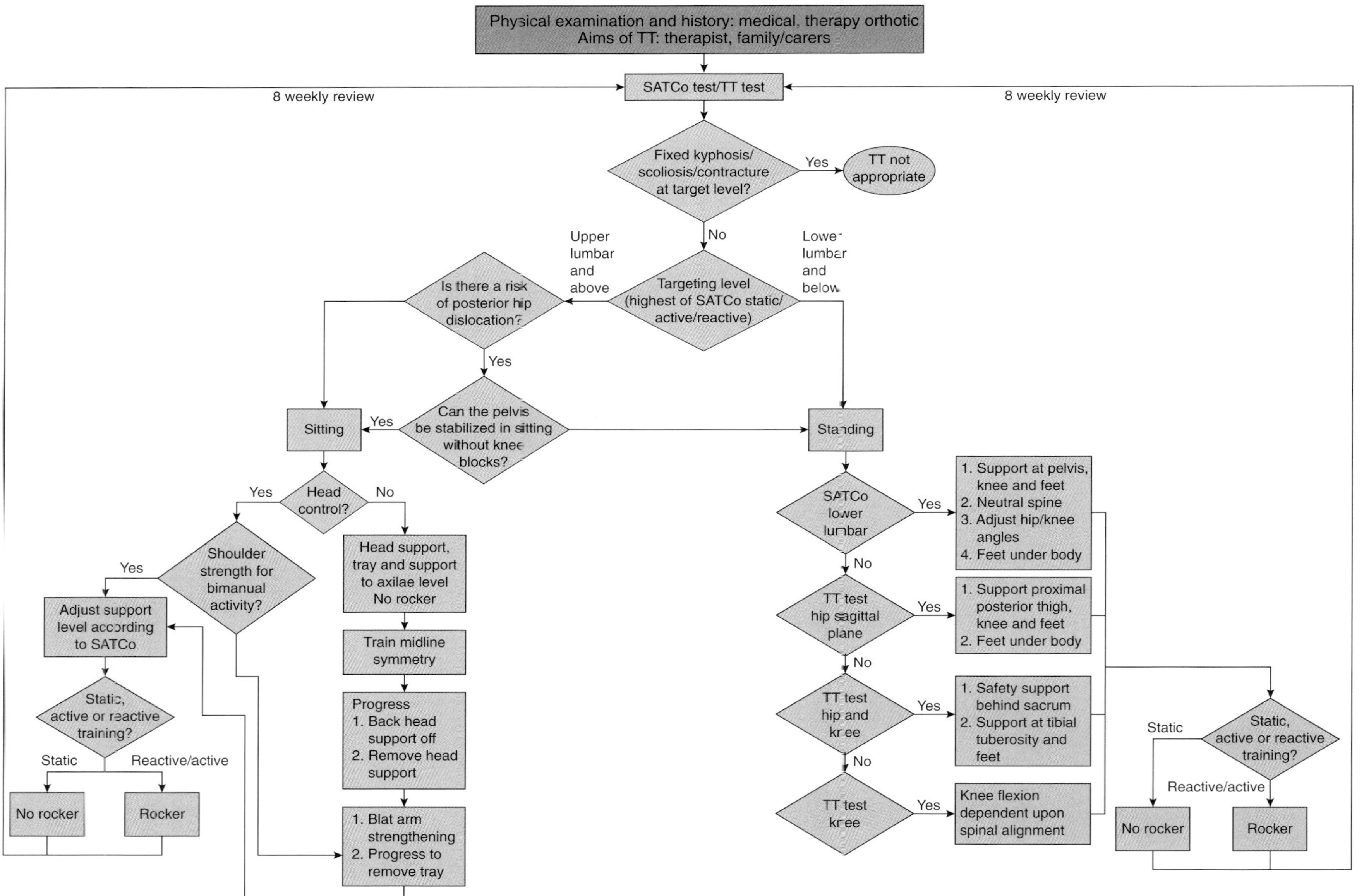

Figure 11.27 An algorithm to assist in decision-making related to targeted segmental trunk training. (Curtis DJ. PhD Thesis: Head and Trunk Postural Control in Moderate to Severe Cerebral Palsy: A Segmental Approach to Analysis and Treatment. Faculty of Health and Medical Sciences, University of Copenhagen, Copenhagen, Denmark, Submitted February 2014.)

improved postural sway of head and trunk 6 months after therapy. In this research, however, segmental training did not show improvements on the SATCo or functional outcomes compared to customary therapy. Factors like sample heterogeneity, dosage, training intensity, and the comparison between a targeted training as a home-therapy program versus clinically supervised therapy may have masked the lack of functional improvements. Indeed, the SATCo has been shown to be sensitive and responsive to change when examining motor improvements in response to therapy in children with spinal cord injury (Argetsinger et al., 2019).

Sensory Systems

Treating Underlying Sensory Impairments

As discussed in Chapter 5, the use of sensory stimulation to facilitate activation of the motor systems is not a new concept. Many types of sensory stimulation have been used, including icing, vibration, tapping, and sensory transcutaneous electrical stimulation. What evidence do we have that treatments targeting sensory impairments will improve balance control? Does combining sensory stimulation with functional task training improve outcomes? Finally, who is most likely to benefit from sensory training?

Bernard-Demanze et al. (2009) performed a study to reduce sway in older adults with decreased sensation on the plantar surface of the foot. They examined the effects of 10 minutes of plantar stimulation performed in the seated position on COP measures in quiet stance in older adults with and without plantar sole deficits and a group of young adults. Plantar stimulation was designed to stimulate slowly adapting receptors in the plantar surface of the feet. Mediolateral sway was significantly decreased in the older adults with the sensory deficit, though training did not significantly affect sway in individuals with no sensory deficit. Results suggest that sensory stimulation of the feet may be effective (at least in the short term) in improving quiet stance balance, but only in those who have impaired sensation. The dose needed to impact balance in the short term was 10 minutes (less time had no effect); however, further research is needed to determine optimal dose for long-term effects of this type of stimulation. Ko and colleagues (2016) did a randomized controlled study in CP and found that the use of whole-body vibration in addition to conventional therapy improves joint position sense at the ankle and gait control (speed and step width).

A systematic review examining the effect of sensory TENS on motor recovery following a stroke concluded that only when it was combined with active functional task training did sensory TENS improve recovery (Laufer & Elboim-Gabyzon, 2011). These studies suggest that in order to be effective, treatments aimed at underlying sensory or motor impairments must be done in conjunction with appropriate functional task practice.

For example, as shown in the postural control segment in the video "Treatment of Stroke," when treating balance in Genise our patient who is 1 month poststroke, we begin with treatments aimed at underlying sensory and motor impairments. In the seated position, we use mobilization techniques to improve range of motion in her hemiparetic foot and ankle and then, based on research evidence from Bernard-Demanze, provide sensory stimulation to the plantar surface of her paretic foot. Treatments aimed at the impairment level are immediately followed by practice of functional tasks including sit-to-stand and quiet stance, both of which require use of lower extremities for balance control. Stance balance tasks include both quiet standing (steady-state balance) and small nudges to encourage use of in-place strategies for recovery of balance (reactive balance) and larger nudges or perturbations to encourage stepping or reaching (also reactive balance). In addition, she practices functional tasks that require anticipatory postural adjustments, such as reaching, leaning over, and lifting objects, as well as stepping up to different height steps with her paretic and nonparetic limb. At 1 month poststroke, Genise's balance in sitting is quite good (with the exception of her inability to reach for support with her paretic arm). Thus, balance training at this stage focuses primarily on training balance in stance and gait.

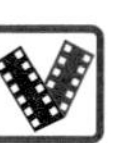

Functional Balance Training: Improving Sensory Strategies

Learning to meet the stability demands of functional tasks under ideal sensory conditions is not sufficient to ensure function in complex environmental conditions. This requires learning to adapt sensory organization strategies to changing sensory conditions. Thus, the goal when retraining sensory organization strategies is to help the patient learn to effectively organize and select appropriate sensory information for postural control. Treatment strategies generally require the patient to maintain balance during progressively more difficult balance tasks while the clinician systematically varies the availability and accuracy of one or more senses for orientation (Shumway-Cook & Horak, 1989, 1990).

Patients who show increased reliance on vision for orientation are asked to perform a variety of balance tasks when visual cues are absent (eyes closed or blindfolded) or reduced (blinders or diminished lighting). Alternatively, visual cues can be made inaccurate for orientation through the use of glasses smeared with petroleum jelly (Fig. 11.28) or Frenzel glasses. Decreasing a patient's sensitivity to visual motion cues in their environment can be done by asking the patient to maintain balance during exposure to optokinetic

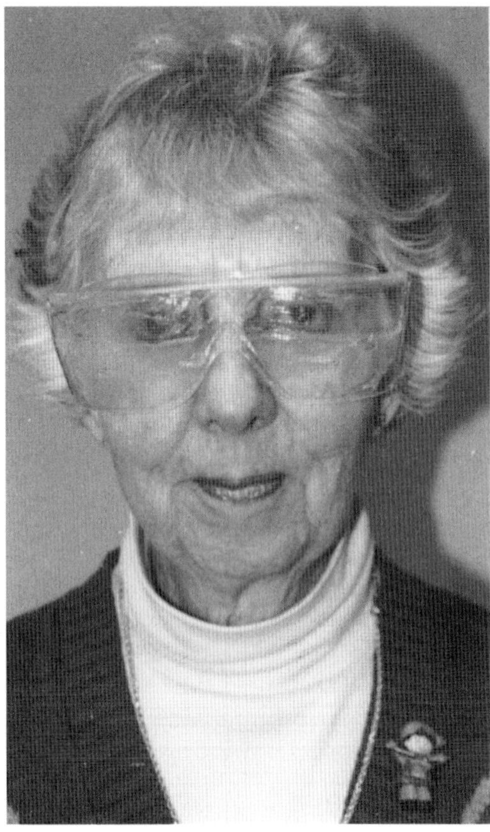

Figure 11.28 Training sensory adaptation for postural control. Petroleum jelly–covered glasses are used to obscure but not completely remove visual cues for postural control.

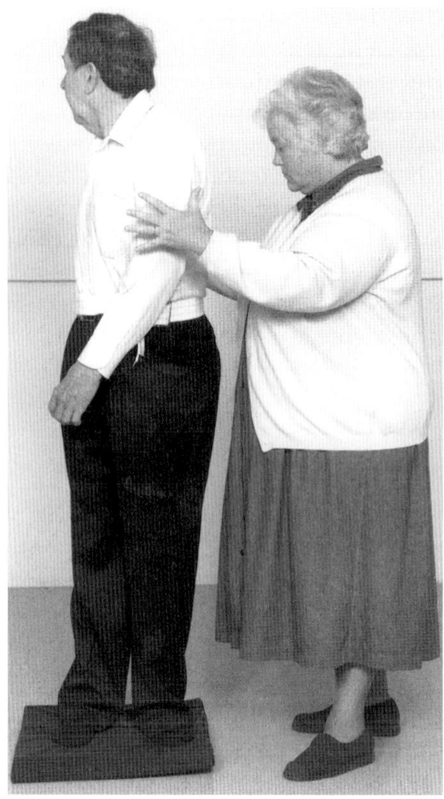

Figure 11.29 Training sensory adaptation for postural control. The patient is asked to turn the trunk while standing on foam, which is purported to reduce the availability of somatosensory inputs for postural control and thus increases the weighting of vision or vestibular inputs for postural control.

stimuli, such as moving curtains with stripes, moving large cardboard posters with vertical lines, or even moving rooms (see Chapter 7).

Patients who show increased reliance on somatosensory inputs from the feet in contact with the surface are asked to perform tasks while sitting or standing on surfaces providing decreased somatosensory cues for orientation, such as carpet or compliant foam surfaces, or on moving surfaces, such as a tilt board. Finally, to enhance the patient's ability to use the remaining vestibular information for postural stability, exercises are given that require the patient to balance while both visual and somatosensory inputs for orientation are simultaneously reduced, such as standing on compliant foam, thick carpet, or an inclined surface with eyes closed. Figure 11.29 shows a patient asked to turn his trunk while standing on foam, which is purported to reduce the availability of somatosensory inputs for postural control and thus to increase the weighting of vision or vestibular inputs for postural control. In Figure 11.30, the subject wears petroleum jelly–covered glasses and stands on foam while reaching for a glass of water. The rationale for this exercise is to increase reliance on vestibular inputs for postural control by reducing the availability of both somatosensory and visual inputs

Research Evidence. Is there research evidence to suggest that practicing tasks under altered sensory contexts can improve the way people organize and select sensory information for balance control? The answer appears to be "yes," in both geriatric and neurologic populations. A number of studies have demonstrated improvements in the organization of sensory information for postural control through training in older adults (Hu & Woollacott; 1994a, 1994b); adults with vestibular dysfunction (Cass et al., 1996), stroke (Bayouk et al., 2006; Bonan et al., 2004; Smania et al., 2008), and MS (Cattaneo et al., 2007); and children with sensorineural hearing loss and vestibular impairment (Rine et al., 2004).

A study by Hu and Woollacott (1994a, 1994b) used a balance-training protocol that focused on the use of different sensory inputs and the integration of these inputs under conditions in which sensory inputs were reduced or altered. Subjects (65 to 87 years of age) participated in five 1-hour training sessions per week for 2 weeks. The training conditions consisted of standing on a force plate under the following sensory conditions: normal support surface, eyes open, and head neutral; normal surface, eyes closed, and head neutral; normal support surface, eyes open, and head extended; and normal surface, eyes closed, and head extended; then,

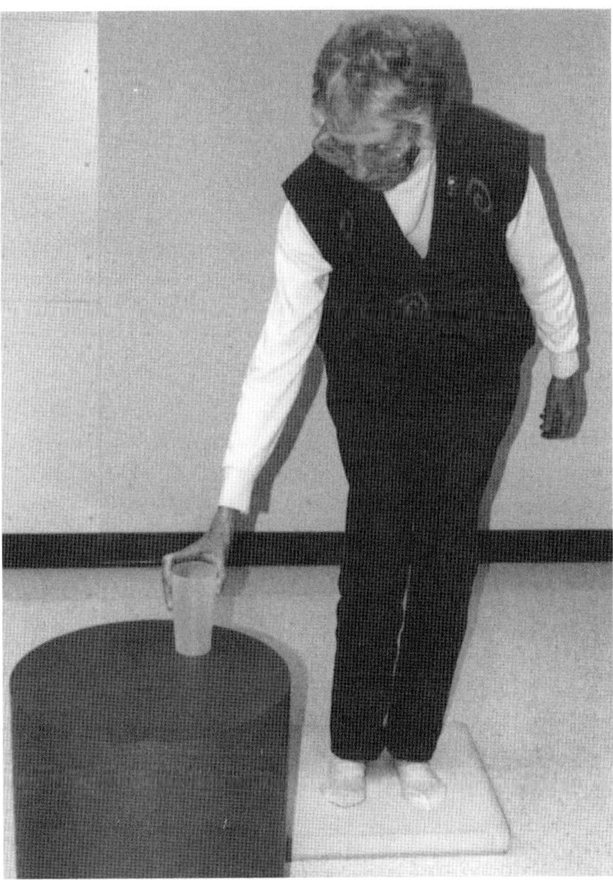

Figure 11.30 Training sensory adaptation for postural control. The patient wears petroleum jelly–covered glasses and stands on foam while reaching for a glass of water. The rationale for this exercise is to increase reliance on vestibular inputs for postural control by reducing the availability of both somatosensory and visual inputs.

all trials were repeated on a foam surface. They found significant improvements in the sway of the training group between the first and the last day of training in five of the eight training conditions (the four foam surface conditions and eyes closed and head extended on the normal surface).

Bayouk et al. (2006) examined the effects of a task-oriented exercise program with and without altered sensory input on postural stability in subjects with stroke. Sixteen patients participated in an 8-week training program; half performed task-oriented training with sensory manipulation (e.g., practicing tasks with eyes open or closed while standing on a firm or foam surface), while half performed the same set of exercises without sensory manipulation. Both groups significantly improved on the 10-minute walk test; however, only the group that practiced under altered sensory conditions showed an improved ability to stand under altered sensory conditions. The authors suggest that "balance senses have to be specifically targeted when designing balance-retraining programs for hemiparetic subjects" (Bayouk et al., 2006, p. 57). Other researchers have also reported that sensory manipulation, including changing vision (Bonan et al., 2004), or a combination of both vision and somatosensory inputs (Smania et al., 2008) was more effective in improving balance than similar training without sensory manipulation in patients with impaired balance following stroke.

Similarly, in a randomized clinical trial, Cattaneo and colleagues (2007) compared the effect of balance exercises with and without sensory manipulation (e.g., visual manipulation [eyes open and closed], somatosensory manipulation [firm vs. foam surface], and vestibular manipulation [combinations of head and eye movements]) in two groups of individuals with MS. Both groups improved performance on the BBS and the Dynamic Gait Index (DGI) (a measure of dynamic balance), with the greatest improvements found in the group receiving balance training with sensory manipulation.

Augmenting Sensory Inputs to Improve Balance Control

Treatments to improve sensory strategies for balance control have focused primarily on reducing or distorting sensory inputs from one sensory system in order to increase the relative weight and thus the selection of alternative sensory inputs for balance control. Augmenting sensory inputs for postural control during functional task training has also been used to improve the control of balance. As discussed in Chapter 7, augmenting somatosensory inputs by touching the index finger to a stationary surface improved stance postural control in persons with vestibular deficits (Jeka, 1997) and those with peripheral neuropathy (Dickstein et al., 2001).

Researchers have used augmented sensory feedback systems to improve postural control in persons with peripheral and central nervous system pathology. For example, providing real-time visual feedback related to body (COP) or head or trunk movements during quiet stance improved performance among many patient groups, including individuals with vestibular disorders (Cakrt et al., 2010), stroke (Walker et al., 2000), and MS (Prosperini et al., 2010) and children with cerebral palsy (Ledebt et al., 2005).

Feedback devices using other sensory modalities including auditory (Dozza et al., 2005; Nicolai et al., 2010), electrotactile (Cakrt et al., 2012; Danilov et al., 2006), and vibrotactile (Haggerty et al., 2012; Lee et al., 2012; Sienko et al., 2013) also improved performance during both quiet and perturbed stance. For example, among individuals with vestibular dysfunction, trunk-based vibrotactile feedback provided during functional task training decreased body sway, improved Sensory Organization Test scores, and decreased dizziness (Harada et al., 2010; Wall & Kentala, 2005). Persons with Parkinson's disease who underwent a single session of balance training in conjunction with trunk-based vibrotactile feedback improved balance during stance and gait more than did those who received balance training alone (Nanhoe-Mahabier et al., 2012). Two weeks of functional balance training combined with a tongue-based electrotactile feedback system related to sway (stimulation on the tongue indicated direction of sway) significantly improved balance control in standing with eyes closed in persons with progressive cerebellar degeneration (Cakrt et al., 2012).

Among persons with diabetic peripheral neuropathy, use of therapeutic shoes, inserts, and ankle–foot orthoses that provide tactile and proprioceptive stimulation to increase feedback from cutaneous receptors in the foot and ankle has been shown to improve balance and reduce risk for falls (Aruin & Rao, 2010; Hijmans et al., 2007). Researchers have also used vibratory shoe inserts to improve utilization of somatosensory inputs from the lower extremity for postural control (Priplata et al., 2002). This approach is based on studies in a variety of systems showing that certain levels of noise (background vibration) can enhance the detection and transmission of weak signals (a process referred to as "stochastic resonance"). Introducing vibrotactile noise has been shown to improve detection of mechanical and tactile receptors in older adults (Priplata et al., 2003), patients with stroke (Liu et al., 2002), and patients with diabetic neuropathy (Priplata et al., 2006).

Is one form of feedback better than another? There are very few controlled studies examining the relative effectiveness of different modalities of sensory feedback on balance control in specific populations. A study by Bechly and colleagues (2013) compared the effects of discrete visual, vibrotactile, multimodal, and continuous visual feedback on the stance balance performance (mediolateral and anteroposterior body tilt) in individuals with and without vestibular dysfunction during a quiet stance balance task. Participants were asked to stand quietly and keep sway within a "no-feedback" zone. All modalities provided feedback in the direction of body tilt and were activated only when body tilt approximately exceeded a "no-feedback zone" threshold in that direction. Feedback was deactivated when the subject moved his body back within the no-feedback zone (see Fig. 11.31 to see the research setup). As shown in Figure 11.32, all forms of feedback improved performance; however, the group with vestibular deficits (labeled VP) showed the most improvement in trunk tilt (Fig. 11.31A) and time spent in the "no-feedback" zone (Fig. 11.32B), when provided with continuous visual feedback. The authors suggest that since individuals with vestibular deficits benefit from all types of feedback, the type of feedback selected for rehabilitation training program could be based on an individual's preference (Bechly et al., 2013). Whether the finding that all forms of feedback are equally effective in improving stance postural control generalizes across patient populations is unclear. In addition, the research examining the use of augmented feedback training to improve

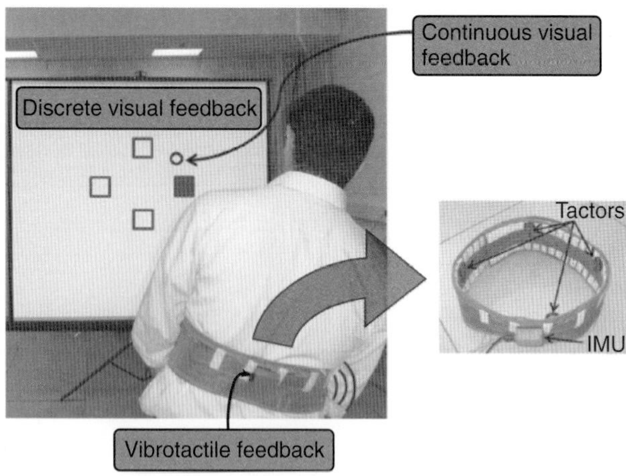

Figure 11.31 Experimental setup, including discrete visual feedback display, continuous visual feedback display, and vibrotactile feedback device. (Reprinted from Bechly KE, Carender WJ, Myles JD, et al. Determining the preferred modality for real-time biofeedback during balance training. *Gait Posture*. 2013;37:393, with permission).

balance function among older adults has mixed results (see Zijlstra et al. [2010] for a review).

How could this evidence be used to improve balance in our case studies? There is evidence to support the use of augmented sensory feedback during task-specific balance training in almost all of our patients. Based on research by Nanhoe-Mahabier and colleagues (2012), vibrotactile feedback regarding trunk position combined with functional task training may improve balance in Mike, our patient with Parkinson's disease, more than task training alone. There is considerable evidence that augmented sensory feedback (visual, auditory, and vibrotactile) done in conjunction with functional balance training will improve balance in sitting, standing, and walking in Jean and Genise, our patients with stroke. In addition, vibrotactile shoe inserts to compensate for reduced somatosensory inputs from the hemiparetic leg may improve balance.

We know that balance training combined with electrotactile feedback regarding body position significantly improves balance in patients like John, with progressive cerebellar degeneration (Cakrt et al., 2012). Whether feedback from other sensory systems (visual, auditory, and vibrotactile) will also impact balance is less clear.

Use of visual feedback in conjunction with task-specific balance training has been shown to improve balance performance in children, like Thomas, who have cerebral palsy, although the added benefits of visual feedback beyond those expected from training alone is unclear (Ledebt et al., 2005). In this new technological era, more sophisticated equipment such as movement-based video games, transcranial direct stimulation, or virtual reality are being incorporated more frequently in therapeutic programs. Lazzari and colleagues (2017) investigated in a randomized controlled trial the effectiveness of virtual reality combined

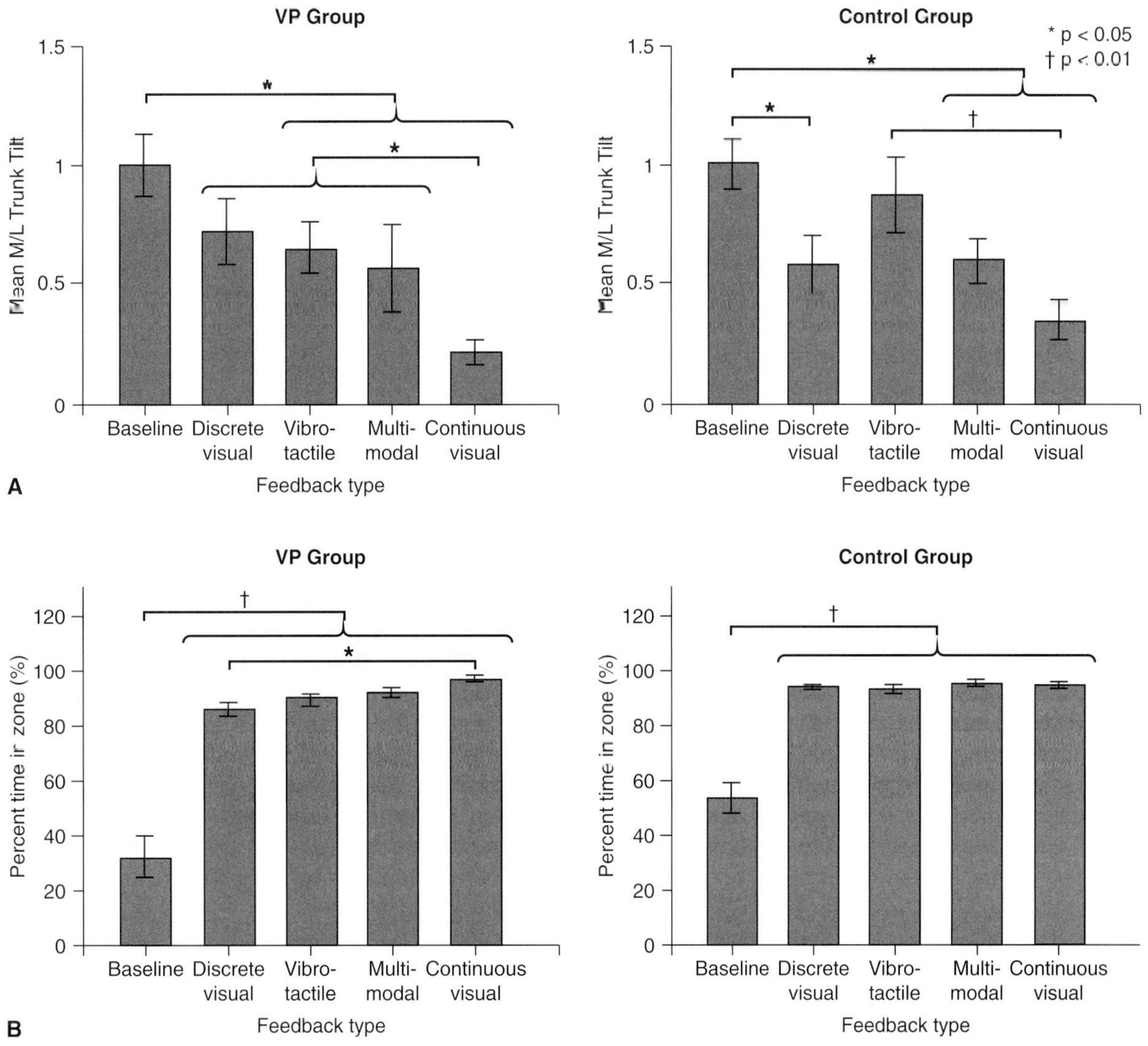

Figure 11.32 Postural sway feedback results for individuals with vestibular deficits (VP group): **(A)** normalized mean M/L body tilt and **(B)** percent time spent in the no-feedback zone; statistical significance represented by * for p <0.05 and y for p <0.01. (Adapted from Bechly KE, Wendy J, Carender WJ, et al. Determining the preferred modality for real-time biofeedback during balance training. *Gait Posture*. 2013;37:395.)

with transcranial direct current stimulation to train balance control in children with CP (experimental group). The children with CP included in the control group received virtual reality but with sham stimulation. The authors found significant improvements in the experimental group for the Pediatric Balance Scale, TUG Test, and improved balance control (COP) during postural stance, which suggest that transcranial direct stimulation has a potentiation motor effect when combined with mobility training—in this case virtual reality.

Cognitive Systems

Training Attention in Isolation: Effects on Balance

As discussed in Chapter 10, impaired attention is a significant factor contributing to instability and falls in dual-task conditions in both geriatric and neurologic populations. Can nonmotor dual-task training of attentional control in the absence of functional balance training impact balance? Preliminary evidence suggests this may be the case. Li and colleagues (2010) randomly assigned 20 healthy older adults to either five 1-hour sessions of cognitive dual-task training over 2 days or a control group. Cognitive training involved making two-choice decisions to visually presented stimuli under single- and dual-task conditions. Outcome measures included tests of cognition, balance, and mobility (single-support balance, Sensory Organization Test using dynamic posturography, five times sit-to-stand, 40-foot walk) under single- and dual-task (in conjunction with n-back test) conditions. Compared to the control group, training benefits were found in both single-support standing balance (single-task conditions only) and double-support standing balance (firm surface, dual-task conditions only).

There were no benefits either to the sit-to-stand task or to walking speed.

Similar results were reported by Smith-Ray and colleagues (2014). In their pilot study, 45 community-dwelling African American older adults with a history of falls were randomly assigned to either cognitive training (n = 23) or a control (no intervention) group (n = 22). Cognitive training involved a computer-based class that met 2 days a week for 60 minutes over 10 weeks, with classes held at senior or community center. Compared to the controls, the group receiving cognitive training showed significant improvements on the BBS and faster gait speed on the single-task 10-meter walk test (10MWT). Interestingly, there were no significant differences in dual-task walking performance between the two groups (Smith-Ray et al., 2014).

These studies, though limited by small sample size, nonetheless provide preliminary evidence that for older adults, training dual-task control using nonmotor tasks may improve balance in some but not all functional tasks. Further research is needed to verify and expand findings to persons with neurologic pathology. If robust, this approach offers a unique way to train dual-task balance control in patients with very limited capacity to participate in task-specific balance training, either due to fatigue or because of a high risk for falls.

Cognitive Strategies

The growing evidence that instability and falls increase during the performance of multiple tasks in both neurologic and geriatric populations suggests the need for training balance under both single- and dual-task conditions. Training balance under dual-task conditions involves practicing tasks requiring steady-state, anticipatory, and reactive balance control while simultaneously varying the cognitive demands through the use of secondary tasks. This aspect of balance rehabilitation is relatively new; thus, we have limited evidence to guide and support the use of dual-task training in balance rehabilitation.

Research Evidence. Silsupadol et al. (2006, 2009a, 2009b) described the outcomes of three approaches to training balance—single task, dual task with fixed-priority instructions, and dual task with variable-priority instructions—in older adults with balance impairment. Outcome measures for this series of studies included the BBS, the DGI, the single- and dual-task TUG, and the ABC scale. In addition, laboratory measures of walking under single- and dual-task conditions (novel tasks not specifically trained) were also analyzed. Participants were older adults who volunteered for balance training because of a self-reported history of falls in the previous year or concern about impaired balance in the absence of neurologic or musculoskeletal diagnoses. Participants were randomly assigned to one of the three balance-training approaches. Balance training was done three times a week for 4 weeks. For all participants, balance training was based on a systems theory of postural control and used a progression of activities designed to improve steady-state, anticipatory, and reactive balance control. In addition, training targeted sensory and motor components of postural control.

Examples of the balance-training strategies used are summarized in Table 11.7. Dual-task training was done under either a fixed (maintain attention on both tasks all the time) or variable (attentional focus was on balance activities for half of each session and on secondary tasks for the other half) instructional set. A summary of the types of secondary tasks used in this study is also found in Table 11.7. All three forms of balance training improved balance on the BBS (p <0.001, effect size = 0.72) and gait speed on the 10-m walk (p = 0.02, effect size = 0.27). However, only participants who received dual-task training improved gait speed under dual-task conditions (Silsupadol et al., 2009a). In addition, using a variable-priority instructional set during dual-task balance training was more effective at improving balance under dual-task training conditions than either single-task or fixed-priority training strategies. The use of a variable-priority strategy during dual-task training appears to improve both single-task automatization and the ability to coordinate multiple tasks (Silsupadol et al., 2009b). The authors conclude that training balance under single-task conditions may not generalize to balance control under dual-task conditions. In addition, explicit instructions regarding attentional focus may significantly impact the results of dual-task balance training.

Kim and colleagues (2014) compared single- to dual-task training in a group of 20 patients, on average 16 to 19 months poststroke, using the treatment paradigm from Silsupadol and colleagues. Patients were randomly assigned to receive gait training under single- (n = 10) or dual-task (n = 10) conditions. Outcome measures including the Stroop test, TUG test performed under single- and dual-task conditions, 10MWT, Figure-of-8 Walking Test (F8WT), and DGI were performed before the intervention, immediately postintervention, and then again 2 weeks postintervention. Training was 30 minutes a day, 3 days a week for a total of 4 weeks. Variable-priority instructions were used during the dual-task training. Similar to Silsupadol's results with balance-impaired older adults, the patients with stroke who received the dual-task training were significantly better on all outcome measures (except the F8WT). For example, the single-task training group showed no change in TUG performance under dual-task conditions (pretraining, 42 ± 24 s; immediately posttraining, 40 ± 22 s; 2 weeks posttraining, 40 ± 23 s) while the dual-task trained group showed a significant improvement (pretraining, 34 ± 20 s; posttraining, 24 ± 15 s; 2 weeks posttraining, 25 ± 16 s). In addition, performance on the cognitive task (Stroop test) improved in the dual-task group but not in the single-task training group.

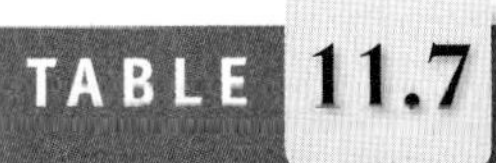

TABLE 11.7 List of Activities Used during Balance Retraining under Single- and Dual-Task Conditions

Balance activities	Secondary tasks
Stance Activities	**Secondary Task Activities**
1. Semitandem, eyes open, arm alternation	• Spell words forward
2. Semitandem, eyes closed, arm alternation	• Spell words backward
3. Draw letters with right foot	• Name any words starting with letters A to K
4. Draw letters with left foot	• Name any words starting with letters L to Z
5. Perturbed forward standing while holding a ball	• Remember prices (e.g., bill payment)
6. Perturbed backward standing while holding a ball	• Remember prices (e.g., groceries)
Gait Activities	• Count backward by 'threes'
	• Remember words
7. Walk forward/backward, normal base of support	• Tell the opposite direction of a ball toss
8. Walk forward/backward, narrow base of support	• Visual imaginary task (tell the road directions from home to the lab)
9. Walk narrow base of support, step, forward avoiding the obstacles (holding a basket)	• Recount daily activities
10. Walk narrow base of support, step, sideways, backward avoiding the obstacles (holding a basket)	
11. Walk and kick a ball to hit the cans	
12. Walk and reach and trunk twisting	

Source: Adapted from Silsupadol P, Shumway-Cook A, Woollacott M. Training of balance under single and dual task conditions in older adults with balance impairment: three case reports. *Phys Ther*. 2006;86:269–281, with permission of the American Physical Therapy Association.

Recent research in healthy individuals points out that balance training with particular emphasis on the vestibular system can improve cognition (Rogge et al., 2017). In this study, the experimental group practiced a one- or two-leg balance circuit on different surfaces that was skill progressed, while a control group practicing relaxation techniques. As was expected, only the experimental group improved in balance performance. However, the balance group also improved in memory and spatial cognition tests compared to controls, without the need to improve cardiovascular endurance, which would require a greater level of physical training intensity.

PUTTING IT ALL TOGETHER

In our task-oriented approach to retraining the patient with postural control problems, therapeutic strategies are used to (a) improve impairments in underlying systems critical to postural control (e.g., exercises and activities to improve motor impairments such as strength and range of motion, sensory stimulation to prime sensory systems in preparation for task-specific balance training, and cognitive training to improve dual-task balance control); (b) engage in functional task-specific practice to develop and refine sensory, motor, and cognitive strategies used for postural control; and (c) learn to control balance during changing environmental conditions, thus maximizing the person's ability to participate in the social roles, tasks, and activities that are essential to the quality of their lives.

At the heart of balance training is practicing progressively more challenging tasks and activities that facilitate the development of postural behaviors needed for the (re)acquisition of skilled functional movement. Task-specific practice is done in combination with interventions targeting underlying sensory, motor, and cognitive impairments. The selection and sequencing of tasks, activities, and contexts, integrated into a schedule of practice consistent with motor learning principles, is a powerful tool in retraining balance. For example, in initial stages of balance retraining, when the patient has minimal ability to control the body's COM, the patient may practice tasks with minimal demands for postural control in "closed" environments (e.g., constant and predictable conditions), such as sitting or standing on a firm flat surface with and without support. As an option, the therapist may decide to provide external augmented feedback to the patient in order to enhance motor performance, keeping in mind that such feedback should be progressively discontinued for transitioning the individual to a new learning stage of the postural task. As postural control improves, more challenging tasks with increasing postural demands are introduced, such as sitting or standing unsupported (steady-state postural control), sitting or standing unsupported while turning the head or reaching for an object (anticipatory postural control), or recovery of a stable seated or standing position following displacements (reactive balance). Tasks are practiced in "open" environments (e.g., changing and less predictable), such as on an unstable or foam surface while catching objects thrown from different directions or while performing a secondary task, like holding a cup of water. Retraining balance within mobility tasks is discussed in Chapter 15.

It is important to realize that one does not work on these goals sequentially but rather in parallel. Thus, therapeutic strategies for achieving these goals are intertwined; this reciprocal interweaving of exercises, tasks, and activities supports the goal of recovery of postural control, enabling the reestablishment of functional independence and participation. Figure 11.33 illustrates how this type of practice might be integrated into a single therapy session with Genise, our patient who has had a stroke.

In addition, rehabilitation of the patient with postural-control problems needs to be organized around learning theory. This will help to ensure that improvements in performance gained through therapy are converted to permanent changes in behavior and retained in varied and novel environments. Patients need to practice the desired behavior (in the case of balance, orientation, and the effective control of the COM within the context of a goal-directed functional task) providing sufficient therapeutic dosage (e.g., duration

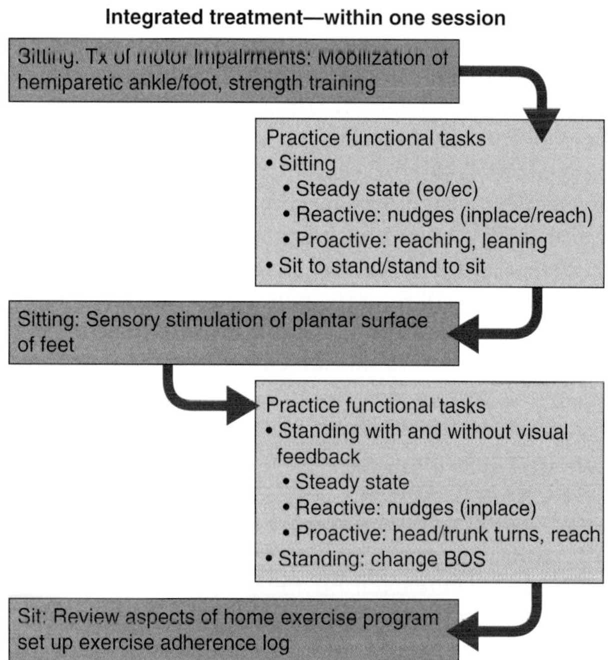

Figure 11.33 An example of a single treatment session designed to improve balance in Genise, 1 month poststroke, using a task-oriented approach.

and intensity) to induce neural plasticity within the nervous system and long-lasting functional improvements.

How much practice is enough to induce neural change? Views on this issue are changing. Traditionally, practice was restricted to the hours a patient spent in therapy sessions. With increasing awareness that more practice is needed to induce permanent change, patients were given "homework," that is, exercises, tasks, and activities to be practiced for varying amounts of time (usually 30 to 60 minutes) daily.

Using upper extremity training as a paradigm to study motor learning, it has been found that a high frequency and intensity of practice is critical to induce permanent changes in functional movement behaviors in patients following a neurologic injury. Edward Taub, a psychologist at the University of Alabama, developed Constraint-Induced (CI) Movement Therapy, an approach to retraining upper-limb function based on the concept of learned nonuse (Taub, 1980, 1993). Working with colleagues, he found that significant changes in both the frequency and the quality of functional movement of the paretic arm occurred after 10 days of intensive therapy, involving 6 hours of forced use of the paretic limb (the noninvolved limb was constrained in a sling) (Liepert et al., 1998; Miltner et al., 1999; Taub et al., 1998). These authors noted in an additional research study that the same improvement in function can be found with conventional therapy delivered over the same period, suggesting that the critical variable in recovery may not be the nature of the therapy but rather the frequency and intensity with which it is delivered (Liepert et al., 1998). Recent research suggests that intensity during skill practice and systematic task progression are cornerstone therapeutic ingredients to promote neuroplastic changes and long-lasting functional improvements (Friel et al., 2016; Hung et al., 2017).

Motor learning theory also tells us that in order to optimize motor schemas, practice needs to be under varied conditions. Retraining under varied conditions helps a patient learn the "rules" for postural control rather than a single way for controlling the COM. This ensures that the individual will be able to maintain stability in the face of new and changing task and environmental conditions.

Evidence-based balance rehabilitation means integrating the best available research evidence with clinical expertise and a patient's preferences regarding treatment. Research related to treatment of instability can help guide a clinician to make choices regarding how to treat impaired balance. Research can provide a rationale for treatment selection and help determine probable outcomes in a patient. Lab Activity 11.3 provides a framework for developing a treatment program for the case of Genise. Complete the table proposed in Lab Activity 11.3, identifying the specific individual system to be targeted (column 1), the task or activity to be practiced (column 2), the environmental conditions (including both sensory conditions and cognitive load) under which practice will

LAB ACTIVITY 11.3

Objective: To apply a task-oriented approach to retraining posture and balance to a patient with poststroke hemiparesis. To identify the research evidence to support clinical decisions regarding specific treatment interventions

Procedure: Reread the case study on Genise T. presented in Figure 11.18 and your assignment from Lab Activity 11.2. Review the list of functional problems, strategies, and impairments you outlined.

Assignment

1. Create a table identifying the various treatments you will use to improve balance in Genise. List the specific individual system to be targeted (column 1), the task or activity to be practiced (column 2), the environmental conditions under which practice will occur (column 3), and the research evidence that supports this aspect of treatment. For example, you may decide to do progressive resistance strength training with Genise because weakness is an underlying impairment contributing to her impaired balance and function. In this case, the individual component listed in the table is Motor: Strength, the task is strength training, and the specific environmental conditions you choose may be free weights at 60% 1 repetition maximum (RM). Several research studies support your decision to incorporate progressive resistive strength training with Genise, including the meta-analysis by Ada et al. (2006). Is strength training alone enough to ensure recovery of balance? What other aspects of balance will you train? What research supports your decision?

Individual Component of Balance	Task or Activity	Environmental Conditions	Research Evidence
Motor: Strength	Progressive resistance strength training	Free weights, 60% of 1 RM	Ada et al. (2006)

occur (column 3), and the research evidence that supports this aspect of treatment (column 4).

Research Evidence for a Task-Oriented Approach to Balance Rehabilitation

What evidence do we have that task-oriented training improves balance and the performance of functional activities in both geriatric and neurologic populations? Despite the growing research in this area, it can be difficult to draw conclusions because of differences in how task-oriented intervention is defined. In some cases, task-oriented therapy is defined by the repetitive practice of functional tasks, with no interventions targeting underlying impairments such as strength. In other cases, a task-oriented approach to therapy uses multidimensional exercises, including strength, flexibility, balance, functional-task practice, and endurance training. Because of these varying definitions, meta-analyses comparing task-oriented therapy to other forms of intervention can be difficult to interpret.

Several studies have demonstrated the positive effects of a multidimensional exercise program on balance and mobility function in community-living older adults. Shumway-Cook and colleagues (1997b) used a multidimensional exercise program including combinations of lower-extremity strength and flexibility exercises, balance training within the context of repetitive functional-task practice, and participation in an aerobic activity (usually a progressive walking program) to improve balance and mobility function in balance-impaired older adults. Activities targeted improving steady-state balance in sitting, standing, and walking; anticipatory balance activities, including reaching, lifting, turning, changing the base of support (narrow base of support, single-limb stance, tandem stance), stepping over and around obstacles, walking forward and backward at different speeds, and walking on different surface types and configurations with and without packages; reactive balance (perturbations of varying sizes, speeds, and directions performed while sitting and standing); and sensory training (varying availability of visual and somatosensory cues). Exercises became progressively more challenging over the 8-week program. Compared to the nonexercising control group, the group that exercised had significant improvement on all balance measures, including the BBS, DGI, and POMA.

Similar results have been reported in other studies. Wolf et al. (2001) undertook a randomized controlled trial to investigate the effects of a multidimensional exercise program based on a systems theory of postural control to improve balance in older adults (≥75 years of age). They found that 12 sessions of individualized balance training (over 4 to 6 weeks) significantly improved performance on the BBS and the DGI, which was maintained at 1 month but was not maintained at 1 year.

Judge et al. (1993) studied community-dwelling older adults (62 to 75 year) in a training program that combined lower-extremity resistance training, brisk walking, and Tai Chi training versus flexibility training alone (three times per week for 6 months). They found that balance performance did improve in the Tai Chi/resistance training group but not in the flexibility group. Single-leg-stance center of force displacement decreased by 18% in the Tai Chi/resistance training group ($p = 0.02$).

A number of studies have examined the effectiveness of exercise on improving balance and functional performance in persons with different types of neurologic pathology. Vearrier and colleagues (2005), using a task-oriented approach, delivered an intensive massed practice (6 hours/day for 2 consecutive weeks) to retrain balance in 10 patients with chronic stroke disability. In addition to significant improvements in the steady-state and anticipatory aspects of balance control, patients also showed significant improvements in their ability to recover from unexpected perturbations to stance. Weight-bearing symmetry improved, and patients significantly reduced the number of falls following training.

Duncan and colleagues (1998) compared the effects of a 12-week multidimensional home-based exercise program (resistance strength training, balance exercises, functional training of upper extremities, and an aerobic component of progressive walking or progressive bicycling) to usual care in patients with poststroke hemiparesis. Both groups showed equivalent improvements on many measures, including the BBS, 6-minute walk test, Barthel Activities of Daily Living, and other tests; however, the home-based exercise group performed significantly better than did the usual-care group on the Fugl–Meyer Test (lower-extremity function portion) and in gait velocity.

Marigold et al. (2005) compared two types of community-based group exercise on functional balance, mobility, postural reflexes, and falls in 61 older adults with chronic stroke (>6 months after stroke). Thirty patients were randomly assigned to an agility program involving a series of progressively more difficult balance tasks, including standing in various postures, walking with various challenges, and standing perturbations (instructor pushing participant). Tasks were performed with eyes open and eyes closed and when standing on both firm and foam surfaces.

A second set of 31 patients were randomly assigned to a stretching or weight-shifting program focused on slow, low-impact movements that incorporated Tai Chi–like movements stressing increased weight bearing of the paretic lower limb. Both exercise interventions were effective in improving performance on all outcome measures, including the BBS, TUG, and ABC, and these improvements were maintained at 1 month after testing. On the platform recovery measures, only the agility group improved onset latencies of postural muscles in the paretic limb, and this was associated with a concomitant decrease in falls.

Hammer et al. (2008) completed a systematic review of 14 randomized controlled studies related to balance training after stroke. This review concluded that balance following stroke could be improved at all stages of recovery. In addition, a variety of interventions were effective in improving balance after stroke.

Impaired balance and walking is a significant problem among patients with cerebellar pathology. Gill-Body and colleagues (1997) examined the effect of a 6-week staged, home-based intervention approach that provided progressive challenges to body stability in standing and walking in two patients with cerebellar dysfunction (a 36-year-old woman with a 7-month history of unsteadiness and dizziness following surgical resection of a recurrent astrocytoma in the cerebellar vermis and a 48-year-old man with a 10-year history of progressive balance problems due to cerebrotendinous xanthomatosis and diffuse cerebellar atrophy). Table 11.8 shows the rehabilitation treatment program and its rationale, used with the female patient who had a resected cerebellar tumor.

Both patients reported improved steadiness during stance and gait (significant improvements on the Dizziness Handicap Index). In addition, there was a concomitant improvement on both clinical and laboratory tests of balance. Kinematic analysis showed a decrease in sway in the standing position. Posturography tests showed that the ability to stand under altered sensory conditions improved, as did the ability to respond to external perturbations to balance. Patients were able to more quickly take a step as needed and, in addition, were better able to scale the magnitude of postural responses to perturbations of differing sizes. The authors conclude that patients with cerebellar lesions (whether acute or chronic) can significantly improve postural stability following a structured exercise program (Gill-Body et al., 1997).

Results from research in both geriatric and neurologic populations are remarkably similar. It appears that exercise is an effective way to improve balance and that these improvements are associated with enhanced performance on functional tasks and a reduction in falls. Multidimensional exercises appear to be more effective in improving balance than exercises targeting a single system (e.g., strength, flexibility, or

TABLE 11.8 Rehabilitation Treatment Program for a Patient with Imbalance Caused by a Resected Cerebellar Tumor

Rationale	Treatment activity
Phase 1	
Promote use of VOR and COR for gaze stability	Visual fixation, EO, stationary target, slow head movements
Promote use of saccadic eye movements for gaze stability	Active eye and head movements between two stationary targets
Promote VOR cancelation	EO, moving target with head movement, self-selected speed
Improve ability to use somatosensory and vestibular inputs for postural control	Static stance, EO and EC, feet together, arms close body, head movements
Improve ability to use vestibular and visual	Static stance on foam surface, EC intermittently, feet 2.54–5.08 cm inputs for postural control (1–2 inch) apart
Improve postural control using all sensory inputs	Gait with narrowed base of support, EO, wide turns to right and left
Improve postural control using visual and vestibular inputs	March in place, EO, on firm and foam surfaces, prolonged pauses in unilateral stance
Phase 2	
Promote use of VOR and COR for gaze stability	Visual fixation, EO, stationary and moving targets, slow and fast speeds, simple static background; imaginary visual fixation, EC
Promote use of saccadic eye movements for gaze stability	Active eye and head movements between two targets, slow and fast speeds
Promote VOR cancelation	EO, moving target with head movement, fast and slow speeds
Improve ability to use somatosensory and vestibular inputs for postural control	Semitandem stance, EO and EC, arms crossed
Improve ability to use vestibular inputs for postural control	Stance on foam, EC intermittently, feet 2.54–5.08 cm apart
Improve postural control using visual and vestibular inputs	Gait with EO with sharp 180-degree turns to the right and left, firm and padded surfaces
Improve postural control using vestibular and somatosensory inputs	March in place, EC, prolonged pauses in unilateral stance
Improve postural control using all sensory	Walking sideways and backward; standing EO and EC, heel touches inputs forward, toe touches backward
Improve postural control with head moving using all sensory inputs	Gait with EO, normal base of support, slow head movements
Phase 3	
Promote use of VOR and COR for gaze stability	Visual fixation, EO, stationary and moving targets, various speeds, complex static and dynamic backgrounds; imaginary visual fixation, EC
Promote use of saccadic eye movements for gaze stability	Active eye and head movements between two targets, various speeds
Promote VOR cancelation	EO, moving target with head movement, various speeds, complex static and dynamic backgrounds

(continued)

TABLE 11.8 Rehabilitation Treatment Program for a Patient with Imbalance Caused by a Resected Cerebellar Tumor *(continued)*

Rationale	Treatment activity
Improve ability to use somatosensory and vestibular inputs for postural control	Semitandem stance with EC continuously and with EO on firm and padded surfaces
Improve postural control using vestibular and somatosensory inputs	Gait with EC with base of support progressively narrowed, firm and padded surfaces; march in place slowly, EO and EC on firm and foam surfaces
Improve postural control using visual and vestibular inputs	Gait with EO, rapid sharp turns to right and left, firm and padded surfaces
Improve postural control when head is moving using all sensory inputs	Gait with normal base of support, EO, fast head movements
Improve postural control using all sensory inputs	Braiding; active practice of ankle sway movements; bending and reaching activities

COR, cervicoocular reflex; EO, eyes open; EC, eyes closed; VOR, vestibuloocular reflex.

Source: Reprinted from Gill-Body KM, Popat RA, Parker SW, et al. Rehabilitation of balance in two patients with cerebellar dysfunction. *Phys Ther.* 1997;77:534–552, with permission.

aerobic conditioning). Finally, effective interventions for improving balance include activities that target specific components of postural control; in addition, activities should be systematically progressed to increase the challenge to balance over the duration of intervention.

Improving Participation—Evidence-Based Fall Prevention

As discussed earlier, the overall goal of task-oriented balance rehabilitation is to improve participation outcomes, reflected in an improved ability to participate in the social roles, tasks, and activities that are important in the daily life of the patient. Improved participation can be demonstrated by increased frequency and independence in performing daily tasks and activities. Improved participation may also be reflected in a reduced frequency of falls, as well as increased confidence. Because of the social and economic impact of falls, considerable research has focused on strategies to reduce the risk for falls among older adults. Less research is available on the impact of therapeutic interventions to reduce falls among patients with neurologic pathology.

Research Evidence

There have been several systematic reviews examining the effects of various therapeutic interventions, including exercise and balance training, on reducing falls in older adults (Campbell & Robertson, 2007; Gillespie et al., 2009; Howe et al., 2007; Rubenstein & Josephson, 2001; Sherrington et al., 2008). The Cochrane review by Gillespie et al. (2009) included 111 randomized clinical trials and examined the effect of different types of interventions on both the rate of falls (falls per person-year shown as the rate ratio) and the number of participants sustaining at least one fall during follow-up (risk ratio). This review included 43 clinical trials related to exercise.

The main findings from the review included the following: (a) Assessment and multifactorial intervention reduced the rate of monthly falls (rate ratio, 0.75; 95% confidence interval [CI], 0.65 to 0.86) but not the number of people who fell; (b) home safety interventions did not reduce either the rate of falls or the number of people who fell but were effective in people with severe visual impairment and in others at higher risk of falling; and (c) medication management, including withdrawal of psychotropic medications, reduced the rate of falls (rate ratio, 0.34; 95% CI, 0.16 to 0.73) but not the risk of falling. The review also reported the effects of different types of exercise programs on fall rate and risk for falls. Multiple-component group exercise reduced both the rate of falls (rate ratio, 0.78; 95% CI, 0.71 to 0.86) and the number of people at risk for falls (risk ratio, 0.83; 95% CI, 0.72 to 0.97), as did Tai Chi (rate ratio, 0.63; 95% CI, 0.52 to 0.78; risk ratio, 0.65; 95% CI, 0.51 to 0.82). In addition, individually prescribed multiple-component home-based exercise significantly reduced both the rate of falls (rate ratio, 0.66; 95% CI, 0.53 to 0.82) and the number of persons falling (risk ratio, 0.77; 95% CI, 0.61 to 0.97).

While the review found evidence to support the role of exercise in fall prevention among older adults, it also cautioned that it may not be possible to prevent falls completely; however, among people who fall frequently, it may be possible to reduce the number of falls. In addition, the report concluded that at this time there was no evidence to support the efficacy of any intervention on falls among persons with stroke or Parkinson's disease or after a hip fracture.

Several studies have found that a single intervention such as exercise can be as effective in reducing falls as complex multifactorial interventions (Campbell & Robertson, 2007; Gardner et al., 2000; Sherrington et al., 2008). However, these reviews are consistent in suggesting that exercise by itself is effective in reducing the rate of falls only if (a) it targets people whose primary risk factors are improved by exercise (e.g., impaired balance, gait, and lower-extremity strength) and (b) it is of sufficient intensity to modify these risk factors (Gardner et al., 2000; Sherrington et al., 2008). How much exercise, and what type, is needed to reduce falls? Critical attributes of successful fall-prevention exercise trials included a total dose (a combination of frequency of exercise on a weekly basis with total duration) of greater than 50 hours of training and the presence of highly challenging balance training.

These systematic reviews suggest that exercise (including combinations of balance, strength, and endurance training) can improve balance and reduce falls in community-living older adults. In order to be effective, exercise has to be of sufficient duration and intensity (although optimal range and intensity have yet to be completely defined) and targeted to people whose primary risk factors for falls can be reduced by exercise.

SUMMARY

1. A task-oriented approach to examining postural control uses a variety of tests, measurements, and observations to (a) document functional abilities related to posture and balance control; (b) examine sensory, motor, and cognitive strategies used to maintain or regain stability; and (c) determine the underlying impairments contributing to abnormal postural control. In addition, an important part of examination is understanding the impact of impaired balance on the person's ability to participate in the social roles, activities, and tasks important to their lives.
2. Following completion of the examination, the clinician must interpret results, identifying functional limitations and underlying impairments, and establish the goals and plan of care.
3. The plan of care for retraining postural control in the patient with a neurologic deficit will vary widely, depending on the constellation of underlying impairments and the degree to which the patient has developed compensatory strategies that are successful in achieving postural demands in functional tasks.
4. The goals of a task-oriented approach to retraining postural control include treatments to resolve or prevent impairments and functional training to improve steady-state, reactive, and anticipatory balance control. Functional balance training is designed to develop effective task-specific sensory, motor, and cognitive strategies and adapt those strategies to changing environmental contexts, thereby maximizing the recovery of participation and minimizing disability.
5. The application of research evidence to the clinical management of patients with postural disorders requires familiarity with the growing body of research and understanding the application of this research to the specific needs of individual patients.

ANSWERS TO LAB ACTIVITY ASSIGNMENTS

Lab Activity 11.1

1. The BBS is heavily weighted toward tasks requiring steady-state and anticipatory postural control. Steady-state balance in sitting and standing is tested in items 2 and 3.
2. Anticipatory postural control could be inferred from items 1, 4, 5, 7, 8, 9, 10, 11, 12, 13, and 14. One item (6) manipulates vision, testing a sensory component of postural control. Items 7, 13, and 14 examine balance with a reduced base of support, which increases the demands for mediolateral stability, and is often associated with a shift in movement strategy.
3. There is no task (such as the nudge test in Tinetti's POMA test) that requires reactive postural control. In addition, most items are performed while standing; hence, stability during walking tasks is not tested. This does not mean that the BBS is a poor test; it just indicates the limitations of the test with respect to the systems conceptual framework.

Lab Activity 11.2

1. A review of her examination and the case study video findings at 1 month poststroke suggests that Genise's functional limitations are primarily found in stance and gait (although her mobility problems will be discussed in the mobility section of the book), while seated activities can be performed without loss of balance.
2. Based on a BBS score of 19, her estimated fall risk would be 99%. She is independent in sitting and is able to transfer and move from sit to stand and back independently using her arms. She requires close supervision for many items performed in standing (e.g., standing eyes closed, reaching or leaning over) and is unable to perform tasks such as standing feet together, stool touch, one-leg stance, and heel-to-toe stance.
3. At 1 month poststroke, postural control in sitting is good; she shows good steady-state and anticipatory balance. She is able to recover from small perturbations in all directions independently but is unable

to reach for support with her paretic arm to recover balance from a large perturbation to her paretic side.

4. Problems in stance include reduced steady-state, reactive, and anticipatory balance control. She is able to stand for 30 seconds with eyes open and closed; however, she requires close supervision. She stands asymmetrically, with her weight shifted to the left. She has significantly impaired reactive balance and is unable to recover from small or large perturbations without the physical assistance of another person. She has impaired anticipatory balance and requires close supervision when reaching or leaning over without her assistive device.
5. She is able to stand on a firm surface with eyes open and closed for 30 seconds but requires close supervision. She is unable to maintain stability on a foam surface with eyes open (or closed), suggesting she may rely on somatosensory inputs for postural control. This suggests that she might have problems maintaining stability when on uneven surfaces, inclines, or moving surfaces.

With a better understanding of the functional limitations she is experiencing and the components of balance control that may be contributing to her balance problems, we can turn to establishing a plan of care that incorporates a balance-retraining program to improve her balance, enhance function, and reduce her risk for falls.

Lab Activity 11.3

1. The following is an example of how evidence-based balance training is applied to Genise, our patient who is at 1 month poststroke. It is important to remember that there is no single correct way to train balance in Genise. It is essential that all aspects of postural control be included in her rehabilitation program (e.g., steady state, anticipatory, and reactive) and that a range of tasks and conditions be used to help her develop a variety of postural control strategies so that she is able to maintain balance in a wide variety of tasks and conditions. The specific order, duration, and timing of each activity may vary from therapist to therapist.

We begin by determining Genise's main concern and goals related to her balance. She expresses concern that she be able to perform the activities done during standing and while walking (dressing, grooming, transferring, etc.) safely (with confidence that she will not fall) and without assistance. She is confident in her ability to maintain balance while performing sitting activities, and this is consistent with her performance on the tests and measures used to evaluate balance.

So our approach to training balance will primarily focus both on improving underlying impairments (her weakness and reduced range of motion) and on practicing functional tasks in standing and walking, as she appears to have fairly good balance in the seated position (the specifics of training mobility will be discussed in later chapters).

Activities will progress from more "static" balance activities, such as practice maintaining a steady position in sitting and standing (steady-state balance) without support in a simple, fairly predictable environment (flat surface/well lit), to more dynamic activities performed in less predictable environments (on unstable surfaces) and under varying visual conditions (low light and in the presence of external visual motion cues). She will practice a variety of skilled functional activities that are goal directed and that involve varying requirements for anticipatory (reaching, lifting, turning, weight shift, stepping, sit-to-stand, stand to sit, etc.) and reactive (responding to unexpected perturbations in different directions, speeds, and amplitudes) postural control.

We will systematically vary the conditions under which she practices functional tasks, including varying the sensory and cognitive demands. This will allow her to solve stability problems under varying conditions, developing flexibility and adaptability critical to her ability to maintain stability when she performs functional tasks in her own environment.

We will try to incorporate motor learning principles into her training. Initially, we will have her practice functional tasks in a blocked manner (practicing each task for a time, before switching to a different task). As she improves, we will shift to a more random practice pattern (alternating the types of tasks she practices), modifying the conditions under which she practices as well (variable practice). As she is reacquiring balance ability, we will vary the timing and extent of the external feedback she is given. Initially, we may provide continuous feedback using verbal and manual cues, perhaps providing her a mirror to augment visual cues related to postural stability in sitting and standing as well. As she progresses, we will fade the external cues given, allowing her to develop intrinsic feedback mechanisms for postural control. Examples of some of the treatment strategies used to improve postural control in Genise at 1 month poststroke may be found in her video segment of postural control named "Treatment of Stroke."

There is considerable research to support our clinical decision-making regarding this approach to treatment. Table 11.7 presents some examples. What other research can you find to support your evidence-based balance rehabilitation program?

PART III

Mobility Functions

"*A key feature of our independence as human beings is mobility.*"

CHAPTER 12

Control of Normal Mobility

Learning Objectives

Following completion of this chapter, the reader will be able to:

1. Define the major requirements of locomotion, as well as the goals of each phase of locomotion.
2. Define mobility within the context of the International Classification of Functioning, Disability and Health (ICF).
3. Describe the major kinematic, kinetic, and electromyographic parameters that contribute to a normal gait pattern.
4. Describe the contributions of neural (sensory, motor, and higher cognitive) and nonneural subsystems to the control of gait.
5. Define the requirements of other forms of mobility, including stair climbing and transfers.

INTRODUCTION

A key feature of our independence as human beings is mobility. We define *mobility* as the ability to independently and safely move oneself from one place to another. Mobility incorporates many types of tasks, including the ability to move and change position while in bed, to stand up from a bed or chair, to walk or run, and to navigate through often quite complex environments. During rehabilitation, a primary goal of treatment is to help patients regain as much independent mobility as possible. Often, regaining mobility is the primary goal of a patient. This is reflected in the constantly asked question, "Will I walk again?"

In this chapter, we discuss many aspects of mobility, including gait, transfers, bed mobility, and stair walking, examining the contribution of the individual, task, and environment to each of these abilities. We begin with a discussion of mobility within the context of the International Classification of Functioning, Disability and Health (ICF) framework. We then discuss the control of gait, including the requirements for successful locomotion and the contributions of motor, sensory, and cognitive systems to the control of gait. We also discuss mechanisms essential for adapting gait to changing task and environmental conditions. Finally, we consider other forms of mobility, including the initiation of gait, stair climbing, and transfers.

Mobility in the International Classification of Functioning, Disability and Health Framework

Mobility fits into the ICF framework in a number of ways (see Fig. 12.1). Mobility is one of the nine domains within the component *Activity and Participation*. Mobility in the component of *Activity and Participation* includes changing and maintaining body position; carrying, moving, and handling objects; walking and moving; and moving around using transportation. The activity of walking is characterized by the distance walked (short <1 km vs. long >1 km), the ability to negotiate different surfaces (such as slopes and uneven and moving surfaces), and both static and dynamic obstacles. Mobility also includes moving around the environment. This includes the ability to move (walk) in and around different locations (within the home, within buildings other than home, and outside the home and other buildings).

The gait pattern is considered a body function and thus found within the component of *Body Structure and Function*. Contextual factors also impact mobility, including both environmental factors, such as terrain characteristics, and personal factors, such as age, sex, and self-efficacy.

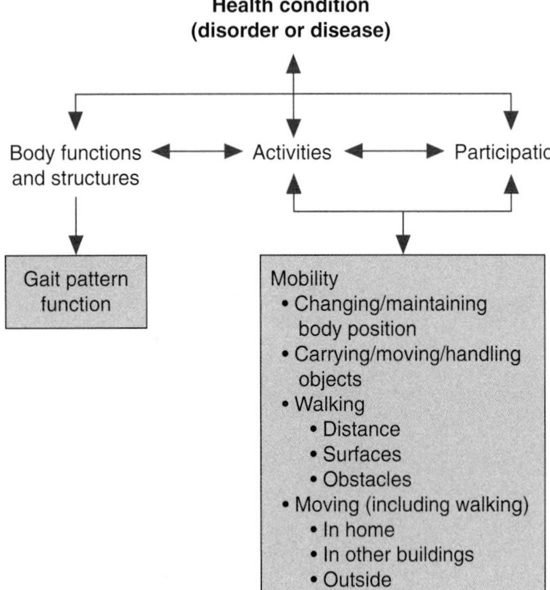

Figure 12.1 Mobility in the International Classification of Functioning, Disability and Health.

Mobility is an extraordinarily complex function, with many components. While considerable research has focused on mobility, the primary focus has been on characterizing the normal gait pattern and understanding the underlying control mechanisms for gait. Less effort has been directed at understanding mobility from the perspective of activity and participation, leading one prominent gait researcher to say "we know a lot about gait, but very little about mobility" (Patla, personal communication, 2004).

MOTOR SYSTEMS AND GAIT

At first glance, it may seem as though gait is a simple fairly straightforward behavior, but in fact, it is remarkably challenging. It involves the entire body and therefore requires the coordination of many muscles and joints. Navigating through complex and often cluttered environments requires the use of sensory inputs to assist in the control and adaptation of gait. Finally, locomotor behavior includes the ability to initiate and terminate locomotion, to adapt gait to avoid obstacles, and to change speed and direction as needed (Patla, 1991). Because of these complexities, understanding both the control of normal gait and the mobility problems of patients with neurologic impairments can seem like an overwhelming task.

To simplify the process of understanding the control of gait, we describe a framework for examining gait that we have found useful. The framework is built around understanding the essential requirements of locomotion and how these requirements are translated into goals accomplished during the different phases of gait. When examining both normal and abnormal gait, it is important to keep in mind both the essential requirements of gait and the conditions that must be met during the stance and swing phases of gait to accomplish these requirements.

Essential Requirements of Locomotion: Progression, Postural Control, and Adaptation

Locomotion is characterized by three essential requirements: progression, postural control, and adaptation (Das & McCollum, 1988; Patla, 1991). Progression is ensured through a basic locomotor pattern that produces and coordinates rhythmic patterns of muscle activation in the legs, trunk, and arms that successfully move the body in the desired direction. Progression also requires the ability to initiate and terminate locomotion, as well as to guide locomotion toward end points that are not always visible (Patla, 1997).

The second requirement for locomotion is that of postural control. Postural control involves the organization of multiple systems in the body to achieve both orientation and stability. Orientation involves aligning body segments relative to one another and the environment to achieve the requirements of locomotion under all task and environmental conditions. Stability involves controlling the center of mass relative to the moving base of support and includes three aspects: steady-state, reactive, and anticipatory balance control. Steady-state balance control in gait refers to maintaining orientation and stability when walking under constant velocity conditions. Reactive balance control is used to recover stability following an unexpected perturbation to the center of mass while walking. Anticipatory balance control includes activating muscles to counter potentially destabilizing internal forces generated during the gait cycle as well as potentially destabilizing external forces. For example, carrying a heavy object while walking requires modifications to gait in order to maintain stability. Some researchers have used the term "proactive balance control" during gait to refer to the use of vision in guiding locomotion relative to a changing environment (e.g., stepping over an obstacle) (Patla, 1997). In this chapter, we use the terms "anticipatory" and "proactive" interchangeably to include modifications made to counter both internal and external destabilizing forces. During normal steady-state gait, progression and balance control work together synergistically to ensure stable forward movement when walking; thus, they will be discussed together in the steady-state gait section.

Walking in daily life is rarely characterized by bouts of steady-state gait. Instead, walking in daily life is characterized by short bouts of walking lasting less than 30 seconds and requiring fewer than 40 steps (Orendurff et al., 2008). In addition, walking in daily life is characterized by stops; starts; changes in direction; the ability to negotiate terrain changes including inclines, stairs, and curbs; and the ability to accelerate or decelerate to avoid colliding with static and dynamic objects in the environment (Shumway-Cook et al., 2002). Thus, the third essential requirement of locomotion (mobility) in daily life is the ability to adapt gait, specifically the strategies used to accomplish progression and postural control, to changing task and environmental demands. This is shown in Figure 12.2. Reactive and anticipatory (proactive) postural controls ensure that stability is maintained in the face of both internal and environmental challenges to balance (e.g., recovering stability following a trip [reactive balance] or modifying gait in advance of an obstacle to avoid a trip [proactive balance]). Since both reactive and proactive balance control are essential to the ability to adapt gait to changing task and environmental demands, they are discussed under the adaptation section of this chapter. As shown in Figure 12.2, to be effective, the gait pattern must accomplish the requirements of progression and postural control. However, mobility (walking) in daily life requires that the gait pattern strategies used to meet the progression and postural control requirements be adapted to changing task and environmental conditions. Each of these goals must be met in the different phases of gait.

Human gait can be subdivided into stance (or support) and swing phases. During the support phase of gait, we need to generate both horizontal forces against the support surface to move the body in the desired direction (progression) and vertical forces that support the body mass against gravity (postural control). In addition, strategies used to accomplish progression and postural control must be flexible to accommodate changes in speed and direction or alterations in the support surface (adaptation).

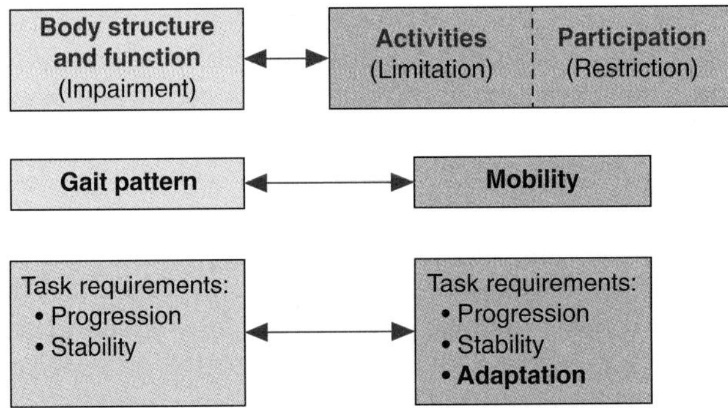

Figure 12.2 The two requirements of an effective gait pattern (a component of *Body Structure and Function*) are progression and postural stability. Mobility (a domain of *Activities and Participation*) has a third requirement—adaptation—the ability to modify the gait pattern (including strategies for accomplishing progression and postural stability) to meet changing task and environmental demands.

During the swing phase of gait, advancement of the swing leg helps to accomplish the progression requirement of gait, while repositioning the limb in preparation for weight acceptance serves the requirement for postural control. Both the progression and postural control goals require sufficient foot clearance so that the toe does not drag on the supporting surface during swing. In addition, strategies used during the swing phase of gait must be sufficiently flexible to allow the swing foot to avoid any obstacles in its path (adaptation).

The movement strategies used by normal subjects to meet the task requirements of locomotion have been well defined. Kinematic studies describing body motions suggest a similarity in movement strategies across subjects. This is consistent with intuitive observations that we all walk somewhat similarly. In contrast, studies that have described the muscles and forces associated with gait suggest that there is a tremendous variability in the way these gait movements are achieved. Thus, there appears to be a wide range of muscle activation patterns used by normal subjects to accomplish the task requirements of gait.

Characterizing Steady-State Gait

Though walking in daily life is rarely done under steady-state conditions (long bouts of constant velocity walking), most research designed to characterize the normal gait pattern is done under steady-state conditions. The normal human perception–action system has developed elegant control strategies for meeting the essential requirements for steady-state gait. The following sections describe the motor strategies used to accomplish the progression and postural control requirements of steady-state gait. Later sections discuss the motor strategies used to modify gait in response to both expected and unexpected perturbations.

Although other gait patterns are possible (i.e., we can skip, hop, or gallop), humans normally use a symmetrical alternating gait pattern, probably because it provides the greatest stability for bipedal gait with minimal control demands (Raibert, 1986). Thus, normal locomotion is a bipedal gait in which the limbs move in a symmetrical alternating motion, which can be described by a phase lag of 0.5 (Grillner, 1981).

A phase lag of 0.5 means that one limb initiates its step cycle as the opposite limb reaches the midpoint of its own cycle (Fig. 12.3). Thus, if one complete stride cycle is defined as the time between two ipsilateral foot strikes (right heel contact to right heel contact) (Fig. 12.3), then the contralateral limb begins its cycle midway through the ipsilateral stride cycle.

Traditionally, all descriptions of gait, whether kinematic, electromyographic (EMG), or kinetic, are described with reference to different aspects of the gait cycle. For a review of the technology used to analyze these various aspects of gait, refer to the technology

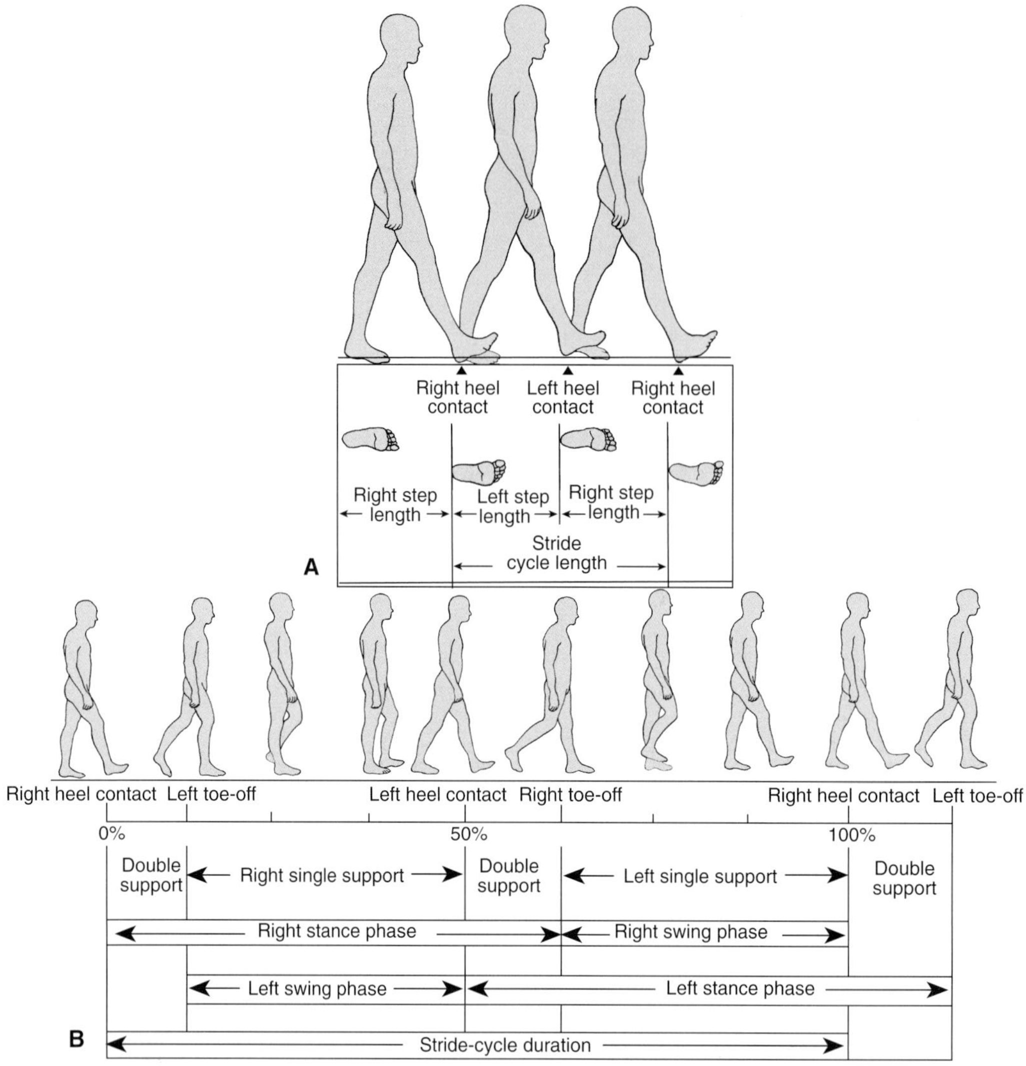

Figure 12.3 Temporal and distance dimensions of the gait cycle. **(A)** Step length and stride length characteristics. **(B)** Swing and stance phase characteristics. (Adapted from Inman VT, Ralston H, Todd F. *Human walking*. Baltimore, MD: Williams & Wilkins, 1981, with permission.)

boxes found in Chapter 7. An understanding of the various phases of gait is necessary for understanding descriptions of normal locomotion.

Phases of the Step Cycle

As we mentioned previously, the gait cycle consists of two main phases: stance, which starts when the foot strikes the ground, and swing, which begins when the foot leaves the ground (Fig. 12.3). The average duration of one gait cycle is 0.98 to 1.07 seconds (Murray et al., 1964). At freely chosen walking speeds, adults typically spend approximately 60% of the cycle uration in stance and 40% in swing. As shown in Figure 12.3, approximately the first and the last 10% of the stance phase are spent in double-support, the period of time when both feet are in contact with the ground. Single-support phase is the period when only one foot is in contact with the ground, and in walking, this consists of the time when the opposite limb is in swing phase (Murray et al., 1984; Rosenrot et al., 1980).

The stance phase is often further divided into five subphases: (1) initial contact, (2) the loading response (together taking up about 10% of the step cycle, during double-support phase), (3) midstance, (4) terminal stance (about 40% of the stance phase, which is in single-support), and (5) preswing (the last 10% of stance, in double-support). The swing phase is often divided into three subphases: initial swing, midswing, and terminal swing (all of which are in single-support phase and, in total, make up 40% of the step cycle) (Enoka, 2002; Perry & Burnfield, 2010).

Temporal and Distance Factors

Gait is often described with respect to temporal and distance parameters such as velocity, step length, step frequency (called "cadence"), and stride length (Fig. 12.3).

Velocity of gait is defined as the average horizontal speed of the body measured over one or more strides. In the research literature, it is usually reported in the metric system (e.g., meters per second) (Perry & Burnfield, 2010). In contrast, in clinics in the United States, gait is usually described in nonmetric terms (feet) and in either distance or time parameters. For example, one might report that the patient is able to walk 50 feet or that the patient is able to walk continuously for 5 minutes. Because of this difference in convention between many clinics and the lab, we offer information in both metric and nonmetric terms.

Cadence is the number of steps per unit of time, usually reported as steps per minute. Step length is the distance from one foot strike to the foot strike of the other foot. For example, the right step length is the distance from the left heel to the right heel when both feet are in contact with the ground. Stride length is the distance covered from one heel strike to the next heel strike by the same foot. Thus, right stride length is defined by the distance between one right heel strike and the next right heel strike.

Normal and abnormal gait are often described with reference to these variables. When performing a clinical assessment, there is an advantage to measuring step length, rather than stride length. This is because you will not be able to note any asymmetry in step length if you evaluate only stride length.

How fast do people normally walk? Normal young adults tend to walk about 1.46 meters per second (3.26 miles per hour), have a mean cadence (step rate) of 1.9 steps per second (112.5 steps per minute), and have a mean step length of 76.3 cm (30.05 inches) (Craik, 1989).

How do variables such as step length and cadence vary as a function of gait velocity? Complete Lab Activity 12.1 to find out. Walking velocity is a function of step length and step frequency or cadence. When people increase their walking speed, they typically lengthen their step and increase their pace. Although normal adults have a wide range of walking speeds, self-selected speeds tend to center around a small range of step rates, with averages of about 110 steps per minute for men and about 115 steps per minute for women (Finley & Cody, 1970; Murray et al., 1984). Preferred step rates appear to be related to minimizing energy requirements (Ralston, 1976; Zarrugh et al., 1974). In fact, it has been found that in locomotion, we exploit the pendular properties of the leg and the elastic properties of the muscles. Thus, swing phase requires little energy expenditure. A person's comfortable or preferred walking speed is at the person's point of minimal energy expenditure per unit distance. At slower or higher speeds, passive pendular models of gait break down, and much more energy expenditure is required (Mochon & McMahon, 1980).

LAB ACTIVITY 12.1

Objective: To learn how to calculate temporal and distance parameters of gait.

Procedure: Materials needed for this lab: roll of white paper (1/2 m wide), moleskin cut into 1-inch triangle and square shapes, one bottle each of water-soluble red and blue ink, masking tape, cotton swabs, and a stopwatch. Tape a strip of paper 6-meter long to the floor at the beginning of each trial. Seat the subject on a chair at one end of the paper. Place one triangle and one square of moleskin approximately at the midline of the sole of each shoe, on the toe and heel, respectively. Saturate the moleskin on the right shoe with red ink and the moleskin on the left shoe with blue ink. Have your subject walk down the paper pathway at a comfortable pace. Use the stopwatch to record the time needed to walk the entire length of the paper. Repeat these procedures, asking subject to walk at their fastest pace. You may wish to repeat the lab activity, asking the subject to walk with a variety of assistive devices, such as a cane or walker.

Assignment

From the ink prints on the paper calculate the following for each leg:

1. Step length: vertical distance between heel marker of one foot and the next heel marker of the opposite foot.
2. Stride length: vertical distance between heel marker of one foot and heel marker of the same foot on the next successive step.
3. Step width: horizontal distance between center of heel markers of one foot and the next foot.
4. Cadence: number of steps taken per unit of time (the amount of time taken to walk across the paper divided by the total number of steps).
5. Establish norms (means and standard deviations) for each of these parameters for the subjects tested. Compare your norms with those presented in this chapter. How do spatial and temporal factors change as a function of gait speed? How do they change if an assistive device is used for gait?

(Adapted from Boenig DD. Evaluation of a clinical method of gait analysis. *Phys Ther.* 1977;7:795–798.)

As we increase walking speed, the proportion of time spent in swing and stance changes, with stance phase becoming progressively shorter in relation to swing (Herman et al., 1976; Murray, 1967). Finally, the stance and swing proportions shift from the 60/40 distribution of walking to the 40/60 distribution, as running velocities are reached. Double-support time also disappears during running.

As walking speed slows, stance time increases, while swing times remain relatively constant. The double-support phase of stance increases most. For example, double-support takes up 25% of the cycle time with step durations of about 1.1 seconds and 50% of the cycle time when cycle duration increases to about 2.5 seconds (Herman et al., 1976). In addition, variability increases at lower speeds, probably because of decreased postural stability during the single-support period, which also lengthens with slower speeds.

Within an individual, joint-angle patterns and EMG patterns of lower-extremity muscles are quite stable across a range of speeds, but the amplitude of muscle responses increases with faster speeds (Murray et al., 1966; Winter, 1983b; Zarrugh et al., 1974). In contrast, joint torque patterns appear more variable, though they also show gain increases as walking velocity increases.

Kinematic Description of Steady-State Gait

Another way of describing normal versus abnormal gait is through the kinematics of the gait cycle, that is, the movement of the joints and segments of the body through space. Figure 12.4 shows the normal movements of the pelvis, hip, knee, and ankle in the sagittal, frontal, and transverse planes (Perry, 1992).

The elegant coordination of motion at all the joints ensures the first requirement of gait: the smooth forward progression of the center of body mass (COM). While motion at each individual joint is quite large, the coordinated action of motion across all the joints results in the smooth forward progression of the body.

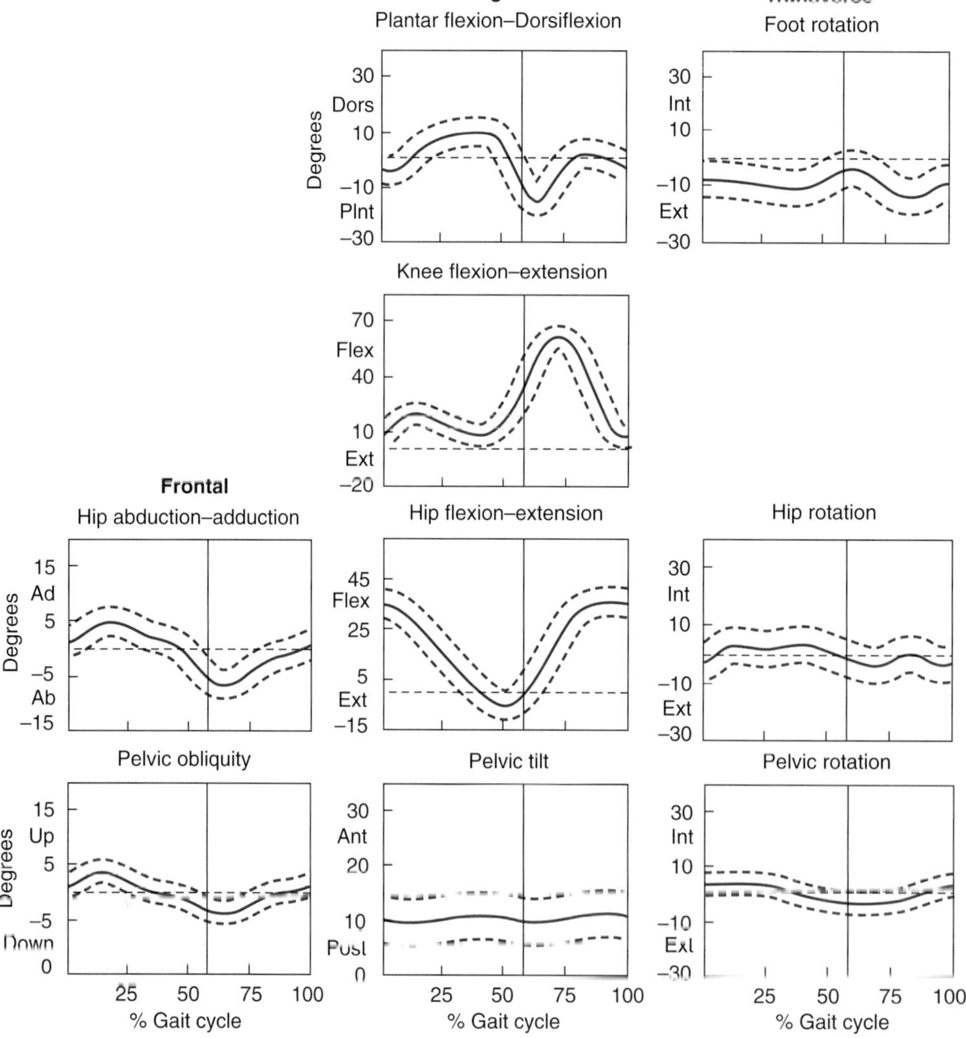

Figure 12.4 Normal movements of the pelvis, hip, knee, and ankle in sagittal, frontal, and transverse planes during the gait cycle. (Adapted from DeLuca PA, Perry JP, Ounpuu S. The fundamentals of normal walking and pathological gait. *AACP and DM Inst. Course 2*. London, UK: Mac Keith Press, 1992.)

Walking is energy efficient, but what is responsible for this efficiency? Saunders et al. (1953) suggested that complementary motion at the different joints minimizes the vertical displacement of the body's COM and thereby optimizes energy expenditure. However, Farley and Ferris (1998) suggest that it is not minimizing vertical COM motion that reduces the metabolic cost of walking, but the smooth mechanical transfer of kinetic and gravitational energies. In fact, the COM must fluctuate in a sinusoidal fashion to achieve efficient transfer of mechanical energy. Research has shown that during walking, the body vaults over a relatively stiff stance limb and that the COM reaches its highest point at the middle of the stance phase. Thus, the gravitational potential energy of the COM is at its highest during the midstance phase. In contrast, the kinetic energy of the COM reaches its minimum value at midstance, since the horizontal ground reaction force decelerates the body during the first half of the stance phase and accelerates it during the second half (Farley & Ferris, 1998).

In summary, the step cycle is made up of a complex series of joint rotations, which when coordinated into a whole, provide for a smooth forward progression of the COM and reduce the metabolic cost of walking.

Clinical gait assessment relies in part on the observation and description of body motion and joint kinematics. To practice your ability to observe and describe the movements associated with normal and atypical gait patterns, practice Lab Activity 12.2.

Muscle Activation Patterns in Steady-State Gait: Progression and Postural Control

Next, we examine the muscle responses during locomotion in terms of their function at each point in the step cycle (Basmajian & De Luca, 1985; Perry & Burnfield, 2010). Despite the variability between subjects and conditions in the EMG patterns that underlie a typical step cycle, certain basic characteristics have been identified.

In general, muscles in the stance limb act to support the body (postural control) and propel it forward (progression). Muscle activity in the swing limb is largely confined to the beginning and end of the swing phase, since the leg swings much like a jointed pendulum under the influence of gravity (McMahon, 1984). Muscles activated during the different phases of the step cycle are shown in Figure 12.5.

Remember, there are two goals to be accomplished during the stance phase: (a) postural control, securing the stance limb against the impact force of foot strike and supporting the body against the force of gravity, and (b) progression, involving force generation, to propel the body forward into the next step.

Stance Phase. To ensure postural stability at heel strike, eccentric activation of the tibialis anterior (TA) decelerates the foot (Fig. 12.5A), opposing and slowing the plantarflexion that results from foot strike. Activation of the gluteus maximus (hip extensors) minimizes

LAB ACTIVITY 12.2

Objective: To begin learning how to observe the kinematics of gait.

Procedure: You will need to do this lab in a large room, where your partner can walk for 20 to 30 feet, and you can observe them from the side (sagittal plane). Your partner will need to wear shorts. Have your partner walk back and forth. Choose a reference leg, and observe the following from the sagittal plane:

- Observe the stance versus the swing phase of gait.
- Within the stance phase, identify the following events: heel strike, midstance, and push-off.
- Within the swing phase, identify the following events: early swing and late swing.
- Observe the hip at these five points in the gait cycle and determine whether the hip is flexed, extended, or in a neutral position (i.e., thigh segment is vertical).
- Observe the knee at these five points in the gait cycle, and determine whether the knee is flexed or extended.
- Observe the ankle at these five points in the gait cycle, and determine whether the ankle is dorsiflexed, plantarflexed, or neutral (90 degrees).

Assignment

1. You are going to create a graph that plots angular change at each of the three joints as a function of the events observed in the gait cycle. Create a graph for each joint similar to the ones shown in Figure 12.2. On the *x*-axis, mark the five events you were observing across the step cycle. On the *y*-axis is the angular displacement of the joint. Neutral joint position is represented by a line. Flexion of the joint is above the line, while extension is below the line. Roughly graph the motions you observed at each of the three joints on the graphs. Now compare your results with those found in Figure 12.2. How closely do your graphs approximate those shown in Figure 12.2? If your graphs differ significantly from those shown in the figure, again observe your partner walking, and determine why there is a discrepancy between the two. Is your partner walking with an atypical gait pattern? Or, alternatively, were there errors in your observations?

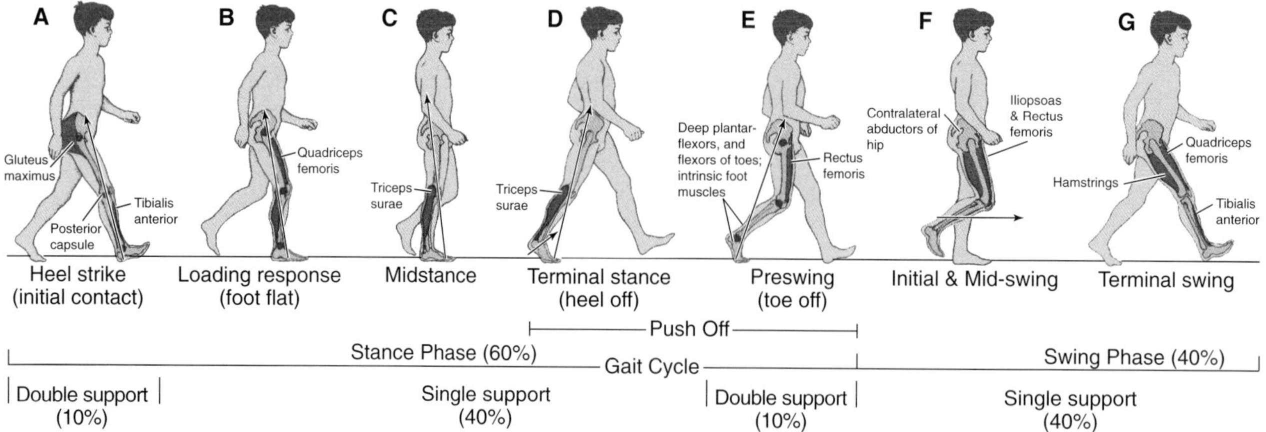

Figure 12.5 EMG patterns associated with the adult step cycle. (Reprinted from Moore KL, Dalley AF, Agur AMR. *Clinically oriented anatomy,* 8th ed. Baltimore, MD: Lippincott Williams & Wilkins, 2017, Figure 7.23 with permission.)

forward motion of the head, arm, and trunk segments that would otherwise occur in response to the loss of forward momentum associated with foot strike. During the loading response (Fig. 12.5B), eccentric activation of the quadriceps controls the small knee flexion wave that is used to absorb the impact of foot strike. In addition, activation of extensor muscles at the hip, knee, and ankle keeps the body from collapsing into gravity; however, by midstance (Fig. 12.5C), only the triceps surae is active, with the quadriceps and pretibial muscles becoming predominantly inactive.

The second goal of the stance phase of gait is generating a propulsive force to keep the body in motion. There is debate among researchers as to the primary strategy used to propel the body forward during locomotion (Chen & Patten, 2008; Kepple et al., 1997; Neptune et al., 2001; Perry, 1992; Perry & Burnfield, 2010; Sadeghi et al., 2000; Winter, 1990). Several authors have suggested that generating propulsive forces for progression involves primarily the concentric contraction of the plantarflexors (gastrocnemius and soleus) during terminal stance (Fig. 12.5D) with the assistance of the hip flexors during preswing (Fig. 12.5E), which provides pull-off (Chen & Patten, 2008; Eng & Winter, 1995; Kepple et al., 1997; Winter, 1990). The "active push-off" theory hypothesizes that the energy generated by the plantarflexor group is transferred to the trunk to provide support and forward progression (Chen & Patten, 2008; Kepple et al., 1997; Neptune et al., 2001; Winter, 1990). The hip extensors are also recognized as a source of both balance and propulsion. Late in the stance phase, hip and knee extensors give the body a "push from behind," though the contribution of these muscles appears less important than the plantarflexors and hip flexors (Gottschall & Kram, 2003; Kepple et al., 1997; Winter, 1990). The extensors, however, do play an important role in controlling the movement of the head, arms, and trunk during push-off and preventing collapse of the stance limb (Eng & Winter, 1995; Sadeghi et al., 2000; Winter, 1990).

In contrast to the active push-off theory, some researchers suggest that forward velocity during walking is generated by a roll-off rather than a push-off (Neptune et al., 2001; Perry, 1992; Perry & Burnfield, 2010). The "controlled roll-off" theory describes forward progression during single-leg stance as a controlled fall. Further information regarding the research investigating push-off versus roll-off may be found in the Extended Knowledge 12.1.

Swing Phase. The primary goal to be accomplished in the swing phase of gait is to reposition the limb for continued forward progression. This requires both accelerating the limb forward and making sure the toe clears the ground. Much of the energy for swing initiation occurs during the preswing phase of gait (Chen & Patten, 2008; Fox & Delp, 2010; Neptune et al., 2001). Preswing (Fig. 12.5E) has been identified as a key portion of the gait cycle because the muscle forces produced during preswing determine knee flexion velocity at toe-off, and this is correlated with swing-phase peak knee flexion (Fox & Delp, 2010; Reinbolt et al., 2008). Preparation for swing begins in double-support, with most of flexion acceleration occurring before the toe leaves the ground; this results in a peak knee flexion velocity around toe-off (Fox & Delp, 2010). During initial and midswing (Fig. 12.5F) hip flexors (iliacus and psoas), with the assistance of the biceps femoris (BFi), accelerate the knee into flexion (Fox & Delp, 2010). Forward acceleration of the thigh in the early swing phase is also associated with a concentric contraction of the quadriceps. By midswing, however, the quadriceps muscles are virtually inactive as the leg swings through, much like a pendulum driven by an impulse force at the beginning of swing phase. However, the iliopsoas contracts to aid in this forward motion, as shown in Figure 12.5F. The hamstrings become active in terminal swing (Fig. 12.5G) to slow the forward rotation of the thigh, in preparation for foot strike. Knee extension at the

Extended Knowledge 12.1

Propelling the Body During Gait: Push-Off versus Roll-Off

As discussed in the text, there is debate among researchers as to whether propelling the body is accomplished through an active push-off versus a more passive roll-off. The active push-off theory suggests that generating propulsive forces for progression involves primarily the concentric contraction of the plantarflexors (gastrocnemius and soleus) during terminal stance with the assistance of the hip flexors during preswing, which provides pull-off (Chen & Patten, 2008; Eng & Winter, 1995; Kepple et al., 1997; Winter, 1990). In contrast to the active push-off theory, researchers have suggested that forward velocity during walking is generated by a roll-off rather than a push-off (Neptune et al., 2001; Perry, 1992; Perry & Burnfield, 2010). The "controlled roll-off" theory describes forward progression during single-leg stance as a controlled fall. In this theory, the primary action of the ankle plantarflexors during the controlled roll-off is to decelerate tibia rotation and prevent knee flexion as the body rotates over the stance leg. Forward progression is accomplished passively, not actively, because the body moves forward as a result of momentum and inertia (Neptune et al., 2001; Perry, 1992; Perry & Burnfield, 2010).

To clarify the role of the ankle-joint muscles in forward progression, Winter examined the power output at the ankles and knees during walking and found that the generation of forward velocity was associated with a plantarflexor push-off rather than a passive roll-off (Kepple et al., 1997; Winter, 1983a). This was supported by research by Gottschall and Kram (2003), who showed that the generation of propulsive forces by the gastrocnemius makes up about half of the metabolic cost of walking.

The ability of the body to move freely over the foot, in conjunction with the concentric contraction of the gastrocnemius, also means that the COM of the body will be anterior to the supporting foot by the end of stance; this creates the forward fall, noted by Perry (1992), which is also critical to progression.

This research suggests that the generation of propulsive forces is a primary factor in generating forward progression of the body; however, roll-off associated with a forward fall position contributes as well.

end of swing in preparation for loading the limb for stance phase occurs, not as the result of muscle activity but as the result of passive nonmuscular forces (Winter, 1984).

During swing, foot clearance is accomplished through flexion at the hip, knee, and ankle, which results in an overall shortening of the swing limb as compared with the stance limb. Again, flexion of the hip is accomplished through activation of the quadriceps muscles. Flexion at the knee is accomplished passively, since rapid acceleration of the thigh will also produce flexion at the knee. Activation of the pretibial muscles produces ankle dorsiflexion late in the swing phase to ensure toe clearance and to prepare for the next footfall.

Joint Kinetics of Steady-State Gait: Progression and Postural Control

Thus far, we have examined the kinematics or movements of the body during the step cycle and looked at the patterns of muscle activity in each of the phases of gait. What are the typical forces that these movements and muscle responses create during locomotion? The dominant forces at a joint do not necessarily mirror the movements of the joint, as you will see in the discussion that follows.

Determination of the forces generated during the step cycle is considered a kinetic analysis. The kinetic or force parameters associated with the normal gait pattern are less stereotyped than the kinematic or movement parameters. The active and passive muscle forces (called "joint moments") that generate locomotion are themselves quite variable.

Stance Phase. Remember, the goals during stance phase include stabilizing the limb for weight acceptance and shock absorption and generating propulsive forces for continued motion. Figure 12.6 shows the averaged joint-angle changes at the ankle, knee, and hip in the sagittal plane (top part of Fig. 12.6) and joint moment changes observed during one stride cycle (bottom part of Fig. 12.6). Note that the support moment (top trace of joint moment graph) during the stance phase of the step cycle (0%–60% of stride) is the algebraic sum of the joint moments at the hip, knee, and ankle (lower traces) (Winter, 1990). This net extensor moment keeps the limb from collapsing while bearing weight, allowing stabilization of the body and thus accomplishing the postural control requirements of locomotion.

However, researchers have shown that people use a wide variety of force-generating strategies to accomplish this net extensor moment. For example, one strategy for achieving a net extensor moment involves combining a dominant hip extensor moment, to counter a knee flexor moment. Alternatively, a knee and ankle extensor moment can be combined to counterbalance a hip flexor moment and still maintain the net extensor support moment (Winter, 1980, 1984, 1990; Winter et al., 1990). There is a clear tradeoff in the forces generated between the plantarflexors during push-off and the ipsilateral hip flexors during terminal stance and early swing, and the contralateral hip extensors during early midstance. Higher ankle power output simultaneously alleviates mechanical power demands on the ipsilateral hip flexors but increases demands in the contralateral hip extensors. Decreasing ankle power output has the opposite effects. Thus, the positive and negative force generation by the trailing and

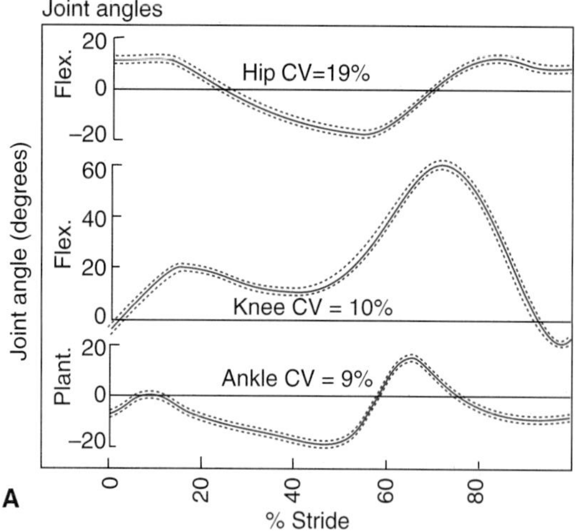

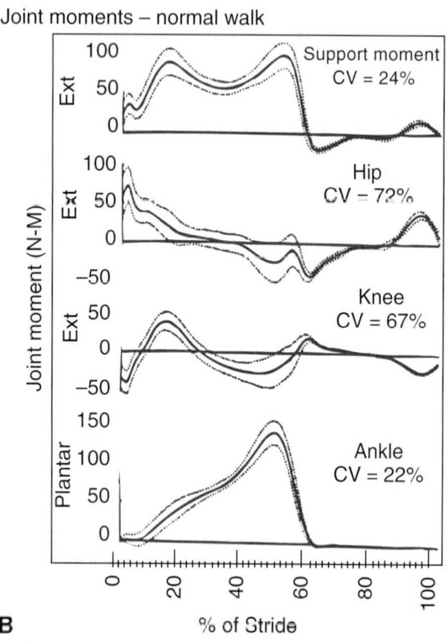

Figure 12.6 (A) Joint-angle changes occurring in the hip, knee, and ankle associated with the adult step cycle. **(B)** Individual joint moments (ankle, knee, hip) and the net support moment associated with the adult step cycle during normal walking (normal walk). CV, coefficient of variation; N-M, Newton-meters. Stance phase is approximately the first 60% of the cycle. (Adapted from Winter DA. Kinematic and kinetic patterns of human gait: variability and compensating effects. *Hum Mov Sci.* 1984;3:51–76, with permission.)

leading legs, respectively, is tuned in timing and magnitude to efficiently accelerate the body's COM (Fickey et al., 2018).

Why is it important to have this flexibility in the individual contributions of joint torques to the net extensor moment? Apparently, this motor flexibility in how torques are generated is important to controlling balance during gait.

Winter and his colleagues have studied gait extensively and suggest that balance during steady-state (unperturbed) gait is very different from the task of balance during quiet stance (Winter et al., 1991). In walking, the center of gravity does not stay within the support base of the feet, and thus the body is in a continuous state of postural imbalance. The only way to prevent falling is to place the swinging foot ahead of and lateral to the center of gravity as it moves forward.

In addition, the mass of the head, arms, and trunk (the HAT segment) must be regulated with respect to the hips, as the HAT segment represents a large inertial load to keep upright. Winter and colleagues proposed that the dynamic balance of the HAT segment is the responsibility of the hip muscles, with almost no involvement of the ankle muscles. They suggested that this is because the hip has a much smaller inertial load to control, that of the HAT segment, as compared with the ankles, which would have to control the entire body. Thus, they proposed that balance during ongoing gait is different from stance balance control, which relies primarily on ankle muscles (Winter et al., 1991).

They note that the hip muscles are also involved in a separate task, that of contributing to the extensor support moment necessary during stance, and view the muscles controlling the HAT segment and those controlling the extensor support moment as two separate synergies. We mentioned previously that the net extensor moment of the ankle, knee, and hip joints during stance was always the same, but that the individual moments were highly variable from stride to stride and individual to individual. One reason for this variability is to allow the balance control system to continuously alter the anteroposterior (AP) motor patterns on a step-to-step basis. However, the hip balance adjustments must be compensated for by appropriate knee moments in order to preserve the net extensor moment essential for the stance phase of gait (Winter, 1990; Winter et al., 1991).

Does walking speed affect COM displacement? This is an important issue to explore, as many patient populations use a reduced walking speed, which may actually increase COM displacements and potentially make them more unstable. In order to answer this question, Orendurff and colleagues (2004) examined COM excursion in normal adults during several walking speeds. They found that the mean (±SD) mediolateral (ML) COM displacement was 6.99 ± 1.34 cm at the slowest walking speed (0.7 meters per second) and was reduced significantly, to 3.85 ± 1.41 cm, at the fastest speed (1.6 meters per second). Thus, even normal individuals show substantial ML COM displacement at slow speeds.

Swing Phase The major goal during swing is to reposition the limb, making sure that the toe clears the ground and to place the foot in an ideal position to accept and bear weight for the next gait cycle. Researchers have found that the joint moment patterns during the swing phase are less variable than during the stance phase, indicating that adults use fairly similar force-generating patterns to accomplish this task. This is illustrated by the large standard deviations around the mean joint torques during stance (0%–60% of stride) as compared with the small standard deviations in swing (60%–100% of stride), shown in Figure 12.6, bottom graph.

At normal walking speeds, early in swing, there is a flexor moment at the hip that contributes to flexion of the thigh. Early hip flexion is assisted by gravity, reducing the need for a large flexor hip joint moment. In adults, the foot is then automatically raised in midswing to a preferred, optimal amount of clearance height, which is associated with less metabolic cost compared to higher or lower foot lifts (Wu & Kuo, 2016).

Once swing phase has been initiated, it is often sustained by momentum. Then, as swing phase ends, an extensor joint moment may be required to slow the thigh rotation and prepare for heel strike (Woollacott & Jensen, 1996). Thus, even though the thigh is still flexing, there is an extensor moment on the thigh at this point.

What controls knee motions during swing? Interestingly, during swing, joint torque at the knee is basically used to constrain knee motion rather than to generate motion. In early swing, an extensor moment slows knee-joint flexion and contributes to reversal of the knee joint from flexion to extension. Later in swing, a flexor knee-joint moment slows knee extension to prepare for foot placement (Cavanagh & Gregor, 1975; Winter, 1990, 1993).

At the end of swing phase and during the initial part of stance phase, a small dorsiflexing moment occurs at the ankle, which helps control plantarflexion at heel strike. So even though the ankle motion is one of plantarflexion, the ankle-joint force is a dorsiflexion moment.

Moving through the stance phase, the ankle plantarflexion moment increases to a maximum point just after knee flexion, when the ankle begins to plantarflex. The ankle-joint torque is the largest of all the moments of the lower limb and is the main contributor to the acceleration of the limb into swing phase.

Thus, in many of the previous examples, we see that the joint torque is opposite to that of the limb movement itself. In other words, the joint torque shows us that the combined forces may be acting to brake the movement or control footfall, rather than simply accelerate the limb.

We have discussed how the progression and postural control requirements are met in steady-state (nonperturbed) gait. However, very little of daily life mobility occurs under steady-state (nonperturbed) conditions. Instead, real-life mobility requires modifying gait, both the progression and stability requirements, in response to both expected and unexpected disruptions to walking. The following sections discuss two other components necessary to walking function in daily life: reactive postural control strategies and proactive strategies used to adapt gait to changing task and environmental demands.

Adaptation of Gait: Contributions of Reactive and Proactive Balance Control in Gait

Adapting gait to changes in task and environmental demands is a critical aspect of mobility in daily life. The mobility domain, within Activities and Participation of the ICF (see Fig. 12.2), is characterized by the ability to perform complex walking tasks, such as walking over obstacles, changing speed and direction, and walking under different terrain conditions. Adapting gait is the hallmark of functional mobility.

Adaptation of gait involves adapting the strategies used to accomplish both the progression and postural control requirements in the face of changing task and environmental conditions. Adapting the progression requirement of gait involves modifying force generation strategies used to move the body in the desired direction. Adapting the postural control requirement involves the use of both reactive balance strategies that aid in the recovery of stability after an unexpected perturbation and proactive (or anticipatory) balance strategies that are activated in advance of potential disturbances to gait, in order to avoid loss of stability. Disturbances may result from external sources, for example, obstacles in the environment, or internal sources such as carrying a load. Adaptation of both the progression and postural control requirements of gait involves both short-term changes and long-term modifications to gait needed in the face of more sustained changes in the task or environment.

Reactive Balance Control in Gait

Research has shown that compensatory automatic postural adjustments, similar to those used for recovering stance balance, are integrated into the step cycle during recovery from an unexpected perturbation to gait. Studies were performed in which subjects walked across a platform that could be perturbed at different points in the step cycle to simulate a slip during walking. Results showed that automatic postural responses were incorporated appropriately into the different phases of the step cycle (Nashner, 1980). For example, postural muscle responses were activated at about 100-ms latencies in the gastrocnemius when this muscle was stretched faster than normal in response to backward surface displacements pitching the body forward. This helped slow the body's rate of forward progression to realign the COM with the backward-displaced support foot. Similarly, responses occurred in the TA muscle when it was shortened more slowly than normal because of forward surface displacements that displaced the body backward. This helped increase the rate of forward progress to realign the body with the forward-displaced foot.

Previous research on the control of steady-state walking has shown that one of the main control issues is keeping the HAT segment well balanced and that the trunk and hip muscles play an active role in this control (Winter et al., 1990). The previous work discussed on reactive control of balance during gait has shown that the distal perturbed leg muscles are important in this type of control (Gollhofer et al., 1986; Nashner, 1980). However, when a slip occurs, there is not only stretch of the ankle musculature but a challenge to upper-body balance as well. Thus, it is possible that proximal hip and trunk muscle activity may be a primary contributor to both steady-state gait and the recovery of balance during slips.

Studies recording from bilateral leg, thigh, hip, and trunk muscles have shown that proximal muscles are not the primary muscles contributing to recovery from balance threats during slips in healthy, young adults. Although proximal muscle activity was often present during the first slip trial in young adults, adaptation tended to eliminate this activity during subsequent trials. However, activity in anterior bilateral lower leg muscles as well as anterior and posterior thigh muscles showed early (90–140 ms), high-magnitude (four to nine times the activity in normal walking), and relatively long-duration bursts (Tang et al., 1998). As shown previously for recovery of balance during quiet stance, muscle response patterns to balance threats during walking were activated in a distal-to-proximal sequence. As shown in Figure 12.7 for a forward slip at heel strike, first the tibialis anterior on the ipsilateral side was activated (TAi), followed by the rectus femoris (RFi) and BFi, and then the gluteus medius (GMEi) and abdominal muscles (ABi) (in initial trials).

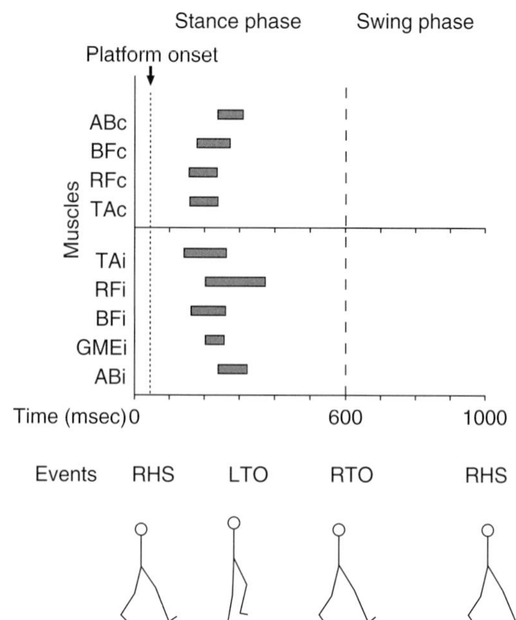

Figure 12.7 The organization of postural muscle responses to a forward slip at heel strike. The horizontal bars indicate the duration of postural activity in these muscles. The stick figures indicate the events during normal walking. AB, rectus abdominis; BF, biceps femoris; c, contralateral side; GME, gluteus medius; i, ipsilateral to the perturbed side; LTO, left toe-off; RF, rectus femoris; RHS, right heel strike; RTO, right toe-off; TA, tibialis anterior. (Adapted from Tang PF, Woollacott MH, Chong RKY. Control of reactive balance adjustments in perturbed human walking: roles of proximal and distal postural muscle activity. *Exp Brain Res.* 1998;119:141–152, with permission.)

Similar to the research in stance, arm movements are typically used during balance recovery in gait. Forward arm elevation evoked in response to a slip during locomotion aids to counteract the backward fall of the COM. Arm movements also may be used in a protective role, either with hands being directed to nearby handrails or, if a fall occurs, with arms absorbing force at the point of impact. These are often called "whole-body responses."

When given multiple slip perturbations, young adults adapt their strategy of recovery (Bhatt et al., 2006; Marigold & Patla, 2002). On the first slip (subjects unexpectedly stepped on rollers as they walked), individuals used a rapidly activated flexor synergy, with the TA and BFi being activated, along with a large arm elevation and modified swing trajectory, as noted previously. With repeated slips, individuals modified the strategy, using a more flat-footed landing, a shift of the ML COM closer to the support limb at foot contact with the rollers, which allowed them to attenuate the responses and use a "surfing strategy" as they went across the rollers. This suggests that they incorporated proactive adjustments in subsequent trials as they crossed the slippery surface.

Many falls in older adults occur as the result of trips. How is balance recovery accomplished during trips? Research analyzing responses to a tripping perturbation has found that the type of strategy used to maintain stability depends on when in the swing phase the trip occurs. As shown in Figure 12.8, if the trip occurs early in the swing phase of walking, the most common movement outcome is an elevating strategy of the swing limb with muscle responses occurring at 60 to 140 ms. Figure 12.8 shows the increased flexion at the hip, knee, and ankle (dashed lines) after obstacle contact (shown by the arrow) in the trial in which the subject was tripped, compared with the control trial (solid lines). The elevating strategy consisted of a flexor torque component of the swing limb, with the temporal sequencing of the swing limb BFi occurring prior to the swing limb RFi to remove the limb from the obstacle before accelerating the limb over it. An extensor torque component in the stance limb generated an early heel-off to increase the height of the body.

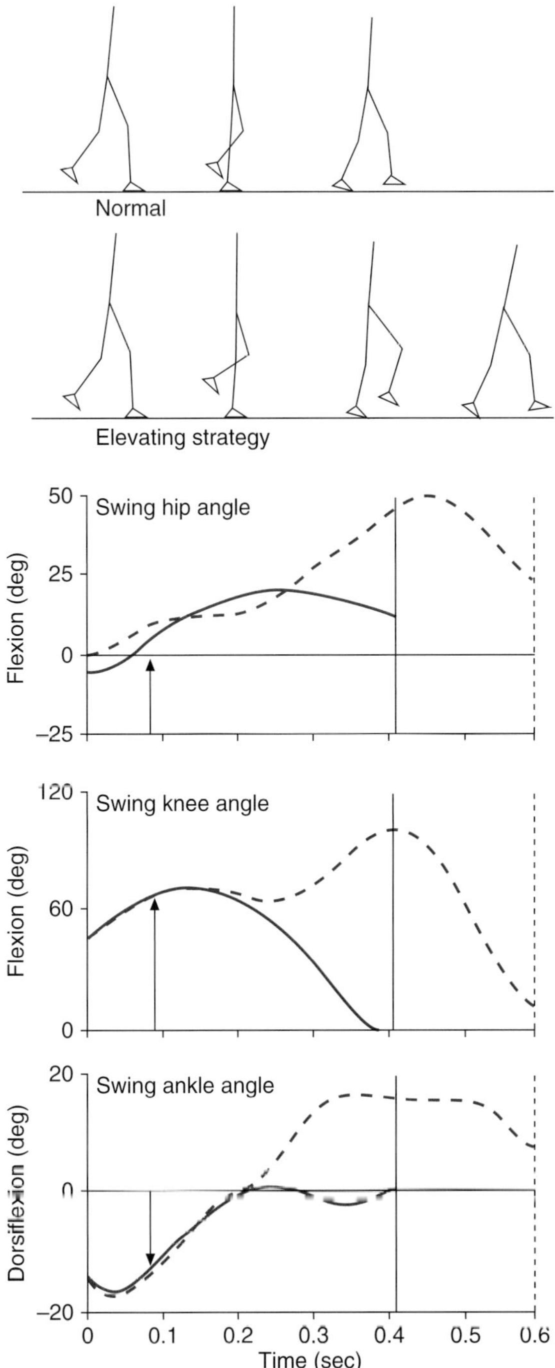

Figure 12.8 Hip, knee, and ankle trajectories of the swing limb observed in response to a trip during early swing phase of walking, showing the elevation strategy. *Solid line* = normal trial; *dashed line* = perturbed trial. Time 0 = toe-off; *arrows* = contact of the foot with obstacle; *vertical solid line* = normal heel contact; *vertical dashed line* = perturbed heel contact. (Adapted from Eng JJ, Winter DA, Patla AE. Strategies for recovery from a trip in early and late swing during human walking. *Exp Brain Res.* 1994;102:344, with permission.)

Use of the elevating strategy would be dangerous if a trip occurred late in the swing phase, as flexion of the swing limb as it is approaching the ground would increase, not decrease, instability; thus, a lowering strategy was used by subjects, as shown in Figure 12.9.

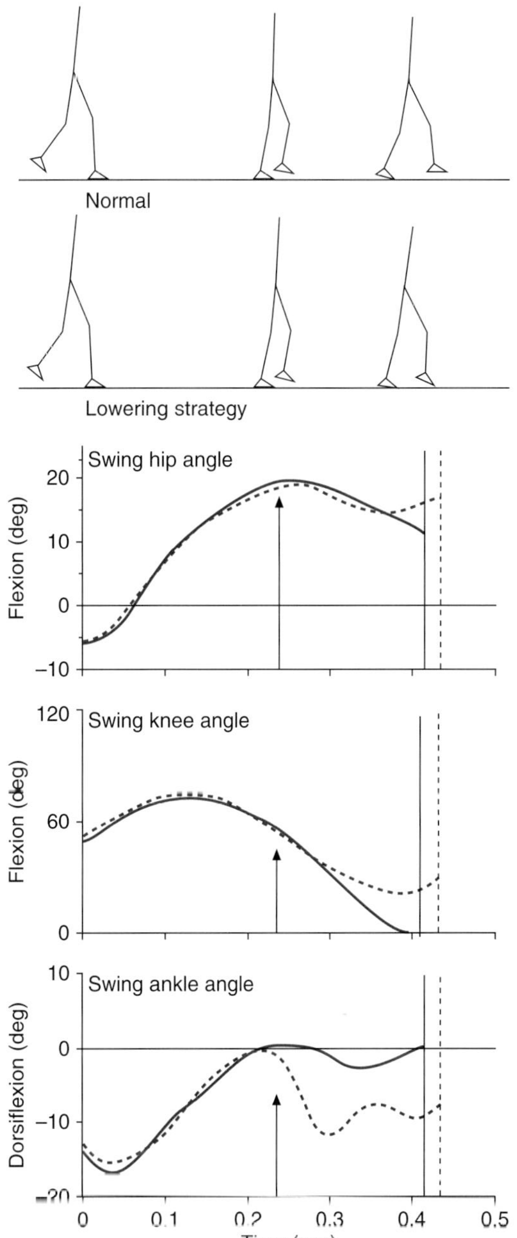

Figure 12.9 Hip, knee, and ankle trajectories of the swing limb observed in response to a trip during the late swing phase of walking, showing the lowering strategy. *Solid line* = normal trial; *dashed line* = perturbed trial. Time 0 = toe-off; *arrows* = contact of the foot with obstacle; *vertical solid line* = normal heel contact; *vertical dashed line* = perturbed heel contact. (Adapted from Eng JJ, Winter DA, Patla AE. Strategies for recovery from a trip in early and late swing during human walking. *Exp Brain Res.* 1994;102:345, with permission.)

Note the early plantarflexion of the ankle. The lowering strategy was accomplished by inhibitory responses in the swing limb vastus lateralis and an excitatory response of the swing limb BFi, resulting in a shortened step length (Eng et al., 1994).

In a study examining recovery from trips in more detail (Schillings et al., 2000), researchers asked individuals to walk on a treadmill, and at different times in the swing phase a rigid obstacle unexpectedly blocked the forward movement of the foot. As noted previously, all subjects showed an elevation strategy for early swing and a lowering strategy for late swing perturbations. The muscle responses used for the elevation strategy included the ipsilateral BFi, causing extra knee flexion, and the TA, causing ankle dorsiflexion. Later RFi responses were associated with knee extension as the foot was placed back on the treadmill. In the lowering strategy, the foot was placed quickly on the treadmill and was lifted over the obstacle in the subsequent swing phase. Foot placement was controlled by the ipsilateral RFi and BFi, associated with knee extension and deceleration of forward sway. Activation of the ipsilateral TA preceded the main ipsilateral soleus response.

Midswing perturbations could activate either elevation or lowering strategies. The first response was typically a short-latency stretch reflex, caused by the impact of the collision with the foot. This was not functionally related to the subsequent behavioral strategy. The first responses associated with elevation or lowering strategies occurred at about 110 ms.

Roeles and colleagues (2018) examined recovery of gait stability following various types of perturbations: two medio-lateral platform perturbations to the non-dominant and dominant sides, two anterior–posterior unilateral belt perturbations of the non-dominant side (one perturbation accelerated the belt and the other decelerated it), a visual perturbation consisting of darkening of the room, and an auditory perturbation in the form of a lasting air horn noise. All mechanical perturbations (medio-lateral and anterior–posterior perturbations) altered gait patterns while sensory perturbations did not. The medio-lateral perturbation toward the contralateral leg (i.e., platform movement to the right at left heel strike or to the left at right heel strike) induced the highest body perturbation requiring adults to take a cross-step to prevent falling. Similarly, the decelerating anterior–posterior perturbation decreased postural stability and required adults to take faster, shorter, and wider steps. The authors conclude that slips and trips leading to contralateral sway or deceleration of gait are the most disturbing to spatio-temporal gait patterns and may increase the risk of falls.

Finally, the nervous system takes advantage of passive dynamics to control the recovery from a trip during the swing phase of gait. Kinematic data were analyzed using inverse dynamics techniques (see Technology Tool 12.1) to determine the joint moment and mechanical power (kinetic) profiles and to partition the joint moments into active and passive components. Results showed that the nervous system used the passive dynamics of the musculoskeletal system to aid in balance recovery. Active control of one joint, the knee joint, passively contributed to the flexion at the hip and the ankle joints following a trip in early swing (Eng et al., 1997). Thus, it is important to consider both the passive and the active joint moments produced during balance recovery, in addition to the response patterns of involved muscles, in order to understand the interactions between passive and active components of the control systems.

Proactive Strategies

Proactive balance strategies are used to modify and adapt gait in two different ways: prediction and visually activated strategies. Prediction is used to minimize the destabilizing forces arising from our own movements, since forces generated by one body segment exert reactive forces on other segments. For example, when walking, the alternating push-off and braking forces of the lower limbs if not countered would cause the large mass of the trunk to move backward (during push-off) and forward (during initial contact). In healthy young adults, the trunk is stabilized by predictive postural adjustments that are initiated in advance of or coincident with the destabilizing force; this predictive control is the result of experience (Frank & Patla, 2003). Proactive strategies

TECHNOLOGY TOOL 12.1 Kinetic Analysis: Inverse Dynamics

Inverse dynamics is a process that allows researchers to calculate the joint moments of force (torque) responsible for movement—in this case, locomotion. Researchers begin by developing a reliable model of the body using anthropometric measures such as segment masses, center of mass, joint centers, and moments of inertia. Because these variables are difficult to measure directly, they are usually obtained from statistical tables based on the person's height, weight, and sex (Winter, 1990).

Using extremely accurate kinematic information on the limb trajectory during the step cycle, in combination with a reliable model, researchers can calculate the torque acting on each segment of the body. They can then partition the net torque into components due to gravity, the mechanical interaction among segments (motion-dependent torques), and a generalized muscle torque. This type of analysis allows researchers to assess the roles of muscular and nonmuscular forces in the generation of the movement (Winter et al., 1990).

include visually activated strategies to modify gait in response to potential threats to stability in the environment. Most visually activated proactive strategies can be successfully carried out within a step cycle. An exception occurs when changing directions, and this requires planning one step cycle in advance. It has been suggested that there are various rules associated with changing the placement of the foot. For example, when possible, step length is increased, rather than shortened, and the foot is placed inside rather than outside an obstacle, as long as the foot does not need to cross the midline of the body. Adapting strategies for foot placement does not involve simply changing the amplitude of the normal locomotor pattern but is complex and task specific (Patla, 1997). The next sections discuss research on visually activated proactive strategies used to adapt gait and maintain stability in the face of commonly encountered conditions in the environment.

Obstacle Crossing. Controlling balance when walking over obstacles requires increased control as compared with normal locomotion, as imbalance of the body may occur and cause a fall. In order to determine the motion of the COM when stepping over obstacles of different heights, Chou and colleagues (2001) asked young adults to step over obstacles of 2.5% to 15% of their body height, while walking at their own comfortable walking speed. They found that stepping over higher obstacles caused significantly greater ranges of COM motion in both the AP and vertical directions (but not the ML direction), along with a greater AP distance between the COM and center of pressure (COP). Minimizing shifts in ML COM during obstacle crossing may reflect a control strategy used by healthy individuals to keep the COM well within safe limits for balance control. Balance-impaired older adults and patient populations appear to have more difficulty with controlling ML COM motion during obstacle crossing (see Chapters 13 and 14).

The decision to step over an obstacle rather than move around it is related to object size as compared with body size. For example, when the ratio of obstacle size to leg length is 1:1, subjects prefer to go around it (Warren, 1988). It is probable that this choice relates to stability issues, as the risk of tripping increases as we step over obstacles of increased height.

Characteristics of an obstacle also influence how gait is modified to avoid obstacle collision. For example, perceived fragility of an obstacle influences the amount of toe clearance, with clearance being larger for the more fragile objects (Patla, 1997).

Adapting to Surface Conditions. How do humans modify gait when walking or running on different surface conditions? In a study to determine how strategies for dealing with slippery floors are altered when subjects know in advance of a possible hazard, Cham and Redfern (2002) asked individuals to walk across either dry (baseline conditions) or water-, soap-, or oil-covered floors, for which they did not know the identity of the possible contaminant in advance. They found that when individuals anticipated a slippery surface, they produced peak required coefficient of friction values that were 16% to 33% less than during baseline conditions, in order to reduce the potential for a slip. This was accomplished by reductions in stance duration and loading speed on the supported foot, taking shorter stride lengths, and using a slower angular velocity at heel strike. Interestingly, during a recovery condition in which subjects knew the floor was again dry, gait characteristics did not return to normal, but showed 5% to 12% reductions in coefficient of friction values.

In a study looking at gait adaptability in healthy adults, researchers found immediate changes in the dynamics of walking when participants were first exposed to an uneven wooden terrain (Kent et al., 2019). Variability in COM excursion range and peak COM velocity were higher during the first 60 strides of walking on uneven terrain compared to flat terrain. In addition, at first adults adopted a more cautious and restrictive gait pattern by increasing their step width and decreasing their step length. Following a practice period of walking on the uneven terrain, COM excursion range and peak COM velocity remained high, but adults were able to refine their gait patterns and reduce their restrictive strategy by decreasing step width and increasing step length.

How do humans modify walking on surfaces with a different compliance or compressibility? If humans used the same muscle stiffness for all surfaces, the dynamics of walking and running would be strongly affected by surface stiffness or compliance. Marigold and Patla (2005) showed that humans adjust muscle activity and subsequent limb movements to control the stability of walking dynamics on compliant surfaces. They tested adults walking along a walkway where they had to step unexpectedly on either compliant surfaces with different levels of density of foam or a firm surface. Consistent with previous studies on slipping and tripping, the authors found that adults responded to the first unexpected compliant surface with a long-latency reflex (between 97 and 175 ms) and modulated muscle activity depending on the phase of the gait cycle. For example, the perturbed-limb ankle muscle amplitude (TA, soleus, and gastrocnemius) increased during the early response on the compliant surface, suggesting a stiffening response of the muscles that control the ankle to stabilize the limb that is in contact with the compliant surface. Moreover, adults lowered their COM more while stepping on the compliant surface than on the firm surface and they inclined their trunks forward at toe-off and increased the flexion of the knee to ensure an adequate toe-off while walking on compliant surfaces (Fig. 12.10). Thus, the central nervous system must not only deal

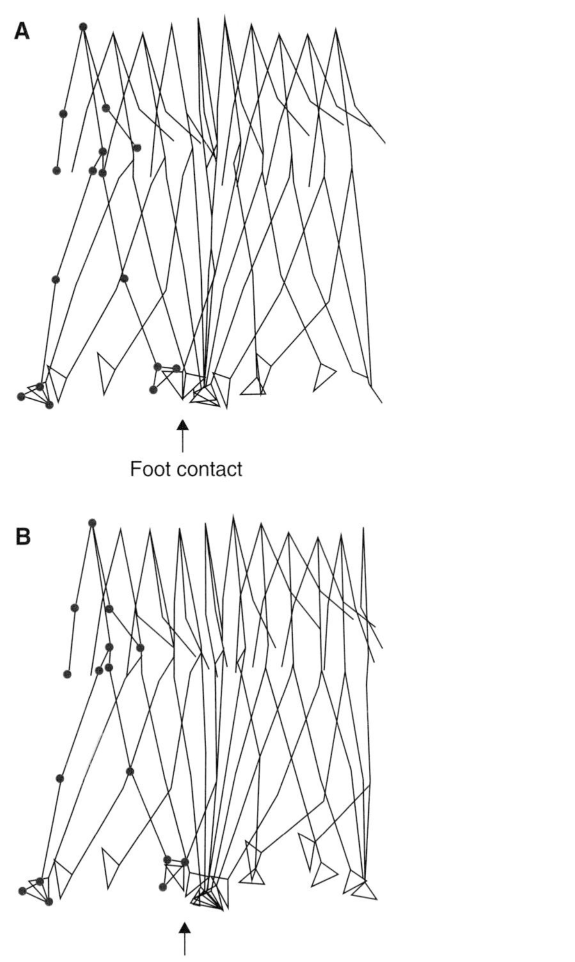

Figure 12.10 Typical stick figures of body postures during the control trials **(A)** and during the first compliant-surface trial **(B)** The darker lines represent the left side of the body (i.e., perturbed limb) and the lighter lines represent the right side of the body (i.e., unperturbed limb). (Adapted with permission from Marigold DS, Patla AE. Adapting locomotion to different surfaces compliances: Neuromuscular Responses and Changes in Movement Dynamics. *J Neurophysiol.* 2005;94:1744.)

with the postural imbalance secondary to the initial step onto an unstable surface but also adjust the mechanics and dynamics of the lower extremity and body through the entire the gait cycle to stabilize the walking pattern before stepping off onto a firm surface. Work by Ferris et al. (1998) on *running* showed similar results. They found that the central nervous system modulates joint displacements and joint moments according to surface stiffness, probably in order to keep COM movement and ground contact time the same. Research on animals has shown that this is done within one step of moving on to the new surface. Research on human stretch reflex and Golgi tendon organ (GTO) contributions to the step cycle suggests that proprioceptive feedback may be a factor contributing in this stiffness modulation (Pearson et al., 1992; Stein, 1991). However, research has also shown that when lower-limb reflexes are temporarily blocked by ischemia, adults run with a normal ground contact time, suggesting that leg stiffness is unchanged (Dietz et al., 1979). Thus, there may be multiple contributions to stiffness regulation.

Adapting to Inclines. Research has verified that inclined surfaces are routinely encountered when walking in the community and cannot be avoided (Shumway-Cook et al., 2002). The ability to modify gait in response to changes in surface incline is thus necessary to avoiding mobility disability. Research indicates that young adults show greater joint angular motion and increased muscle activity in their lower limbs when walking on inclines or slopes when compared to walking on level surfaces. These changes are accompanied by an increase in step length and reduced cadence when walking uphill and a decrease in step length and increased cadence when walking downhill. These modifications allow young adults to successfully negotiate an uphill or downhill surface (Kawamura et al., 1991; Lay et al., 2006; McIntosh et al., 2006; Sun et al., 1996).

Turning During Walking. Making postural transitions during the performance of complex walking tasks, such as changing walking direction, is another aspect of community mobility that cannot be avoided and requires adjusting the body to control for the postural imbalances, especially in the ML direction (Shumway-Cook et al., 2002). Making a sudden turn while walking is a precipitating factor in falls in both geriatric and neurologic populations (see Chapter 14 for more details). When compared with walking straight, turning behavior entails additional motor coordination and changes in muscle activity. For example, Courtine and Schieppati (2004) revealed three basic features of curved walking: (a) the stride length of the inner leg decreases with respect to the stride length of the outer leg; (b) the outer and inner feet move away from and closer to the body midpoint trajectory, respectively; and (c) both feet are rotated toward the inner part of the curved trajectory. Moreover, EMG studies demonstrate different muscle activities during turning compared to walking, such as an increase in soleus amplitude during stance in the outer leg and a decrease in the inner leg, and an increase in TA activity in both legs during the swing phase (Courtine & Schieppati, 2003). In addition, the deceleration of walking before the turn involves activation of muscles in a sequence similar to the "ankle strategy" for balance control, starting at the distal soleus muscle and moving proximally to the hamstrings and erector spinae, showing that balance synergies may be used in a variety of tasks (Hase & Stein, 1999). In fact, researchers have identified task-specific and common muscle synergies that occur during straight walking, turning left, and turning right, suggesting that the central nervous system not only shares and modulates the same motor strategy

LAB ACTIVITY 12.3

Objective: To understand the movements essential to the initiation of gait.

Procedure: Get up and stand next to a wall, with your shoulder touching the wall. First try to start walking with the foot that is next to the wall. Then try to start walking with the foot that is away from the wall.

Assignment

In each condition (e.g., gait initiation with the leg nearer vs. farther from the wall), note the following:

1. What muscles contract and relax?
2. Which way does the body move in the process of preparing to take a step?
3. Under which condition is it easiest to initiate gait?
4. When you tried to initiate gait with the leg farther away from the wall, did you notice that you had more problems?
5. Why?

between similar types of behaviors but also develops task-specific strategies to adapt to different biomechanical demands (Choi et al., 2019).

Initiating Gait

How do we initiate walking? Before we describe the initiation of gait, complete Lab Activity 12.3. Research studies confirm what you no doubt noticed from your own experiment: the initiation of gait from quiet stance begins with the relaxation of specific postural muscles, the gastrocnemius and the soleus (Carlsoo, 1966; Herman et al., 1973). In fact, the initiation of gait has the appearance of a simple forward fall and regaining of one's balance by taking a step. This reduction in the activation of the gastrocnemius and soleus is followed by activation of the TA, which assists dorsiflexion and moves the COM forward in preparation for toe-off. But, as you noticed, and as research on gait confirms, the initiation of gait is more than a simple fall.

In tracing the COP during the initiation of gait in normal adults, the following sequence of events is evident. Prior to movement onset, the COP is positioned just posterior to the ankle and midway between both feet, as shown in Figure 12.11. As the person begins to move, the COP first moves posteriorly and laterally toward the swing limb and then shifts toward the stance limb and forward.

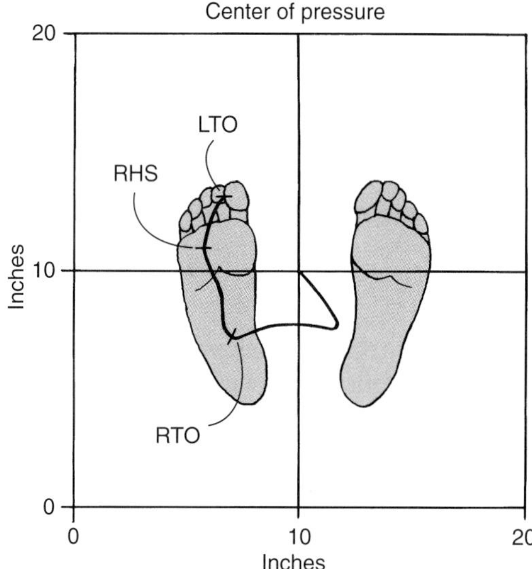

Figure 12.11 Trajectory of the COP during the initiation of gait from a balanced, symmetric stance. Prior to movement, the center of pressure is located midway between the feet. COP, center of pressure; LTO, left toe off; RHS, right heel strike; RTO, right toe off. (Adapted from Mann RA, Hagy JL, White V, et al. The initiation of gait. *J Bone Joint Surg Am*. 1979;61:232–239, with permission.)

Movement of the COP toward the stance limb occurs simultaneously with hip and knee flexion and ankle dorsiflexion as the swing limb prepares for toe-off. Toe-off of the swing limb occurs when the COP shifts from lateral to forward movement over the stance foot (Mann et al., 1979).

What neural patterns are correlated with these shifts in COP? As the COP moves posteriorly and toward the swing limb, both limbs are stabilized against backward sway by activation of anterior leg and thigh muscles: the TA and the quadriceps. Subsequent activation of the TA then causes dorsiflexion in the stance ankle, pulling the lower leg over the foot, as the body moves forward in preparation for toe-off. Anterior thigh muscles are activated to keep the knee from flexing so that the leg rotates forward as a unit. Activation of hip abductors counters lateral tilt of the pelvis toward the swing limb side as this limb is unloaded. Also, activation of the peroneal muscles stabilizes the stance ankle. After toe-off, the gastrocnemius and hamstrings muscles in the stance leg are used for propelling the body forward (Herman et al., 1973; Mann et al., 1979).

How long after initiation does it take to reach a steady velocity in gait? Steady state is reached within one to three steps, depending on the magnitude of the velocity one is trying to achieve. Over subsequent steps, joint moment patterns are further refined toward the joint moment characteristics of steady-state gait. The ankle contributes to the extensor moment pattern, providing most of the energy needed for propelling the body forward. Simultaneously, the hip contributes to the abductor moment pattern to stabilize the trunk, which facilitates the lateral movement of the COM toward midline (Breniere & Do, 1986; Cook & Cozzens, 1976; Smith & Wong, 2019).

CONTROL MECHANISMS FOR GAIT

How is a coordinated gait pattern achieved? What are the control mechanisms that ensure that the task requirements for successful gait are met? Much of the research examining the neural and nonneural control mechanisms essential for locomotion has been done with animals. It is through this research on locomotion in animals that scientists have learned about pattern formation (PF) in locomotion, the integration of postural control to the locomotor pattern, the contribution of peripheral and central mechanisms to adaptation and modulation of gait, and the role of the various senses in controlling locomotion.

The following section reviews some of the research on locomotor control in animals, relating it to experiments examining the neural control of locomotion in humans.

Pattern Generators for Gait

Research in the past 30 years has greatly increased our understanding of the nervous system control of the basic rhythmic movements underlying locomotion. Results of these studies have indicated that central pattern generators (CPGs) within the spinal cord play an important role in the production of these movements (Grillner, 1973; Smith, 1980; Wallen, 1995). A rich history of research has enhanced our understanding of the neural basis of locomotion. For a review of this history, see Extended Knowledge 12.2.

The three preparations that are most often studied when examining the control of locomotion are the spinal, the decerebrate, and the decorticate preparations, as shown in Figure 12.12. We will first discuss experiments using the spinal preparation. To produce locomotor behavior with this preparation, one needs an external stimulus. This can be either electrical or pharmacological.

Studies have found that muscle activity in spinalized and deafferented cats is similar to that seen in normal cats walking on a treadmill (Grillner & Zangger, 1979), with the extensor muscles of the knee and ankle activated prior to paw contact in stance phase. This demonstrates that extension is not simply a reflex in response to contact, but is part of a central program. In addition, the spinalized cat is capable of fully recruiting motor units within the spinal cord when increasing gait from a walk to a gallop (Smith et al., 1979).

Can a spinalized cat adapt the step cycle to clear obstacles? Yes. If a glass rod touches the top of the cat's paw during swing phase, it activates a flexion response in the stimulated leg, with simultaneous extension of the contralateral leg. This lifts the swing leg up and over the obstacle and gives postural support in the opposite leg. Interestingly, the same stimulation of the dorsal surface of the paw during stance causes increased extension, probably to get the paw quickly out of the way of the obstacle. Thus, the identical stimulus to the skin activates functionally separate sets of muscles during different phases of the step cycle, to compensate appropriately for different obstacles perturbing the movement of the paw (Forssberg et al., 1977).

Extended Knowledge 12.2

Historical Research on Locomotion

In the late 1800s, Sherrington and Mott (Mott & Sherrington, 1895; Sherrington, 1898) performed some of the first experiments to determine the neural control of locomotion. They severed the spinal cord of animals to eliminate the influence of higher brain centers and found that the hindlimbs continued to exhibit alternating movements.

In a second set of experiments, in monkeys, they cut the sensory nerve roots on one side of the spinal cord, eliminating sensory inputs contributing to stepping on one side of the body. They found that the monkeys did not use the limbs that had undergone deafferentation during walking. This led them to the conclusion that locomotion required sensory input. A model of locomotor control was created that attributed the control of locomotion to a set of reflex chains, with the output from one phase of the step cycle acting as a sensory stimulus to reflexly activate the next phase.

Thomas Graham Brown (1911) performed an experiment only a few years later showing the opposite result. He found that by making bilateral dorsal (sensory) root lesions in animals whose spinal cord had been transected (called "spinalized animals"), he could see rhythmic walking movements.

Why did the two labs get different results? It appears that it is because Sherrington cut sensory roots on only one side of the spinal cord, not both. In later experiments, Taub and Berman (1968) found that animals did not use a limb when the dorsal roots were cut on one side of the body, but they would begin to use the limb again when dorsal roots on the remaining side were sectioned. Why? Since the animal has appropriate input coming in from one limb and no sensation from the other, the animal prefers not to use the limb that has no sensation. Interestingly, researchers have found that they can make animals use a single limb that has undergone deafferentation by restraining the intact limb. These results are the rationale behind a therapy approach called the "constraint-induced (or forced-use) paradigm." In this approach, patients with hemiplegia are forced to use their hemiplegic arm, since the intact side is restrained (Taub et al., 1993, 2004; Wolf et al., 1989b).

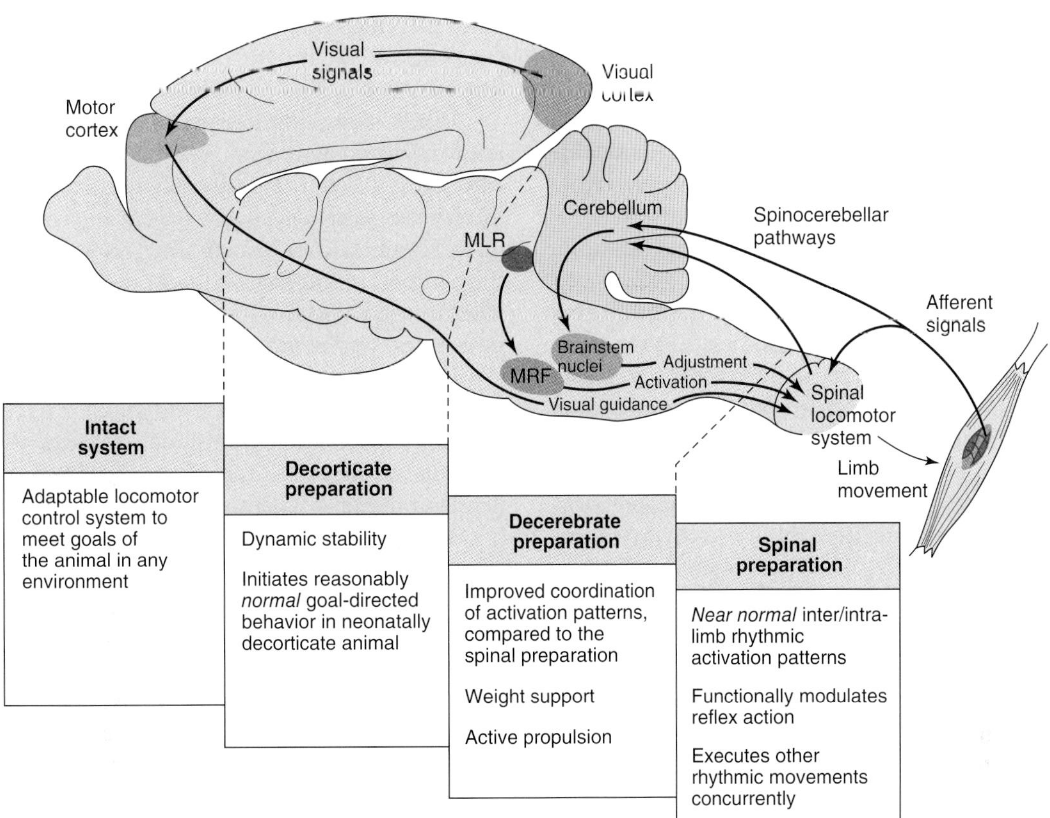

Figure 12.12 The brain and spinal cord, showing the different sites of lesions used in the study of the contributions of different neural subsystems to gait. See text for details. MLR, mesencephalic locomotor region; MRF, medial reticular formation. (Adapted from Patla AE. Understanding the control of human locomotion: a prologue. In: Patla AE, ed. *Adaptability of human gait*. Amsterdam: North-Holland, 1991:7, with permission.)

CPG Organization

Graham Brown proposed that there was a CPG creating the rhythmic alternating flexor and extensor activity in spinal locomotion, which was later called the "half-center" model for gait control. The organization of the half-center CPG involves the following principles. First, each of the limbs is separately controlled by its own CPG. Second, CPGs have two groups of excitatory interneurons—the half-centers—that control the activity of flexor and extensor motor neurons. Third, inhibitory connections between the half-centers allow only one center to be active at a time. Fourth, a fatigue process gradually reduces excitation in the active half-center, allowing phase switching to happen when the reduction in the excitability of one half-center falls below a critical value and the opposing center is released from inhibition. Finally, inhibition of antagonist and agonist motor neurons is tightly coupled (McCrea & Rybak, 2008).

More recently, a two-level CPG model has been proposed to address a number of limitations of Graham Brown's model. This model includes both a rhythm generator (RG) and a PF network. An important characteristic of the model is its ability to independently regulate gait speed (step cycle periods and phase durations) at the RG level and level of motor neuron activity at the PF level (as this has its own independent mesencephalic locomotor region [MLR] input). This creates a flexible network for both sensory and descending control of gait that the one-level CPG was not able to accommodate (McCrea & Rybak, 2008).

The pattern generating circuits in the brainstem reticular formation and spinal cord have been characterized in great detail in order to understand how network units are precisely coordinated to achieve proper timing of the different muscle groups in locomotion. Studies have shown that different modulatory systems act on the spinal networks to change the rate of burst activity (Grillner et al., 1995; Pearson & Gordon, 2000).

CPG in Humans. Do spinal CPGs also contribute to the control of gait in humans? A large amount of evidence from spinal cord-injured individuals during partial weight support treadmill walking suggests that CPGs contribute to pattern generation during gait (Dietz, 1997; Zehr & Duysens, 2004). Zehr and Duysens (2004) note that modulation of motor activity correlated with changes in peripheral feedback during gait can also infer CPG activity in humans, and thus activity in a feedback pathway can be used as a probe of CPG activity. As a result of this logic, the modulation of cutaneous reflexes during locomotion in humans has been used to infer the presence of activity of a CPG in humans.

As might be expected, in humans, the most convincing evidence for CPGs comes from neonates, as descending pathways from the brain are not developed. For example, stepping is observed in newborns, though they do not have mature pyramidal tracts; in addition, newborns have reflexes to perturbations during walking (Pang & Yang, 2000, 2001, 2002; Pang et al., 2003). In addition, research evidence indicates that limb loading (activating GTOs) and hip position (activating muscle spindles) regulate stepping patterns in newborns as they also do in spinalized cats (Pang & Yang, 2000; Yang et al., 1998; Zehr & Duysens, 2004).

Although spinal pattern generators are able to produce stereotyped locomotor patterns and perform certain adaptive functions, descending pathways from higher centers and sensory feedback from the periphery allow the rich variation in locomotor patterns and adaptability to task and environmental conditions.

Descending Influences

Descending influences from higher brain centers are also important in the control of locomotor activity. Using resting state functional magnetic resonance imaging (fMRI), researchers have shown that among healthy adults, connectivity of midbrain and cerebellar locomotor regions is associated with walking capacity (Boyne et al., 2018). In fact, walking capacity is more strongly associated with connectivity of these brain regions than with other phenotypic variables such as age or sex. Studies have also shown that the motor cortex and corticospinal tract contribute directly to the muscle activity observed in steady-state walking, and this cortical activity is even more pronounced when the placement of the foot is visually guided (Jensen et al., 2018; Petersen et al., 2012). Nevertheless, much of the research on identifying the roles of higher centers in controlling locomotion has been conducted through transecting the brain of animals along the neuraxis and observing the subsequent locomotor behavior (Pearson & Gordon, 2000).

Research Using Decerebrate Preparations

The second type of preparation used to study the control of gait, the decerebrate preparation, leaves the spinal cord, brainstem, and cerebellum intact. Using this preparation, researchers have discovered that an area in the brainstem called the "MLR" (Fig. 12.12) is important in the descending control of locomotion (see Chapter 3 for more information on its control of posture and locomotion). Decerebrate cats will not normally walk on a treadmill but will begin to walk normally when tonic electrical stimulation is applied to the MLR (Shik et al., 1966). Neurons from the MLR activate the medial reticular formation (MRF in Fig. 12.12), which then activates the spinal locomotor system. Weight support and active propulsion are locomotor characteristics seen in this preparation.

When spinal pattern-generating circuits are stimulated by tonic activation, they produce, at best, a bad caricature of walking due to the lack of important modulating influences from the brainstem and cerebellum. This is because normally, within each step cycle, the cerebellum receives afferent feedback from sensory receptors related to locomotion (via spinocerebellar pathways) and sends modulating signals to the brainstem that are relayed to the spinal cord (see Fig. 12.12) via brainstem nuclei (vestibulospinal, rubrospinal, and reticulospinal pathways), which act directly on motor neurons, to fine-tune the movements according to the needs of the task (Grillner & Zangger, 1979).

The cerebellum also may have a very important role in modulation of the step cycle. Experiments suggest that two tracts are involved in this modulation. First, the dorsal spinocerebellar tract is hypothesized to send information from muscle afferents to the cerebellum and is phasically active during locomotion. Second, the ventral spinocerebellar tract is hypothesized to receive information from spinal neurons concerning the CPG output and to send this information also to the cerebellum (Arshavsky et al., 1972a, 1972b).

It is also possible that the cerebellum has an additional role in the modulation of the step cycle. It has been shown that automatic aspects of gait control are regulated by the medial zone of the cerebellum, which receives input from somatosensory, visual, and vestibular systems and sends outputs to the reticular formation of the brainstem. The intermediate zones largely regulate gait through somatosensory input from the limbs, while the lateral cerebellum may adjust gait in novel contexts and when visual guidance is critical (Takakusaki et al., 2008).

Results of this and other research suggest that the cerebellum may also modulate activity, not to correct error but to alter stepping patterns. For example, as an animal crosses uneven terrain, the legs must be lifted higher or lower depending on visual cues about the obstacles encountered. The muscle response patterns may be modulated through the following steps. First, the locomotor rhythm is conveyed to the cerebellum. The cerebellum extrapolates forward in time to specify when the next flexion (or extension) is to occur. The cerebellum would then facilitate descending commands that originate from visual inputs to alter the flexion (or extension) phase at precisely the correct time (Keele & Ivry, 1990).

Research Using Decorticate Preparations

The decorticate preparation also leaves the basal ganglia intact, with only the cerebral cortex removed. As mentioned in Chapter 3, basal ganglia–brainstem–spinal cord pathways contribute to automatic control of movements such as locomotion and postural tone mainly via pathways originating in the substantia nigra and the mesencephalic area of the reticulospinal systems. These pathways appear to maintain appropriate postural muscle tone as well as to modulate rhythmic stepping movements and to initiate locomotion (Takakusaki, 2017). In this preparation, an external stimulus is not required to produce locomotor behavior, and this behavior is reasonably normal and goal directed.

Locomotor Control with the Intact Nervous System

Though the previously discussed studies show the contributions of lower nervous system centers to gait control, the cortex is very important in skills such as walking over uneven terrain. In this preparation, vision may have a major role in modulating locomotor outputs (see Fig. 12.12). As reviewed in Chapter 3, the two major pathways involved in visual processing from the primary visual cortex go to the posterior parietal cortex and inferotemporal cortex, often called the "where and what" pathways or, alternatively, the "perception and action" pathways (Milner & Goodale, 1993). These pathways help us to visually recognize objects and events from different viewpoints and to process this information from an egocentric perspective, so that we can move efficiently in space. In addition, visual input to the superior colliculus is involved in orienting to novel stimuli in the visual field. It is of interest that walking subjects are aware of the objects around them and alter their steps even when no visual information is currently available about obstacle locations. In addition, cats that have stepped over an obstacle in the past remember the location of that obstacle and use this information to guide stepping. However, if cats have parietal cortex lesions, they can no longer adjust their limbs to negotiate obstacles successfully. Intentional gait modification requires motor programming in the premotor cortices. Such motor programs utilize information about the body, sometimes referred to as the body schema, which is preserved and updated in the temporoparietal cortex (Takakusaki, 2013). Basal ganglia and cerebellar loops may serve the purpose of processing limb trajectories to achieve accurate foot placement, and thus might be the neural structures involved in locomotor movements that require volitional control, cognition, and attention (Lajoie & Drew, 2007; McVea & Pearson, 2009; Middleton & Strick, 2000; Takakusaki et al., 2008).

It has been hypothesized that the hippocampus is the site that codes topological information, while the parietal cortex (receiving visual and somatosensory information) provides a metric representation of three-dimensional space. The frontal cortex, along with the basal ganglia, would then transform this information into appropriate spatially directed locomotor movements in an egocentric frame (Paillard, 1987; Patla, 1997).

Evidence regarding cortical control of locomotion in primates shows that injections of muscimol into the hindlimb region of the motor cortex (M1) cause local paresis of the contralateral hindlimb when walking. This same injection into trunk and hindlimb areas of the supplementary motor area (SMA), which has connections to the reticular formation, disturbs postural control rather than paralyzing the limb. It is also likely that premotor cortex and SMA contribute to planning and programming of locomotion, in addition to postural control, as patients with lesions in these areas show problems with gait initiation and with freezing of gait. This may be because corticoreticular pathways are important for postural preparation before gait initiation (Takakusaki et al., 2008) (see Chapter 3 for more detailed information on locomotor pathways).

It is now possible to record cerebral activity during the gait cycle through neuroimaging techniques like single-photon emission tomography (SPECT), measuring regional cerebral blood flow, and near-infrared spectroscopy (NIRS), measuring oxygenated versus deoxygenated hemoglobin levels. SPECT studies during gait have shown increased activity in the SMA, medial primary sensorimotor area, striatum, cerebellar vermis, visual cortex, and dorsal brainstem (Fukuyama et al., 1997; Hanakawa et al., 1999). NIRS techniques have also shown that activity increases in the prefrontal and premotor cortex as locomotor speed increases, while sensorimotor cortex activity was not influenced by speed (Bakker et al., 2007; Suzuki et al., 2004). This research is in its infancy, but it reminds us of the many brain regions that contribute to the control of gait.

Musculoskeletal Contributions to Gait

So far, we have looked at neuromuscular contributions to the control of gait, but there are also important musculoskeletal contributions. Biomechanical analyses of locomotion in cats have determined the contributions of both muscular and nonmuscular forces to the generation of gait dynamics (Hoy & Zernicke, 1985, 1986; Hoy et al., 1985; Smith & Zernicke, 1987). This involves a type of kinetic analysis called *inverse dynamics*. To understand more about inverse dynamics, refer to the Technology Tool 12.1.

When an inverse dynamics analysis of limb dynamics is used, it is possible to determine the relative importance of the muscular and nonmuscular contributions (Hoy & Zernicke, 1985; Wisleder et al., 1990). For example, during locomotion in the cat, there are high passive extensor torques at a joint, which must be counteracted by active flexor torques generated by the muscles, when the animal is moving at one speed, or in one part of the step cycle. When the speed is increased, or the animal moves to a different part of the cycle, the passive torques that must be counteracted change completely. How does the dialogue between the passive properties of the system and the neural pattern-generating circuits occur? This is still unclear, although the discharge from somatosensory receptors plays a role (Hoy et al., 1985; Smith & Zernicke, 1987; Wisleder et al., 1990). Changes in the passive properties of the musculoskeletal system that occur secondary to primary neuropathology can influence gait in geriatric and neurologic populations. This will be discussed in Chapter 14.

To summarize the research on the neural control of normal locomotion, studies have shown that there is a continuous interaction between the CPGs and descending signals. Higher centers contribute to locomotion through feedforward modulation of patterns in response to the goals of the individual and to environmental demands. As noted briefly previously, the nervous system takes into account nonneuromuscular forces in the control of gait. In addition, sensory inputs are critical for feedback and feedforward modulation of locomotor activity in order to adapt it to changing environmental conditions.

SENSORY SYSTEMS AND THE CONTROL OF GAIT

Sensory information from all the senses plays a critical role in all three of the main determinants of gait: progression, postural control, and adaptation. Differentiating the contribution of sensory information to these three determinants can be difficult, because of the interactions among the three determinants. For example, as you will see in the following, somatosensory feedback, specifically information from the hip flexors in terminal stance, plays a role in progression by activating the swing phase of gait. Somatosensory inputs, in this case from cutaneous receptors, also contribute to recovery of gait stability following contact with an obstacle. In animals, when all sensory information is taken away, stepping patterns tend to be very slow and stereotyped. The animal can neither maintain balance nor modify its stepping patterns to make gait truly functional. Gait ataxia is a common consequence among patients with sensory loss, particularly loss of proprioceptive information from the lower extremities (Sudarsky & Ronthal, 1992).

Somatosensory Systems

As noted earlier in the chapter, researchers have shown that animals that have both been spinalized and undergone deafferentation can continuously generate rhythmic alternating contractions in muscles of all the joints of the leg, with a pattern similar to that seen in the normal step cycle (Grillner & Zangger, 1979). Does this mean that sensory information plays no role in the control of locomotion? No. Although these experiments have shown that animals can still walk in the absence of sensory feedback from the limbs, the movements show characteristic differences from those in the normal animal. These differences help us to understand the role that sensory input plays in the control of locomotion (Smith, 1980).

First, during normal steady-state gait, sensory information from the limbs contributes to appropriate stepping frequency. For example, the duration of the step cycle is significantly longer in cats that have undergone deafferentation than in a chronic spinalized cat (i.e., spinalized previously and allowed to recover) without deafferentation.

Second, as mentioned earlier, joint receptors and muscle spindle afferents (from the stretched hip flexors) contribute to the onset of swing phase (Grillner & Rossignol, 1978; Pearson, 1995; Smith, 1980). Studies of decerebrate cats have shown that input from muscle spindles can reset the locomotor rhythm. Activation of both ankle extensor Ia afferents and group II flexor afferents resets the rhythm to extension in fictive locomotion. In addition, small movements about the hip joint produce entrainment of the locomotor rhythm. This continues after anesthetizing the joint capsule, and it gradually is reduced in strength when more hip muscles are denervated. This and other research suggests that muscle spindle afferents from hip flexors influence the rhythm-generating neurons by exciting hip flexor activity. Figure 12.13 shows how hip extension controls the transition from stance to swing. The hip flexor muscle spindle afferents (shown in the diagram of a cat whose hip is oscillating in flexion and extension) are stretched sufficiently at the end of stance phase to excite their own muscle (hip flexor) and inhibit the hip extensors, thus aiding in the stance to swing phase transition (Kriellaars et al., 1994; Pearson & Gordon, 2000).

This information has been used to aid individuals in relearning gait after a stroke. Gait has been retrained using partial body weight support during treadmill walking and the hip extension as the leg is drawn backward during stance phase on the treadmill aids in the activation of hip flexors to initiate swing phase.

The GTO afferents (the Ib afferents) from the leg extensor muscles can also strongly influence the timing of the locomotor rhythm during steady-state gait, by inhibiting flexor burst activity and promoting extensor activity. A decline in their activity at the end of the stance phase may be involved in regulating the transition from stance to swing (Pearson, 2004).

In addition, GTO afferents contribute to the adaptation of gait to changing terrain characteristics. They provide a mechanism for automatically compensating for changes in loads carried by extensor muscles. For example, when one walks up an incline, the load increase on the extensor muscles would increase the feedback from the GTOs and automatically increase the activity in the extensor motor neurons. Note that this activity of the GTOs is exactly the opposite of their activity when they are activated passively, when the animal is at rest. At rest,

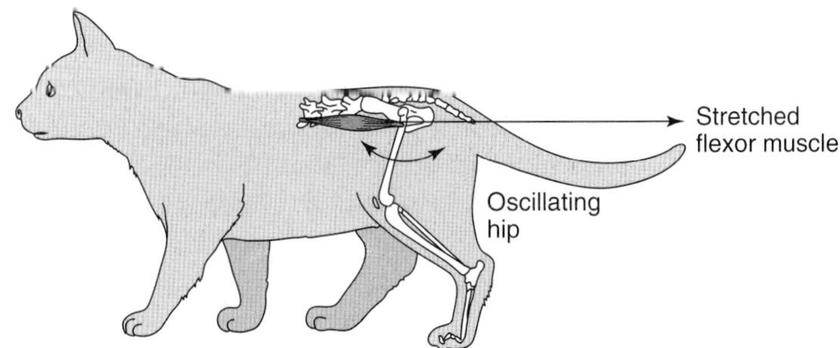

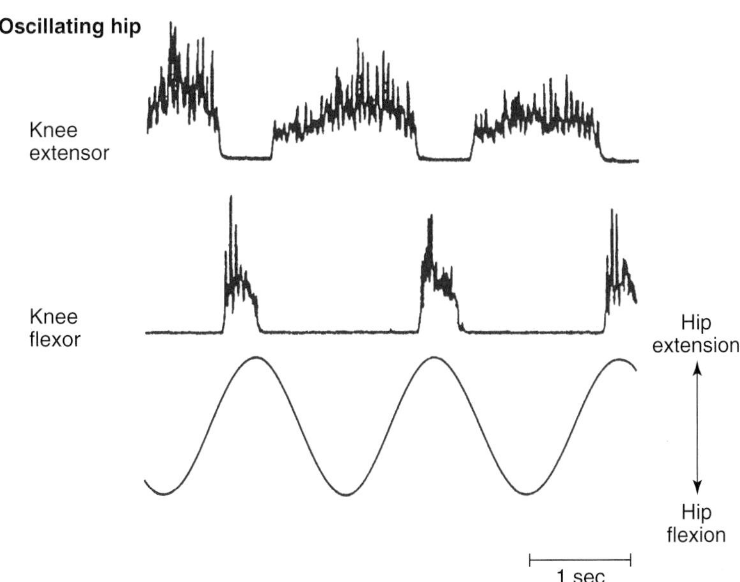

Figure 12.13 Cat whose hip is being oscillated in flexion and extension. The flexor muscle is stretched during extension (e.g., in the stance phase of locomotion), and flexor muscle spindle afferents then excite the flexors and inhibit the extensors. (Reprinted from Pearson K, Gordon J. Locomotion. In: Kandel E, Schwartz JH, Jessell TM, eds. *Principles of neural science,* 4th ed. New York, NY: McGraw-Hill, 2000:748, with permission Fig. 37.8.)

the GTOs inhibit their own muscle and excite the antagonist muscles, while during locomotion, they excite their own muscle and inhibit antagonists (Pearson & Gordon, 2000; Pearson et al., 1992).

Third, cutaneous information has an important role in postural control, specifically reactive balance. For example, cutaneous information from the paw of the chronic spinalized cat has a powerful influence on the spinal pattern generator and ensures recovery of stability when the animal's paw hits an obstacle, as discussed previously (Forssberg et al., 1977).

It is of interest that in human research (normal adults), it is difficult to produce a strong effect on gait transition when performing loading and unloading experiments on the extensor muscles, unlike what was noted previously in the cat (Stephens & Yang, 1999). Why do we see this difference? It is probably the case that these cues do not operate in isolation in humans, and other influences may override the unloading effect (Zehr & Duysens, 2004). However, it appears that cutaneous input and stretch reflexes are more tightly controlled during human gait than are loading reflexes. For example, human research, similar to animal research, has shown that these reflexes are enhanced during gait as compared with quiet stance and are highly modulated in locomotion during each phase of the step cycle; this allows them to adapt functionally to the requirements of each phase (Stein, 1991; Zehr et al., 1997).

As was shown in research on cats, cutaneous reflexes actually showed a complete reversal from excitation to inhibition during the different phases of the step cycle. For example, in the first part of swing phase, when the TA is active, the foot is in the air and little cutaneous input would be expected, unless the foot strikes an object. If this happens, a rapid flexion would be needed to lift the foot over the object to prevent tripping. This is when the reflex is excitatory to the TA. However, in the second TA burst, the foot is about to contact the ground, which is a time when a lot of cutaneous input would occur. Limb flexion would not be appropriate at this time, since the limb is needed to support the body. In addition, at this time, the reflex shows inhibition of the TA (Stein, 1991; Zehr & Duysens, 2004). It is interesting that humans have both short-latency and middle-latency (75–80 ms) responses to cutaneous stimulation, unlike cats, who show most evidence for short-latency responses. In humans, it is the middle-latency responses that show the phase-dependent modulation.

Stretch reflexes in the ankle extensor muscles are small in the early part of the stance phase of locomotion, since this is the time that the body is rotating over the foot and stretching the ankle extensors. A large reflex at this phase of the step cycle would slow or even reverse forward momentum.

On the other hand, the stretch reflex is large when the COM is in front of the foot during the last part of stance phase, since this is the time when the reflex can help in propelling the body forward. This phase-appropriate modulation of the stretch reflex is well suited to the requirements of the task of locomotion as compared with stance. Stretch reflex gains are reduced in running, probably because a high gain reflex response would destabilize the gait in running. Stretch reflex gain changes alter quickly (within 150 ms) as a person moves from stance to walking to running (Stein, 1991).

It is important to note that modulation of stretch reflex amplitudes is sometimes different from that seen in cutaneous reflexes. For example, BFi stretch reflexes are facilitated at the end of swing, supporting the hypothesis that part of this muscle's activation at this time is due to stretch reflex input. This is at a time when cutaneous reflexes to this muscle are suppressed (Zehr & Duysens, 2004).

Up to now, we have talked about phase-dependent modulation of medium-latency reflexes and their importance in the control of gait; however, task-dependent reflex modulation is also thought to be an important factor in maintaining stable locomotion. Task-dependent modulation occurs when there is a change in task demands. For example, cutaneous reflexes in leg muscles are modulated with increased risk of instability during walking. Increasing threats to stability, for example, walking on a treadmill with arms crossed, increases cutaneous reflex amplitude, while walking under more stable condition (e.g., while walking on a treadmill and holding onto handles) significantly reduces reflex amplitudes (Haridas et al., 2005). There is evidence to suggest that task- and phase-dependent reflex modulation is mediated by descending cortical influences (Haridas et al., 2005; Pijnappels et al., 1998).

Finally, somatosensory information appears to be very important in ensuring normal interlimb coordination. In neurologically intact adults, regulation of rhythmic arm and leg movement during human locomotion is supported by interlimb reflexes that depend on propriospinal connections and interneuronal networks coupling the lumbar and cervical spinal cord (Dietz et al., 2001; Haridas & Zehr, 2003; Juvin et al., 2005; Lamont & Zehr, 2007; Mezzarane et al., 2011; Nathan et al., 1996; Zehr & Duysens, 2004; Zehr et al., 2007a, 2007b). Nerve stimulation applied at either the hand or the ankle results in phase-dependent modulation of interlimb reflexes in muscles in all four limbs, which contributes to the maintenance of postural stability during gait (Haridas & Zehr, 2003). Neural pathology that interrupts the regulation of interlimb coordination has a significant effect on the control of gait (Kautz & Patten, 2005; Tseng & Morton, 2010; Zehr & Loadman, 2012).

Vision

Work with humans suggests that there are a variety of ways in which vision modulates locomotion in a feedback manner. First, visual flow cues help us determine our speed of locomotion (Lackner & DiZio, 1988). Studies have shown that if one doubles the rate of optic flow past subjects as they walk, 100% of them will increase their stride length. In addition, about half will perceive that the force exerted during each step is less than normal. However, other subjects will perceive that they have nearly doubled their stepping frequency (Lackner & DiZio, 1992).

Visual flow cues also influence the alignment of the body with reference to gravity and the environment during walking. For example, when researchers tilted the room surrounding a treadmill on which a person was running, it caused the person to incline the trunk in the direction of the tilted room to compensate for the visual illusion of body tilt in the opposite direction (Lee & Young, 1986). Is this effect similar during overground walking? Martelli and colleagues (2019) looked at the extent to which healthy adults modify and adapt gait during overground walking using a virtual reality headset. Adults displayed shorter steps and higher variability in step width while walking in the virtual environment. Multidirectional perturbations of the visual field lead to further disruptions—adults displayed shorter, wider, and more variable steps. However, these gait modifications were reduced over time, suggesting that adults may rely more on other sensory systems than vision for regulating gait patterns.

How do we sample the environment for proactive visual control? Visual processing time is shared with other tasks, and thus, the terrain is typically sampled for less than 10% of our travel time when walking over even surfaces. However, when uneven surfaces are simulated by requiring subjects to step on specific locations, visual monitoring goes up to about 30% (Patla, 1997; Patla et al., 1996). In an experiment in which individuals were asked to wear opaque liquid crystal glasses and press a handheld switch to make the glasses transparent when they wanted to sample the environment, results showed that even in a novel environment, individuals could walk safely while sampling less than 50% of the time. Visual sampling was increased when specific foot placement was required or if there was a hazard in the path (Patla et al., 1996).

To what extent do we use central versus peripheral vision in proactive control of gait? To answer this question, researchers asked participants to wear goggles that could occlude the upper, lower, or circumferential peripheral visual field, while they were walking over obstacles. The researchers found that even without cues from the lower or peripheral visual field, the participants could complete the task safely, suggesting that subjects used central visual information in a feedforward manner to help them negotiate the obstacles. However, participants were much more variable in their performance under the peripheral occlusion conditions, increasing minimum foot clearance and decreasing walking speed and step length, suggesting that peripheral visual information is used for online control of the legs during obstacle crossing (Graci et al., 2009, 2010).

Vestibular System

An important part of controlling locomotion is stabilizing the head, since it contains two of the most important sensors for controlling motion: the vestibular and visual systems (Berthoz & Pozzo, 1994). The otolith organs, the saccule and the utricle, detect the angle of the head with respect to gravity, and the visual system also provides us with the so-called visual vertical.

Adults appear to stabilize the head, and thus gaze, by covarying both pitch (forward) rotation and vertical displacement of the head to give stability to the head in the sagittal plane (Pozzo et al., 1990, 1992). The head is stabilized with a precision (within a few degrees) that is compatible with the efficiency of the vestibuloocular reflex, an important mechanism for stabilizing gaze during head movement.

It has been hypothesized that during complex movements, like walking, postural control is not organized from the support surface upward, in what is called a "bottom-up mode," but is organized in relation to the control of gaze, in what is called a "top-down mode." Thus, in this mode, head movements are independent from the movements of the trunk. It has been shown that the process for stabilizing the head is disrupted in patients with bilateral labyrinthine lesions (Berthoz & Pozzo, 1994), suggesting the vestibular system plays an important role in controlling gait.

Anson and colleagues (2019) confirmed the importance of vestibular function in controlling gait. They showed that a decreases in the horizontal semicircular canal function (rotatory information) results in longer stride length, longer stance time, and slower cadence. However, otolith function (linear acceleration information) does not seem to be associated with any specific gait parameter.

How do we navigate in a large-scale spatial environment? Humans use what is called a "piloting strategy," which requires a mental representation of the spatial environment. These cognitive maps include both topological information (relationships of landmarks in the environment) and metric information (specific distances and directions). Topological information is needed when obstacles constrain our travel path. The fact that most animals can also accurately take shortcuts to reach a goal supports the concept that metric information is also used in navigation (Patla, 1997).

COGNITIVE SYSTEMS AND GAIT

As mentioned in Chapter 7, although posture and gait are often considered to be automatic, they require attentional processing resources, and the amount of resources required varies depending on the difficulty of the cognitive as well as the postural or locomotor task. Experiments using a dual-task design have led researchers to propose a hierarchy of cognitive, postural, and gait tasks based on attentional processing requirements of the tasks. The least resources are required for nondemanding tasks. For postural tasks, this includes sitting or standing with feet shoulder width apart; attentional demands increase when standing in tandem Romberg position, walking (Lajoie et al., 1993), during obstacle avoidance while walking (Chen et al., 1996), and during recovery from external perturbations (Brown et al., 1999; Rankin et al., 2000).

Dual-Task Performance during Steady-State Gait

In a study by Lajoie et al. (1993), young adults were asked to perform an auditory reaction time task while sitting, while standing with a normal versus a reduced base of support, and during walking (comparing single- vs. double-support phase). Reaction times were fastest for sitting and slowed for the standing and walking tasks. Reaction times were slower in the single-support phase as compared with the double-support phase of the step cycle.

Lajoie et al.'s study focused on examining the attentional demands associated with gait (i.e., its effect on the performance of a secondary task) and reported no change in gait parameters associated with the performance of a simple reaction time task in young adults. The increase in reaction time when walking, while not affecting gait parameters, suggests that walking requires more attention than standing or sitting. Ebersbach et al. (1995) specifically studied the effect of concurrent tasks on the control of gait. They measured gait parameters (stride time, double-support time) under a single-task condition (walking without a concurrent task) and four dual-task conditions presented in random order: (1) memory retention task (digit-span recall), (2) fine-motor task (opening and closing a coat button continuously while walking), (3) a combination task (digit-recall and buttoning task), and (4) finger tapping at 5 Hz or faster. The only dual-task condition that produced a significant decrease in stride time (increased stride frequency) was finger tapping. The other gait parameter measured, double-support time, was significantly affected when the fine-motor and memory tasks were performed synchronously with the walking; no other dual-task condition affected this parameter. Interestingly, the authors noted that performance of the gait task did affect the digit-recall task. The mean digit-span recall was 6.7 (range 6–8) during quiet stance but reduced to 5.8

(range 4–8) during walking. In this study, the significant changes in gait parameters were fairly small, suggesting that performance of a simple cognitive task during unperturbed gait does not present a significant threat to stability in healthy young adults.

However, it is also clear that performance of more complex cognitive tasks, such as cell phone use, does create a threat for injury during walking. Data show that increases in pedestrian injuries related to mobile phone use have paralleled the increase in injuries for drivers and that cell phone use while walking puts pedestrians at risk of accident, injury, or death (Nasar & Troyer, 2013).

It is interesting that this research contrasts previous laboratory-based studies indicating that young adults have only minimal dual-task interference during walking; this new research suggests that cell phone use while walking in the real world causes significant interference with gait associated with increased risk of injury. Deterioration in gait performance in this dual-task context includes reduced gait speed, weaving, and noticing significantly fewer objects in the surrounding environment. In addition, young adults using a cell phone demonstrate more risky behavior when crossing a street than those not distracted by a cell phone conversation or texting (during experiments, this results in more hits by virtual vehicles) (Plummer et al., 2015). Adults seem to place greater value on talking than the task of walking safely, but this appears to be task specific. When the task of walking in addition to talking has increased challenges (e.g., walking over obstacles or carrying a tray), both speech and gait appear to be affected. Nevertheless, adults *are* capable of flexibly allocating resources to the subcomponents of the overall task (Raffegeau et al., 2018). For example, when adults are informed about the probability of slipping or falling, adults adapt their gait during dual-tasking to avoid injury. Soangra and Lockhart (2017) found that both young and old adults adopted a more cautious gait strategy—evidenced by reduced walking speed, shorter step length, increased step width, and reduced heel contact velocity—during dual-task walking (walking while counting backward starting from a random number) followed by a slip perturbation.

Dual-Task Performance during Obstacle Crossing

Chen and colleagues (1996) examined the effect of dividing attention on the ability to step over obstacles efficiently. In this study, individuals were asked to walk down a walkway and to step over a virtual object (a band of light) when a red light turned on at the end of the walkway. On some trials, they were asked to perform a secondary task involving giving a vocal response. The authors measured obstacle contact in single- versus dual-task conditions. Results indicated that obstacle contact was increased when attention was divided.

One interesting question regarding the attentional requirements of obstacle crossing is the time course of attentional demands and when they are the highest. To answer this question, Brown and colleagues (2005) compared the attentional demands associated with steady-state walking and the precrossing and crossing phases of an obstacle task. They found that young adults directed more attention to gait during precrossing than during obstacle crossing.

Though it is clear that obstacle crossing requires attentional resources, the extent to which it affects the performance of the postural versus cognitive task is not understood. Using a dual-task paradigm, Siu et al. (2008a) examined the extent to which young adults were able to respond to a secondary auditory Stroop task (the words "high" vs. "low," spoken in a high vs. low pitch, a task which requires executive attentional network resources) during obstacle crossing as compared to steady-state walking or sitting. They found that as the level of difficulty of the postural task increased, young adults showed a significant reduction in their verbal response time in the auditory Stroop task, but no differences in gait. This confirms previous research showing that postural tasks require attention, and it further shows that young adults use a strategy during dual-task performance of reducing performance on the auditory Stroop task while maintaining gait performance. This confirms the existence of a hierarchy of control for young adults within both postural/locomotor task (obstacle avoidance has the highest attentional requirements) and dual-task (gait stability has a higher priority) conditions, within this context. This is different than the results from studies of cell phone use during gait, where cell phone use received priority in the dual-task conditions. It is thus clear that prioritization of postural and gait control is task dependent and modifiable.

Research has shown that instructions regarding attentional focus modify performance during dual-task walking. Siu and colleagues (2008b) next examined obstacle crossing while performing an auditory Stroop task, under three different instructional conditions: no focus (no specific instructions related to attentional focus), focus on the obstacle, and focus on the Stroop task. The paradigm for this study is explained in Figure 12.14. As shown in Figure 12.15A, attentional focus significantly impacted verbal reaction times in healthy young adults. Specifically, when told to focus on the Stroop task (FS condition), reaction times were much faster compared to the focus on the obstacle (FO) condition. Changes in performance related to instructional focus were also seen in the obstacle task. As shown in Figure 12.15B, when told to FO, trailing limb toe clearance was significantly greater than when participants focused on either the Stroop task or both tasks equally. Similar to previous research, Siu and colleagues (2008a) demonstrated that attentional demands

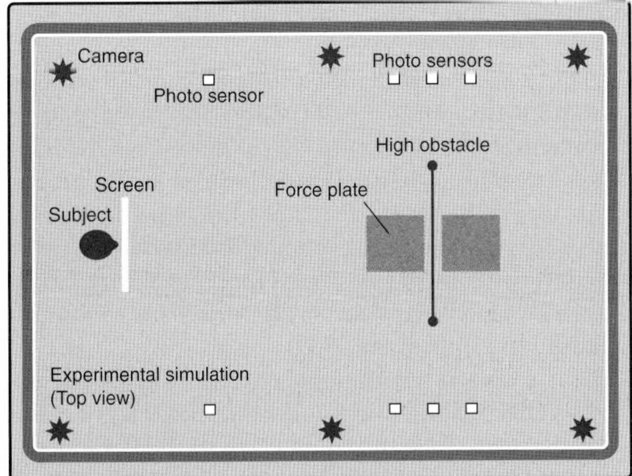

Figure 12.14 Paradigm used to study the effect of a secondary task on obstacle crossing while walking. A screen is used to initially block visual information regarding the obstacle. The screen is removed and the person walks while performing the auditory Stroop task and steps over the obstacle. Force plates on both sides of the obstacle measure forces. Cameras measure the kinematics of walking under the multiple conditions.

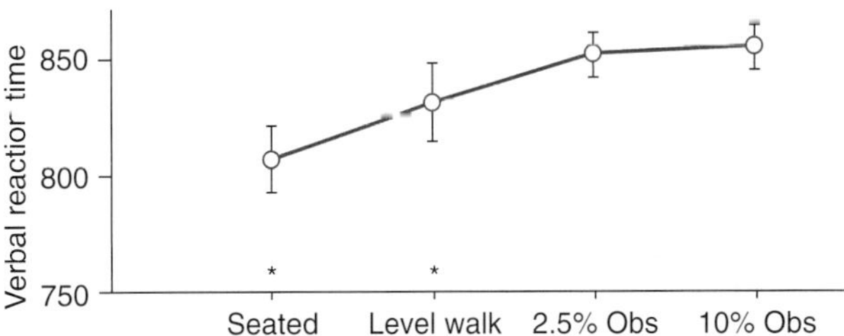

Figure 12.16 Attentional demands (as indicated by longer verbal reaction times) are higher during obstacle crossing compared to sitting or level walking, with attentional demands increasing slightly as obstacle height increases. (Adapted from Winter DA. Kinematic and kinetic patterns of human gait: variability and compensating effects. *Hum Mov Sci*. 1984;3:51–76, with permission.)

were higher during obstacle crossing compared to sitting or level walking (see Fig. 12.16), with attentional demands increasing as obstacle height increased.

STAIR WALKING

Stair walking accounts for the largest percentage of falls occurring in public places, with four out of five falls occurring during stair descent. Understanding the sensory and motor requirements associated with stair walking is critical to retraining this skill. Stairs represent a significant hazard even among individuals without disability. Stair walking is similar to level walking in that it involves stereotypical reciprocal alternating movements of the lower limbs (Craik et al., 1982; Simoneau et al., 1991). Like locomotion, successful negotiation of stairs has three requirements: (a) the generation of primarily concentric forces to propel the body upstairs or eccentric forces to control the body's descent downstairs (progression), (b) controlling the COM within a constantly changing base of support (stability), and (c) the capacity to adapt strategies used for progression and stability to accommodate changes in stair environment, such as height, width, and the presence or absence of railings (adaptation) (McFadyen & Winter, 1988).

Sensory information is important for controlling the body's position in space (stability) and to identify critical aspects of the stair environment so that appropriate movement strategies can be programmed (adaptation). Researchers have shown that normal subjects change movement strategies used for negotiating

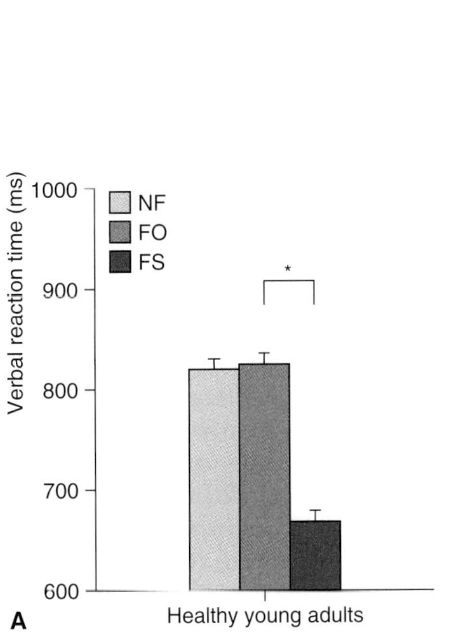

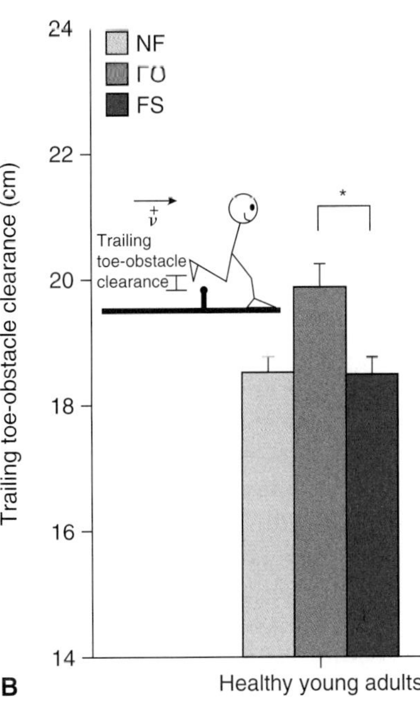

Figure 12.15 Changes in performance related to instructional focus during dual-task obstacle walking. Instructions to focus on the Stroop task (FS) resulted in faster verbal reaction times **(A)** compared to focus on the obstacle (FO) condition. Trailing limb toe clearance **(B)** was greater when the focus on attention was on the obstacle task (FO) compared to the other two conditions. (Reprinted from Moore KL, Dalley AF, Agur AMR. *Clinically oriented anatomy*, 8th ed. Baltimore, MD: Lippincott Williams & Wilkins, 2017, Figure 7.23 with permission.)

stairs when sensory cues about stair characteristics are altered (Craik et al., 1982; Simoneau et al., 1991).

Similar to gait, stair climbing has been divided into two phases: a stance phase lasting approximately 64% of the full cycle and a swing phase lasting 36% of the cycle. In addition, each phase of stair walking has been further subdivided to reflect the objectives that need to be achieved during each phase.

Ascent

During ascent, the stance phase is subdivided into weight acceptance, pull-up, and forward continuance, while swing is divided into foot clearance and foot placement stages.

During stance, weight acceptance is initiated with the middle to front portion of the foot. Pull-up occurs because of extensor activity at the knee and ankle, primarily concentric contractions of the vastus lateralis and soleus muscles. Stair ascent differs from level walking in two ways: (a) forces needed to accomplish ascent are two times greater than those needed to control level gait, and (b) the knee extensors generate most of the energy to move the body forward during stair ascent. Finally, during the forward continuance phase of stance, the ankle generates forward and lift forces; however, ankle force is not the main source of power behind forward progression in stair walking. In controlling balance during stair ascent, the greatest instability comes with contralateral toe-off, when the ipsilateral leg takes the total body weight and the hip, knee, and ankle joints are flexed (McFadyen & Winter, 1988).

The objectives of the swing phase of stair climbing are similar to those of level gait and include foot clearance and placing the foot appropriately so weight can be accepted for the next stance phase. Foot clearance is achieved through activation of the TA, dorsiflexing the foot, and activation of the hamstrings, which flex the knee. The RFi contracts eccentrically to reverse this motion by midswing. The swing leg is brought up and forward through activation of the hip flexors of the swing leg and motion of the contralateral stance leg. Final foot placement is controlled by the hip extensors and ankle dorsiflexors (McFadyen & Winter, 1988).

Descent

Walking upstairs is accomplished through concentric contractions of the RFi, vastus lateralis, soleus, and medial gastrocnemius. In contrast, walking downstairs is achieved through eccentric contractions of these same muscles, which work to control the body with respect to the force of gravity. The stance phase of stair descent is subdivided into weight acceptance, forward continuance, and controlled lowering, while swing has two phases: leg pull-through and preparation for foot placement (Craik et al., 1982; McFadyen & Winter, 1988).

The weight-acceptance phase is characterized by absorption of energy at the ankle and knee through the eccentric contraction of the triceps surae, RFi, and vastus lateralis. Energy absorption during this phase is critical, since ground reaction forces as much as two times body weight have been recorded when the swing limb first contacts the stair. Activation of the gastrocnemius prior to stair contact is responsible for cushioning the landing (Craik et al., 1982).

The forward continuance phase reflects the forward motion of the body and precedes the controlled lowering phase of stance. Lowering of the body is controlled primarily by the eccentric contraction of the quadriceps muscles and, to a lesser degree, the eccentric contraction of the soleus muscle.

During swing, the leg is pulled through, because of activation of the hip flexor muscles. However, by midswing, flexion of the hip and knee is reversed, and all three joints extend in preparation for foot placement. Contact is made with the lateral border of the foot and is associated with TA and gastrocnemius activity prior to foot contact.

Adapting Stair-Walking Patterns to Changes in Sensory Cues

Researchers have shown that neurologically intact people adapt the movement strategies they use for going up and down stairs in response to changes in sensory information about the task. Adults primarily use peripheral vision with occasional downward gaze shifts to walk downstairs (Miyasike-daSilva & McIlroy, 2016). Thus, when normal subjects wear large collars that obstruct their view of the stairs, anticipatory activation of the gastrocnemius prior to foot contact is reduced. This anticipatory activity is further reduced when the subject is blindfolded. In this study, subjects still managed a soft landing by changing the control strategy used to descend stairs. Subjects moved more slowly, protracting swing time and using the stance limb to control the landing (Craik et al., 1982).

Foot clearance and placement are critical aspects of movement strategies used to safely descend stairs. Good visual information about stair height is critical. When normal subjects wear blurred-vision lenses and are unable to clearly define the edge of the step, they slow down and modify movement strategies so that foot clearance is increased and the foot is placed further back on the step to ensure a larger margin of safety (Simoneau et al., 1991). Thus, information from the visual system about the step height appears to be necessary for optimal programming of movement strategies used to negotiate stairs.

MOBILITY OTHER THAN GAIT

Although mobility is often thought of solely in relationship to gait or locomotion, there are many other aspects of mobility that are essential to independence in activities of daily living. The ability to change positions, whether moving from sitting to standing, rolling, rising from a bed, or moving from one chair to another, is a fundamental part of mobility. These various types of mobility activities are often grouped together and referred to as "transfer tasks."

Retraining motor function in the patient with a neurologic impairment includes the recovery of these diverse mobility skills. This requires an understanding of (a) the essential characteristics of the task, (b) the sensory motor strategies that normal individuals typically use to accomplish the task, and (c) the adaptations required for changing environmental characteristics.

All mobility tasks share three essential task requirements: motion in a desired direction (progression), postural control (orientation and stability), and the ability to adapt to changing task and environmental conditions (adaptation). The following sections briefly review some of the research on these other aspects of mobility function. As you will see, compared to the tremendous number of studies on normal gait, there have been relatively few studies examining these other aspects of mobility function.

Transfers and Bed Mobility

Transfers and bed mobility represent important aspects of mobility function. One cannot walk if one cannot get out of a chair or rise from a bed. Inability to safely and independently change positions represents a great hindrance to the recovery of normal mobility. Several researchers have studied transfer skills from a biomechanical perspective. As a result, we know quite a bit about typical movement strategies used by neurologically intact adults when performing these tasks. However, use of a biomechanical approach has provided us with little information about the perceptual strategies associated with these various tasks. In addition, because most often research subjects are constrained to carry out the task in a unified way, we have little insight into ways in which sensory and movement strategies are modified in response to changing task and environmental demands.

Sit-to-Stand

Sit-to-stand (STS) behaviors are fundamental for functional independence. Dall and Kerr (2010) showed that adults perform on average 60 STS behaviors each day! While the biomechanics of STS have been described, there are many important questions that have not yet been studied by motor control researchers. For example, how do the movements involved in STS vary as a function of the speed of the task, the characteristics of the support, including height of the chair, the compliance of the seat, or the presence or absence of hand rests? In addition, do the requirements of the task vary depending on the nature of the task immediately following? That is, do we stand up differently if we are intending to walk instead of stand still? What perceptual information is essential to establishing efficient movement strategies when performing STS?

The essential characteristics of the STS task include the following: (a) generating sufficient joint torque needed to rise (progression), (b) ensuring stability by moving the COM from one base of support (the chair) to a base of support defined solely by the feet (stability), and (c) the ability to modify movement strategies used to achieve these goals depending on environmental constraints such as chair height, the presence of armrests, and the softness of the chair (adaptation).

The STS task has been divided into different phases—2, 3, or 4—depending on the researcher. Each phase has its own unique movement and stability requirements. A four-phase model of the STS task is shown in Figure 12.17 (Millington et al., 1992; Schenkman et al., 1990). This figure also shows the movements of the joints and the muscle activity used by a normal subject when completing this task.

The first phase, called the "weight shift" or "flexion momentum" stage, begins with the generation of forward momentum of the upper body through flexion of the trunk. The body is quite stable during this phase, since the COM, although moving forward, is

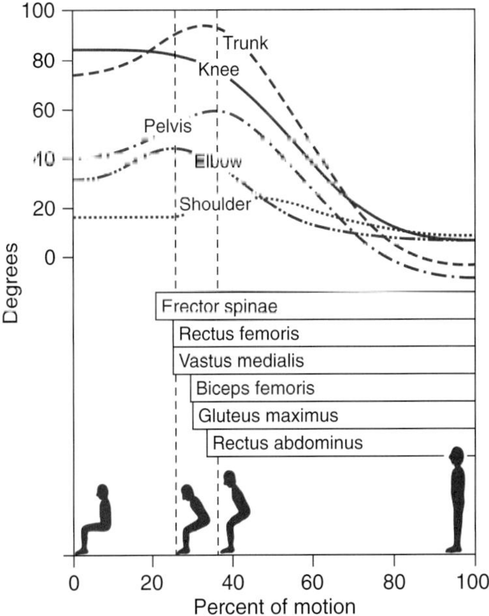

Figure 12.17 Four phases of the sit-to-stand (STS) movement, showing the kinematic and EMG patterns associated with each phase. (Adapted from Tang PF, Woollacott MH, Chong RKY. Control of reactive balance adjustments in perturbed human walking: roles of proximal and distal postural muscle activity. *Exp Brain Res.* 1998;119:141–152, with permission.)

still within the base of support of the chair seat and the feet. Muscle activity includes activation of the erector spinae, which contract eccentrically to control forward motion of the trunk (Millington et al., 1992; Schenkman et al., 1990).

Phase 2 begins as the buttocks leave the seat and involves the transfer of momentum from the upper body to the total body, allowing lift of the body. Phase 2 involves both horizontal and vertical motion of the body and is considered a critical transition phase. Stability requirements are precise, since it is during this phase that the COM of the body moves from within the base of support of the chair to that of the feet. The body is inherently unstable during this phase because the COM is located far from the center of force. Because the body has developed momentum prior to liftoff, vertical rise of the body can be achieved with little lower-extremity muscle force. Muscle activity in this phase is characterized by coactivation of hip and knee extensors, as shown in Figure 12.17 (Schenkman et al., 1990).

Phase 3 of the STS task is referred to as the "lift" or "extension" phase and is characterized by extension at the hips and knees. The goal in this phase is primarily to move the body vertically; stability requirements are less than in phase 2 since the COM is well within the base of support of the feet. The final phase of STS is the stabilization phase; it is the period following complete extension when task-dependent motion is complete and body stability in the vertical position is achieved (Schenkman et al., 1990).

STS requires the generation of propulsive impulse forces in both the horizontal and the vertical directions. However, the horizontal propulsive force responsible for moving the COM anteriorly over the base of support of the foot must change into a braking impulse to bring the body to a stop. Braking the horizontal impulse begins even before liftoff from the seat. Thus, there appears to be a preprogrammed relationship between the generation and braking of forces for the STS task. Without this coordination between propulsive and braking forces, the person could easily fall forward upon achieving the vertical position.

Horizontal displacement of the COM appears to be constant, despite changes in the speed of STS. Controlling the horizontal trajectory of the COM is probably the invariant feature controlled in STS to ensure that stability is maintained during vertical rise of the body (Millington et al., 1992).

This strategy could be referred to as a "momentum-transfer strategy," and its use requires (a) adequate strength and coordination to generate upper-body movement prior to liftoff, (b) the ability to eccentrically contract trunk and hip muscles in order to apply braking forces to slow the horizontal trajectory of the COM, and (c) concentric contraction of hip and knee muscles to generate vertical propulsive forces that lift the body (Schenkman et al., 1990).

Accomplishing STS using a momentum-transfer strategy requires a trade-off between stability and force requirements. The generation and transfer of momentum between the upper body and the total body reduces the requirement for lower-extremity force because the body is already in motion as it begins to lift. On the other hand, the body is in a precarious state of balance during the transition stage, when momentum is transferred.

An alternative strategy that ensures greater stability but requires greater amounts of force to achieve liftoff includes flexing the trunk sufficiently to bring the COM well within the base of support of the feet prior to liftoff. However, the body has zero momentum at liftoff. This strategy has been referred to as a "zero-momentum strategy," and it requires the generation of larger lower-extremity forces in order to lift the body to vertical (Schenkman et al., 1990).

Another common strategy used by many older adults and people with neurologic impairments involves the use of armrests to assist in STS. Use of the arms assists in the stability and force generation requirements of the STS task.

Understanding the different strategies that can be used to accomplish STS, including the trade-offs between force and stability, will help the therapist when retraining STS in the patient with a neurologic deficit. For example, the zero-momentum strategy may be more appropriate to use with a patient with cerebellar pathology who has no difficulty with force generation, but who has a major problem with controlling stability. On the other hand, the patient with hemiparesis, who is very weak, may need to rely more on a momentum strategy to achieve the vertical position. The frail older person who is both weak and unstable may need to rely on armrests to accomplish STS.

Supine to Stand

The ability to assume a standing position from a supine position is an important milestone in mobility skills. This skill is taught to a wide range of patients with neurologic impairments, from young children with developmental disabilities first learning to stand and walk to frail older people prone to falling. The movement strategies used by normal individuals moving from a supine to a standing position have been studied by a number of researchers. An important theoretical question addressed by these researchers relates to whether rising to standing from supine follows a developmental progression and whether by the age of 4 or 5 years the mature, or adult-like, form emerges and remains throughout life (VanSant, 1988a). By performing Lab Activity 12.4, you can come to your own conclusions about some of these questions.

Researchers have studied supine-to-standing movement strategies in children, ages 4 to 7 years, and young adults, ages 20 to 35 years (VanSant, 1988b). These

LAB ACTIVITY 12.4

Objective: To observe the strategies used to move from a supine to a standing position in healthy adults.

Procedures: For this lab, you will need a stopwatch, four or five partners, and room to observe each individual moving from a supine (flat on the floor) to a standing position. Time each person as they move from a supine to a full standing position. Observe the movement patterns used by each individual to arise. Pay specific attention to the use of arms, symmetry of foot placement, and trunk rotation.

Assignment

1. Were all subjects able to rise independently without physical assistance of another? How did times vary across subjects? How many different strategies were observed among the subjects? Did any two subjects move in the same way? How do your results compare with VanSant's (1988b) results shown in Figure 12.13? What are the primary muscles that are active in each of the strategies? How would weakness or loss of joint range of motion affect each of these strategies?

researchers found that while there was a slight tendency toward age-specific strategies for moving from supine to standing, there was also great variability among subjects of the same age. Their findings do not appear to support the traditional assumption of a single mature supine-to-standing pattern, which emerges after the age of 5 years.

The three most common movement strategies for moving from supine to standing are shown in Figure 12.18. When analyzing strategies used for moving from supine to standing, the body is divided into three components—upper extremities, lower extremities, and axial—which includes the trunk and the head. Movement strategies are then described in relationship to the various combinations of movement patterns within each of these segments. The research on young adults suggests that the most common pattern used involves symmetrical movement patterns of the trunk and extremities, and the use of a symmetrical squat to achieve the vertical position (Fig. 12.18A). However, only one-fourth of the subjects studied used this strategy.

The second most common movement pattern involved an asymmetric squat on arising (Fig. 12.18B), while the third most common strategy involved asymmetric use of the upper extremities, a partial rotation of the trunk, and assumption of stance using a half-kneel position (Fig. 12.18C).

Additional studies have characterized movement patterns used to rise from supine in middle-aged adults, ages 30 to 39 years, and found some differences in movement strategies as compared with younger adults (Green & Williams, 1992). In addition, this study looked at the effect of physical activity levels on strategies used to stand up. Results from the study found that strategies used to stand up are influenced by lifestyle factors, including level of physical activity.

Many factors probably contribute to determining the type of movement strategy used to move from supine to standing. Traditionally, nervous system maturation, specifically, the maturation of the righting reactions, was

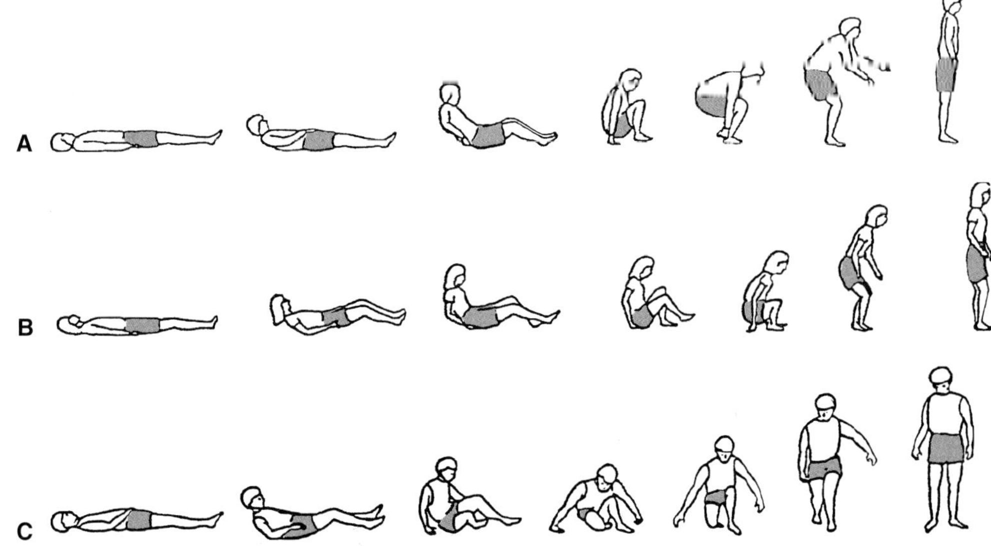

Figure 12.18 The three most common movement strategies identified among young adults for moving from a supine to a standing position. **(A)** Strategy involving symmetrical trunk and symmetrical squat. **(B)** Strategy involving symmetrical trunk and asymmetrical squat. **(C)** Strategy involving asymmetrical trunk movement. (Adapted from VanSant AF. Rising from a supine position to erect stance: description of adult movement and a developmental hypothesis. *Phys Ther.* 1988;68:185–192, with permission of the American Physical Therapy Association. This material is copyrighted, and any further reproduction or distribution requires written permission from APTA.)

considered the most significant factor affecting the emergence of a developmentally mature supine-to-standing strategy. However, other factors such as strength have been shown to influence the switch from an asymmetric rotation to a symmetric sit-up strategy, specifically the ability to generate sufficient abdominal and hip flexor strength. Developmental changes in moving from supine to standing are considered further in Chapter 13, on age-related aspects of mobility.

Rising from Bed

Clinicians are often called on to help patients relearn the task of getting out of bed. In therapeutic textbooks on retraining motor control in patients with neurologic impairments, therapists are often instructed to teach patients to move from supine to side-lying, then to push up to a sitting position and from there, to stand up. These instructions are based on the assumption that this pattern represents that typically used to rise from a bed (Bobath, 1990; Carr & Shepherd, 1992).

To test this assumption, researchers examined movement patterns used by young adults to rise from a bed (McCoy & VanSant, 1993; VanSant, 1988b). These studies report that movement patterns used by individuals without disability to rise from a bed are extremely variable. Eighty-nine patterns were found among 60 subjects. In fact, no subject used the same strategy consistently in 10 trials of getting out of bed.

Figure 12.19 shows one of the most common strategies used by young adults to rise from a bed. Essential components of the strategy include pushing with the arms (or grasping the side of the bed and then pushing with the arms), flexing the head and trunk, pushing into a partial sit position, and rolling up to standing. Another common strategy found was a push-off pattern with the arms, rolling to the side and coming to a symmetrical sitting position prior to standing up.

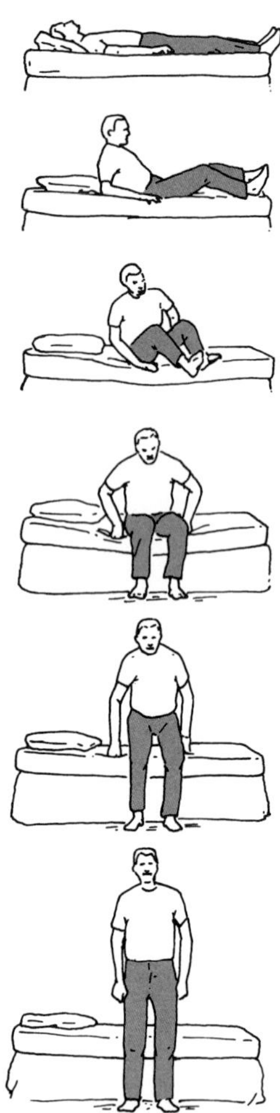

Figure 12.19 Most common movement strategy used by young adults for getting out of bed. (Adapted from Ford-Smith CD, VanSant AF. Age differences in movement patterns used to rise from a bed in subjects in the third through fifth decades of age. *Phys Ther*. 1992;73:305, with permission of the American Physical Therapy Association. This material is copyrighted, and any further reproduction or distribution requires written permission from APTA.)

While the authors of the studies on movement patterns to rise from bed have not specifically stated the essential features of this task, its similarity to the STS task suggests that they share the same invariant characteristics. These include (a) the need to generate momentum to move the body to vertical, (b) stability requirements for controlling the COM as it changes from within the support base defined by the horizontal body to that defined by the buttocks and feet and finally to a base of support defined solely by the feet, and (c) the ability to adapt how one moves to the characteristics of the environment.

In trying to better understand why people move as they do, and in preparation for understanding why patients move as they do, it might be helpful to reexamine descriptions of movement strategies used to rise from a bed in light of these essential task characteristics. In doing so, it would be possible to determine common features across diverse strategies that are successful in accomplishing invariant requirements of the task. It would also be possible to examine some tradeoffs between movement and stability requirements in the different strategies. For example, in the roll-off strategy, is motion achieved with greater efficiency at the expense of stability? Alternatively, the come-to-sit pattern may require more force to keep the body in motion, but stability may be inherently greater.

This research demonstrates the tremendous variability of movement strategies used by neurologically intact subjects when getting out of bed. It suggests the importance of helping patients with neurologic impairments to learn a variety of approaches to getting out of bed.

Rolling

Rolling is an important part of bed mobility skills and an essential part of many other tasks, such as rising from bed. Movement strategies used by nonimpaired adults to roll from supine to prone are very variable.

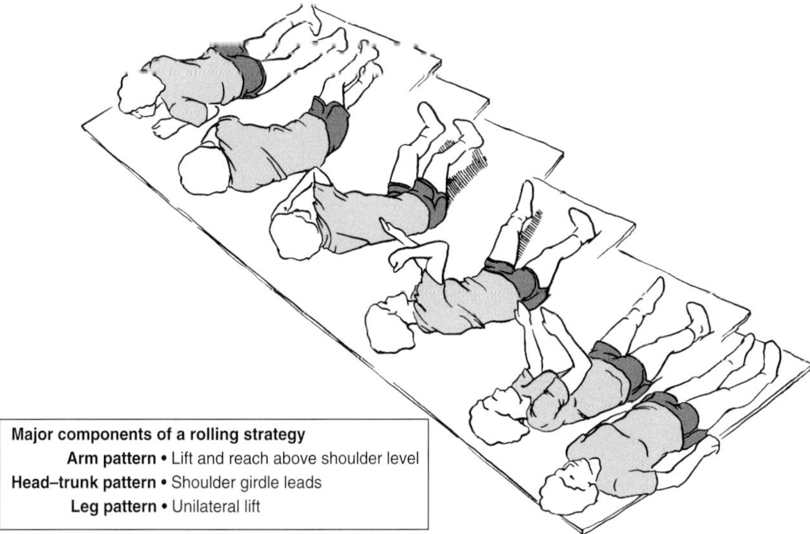

Figure 12.20 Most common movement strategy used by young adults when rolling from a supine to a prone position. (Adapted from Richter RR, VanSant AF, Newton RA. Description of adult rolling movements and hypothesis of developmental sequences. *Phys Ther.* 1989;69:63–71, with permission of the American Physical Therapy Association. This material is copyrighted, and any further reproduction or distribution requires written permission from APTA.)

Figure 12.20 shows one of the most common movement patterns used by adults to roll from a supine to a prone position (Richter et al., 1989). Essential features of this strategy include a lift-and-reach arms pattern, with the shoulder girdle initiating motion of the head and trunk, and a unilateral lift of the leg.

A common assumption in the therapeutic literature is that rotation between the shoulders and pelvis is an invariant characteristic in rolling patterns used by normal adults (Bobath, 1965); however, in this study on rolling, many of the adults tested did not show this pattern. Similar to the findings from studies on rising from a bed, the great variability used by normal subjects to move from a supine to a prone position suggests that therapists may use greater freedom in retraining movement strategies used by patients with neurologic impairments. Clearly, there is no one correct way to accomplish this movement.

SUMMARY

1. Within the ICF framework, mobility is represented in multiple ways, including in the components of *both Body Structure and Function* (gait pattern function) and as one of nine domains in *Activities and Participation*.
2. There are three major requirements for successful locomotion: (a) progression, defined as the ability to generate a basic locomotor pattern that can move the body in the desired direction; (b) postural control, defined as the ability to control the body's position in space to accomplish both orientation and all aspects of stability, including steady-state, reactive, and anticipatory balance control; and (c) adaptability, defined as the ability to adapt gait (progression and postural control) to meet the individual's goals and the demands of the environment.
3. Normal locomotion is a bipedal gait in which the limbs move in a symmetrical alternating relationship. Gait is divided into a stance and swing phase, each of which has its own intrinsic requirements.
4. During the support phase of gait, horizontal forces are generated against the support surface to move the body in the desired direction (progression), while vertical forces support the body mass against gravity (stability). In addition, strategies used to accomplish both progression and stability must be flexible in order to accommodate changes in speed, direction, or alterations in the support surface (adaptation).
5. The goals to be achieved during the swing phase of gait include advancement of the swing leg (progression) and repositioning the limb in preparation for weight acceptance (stability). Both the progression and stability goals require sufficient foot clearance, so the toe does not drag on the supporting surface during swing. In addition, strategies used during the swing phase of gait must be sufficiently flexible in order to allow the swing foot to avoid any obstacles in its path (adaptation).
6. Gait is often described with respect to temporal distance parameters such as velocity, step length, step frequency (cadence), and stride length. In addition, gait is described with reference to changes in joint angles (kinematics), muscle activation patterns (EMG), and the forces used to control gait (kinetics).
7. Many neural and nonneural elements work together in the control of gait. Although spinal pattern generators are able to produce stereotyped locomotor patterns and to perform certain adaptive functions, descending pathways from higher centers and sensory feedback from the periphery allow the rich variation in locomotor patterns and adaptability to task and environmental conditions.
8. One of the requirements of normal locomotion is the ability to adapt gait to a wide-ranging set of environ-

ments, and this involves using sensory information from all the senses, both reactively and proactively.

9. An important part of controlling locomotion is stabilizing the head, since it contains two of the most important sensors for controlling motion: the vestibular system and visual system. In neurologically intact adults, the head is stabilized with great precision, allowing gaze to be stabilized through the vestibuloocular reflex.
10. Stair walking is similar to level walking in that it involves stereotypical reciprocal alternating movements of the lower limbs and has three requirements: the generation of primarily concentric forces to propel the body upstairs, or eccentric forces to control the body's descent downstairs (progression); controlling the COM within a constantly changing base of support (stability); and the capacity to adapt strategies used for progression and stability to accommodate changes in stair environment, such as height, width, and the presence or absence of railings (adaptation).
11. Although mobility is often thought of in relation to gait, many other aspects of mobility are essential to independence. These include the ability to move from a sitting to a standing position, rolling, rising from a bed, or moving from one chair to another. These skills are referred to as "transfer tasks."
12. Transfer tasks are similar to locomotion in that they share common task requirements: motion in a desired direction (progression), postural control (stability), and the ability to adapt to changing task and environmental conditions (adaptation). Researchers have found great variability in the types of movement strategies used by neurologically intact young adults when performing transfer tasks.
13. Understanding the stability and strength requirements for different types of strategies used to accomplish transfer tasks has important implications for retraining these skills in neurologically impaired patients with different types of motor constraints.

ANSWERS TO LAB ACTIVITY ASSIGNMENTS

Lab Activity 12.1

1. Step length: mean step length of about 76.3 cm (30.05 inches).
2. Stride length: approximately twice the step length, unless the participant has an asymmetric gait.
3. Step width: about 8 to 9 cm.
4. Cadence: mean cadence (step rate) of about 1.9 steps per second (about 112.5 steps per minute).
5. There is a linear relationship between step length and step frequency over a wide range of walking speeds. However, once an upper limit to step length is reached, continued elevation in speed comes from step rate. Stance phase shortens as walking speed increases. Also, the addition of an assistive device most often decreases gait velocity even among non-impaired individuals.

Lab Activity 12.2

1. For answers, see Figure 12.2. Determine whether your numbers are similar to those in the individual graphs.

Lab Activity 12.3

1. Gastrocnemius and soleus relax and tibialis anterior contracts.
2. COP first moves posteriorly and laterally toward the swing limb and then shifts toward the stance limb and forward.
3. With the leg closer to the wall.
4. Yes.
5. You could not easily shift your weight in preparation for stepping.

Lab Activity 12.4

1. Answers will vary.

CHAPTER 13

Development of Mobility

Learning Objectives

Following completion of this chapter, the reader will be able to:

1. Describe the time course of emergence during development of the three major requirements of locomotion—progression (pattern generation), postural control (both orientation and stability), and adaptation (to changing task and environmental conditions).
2. Describe the major kinematic, kinetic, and electromyographic changes that occur during the development and maturation of independent gait in children.
3. Describe the contributions of neural (sensory, motor, and higher cognitive) and nonneural subsystems to the development of gait in children.
4. Discuss the changes during development associated with other forms of mobility, including rolling, prone progression, sit-to-stand, and supine to stand.

INTRODUCTION

It is wonderful to see children develop their first mobility skills as they begin to crawl, creep, walk, and run—finally navigating expertly through complex environments. How do these skills develop? When do they first begin to emerge? What amount of practice does it take for an infant to begin to walk proficiently? What key features of normal locomotor development should we incorporate into our measurement tools and training sessions so that we can better understand and train mobility skills in the child who shows delayed or disordered development of mobility?

This chapter discusses the development of mobility skills within the International Classification of Functioning, Disability and Health (ICF) framework. Thus, we look at changes in the gait pattern during development within the component of *Body Structure and Function*. We also discuss characteristics of the activity of walking (distance walked, negotiation of obstacles, etc.) and how it relates to participation, including moving around different locations in the home and outside the home. We review the development of mobility skills in typically developing children and summarize research from different theoretical perspectives that explore the factors contributing to the emergence of this complex ability.

DEVELOPMENT OF MOTOR SYSTEMS AND GAIT

Independent locomotion may at first seem to be a fairly simple and automatic skill, but it is really a very intricate motor task. One researcher has observed infants' normal activities while learning to walk and found that they averaged 2,368 steps and 17 falls per hour! That is the equivalent of 14,000 steps daily, traveling the length of 46 football fields and having 100 falls! Albeit immense, infants practice walking in large amounts of short, variable bouts. Infants frequently start and stop walking without reaching a destination or goal, most often after taking three or fewer steps (Cole et al., 2016). In addition, infants take steps in every direction, including both curving and twisting paths (Lee et al., 2018). Figure 13.1 shows an example of a typical 13-month-old's walking path during the first 10 minutes of spontaneous play in a laboratory playroom. Adolph's conclusion is that infants learn to walk by acquiring incredible amounts of time-distributed variable practice, over weeks and months of walking experience, traveling further and falling less (Adolph et al., 2012).

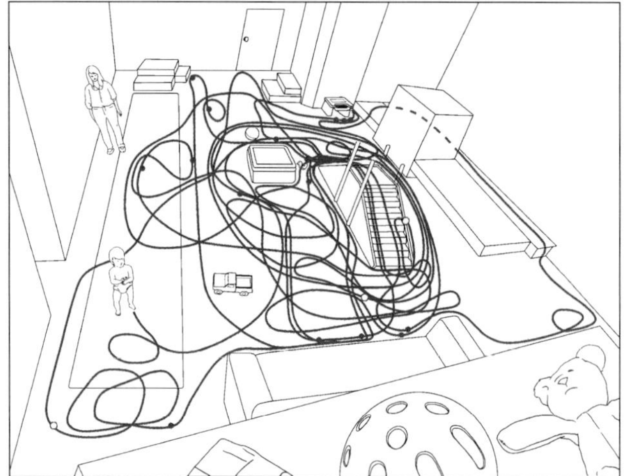

Figure 13.1 Example of a typical 13-month-old natural walking path during the first 10 minutes of spontaneous play. Overlapping lines indicate revisits to the same location. Filled circles represent rest periods longer than 5 seconds. Open circles denote falls. (Reprinted from Adolph, K.E., Cole, W.G., Komati, M., et al. How do you learn to walk? Thousands of steps and dozens of falls per day. *Psychol Sci.* 2012;23:1389, with permission.)

A child learning to walk needs to activate a complex pattern of muscle contractions in many body segments to produce a coordinated stepping movement, meeting the goal of progression. To accomplish the goal of postural control (both orientation and stability), the child must be strong enough to support body weight and stable enough to compensate for shifts in the center of body mass (COM) while walking. Finally, the child must develop the ability to adapt gait to changing task and environmental circumstances, allowing navigation around and over obstacles and across uneven surfaces (Thelen & Ulrich, 1991).

In the following section, we summarize research evidence suggesting that in the development of locomotion, the three requirements of gait—progression, postural control, and adaptation—emerge sequentially during the first years of life. How does this complex behavior develop? What are the origins of this behavior during prenatal development?

Development of Steady-State Gait

Prenatal Development

Researchers have actually traced the origins of locomotor rhythms back to embryonic movements that begin to occur in the first stages of development. Ultrasound techniques have been used to document the movements of human infants prenatally. This research has shown that all movements except those observed in the earliest stages of embryonic development (7–8 weeks) are also seen in neonates and young infants. Isolated leg and arm movements develop in the embryo by 9 weeks of age, while alternating leg movements, similar to walking movements seen after birth, develop by about 16 weeks of embryonic age (De Vries et al., 1982; Prechtl, 1984).

Control Mechanisms in Prenatal Gait. Animal research has also explored the prenatal development of locomotor circuitry. Detectable limb movements appear to emerge in a cephalocaudal sequence, with movements in the forelimbs preceding those in the hindlimbs (Bradley & Smith, 1988). Intralimb coordination develops prior to interlimb coordination, with the first detectable movements occurring at proximal joints and moving distally with development. Finally, interlimb coordination develops, first with alternating patterns and then with synchronous patterns (Stehouwer & Farel, 1984).

Steady-State Gait in the Newborn and Emergence of Independent Walking

Many newborn animals, such as rats, do not normally show coordinated locomotor movements until about 1 week after birth (Bradley & Bekoff, 1989). If, however, rats are placed in water at birth, they swim, demonstrating the maturity of their locomotor system. In addition, adult forms of locomotion can be elicited in 3-day-old kittens by placing them on a treadmill (Bradley & Smith, 1988). However, gait in kittens is uncoordinated, because of their poor postural abilities.

These results suggest that a primary constraint on emerging locomotor behavior is the immaturity of the postural control system and thus the inability to achieve and maintain upright stability. In addition, these findings remind us to be careful about assuming that because a behavior is not evident, there is no neural circuitry for it.

Factors Contributing to Newborn Stepping and Its Disappearance: Pattern Generators and Self-organizing Systems. Because locomotor patterns have been developing for some months prenatally, it is not surprising to find that stepping behavior can be elicited in newborns under the right conditions (Forssberg, 1985; Prechtl, 1984; Thelen et al., 1989). For example, when newborn infants are held under the arms in an upright position, tilted slightly forward, with the soles of the feet touching a surface, they often perform coordinated movements that look much like erect locomotion. Surprisingly, stepping becomes progressively more difficult to elicit during the first month of life, tending to disappear in most infants by about 2 months of age and reappear with the onset of self-generated locomotion many months later.

This pattern of appearance and disappearance of newborn stepping was found in a study that examined 156 children longitudinally (Forssberg, 1985). It was found that 94 infants stepped at 1 month, 18 stepped at 3 months, and only 2 stepped at 4 and 5 months. Then, at 10 months, after a 4- to 8-month period of no stepping, all 156 infants stepped with support and 18 stepped without support. Thus, the stepping pattern appeared to be temporarily lost in 98% to 99% of the infants.

What causes these changes? Different theoretical approaches explain changes in infant behavior in very different ways. From a reflex hierarchy perspective, newborn stepping is thought to result from a stepping reflex. Its disappearance is assumed to be mainly the result of inhibition by maturing higher neural centers. Figure 13.2 illustrates seven phases in the development of infant locomotion, beginning with the observation of this reflex (phase 1) and its disappearance (phase 2), continuing with its reappearance (phase 3) and the emergence of assisted locomotion (phase 4), and concluding with three phases of erect independent walking, in which the hands gradually move from a high guard position (phase 5) down to the side (phase 6) and the trunk and head become more erect (phase 7) (McGraw, 1945).

In contrast to a reflex hierarchical model, researchers using a dynamic systems approach have examined the emergence of stepping in relation to the contributions of multiple neural and nonneural systems. In particular, these studies have explored the conditions leading to the emergence of newborn stepping and the changes that cause its disappearance. Esther Thelen, a psychologist, and her colleagues have applied a dynamic systems approach to the study of locomotor development (Thelen et al., 1989). This approach views locomotion as an emergent property of many interacting complex processes, including sensory, motor, perceptual, respiratory, cardiac, and anatomical systems. According to a dynamic systems approach, moving and developing systems have certain self-organizing properties; that is, they can spontaneously form patterns that arise simply from the interaction of the different parts of the system.

A dynamic systems model stresses that actions always occur within specific contexts. As a result, a given neural code will produce very different behavioral outcomes, depending on the contributions of the other elements of the system, as in the position of the child with relation to gravity. Thus, dynamic systems researchers suggest that the specific leg trajectory seen in newborn stepping is not coded precisely anywhere in the nervous system. Instead, the pattern emerges through the contributions of many elements. These include the neural substrate, anatomical linkages, body composition, activation or arousal level, and the gravitational conditions in which the infant is kicking (Thelen et al., 1989).

From a dynamic systems perspective, the disappearance of the neonatal stepping pattern at about 2 months of age results from changes in a number of components of the system that reduce the likelihood of seeing this behavior. For example, body build changes greatly in the first 18 months of life. Infants add a lot of body fat in the first 2 months of life and then slim down toward the end of the first year. It has been suggested that the stepping pattern goes away at 2 months

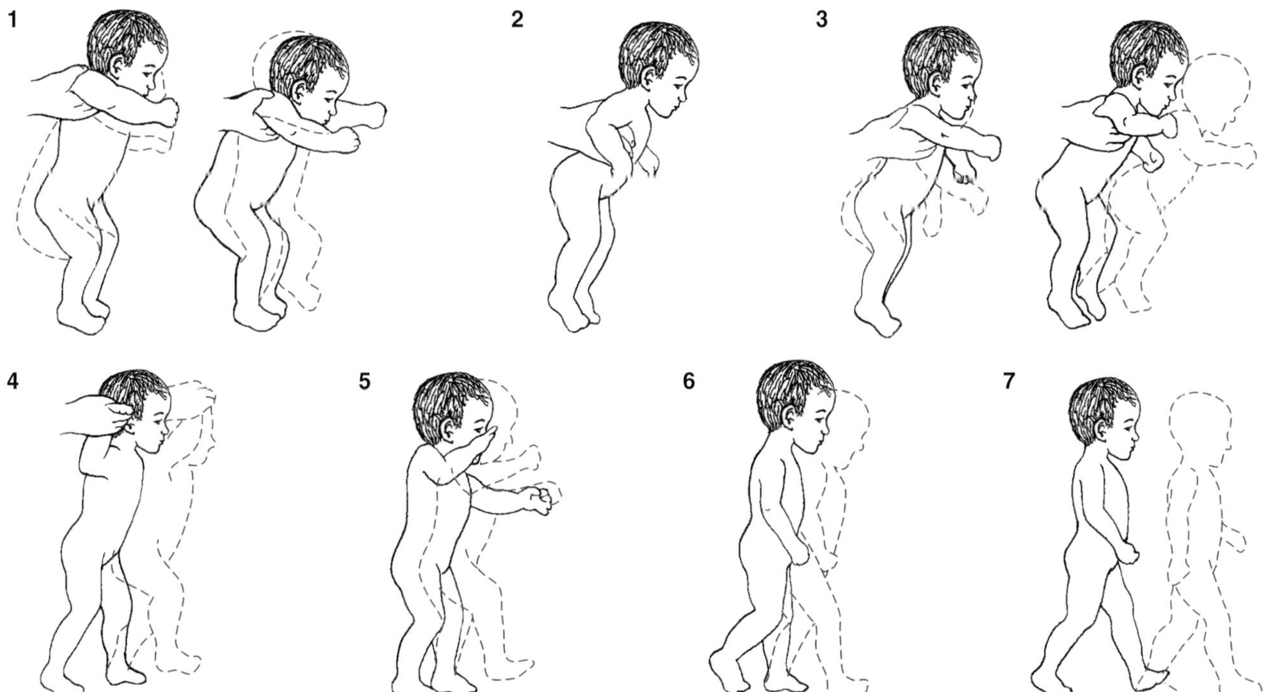

Figure 13.2 The seven phases of erect locomotion according to McGraw. *1*, Stepping reflex; *2*, its disappearance; *3*, its reappearance; *4*, assisted locomotion; *5–7*, three phases of erect independent walking in which the hands gradually move from a high guard position (*5*) down to the side (*6*) and the trunk and head become more erect (*7*). (McGraw MB. Neuromuscular development of the human infant as exemplified in the achievement of erect locomotion. *J Pediatr.* 1940;17:747–771; Figure 1.)

because infants have insufficient strength to lift the heavier leg during the step cycle (Thelen et al., 1989).

Thelen and colleagues (1984) showed that 4-week-old infants who have more body fat step less frequently than infants with less weight gain. Moreover, when infants' legs are weighted to simulate the weight gained over the first 4 weeks of life, infants who normally take steps do so at a smaller rate and with weaker flexion movements. When 4-week-old infants are submerged up to their trunk in water, thus making them more buoyant and counteracting the effects of gravity, stepping increases in frequency (Thelen et al., 1984). All of her studies suggests that the infant's weight is a factor that affects the step cycle. Further support for the weight hypothesis related to the disappearance of newborn stepping comes from research examining newborn kicking patterns. Supine kicking has the same kinematic spatial and temporal patterning as newborn stepping. Both behaviors involve a quasi-synchronous hip–knee–ankle flexion, followed by a forward swing and extension of the limb (Sylos-Labini et al., 2020). The swing phase of locomotion is similar to the flexion and extension phases of the kick, while the stance phase is similar to the pause between kicks. As stepping speeds up, the stance phase is reduced, and as kicking speeds up, the pause phase is reduced (Thelen et al., 1989).

Nevertheless, newborn kicking and stepping involve distinct neuromuscular patterns—newborn kicking involves variable temporal activation patterns of the limb muscles whereas ground-stepping involves only two temporal activation patterns, each associated with a stable muscle synergy: one for limb extension during stance and the other one for limb flexion during swing (Sylos Labini et al., 2020). This suggests that both supine kicking and newborn stepping may involve distinct pattern generators. Regardless of the neural circuitry involved in newborn supine kicking and stepping, kicking continues during the period when newborn stepping disappears. One long-standing explanation for the persistence of supine kicking is that it does not require the same strength as stepping, since the infants are not working against gravity (Thelen et al., 1984). Likewise, Barbu-Roth and colleagues (2015) showed the persistence of 4-week-old infants' stepping movements in the air in contrast to their disappearance when infants were supported with their feet contacting a surface. The authors support the idea that infants' lower limbs at 4 weeks are relaxed and leads to a more flexed posture when they are in contact with a surface, making tactile stepping difficult to elicit. Nonetheless, with a few minutes of daily practice of upright stepping to strengthen their legs, infants do not show the typical decline in step frequency at 8 weeks (Zelazo et al., 1972).

Locomotion in human neonates may be similar to that of quadrupeds who walk on their toes, like cats, dogs, and horses. For example, newborns show high knee and hip flexion and do not have heel strike. Since extensor muscle activity occurs prior to foot touch-down, it appears to be driven by an innate locomotor pattern generator, as has been found in quadrupeds, rather than being reflexly activated by the foot in contact with the ground. It has also been suggested that the neural network for stepping must be organized at or below the brainstem level, since anencephalic infants (infants born without a cerebral cortex) can perform a similar pattern of infant stepping (Peiper, 1963).

Interestingly, some researchers believe that the abnormal gait patterns found in many patients with neurologic pathology are actually immature locomotor patterns. Thus, children with cerebral palsy, children with developmental delays, and children who habitually toe-walk may persist in using an immature locomotor pattern, while adults with acquired neurologic disease may revert to immature locomotion because of the loss of higher center modulation over the locomotor pattern generator (Forssberg, 1985).

Characterizing the Development of Steady-State Gait: Electromyography and Kinematics

Other researchers (Forssberg, 1985; Okamoto et al., 2001) have examined in more detail the contribution of the nervous system to the emergence of locomotion. Forssberg (1985) postulated that human locomotion is characterized by the interaction of many systems with certain hierarchical components. His research suggests that an innate pattern generator creates the basic rhythm of the step cycle, which can be seen in newborn stepping. In the first year, the gradual development of descending systems from higher neural centers gives the child the ability to control this locomotor activity. Systems for posture or equilibrium control, organized at a higher level than those controlling the pattern generator, develop over a longer period.

According to this research, the emergence of walking with support is not the result of critical changes in the stepping pattern per se but appears to be due to maturation of the postural control system. In addition, the gradual emergence of mature gait over the next year is hypothesized to result from a new higher-level control system influencing the original lower-level network and modifying it (Forssberg, 1985).

Forssberg's research, using electromyography (EMG) and motion analysis, has examined how the locomotor pattern changes over the first 2 years of development. Studies using motion analysis techniques have shown a gradual transformation of the locomotor movement from a synchronous pattern of joint movements in newborn stepping to a more adult-like pattern of joint motion by the end of the first year of development. The transformation to adult-like gait patterns happens during the latter part of the second year. At this point, heel

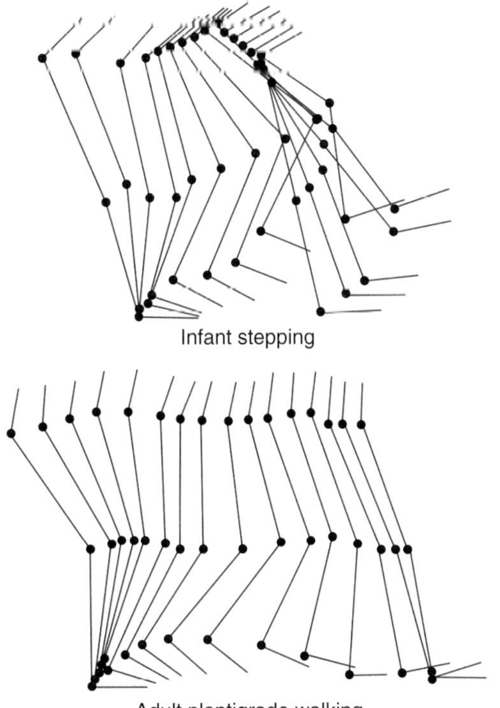

Figure 13.3 Stick figures taken from motion analysis of one step cycle of walking in an infant versus an adult. Note the high amounts of hip flexion in the infant. (Source: Forssberg H. Ontogeny of human locomotor control: 1. Infant stepping, supported locomotion and transition to independent locomotion. *Exp Brain Res.* 1985;67:481.)

strike begins to occur in front of the body. Figure 13.3 shows the kinematics of neonatal versus adult stepping movements. Note that the infant shows high levels of hip flexion as compared with the adult.

The EMG analysis supported the findings of the motion analysis. For example, in the neonate, the motor pattern was characterized by a high degree of synchronized activity. In other words, the extensor muscles of different joints were active simultaneously, and there was much coactivation of agonist and antagonist muscles at each joint. As with the movement patterns, the EMG patterns also began to look more mature during the latter part of the second year, with asynchronous patterns emerging at the different joints (Forssberg, 1985).

Another set of longitudinal studies explored the developmental changes in control of the leg muscles from newborn stepping through the first 4 months of life and from the onset of independent walking through 3 years of age (Okamoto & Okamoto, 2001; Okamoto et al., 2001) and supported and extended the results of Forssberg. The researchers found that neonatal stepping showed cocontraction patterns of agonists and antagonists, especially during the stance phase. They found that EMG patterns began to change to reciprocal patterns in infant stepping after the first month, but excessive muscular contraction accompanying the infants' slightly squatted posture as well as forward lean was still present. Results showed that strong leg extensor activation before floor contact, not seen in the neonatal period, began to appear in the young infant period from 1 to 3 months of age.

Okamoto and colleagues (Okamoto & Okamoto, 2001; Okamoto et al., 2001) noted that the EMG characteristics of infant gait up to about 1 month after learning to walk were clearly distinct from those in the adult. For example, in the stance phase from foot contact until push-off, the vastus medialis appeared to be critical for maintaining stability, with a slightly squatted position being used to lower the center of gravity (COG). Subsequently, reciprocal or cocontraction patterns of activity in the rectus femoris and biceps femoris or in the tibialis anterior and gastrocnemius were associated with the return of the body's COM toward its initial position. Finally, toward the end of the swing phase, the vastus medialis and gastrocnemius were strongly activated for active leg extension, possibly used to prevent falling. The authors suggest that this excessive muscle activation in infant walking may be due to weak muscle strength and an immature balancing system. Like Forssberg, Okamoto and colleagues suggest that the gradual changes of leg muscular activity from newborn stepping through more mature walking are due to the development of subsystems underlying postural control and muscle strength, thus modulating the neonatal stepping reflex.

Postural Control during the Emergence of Walking: Kinematics and Electromyography. One of the rate-limiting factors hypothesized to constrain the emergence of independent locomotion is the development of postural control, and it has been hypothesized that one factor contributing to unusual EMG and kinematic characteristics of newly walking toddlers is their postural instability. In order to determine the extent to which instability can explain why toddlers walk with a different gait, Ivanenko et al. (2005) compared kinematics and EMGs in toddlers performing their first independent steps with versus without hand or trunk support. They found that hand support significantly improved postural stability and reduced the percentage of falls, step width, lateral hip deviations, and trunk oscillations. However, in spite of these improvements, many kinematic and EMG patterns were unaffected by increased postural stability. In particular, they found that the covariance of the angular motion of the lower limb segments, the pattern of bilateral coordination of the vertical movement of the two hip joints, the high variability of the foot path, the single peak trajectory of the foot in the swing phase, and characteristic EMG bursts at foot contact remained similar in both supported and unsupported walking. The toddler pattern was, rather, found to show features similar to those of an adult stepping in place. They also found that characteristics of walking kinematics did not basically change until the occurrence of a child's first unsupported steps; then, they quickly matured. They thus proposed that many of the idiosyncratic features of newly walking toddlers are not due to poor balance control but may represent an innate kinematic template of stepping (Ivanenko et al., 2005). Indeed, various studies have proved that the neonate's early manifestation of ground-stepping activation patterns and kinematic parameters (e.g., foot placement characteristics and arm-leg coordination) are similar to more mature forms of locomotion, further supporting the claim that there is an innate template of locomotor patterns (La Scaleia et al., 2018; Sylos-Labini et al., 2017, 2020).

So, what are the elements that contribute to the emergence of locomotion in the infant? Remember that in development, some elements of the nervous and musculoskeletal systems may be functionally ready before others, but the systems must wait for the maturation of the slowest component before the target behavior can appear. A small increase or change in the development of the slowest component can act as the control parameter, becoming the impetus that drives the system to a new behavioral form.

The research we just discussed shows that many of the components that contribute to independent locomotion are functional before the child takes any independent steps. Function of the locomotor pattern generator is present in a limited capacity at birth and is improved during the second half of the first year, as the tight intralimb synergies become dissociated and capable of more complex modulation and control. As we noted in Chapter 8 on the development of postural control, infants are able to use optic flow information at birth to modulate head movements and at least by 5 to 6 months of age for modulation of stance. Motivation to navigate toward a distant object is clearly present by the onset of creeping (Atun-Einy et al., 2013; Hoch et al., 2020), and voluntary control over the limbs is certainly present by this time for many behaviors (Thelen et al., 1989).

So, what is the constraint that keeps upright bipedal locomotion from emerging before 9 to 12 months of age? Most researchers believe that it is primarily due to limitations in balance control and possibly also limitations in strength (Forssberg, 1985; Thelen et al., 1989; Woollacott, 1989). Of course, balance control and the stepping pattern continue to mature after the emergence of independent walking (Ivanenko et al., 2005).

For example, when an infant is creeping, one foot at a time can be picked up, so there is always a tripod stance available and, thus, balance is much less demanding. Normal infants who are about to take their first steps have developed motor coordination within the locomotor pattern generator; they also have functional visual, vestibular, and somatosensory systems and the motivation to move forward. Infants may also have sufficient muscle strength at least to balance, if not for use in propelling the body forward. But they will not be able to use these processes in effective locomotion until the postural control system can effectively control the COM, thus avoiding a fall. When these processes hit a particular threshold for effective function, then the dynamic behavior of independent bipedal locomotion can emerge.

Changes in Temporal Distance Factors during Early Walking (Progression and Postural Control)

Studies of changes in EMG characteristics and kinematics from the onset of walking through the mastery of mature forms of gait have been performed by many laboratories (Dierick et al., 2004; Okamoto & Kumamoto, 1972; Okamoto & Okamoto, 2001; Sutherland et al., 1980).

As noted previously, in the first days of independent walking, stepping patterns are immature. For example, the push-off motion in the stance phase is absent, the step width is very wide, and the arms are held high. The infant appears to generate force to propel the body forward by leaning forward at the trunk, twisting their trunk to swing the contralateral leg forward, or by taking small discrete steps (Snapp-Childs & Corbetta, 2009). The swing phase is short because the infant is unable to balance on one leg. Moreover, infants' first steps are characterized by increased flexion in the hip and knee during stance (a "squatted" position thought to be related to poor balance) resulting in a dominance of extending moments around the hip and knee and plantarflexion moments at the ankle (Hallemans et al., 2006).

By 10 to 15 days of independent walking, the infant begins to reduce cocontraction, and at 50 to 85 days after the onset of walking, the muscle patterns begin to show a reciprocal relationship. Okamoto and Kumamoto (1972) note that if infants are supported during walking, the reciprocal relationship between muscles emerges, but with the additional requirement of stabilizing the body while walking independently, the coactivation returns. This is in contrast to the results of Ivanenko et al. (2005), noted previously, that indicated that most EMG and kinematic patterns were unaffected by giving additional postural support to new walkers.

Other common gait characteristics in the first year of walking include a high step frequency, absence of the reciprocal swinging movements between the upper and lower limbs, a flexed knee during stance phase, and an increased hip flexion, pelvic tilt, and hip abduction during swing phase. There is also ankle plantarflexion at foot strike and decreased ankle flexion during swing, giving a relative foot drop (Sutherland et al., 1980). By 2 years of age, the pelvic tilt and abduction and external rotation of the hip are diminished. At foot strike, a knee-flexion wave appears, and reciprocal swing in the upper limb is present in about 75% of the children. The relative foot drop disappears as the ankle dorsiflexes during swing. By the end of 2 years, the infant begins to show a push-off in stance. During the years from 1 until 7, the muscle amplitudes and durations gradually reduce toward adult levels. By the age of 7, most muscle and movement patterns during walking look very similar to those of adults (Sutherland et al., 1980).

Sutherland et al. (1980) list five important characteristics that determine mature gait: (a) duration of single-limb stance, (b) walking velocity, (c) cadence, (d) step length, and (e) the ratio of pelvic span to step width.

Duration of single-limb stance increases steadily from 32% in 1-year-olds to 38% in 7-year-olds (39% is a typical adult value). Walking velocity and cadence decrease steadily, while step length increases. Step length is short in the newly walking child, due to lack of stability of the supporting limb, and lengthens with increasing balance abilities. Finally, the ratio of pelvic span, which is defined as body width at the level of the pelvis to step width increases until age 2.5, after which it stabilizes. By 3 years of age, the gait pattern is essentially mature, although small improvements continue through age 7 (Sutherland et al., 1980).

Is Learning to Walk a Two-Stage Process? Bril and Breniere studied locomotion in early and more mature walkers and hypothesized that learning to walk is a two-stage process (Breniere & Bril, 1998; Bril & Breniere, 1993). In the initial phase (3–6 months after the onset of walking), infants learn to control balance, while in the second phase (lasting through 5 years of independent walking), the locomotor pattern (progression) is progressively refined.

Another study observing infants' everyday exploration of their home environments corroborate lab data showing that fall frequency, frequency of stops, gait cadence, and time of stance phase, swing phase, and double support all decrease with walking experience (Marencakova et al., 2019).

Like Sutherland, they studied children longitudinally during the first 6 years of life to see how gait patterns change as independent locomotion develops. Significant changes in emerging gait patterns are summarized in Figure 13.4. Figure 13.4A illustrates the decrease in the duration of the double-support (DS) phase of gait (related to improving postural control) that shows a dramatic drop in the first 4 months of walking and then continues to drop until about 35 months of independent walking. Figure 13.4B shows the dramatic increase in step length that occurs in the first 4 months of walking, along with a decrease in step width (also related to improving postural stability) that continues through about 10 months of walking experience. They noted that in newly walking children, walking velocity was very low, with the duration of the swing phase being very short and that of the DS phase being long, probably because the children needed a long DS phase to regain balance. Studies observing infants' natural walking confirm laboratory data. With walking experience, infants' steps become faster, longer, and narrower (Lee et al., 2018).

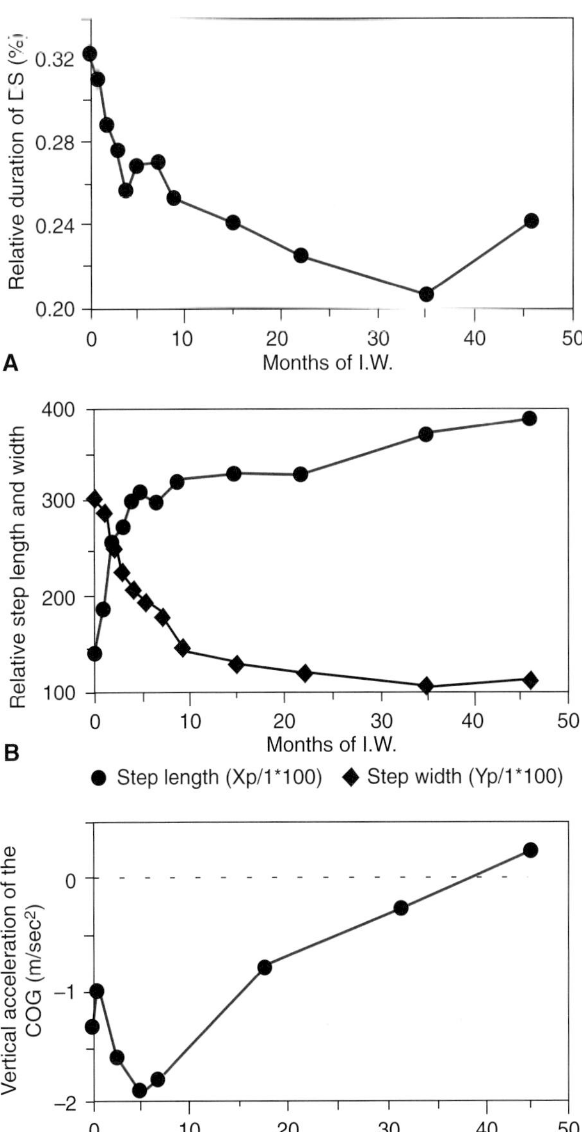

Figure 13.4 Changes in different walking parameters during the first 4 years of walking. **(A)** Relative duration of the double-support (DS) phase. **(B)** Changes in relative step length and width. **(C)** Changes in vertical acceleration of the center of gravity (COG). *IW*, independent walking; *Xp*, step length; *Yp*, step width. (Reprinted from Bril B, Breniere Y. Posture and independent locomotion in childhood: learning to walk or learning dynamic postural control? In: Savelsbergh GJP, ed. *The development of coordination in infancy*. Amsterdam, Netherlands: North-Holland, 1993:337–358, with permission.)

Bisi and Stagni (2015) further examined whether changes in gait patterns during the initial phase of walking is a strict continuous process. They showed that after 2 months of independent walking, there was a developmental shift in certain gait temporal parameters due to an increase in postural control. For example, cadence first increases and then decreases after 2 months of independent walking, whereas acceleration shows a constant decrease. The authors conclude that after 2 months of independent walking, infants' increase in walking velocity is most likely due to an increase in step length rather than to cadence.

Control of Vertical Center of Mass Motion during Walking: Contributions of Muscle Strength and Increased Postural Control. The authors asked what factors might constrain the development of postural abilities during walking (Breniere & Bril, 1998). They proposed that high levels of strength are required to control gravitational forces that tend to destabilize the upper body. In fact, it has been predicted that requirements of musculotendinous forces at the hip may reach six to eight times body weight at certain points in the stance phase of gait (McKinnon & Winter, 1993). Thus, Breniere and Bril (like Okamoto & Okamoto, 2001) hypothesized that newly walking children may lack the muscular strength to control balance. In order to test this hypothesis, the authors measured vertical COG acceleration, under the assumption that vertical ground reaction forces reflect the ability of the musculoskeletal system to compensate for body weight.

In adults, the vertical acceleration of the COM at heel strike is positive, indicating that they have both the muscular capacity and the control to counter destabilizing forces associated with initial contact. In contrast, Breniere and Bril (1998) found (as shown in Fig. 13.4C) that at the onset of independent walking in infants, the vertical acceleration of the COM at heel strike was always negative, indicating an initial deficit in muscular capacity. In the first 5 months of independent walking, the infants increased walking velocity substantially, due in large part to increases in step length. This increases the vertical instability, and interestingly, the vertical acceleration of the COM becomes even more negative. Thus, during this period, muscle strength appears to remain low compared with balance requirements. As shown in Figure 13.4C, by about 6 months of independent walking, the vertical acceleration of the COM at heel strike finally showed a change in direction toward positive values, indicating a change in postural control. Now, the infants stopped "walking by falling" and began controlling this forward "fall" during walking. The vertical acceleration of the COM at heel strike finally reached 0 value at about 3 to 4 years of walking experience (4–5 years of age), showing that they could control the inertial and gravity forces induced by walking (Fig. 13.4C). By 5 years of walking experience, three of the five children showed positive values similar to those of adults (Breniere & Bril, 1998). Since the changes in step width, step length, and DS phase relate to the mastery of balance control, their findings support the idea that it is during the first phase of walking that a child learns to integrate postural control into locomotor movements.

Another way of characterizing these refinements in the control of the COM during the development of mature walking is by measuring its pendular movement, associated with the COM of the body vaulting over the stance leg in an arc. This is called the "inverted pendulum mechanism of bipedal walking." Researchers have explored whether the pendulum mechanism is innate or, alternatively, is acquired with walking experience (Ivanenko et al., 2004). The kinematics of locomotion from infants taking their first unsupported steps (at about 1 year of age) was compared with that in older children and adults. As in the study of Bril and Breniere, discussed previously, results indicated that the pendulum mechanism was not implemented at the onset of unsupported locomotion.

To determine whether differences were due to the infants walking much more slowly than older children, the researchers normalized the locomotor speed and found that the percentage of recovery of mechanical energy in children older than 2 years was roughly similar to that of adults, while the percentage of recovery in toddlers was about 50% lower. They found that pendulum-like behavior along with a fixed coupling of the angular motion of the lower limb segments rapidly moved toward mature values within a few months of independent walking, suggesting that independent walking experience could be a functional trigger for these developmental changes. They concluded that the emergence of the pendulum mechanism is not an inevitable mechanical consequence of a system of linked segments but requires active neural control and an appropriate pattern of intersegmental coordination (Ivanenko et al., 2004).

Control of Lateral Center of Mass during Walking: Contributions of Increased Postural Control. Because control of the COM during walking has been found to be a good indicator of stability, one study further examined changes in the vertical and lateral displacement of the COM in walking during development in children from 1 to 9 years. Results showed that vertical and lateral amplitudes of the COM (when controlled for leg length) were greater for children before 4 years of age and that the forward amplitude was greater for children before 7 years of age. The authors concluded that the development of COM displacement during gait is a gradual process, evolving through 7 years of age (Dierick et al., 2004).

Hallemans and colleagues (2018) examined 1- to 10-year-old children's spatial margin of stability—defined as the minimum distance between the center of pressure and the "extrapolated COM" (vector sum of the COM position and a proportion of its velocity) along the mediolateral axis. In their study, they found that spatial margin of stability was positively correlated

TABLE 13.1 Developmental Sequence for Walking

I. WALKING
- A. Initial stage
  1. Difficulty maintaining upright posture
  2. Unpredictable loss of balance
  3. Rigid, halting leg action
  4. Short steps
  5. Flat-footed contact
  6. Toes turn outward
  7. Wide base of support
  8. Flexed knee at contact followed by quick leg extension
- B. Elementary stage
  1. Gradual smoothing of pattern
  2. Step length increased
  3. Heel–toe contact
  4. Arms down to sides with limited swing
  5. Base of support within the lateral dimensions of trunk
  6. Out-toeing reduced or eliminated
  7. Increased pelvic tilt
  8. Apparent vertical lift
- C. Mature stage
  1. Reflexive arm swing
  2. Narrow base of support
  3. Relaxed, elongated gait
  4. Minimal vertical lift
  5. Definite heel toe contact

II. COMMON PROBLEMS
- A. Inhibited or exaggerated arm swing
- B. Arms crossing midline of the body
- C. Improper foot placement
- D. Exaggerated forward trunk lean
- E. Arms flopping at sides or held out for balance
- F. Twisting of trunk
- G. Poor rhythmic action
- H. Landing flat-footed
- I. Flipping the foot or lower leg in or out

Reprinted with permission from Gallahue DL, JC Ozmun. *Understanding motor development: infants, children, adolescents,* 6th ed. Boston, MA: McGraw Hill, 2006:208.

with normalized step width and negatively correlated with normalized stride length (SL) and swing duration. The authors conclude that spatial margin of stability is linked to children's gait control—a larger spatial margin of stability induces a larger lateral divergence of the COM and this would be compensated by a larger and/or a quicker step (an increased step width and/or a reduced swing time).

Table 13.1 summarizes some of the characteristic changes in the step cycle from the initiation of independent walking through the development of mature patterns at about the age of 3 (Gallahue, 1989). These changes can be seen more graphically in Figure 13.5. To better understand changes in gait associated with development, complete Lab Activity 13.1.

When looking at the three requirements for successful locomotion, a rhythmic stepping pattern (progression), the control of balance (stability), and the ability to modify gait (adaptation), clearly, a rhythmic stepping pattern develops first. It is present in limited form at birth and is refined during the first year of life. Postural stability develops second, toward the end of the first year and the beginning of the second year of life and continues to improve throughout childhood. As we discuss in the next section, it appears that adaptability is refined in the first years after the onset of independent walking.

Development of Adaptation

How do children learn to adapt their walking patterns so they can navigate over and around obstacles, on different surfaces, and while performing other tasks? As we mentioned in Chapter 12, both reactive and proactive strategies are used to modify gait to changes in the task and environmental demands.

Development of Reactive Balance Strategies during Gait

Reactive strategies for adapting gait relate to the integration of compensatory postural responses into the gait cycle. Researchers have looked at compensatory postural muscle responses to perturbations during locomotion and have compared them with those during perturbed quiet stance.

In response to fast-velocity stance perturbations, children respond with both an automatic postural response and a monosynaptic reflex response. As children mature, the stretch reflex response gets smaller in amplitude, while the postural response gets faster. In very young children, there is considerable coactivation of antagonist muscles (Berger et al., 1985).

Perturbations during gait produce a monosynaptic reflex response in children from 1 to 2.5 years but

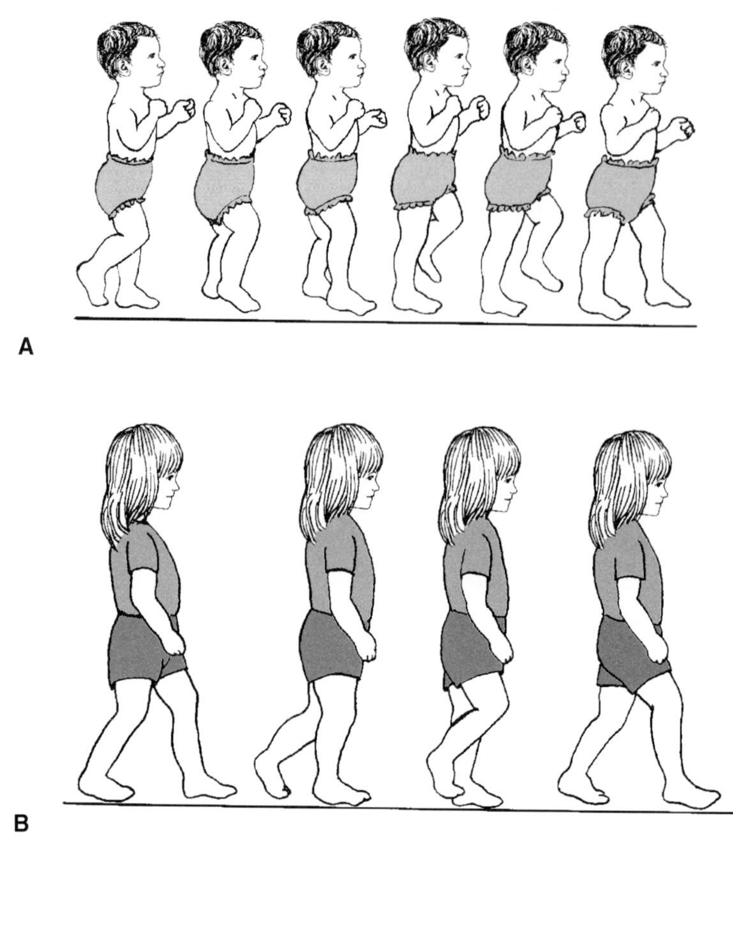

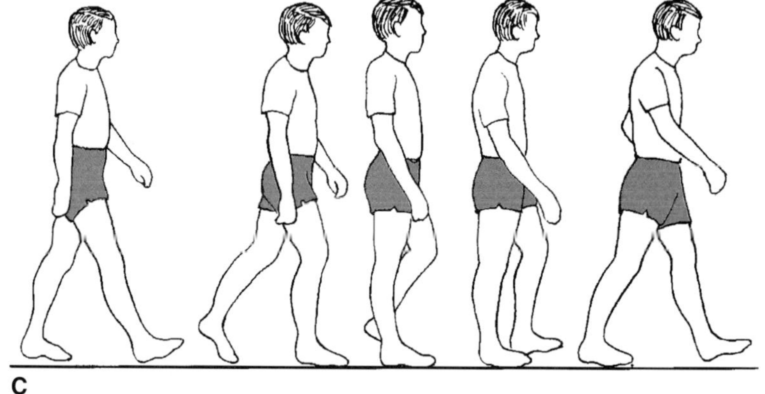

Figure 13.5 Body motions associated with developing gait. **(A)** Initial forms of gait. **(B)** Elementary forms of gait. **(C)** Mature forms of gait. (Adapted with permission from Gallahue DL, JC Ozmun. *Understanding motor development: infants, children, adolescents,* 6th ed. Boston, MA: McGraw Hill, 2006:208.)

not in older children, as shown in Figure 13.6. This figure shows a large monosynaptic reflex before the automatic postural response in the 1-year-old, which is reduced in the 2.5-year-old, and has disappeared in the 4-year-old and adult. Similar to stance perturbations, automatic postural responses to gait perturbations become faster with age, with mature responses occurring by about 4 years. Coactivation of antagonist muscles also is reduced with age.

Changes in the characteristics of compensatory postural activity are associated with increased stability during gait and increased ability to compensate for perturbations to gait (Berger et al., 1985). This study suggests that children as young as a year old who are capable of independent locomotion can integrate compensatory postural activity into slow walking when gait is disturbed, although their responses are immature.

Compensatory Stepping Skills during Balance Recovery. The ability to step independently is a fundamental skill required both for locomotion and for balance recovery when threats to balance are large, requiring a step. Interestingly, it appears that the

LAB ACTIVITY 13.1

Objective: To examine the kinematics of developing gait.

Procedures: Observe gait patterns in one or two infants of the following ages: 8 to 10 months (prewalkers), 12 to 18 months (new walkers), and 18 to 24 months (experienced walkers). Document age-related changes in spatial and temporal aspects of gait across these age groups. Also, observe and describe the following gait characteristics in each child: (a) ability to maintain an upright posture, (b) ability to control stability (How often does the child fall within a fixed time period?), (c) initial contact at foot strike, and (d) position of arms.

Assignment

1. Compare your descriptions among the children observed. How do each of the parameters change with age and walking experience?
2. Compare your descriptions of the development of gait to those described in Table 13.1. When do gait parameters begin to approximate those of adults?

ability to take independent steps in walking does not automatically translate into the ability to use a step for balance recovery. In a study examining the emergence of the ability to step in response to increasing velocities of balance threats, "standers" (children who could stand but not walk), new walkers (children capable of three steps but with less than 2 weeks of walking experience), intermediate walkers (children with 1–3 months of walking experience), and advanced walkers (children with 3–6 months of walking experience) were given backward support surface translations. Results showed that the ability to adapt balance responses to increasing balance threats is not present in new standers and new walkers, since almost no children in these two categories were able to take a step to recover balance. Stepping to recover balance begins to develop in infants with 1 to 3 months of walking experience and is relatively refined by 6 months of walking experience (Roncesvalles et al., 2000). Nevertheless, when examining 13- to 19-month-old infants' falls during spontaneous free play, reactive behaviors seem to remain consistent across development. Just prior to a loss of balance, infants take reactive steps, flex their knees, hold on to nearby supports, and outstretch their arms to arrest the fall. Infant reactive responses are rapid, averaging less than half a second after losing balance but before the body hits the ground, and typically involves a combination of multiple reactive behaviors (Han & Adolph, 2020).

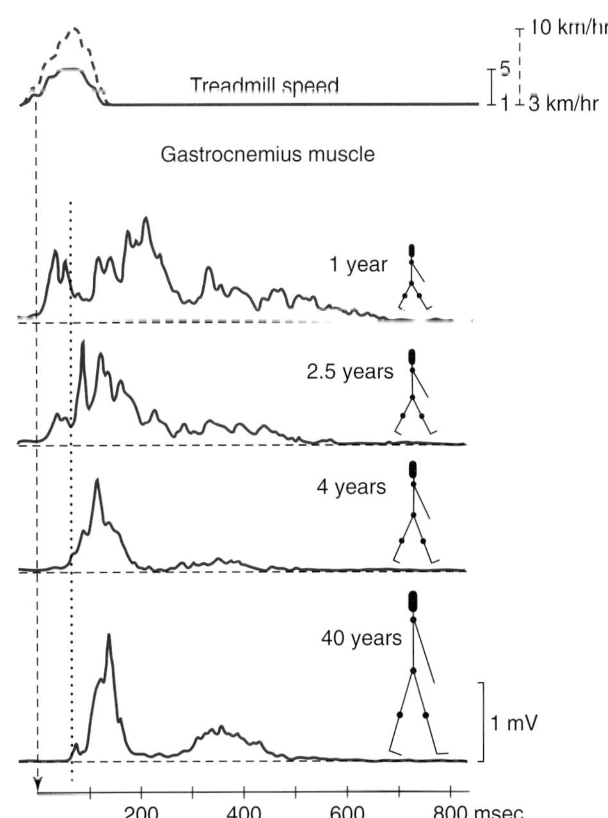

Figure 13.6 Examples of the gastrocnemius EMG responses of individual children of 1, 2.5, and 4 years of age and of an adult when their balance is perturbed during walking on a treadmill by briefly increasing treadmill speed. The *leftmost vertical line* is the onset of the treadmill acceleration, and the *dotted line* to its right is the onset of the automatic postural EMG response. Note that there is a large monosynaptic reflex in the youngest children, before the automatic postural response. This disappears by 4 years of age. (Reprinted from Berger W, Quintern J, Dietz V. Stance and gait perturbations in children: developmental aspects of compensatory mechanisms. *Electroencephalogr Clin Neurophysiol*. 1985;61:388, with permission.)

Development of Proactive Strategies during Gait

Proactive strategies for adapting gait use sensory information to modify gait patterns in advance of encountering obstacles to gait. When do children begin integrating these strategies into the step cycle? It has been suggested that children first learning to walk acquire feedback control of balance before feedforward control (Hass & Diener, 1988). The results of experiments by Bril and Breniere (1993) support this idea, as children seem to spend the first 4 to 5 months of walking learning to master steady-state balance and integrating balance mechanisms into the step cycle.

Anticipatory Head Movements when Changing Gait Direction. There is little research on the development of proactive strategies during gait. However, Grasso et al. (1998) examined the ability of children from 3.5 to 8 years to use anticipatory head movements when turning a 90-degree corner while walking. The results showed that predictive head orientation movements occurred in all the 3.5-year-old children in at least one trial, beginning at about 1 second before the turn, as it did in the older children and adults. However, the peak of the head rotation coincided with turning the 90-degree corner for the children, while it occurred about 250 ms earlier in adults. The results suggest that proactive strategies for goal-directed walking are in use early in the development of gait, although they do not mature until later in childhood.

Obstacle Avoidance during Gait. Studies by McFadyen and others (McFadyen et al., 2001; Vallis & McFadyen, 2005) have examined the ability of children aged 7 to 12 years to use proactive locomotor control to avoid obstacles. These studies showed that these children use adult-like limb displacements and general dynamic strategies for obstacle clearance. However, when data were normalized to body mass, the amplitudes of muscle power bursts related to anticipatory locomotor adjustments were reduced as compared with those of adults.

They also found that when adults and children altered their mediolateral (ML) COM trajectory, adults reoriented the head and trunk segments at the same time as the COM, while children reoriented the head and trunk before changing COM direction. Finally, adults changed their gait patterns well before obstacle crossing, while children initiated ML adjustments to gait patterns just prior to obstacle crossing. The authors conclude that children partition obstacle avoidance into two tasks, initially steering with proactive movement of the head and trunk segments and then making adjustments to their gait trajectory, through stride and step width changes, to obtain the necessary obstacle clearance just before obstacle crossing. The different head and trunk anticipatory coordination patterns imply that the way children obtain visual information is different from that in adults when avoiding obstacles, and they depend more on visual input to guide their locomotor strategy (Vallis & McFadyen, 2005).

Dominici and colleagues (2010) looked at characteristics of stepping over a variety of nonhorizontal surfaces in newly walking infants. Surfaces included stepping over an obstacle, going up and downstairs, and walking uphill and downhill. Results demonstrated that infants display more exploratory haptic foot placement behaviors compared to adults. For example, they showed that compared to adults, infants' foot paths were less accurately controlled and foot lift during successful obstacle crossing attempts was not dependent on the obstacle height, often touching the edges of the stairs with the foot prior to ascending or descending. Moreover, infants displayed a higher percentage of stumbling steps, and their intersegmental coordination remained constant across support surface conditions. The authors conclude that newly walking infants have yet to gain control of their movements, calibrate their sensorimotor space, and integrate the visual, proprioceptive, and effector system properties in a coherent manner.

Initiation of Gait. Chapter 12, on locomotion in adults, showed that gait initiation involves anticipatory shifts in the center of pressure (COP) backward and toward the stepping foot, which cause a forward and lateral shift of the COG toward the stance leg. Some research has shown that an anticipatory backward shift in the COP is present in children as young as 2.5 years of age and becomes habitual by 6 years of age (Ledebt et al., 1998).

In adults, the anticipatory changes in the COP are accompanied by inhibition of the soleus muscle and activation of the tibialis muscles prior to heel-off (Breniere et al., 1981; Herman et al., 1973). In a study using motion analysis and muscle response patterns to characterize step initiation in both prewalkers and in children with 1 month to 4 years of walking experience (Assaiante et al., 2000), anticipatory postural adjustments before step initiation were not found in prewalkers but were present in children with as little as 1 to 4 months of walking experience. These adjustments included a clear anticipatory lateral tilt of the pelvis and of the stance leg, in order to unload the opposite leg shortly before its swing phase. In addition, there was an anticipatory activation of the hip abductor muscle of the leg in stance phase prior to heel-off, suggesting the control of pelvis stabilization. These anticipatory postural adjustments did not occur consistently until 4 to 5 years of age. Between 1 and 4 years of age, there was a shift from the use of both upper and lower parts of the body (an en bloc strategy) in the lateral shift of the body toward the stance leg, to the inclusion of only the pelvis and leg (articulated operation) in the older children, similar to results from adults. Accompanying these kinematic changes were lower use of hip and knee muscles and greater use of ankle muscles in the older children during the gait initiation process (Assaiante et al., 2000).

Expanding the Repertoire of Steady-State Gait Patterns: Run, Skip, Hop, and Gallop

Running is often described as an exaggerated form of walking. It differs from walking as the result of a brief flight phase in each step. The flight phase that distinguishes a run from a walk is seen at about the second year of age. Until this time, the infant's run is more like a fast walk, with one foot always in contact with the ground. By 4 years of age, most children can hop (33%) and gallop (43%). The development of the gallop precedes the hop slightly. In one study, by 6.5 years, children were skillful at hopping and galloping. However, only 14% of 4-year-olds could skip (step-hop) (Clark & Whitall, 1989).

If central pattern generators (CPGs) control walking, are there separate CPGs for hopping, galloping, and skipping? Probably not. Then, why do they emerge in a fixed order of appearance? It is possible to explain their emergence from the dynamic systems perspective. Remember that walking and running are patterns of interlimb coordination in which the limbs are 50% out of phase with one another. This is the easiest stepping pattern to produce, and thus, it appears earliest. Running appears later than walking, probably because of its increased strength and balance requirements as compared with walking. Galloping requires that the child produce an asymmetrical gait with unusual timing and a differentiation in force production in each limb, and it may have additional balance requirements. Hopping emerges next, possibly because it requires the ability to balance the body's weight on one limb and it requires additional force to lift the body off the ground after landing. Skipping (a step-hop) emerges last, possibly because one locomotor coordination pattern is imbedded into another, and thus, it requires additional coordination abilities (Clark & Whitall, 1989).

It has been proposed that developmental milestones such as walk, run, gallop, hop, and skip are better indicators of balance development than chronological age. For example, in a study that compared EMG (timing and amplitude) and kinetic (COP and torque production) characteristics of reactive postural responses in children, the highest level of significance between groups across development was found when children were grouped by the previously mentioned developmental milestones rather than by chronological age (Sundermier et al., 2001).

Sensory Systems

As discussed in Chapter 12, sensory information from all the senses plays a critical role in all three of the main determinants of gait: progression, postural control, and adaptation. The contribution of individual sensory inputs to the development of gait is reviewed in the following sections.

Visual Contributions to Gait Development

Vision plays an essential role in guiding locomotion, with regard to both the layout of the environment and the body's orientation with respect to the environment. Kretch and Adolph (2017) examined the real-time process of visual and haptic exploration in 14-month-old infants as they walked over a series of bridges varying in width. The authors found that infants organize their exploratory behaviors in a sequential order; infants first looked at the bridge from a distance, which led to gait modifications while approaching narrow bridges and haptic exploration (touching with the feet or hands) at the edge of the bridge. Even though all infants looked, more experienced walkers' initial looks prompted them to touch more on narrow bridges and less on wider bridges. Less experienced infants were less discriminating—after the initial look, infants touched on safe, wide bridges. Less experienced infants also fell more frequently. Thus, infants can gather perceptual information to guide locomotion; however, more experienced walkers know how to interpret perceptual information obtained from vision, causing subsequent haptic exploration to be more efficient and decisions to walk over obstacles of varied risk to be more accurate.

Depriving adults of vision, or alternatively perturbing visual information, affects movement direction, speed, SL, cadence, and foot position. Does it affect children more than adults? In a study testing the effects of visual deprivation on walking in 3- to 6-year-olds, 7- to 11-year-olds, and adults, Hallemans and colleagues (2009a) found that children in both age groups slowed walking speed and deviated from a straight path more than adults when walking blindfolded. These results indicate that compared to adults, children under the age of 11 years of age are less able to substitute vestibular and somatosensory information for the control of locomotion when vision is unavailable.

The authors also examined postural sway and gait speed under eyes-open versus eyes-closed conditions and found a significant inverse correlation; under the eyes-closed condition, reduced gait speed was associated with increased postural sway, suggesting that reductions in gait speed were compensatory to postural instability.

When comparing kinematics of gait in eyes-open versus eyes-closed conditions, both adults and the two groups of children showed more backward lean of the trunk, reduced pelvic movement and adduction, increased flexion of the knee related to flatfoot floor contact, and reduced ankle plantarflexion at push-off. The researchers conclude that these changes in gait characteristics in the absence of vision result from a more cautious walking strategy, possibly related to postural control limitations (Hallemans et al., 2009b).

Vestibular Contributions to Gait Development

Does maturation of the semicircular canals or the otoliths in the vestibular system contribute to improvements in walking in infants and toddlers? To answer this question, a study tested children 6 to 25 months of age, prior to independent walking, during the transition to independent walking, and during the first year of independent walking. The researchers found that semicircular canal vestibuloocular reflexes (VORs) did not change significantly as infants learned to walk; in contrast, otolith VOR characteristics did. Thus, they concluded that development in otolith function could be a key contributor to the emergence of walking (Wiener-Vacher et al., 1996).

Stabilizing the Head and Trunk during Gait: Shifting Use of Somatosensory, Visual, and Vestibular Systems

An important part of controlling locomotion is learning to stabilize the head. Adults stabilize the head with great precision, allowing a steady gaze. Thus, control of the head, arm, and trunk (HAT) segments is a critical part of controlling mobility. How do children control the trunk, arms, and head during locomotion to ensure stabilization of the head and gaze?

Assaiante and Amblard (1995; Assaiante et al., 2005) performed experiments in children from early walkers through children 10 years of age to explore changes in control of these body segments. They suggest that balance and progression during gait can be organized according to one of two stable reference frames, either the support surface on which the subject stands and moves or the gravitational reference of vertical.

They noted that when using the support surface as reference, the subject organized balance responses from the feet upward toward the head, using mainly proprioceptive and cutaneous cues. In contrast, when the subject stabilized the head using vision and vestibular information, balance was organized from the head down toward the feet. These researchers explored the changing use of these two strategies in balance control during locomotor development in children.

They also noted that the head can be stabilized on the trunk in one of two modes, in an en bloc mode, in which it moves with the trunk, or in an articulated mode, in which it moves freely, minimizing movements away from vertical. This study explored locomotor strategies through kinematic analysis of walking in infants and children up to 8 years of age.

The authors found that from the acquisition of stance until about 6 years of age, children organize locomotion in a bottom–up manner, using the support surface as a reference and controlling head movements in an en bloc mode, which serves to reduce the degrees of freedom to be controlled. During this period, the children gradually learn to stabilize the hips, then the shoulders, and finally the head. At about 7 years of age, with mastery of control of the head, there is a transition, and the head control is changed to an articulated mode, and top–down organization of balance during locomotion becomes dominant. The authors hypothesized that at 7 to 8 years of age, information specifying head position in relation to gravity becomes more available to the equilibrium control centers and thus allows the child to use an articulated mode of head control. They suggest that there may be a transient dominance of vestibular processing in locomotor balance at this age (Assaiante & Amblard, 1995; Assaiante et al., 2005).

Research by Ledebt et al. (1995) has shown that hip stabilization in space is present at the onset of walking while head and trunk stabilization improve considerably during the following 3 to 4 months, after which they do not change for about a year.

As noted previously, studies of the development of canal and otolith VORs have shown that their developmental time courses are very different. The canal VOR is relatively stable in young walkers. However, the onset of walking is a transition point in otolith VOR development, with clear changes in the slow-phase velocity of the VOR. It has thus been proposed that otolith VOR development may play a critical role in the development of postural control during the first months of walking. The authors noted that although the canal VOR does not change during this period, it is very different from that of older children, suggesting that it is still immature. They propose that this may be related to the fact that new walkers adopt a stiff neck posture during walking, a strategy also used by adults with bilateral vestibular deficits. This strategy reduces the amplitude of head rotations in the pitch and roll planes in order to limit instability in the movement of the visual field due to problems with gaze stabilization (Wiener-Vacher et al., 1996).

Sensory Adaptation: Perceiving Affordances for Locomotion

When infants begin to crawl, cruise, and walk, they need to learn to take advantage of the environments and surfaces that afford safe locomotion and to avoid contexts that are not safe (e.g., cliffs or steep stairs). What constitutes a safe environment changes as the infant gains new locomotor skills and learns to navigate steeper slopes and narrower surfaces with agility. How do infants acquire these perceptual skills? Researchers have studied this by changing surface properties that infants move over, including the friction, surface rigidity, slant, bridge width over a steep drop, cliff edges, height of stairs and pedestals, and availability of handrails (Berger & Adolph, 2007). Figure 13.7 shows examples of some of the contexts that have been studied.

Figure 13.8 shows both cross-sectional and longitudinal data indicating that infants learn to perceive affordances for locomotion through crawling and walking experience. For example, in their first weeks of both crawling and walking, infants attempted to navigate slopes that were well beyond their ability. (Positive numbers on the x-axis of the graph show that the slope is well beyond their ability to navigate.) With experience, this behavior decreased, as perceptual judgments became similar to actual motor ability. Interestingly, results showed no transfer between crawling and walking postures. For example, infants who were new walkers avoided a 36-degree descent in crawling but would plunge down the same slope when walking (Adolph & Berger, 2006).

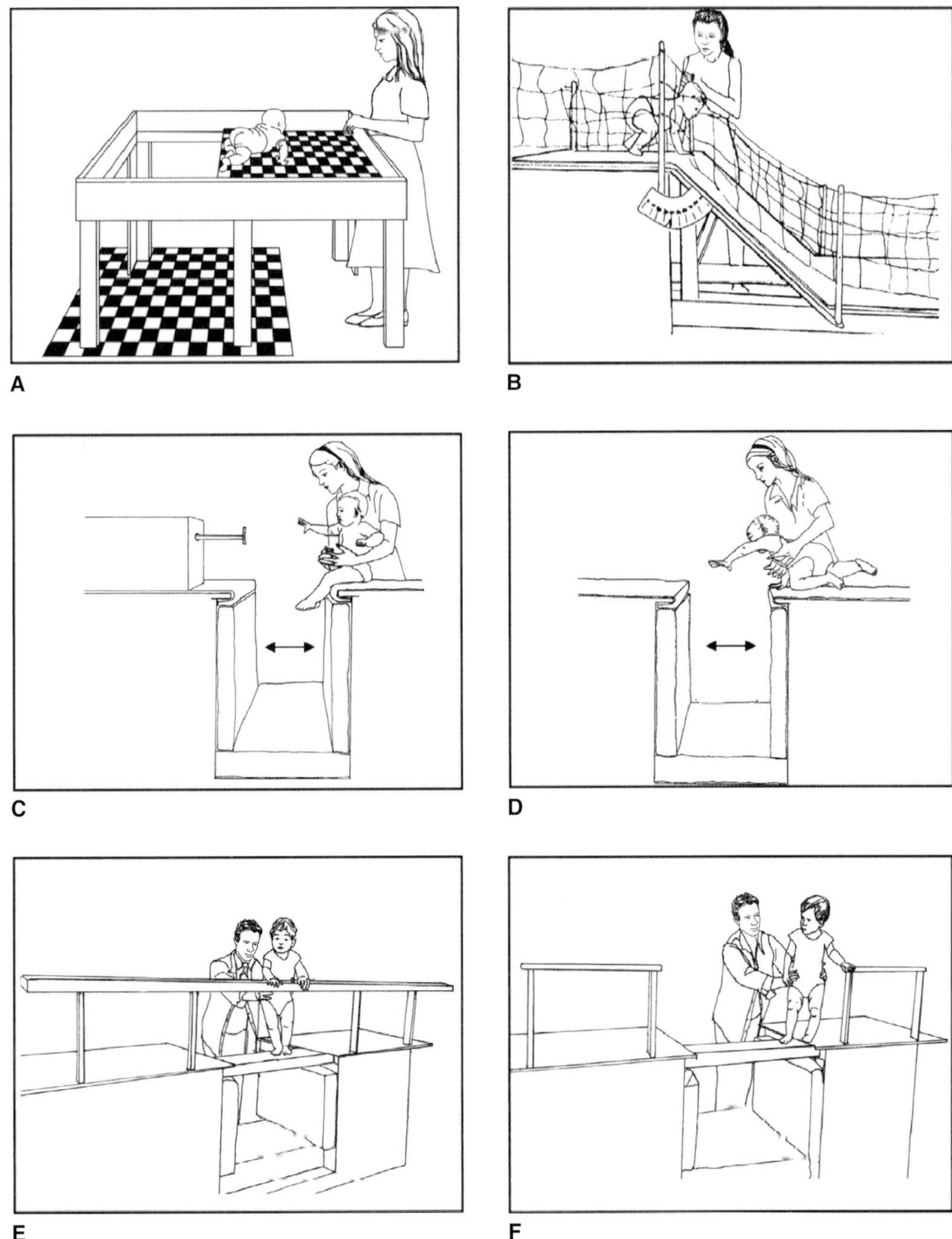

Figure 13.7 Examples of paradigms that have been used to test infants' perception of affordances for locomotion: **(A)** A crawling infant approaching a "visual cliff" with an apparent drop off. **(B)** A crawling infant at the top of a changeable slope. **(C)** A sitting infant reaching forward over an adjustable gap in the surface. **(D)** A crawling infant approaching a gap in the support surface. **(E)** A walking infant using a handrail to help balance on a narrow bridge. **(F)** A walking infant exploring a narrow bridge. (Reprinted with permission from Adolph KE, Berger SE. Motor development. In: Damon W, Lerner R, series eds.; Kuhn D, Siegler RS, vol. eds. *Handbook of child psychology, vol. 2. Cognition, perception, and language,* 6th ed. New York, NY: Wiley, 2006:192. Copyright © 2006 John Wiley & Sons, Inc. Reproduced with permission of John Wiley & Sons, Inc.)

Cognitive Systems

As mentioned in Chapter 12, walking is not completely automatic and thus, when adults perform a second cognitive or motor task while walking (tested in dual-task paradigms), either one or both tasks may be affected. How does dual-task control of walking develop in children?

Walking while Performing a Manual Task

Though balancing while walking requires a large portion of an infant's limited attentional resources, they nevertheless start mastering dual-task control by carrying objects when they are first beginning to walk. In a study on 13-month-old infants, who were in the transition period between crawling and walking,

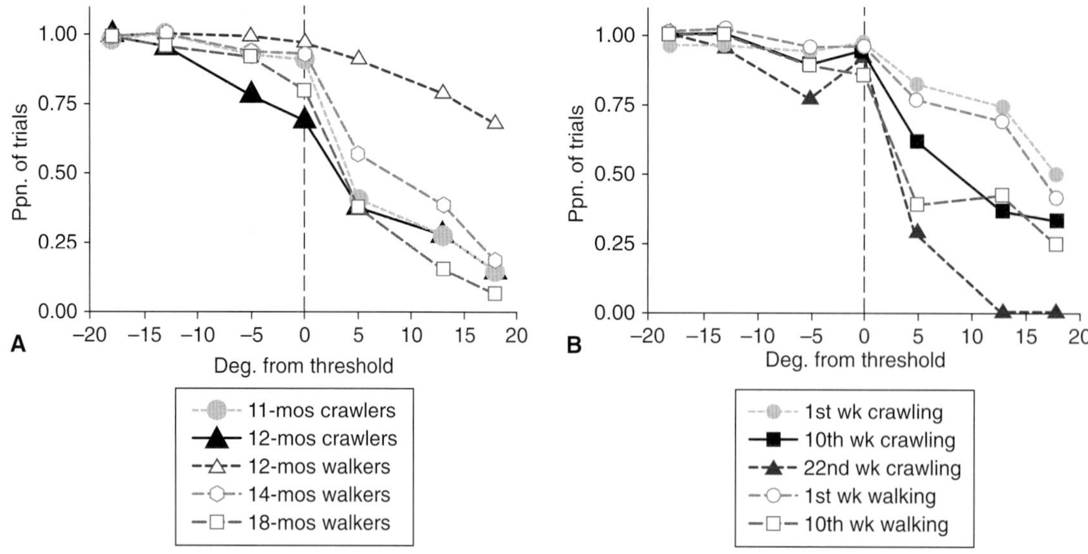

Figure 13.8 Perceptual judgments of infants as indicated by attempts (proportion of trials) to crawl and walk down slopes. **(A)** Cross-sectional data. **(B)** Longitudinal data. Data are normalized to each infant's motor threshold (indicated by 0 on the *x*-axis). Negative numbers on the *x*-axis indicate safe slopes that were shallower than the infants' motor thresholds. Positive numbers indicate risky slopes steeper than the infants' motor thresholds. Graphs show that perceptual errors (attempts to locomote on risky slopes) depend on the motor experience of the infant within a posture, not on their age or the specific locomotor posture. (Reprinted with permission from Adolph KE, Berger SE. Motor development. In: Damon W, Lerner R, series eds.; Kuhn D, Siegler Rs, vol. eds. *Handbook of child psychology, vol. 2. Cognition, perception, and language,* 6th ed. New York, NY: Wiley, 2006:194. Copyright © 2006 John Wiley & Sons, Inc. Reproduced with permission of John Wiley & Sons, Inc.)

Karasik et al. (2012) observed that almost all infants (90%) carried objects. Among the crawlers, 81% carried objects, while all of the walkers carried objects. More experienced walkers walk more, and thus carry objects more frequently than new walkers. However, when normalizing the rate of holding an object by the overall frequency of walking, spontaneous carrying continues unabated across infant development (Heiman et al., 2019). Moreover, infants spontaneously explore objects by looking and/or manipulating while walking—the infant equivalent of walking while texting—but exploration is more frequent while standing than walking (Heiman et al., 2019). It is interesting that less than 3% of carrying bouts resulted in a fall, and falls were equally rare when infants were not carrying an object. Thus, infant walkers are capable of integrating an attentionally demanding secondary task such as carrying an object, without the cost of falling, and are able to selectively choose to explore objects during a less demanding balance task (a stationary position rather than walking).

How does this type of dual-task performance change as children mature? In studies on children who were 4 to 6 years, 7 to 9 years, and 10 to 13 years, participants were asked to walk while carrying a large box, keeping it level. Researchers examined the effect of the secondary task on both bimanual coordination and gait characteristics. They found that only the youngest group (4–6 years) showed differences in gait (a reduction in SL and decreased and more variable ground reaction forces) when walking under the dual-task conditions. The youngest group also showed lower ability to maintain the box level, less coordinated hand movements, and more elbow and shoulder joint excursion in the dual-task walking condition than the older groups. The authors note that these changes in gait characteristics suggest that the youngest children do not have the attentional resources to maintain gait while performing the manual task (Gill et al., 2017; Hung et al., 2013).

Walking while Performing a Cognitive Task

Within the domain of dual-task research, manual tasks are typically considered to require less attentional resources than more complex cognitive tasks. Thus, researchers have explored the effects of more attentionally demanding cognitive tasks on gait performance during development as well.

One study examined the effect of different levels of cognitive load and different walking speeds on walking patterns. In this study, Schaefer and colleagues (2015) compared the treadmill walking performance of 7-year-olds, 9-year-olds, and young adults when carrying out a cognitive task (the N back task, in which they must say whether a number from 1 to 9 is the same as a number they heard two or three positions back in the sequence). Walking performance was measured by determining the variance of the lower body gait pattern under the different cognitive conditions. Results showed that, though cognitive load did not influence walking variability in the young adults, both groups of children were affected by cognitive load. However, gait variability actually decreased when children were working on the easier cognitive task as compared to no task, and variability increased when cognitive load was high.

This resulted in a U-shaped relationship between gait variability and dual-task performance difficulty. The U-shaped relationship regarding performance in dual-task settings has been shown in dual-task experiments performed in stance as well. Decreased gait variability when performing an easy secondary task is thought to result from an external focus of attention allowing gait to become more automatic. However, when the secondary task becomes more difficult, gait variability is increased. In this experimental condition, cognitive performance did not change during walking as compared to the control condition (sitting, performing the cognitive task alone).

In another study examining dual-task costs of locomotion, Boonyong et al. (2012) asked 5- to 6-year-old children, 7- to 16-year-old children, and young adults to walk under single- or dual-task conditions, while performing the auditory Stroop task, a test of executive attention function. Results indicated that the 5- to 6-year-olds had greater dual-task costs, including slower gait velocity (GV) and changes in SL and time, compared to older children or young adults, as you see in Figure 13.9A. There were no differences for any of the groups in dual-task costs for reaction time on the auditory Stroop task, though the 7- to 16-year-olds had greater accuracy costs in the dual-task condition. Results suggest that children below 7 years of age prioritize the cognitive task over gait in a dual-task condition and do not yet have sufficient attentional resources to perform the two tasks simultaneously without a decrement in performance.

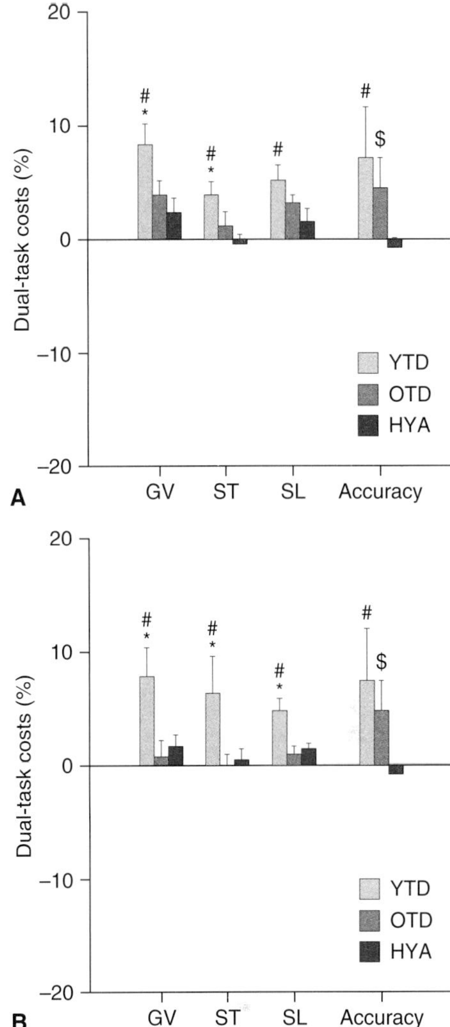

Figure 13.9 Graphs showing dual-task costs for 5- to 6-year-olds (*YTD*), 7- to 16-year-olds (*OTD*), and young adults (*HYA*). **(A)** Dual-task costs for walking, including gait velocity (*GV*), stride time (*ST*), stride length (*SL*), and cognitive task accuracy. Note that the 5- to 6-year-olds showed higher dual-task costs for gait characteristics than the older children or adults. However, older children showed increased dual-task costs for accuracy. **(B)** Dual-task costs for obstacle crossing. Note that the 5- to 6-year-olds also showed significantly higher costs than either the older children or the adults. Both young and older children showed higher costs for cognitive task accuracy than adults. *, Significant difference between YTD and OTD. #, Significant difference between YTD and HYA. $, Significant difference between OTD and HYA. (Adapted from Boonyong S, Siu KC, van Donkelaar P, et al. Development of postural control during gait in typically developing children: the effects of dual-task conditions. *Gait Posture*. 2012;35(3):432, Figure 4.)

Obstacle Crossing while Performing a Cognitive Task

In an extension of the study described in the previous section, Boonyong et al. (2012) asked the same groups of children and young adults to cross an obstacle while performing the auditory Stroop task, to determine if adding the extra difficulty of obstacle crossing to the gait task would challenge attentional resources further. As observed for level walking, the 5- to 6-year-olds showed significantly greater dual-task cost for GV, SL, and stride time (ST) compared to older children or young adults (Fig. 13.9B). In addition, both 5- to 6-year-olds and 7- to 16-year-olds showed increased dual-task costs for the auditory Stroop task compared to young adults. Thus, with obstacle crossing, both gait and the cognitive task were impaired in the younger group, in part due to limited attentional resources.

Did the children also use a different strategy when performing a secondary task during obstacle crossing compared to the young adults? Yes. While both groups of children performed the two tasks in series (e.g., waited to respond to the Stroop task until after they had crossed the obstacle and taken a few steps), the young adults performed the two tasks at about the same time. Figure 13.10 shows these differences between the groups. Results suggest that under dual-task conditions, children deal with limited information-processing resources by performing tasks sequentially, rather than in parallel, as do adults.

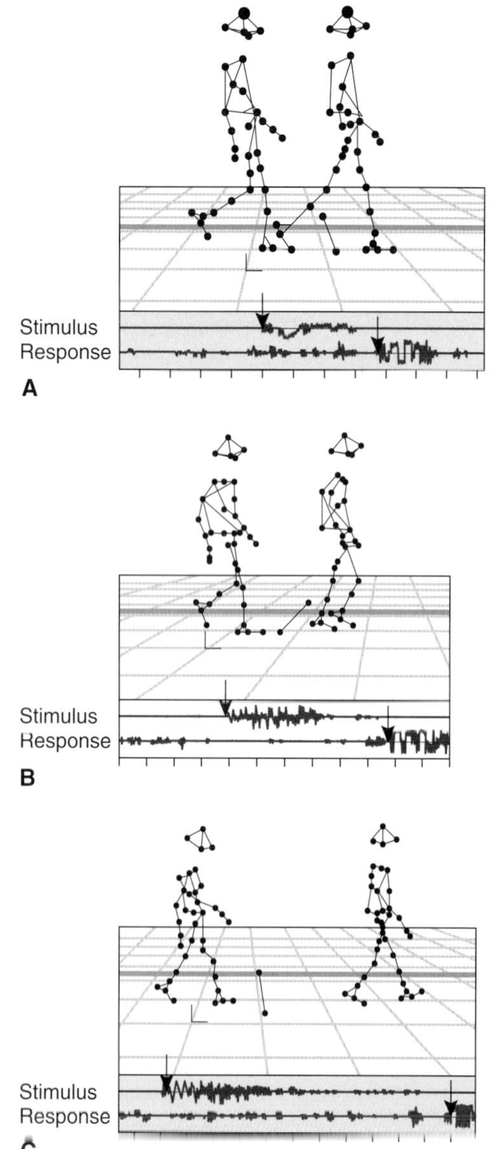

Figure 13.10 Example pictures of obstacle crossing with a concurrent auditory Stroop task in healthy young adults **(A)** and older (7–16 years) **(B)** and younger (5–6 years) **(C)** typically developing children, demonstrating the differences in the point in the obstacle crossing at which a person in each group responded to the auditory stimulus in Stroop task. The first *arrow* indicates the onset of the auditory Stroop stimulus, while the second *arrow* indicates the onset of the verbal response. Note that the adult is crossing the obstacle when giving the verbal response. In contrast, the youngest child **(C)** is well beyond the obstacle when giving the verbal response. (Adapted from Boonyong S, Siu KC, van Donkelaar P, et al. Development of postural control during gait in typically developing children: the effects of dual-task conditions. *Gait Posture*. 2012;35(3):433, Figure 5.)

DEVELOPMENT OF OTHER MOBILITY SKILLS

The first part of this chapter describes the emergence of independent locomotion. We now turn briefly to a review of some of the information on the emergence of other mobility behaviors during development, including rolling, prone progression, and movement from lying in a supine position to standing.

There are two approaches to describing motor development in infants and children. One approach relies on normative studies that describe the age at which various motor behaviors emerge. Normative studies have given rise to norm-referenced scales that compare an infant's motor behavior with the performance of a group of infants of the same age. Normative studies can provide clinicians with rough guidelines about the relative ages associated with specific motor milestones. However, they have universally reported that there is incredible variability in the time at which normal children achieve motor milestones (Palisano, 1993).

Another approach to describing motor development is with reference to the stages associated with the emergence of a single behavior, such as rolling or coming to standing. Stages within the emergence of a skill are often used by clinicians as the basis for a treatment progression, with the assumption that a mature and stable adult-like pattern is the last stage in the progression. However, some research has raised doubts about the concept that there is a consistent stable sequential pattern during the emergence of a particular motor behavior (Fishkind & Haley, 1986; Horowitz & Sharby, 1988).

Given these cautions about timing, variability, and the sequential nature of the emergence of motor skills, we review some of the studies that have examined the stages in the emergence of rolling, prone progression, and the assumption of the vertical position from supine. As we mentioned in Chapter 8, on development of postural control, much of the information we have on the emergence of motor behavior in children is largely the result of efforts in the 1920s to 1940s by two developmental researchers, Arnold Gesell and Myrtle McGraw, who observed and recorded the stages of development in normal children (McGraw, 1945).

Development of Rolling

Rolling is an important part of mobility skills because rotation or partial rotation is a part of movement patterns used to achieve supine-to-sitting or supine-to-standing behavior. Babies first roll from the side-lying to the supine position at 1 to 2 months of age and from the supine to the side-lying position at 4 to 5 months. Infants roll from prone to supine at 4 months of age and then from supine to prone at 6 to 8 months. Infants change their rolling pattern as they mature, from a log-rolling pattern, in which the entire body rolls as a unit, to a segmental pattern. By 9 months of age, most infants use a segmental rotation of the body on the pelvis (McGraw, 1945; Towen, 1976).

Development of Prone Progression

According to McGraw (1945), the prone progression includes nine phases that take the infant from the prone position to creeping and crawling and span the months from birth to 10 to 13 months. Figure 13.11 illustrates the nine phases reported by McGraw and the relative time in which the behavior was seen. The age at which the behavior was seen and the percentage of children in which the behavior was observed are graphed. The first phase is characterized by lower-extremity flexion and extension in a primarily flexed posture. In phase 2, spinal extension begins, as does the development of head control. In the third phase, spinal extension continues cephalocaudally, reaching the thoracic area. The arms can extend and support the chest off the surface. Propulsion movements begin in the arms and legs during phases 4 and 5. In phase 6, the creeping position is assumed. Phase 7 is characterized by fairly disorganized attempts at progression; however, by phases 8 and 9, organized propulsion in the creeping position has emerged.

Keep in mind that McGraw placed great emphasis on the neural antecedents of maturing motor behavior. Indeed, more recent work has shown that 2-day-old newborns can crawl with locomotor patterns similar to those documented during quadrupedal locomotion in animals and human adults, suggesting there is a neural circuitry underlying crawling (Forma et al., 2019). Thus, McGraw's emphasis was on describing stages of motor development that could be related to the structural growth and maturation of the central nervous system (CNS). However, current research has shown that many factors contribute to the emergence of motor skills during development, including but not limited to maturation of the CNS (Thelen & Ulrich, 1991).

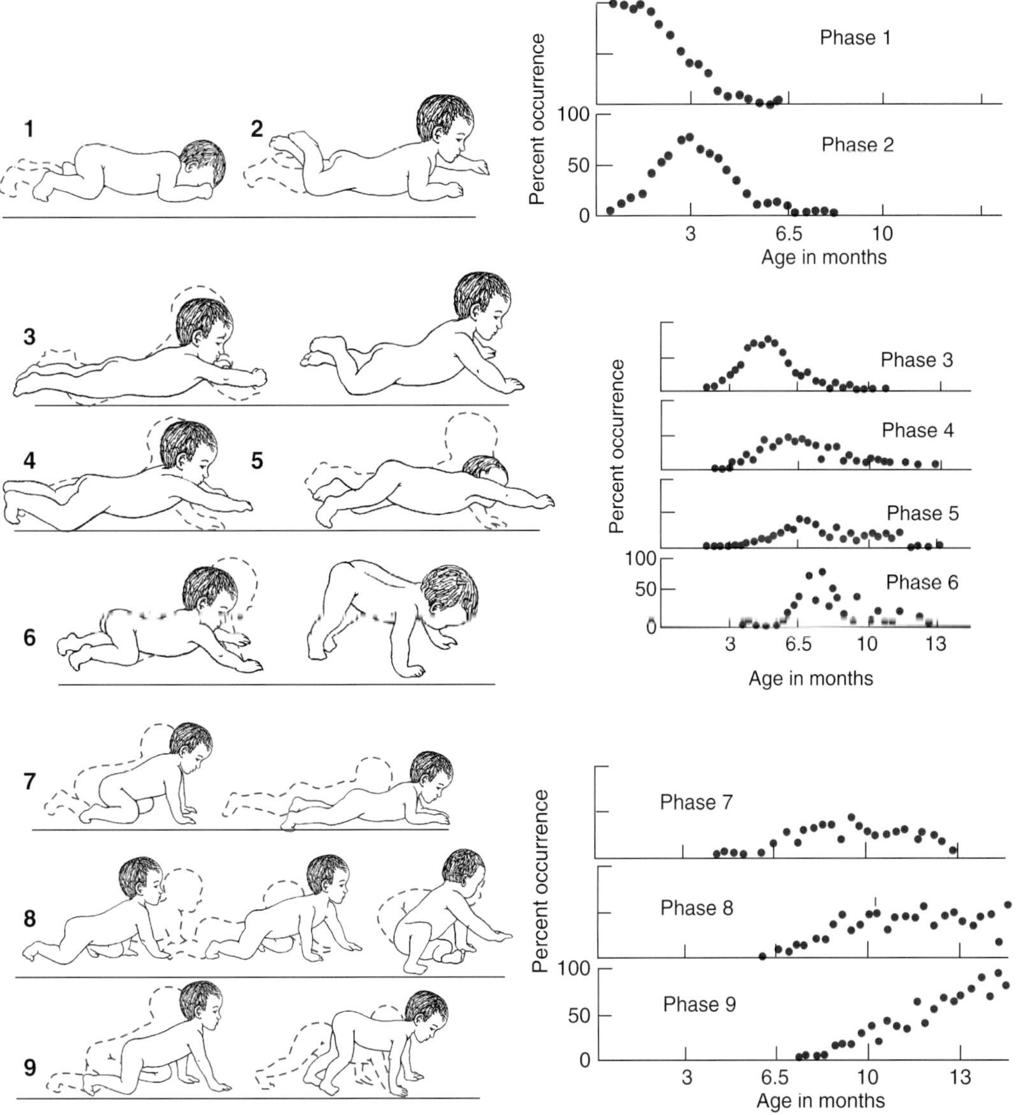

Figure 13.11 Illustration of the nine phases of prone progression as reported by McGraw **(left)**. Graphs, for each phase, showing the ages at which the behavior was seen (*x*-axis) and the percentage of children in which the behavior was observed (*y*-axis) **(right)**. (Adapted from McGraw M. *The neuromuscular maturation of the human infant*. New York, NY: Hafner Press, 1945.)

Moreover, as described in Chapter 8, motor skill acquisition is characterized by large individual differences in onset ages, the sequence of skills, and the pattern of movements. Infants begin creeping anywhere between 6.1 and 11.3 months (5th and 95th percentiles on the WHO standards). Some infants follow the phases reported by McGraw—first with low propulsion movements before acquiring the creeping position. However, others skip propulsion movements and progress straight to creeping, and still others skip creeping altogether and instead hitch, bum shuffle, or go directly to walking (Adolph, 1998). If infants were to have a crawling period, they would do so by coordinating their arms and legs in various ways (see Fig. 13.12)—some would "army" belly crawl using their belly and thighs for support or would "inchworm" belly crawl by alternating their limbs on their belly; some would crawl on hands and knees or hands and feet with their belly off the floor, and others would do a combination of both using the knee of one leg and the foot of the other; and still others would scoot forward in a seated position (Adolph et al., 1998; Patrick et al., 2012). Thus, although the CNS may be an important factor involved in the acquisition of motor skills, these varied sequences and patterns of movements suggest that infants find their own, unique solutions to a problem: how to get to the other end of the room. Motivation to move may also play a role, especially in the wide age bands for skill acquisition. For example, research has shown that infants with higher "motivation to

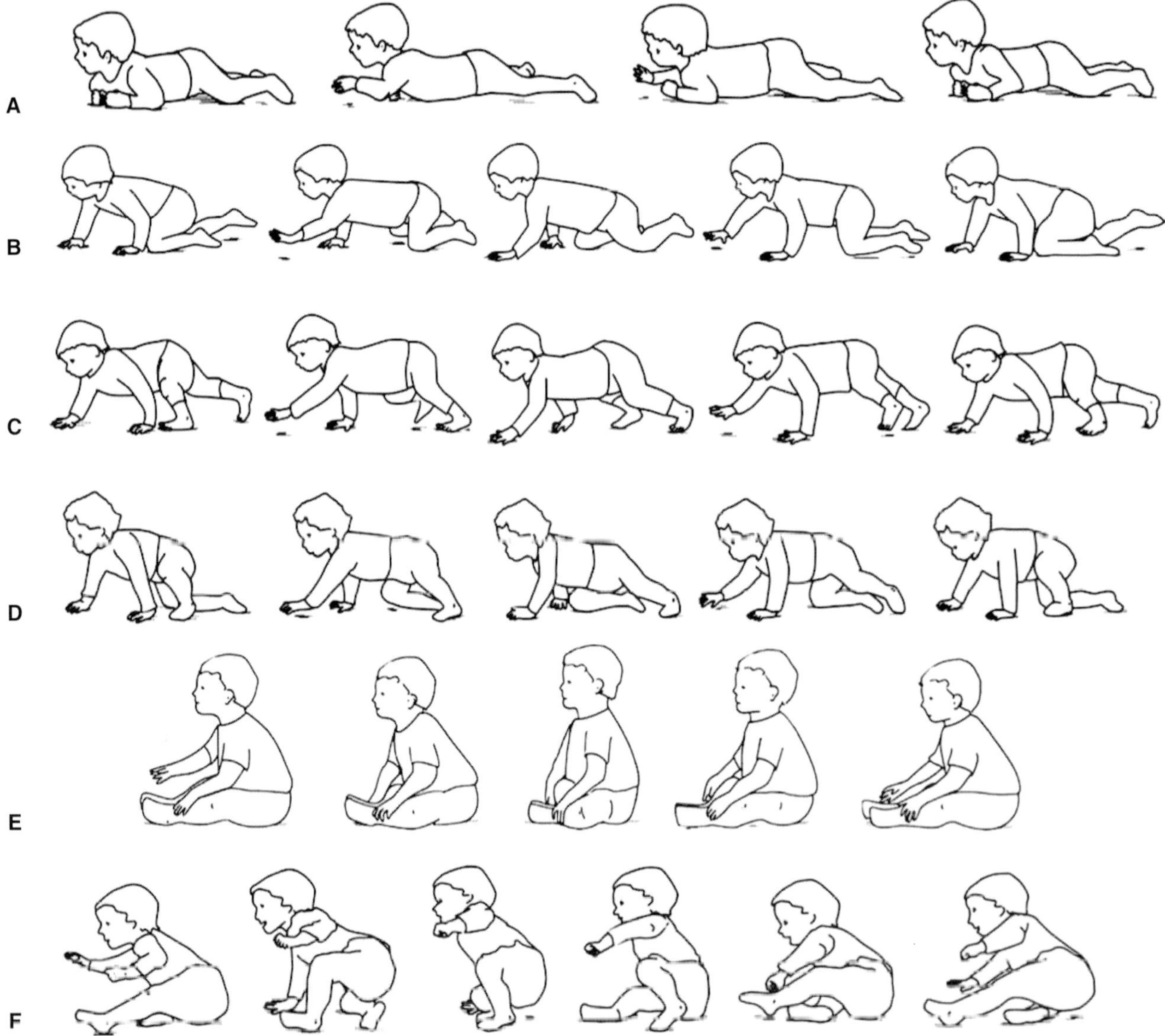

Figure 13.12 Illustration of crawling styles. Each sequence is an example of one crawling style cycle and reads from left to right: belly crawling **(A)**; standard hands-and-knees crawling **(B)**; hands-and-feet crawling **(C)**; step-crawl mix, using left foot and right knee **(D)**; scooting, using flexion of the legs to pull the body forward **(E)**; and step-scoot mix using one hand, one knee, and one foot **(F)**. (Reprinted and adapted from Patrick, S.K., Noah, J.A., & Yang, J.F. Developmental constraints of quadrupedal coordination across crawling styles in human infants. *J Neurophysiol*. 2012;107:3051, with permission.)

move" scores (as indexed by higher spontaneous activity levels, higher persistence, and fewer social encouragements to move) achieve their motor milestones at earlier ages than infants with the lowest "motivation to move" scores (Atun-Einy et al., 2013).

Development of Supine to Stand

Just as the pattern used to roll changes as infants develop, so does the movement pattern used to achieve standing from a supine position. The pattern initially seen in infants moving from supine to standing includes rolling to prone, then moving into an all-fours pattern, and using a pull-to-stand method to achieve the erect position by first using a two-leg strategy followed by a half-kneel strategy (Atun-Einy et al., 2012). With development, the child learns to move from the all-fours position to a plantigrade position and from there to erect stance. By the age of 2 to 3 years, the supine-to-prone portion is modified to a partial roll and sit-up pattern, and by ages 4 to 5, a symmetrical sit-up pattern emerges (Fig. 13.13). This is considered a mature or adult-like movement pattern used for this task (McGraw, 1945). But as you remember from Chapter 12, on normal mobility skills, researchers have found tremendous variability in how adults move from supine to standing. Just as for adults, most likely, strength in the abdominals and hip flexors plays a major role in the type of pattern used by infants when moving from supine to standing (VanSant, 1988a).

Development of Sit-to-Stand

Studies have also examined variations in sit-to-stand behavior in infants and children and have compared children with adults (Cahill et al., 1999; Guarrera-Bowlby & Gentile, 2004). At the ages of 12 to 14 months, infants tend to maintain the trunk and knees more flexed, to maintain the COG low, and thus attain better balance during upright standing (Da Costa & Rocha, 2013). Then, sit-to-stand patterns become more adult like but remain immature. When comparing children of 12 to 18 months, 4 to 5 years, and 9 to 10 years, researchers found that even the youngest children had mastered the basic intersegmental pattern seen in adults. However, the youngest children were not able to perform the movement as efficiently because they ended the movement by either rising up on toes or taking a step forward. In addition, movement time, amplitude, and peak angular velocity of trunk flexion increased with development. Children in the older age groups showed ground reaction force patterns that were similar to those of adults, while younger children reached peak force gradually, with fluctuations. Other studies have shown that children who are 6 to 7 years old have twice the intraindividual variability across trials as adults (Guarrera-Bowlby & Gentile, 2004). It is possible that these changes are related to the development of children's ability to control horizontal momentum and balance (Cahill et al., 1999).

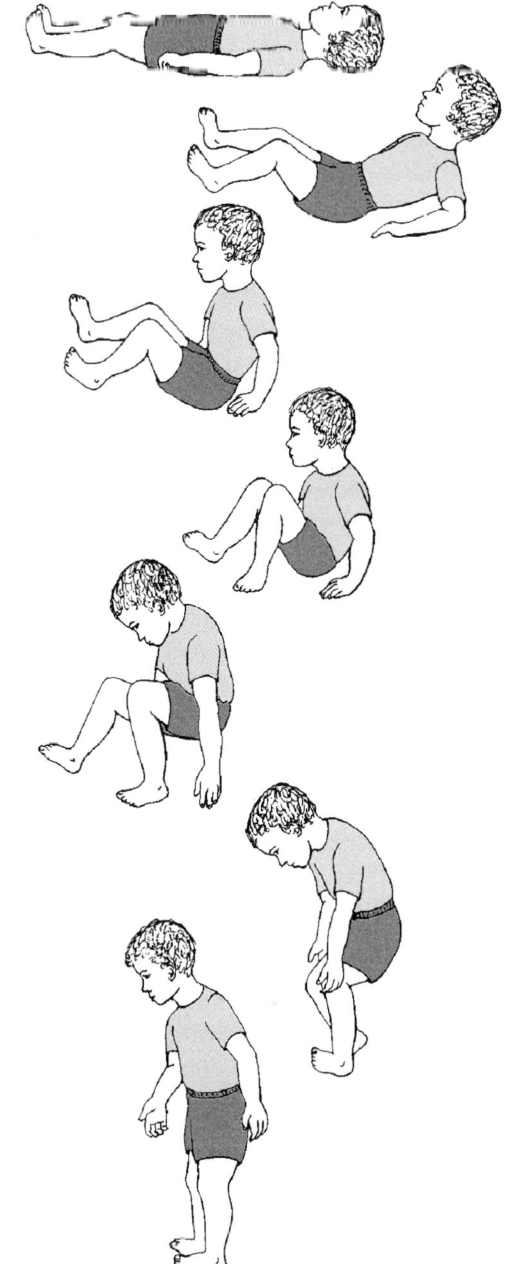

Figure 13.13 Common pattern used to move from supine to standing in children ages 4 to 5. Note that the child uses a symmetrical pattern. (Adapted with permission from Van Sant AF. Age differences in movement patterns used by children to rise from a supine position to erect stance. *Phys Ther.* 1988;68: 1130–1138, with permission of the American Physical Therapy Association. This material is copyrighted, and any further reproduction or distribution requires written permission from APTA.)

In summary, the research studies reviewed support the concept that locomotion is a behavior that emerges through the progressive development of many subsystems. The subsystems contributing to the emergence of mature gait develop at different rates; however, postural control appears to be the most significant rate-limiting factor in the development of independent walking. The emergence of walking results from a combination of maturation within neural processes and a tremendous amount of experience, including on average 14,000 steps daily and hundreds of falls!

SUMMARY

1. There are three requirements for successful locomotion: (a) the ability to generate a rhythmic stepping pattern to move the body forward (progression); (b) postural control, ensuring orientation and stability; and (c) the ability to adapt gait to changing task and environmental requirements (adaptation). In the development of locomotion, these three factors emerge sequentially, with the stepping pattern appearing first, equilibrium control next, followed by adaptive capabilities.
2. The emergence of independent gait is characterized by the development of many interacting systems with certain hierarchical components. An innate pattern generator creates the basic rhythm of the step cycle, which can be seen in newborn stepping. In the first year, the gradual development of descending systems from higher neural centers gives the child increasing control over this locomotor behavior. The control of equilibrium, organized at a higher level than that of the pattern generator, develops over a longer period, as do adaptive systems essential to the integration of reactive and proactive strategies into gait.
3. The development of locomotor behavior begins prenatally and continues until the emergence of mature gait at about 7 years of age. Stepping behavior is present at birth and can be elicited in most infants if they are supported and inclined slightly forward. This early behavior resembles quadrupedal stepping, with flexion of the hip and knee, synchronous joint motion, and considerable coactivation of agonist and antagonist muscles.
4. In many infants, early stepping disappears at about 2 months of age, possibly because of biomechanical changes in the infant's system, such as an increase in relative body weight. Early stepping gradually transforms into a more mature pattern over the first 2 years of life.
5. There seems to be agreement among researchers that the ability to integrate postural control into the locomotor pattern is the most important rate-limiting factor in the emergence of independent walking.
6. The most significant modifications to the gait pattern occur during the first 4 to 5 months of independent walking. Most of these changes reflect the child's growing ability to integrate balance control with locomotion in these first months.

ANSWERS TO LAB ACTIVITY ASSIGNMENTS

Lab Activity 13.1

1, 2. See Table 13.1.

CHAPTER 14

Aging and Mobility

Learning Objectives

Following completion of this chapter, the reader will be able to:

1. Describe the age-related changes in the three major requirements of locomotion—progression (pattern generation), postural control (both orientation and stability), and adaptation (to changing task and environmental conditions).
2. Describe changes in the major kinematic, kinetic, and electromyographic parameters of gait that occur with aging.
3. Describe age-related changes in the contributions to gait of neural (sensory, motor, and higher cognitive) and nonneural subsystems.
4. Discuss age-related changes associated with other forms of mobility, including stair climbing, transfers, sit-to-stand, supine-stand, and rising from bed.

INTRODUCTION

Falls, and the injuries that often accompany them, are a serious problem in the older adult. In fact, falls are the leading cause of injury-related deaths among persons aged 65 years of age or older (CDC, 2018). Fifty-seven percent of adults over 75 years report some degree of fear of falling, which is a significant predictor of their activity restriction (Yardley & Smith, 2002). Consequently, these people begin avoiding situations that require refined balance skills, which leads to further declines in walking and balance skills. Nevertheless, not all older adults have difficulties with mobility skills. Much like the study of balance control, it is important to distinguish between age-related changes in mobility affecting all older adults and pathology-related changes, which affect only a few.

Many of the falls experienced by older adults occur during walking. It is thus important to understand the changes in the systems contributing to normal gait in older adults to fully understand the cause of increased falls in this population. Many researchers now believe that balance control is a primary contributor to stable walking. In addition, decreased balance control is a major factor affecting loss of independent mobility in many older adults. This chapter discusses age-related changes in mobility skills within both the systems framework and the International Classification of Functioning, Disability and Health (ICF) framework. Thus, in addition to examining age-related changes in systems contributing to mobility, we examine changes in the gait pattern within the ICF component of *Body Structure and Function*. We also discuss characteristics of the activity of walking (distance walked, negotiation of obstacles, etc.) and how it relates to participation, including moving around different locations in the home and outside the home.

Gait Dysfunction: Aging or Pathology?

Age-related changes in locomotion may be due to primary or secondary aging phenomena. Primary factors affecting aging include changes in gene expression that result in changes in hormonal function, aging, and death. Also, individuals may have a genetic predisposition to specific diseases, which results in an inevitable decline of neuronal function within a particular system. Secondary factors are experiential and include nutrition, exercise, stress level, and acquired pathologies, among others. The extent to which gait disorders in older adults are due to primary or secondary factors is a very important point to consider as we begin to look at the literature on changes in gait characteristics in older adults (Karasik et al., 2005).

The older clinical literature classified a variety of different walking patterns as "age-related gait disorders." These diverse gait disorders included gait apraxia (slow, halting, short-stepped, shuffling, or sliding gait), hypokinetic–hypertonic syndrome (slow, deliberate gait, but without the shuffling or sliding components described previously), and marche à petits pas (small, quick shuffling steps, followed by a slow cautious, unsteady gait), vestibular dysfunction gait (difficulties in turning), and proprioceptive dysfunction gait (cautious, with a tendency to watch the feet and make missteps) (Craik, 1989).

As was true in the postural control literature, care must be taken when reviewing studies discussing age-related changes in gait. When interpreting the results of a study, one should examine carefully the population studied and ask questions such as, What criteria were used in selecting older participants? Did researchers exclude anyone with pathology under the assumption that pathology is not a part of primary aging? Results will vary tremendously depending on the composition of the group of older adults under study. For example, one study noted that in an unselected group of subjects 60 to 99 years of age, walking velocities were much slower than those for young adults and also slower than those shown in other published studies on older adults (Imms & Edholm, 1981). It is quite possible that the subjects in the study were less fit, and many subjects reported symptoms likely to impair gait. In contrast, a study that screened 1,184 older adults and chose 32 who had no pathology found no differences in the gait parameters between this select group of older nonimpaired adults and young adults (Gabell & Nayak, 1984).

More recent research has begun to indicate that many gait disorders once considered to be "age related," such as gait apraxia, hypokinetic–hypertonic syndrome, and marche à petits pas, are really manifestations of pathology rather than characteristics of a generalized aging process. However, as we note in the following sections, there are distinctive changes in gait that occur in many, even healthy, older adults. In the following section, we discuss age-related changes in the motor systems contributing to gait impairments in both normal and balance-impaired older adults (BIOAs). Our discussion includes impairments in steady-state gait, including deficits in progression and postural control, as well as impairments in the ability to adapt gait to changing task and environmental conditions, including recovery from balance threats and proactive balance in gait, involving navigating through changing environments.

MOTOR SYSTEMS AND GAIT

Gait is an extraordinarily complex behavior that involves coordination of muscles and joints throughout the body in order to achieve the three requirements of gait: progression, postural control, and adaptation.

Age-Related Changes in Steady-State Gait

A primary focus of research on age-related changes to gait has been on characterizing changes in the gait pattern during steady-state gait, including temporal, distance, kinematic, kinetic, and muscle activation patterns.

Temporal and Distance Factors

Studies examining changes in walking patterns with age have used a number of different experimental approaches. In one approach, which we might call a "naturalistic approach," adults were observed walking spontaneously in a natural setting. This paradigm was used to try to minimize the constraints on walking style that are often necessary when quantifying gait parameters in a laboratory setting.

In these studies, researchers observed people of different ages walking along the streets of New York City (Drillis, 1961) or Amsterdam (Molen, 1973). In the first study, of 752 pedestrians in New York City, as age increased from 20 to 70 years, there was a decrease in walking velocity, step length, and step rate (no statistical analysis was reported). In the second study, on 533 pedestrians in Amsterdam, similar results were found. Gender differences were also found; both younger and older women walked with slower velocity, shorter step length, and higher cadence than did men. While there are advantages in allowing subjects to walk in a natural environment, the disadvantages include being unable to control for variables such as different walking goals, taking a stroll versus hurrying to work, and relative health of the subjects (Craik, 1989). Nevertheless, experiments conducted in controlled laboratory settings with older adults show similar results to findings from natural studies—with increasing age, gait speed decreases, stride length decreases, and double support time increases (Hollman et al., 2011).

Age-Related Changes in Kinematics

Later studies of age-related changes in gait focused on a kinematic analysis of stepping patterns in older adults. In one study, subjects were healthy men, with normal strength and range of motion, ranging in age from 20 to 87 years (Murray et al., 1969). Each was tested at his preferred speed and at a fast walking speed. Men over 67 years of age showed significantly ($p < 0.01$) slower walking speeds (118–123 cm/s) than did the young adults (150 cm/s). Stride length was also significantly shorter, especially during fast walking. Vertical movement of the head during the gait cycle was smaller while lateral movement was larger. Stride width tended to be wider for men over 74. Toeing out was also greater for men over 80. Over age 65, the stance phase was longer, with a commensurate shortening of time in the swing phase.

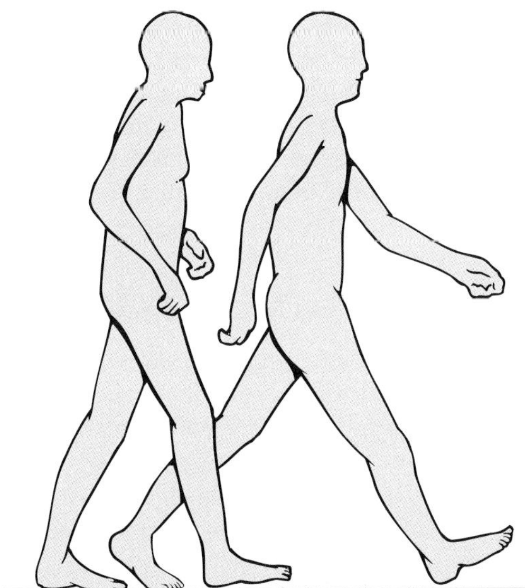

Figure 14.1 Example of the walking pattern of a young adult **(right)** versus a healthy older man **(left)**. Note the reduced step length and arm swing. (Adapted from Murray MP, Kory RC, Clarkson BH. Walking patterns in healthy older men. *J Gerontol.* 1969;24:169–178.)

Finally, hip, knee, and ankle flexion was less than in young adults, and the whole shoulder rotation pattern was shifted to a more extended position, with less elbow rotation as well. Figure 14.1 is adapted from the study of Murray et al. (1969), showing the differences in the limb positions of a younger versus an older man at heel strike. Note the significantly shorter step length and extended arm position. In a second study (Murray et al., 1970), age-related changes in gait patterns were investigated in women, and similar changes were noted, including reduced walking speeds and shorter steps. These changes occurred in the 60- to 70-year-old age group.

Interestingly, the researchers concluded that the older adults studied did not have a pathologic gait pattern. Instead, their walking was reported as guarded, possibly with the aim to increase stability. Gait patterns were similar to those used by someone walking on a slippery surface or someone walking in darkness. However, due to the short step length and wide step width in older adults, researchers have shown that the components of the required coefficient of friction (i.e., the slip risk) is low in the anterior–posterior plane and high in the medio-lateral plane. Consequently, older adults, who walk with a cautious gait, may have a high risk of losing balance in the mediolateral direction (Yamaguchi & Masani, 2019).

All of this sounds like a postural control problem. From reading this description, one might hypothesize that gait changes in the older adult relate more to the loss of balance control than to changes in the step cycle itself (Murray et al., 1969).

How do these slower walking speeds affect function in daily life? Many of the previous studies report that older adults are unable to walk faster than 1.4 m/s. This is the minimal speed required to cross a street safely. Lundgren Lindquist et al. (1983) have shown that none of the 205 subjects studied who were 79 years old could cross a street before the traffic light changed when walking at their preferred speed. Thus, many of the older adults studied would not be considered safe independent community ambulators.

How do the walking characteristics of older adults who fall compare with those with no history of falls? While the previous studies have shown that the gait characteristics of healthy older adults show few differences when compared with those of younger adults, older individuals with a history of falls show significant differences in walking patterns (Hausdorff et al., 1997; Heitmann et al., 1989; Wolfson et al., 1995). Wolfson et al. (1995) have shown that both stride length (nonfallers, 0.82 ± 0.22 m; fallers, 0.53 ± 0.21 m) and walking speed (nonfallers, 0.64 ± 0.21 m/s; fallers, 0.37 ± 0.17 m/s) are significantly reduced in older adults who fall.

Heitmann et al. (1989) have found that older female participants with poor balance performance have increased step width during gait. Other studies have reported that step width measured at the heel was significantly larger in older persons with a history of falls when they walked at a fast speed (6 km/h) when compared with older adults without a history of falls. It was also noted that older adults with a history of falls had balance problems unrelated to gait because they were unable to stand with their feet in tandem position and their eyes open as long as those with no history of falls. Of course, it is likely that older adults with a history of falls have an undiagnosed pathological condition. Therefore, it is important to examine these individuals carefully, to determine if underlying pathology contributes to gait disturbances, when performing studies on older adults who fall (Gehlsen & Whaley, 1990; Heitmann et al., 1989).

Variability in Gait Patterns within the Individual: Does This Contribute to Imbalance? Most studies on age-related deterioration in balance and gait have focused on overall performance differences in older versus young adults. Although these studies have shown substantial and significant differences in performance in older as compared with younger adults, a second performance variable that may also contribute to balance constraints in older adults is the extent to which the individual's performance varies from trial to trial in a repeated task, that is, intraindividual variability. Intraindividual variability may reflect processing fluctuations or lack of processing robustness, indicating "noise" within the physiological system underlying behavioral control (Li et al., 2004). This is an important factor in balance control, as increased variability of center of mass (COM) motion, for example, when an individual is already near their stability limits during gait, could result in the COM moving outside the stability limits and thus result in loss of balance and a subsequent fall.

A number of research labs have begun to explore stride-to-stride variability in older adults who fall. For example, Hausdorff and colleagues (Hausdorff, 2007; Hausdorff et al., 1997) evaluated the variability of gait in community-dwelling older fallers, nonfallers, and young adults. They found that stride-time and swing-time variability were significantly larger in the fallers as compared with both young adult and older adult nonfallers. In contrast, gait speed was similar in the fallers and nonfallers. Although both older adult groups had similar walking speed and muscle strength, the older adults who fell had significant increases in stride variance.

In addition, Studenski and colleagues (Brach et al., 2005) have shown that either too much or too little step-width variability is associated with falls in older adults. They sampled a population of 503 older adults (mean age, 79 years) who were independent walkers and found that individuals with extreme step-width variability (either low or high variability) were more likely to report a fall in the past year than individuals with moderate variability. The association between step-width variability and fall history was not significant in individuals who walked less than 1 m/s.

It has also been shown that walking variability and, specifically, stride-time variability increase when older adults are asked to perform a simultaneous arithmetic task (Beauchet et al., 2005). This increase in variability in dual-task settings is assumed to be due to insufficient attentional processing resources for performing the two tasks simultaneously, causing increased processing noise.

Can gait variability be used to identify persons at risk of falls? Hausdorff et al. (2001) tested the hypothesis that in community-dwelling older adults, altered gait variability would predict future falls. Older adults were assessed at baseline and then followed for 12 months, monitoring fall status weekly. During the 12-month follow-up period, 39% of the participants reported at least one fall. At baseline, gait variability measures were significantly increased in older adults who subsequently fell as compared with those who did not, suggesting that measures of gait variability are *predictive* of future falls.

Researchers examining the progression of gait variability with increasing age have shown that changes in variability are directionally specific and task dependent. Bogen and colleagues (2019) tested 56 70- to 81-year-olds, with a 2-year interval between tests, walking 6.5 m under four different conditions: at preferred speed, at fast speed, during a dual task condition, and on an uneven surface. Trunk accelerations were captured using a body-worn sensor. The authors found that during preferred speed walking, age-related variability increased in the anterior–posterior direction, while during fast speed walking, variability increased in the vertical direction, and finally under dual-task walking, it increased in both the medio-lateral and the vertical directions. However, no changes in gait variability were observed during uneven surface walking. Thus, this study confirms previous cross-sectional studies showing that gait variability increases with age, but the movement plane of variability is task specific.

Age-Related Changes in Musculoskeletal Properties

The studies discussed previously show clear changes in certain kinematic characteristics of the gait cycle in the average older adult. How do these changes relate to changes in muscle response patterns? In a study comparing patterns of muscle activity in younger (19–38 years) and older (64–86 years) women, average electromyographic (EMG) activity levels in gastrocnemius, tibialis anterior, biceps femoris, rectus femoris, and peroneus longus were higher in the older than in the younger age group (Finley et al., 1969).

In addition, there were changes in the activity of individual muscles at specific points in the step cycle. For example, at heel strike, the peroneus longus and gastrocnemius muscles were moderately to highly active in the older women but showed little or no activity in the younger group. The authors suggested that this increased activity resulted from an effort to improve stability during the stance phase of gait. For example, increased coactivation of agonist and antagonist muscles at a joint may be used to improve balance control, by increasing joint stiffness. This strategy is often seen in subjects who are unskilled in a task or who are performing in a situation that requires increased control (Woollacott, 1989).

Other researchers have looked at how certain muscle properties influence functional abilities. For example, Guadagnin and colleagues (2019) studied how decreased tibialis anterior thickness is correlated with decreased lead limb toe clearance during obstacle crossing, and decreased vastus lateralis thickness and muscle quality are correlated with decreased gait speed and step length in older adults. Delabastita and colleagues (2018) performed a systematic review on the influence of Achilles tendon stiffness on functional activities and found that older adults had decreased stiffness, which was related to decreases in their walking performance and balance.

Age-Related Changes in Joint Kinetics

We have just noted several studies indicating that older adults show higher levels of muscle responses and different activation sequences and muscular properties among leg muscles than young adults during walking. But how do these changes influence the dynamics of gait?

Using the method of inverse dynamics, moments of force, as well as the mechanical power generated and absorbed at each joint, can be calculated. This process allows the amount of power generated by muscles to be estimated. Remember from Chapter 12, on locomotion, that an increase in muscle energy is needed to initiate swing while a decrease in energy is needed to prepare for heel strike.

Using inverse dynamics techniques, Winter and colleagues (1990) compared the gait patterns of 15 healthy older adults (62–78 years of age) to those of 12 young adults (21–28 years). They found that older adults had significantly shorter stride length and longer double-support time than did young adults. In addition, in older adult subjects, plantarflexors generated significantly less power at push-off while the quadriceps muscle absorbed significantly less energy during late stance and early swing.

These researchers concluded that the reduction of plantarflexor power during push-off could explain the shorter step length, flatfooted heel strike, and increased double-support duration. Two alternative explanations were proposed for a weaker push-off in older adults. One explanation suggested that a reduction in muscle strength in the ankle plantarflexors in the older adults could be responsible for the weaker push-off. An alternative explanation argued that reduced push-off could be an adaptive change used to ensure a safer gait, since high push-off power acts upward and forward and is thus potentially more destabilizing than when lower power is used at push-off (Winter et al., 1990).

In the study by Winters et al., an index of dynamic balance was computed to determine the ability to coordinate the anterior–posterior balance of the head-arm-trunk (HAT) segment while simultaneously maintaining an appropriate extensor moment in the ankle, knee, and hip during the stance phase. It was found that the older adults showed a reduced ability to covary movements at the hip and knee. This means that older adults had trouble controlling the HAT segment while simultaneously maintaining an extensor moment in the lower stance limb. In evaluating the older group individually, it was noted that two thirds were within the normal young adult range, while one third had very low covariances of moments at the hip and knee. It was concluded that some older adults may have problems with dynamic balance during locomotion, indicative of balance impairments not detected in their medical history or simple clinical tests.

In order to determine whether the decreased joint torques and powers that are found in older adults during gait are due to slower self-selected walking speeds or are true gait-limiting factors, researchers examined these parameters in young and older adults when they were walking at the same speed (Devita & Hortobagyi, 2000). They found that angular impulse (calculated throughout stance from support and ankle torques and during initial half of stance from the knee and hip torques) was the same in both groups, but older adults used 58% more angular impulse and 279% more work at the hip, 50% less angular impulse and 39% less work at the knee, and 23% less angular impulse and 29% less work at the ankle. Thus, the older adults showed a redistribution of joint torques and powers compared with young adults, using hip extensors more and knee extensors and ankle plantarflexors less than young adults when walking at the same speed. It is worth noting that other researchers found conflicting results. For example, Schloemer and colleagues (2017) supported previous findings showing that older adults produce a greater gluteus maximus force during gait than young adults. However, no differences between age groups were observed for ankle plantarflexor forces. The authors highlight that one potential explanation for this discrepancy is the normalization of values to participants' weight and height. Numerous research studies have described changes in gait patterns found among many older adults. These changes are summarized in Table 14.1. To better understand age-related changes to gait, complete Lab Activity 14.1. Compare your findings to the research summarized in Table 14.1.

TABLE 14.1 Summary of Gait Changes in the Older Adult

Temporal or distance factors	Kinematic changes
Decreased velocity	Decreased vertical movement of the center of gravity
Decreased step length	Decreased arm swing
Decreased step rate	Decreased hip, knee, and ankle flexion
Decreased stride length	Flatter foot on heel strike
Increased stride width	Decreased ability to covary hip or knee movements
Increased stance phase	Decreased dynamic stability during stance
Increased time in double support	**Muscle activation patterns**
Decreased swing phase	Increased coactivation (increased stiffness)
	Kinetic changes
	Decreased power generation at push-off
	Decreased power absorption at heel strike

LAB ACTIVITY 14.1

Objective: To examine age-related changes in the spatial, temporal, and kinematic parameters of gait.

Procedures: Find two older adults from your community, one who is very active and well balanced and the other who has reported gait and balance problems. Document changes in spatial and temporal aspects of gait in these two adults. Also observe and describe the following gait characteristics in each adult: (a) ability to maintain an upright posture, (b) ability to control stability (how often does the older adult fall within a fixed time period), (c) initial contact at foot strike, and (d) position of arms.

Assignment

1. Compare the data you have gathered from healthy young adults with the data gathered from your two older subjects. What parameters of gait are similar between the young and the older adults?
2. What parameters differ?
3. How similar or dissimilar are gait parameters between the two older adults?
4. How do your data compare with those described in Table 14.1?

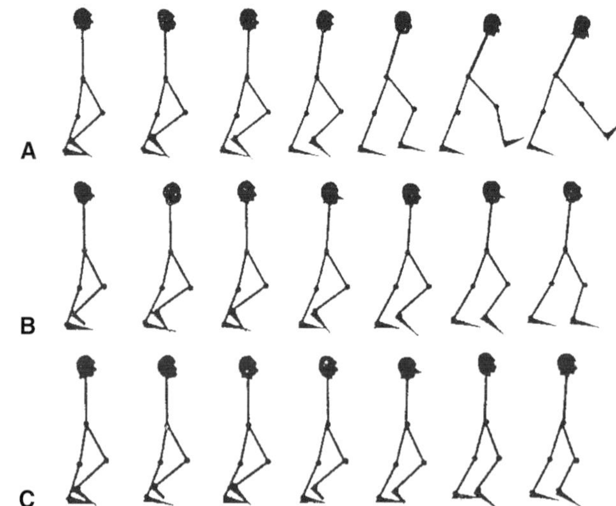

Figure 14.2 **(A)** Stick figure of the response to tripping if a subject had maximum joint torques and torque development rates. **(B, C)** Response to tripping that would be seen if a subject had 75% and 50%, respectively, of joint torques and torque development rates available. For the hypothetical subject in C, the swing foot recontacts the ground, causing an additional trip, with the upper body COM in front of the base of support. (Reprinted from Schultz AB. Muscle function and mobility biomechanics in the elderly: an overview of some recent research. *J Gerontol.* 1995;50A (special issue):60–63, with permission.)

Age-Related Changes in Adaptation of Gait: Reactive and Proactive Balance

Adapting gait is the hallmark of normal mobility function, and a reduced ability to adapt gait in response to both unexpected and expected challenges to gait is a major factor in falls among older adults. Many falls by older adults occur while walking and may be due to slipping and tripping. Several research groups have examined proactive adaptive strategies during gait in older adults. In addition, studies on age-related changes in reactive balance control have been published (Chambers & Cham, 2007; Lockhart et al., 2003; Tang & Woollacott, 1998, 1999).

Age-Related Changes in Reactive Balance

Trips. Research on falls (Gabell et al., 1985; Overstall et al., 1977) has indicated that 35% to 47% of falls in older adults result from tripping over an object. In order to study the determinants of balance recovery from a trip, Chen (1993) used a biomechanical model simulation. He showed that the critical muscles for recovery from a trip are the hip flexors of the swing leg and the ankle plantarflexors of the stance leg. In addition, he found that the rate of torque development, rather than available strength, was critical to balance recovery. Thus, the factor critical to recovery of balance following a trip appears to be how quickly restorative forces can be generated. Figure 14.2 shows the effects of different joint torques and torque development rates on balance recovery after tripping. Figure 14.2A shows a stick figure of the response to tripping if a subject had maximum joint torques and torque development rates, while B and C show a response if a subject had 75% and 50%, respectively, of reference torques and rates available. For subject C, the swing foot recontacts the ground, tripping again, with his upper body COM in front of his base of support, causing an additional perturbation to balance (Schultz, 1995).

A second study (Pijnappels et al., 2005), both supporting and extending these results, was designed to determine whether (a) timing and sequencing of muscle activation and (b) the magnitude and rate of development of muscle activation during recovery after a trip differ between young and older subjects. In this study, young (mean age, 25 years) and older (mean age, 68 years) adults walked over a platform and were tripped several times at different points in the gait cycle. The results showed that after tripping, rapid EMG responses (60–80 ms) were activated in both the hamstrings and gastrocnemius/soleus muscles of the stance leg in both young and older subjects, with the older subjects showing a delay (11 ms) in activation of the soleus muscle. The sequencing of the muscle activity patterns was similar in the two groups; however, the magnitude and rate of development of muscle activity were significantly lower in the older adults. These results and those from previous studies suggest that a lower rate of development of muscle activation in the support limb of older subjects may contribute to inadequate recovery from trips, leading to falls (Pijnappels et al., 2005; Schultz, 1995; Thelen et al., 1996).

In a study designed to determine the risk of falling following a trip, Pavol and colleagues (1999) gave older adults (mean [±SD] age, 72 ± 5 years) a single unexpected trip while walking, by activating without warning the elevation of a concealed mechanical obstacle in their footpath; 22% of the trips resulted in a fall into a harness, while 61% resulted in a full recovery, and 17% resulted in a rope-assisted recovery. Results showed that women fell four times more often than men.

Slips. Slips also account for a high percentage (27%–32%) of falls and subsequent injuries in community-dwelling older adults (Gabell et al., 1985). This phenomenon suggests that although active and healthy older adults preserve a mobility level comparable with that of young adults, these older adults may have difficulty generating efficient reactive postural responses when they slip. A study by Tang and Woollacott (1998) tested the hypothesis that active and healthy older adults use a less effective reactive balance strategy than young adults when experiencing an unexpected forward slip occurring at heel strike during walking. They predicted that less effective balance strategies would be manifested by slower and smaller postural responses, altered temporal and spatial organization of the postural responses, and greater upper-trunk instability after the slip in older adults.

In the study, young adults (n = 33; mean age, 25 ± 4 years) and community-dwelling older adults (n = 32; mean age, 4 ± 14 years) walked down a ramp and across a force plate that moved forward at heel strike, creating a forward slip. Both muscle response characteristics and body segment movements used in the recovery of balance were analyzed.

Tang and Woollacott noted that, behaviorally, older adults were less stable after the slips than young adults. For example, when recovering from a slip, older adults tended to trip more, as the advancing swing limb caught on the surface. Trips occurred 66% of the time in older adults, as compared with 15% in the younger adults. Older adults also showed greater trunk hyperextension and higher arm elevation in response to the slip than the young adults, as shown in Figure 14.3A and B. The figure shows a stick figure drawn from the motion analysis of the movements of a young and an older adult responding to a forward slip at heel strike. Note the backward extension of the trunk and the raising of the arm in the older adult at the onset of the slip. In addition, older adults had an earlier contralateral foot strike and shortened stride length, suggesting a more conservative balance strategy and an attempt to quickly reestablish the base of support after the slip.

What changes in neuromuscular response characteristics could be the cause of these difficulties in regaining balance in the older adults? A summary of the analysis is shown in Figure 14.3C. Older adults (darker bars) showed later onset of contraction and smaller magnitudes in the postural muscles activated in balance recovery (e.g., tibialis anterior, rectus femoris, and abdominal muscles of the perturbed leg) as compared with the younger adults (lighter bars). These delayed and weaker muscle responses thus contributed to the trunk hyperextension and trips seen in the older adults during recovery. In order to compensate for these deficiencies in responses, the older adults showed longer muscle response burst duration (Fig. 14.3C) and the use of the arms to aid in recovery. They also showed a longer coactivation time for the agonist–antagonist muscle pairs at the ankle, knee, and trunk of the perturbed leg, possibly to stiffen the joints as an additional aid in balance control (Tang & Woollacott, 1998). Sawers and Bhatt (2018) found similar results showing that older adults who fell from a laboratory-induced slip recruited fewer muscle synergies with high levels of coactivity consistent with a startle-like response. Other researchers have shown that knee joint muscle strength is also associated with slip-related falls among older adults. The authors found lower knee joint muscle strength capacity among fallers compared to those who did not fall (Ding & Yang, 2016).

How do older adults adapt their responses to balance threats at different phases in the gait cycle? When young adults experience a balance threat at midstance rather than at heel strike, the threat to stability is less, and they reduce the amplitude of responses appropriately. However, when older adults experience a midstance slip, their responses are actually the same size as at heel strike, showing little to no adaptation. Why is this the case? It is possible that their reduced response capacity (i.e., smaller burst magnitudes) at heel strike (see Fig. 14.3C) is the key constraint. They may be showing a normal response at midstance but simply do not have the response capacity to increase the response to appropriate levels for the increased balance threat at heel strike (Tang & Woollacott, 1999).

In another study examining the gait changes in older adults and the effects of these changes on slips and the frequency of falls, Lockhart et al. (2003) asked young and older adults to walk around a circular track and placed a slippery (oily) surface over the force plate at random times, without the participant's awareness. The experimental setup is shown in Figure 14.4. Results showed that the older adults' horizontal heel contact velocity was significantly faster and the step length was shorter. Older adults also slipped longer and faster and fell more often than younger participants. The researchers noted that participants who fell

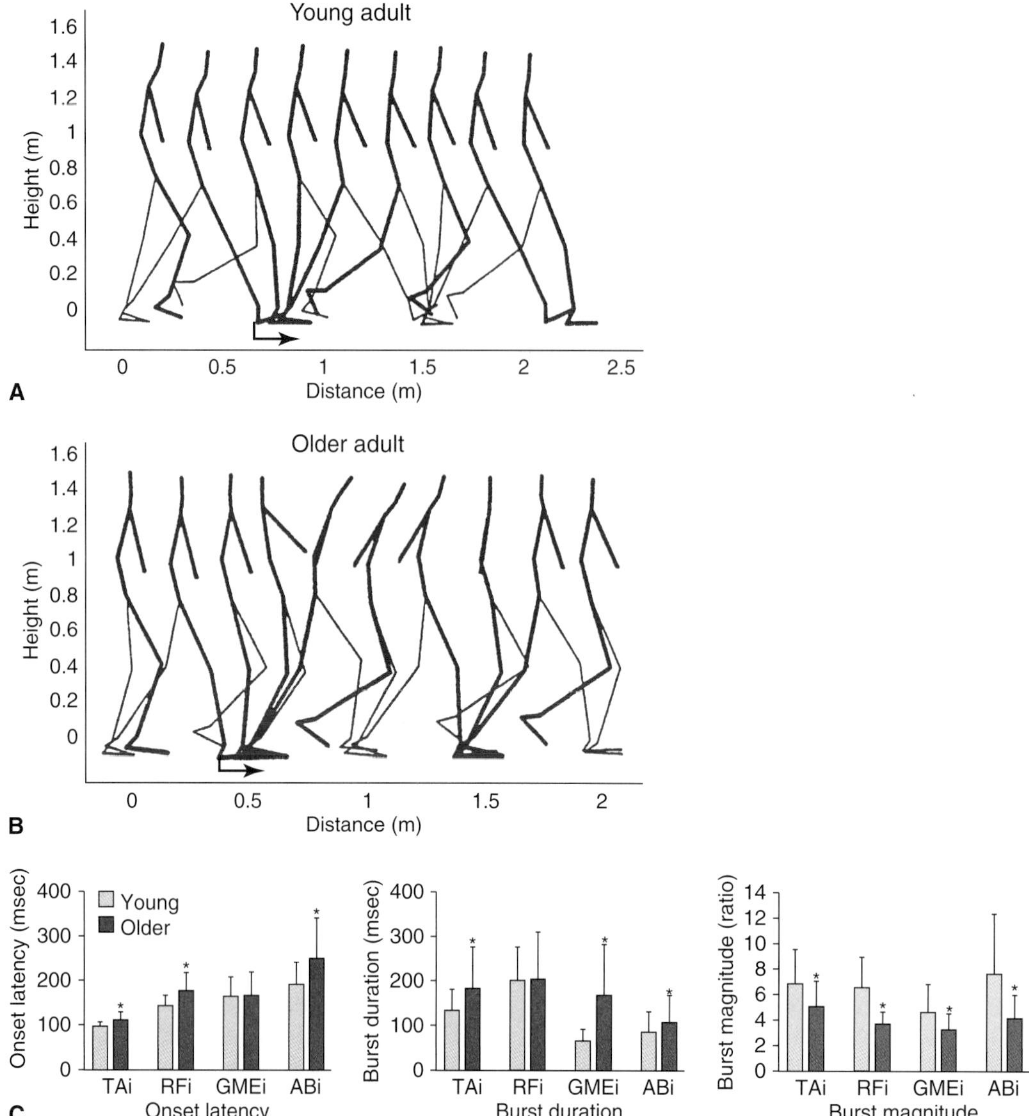

Figure 14.3 Stick figures drawn from the motion analysis of the movements of a young **(A)** and an older adult **(B)** responding to a forward slip (indicated by the *arrow*) at heel strike. Note the backward extension of the trunk and the raising of the arm in the older adult at the onset of the slip. **(C).** Means and standard deviations of onset latencies, burst durations, and burst magnitudes of postural responses in young (*lighter bars*) and older (*darker bars*) adults, for the anterior muscles of the perturbed leg. *ABi*, ipsilateral abdominal; *GMEi*, ipsilateral gluteus medius; *RFi*, ipsilateral rectus femoris; *TAi*, ipsilateral tibialis anterior. (Reprinted from Tang PF, Woollacott MH. Inefficient postural responses to unexpected slips during walking in older adults. *J Gerontol.* 1998;53:M471–M480, with permission.)

had a faster horizontal heel contact velocity than those who did not fall, suggesting that gait changes associated with aging affect the initiation of and recovery from slips. Examination of muscle responses underlying slips on oily surfaces has shown that older adults did not increase the power and duration of their muscle responses when responding to a highly hazardous as compared with a less hazardous slip, unlike young adults. This may be related to reduced lower-extremity strength in older adults (Chambers & Cham, 2007).

When young and older adults were alerted to expect a slippery surface, they added a proactive component to their balance response, coactivating the muscles at the ankle and knee and increasing the power of their muscle responses; however, older adults showed less proactive increase in muscle power than young adults. Subjects also took shorter steps, reducing the foot–floor angle and the vertical heel velocity at heel strike, as well as increasing knee flexion and hip moment, which resulted in a decrease in the potential of a slip and fall (Chambers & Cham, 2007).

In summary, these studies suggest that impaired reactive balance control reducing the ability to recover from unexpected perturbations to gait is a significant factor contributing to both loss of mobility function and increased risk for falls in many older adults. The degree to which impaired reactive balance control is truly "age related" versus the result of underlying pathology in

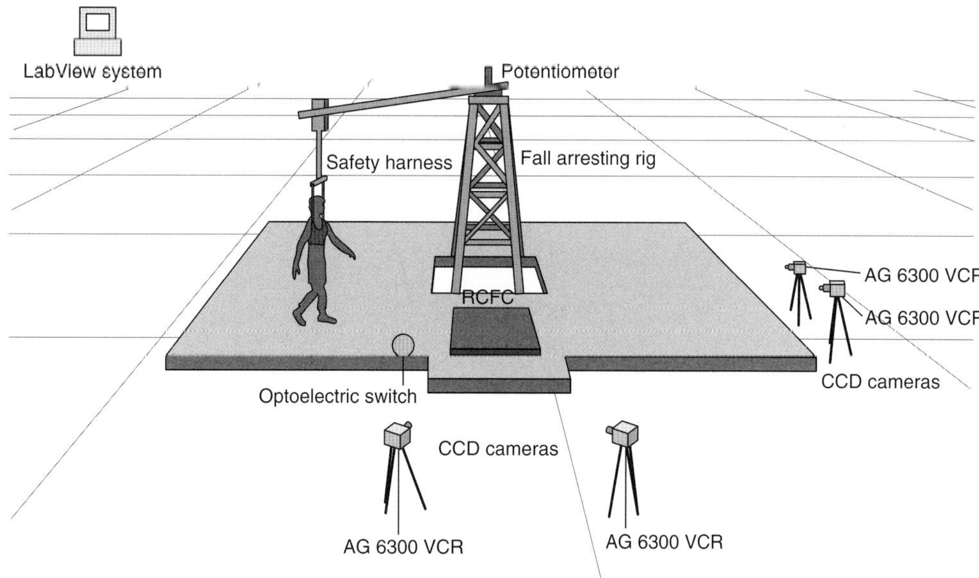

Figure 14.4 Layout of experiment examining age-related gait changes associated with slips and falls. The participant was in a safety harness and walked a 20-m circular track into which was incorporated a force plate. The force plate was covered with outdoor carpet for control trials and oily vinyl tile for the unexpected slip trials. Charge-coupled device (*CCD*) cameras recorded the kinematic data for each trial. A remote-controlled floor changer (*RCFC*) was used to change the test floor surfaces unexpectedly. (Reprinted from Lockhart TE, Woldstad JC, Smith JL. Effects of age-related gait changes on the biomechanics of slips and falls. *Ergonomics.* 2003;46:1140, with permission.)

the nervous system is unclear. The following section examines changes in proactive balance control that affect functional mobility in older adults.

Age-Related Changes in Proactive Balance Control

As discussed in Chapter 12, proactive strategies used to modify and adapt gait include both visually activated strategies that modify gait in response to environmental challenges to walking as well as predictive strategies used to modify gait parameters to minimize the destabilizing effects associated with tasks like carrying an object while walking.

A common everyday situation requiring proactive predictive strategies is turning to change direction while walking. Researchers have documented two main types of turning strategies (Hase & Stein, 1999) depending on which leg is used in front for braking (see Fig. 14.5): step turns (turning away from the inside limb, for example, landing on the right foot and taking a left step before turning to the right) and spin turns (turning toward the inside limb, for example, landing on the right limb, spinning the body around the right foot, and turning to the right). The step turn is easy and stable because the base of support during the turn is much wider than in the spin turn. Dixon and colleagues (2019) tested older adults' turning strategy on two surfaces (flat and uneven) and under two conditions. One condition was preplanned (participants were told whether to turn right, left, or walk straight before the start of the trial) and the other condition was late cued (participants were unaware whether to walk straight, turn right, or turn left before the start of the trial). They found that older adults preferred a step turn as opposed to a spin turn when walking under the preplanned condition. Thus, when time is not constrained, older adults choose the more stable turning strategy.

Modulating Step Length. What is the minimum time required to implement an obstacle avoidance strategy in a younger versus an older adult? In one study, healthy young and older adults were asked to walk along a walkway and, when cued by a light at specific points along the walkway, to either lengthen or shorten their stride to match the position of the light (Patla et al., 1992b).

Compared with young adults, older adults had more difficulty in modulating their step length when the cue was given only one step duration ahead. Young adults succeeded 80% of the time, while older adults succeeded 60% of the time when lengthening the step and only 38% of the time when shortening the step. Both groups were equally successful when the cue was given two step durations in advance (Patla et al., 1992b).

The authors suggest that older adults have more difficulty in shortening a step because of balance constraints. Shortening the step requires regulating the forward pitch of the HAT segment, which, if not controlled, could result in a fall. Remember that in the review of Winter's study presented earlier older adults had more trouble than young adults in controlling dynamic balance during gait.

Nevertheless, modifying step length might be challenging for older adults only when there is a time constraint (e.g., adapting gait when cued by a light).

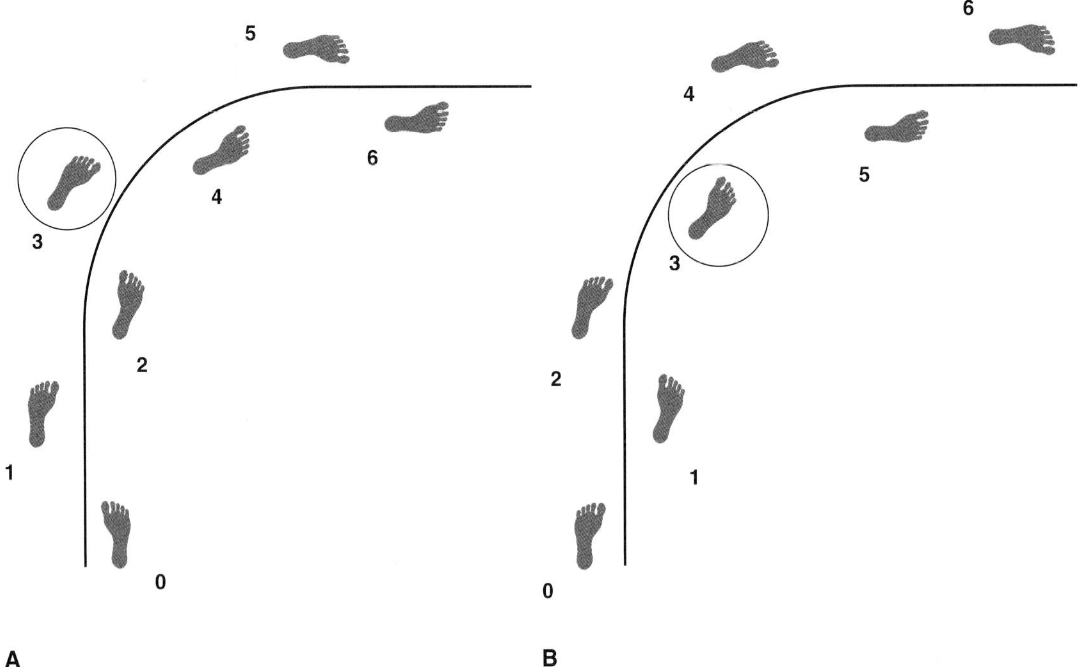

Figure 14.5 Schematic representation of a 90° turn. **(A)** Step turn, turning away from the inside limb with the right foot by taking an outside step (step number 3) with the left foot before turning to the right. **(B)** Spin turn, turning toward the inside limb by spinning the body around the right foot (step number 3) before turning to the right. (Adapted from Dixon PC, Smith T, Taylor MJD, et al. Effect of walking surface, late-cueing, physiological characteristics of aging, and gait parameters on turn style preference in healthy, older adults. *Hum Mov Sci*. 2019;66:507, with permission.)

A study by Andel and colleagues (2018) characterized age-related changes in younger and older participants when initiating an adjustment of their steps. They also examined the strategy used when regulating steps (lengthening, shortening, or a mixed strategy) and the strength of perceptual-motor coupling when stepping up a curb. They found that variability in foot placement was lower for older adults and that younger and older adults used different step length adaptation strategies. Younger adults preferred to lengthen their steps when making an adjustment, whereas older adults more often chose a shortening strategy to place their foot on top of the curb. Moreover, older adults showed a stronger perceptual-motor coupling—the extent to which deviations from the average step length during the approach was related to the adjustment required. The adjustment required was measured as the difference between the location of the foot during the approach (e.g., the second step before the curb) and the mean location of that foot for that step, across multiple trials (i.e., the mean location of the foot during the second step before the curb). The authors argue that the age-related differences in perceptual-motor coupling can be linked to older adults' decreased ability to adapt actions on the fly. Young adults can choose from a variety of actions to step up on the curbs; however, older adults are more constrained by their action capabilities, which in turn increases the task demands, requiring them to perform actions with a strong perceptual-motor coupling. These results suggest that the older adult may need to begin making modifications to gait patterns in the step prior to a step requiring obstacle avoidance. This may be one cause of increased visual monitoring.

Obstacle Crossing. Trips during obstacle crossing are a major cause of falls in older adults. A review of studies examining obstacle-crossing performance showed that when time is not constrained, older adults adopt a slower more conservative strategy when stepping over obstacles, allowing them to adjust foot placement and reduce the risk of tripping. In contrast, when time is constrained and they must move quickly, older adults have more frequent obstacle contacts during crossing than young adults (Galna et al., 2009). The authors suggest that it is under these constraints that increased obstacle contact is a cause of trips and falls in older adults.

What strategies do older adults use to avoid obstacles during walking? To answer this question, researchers analyzed the gait of 24 young and 24 older (mean age, 71 years) healthy adults while they stepped over obstacles of varying heights. Obstacles were made the height of a 1-inch or 2-inch door threshold or a 6-inch curb, and performance was compared with a baseline condition (tape marked on the walkway). No age-related changes in foot clearance over the obstacles were found, but older adults used a significantly more conservative strategy when crossing obstacles. Older adults used a somewhat slower approach speed, a significantly slower crossing speed, and a shorter step length. Also, 4 of the 24 older adults inadvertently stepped on an obstacle, while none of the young adults did (Chen et al., 1991). Muir and colleagues (2020) compared adults' inadvertent failed trials to successful trials to identify the gait characteristics associated with failure. The authors found that young and middle-aged adults were more likely to fail with the trail limb, while older adults were more likely to fail with their lead limb. A lead limb trip may result in higher fall risk as it is more difficult to recover than a trail limb trip (a common trip during everyday activities).

Other research on changes in obstacle-avoidance ability has focused on the control of the COM during obstacle crossing (Hahn & Chou, 2004). During obstacle crossing, older adults showed anterior-direction COM velocities that were significantly slower than those of young adults. They also showed reduced anteroposterior distances between the COM and the center of pressure (COP), which indicates a conservative strategy, reducing the mechanical load on the supporting limb. The authors note that this strategy may be the result of reduced muscle strength in the older adults.

Chou and colleagues (2003) have also studied COM motion during obstacle crossing in older adults with imbalance to determine whether excessive lateral COM motion may be a cause of their instability in these situations and thus to identify persons at great risk of imbalance and falls. Although older adults with imbalance did not have differences in temporal distance gait parameters such as walking velocity and stride length, they did show greater and faster lateral motion of the COM when crossing over obstacles that were 15% of body height. Figure 14.6 shows the mediolateral COM position and velocity trajectories for a healthy (*solid line*) and balance-impaired (*dashed line*) older adult. Note the large deviation of COM position and velocity as the individual with imbalance crosses the obstacle.

In fact, the authors found that COM motion distinguished older adults with balance disorders from healthy older adults better than the motion of markers at the hip, trunk, or pelvis, because of large variations in individual segment motion. These results suggest that information about an older adult's ability to control the COM trajectory during obstacle crossing could help identify persons at risk for falls and allow for interventions before falls occur (Chou et al., 2003; Hahn & Chou, 2003).

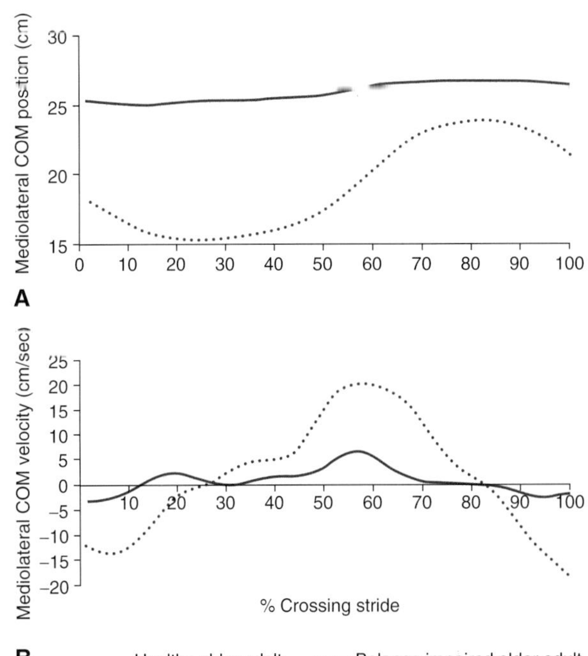

Figure 14.6 Mediolateral COM position **(A)** and velocity **(B)** data from a single trial of a representative healthy older adult (HOA) (*solid line*) and a balance-impaired older adult (BIOA) (*dashed line*) while crossing an obstacle of 15% body height. (Reprinted from Chou L-S, Kaufman KR, Hahn ME, et al. Mediolateral motion of the center of mass during obstacle crossing distinguishes elderly individuals with imbalance. *Gait Posture.* 2003;18:129, with permission.)

Role of Pathology in Gait Changes in Older Adults

What is the role of secondary aging factors, particularly the role of pathology, in gait abnormalities observed in older adults? In many studies examining apparently healthy older adults, participants are considered pathology free if they do not have a known neurologic, cardiovascular, or musculoskeletal disorder. Yet, when this population is examined carefully, many show subtle pathologies. For example, in a study on idiopathic gait disorders among older adults, Sudarsky and Ronthal (1983) found that, on closer medical evaluation, this type of gait pattern could actually be attributed to a number of specific disease processes. This suggests that in many instances, pathological conditions may be an underlying contributing factor to changes in gait pattern seen in older adults. Pathology within a number of systems can potentially affect locomotor skills in the older adult.

In a study examining the effects of multiple impairments on severe walking disability, researchers analyzed data from 1,002 women 65 years of age or older who performed tests of both muscle strength (handheld dynamometer test of knee extension strength) and balance (feet together, semitandem, and tandem Romberg) in their homes. The results showed that the risk of being severely walking disabled was 10 times greater for persons having both strength and balance impairments as compared with those with only one impairment. Thus, an effective method for reducing walking disabilities could be the prevention or remediation of multiple impairments, with improvement in just one impairment having a substantial impact on the probability of having a walking disability (Rantanen et al., 1999).

AGE-RELATED CHANGES IN SENSORY SYSTEMS AND GAIT

As noted in Chapter 9 on changes in postural control in the older adult, pathologies within visual, proprioceptive, and vestibular systems are common among many older adults, reducing the availability of information from these senses for posture and gait. If reduction in sensory function is part of normal aging, it will be important to determine ways to optimize environmental factors and use training to improve stability during walking in older adults.

Somatosensation

As reduced somatosensation associated with peripheral neuropathy is often associated with the aging process, especially in older adults with diabetes, studies have examined its effects on walking characteristics. One study examined both usual and fast-speed walking characteristics in older adults (895 women, aged 65 years and older) who had peripheral nerve dysfunction (Resnick et al., 2000). Results indicated that peripheral nerve dysfunction was associated with slowing in both usual and fast-paced walking speeds. Another study by Lipsitz et al. (2018) looked at the relationship between older adults' ability to detect stimulation of the great toe and slowing of gait speed and development of falls over a 5-year period. Subjects whose sensory function showed a consistent decline over the 5 years also demonstrated a significant decline in gait speed and were at greatest risk of falls.

Vision

Poor vision has also been shown to be associated with poor walking performance in community-dwelling older adults. Tests of performance on both the Timed Up and Go (TUG) Test and walking speed showed significant correlations with functional vision in older adults (Aartolahti et al., 2013). In addition, proactive adaptation during gait, discussed previously, depends in large part on the ability to use visual information to alter gait patterns in anticipation of upcoming obstacles (Patla, 1993). Patla et al. (1992a) studied whether a possible cause of poor locomotor abilities in older adults might be a reduced ability to sample the visual environment during walking. They wanted to know whether visual sampling of the environment changed with age.

In their experiment, subjects wore opaque liquid crystal eyeglasses and pressed a switch to make them transparent whenever they wanted to sample the environment. Subjects walked across a floor that either was unmarked or had footprints marked at regular intervals, on which the subjects were supposed to walk. When subjects were constrained to land on the footprints, the young subjects sampled frequently, though for shorter intervals than older subjects, who tended to sample less often, but for longer time periods. Thus, older adults monitor the terrain during walking much more than do young adults (Patla, 1993).

Vestibular

Studies have also examined vestibular function in older adults, measuring vestibular decline using the vestibular evoked myogenic potentials. Results have shown that age-related slowing in walking speed, especially walking speed on a narrow walkway, is in part a function of decreased magnitude of the saccule response, associated with age.

AGE-RELATED CHANGES IN COGNITIVE SYSTEMS AND GAIT

The ability to divide attention between two or more tasks is an important aspect of locomotion during many activities of daily life. For example, an older adult may be required to walk across a street while talking to a friend and simultaneously looking both ways to avoid oncoming traffic. A number of studies have examined the ability of older adults to simultaneously perform locomotor and other cognitively demanding tasks, in order to determine whether attentional problems could be a factor contributing to falls. In Chapters 7, 9, and 12, we defined attention and discussed the research on the attentional requirements of balance and locomotion and the changes in the attentional requirements of balance in older adults. In this chapter, we will focus on changes in the attentional requirements of locomotion in healthy adults and BIOAs.

It has been suggested that as the functional capacity of older adults is stressed while walking and performing a secondary motor or cognitive task, problems in gait or in the performance of a secondary task will be revealed, due to either (a) a limited capacity to perform either task, requiring more attentional resources, or (b) limitations in the information-processing capacity of the older adults, causing problems in allocating attention efficiently between the two tasks.

Age-Related Changes in Dual-Task Performance during Steady-State Gait

In order to determine whether older adults show problems with attention when performing a secondary task while walking at a constant velocity (steady-state gait), Eichhorn et al. (1998) asked older (mean age, 73 years) and young (mean age, 24 years) adults to respond vocally to a tone cue (say "soft" to a low and "loud" to a high tone) as quickly as possible while walking at their preferred pace. They found that the reaction time of the older adults on the auditory task was significantly reduced when walking, while that of the younger adults was not. Thus, older adults showed problems performing both tasks efficiently when they were performed simultaneously. Other studies have shown that the type of cognitive task is an important determinant of dual-task interference with walking. For example, a simple push-button reaction time task did not affect gait performance in older recurrent fallers, while a visuospatial reaction time task significantly slowed gait in a dual-task setting (Faulkner et al., 2007). Similarly, Beauchet and colleagues (2005) measured gait performance in frail older adults while walking alone, performing a simple arithmetic task, or performing a task of verbal fluency. Walking time and number of steps increased under both dual-task conditions compared to walking alone. However, lateral gait instability (number of times the subject stepped over a lateral line) increased in the arithmetic but not in the verbal fluency task. Thus, performing a cognitive task while walking interferes with walking performance, but this effect is dependent on the type of cognitive task.

In a study examining the effect of age on dual-tasks costs, young, middle-aged, and older adults were asked to memorize word lists while sitting, standing, or walking. Dual-task interference was present during walking and was characterized by reduced memory accuracy and walking speed and accuracy. Some decrements, including memory accuracy and walking speed, were already present in 40- to 50-year-olds, while others (walking accuracy) were apparent only in the 60- to 70-year-olds. The authors propose that as a general phenomenon of aging, sensory/motor aspects of performance require more cognitive control as individuals age, because of frailty, sensory deficits, and problems in sensory integration (Lindenberger et al., 2000).

Does dual-task walking in a lab setting resemble everyday natural walking? Yes, indeed! Hillel and colleagues (2019) measured gait during usual walking and dual-task walking in the lab with gait during daily-living in 150 older adult fallers. As expected, in-lab gait speed, step regularity, and stride regularity were worse during dual-task walking compared to usual walking. Moreover, usual walking values measured in the lab were better than those found in typical daily living. Interestingly, dual-task walking values were similar in both lab and daily life conditions. Thus, the authors conclude that cognitive-motor and motor-motor dual and multitasking are common in daily life (e.g., walking while talking, while using a cellphone, while carrying a bag, or while negotiating traffic).

Age-Related Changes in Dual-Task Performance during Obstacle Crossing

In order to determine the attentional requirements of more difficult walking tasks, studies have examined dual-task performance during obstacle crossing. In one of these studies, Chen et al. (1996) asked healthy older (mean age, 72 years) and young (mean age, 24 years) adults to walk down a walkway and step over a virtual object (a band of light) while responding vocally when a red light was turned on at the end of the walkway. Figure 14.7 shows the experimental setup. They found that both young and older adults showed increased obstacle contact when performing the secondary task, but this was greater in the older adults. Thus, decrements in obstacle avoidance occur in both younger and older adults when performing a secondary cognitive task, but older adults show higher decrements. This decreased ability to avoid obstacles when performing a secondary cognitive task could contribute to many falls in older adults.

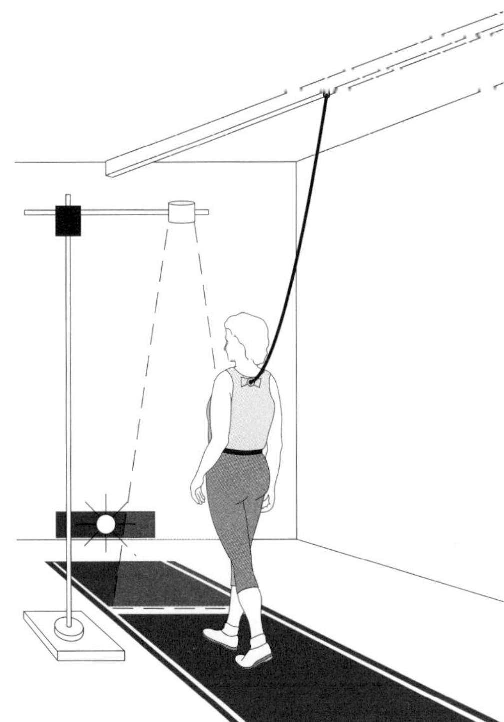

Figure 14.7 Experimental setup for study of attentional demands associated with performing a secondary task while avoiding an obstacle. Young and older adults walked down a walkway and stepped over a virtual object (a band of light) while responding vocally when a red light was turned on at the end of the walkway. (Adapted from Chen HC, Schultz AB, Ashton-Miller JA, et al. Stepping over obstacles: dividing attention impairs performance of old more than young adults. *J Gerontol.* 1996;51A:M116–M122, with permission.)

Not only do older adults have more obstacle contact as compared with young adults when performing obstacle crossing in a dual-task situation, the previously discussed research has shown that the secondary task is affected as well. Older adults also show higher error rates than young adults on the secondary task, suggesting that the attentional demands of obstacle avoidance increase with age as well.

Brown et al. (2005) have also shown that the attention directed toward obstacle avoidance in the pre-crossing phase was more than in the crossing phase in young adults. However, for older adults, both precrossing and crossing phases of obstacle negotiation required equal attention, suggesting decreased balance control during the crossing phase in older adults.

One difficulty that older adults, and especially BIOAs, may have during dual-task performance is decreased ability to flexibly allocate attention between the walking and a secondary cognitive task. For example, it may be important, when crossing a street, to shift attention between the walking task (while avoiding other pedestrians or cars) and a second task, such as watching the "walk–don't walk" signal or listening to the conversation of a friend. In order to better understand problems that older adults may have in allocating attention between two tasks, Siu et al. (2009) asked healthy older adults and BIOAs to perform an obstacle-crossing task and an auditory Stroop task (a task of executive attention) while focusing on both tasks equally or allocating attention primarily to walking or to the Stroop task.

They found that healthy older adults were able to shift their focus to the obstacle-avoidance task or auditory Stroop task under different instructional sets, as indicated by faster reaction times when focusing on the Stroop task and higher trailing limb obstacle clearance when focusing on the gait task. However, the balance impaired showed no significant difference in performance for the Stroop or the obstacle-crossing tasks across the three instructional conditions (Fig. 14.8A and B). Thus, BIOAs may be at risk for falls or other injuries in dual-task conditions due to their inability to flexibly allocate attention between cognitive tasks and walking performance.

In support of the previously discussed studies, research has shown that executive attentional function is essential for successful dual-task performance. For example, the InCHIANTI study showed that poor performance on the Trail Making Test, a test of executive function, was related to reduced gait speed over an obstacle course and to a variety of dual-task physical tests (Coppin et al., 2006). Liu-Ambrose and colleagues (2009) examined the extent to which different aspects of executive function contribute to reduced dual-task walking abilities in older adults. They found that deterioration in set shifting abilities was significantly associated with poor dual-task gait performance. However, executive function played a role in dual-task performance only when cognitive load was high. They also found that balance confidence was independently associated with dual-task gait performance in community-dwelling older women.

Cognitive Influences on Gait: Fear of Falling in Older Adults

Studies have shown that after repeated falls, older persons develop a fear of falling, and this fear may contribute to changes in gait characteristics as well. For example, it has been shown that preferred walking pace, anxiety level, and depression are good predictors of the extent of fear of falling in community-dwelling older adults (Tinetti et al., 1990). Older adults who avoid activities because of a fear of falling tend to walk at a slower pace and to have higher levels of anxiety and depression as compared with adults who have little fear of falling. This has led several investigators to propose that slowed gait velocity among older adults reflects a conscious strategy to ensure safe gait, rather than the consequence of specific constraints on walking speed (Craik, 1989; Murray et al., 1969; Winter et al., 1990).

In other studies examining balance control in older adults with a fear of falling, researchers were not sure whether these adults had real problems with

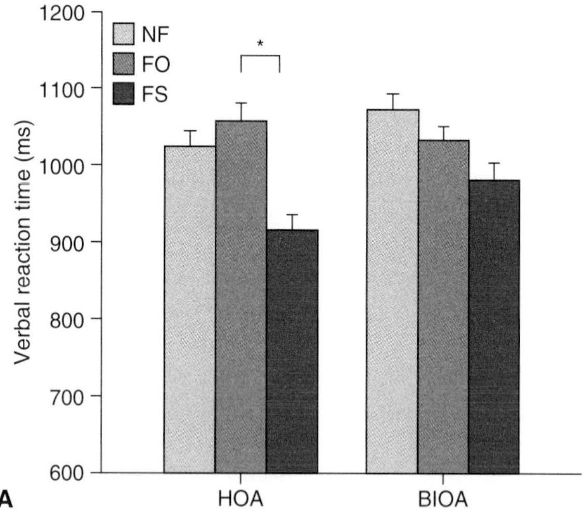

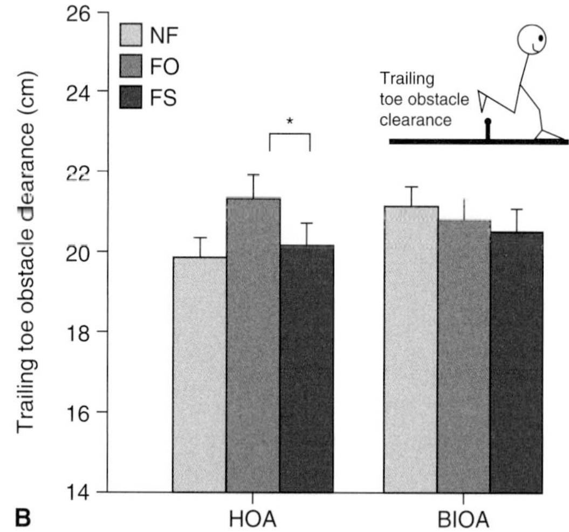

Figure 14.8 Dual-task performance of healthy older adults (HOA) and balance-impaired older adults (BIOA), including verbal response time on the Stroop task **(A)** and toe-obstacle clearance in the trailing limb (TTOC) **(B)**, in three instructional conditions: no priority focus (*NF*), variable priority focus on the obstacle (*FO*), and variable priority focus on the Stroop task (*FS*). (Adapted from Siu KC, Chou LS, Mayr U, et al. Attentional mechanisms contributing to balance constraints during gait: the effects of balance impairments. *Brain Res.* 2009;1248:62, Figure 3.)

balance control or whether the fear of falling itself was affecting stability in an artifactual way (Maki et al., 1991). Thus, it is possible that cognitive factors, such as fear of falling, may contribute to changes in gait patterns in older adults.

AGE-RELATED CHANGES IN OTHER MOBILITY SKILLS

Gait Initiation and Backward Gait

Gait initiation requires dynamic balance control, since it is a transitional phase between static standing balance and dynamic balance requirements associated with walking. One way of examining the ability to control gait initiation is to measure both center of gravity (COG) changes, reflecting body position, and COP changes, reflecting both weight shifts and muscular control during dynamic postural changes. Gait initiation requires the separation of the COG and the COP in order to push off and begin gait. This separation between the COG and COP, known biomechanically as the "COG–COP moment arm," helps predict an individual's ability to tolerate dynamic unsteadiness. Thus, a small moment arm would indicate that the COP and COG are being kept closely aligned during gait initiation, minimizing dynamic unsteadiness. Chang and Krebs (1999) have shown that the length of COG–COP moment arm during gait initiation clearly differentiates healthy older adults, who show a COG–COP moment arm of 21 ± 8 cm, from BIOA who show a moment arm of 15 ± 3 cm. This shortened moment arm could be due to either the result of muscle weakness (a primary impairment) or a compensatory strategy used to minimize dynamic unsteadiness.

Since backward walking is used in rehabilitation programs to improve balance, strength, and coordination, a study by Laufer (2005) compared the ability of older adults to perform backward walking with that of young adults. It was found that older adults showed significantly decreased stride length for backward walking as compared with young adults. In addition, they could increase velocity only by increasing cadence, while young adults used both cadence and stride length increases to increase velocity.

Stair Walking

Research has documented that falls on stairs account for approximately 10% of all fall-related deaths (Startzell et al., 2000), with stair descent being four times more hazardous than stair ascent (Tinetti et al., 1988). The main reason why walking down stairs is so challenging is because one needs to maintain the lowering velocity of the body's center of mass within safe limits, which can be problematic for older adults due to a reduced range of motion in all involved joints (ankle and knee) and a reduced ability to generate adequate joint moments at the extremes in joint ranges of motion. To compensate for these impairments, older adults adopt a strategy of reducing the body's center of mass velocity to lessen the eccentric landing demands and rely on the leading-limb eccentric plantarflexion during landing of a high downward step (Foster et al., 2019).

To understand the role of vision in during stair walking in older adults, characteristics of stair descent were studied in a group of 36 healthy women between the ages of 55 and 70 (Simoneau et al., 1991). Participants were asked to walk down a set of stairs under conditions of poor or distorted visual inputs; for example, (a) stairs were painted black, (b) vision of the stair was blurred (stairs were painted black and the subject wore a headband with a light-scattering plastic shield), or (c) stairs were painted black with a white stripe at the edge of each tread. A striped corridor surrounded the stairs.

The results of high-speed film analysis showed significantly slower cadence, larger foot clearance, and more posterior foot placement while subjects walked under the blurred condition as compared with the other two conditions. The authors further observed that foot clearance was larger than that obtained during pilot work from their laboratory on young adults. They concluded that older subjects walked with larger foot clearance during stair descent as compared with young adults and that gait patterns during stair descent were affected by visual conditions. It has also been shown that when going down stairs, older adults show a greater medial inclination angle during the stair-to-floor transition phase as compared with young adults. This inability to regulate body sway during the stair-to-floor transition could increase the risk of falling in older adults (Lee & Chou, 2007).

Sit-to-Stand

The task of rising from a seated position is often associated with falling in older adults (Tinetti et al., 1986). Research indicates that 8% of community-dwelling older adults over 65 years of age show some problems in rising from a chair or bed. As a result, several studies have examined the sit-to-standing task in older adults (Alexander et al., 1991; Millington et al., 1992; Pai et al., 1994).

One study compared movement strategies, forces used, and the time taken to rise from sitting among young adults, older adults able to rise without armrests (old able), and older adults unable to rise without armrests (old unable). Average rise times from a chair were similar in the young and old able groups (1.56 vs. 1.83 seconds) but significantly longer in the old unable group (3.16 seconds). In addition, the hand forces used by the old able group were significantly less than those used by the old unable group.

The old able were different from the young mainly in the amount of time they spent in the initial phase of rising from the chair, which included the time from start to lifting off from the seat. They flexed their legs and trunks more during trials in which they used no hands to help themselves rise. Other studies (Mourey et al., 2000; Pai et al., 1994) showed that the peak vertical momentum of the center of mass, the maximal COM velocity in the horizontal axis, and the COM velocity at the instant of lifting off were lower in older adults compared with young subjects. This was probably due to lower levels of muscle strength in the older adults.

In a study by Papa and Cappozzo (2000), different sit-to-stand motor strategies were identified for young versus community-dwelling older adults. The strategies were associated with both a different initial posture (ankle dorsiflexion angle) and speed of execution of the motor task. Prior to lifting off from the seat, the older adult group tended to flex the trunk more than the younger group, bringing the COM closer to the base of support. They also used a higher movement velocity, thus gaining higher momentum. After lifting off from the seat, the older adults rotated the body forward and, only after having brought their COM over the base of support, effectively started elevation. Results showed that both global muscular effort and coordination associated with the achievement of balance and raising the COM were lower. However, maximal speed was also lower. The authors suggested that this may indicate that the older adults had a lower functional reserve than did the young individuals, thus choosing an optimal strategy for their limited reserve capacity.

Dubost et al. (2005) examined stand-to-sit characteristics in older versus young adults. The results showed that older adults tended to minimize the forward body displacement during sitting down. The authors suggested that this strategy was an adaptive mechanism to decrease the risk of anterior disequilibrium during sitting.

Rising from a Bed

Are there age-related differences in the movement patterns used in rising from a bed? To answer this question, adults ranging from 30 to 59 years of age were videotaped while rising from a bed (Ford-Smith & VanSant, 1993). As had been reported for young adults, there was considerable variability in patterns for rising from a bed among the slightly older group, aged 50 to 59. As was mentioned in Chapter 12, the most common patterns of bed rising in the 30- to 39-year-old group involved a grasp-and-push pattern with the upper extremities, a roll-off or come-to-sit pattern, and a synchronous lifting of the lower limbs off the bed, with one limb extending to the floor in front of the other. The slightly older group, consisting of 50- to 59-year-olds, tended to use a more synchronous lifting pattern, with both legs moved to the floor simultaneously, as shown in Figure 14.9. No studies have been published to date on patterns used by the older adults when rising from the bed. Since many older adults report falls at night associated with getting out of bed, such a study is essential.

Supine to Standing

Moving from a supine to a standing position is an important task, even in older adults. The ability to stand up after a fall is a key element for functional independence. A number of studies have examined patterns of supine-to-standing movements across the life span and have shown that there is a progression across childhood to adulthood from asymmetrical to symmetrical movement patterns, with older adults more likely to show asymmetrical patterns like those seen in children (VanSant, 1990). One study investigated the relationship of age, activity level, lower-extremity strength, and range of motion to the movement patterns and time required to rise to a standing position from the floor (Thomas et al., 1998). They confirmed previous results regarding movement patterns and found that symmetrical movement patterns were associated with younger age, greater plantarflexion and hip extension strength, and greater dorsiflexion range of motion. This suggests that symmetrical patterns like those seen in young adults require higher levels of extensor muscle strength; however, alternative asymmetrical standing strategies are available to older adults with extensor weakness.

COMPARING GAIT CHARACTERISTICS OF INFANTS AND OLDER ADULTS: TESTING THE REGRESSION HYPOTHESIS

It has been suggested that changes in the gait pattern among older adults are related to the reemergence of immature walking patterns seen in young infants. Thus, it has been hypothesized that, as aging occurs, there is a regression to immature reflex patterns that characterized movement in young infants. This regression is thought to result from loss of higher-center control over the primitive reflexes that reemerge in the very old (Shaltenbrand, 1928). What are the similarities and differences between the gait characteristics of the very young and the very old?

Both groups show a shorter duration of single-limb stance and a greater relative duration of double support. This has been interpreted in both groups as an indication of decreased balance abilities (Bril & Breniere, 1993; Gabell & Nayak, 1984; Murray et al., 1969; Sutherland et al., 1980).

The gait of young walkers has also been described as having a wide base of support along with toeing out, a characteristic observed in the older adults as well (Bril & Breniere, 1993; Murray et al., 1969). It has been

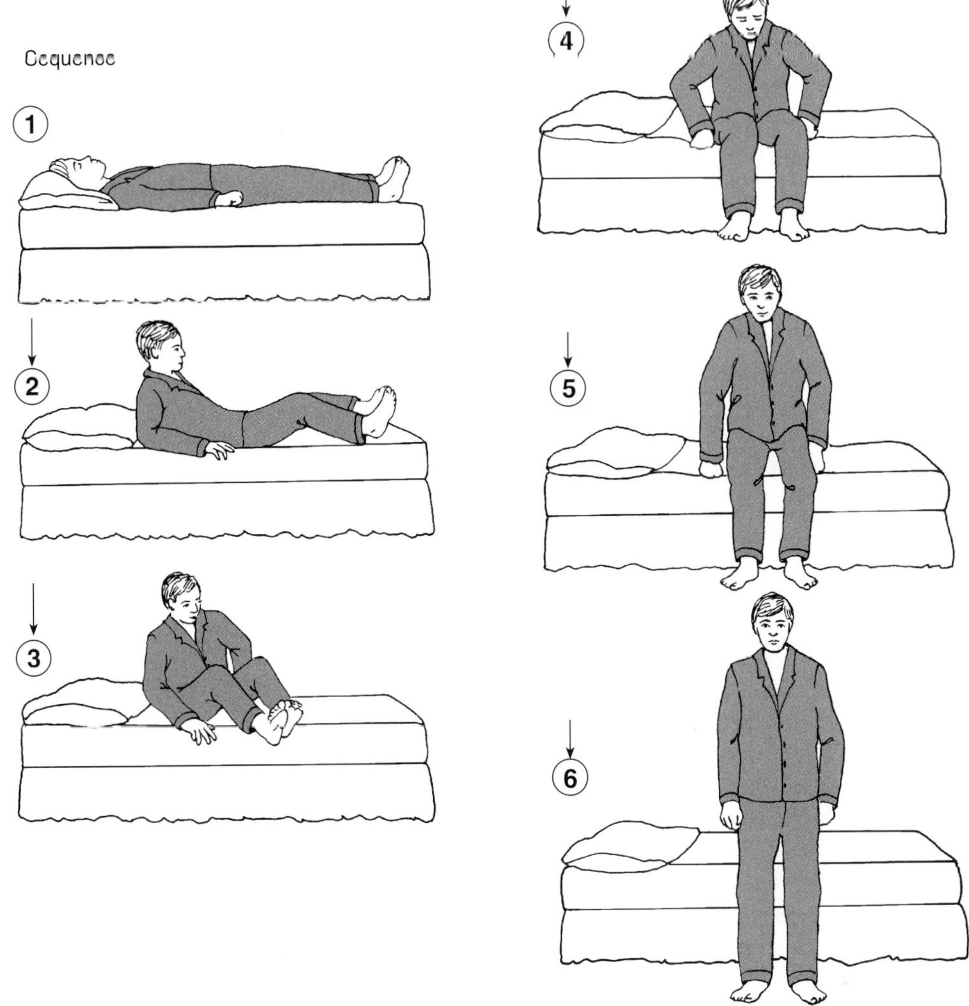

Figure 14.9 Frequent pattern of rising from a bed seen in 50- to-59-year-old subjects. (Adapted with permission from Ford-Smith CD, VanSant AF. Age differences in movement patterns used to rise from a bed in subjects in the third through fifth decades of age. *Phys Ther*. 1993;73:305, with permission of the American Physical Therapy Association. This material is copyrighted, and any further reproduction or distribution requires written permission from APTA.)

suggested in both groups that an increased base of support is used to ensure better balance control.

Finally, both young children (Forssberg, 1985) and older adults (Finley et al., 1969) show coactivation of agonist and antagonist muscles during gait. This again has been described as a way of increasing joint stiffness, which helps in balance control (Woollacott, 1986).

Clearly, there are many similarities in the gait characteristics of young children and older adults. These similarities appear to relate to difficulties with balance control common to both groups. Thus, it is not necessarily true that similarities between the very old and the very young are due to a reappearance of primitive reflexes. In this case, the reason is a functional one: the two groups, often for very different reasons, have difficulties with the balance system but use similar strategies to compensate for those difficulties.

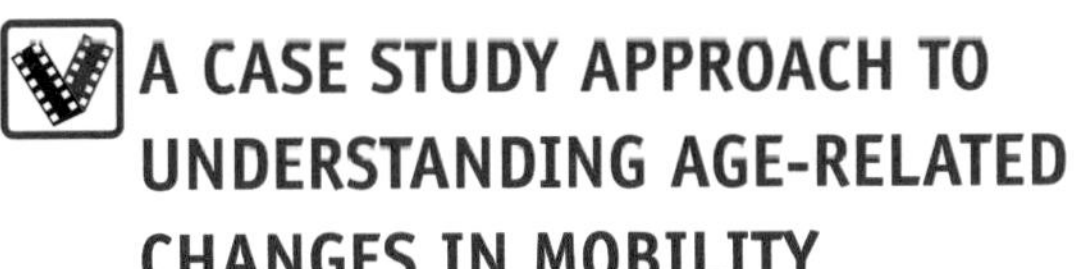

A CASE STUDY APPROACH TO UNDERSTANDING AGE-RELATED CHANGES IN MOBILITY

Bonnie B is our 90-year-old woman with impaired balance and gait, resulting in multiple falls, two of which required hospitalization. She lives alone in an apartment and has a home health aide who assists her with shopping, cooking, cleaning, and laundry. Bonnie's main concerns relate to her declining balance and frequent falls, many of which occur while she is walking. She is very fearful of falling again and restricts her mobility because of this.

As you can see in the Mobility section of her video case study, Bonnie, like many older adults with a history of falls, shows significant differences in her walking pattern as compared with young and healthy older adults (Hausdorff et al., 1997; Heitmann et al., 1989; Wolfson et al., 1985). She shows a decrease in walking velocity, shorter step and stride length, and longer double support time. Bonnie is unable to walk without the use of her four-wheeled walker. With a gait velocity of 0.4 m/s, she is unable to walk fast enough to cross a street safely. In the community, she uses her walker when ambulating for short distances but most often relies on a wheelchair for mobility. Her gait pattern, including stride time, stance time, and swing time, is likely more variable, an indication of her high risk for falls (Hausdorff et al., 1997, 2001).

A kinematic analysis of her walking would find that joint angle excursions at the hip, knee, and ankle flexion are less than in young adults (Winter et al., 1990). She walks with a flexed posture, in part because of her use of a walker.

An EMG analysis of muscle activity during walking would probably find increased coactivation of agonist and antagonist muscles, a strategy to increase joint stiffness and improve balance control. A kinetic analysis would probably find that plantarflexors generated significantly less power at push-off, while the quadriceps muscles absorbed significantly less energy during late stance and early swing (Winter et al., 1990). Reduced plantarflexor torque could be due to muscle weakness or, alternatively, could be a strategy to improve stability during gait (Winter et al., 1990).

As can be seen in the Mobility section of her video, Bonnie has difficulty maintaining balance during complex walking tasks. She has considerable difficulty with obstacle avoidance. She is unable to lift her walker over an obstacle, and this has contributed to several falls in the community. Research has shown that during obstacle crossing, older adults with a history of falls frequently make contact with the obstacle, which increases their risk for falls (Chen et al., 1991).

A reduced ability to recover from slips and trips while walking is a major factor contributing to Bonnie's increased fall risk. Several factors contribute to her reduced ability to recover from a trip. Muscle responses used to recover stability following a slip or trip are likely delayed and weak (Tang & Woollacott, 1998). In addition, she likely has a reduced ability to generate torque quickly in the hip flexors of the swing leg and the ankle plantarflexors of the stance leg, critical muscles for regaining stability following a trip (Chen et al., 1996).

Finally, Bonnie has reduced independence in other mobility tasks, including transfers and stairs. She must use her hands when moving from sitting to standing and often requires several tries in order to stand. In addition, as you see on the video, she is markedly unsteady on rising and requires physical assistance to prevent a fall. She has difficulty on the TUG test, a test of mobility requiring her to stand up from a chair, walk 10 feet, turn around, and walk back to her chair and sit. She completes the test in 24 seconds, considerably slower than the 8 to 10 seconds taken by healthy older adults. When she performs the TUG with the addition of a secondary task, her time slows to 33 seconds, and she is unsteady on her turns. In addition, she demonstrates dual-task interference on the secondary task, making multiple errors on the counting backward task.

Many factors contribute to Bonnie's mobility impairments, including age-related changes in the systems critical to the control of balance and gait. In addition, because of her fear of falls, Bonnie has significantly reduced her activity level. This sedentary lifestyle also contributes to her impaired gait and mobility skills and increases her risk for falls.

SUMMARY

1. Studies characterizing gait patterns in older adults have consistently shown that healthy older adults have reduced walking speed, shorter stride length, and shorter step length than young adults.
2. Proactive locomotor abilities also change with age, with older adults taking more time to monitor the visual environment, taking more time to alter an upcoming step to avoid an obstacle, and using strategies such as slowing of approach and crossover time when stepping over obstacles.
3. Changes in the characteristics of gait patterns in older adults are influenced by balance ability, leg muscle strength, and changes in the availability of sensory information. Cognitive factors such as fear of falling and attentional problems may also be important contributors.
4. When evaluating gait patterns of older people, consideration must be given to the underlying mechanisms contributing to these changes. In this way, one can differentiate between contributions related to pathology versus aging per se. Only after the systems contributing to walking pattern dysfunction are identified can a clinician design effective and appropriate interventions to improve gait and thus help older adults achieve a safe and independent lifestyle.

ANSWERS TO LAB ACTIVITY ASSIGNMENTS

Lab Activity 14.1

1, 2, 3, 4. See Table 14.1 for changes expected for older adults.

CHAPTER 15

Abnormal Mobility

Learning Objectives

Following completion of this chapter, the reader will be able to:

1. Describe abnormal mobility within the International Classification of Functioning, Disability and Health (ICF) framework.
2. Discuss current approaches to classifying gait impairments in individuals with neurologic pathology.
3. Discuss the effects of pathology in motor, sensory, and cognitive systems on steady-state gait.
4. Define mobility disability, and discuss the factors contributing to the recovery of participation in the mobility domain.
5. Discuss the prevalence and cause of other types of mobility problems, including those related to stair climbing, bed mobility, and transfers in people with CNS pathology.
6. Compare and contrast gait abnormalities in individuals with stroke, Parkinson's disease, cerebellar disorders, multiple sclerosis, and cerebral palsy.

INTRODUCTION

Impaired mobility, including disorders of gait, is one of the earliest and most characteristic symptoms of a wide variety of neurologic disorders. Mobility is a critical part of maintaining independence and an essential attribute of quality of life (Patla & Shumway-Cook, 1999). In Chapter 12, we examined normal mobility within the context of the International Classification of Functioning, Disability and Health (ICF) framework. In this chapter, we also use the ICF framework to understand mobility disability resulting from CNS pathology. As shown in Figure 15.1, an abnormal gait pattern is classified as an impairment in body function in the component of *Body Structure and Function*. Within the component of *Activities and Participation*, mobility disability includes limitations in the ability to change or maintain a body posture, walking limitations (characterized by limited speed, distance, or the ability to manage terrain changes), and restricted ability to move in the environment. Environmental factors strongly influence the presence and severity of mobility disability, particularly the ability to move or walk in the environment (Patla & Shumway-Cook, 1999; Shumway-Cook et al., 2002; 2003b; 2005b). Mobility disability has been identified as one of the most debilitating consequences of neurologic pathology, including stroke (Keenan et al., 1984; Lord et al., 2004; Perry et al., 1995; Pound et al., 1998), Parkinson's disease (PD) (Schenkman et al., 2002), multiple sclerosis (MS) (Johansson et al., 2007), and cerebral palsy (CP) (Beckung & Hagberg, 2002).

This chapter discusses components of mobility disability resulting from CNS pathology, including factors contributing to abnormal gait patterns, and considers the relationship between abnormal gait and limitations in walking-related activities and participation. We begin with a discussion of frameworks used for classifying abnormal gait. We then examine the effect of pathology in motor, sensory, and cognitive systems on (a) the strategies used to accomplish progression and postural stability requirements of steady-state gait and (b) the ability to adapt gait to changing task and environmental demands. We then examine factors influencing the recovery of walking, including those that restrict participation in the mobility domain. The chapter concludes with a summary of mobility problems in our case studies in order to provide an understanding of the types of problems found in people with different neurologic diagnoses.

Classification Systems

While an abnormal gait pattern is a common characteristic of many neurologic disorders, the constellation of

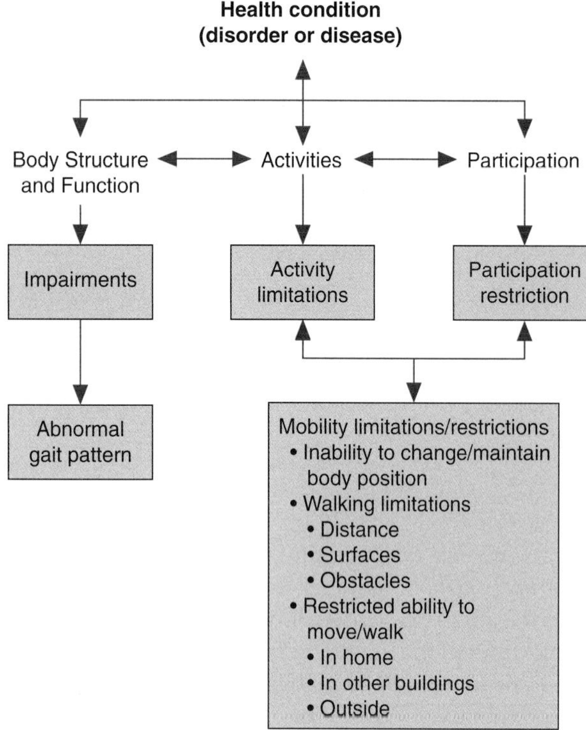

Figure 15.1 Characterizing *Mobility Disability* in the ICF framework.

underlying problems that produces a disordered gait pattern varies from patient to patient, even among patients with the same pathology. The type of gait pattern abnormality observed depends on the type and extent of central nervous system (CNS) pathology, the constellation of resulting impairments, and the extent to which the patient is able to compensate for those impairments.

A number of classification schemes have been proposed; however, there is little consensus on the best framework for classifying gait disorders. Gait classification is designed to organize individuals into homogeneous groups, which can be used to assist clinicians with clinical decision making regarding therapeutic interventions to improve gait (Dobson et al., 2007).

The most common framework for classifying disorders of gait is based on the neurologic diagnosis itself—for example, parkinsonian gait, cerebellar ataxic gait, or spastic hemiparesis gait. A limitation of this approach is the assumption that a specific diagnosis results in a homogeneous gait pattern, an assumption not supported by current research. For example, Rozumalski and Schwartz (2009) found that children with CP who walked with a crouched gait were not a homogeneous group, since the underlying mechanism producing excessive knee flexion included variations in strength, selective motor control, and spasticity. Similarly, Kinsella and Moran (2008) found that while many persons with poststroke hemiplegia walked with an equinus gait pattern (excessive plantarflexion at foot contact), they varied considerably regarding the underlying mechanisms causing this pattern. Thus, there appears to be significant heterogeneity among persons walking with an apparently homogeneous gait pattern.

Researchers have also classified gait according to the primary pathophysiologic mechanism producing disordered gait. For example, Crenna and Inverno (1994) identified four main mechanisms contributing to disordered gait in individuals with CNS pathology: paresis, spasticity, loss of selectivity in motor output, and a nonneural component (changes in mechanical properties of the muscle–tendon system). Knutsson and Richards (1979) identified similar impairments constraining gait following stroke. With technological advancements, researchers are starting to use a large amount of quantitative information concerning patients' gait characteristics, such as video, kinematics, kinetics, electromyography, and plantar pressure data, to classify gait (Arman et al., 2016).

As you can see, a wide variety of classification systems have been proposed to help researchers and clinicians understand abnormal gait. In this chapter, we use both a pathophysiologic and a diagnostic framework to discuss disorders of gait. We begin with a pathophysiologic framework to examine how impairments in motor, sensory, and cognitive systems contribute to gait pattern disorders, and we consider some common compensatory strategies used to maintain function in light of these impairments. You will see that while some impairments (e.g., cocontraction) are common across many neurologic diagnoses, others are unique to specific pathologies (e.g., freezing of gait in persons with PD). Finally, we use our case studies to summarize gait problems from a diagnostic perspective. Regardless of the type of classification system used, understanding the effects of sensory, motor, and cognitive impairments on mobility function, as well as the types of patients likely to have these problems, is essential for examining and treating the patient with mobility problems.

MOTOR SYSTEMS AND ABNORMAL GAIT

Motor problems affecting gait include disruptions to both neuromuscular and musculoskeletal systems. In individuals with neurologic pathology, musculoskeletal problems develop secondary to primary neuromuscular problems that limit movement. Problems in the neuromuscular control of gait disrupt the basic gait pattern (affecting both progression and postural control requirements), as well as the ability to adapt the gait pattern to changing task and environmental demands. Neuromuscular problems affecting steady-state gait patterns are discussed first and include paresis or weakness, abnormal tone (with an emphasis on spasticity), loss of selective control or abnormal synergies, and coordination problems. We then discuss the contribution of problems within the motor system to diminished adaptation, including impaired reactive and proactive balance control.

Paresis or Weakness

A reduced ability to generate force, the so-called paretic component, is a primary contributor to disordered gait (Chen & Patten, 2008; Chow & Stokic, 2019; Jonkers et al., 2009; Knarr et al., 2013; Lamontagne et al., 2002; Perry & Burnfield, 2010). Paresis, or weakness, is a primary neuromuscular impairment affecting the number, type, and discharge frequency of motor neurons essential for force production during gait (Duncan & Badke, 1987). Paresis is a primary impairment among patients with corticospinal pathology (see, for example, the case study video of Genise, our patient with acute stroke); however, many patients with neurologic pathology who have limited physical activity share a common impairment related to weakness.

Paresis affects both the neural and nonneural components of force production. The neural component of weakness or paresis results from insufficient supraspinal recruitment of motor neurons in specific leg muscles either during certain parts of the gait cycle or throughout the gait cycle. Nonneural contributions to weakness reflect secondary changes in the muscle fibers themselves that affect the patient's ability to generate tension.

Muscles in gait act both concentrically to generate motion and eccentrically to control motion. Thus, paresis or weakness affects both the ability to generate forces to move the body forward (i.e., affecting the progression requirement of gait) and unrestrained motions resulting from lack of control (i.e., affecting the postural control requirement of gait).

How much does paresis or weakness affect the ability to walk independently? This depends on which muscles are weak, the extent of the weakness, and the capacity of other muscles to substitute for weak muscles in achieving the requirements of gait. The following section briefly reviews the effect of paresis or weakness in select groups of lower-extremity muscles on gait.

Plantarflexors

In their classic study, Knutsson and Richards (1979) examined gait in 26 hemiparetic subjects; nine (about one-third) showed a paretic pattern of gait. The paretic component was reflected in a significant reduction in muscle activity in both the plantarflexors (Fig. 15.2A) and the TA (Fig. 15.2B) in the persons with stroke (*dotted line*) as compared with normal controls (*solid line*). Reduced activation of muscles was associated with strong hyperextension of the knee in the stance phase and lack of knee flexion in the swing phase (Fig. 15.2C). Interestingly, for several of the participants examined, poor muscle recruitment in gait was associated with preserved recruitment when the muscle was activated voluntarily, suggesting that in these patients, injury disturbed the central generation of preprogrammed gait activation but left the capacity to activate muscles voluntarily relatively intact (Knutsson & Richard, 1979).

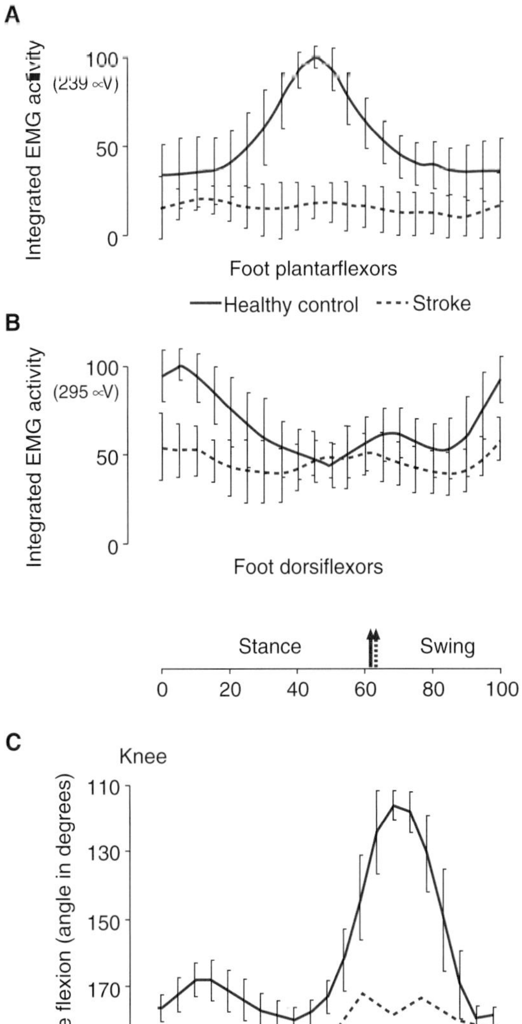

Figure 15.2 Effects of paresis on gait. **(A)** and **(B)** Rectified, integrated EMG activity from ankle plantarflexors and dorsiflexors across the gait cycle in normal healthy controls (HC) (*solid lines*) and a group of subjects with hemiparesis (stroke) (*dotted lines*). EMG in the patient group shows a lack of phasic activation of the plantarflexors and relatively low activity of the dorsiflexors. **(C)** Changes in knee motion in normal subjects (*solid line*) and in patients (*dotted line*). Vertical arrows indicate the transition from stance to swing in healthy controls (*solid arrow*) versus patients with stroke (*dotted arrow*) (Adapted from Knutsson E, Richards C. Different types of disturbed motor control in gait of hemiparetic patients. *Brain*. 1979;102:420, with permission.)

Since the study by Knutsson and Richard, a number of research studies have documented the contribution of plantarflexor weakness to impaired gait following stroke (Bowden et al., 2006; Chen & Patten 2008; Jonkers et al., 2009; Lamontagne et al., 2002; Mulroy et al., 2003; Peterson et al., 2010; 2011) and PD (Svehlík et al., 2009). Chen and colleagues (Chen & Patten, 2008; Chen et al., 2003a) reported that among persons with stroke, reduced leg kinetic energy during preswing was largely the result of reduced ankle plantarflexor work. This can be seen in Figure 15.3,

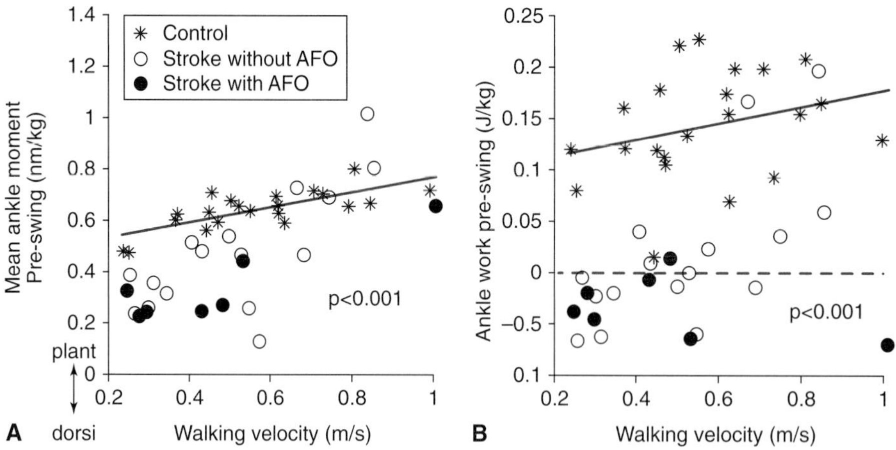

Figure 15.3 Effects of weakness on stance-to-swing transition following stroke. Mean ankle moment **(A)** and ankle work **(B)** during preswing as a function of gait speed in nondisabled controls (*asterisks*) and individuals with hemiparesis with (*filled circles*) and without (*open circles*) an ankle–foot orthosis (*AFO*). Plant, plantarflexor moment (and work) is represented as positive (above zero); dorsi, dorsiflexor moment (and work) is represented as negative (below zero). (Adapted from Chen G, Patten C. Joint moment work during the stance to swing transition in hemiparetic subjects. *J Biomechanics.* 2008;41:880, with permission.)

which compares mean ankle moment (Fig. 15.3A) and ankle work (Fig. 15.3B) during preswing as a function of gait velocity in controls (shown as *stars*) and subjects with stroke (*filled circles* represent subjects who used an ankle–foot orthosis [AFO]; *open circles* are hemiparetic subjects without an AFO). Among the participants with poststroke hemiparesis, plantarflexor work in the paretic limb was very low as compared with the subjects without disability walking at similar slow speeds. Compensation for the reduction in plantarflexor work during preswing occurred through increased knee and hip moments in the paretic limb as well as activity in the nonparetic limb (Bowden et al., 2006; Mahon et al., 2015). Plantarflexor paresis is one of several factors contributing to knee hyperextension in gait following a stroke (Bleyenheuft et al., 2010; Campanini et al., 2013).

Quadriceps

A weak quadriceps will lead to difficulty controlling knee flexion during loading and midstance. The primary compensation for this is hyperextension of the knee during midstance (also known as genu recurvatum), as the forward movement of the body weight will serve as the knee extensor force (Mulroy et al., 2003; Perry & Burnfield, 2010). This compensation is common in patients with stroke or CP (Appasamy et al., 2015; Klotz et al., 2014). Compensation for a weak quadriceps may also involve a forward trunk lean, which brings the body vector anterior to the knee, resulting in knee hyperextension. When hyperextension is continued into preswing, it prevents the knee from moving freely during the swing phase. This can slow progression and result in toe drag. In addition, using hyperextension as a compensatory strategy for stabilizing the knee will, over time, traumatize the internal structure of the knee.

Hip Flexors

Hip flexor weakness primarily affects the swing phase of gait. Hip flexion is used during swing to assist progression by producing a hip flexor moment at the initiation of swing (Chen & Patten, 2008; Neptune et al., 2001; Winter, 1984). Knee flexion is lost in swing when there is inadequate hip flexion; thus, the patient is unable to develop sufficient momentum at the hip to indirectly flex the knee. As a result, toe clearance is reduced or lost. A shortened step is also associated with inadequate hip flexion, and it can affect the position of the foot at heel strike. Thus, limited ability to generate hip flexion during the initiation of swing affects both the progression and postural control requirements of gait.

Impaired hip flexor strength affecting pull-off has been shown in a number of neurologic populations, including stroke (Chen & Patten, 2008) and PD (Svehlík et al., 2009). This may be particularly problematic, since use of the hip flexors to increase pull-off has been shown to be an effective compensatory strategy for persons with significantly reduced plantarflexor force (Nadeau et al., 1997; Olney & Richards, 1996).

There are several compensatory strategies people use to achieve foot clearance during swing despite inadequate hip flexion; these are shown in Figure 15.4. The first uses a posterior tilt of the pelvis and activation of the abdominal muscles to advance the swing limb (Fig. 15.4A). The second uses circumduction, defined as hip hike, forward rotation of the pelvis, and abduction of the hip, to advance the limb (Fig. 15.4B). The other strategies used to advance the limb despite hip flexor weakness include contralateral vaulting (Fig. 15.4C), involving coming up onto the forefoot of the stance limb, or leaning the trunk laterally toward the opposite limb (Fig. 15.4D).

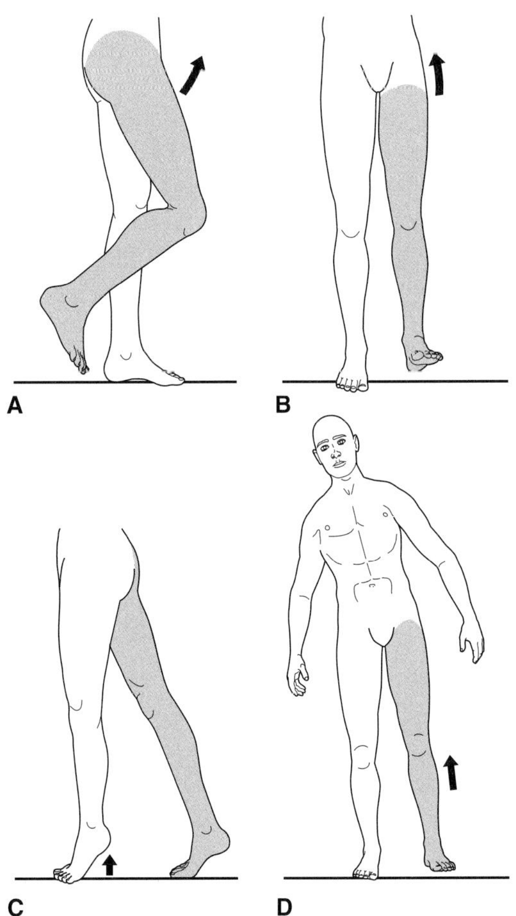

Figure 15.4 Compensatory strategies used to advance the swing leg despite inadequate hip flexion include activation of the abdominal muscles in conjunction with a posterior tip of the pelvis **(A)**, circumduction **(B)**, contralateral vaulting **(C)**, and leaning the trunk laterally toward the opposite limb **(D)**.

Hip Extensors

Activation of the hip extensors is critical to control the head, arms, and trunk (HAT). Hip extensor weakness can result in a forward trunk lean that threatens stability. To compensate for this, participants lean backward to bring the center of mass (COM) behind the hips. However, increased TA activity is needed to prevent falls in the backward direction (Winter, 1984). Following stroke, hip extensor weakness is strongly correlated with reduced gait velocity (Cruz & Dhaher, 2009).

Hip Abductors

Weak hip abductors (gluteus medius) can result in drop of the pelvis on the side contralateral to the weakness, called a "Trendelenburg gait." A common compensation for this is a lateral shift of the COM over the stance leg in conjunction with lateral lean of the trunk toward the stance leg. This shift of the upper body over the stance side moves the ground reaction force (GRF) in the same direction. When the GRF passes directly through the center of the femoral head, the internal moment generated by the hip abductors (that normally produces a stabilizing force) is no longer needed (Gage, 1993; Perry & Burnfield, 2010). This same compensatory mechanism is used when the problem is a painful hip, in order to reduce the proportion of force passing through the hip joint (Gage, 1993). Hip abductor weakness is a contributing factor to hip deformities, including subluxation, in children with CP (Metaxiotis et al., 2000).

Hip abductors also make an important contribution to achieving an appropriate step width, an essential part of ensuring mediolateral stability of the center of body mass (COM). Thus, weakness of these muscles can result in instability in the frontal plane, a factor in increased risk for falls in older adults (Krebs et al., 1998) and patients with neurologic pathology (Basford et al., 2003; Chou et al., 2003).

The effect of paresis on walking function can be seen in the longitudinal case study of Genise, our patient who is recovering from an acute stroke. At 4 days poststroke (first video segment), Genise has profound paresis affecting her right side, causing collapse of the paretic limb when loaded. She is unable to stand or walk without assistance. At 1 month poststroke, she is able to stand and walk with minimal assistance; this is due in part to an increased ability to generate force in her paretic limb and her ability to compensate using her nonaffected leg. In addition, use of an AFO with a plantarflexion stop also helps to minimize knee hyperextension during the stance phase of gait.

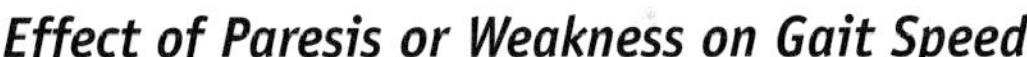

Effect of Paresis or Weakness on Gait Speed

Many researchers have shown that paresis or weakness has a significant effect on gait speed (Chen & Patten, 2008; Chow & Stokic, 2019; Kim & Eng, 2003; Lamontagne et al., 2002; Nadeau et al., 1997; Olney et al., 1986; 1991). Olney and colleagues (1986; 1991) demonstrated that following stroke, reduced amplitude in the plantarflexors at push-off and hip flexors at pull-off was correlated with slower gait speed. These findings were consistent with Nadeau et al. (1997) and Kim and Eng (2003), both of whom showed strong correlations between gait speed and isokinetic torques of the flexor and extensor muscles at the ankle, knee, and hip.

While a relationship between gait speed and lower-extremity power has also been shown in older adults with mobility disability in the absence of a neurologic diagnosis (Bean et al., 2002; Cuoco et al., 2004), it may not apply to persons with PD. While Sofuwa et al. (2005) found a significant reduction in ankle (push-off) and hip flexor (pull-off) power generation in the PD group, there was no correlation between ankle power and gait speed.

In summary, a reduced ability to generate force is a major factor contributing to disordered gait in persons with neurologic pathology. Paresis and weakness affect both control of movement through loss of eccentric contractions and generation of movement through loss of concentric contractions, and this seems to be a significant factor in reduced gait velocity in many patients. The degree to which weakness impacts gait speed may depend not just on the severity of impairment in affected limbs but the capacity of nonparetic muscles to compensate.

Spasticity

Because spasticity is a frequent accompaniment of neurologic disorders, many researchers have looked at its effect on gait. Spasticity can have an impact on gait in two ways. First, spasticity results in the inappropriate activation of a muscle at points during the gait cycle when it is being rapidly lengthened. In addition, spasticity alters the mechanical properties of a muscle, producing increased stiffness (a musculoskeletal problem) (Dietz et al., 1986). Increased stiffness affects the freedom of body segments to move rapidly with regard to one another; this limits the transfer of momentum during gait, affecting the progression requirements of locomotion.

In order to determine the contribution of spasticity to disordered gait, a number of researchers have examined activation levels of muscles in response to stretch during perturbed and nonperturbed gait. Some studies have examined activation of spastic muscles during lengthening contractions in unperturbed gait (Crenna, 1998; Knutsson & Richards, 1979; Lamontagne et al., 2002; Sinkjaer et al., 1996). Others have used perturbations to gait to study spasticity in gait, either by rapidly stretching the calf muscles using mechanical devices fixed to the subject's leg (Anderson & Sinkjaer, 1996) or by abruptly changing belt speed during treadmill walking (Berger et al., 1984b).

Regardless of the methods used, a key to understanding the contribution of spasticity to disordered gait requires knowing when muscles undergo lengthening during the gait cycle. This allows the researcher to examine the activity of spastic muscles during critical lengthening periods. For example, Figure 15.5A summarizes data from 10 healthy children showing the lengthening phases in representative lower limb muscles. As can be seen in this graph, the quadriceps are lengthened twice over the gait cycle, in early-stance phase, during knee yielding associated with loading, and when the knee flexes during toe-off. One would expect, therefore, that the effect of a spastic quadriceps muscle would be greatest during these two points in the gait cycle. In contrast, the hamstrings have one lengthening period in late swing, associated with knee extension in preparation for initial contact. Therefore, one would expect the effect of spasticity in the hamstrings to be heightened activation of this muscle during late swing.

Among children with spastic CP, there is heightened activity in spastic muscles undergoing lengthening; however, spasticity is not the sole contributor to disordered gait. This is best illustrated in Figure 15.5B, which shows the activation of four representative muscles in a child with spastic diplegia. In this figure, the red boxes indicate when a muscle is active, with the black bar underneath indicating the period in which this muscle is active in normal children. The open boxes represent an absence of muscle activity that is normally seen (see, for example, Quad L1), and the pink boxes represent muscle activity that is found in children with CP but never in the normal control children (see, for example, medial hamstrings activity during stance). Thus, one can see from looking at this figure that spasticity (increased activity in a muscle undergoing lengthening) is not the only component contributing to disordered gait; other contributing factors include decreased activation of muscles that are normally active and activation of muscles (nonstretch related) not typically active (Crenna, 1998).

The following section briefly reviews the effects of spasticity in certain key muscles.

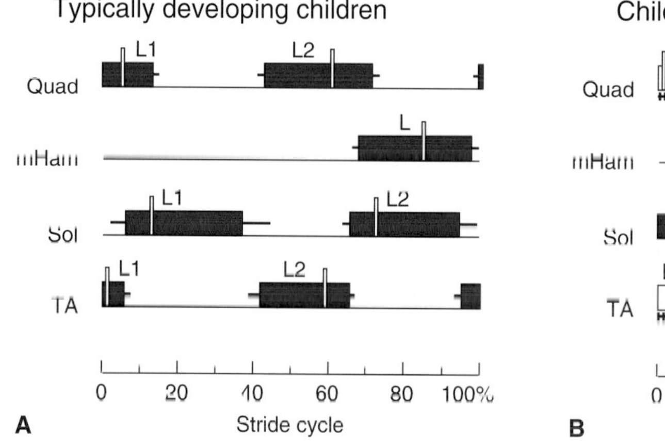

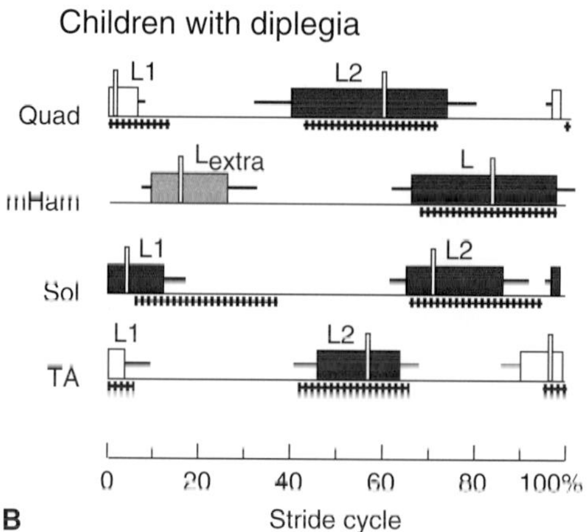

Figure 15.5 Muscle activity in representative lower limb muscles, including the quadriceps (*Quad*), medial hamstrings (*mHam*), soleus (*Sol*), and tibialis anterior (*TA*) in normal healthy children **(A)** and children with spastic cerebral palsy **(B)**. (Adapted from Crenna P. Spasticity and "spastic" gait in children with cerebral palsy. *Neurosci Biobehav Rev*. 1998;22:573, with permission.)

Plantarflexor Spasticity

Spasticity in the ankle plantarflexors (triceps surae [TS]) is a common problem following neurologic injury, and it has been reported in patients with stroke and CP and following traumatic brain injury (Crenna & Inverno, 1994; Knutsson & Richards, 1979; Perry, 1992).

In the Knutsson and Richards study (1979), one-third of patients with poststroke gait disorders showed a "spastic" pattern of gait, characterized primarily by abnormal activation of the TS muscles during the early part of the stance phase of walking. Figure 15.6A compares EMG activation of the TS (upper graphs) in nonimpaired participants (labeled normal) and persons with stroke (hemiparetic) who have spasticity. Following initial contact, stretching of the TS resulted in the early activation of the muscles, albeit at a reduced amplitude (see differences in the y-axis). The resultant shortening of the muscle before the body had passed ahead of the foot pulled the lower leg backward and produced knee hyperextension; thus, plantarflexion spasticity is another factor contributing to knee hyperextension following stroke. This is seen in the graph of knee angle during the gait cycle, in the lower part of the figure. Figure 15.6B is a stick figure of lower limb motion in a control participant (left) versus a person with hemiparesis (right). It illustrates the effect of premature contraction of the TS in the hemiparetic limb, which impedes muscle lengthening and forward rotation of the tibia, resulting in knee hyperextension as the body moves forward. This reduces the ability of the TS to build tension for push-off.

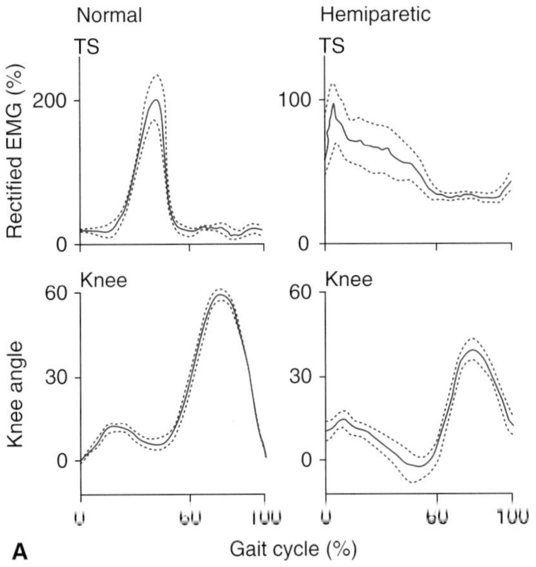

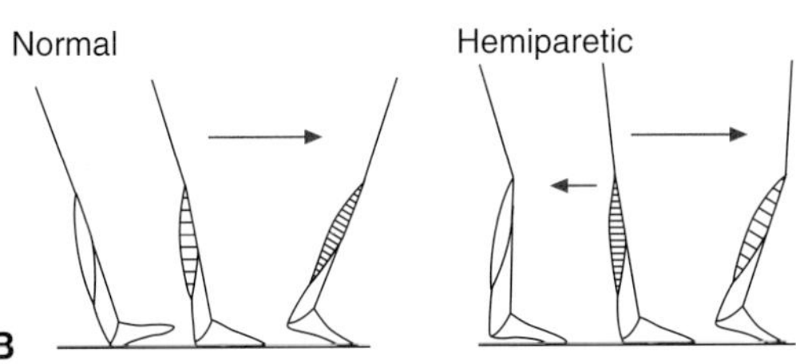

Figure 15.6 Effect of spastic TS on gait in patients with hemiplegia. **(A)** Averaged EMG activity (normalized to 239 mV) of the TS during the gait cycle in 10 normal control subjects and 9 patients with spastic hemiparesis, along with the corresponding knee angular changes. Note the high activation of TS during the entire stance phase (0% to 60%) in the patients with hemiparesis. **(B)** Effect of early TS activation on knee position in normal and hemiparetic gait (note the hyperextension of knee). (Adapted from Knutsson E. Can gait analysis improve gait training in stroke patients? *Scand J Rehab Med Suppl.* 1994;30:78, with permission.)

Consistent with the findings of Knutsson and Richards (1979), Lamontagne et al. (2002) also showed premature activation of the plantarflexor muscles (medial gastrocnemius [MG]) in the spastic hemiparetic limb, which occurred during peak lengthening velocity in the stance phase of gait in two-thirds of the individuals with hemiparesis. Interestingly, the authors did not find excessive activation of the MG when it was lengthened during the swing phase of gait, suggesting that locomotor spasticity is phase dependent. Locomotor spasticity was inversely related to gait speed, suggesting that early premature activation of the MG in response to lengthening velocity impairs ankle push-off in late stance.

Crenna and Inverno (1994) identified spasticity as one of four factors contributing to disordered gait in children with spastic forms of CP (diplegia and hemiplegia). Crenna and Inverno reported an excessive activation of the plantarflexors (soleus muscle) when they were being lengthened in early stance but not during swing phase lengthening. Phase-dependent effects of locomotor spasticity in children with spastic forms of CP can be seen in Figure 15.7. In children, like adults, spasticity is associated with reduced gait speed. However, since the effects of spasticity are increased at faster gait speeds, walking at slower gait velocity may be an attempt to decrease the effect of spasticity on gait kinematics (Van der Krogt et al., 2009).

In summary, spasticity in the plantarflexors can contribute to pathologic gait patterns in both the stance and swing phases of gait. Research has shown that in stance phase, plantarflexor spasticity will affect foot position at initial contact, thus having an impact on the stability component of gait. Spastic plantarflexors limit dorsiflexion and thus prevent heel strike at initial contact. When initial contact is made with a flat foot, the GRF vector is anterior to the knee, producing knee hyperextension (see Fig. 15.8A). Spastic plantarflexors affect forward foot clearance during swing; the subsequent consequence is toe drag (Fig. 15.8B). In terminal swing, spastic plantarflexors resist extension at the knee and dorsiflexion of the foot, critical to positioning the leg for heel strike at initial contact. Compensatory strategies include a shortened stride length and reduced gait velocity.

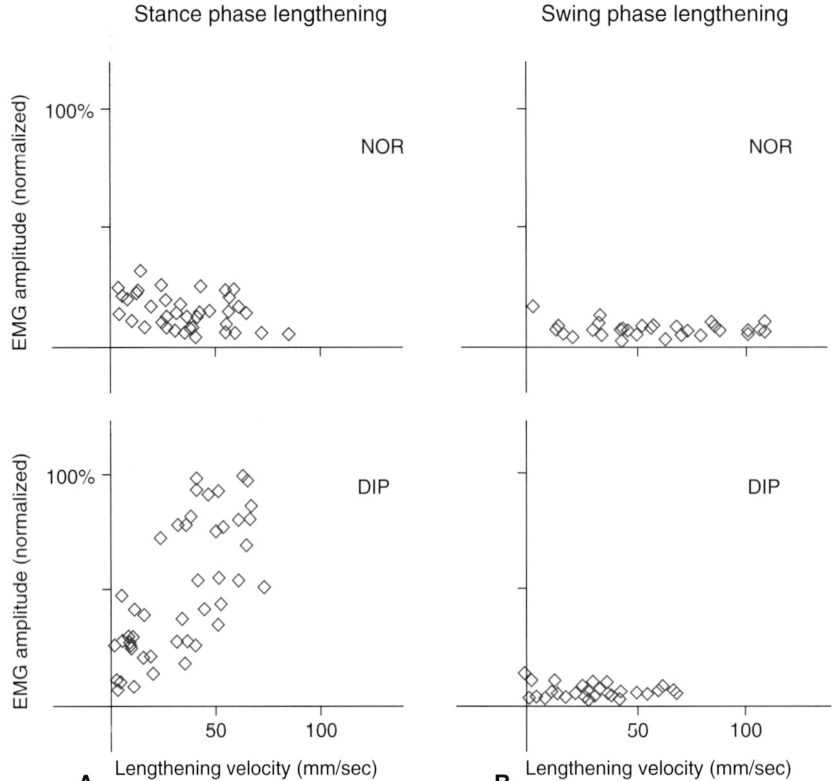

Figure 15.7 Comparison of activity of the soleus muscle when it is being lengthened in early stance **(A)** and in swing **(B)** in a normal control child (*NOR*) and a child with spastic diplegia (*DIP*). Note the excessive activation of the soleus muscle in the child with diplegia during the stance but not swing phase of gait. (Adapted from Crenna P, Inverno M. Objective detection of pathophysiological factors contributing to gait disturbance in supraspinal lesions. In: Fedrizzi E, Avanzini G, Crenna P, eds. *Motor development in children.* New York, NY: John Libbey, 1994:110, with permission.)

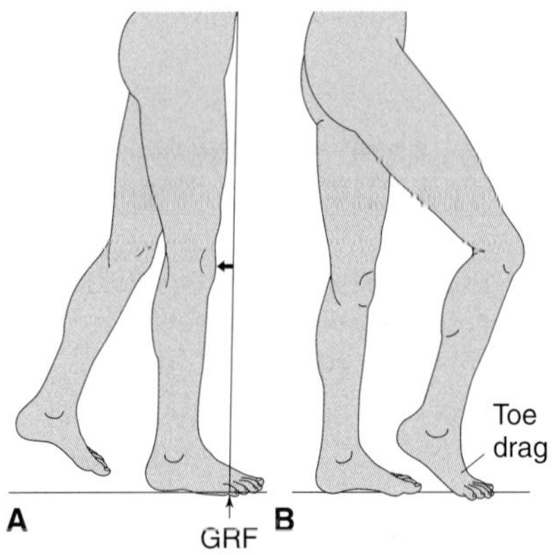

Figure 15.8 The effect of plantarflexor spasticity in gait. **(A)** When initial contact is made with a flat foot, the ground reaction force (*GRF*) vector is anterior to the knee, producing knee extension. **(B)** Spastic plantarflexors affect forward foot clearance during swing; the subsequent consequence is toe drag.

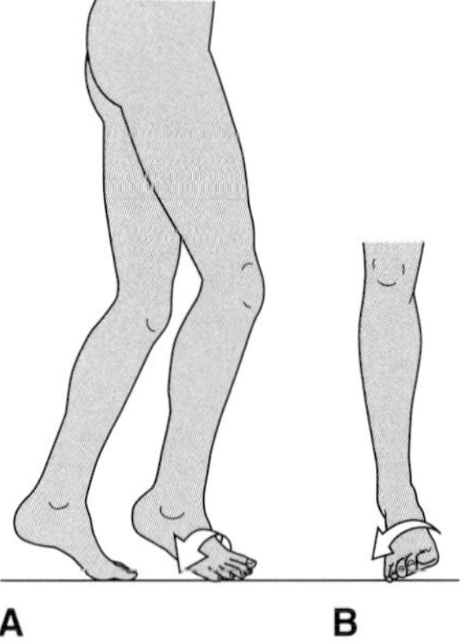

Figure 15.9 A combination of excessive activity of the TS and posterior tibialis muscle produces inversion and an equinovarus foot position, illustrated from both the sagittal **(A)** and frontal **(B)** planes.

A combination of excessive activity of the TS and posterior tibialis muscles produces coronal plane problems of the foot, including inversion and an equinovarus foot position (shown in Fig. 15.9A and B). This is seen clinically as the elevation of the first metatarsal head from the floor, with the subsequent foot contact made on the lateral border of the foot only.

In contrast, in equinovalgus gait, foot contact is made with the medial border of the foot. Equinovalgus gait can result from excessive activation of the TS in conjunction with the peroneus brevis muscle. An alternative cause of valgus gait is weakness or inaction by the ankle invertors, for example, a weak or inactive soleus. Thus, a flaccid paralysis can also lead to a valgus foot posture.

Quadriceps Spasticity

Like plantarflexor spasticity, quadriceps spasticity can also result in excessive knee extension in the stance phase of gait. Remember that during weight acceptance, there is a brief flexion of the knee that assists in absorbing the shock of loading. Quadriceps spasticity results in an excessive response to knee flexion and subsequent lengthening of the quadriceps, triggering spasticity that can limit flexion and result in hyperextension of the knee (Montgomery, 1987; Perry & Burnfield, 2010). Unlike plantarflexor spasticity, there does not appear to be a relationship between knee extensor spasticity and gait speed in patients with stroke (Bohannon & Andrews, 1990; Norton et al., 1975).

Quadriceps spasticity can also lead to a stiff-knee gait during the swing phase (Goldberg et al., 2004) (as shown in Fig. 15.4). This type of gait is common in hemiparetic stroke patients and in children with CP, where a reduction in knee flexion during swing is coupled by excessive hip circumduction (Kerrigan et al., 2000). Finley and colleagues (2008) applied single-joint angular perturbations to the hip and knee to examine the possible occurrence of multijoint reflexes of the leg in individuals with stroke. Their results showed that abduction stretches elicited an excitatory response in the hip adductors and in the rectus femoris, a knee extensor and hip flexor. These responses were reciprocal, such that a stretch of the rectos femoris also caused reflex excitation of the hip adductors. Thus, the authors conclude that these multijoint reflexes occurring after stroke may be contributing to the abnormal coupling between the hip and knee joints in hemiparetic gait.

Hamstrings Spasticity

Hamstrings spasticity producing excessive knee flexion is a frequent problem in certain types of CP; it manifests as a crouched-gait pattern, as shown in Figure 15.10. In the terminal swing phase of gait, excessive activation of the hamstrings muscles prevents the knee from fully extending, resulting in knee flexion at initial contact (Fig. 15.10A). Excessive knee flexion persists throughout the stance phase of gait (Fig. 15.10B), increasing the demand on the quadriceps muscles to prevent collapse of the limb into flexion.

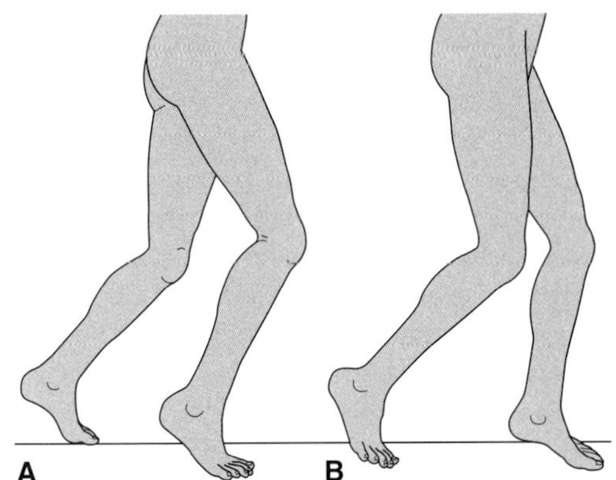

Figure 15.10 Hamstrings spasticity producing excessive knee flexion in both the terminal swing phase and the initiation of stance **(A)** and throughout the stance phase of gait **(B)** is a frequent problem in certain types of cerebral palsy and manifests as a crouched-gait pattern.

Hip Adductor Spasticity

Hip adductor spasticity produces a contralateral drop in the pelvis during stance, as the femur is drawn in medially. Adductor spasticity can result in scissors gait, which is characterized by excessive adduction. During the swing phase of gait, as the hip flexes, excessive adduction produces a severe medial displacement of the entire limb. This results in a reduced base of support, affecting the stability requirement of gait. In severe cases, the adducted swing leg catches on the stance limb and impedes progression (Montgomery, 1987; Perry & Burnfield, 2010).

In summary, spasticity contributes to disordered gait through the inappropriate activation of a muscle during the portions of the gait cycle during which it is lengthened and through changes in stiffness resulting from alterations in the mechanical properties of the muscle itself. You can see examples of spastic gait disorders in the Mobility section of the video case studies for Jean, our patient with chronic stroke, and Thomas, our child with spastic diplegia.

Loss of Selective Control and the Emergence of Abnormal Synergies

As discussed in Chapter 5, inability to selectively recruit muscles is a significant factor contributing to abnormal gait in many patients with CNS pathology, especially those with corticospinal lesions. Inability to recruit muscles selectively is often associated with abnormal coupling of muscles, resulting in stereotypical movement strategies, called "abnormal synergies" or "synkinesia" (Roche et al., 2015). Abnormal synergies manifest in gait as either total extension (Fig. 15.11A) or total flexion (Fig. 15.11B) patterns. This can be seen in the EMG traces as simultaneous activation of either extensors (A) during the stance phase of gait or flexors (B) during the swing phase.

Knutsson and Richards (1979) reported that mass patterns of flexion and extension were one of four characteristic gait patterns found in persons with hemiparesis following stroke. Roche et al. (2015) also reported an abnormal coupling between hip flexors and ankle dorsiflexors during the swing phase of gait in persons with hemiparetic gait following stroke. Abnormal coupling between hip and ankle flexors results in a reduced ability to extend the knee while flexing the hip during terminal swing.

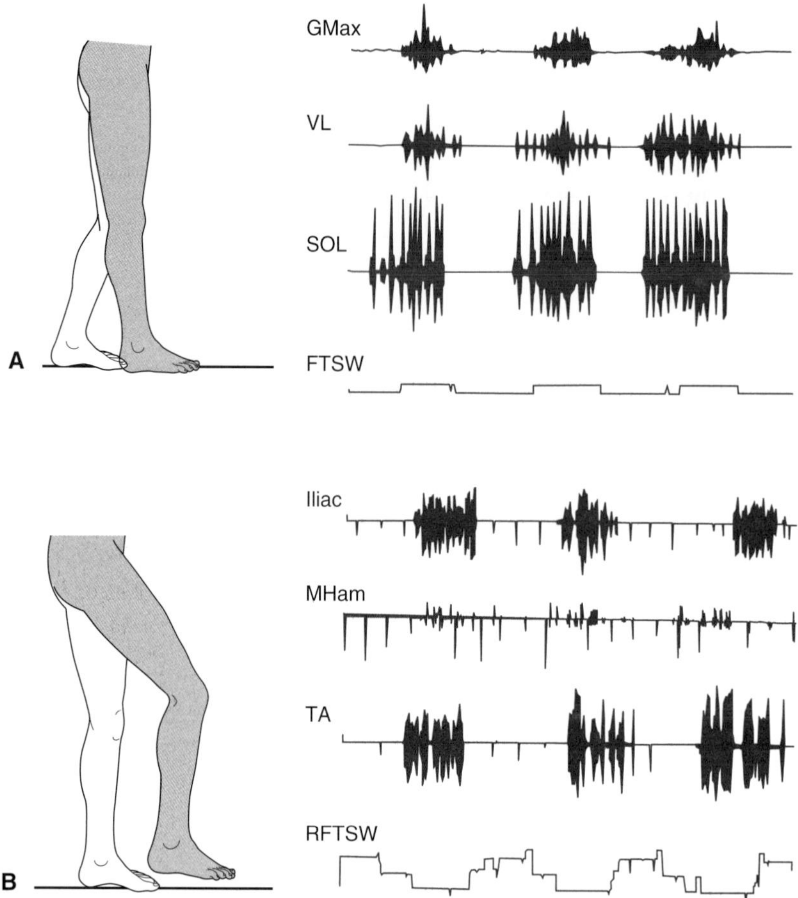

Figure 15.11 Synergies manifest in gait as either total extension **(A)** or total flexion **(B)** patterns. The right panels are EMG traces of extensor muscles **(A)** and flexor muscles **(B)**, while the left panels illustrate the behavior observed: excessive extension in stance **(A)** and flexion in swing **(B)**. *FTSW*, footswitch; *GMax*, gluteus maximus; *Iliac*, iliacus; *MHam*, medial hamstrings; *RFTSW*, right footswitch; *SOL*, soleus; *TA*, tibialis anterior; *VL*, vastus lateralis. (Adapted from Perry J. *Gait analysis: normal and pathological function.* Thorofare, NJ: Slack, 1992:313, with permission.)

Dyer et al. (2014) reported a shared pattern of activation between ankle extensors and knee extensors throughout the stance phase in the paretic leg of individuals with stroke but not among controls. In addition, the amplitude of the coupling between lower-extremity extensor muscles measured during gait was higher than the levels measured in a standing position under static conditions, suggesting that the coactivation of leg extensors on the paretic side might be higher during a dynamic task such as gait than during a static task.

The prevalence of synergistic mass patterns is associated with reduced stability and poor locomotor recovery following stroke (Chen et al., 2003a; DeQuervain et al., 1996; Richards & Olney, 1996). Jean, our patient with chronic stroke, has problems with abnormal synergies, which can be seen in her video case study, in both the Impairment and Mobility sections.

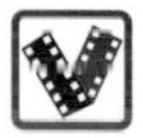

Coordination Problems

Coordination problems resulting in impaired coupling among body segments are a major factor contributing to impaired gait in patients with CNS pathology. Impaired coordination can manifest as (a) increased activation of muscles that is unrelated to spasticity mediated stretch, (b) abnormal phasing of multijoint movement leading to poor intersegmental coordination, and (c) coactivation of agonist and antagonist muscles.

Non–Stretch-Related Muscle Overactivity

Overactivity of muscles can be as problematic to the control of gait as the inability to recruit muscles for both progression and postural control. For example, overactivity of the hamstrings muscles unrelated to stretch has been reported in both adult patients following stroke (Knutsson & Richards, 1979) and children with CP (refer back to Fig. 15.5, which shows both an inappropriate activation of the hamstrings early in stance as well as prolonged activation of the hamstrings in swing phase of gait in children with spastic forms of CP) (Crenna, 1998; Perry & Burnfield, 2010). It was originally thought that hamstrings overactivity was the result of spasticity resulting in stretch-related overactivity. But researchers have subsequently found that performing a dorsal rhizotomy, which involves selectively cutting the sensory nerve roots, does not decrease hamstrings overactivity in children with CP. This suggests that the basis for hamstrings overactivity is abnormal coordination, not a simple hyperactive stretch reflex (Crenna, 1998; Perry & Burnfield, 2010).

Impaired Coordination

Impaired coordination is a significant factor in abnormal gait among persons with CNS pathology and includes both impaired segmental coordination (coordination within a body segment) and impaired intersegmental coordination (coordination between body segments).

Impaired Segmental Coordination. Impaired segmental coordination involves the inability to control the timing and scaling of muscle activity during gait. Impaired segmental coordination is a common finding in gait disorders due to pathology in the cerebellum (ataxic gait), as well as pathology in the basal ganglia (parkinsonian gait).

Pathology in the cerebellum gives rise to ataxic gait, characterized by staggering, veering, irregular stepping, and high steppage. In patients with cerebellar pathology, ataxic gait is associated with delays in the relative movement of the knee and ankle throughout the gait cycle (Palliyath et al., 1998). Intersegmental coordination problems also result in delays in the timing of peak knee flexion during the swing phase of gait (Palliyath et al., 1998). More detailed information

on characteristics of ataxic gait patterns may be found in the Diagnostic Case Study Approach to Gait, found at the end of this chapter. In addition, an example of ataxic gait may be seen in the Mobility section of our case study, John, who has spinocerebellar degeneration.

Pathology in the basal ganglia resulting in PD is also associated with significant gait problems; however, the degree of abnormality depends on both the progression of the disease and the medication state. The speed and amplitude of leg movements are reduced in both the stance and swing phase of gait; gait is also characterized by reduced push-off and pull-off (Sofuwa et al., 2005). Episodes of freezing (e.g., loss of forward momentum) are a major disruption to gait and occur with disease progression. Episodes of freezing are transient, lasting from seconds to minutes, and most often occur during gait initiation, turns, in narrow spaces, or when approaching obstacles (Fahn, 1995; Giladi et al., 1997). More detailed information on characteristics of parkinsonian gait patterns may be found in the Diagnostic Case Study Approach to Gait, found at the end of this chapter. In addition, an example of PD gait can be seen in the mobility section of the video case study on Mike, our patient with PD.

Impaired Intersegmental Coordination. Impaired intersegmental coordination reflects a reduced ability to coordinate movements between body segments (e.g., between the two lower extremities or between the lower and upper extremities). Normal intersegmental coupling is seen in the synchronization of arm and leg movements in normal gait. Swinging the arms during gait facilitates the movements of the legs and decreases the energetic cost of locomotion by about 8%. In addition, the arms assist in stability by aiding in the recovery of the gait pattern after a perturbation (Meyns et al., 2013). Typically, in individuals without impairment walking at a preferred speed, one arm swing is associated with one leg swing (a 1:1 arm-to-leg swing ratio), which increases to a 2:1 ratio at slower gait speeds. Arm swing appears to be accomplished through both passive and active mechanisms (CPG activation of interlimb coordination). In addition, higherorder regulation of interlimb coordination can be achieved at brainstem and cortical level (Barthelemy & Nielsen, 2010; Debaere et al., 2001). This explains why one figure does not necessarily have to walk with natural swinging arms but can perform other actions as well with the arms (i.e., texting, holding a book, etc.) (Meyns et al., 2013).

CNS pathology affects arm swing during gait, which can constrain walking speed. Pathology affects interlimb coupling, by disturbing the amplitude and timing of arm swing and disrupting the synchronization of arm–leg coordination. In persons with hemiplegia (either due to stroke or CP), the hemiplegic arm swings with decreased amplitude, which is often compensated for by increased arm swing on the less-affected side (Ford et al., 2007a; Meyns et al., 2011). In individuals with PD, a reduced arm swing is present; it often presents asymmetrically and is thought to result from increased rigidity. There is little evidence to suggest that individuals with PD compensate for reduced arm swing on one side of the body by increasing the arm swing on the less-affected side (Huang et al., 2012; Lewek et al., 2010). A characteristic upper limb pattern during gait has also been observed in patients with MS. These patients do not show impaired shoulder movements during gait but instead, they swing their arms with reduced range of motion and increased flexion position of elbows compared to controls (Elsworth-Edelsten et al., 2017).

Abnormal arm swing can be the direct result of impairments such as paresis, spasticity, rigidity, or abnormal synergies, which affect the capacity to move the arm normally. Alternatively, altered arm swing can be an indirect result of changes in trunk motion and posture. For example, children with CP show more trunk movements in all planes (Galli et al., 2011; Romkes et al., 2007), while patients with PD walk with increased trunk flexion and reduced trunk rotation throughout the gait cycle (Winogrodzka et al., 2005; Zijlmans et al., 1996).

In summary, CNS pathology affects both inter- and intrasegmental coupling and has a significant effect on gait in a wide variety of patient populations. The evidence indicating that upper and lower limb movements influence each other during gait supports the importance of including arm movements in rehabilitation of gait, discussed in more detail in Chapter 16.

Coactivation of Agonist and Antagonist Muscles

Normal gait is characterized by a remarkable degree of selectivity of muscle activity. There is a reciprocal recruitment pattern during gait such that coactivation of agonist and antagonist muscles is minimized. Cocontraction is defined as the loss of selective recruitment of physiologically antagonistic muscles. Coactivity among antagonist muscles during gait has been reported in many individuals with supraspinal lesions, including stroke (Knutsson & Richards, 1979; Lamontagne et al., 2002) and CP (Crenna, 1998). Researchers have hypothesized several possible reasons for the presence of coactivation, including (a) pathologically disorganized central programs, (b) additional postural support activity, (c) immature gait programs, and (d) compensatory programming—that is, the use of coactivation to increase stiffness (Crenna, 1998; Knutsson, 1994).

Following stroke, coactivation of lower-extremity muscles has been reported in both the paretic (Knutsson & Richards, 1979) and nonparetic limbs (Lamontagne et al., 2002). Crenna reported that the presence of coactivation of lower-extremity muscles was a common finding among children with spastic-type CP (Crenna, 1998). A comparison of coactivation between the hamstrings (medial hamstrings) and quadriceps (vastus medialis) muscles in a typically developing child versus a child with spastic diplegia is shown in Figure 15.12. Note that the filled areas (activity in both muscles greater than 20% of maximum locomotor output) cover a much greater part of the step cycle in the child with spastic diplegia as compared with the typically developing child. Coactivation is also characterized by both temporal and geometric overlap. Coactivation between the tibialis anterior (TA) and MG has been reported as a factor contributing to equinus ankle characteristics during the swing phase of gait in children with CP (Wakeling et al., 2007).

Musculoskeletal Impairments

In addition to neuromuscular problems, problems in the musculoskeletal system, including weakness, loss of range of motion and contractures, and changes in alignment, also impact the gait of persons with CNS pathology. Passive properties of the muscle–tendon system contribute to development of torque during walking. Thus, abnormal joint stiffness and limited range of motion not only reduce joint motion but also affect the ability of muscles to generate power at various speeds (Patla, 2003).

In both children with CP and adults with hemiplegia, changes in the passive properties of the musculoskeletal system have been found to be relevant factors in disordered locomotion. Among these neurologic populations, both soft tissue contractures and bony constrictions limit joint range of motion, constrain movement, and increase the workload on the muscles, thus affecting a patient's ability to meet the requirements of gait. In general, decreased joint mobility during stance restricts forward motion of the body over the supporting foot, thus affecting progression. In swing, decreased joint mobility reduces foot clearance, affecting progression, and appropriate foot placement

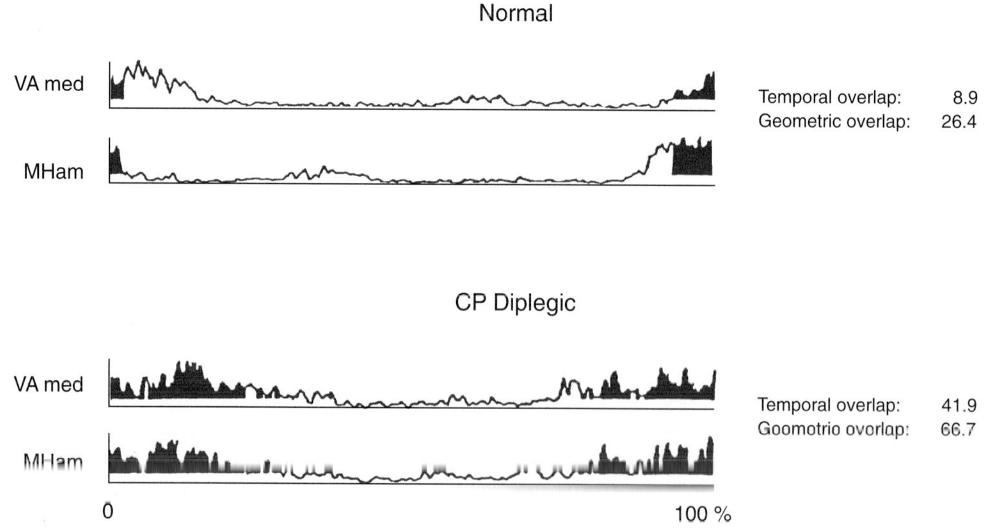

Figure 15.12 Quantitative assessment of cocontraction between quadriceps (*VA med*) and hamstrings (*MHam*) in a child with spastic diplegia and an age-matched typically developing child walking at comparable speed. Filled areas represent coactivation of agonist and antagonist muscles. See text for further explanation. (Reprinted from Crenna P, Inverno M. Objective detection of pathophysiological factors contributing to gait disturbance in supraspinal lesions. In: Fedrizzi E, Avanzini G, Crenna P, eds. *Motor development in children*. New York, NY: John Libbey, 1994:112, with permission.)

for weight acceptance, affecting stability. Limited range of motion also limits a patient's ability to modify movement strategies, thus affecting adaptation. For example, a person with limited ankle and knee flexion will be unable to increase limb flexion during the swing phase of gait to step over an obstacle.

During stance, a smooth progression over the supporting foot requires a minimum of 5 degrees of ankle dorsiflexion; thus, ankle plantarflexor contractures can impair a person's ability to move the limb over the foot (Higginson et al., 2006; Perry & Burnfield, 2010). Plantarflexor contractures limit tibial advancement over the stationary foot during stance. If the contracture is elastic (i.e., able to lengthen in response to body weight), the only result may be an inappropriate foot position at foot contact, since body weight will lengthen the plantarflexors, allowing the tibia to advance (Perry & Burnfield, 2010). However, if the contracture is not elastic, recurvatum results. Recurvatum occurs when the knee has sufficient mobility to move posteriorly past neutral. Knee hyperextension can occur quickly or slowly, and it usually begins in midstance or terminal stance and continues into preswing. Excessive knee extension means the tibia cannot advance over the stationary foot in the stance phase (Perry & Burnfield, 2010). Plantarflexor contractures also affect foot clearance during swing by preventing sufficient ankle flexion to allow toe clearance.

Hip flexion contractures result in inadequate hip extension, which can affect both stability and progression. During midstance, if the hip cannot extend to neutral, the trunk will flex forward, bringing the COM anterior to the hip joint. Gravity will pull the trunk forward into more flexion; this places an additional demand on the hip extensors to prevent collapse of the forward trunk and causes loss of stability (Perry, 1992). Hip flexion contractures have a great effect on terminal stance, as it is during this phase that the hip is normally extended. Lack of hip extension produces an anterior pelvic tilt and an inability to move the thigh posterior to the hip. This results in a shortened step length and reduces forward progression of the body.

In summary, a wide variety of motor impairments contribute to disorders of gait in persons with neurologic dysfunction. These impairments can occur alone or in combination, which can make sorting out their relative contributions difficult. We now turn our attention to impairments affecting the ability to adapt gait to changing task and environmental conditions.

Impaired Adaptation of Gait: Contributions of Impaired Reactive and Proactive Balance Control

Inability to adapt gait to changing task conditions is a significant contributor to abnormal walking function in persons with neurologic pathology. Inability to adapt gait to environmental challenges, such as inclines, curbs, and obstacles significantly, limits participation in mobility-based activities. For example, at the time of discharge from inpatient rehabilitation, only 7% of persons with stroke could manage steps and inclines and walk the distances and speeds required to walk competently in the community (Hill et al., 1997). In addition, while 85% of people with stroke were able to walk independently 6 months after a stroke, only a small proportion were able to independently manage the challenges of community ambulation, such as managing curbs and inclines and crossing a street in the time allotted by a stoplight (Lord et al., 2004). Thus, among persons with CNS pathology, a diminished ability to adapt gait is a critical factor limiting recovery of mobility in the home and community environment. Diminished adaptation results from both impaired reactive balance problems that prevent recovery of stability following an unexpected loss of balance as well as impaired proactive balance essential to countering potentially destabilizing internal and external forces.

Reactive Balance Problems

Reactive balance strategies that are integrated into the gait cycle are necessary to the recovery of stability following an unexpected perturbation, such as a trip or a slip. Impaired reactive balance control is a major factor contributing to instability during both stance and gait in persons with CNS pathology. Impaired stepping in response to a stance perturbation among persons receiving inpatient rehabilitation for stroke was strongly associated with increased rates of falls (Mansfield et al., 2013). At the time of discharge, 99 out of 139 (71%) patients with stroke who could independently ambulate nonetheless had impaired stepping responses and required assistance to recover from a forward fall. Importantly, neither the Berg Balance Scale (BBS) nor usual gait velocity distinguished between those patients able to step and those with impaired stepping reactions (Inness et al., 2014).

Following a stroke, use of a stepping strategy to recover from loss of balance is particularly challenging. Difficulties with speed and precision of paretic limb control limit the patient's ability to step with the paretic limb; thus, compensatory stepping responses are preferentially made with the nonparetic limb. However, stepping with the nonparetic limb is also challenging due to a reduced ability to load the paretic limb without collapse (Lakhani et al., 2011; Mansfield et al., 2011).

Kajrolkar et al. (2014) examined compensatory stepping in response to unexpected perturbations to walking in persons with hemiparetic stroke. The mechanism used to provoke a slip during gait is shown in Figure 15.13. Compensatory stepping in the paretic limb was examined in response to an unexpected slip of the nonparetic limb induced at heel strike. Four of the 10 participants with hemiparetic stroke were able to execute a compensatory recovery step using the paretic limb in response to the slip-induced backward loss of balance. In the recovery

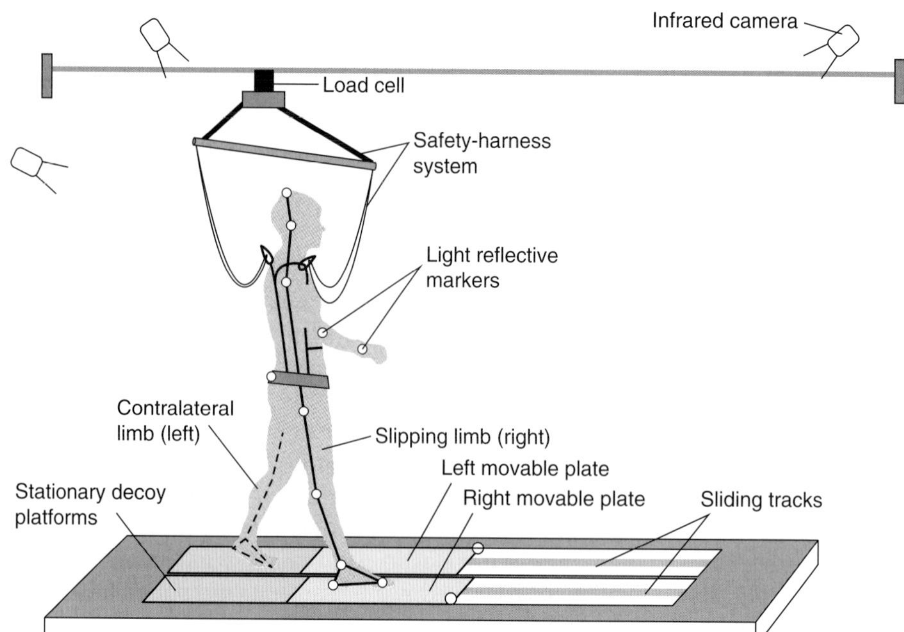

Figure 15.13 A paradigm to study recovery from a slip-induced loss of balance during gait. See text for details. (Adapted from Kajrolkar R, Yang F, Pai YC, et al. Dynamic stability and compensatory stepping responses during anterior gait slip perturbations in people with chronic hemiparetic stroke. *J Biomechanics.* 2014;47: figure 1, page 2753.)

step, the paretic limb landed just posterior to the slipping heel, reestablishing the base of support and restoring dynamic stability (Fig. 15.14B). The remaining six participants used an aborted step strategy to recover stability (Fig. 15.14A). An aborted step response in the paretic limb involved a rapid unloading, followed by an immediate reloading of the limb with no lift-off or step. In response to a second slip perturbation, these six participants showed an increased ability to execute a recovery step rather than an aborted step response, suggesting the ability to adapt responses to repeated exposure (Kajrolkar et al., 2014).

Compensatory responses to unexpected perturbations require not only an appropriate stepping response but also an adequate body configuration for balance recovery. De Kam and colleagues (2018) aimed to determine whether body configuration at the first recovery step following a backward perturbation could predict balance recovery capacity in chronic stroke survivors. They found that leg and trunk inclination angles at stepping-foot contact were stronger determinants of the single-step balance recovery than spatiotemporal parameters of the step. A foot position more posterior to the pelvis and a more forward–tilted trunk were associated with a greater likelihood of successful single-step balance recovery.

These studies suggest that CNS pathology affects the ability to recover from an unexpected perturbation to balance in both stance and gait. Impaired reactive balance is a major contributor to falls in both geriatric and neurologic populations.

Proactive Balance Problems

Walking in daily life is characterized by the performance of complex walking tasks that require adapting gait to changing task and environmental demands (Shumway-Cook et al., 2007). Complex walking tasks, such as stepping over or around obstacles, changing directions, or accelerating or decelerating to avoid collisions with objects and people in the environment, require proactive balance control, including both predictive and visually activated strategies. Performance of complex walking tasks is a good predictor of adverse health outcomes in both geriatric and neurologic populations, including falls, fractures, and incident mobility limitations (Cho et al., 2004; Dargent-Molina et al., 1996; Shumway-Cook et al., 2000). Many researchers have examined the effect of neurologic pathology on the ability to manage a variety of complex walking tasks.

Impaired Obstacle Avoidance. Impaired obstacle crossing has been reported following stroke (Lu et al., 2010; Said et al., 2005; 2008; 2009), traumatic brain injury (Cantin et al., 2007; Catena et al., 2009; Chou et al., 2004; Fait et al., 2009), in patients with PD (Galna et al., 2009; Snijders et al., 2010; Vitorio et al., 2010), and in children with CP (Cappellini et al., 2020; Law & Webb, 2005). Gait impairments during obstacle crossing in these populations include slower gait velocity when approaching and crossing an obstacle, reduced (or alternatively excessive) toe clearance in both the leading and trailing limbs, increased step variability, increased mediolateral instability during crossing, and a reduced ability to modify gait parameters and muscle activity appropriately to changing obstacle height. All of these impairments result in an increased likelihood for striking an obstacle during crossing, increasing the individual's risk for a trip-related fall.

Impaired Turning. The ability to turn while walking is a critical aspect of mobility in daily life. Turning allows

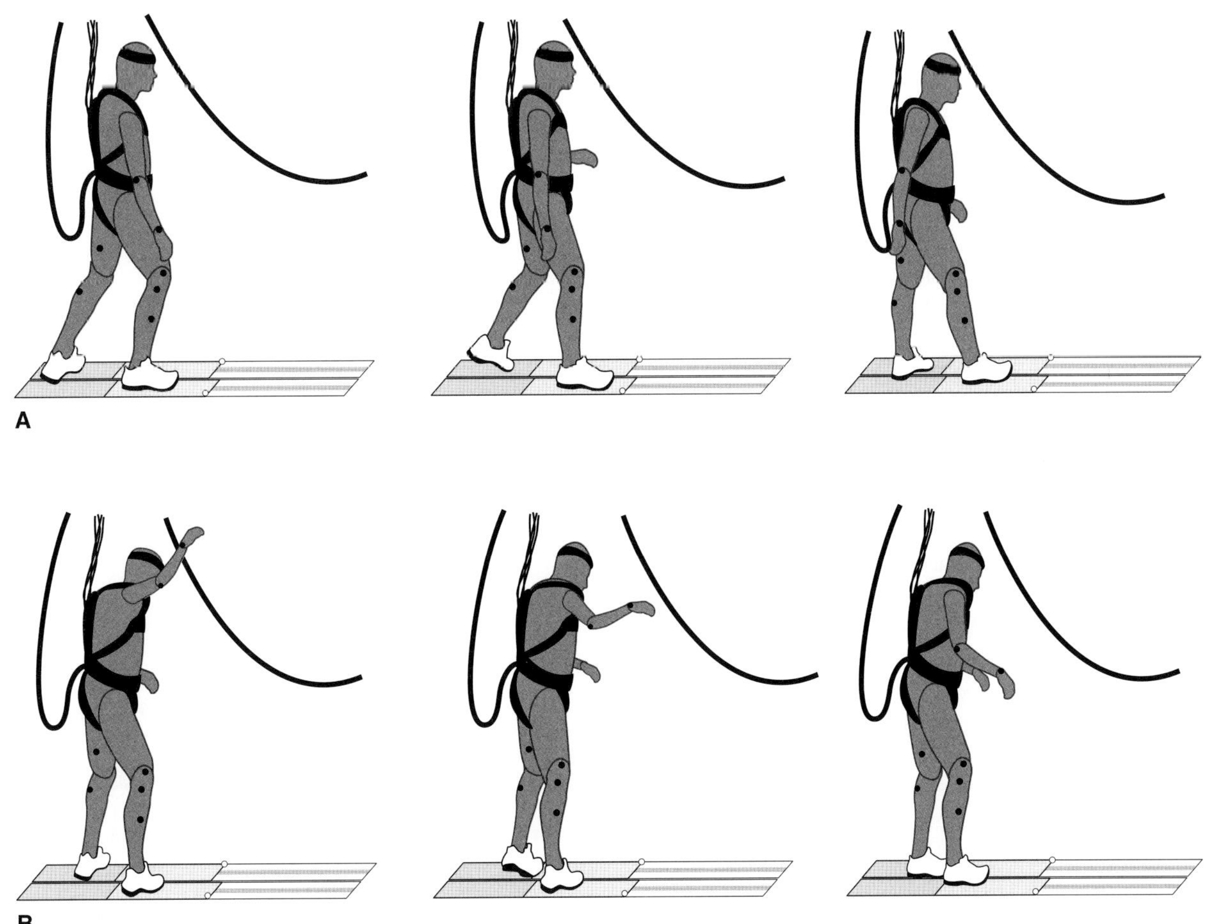

Figure 15.14 Two different strategies used to recover from a forward slip at heel strike. **(A)** Heel strike–induced slip of the right leg results in an aborted step in the hemiplegic (left) leg. **(B)** Heel strike-induced slip of the right (nonparetic) limb results in a recovery step by the paretic (left) leg. (Adapted from Kajrolkar R, Yang F, Pai YC, et al. Dynamic stability and compensatory stepping responses during anterior gait slip perturbations in people with chronic hemiparetic stroke. *J Biomechanics.* 2014;47: Figure 2, page 2754.)

us to avoid obstacles and navigate corners, and accounts for as many as 45% of the steps taken daily (Glaister et al., 2007). Turning while walking is a complex task that presents a significant challenge to individuals with impaired postural control since it requires initiating a state of disequilibrium during single-limb stance in order to change directions. Disequilibrium is created by increasing the distance between the body's COM and the center of pressure (COP); while this distance creates the momentum necessary to turn, it also requires increased neural control to redirect and control this momentum.

Among persons with poststroke hemiplegia, turns toward the paretic side took longer than did turns to the nonparetic side; they were also characterized by shorter, narrower steps, with shorter single-support times compared to those made by age-matched nonimpaired adults (Hollands et al., 2014). Individuals with poststroke hemiplegia reporting falls during turns take longer to initiate turns, are slower, and take more steps when turning compared to individuals with no history of falls (Hollands et al., 2010). Interestingly, when provided with external visual cues prior to a turn, these deficits were eliminated. Thus, the authors hypothesized that falls during turns after stroke may not be due to an inability to produce the necessary movement pattern but may be due to a cognitive–motor interference stemming from limited cognitive resources (Hollands et al., 2010; 2014).

Turns present a significant challenge in PD as well, with more than half of people with PD reporting difficulty with turning (Chou & Lee, 2013). Turns are slower, require more steps, and take longer to initiate in persons with PD compared to nonimpaired controls (Chou & Lee, 2013; Stack & Ashburn, 2008). Shorter, more frequent steps serve to decrease the body's momentum, reduce the distance between the COM and the COP, and in turn decrease the neuromuscular demands associated with turning (Song et al., 2012). Poor intersegmental coordination, as indicated by slower and smaller rotations of the head, trunk, and pelvis and an "en bloc" turn strategy, is observed. Increased postural tone, axial rigidity, and loss of intersegmental flexibility may contribute to an en bloc turning strategy. Turns are also characterized by instability and poor ground clearance, requiring increased use of external support (Chou & Lee, 2013). Instability during turning can be seen even among persons with early-stage PD (Song et al., 2012). Bhatt et al. (2013) compared turning strategies in persons with PD who freeze (freezers) versus those who don't (nonfreezers) and noted that freezers had increased step time variability, failed to increase step width during turns, and were much slower compared to nonfreezers. In addition, episodes of freezing increased in frequency as turn angles become sharper. Freezing of gait during turns can be seen in the mobility section of the video case study of Mike, our participant with PD.

Inability to Adapt to Terrain Changes. Persons with stroke have a diminished ability to modify gait characteristics in response to terrain changes, such as slopes. Phan et al. (2013) investigated spatiotemporal characteristics of gait during self-selected speed across a GAITRite mat placed on level, uphill, and downhill surfaces. Individuals with stroke had significantly slower gait speed and increased variability compared to the control group for all conditions. While nonimpaired individuals maintained speed when walking downhill, individuals with stroke maintained cadence but shortened their step length, resulting in a reduction of speed when walking downhill. Both groups maintained walking speed when walking uphill; however, nonimpaired individuals increased step length and reduced cadence, while those with stroke did not. Results suggest that people with stroke have difficulty adapting their gait to suit the physical features of the environment (Phan et al., 2013).

Studies done on children with CP have shown that these children can adapt to terrain changes, but they use greater postural compensations. For example, Stott and colleagues (2014) compared indoor walking, outdoor walking, and walking up and down a 7° inclined ramp. They found that both children with CP and healthy controls (HC) adapted their gait in a similar way to accommodate for the changes. However, children with CP had greater trunk compensations when walking over the ramp. Children with CP also had greater forward trunk lean during up-slope walking and greater posterior trunk lean during down-slope walking (see Fig. 15.15). Böhm and colleagues (2014) tested children with CP walking on a level, uneven surface. They found that children with CP adapted some gait parameters in a similar fashion to HC; however, their step width was significantly wider. Interestingly, children with CP increased their knee flexion during swing phase more than HC despite children with CP being classified as stiff-knee walkers. Thus, we can conclude that children with CP have the ability to find their own motor solutions to suit the physical features of the environment but require greater adaptations compared to HC.

In summary, impairments to adequately adapt gait and to avoid instability in the face of complex task and environmental conditions is a major factor impairing mobility in a wide variety of patients with CNS pathology. Impaired performance during

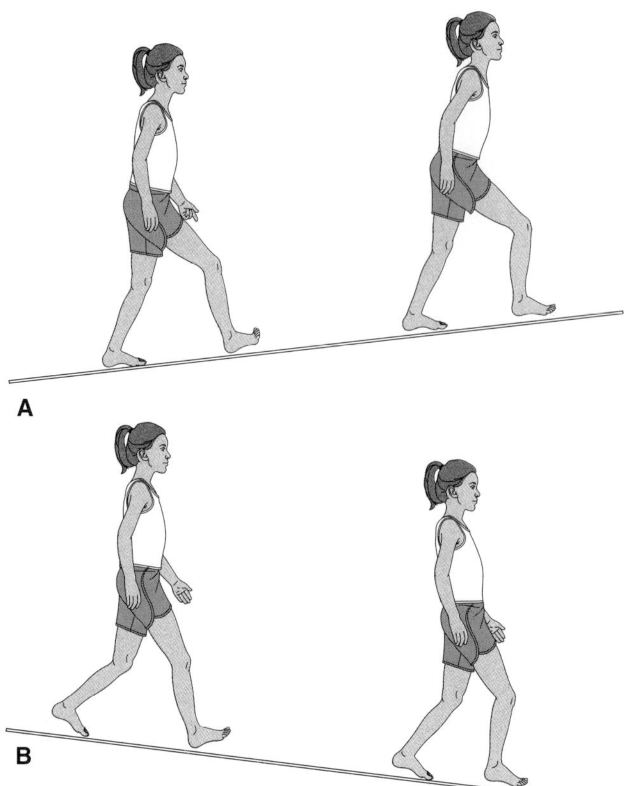

Figure 15.15 Side view of trunk during foot contact for the right leg in up-slope walking **(A)** and down-slope walking **(B)**. Schematics derived from reported median angles for the trunk and right leg. Representation of data for children with typical development are represented on the left and data for children with CP on the right. (Adapted from Stott NS, Reynolds N, McNair, P. Level versus inclined walking: Ambulatory compensations in children with cerebral palsy under outdoor conditions. *Pediatr Phy Ther.* 2014;26:434.)

complex walking tasks includes limitations in obstacle crossing, changing gait speed and direction, carrying objects, walking on uneven or inclined surfaces (Robinson, 2010), and impaired turns or movements of the head (Hong & Earhart, 2010; Huxham et al., 2008; Mak et al., 2008). Impaired ability to adapt gait in response to complex task and environmental demands affects the ability to walk safely in home and community environments and is a major factor in the development of mobility disability (Robinson et al., 2011b; Shumway-Cook et al., 2007).

SENSORY SYSTEMS AND ABNORMAL GAIT

The control of gait is based on the integration of both peripheral sensory inputs and descending supraspinal inputs. Sensation is a critical determinant for maintaining gait in natural environments, in which we are required to constantly modify how we move in response to changes in our surroundings. Sensory inputs play several important roles in the control of locomotion. Sensory inputs serve as a trigger for the initiation of swing. Thus, loss of proprioceptive cues that normally signal hyperextension in the hip and the termination of stance can result in delayed initiation of the swing phase (Smith, 1980). In addition, sensory inputs are necessary in adapting locomotor patterns to changes in environmental demands. This includes signaling unanticipated disruptions to gait as well as the ability to predict and anticipate upcoming obstacles. Thus, the effects of sensory impairments on gait are varied, depending on which sense is affected and the capacity of alternative senses to compensate.

Somatosensory Deficits

Abnormal somatosensory inputs result in gait ataxia. Gait problems in persons with sensory ataxia can be due to interruption of either peripheral or central proprioceptive pathways. When this occurs, the individual is usually no longer aware of the position of the legs in space, or even of the position of the body itself. With mild sensory dysfunction, walking may not appear to be abnormal, if the person can use vision. However, ataxia is worse when visual cues are reduced or inappropriate. Staggering and unsteadiness increase, and some people lose the ability to walk.

Normally, proprioceptively mediated stretch reflexes are modulated throughout the gait cycle. They are facilitated in the gastrocnemius and soleus at the end of stance phase, allowing for compensation for ground irregularities and assisting in push-off, but they are inhibited during the swing phase, to prevent stretch reflex-mediated plantar flexion during ankle dorsiflexion (Sinkjaer et al., 1996). Loss of proprioceptive inputs results in reduced modulation of reflex activity throughout the gait cycle.

Mullie and Duclos (2014) evaluated the role of proprioception in balance control during gait using vibration to the TA, either continuously or only during the stance phase, in individuals with poststroke hemiplegia and nonimpaired controls. While vibration significantly improved balance during walking in the healthy participants, it had no effect on balance or gait parameters in participants with stroke, suggesting that proprioceptive information is not used to control balance during gait following a stroke (Mullie & Duclos, 2014). These findings are similar to those reported on stance postural control; following stroke, there is increased use of visual compared to proprioceptive input in postural control.

Can vision substitute for impaired somatosensation during normal walking? Patla and colleagues (2000) examined visual sampling during steady-state gait in an individual with impaired somatosensation due to a severe peripheral neuropathy. Liquid crystal eyeglasses that turn from opaque to clear in response to a handheld switch were used to examine the frequency and duration of visual sampling during gait. Compared to individuals without impairment, the person with peripheral neuropathy increased visual sampling by about 60%, suggesting an increased reliance on vision to maintain dynamic stability and orientation during locomotion.

Visual Deficits

Vision is critical to visually activated proactive balance strategies during gait. Visual inputs are used to regulate gait on a local level (step-by-step basis) and on a more global level (route finding) (Patla, 2003). On surfaces that are rated as rougher and less stable to walk on, healthy young adults lower their heads to block their lower visual field, increase muscle coactivation, slow their gait, and walk smoother to increase stability and prevent fall risk (Thomas et al., 2020). Loss of vision primarily affects these adaptation aspects. Visually impaired and blind individuals tend to walk more slowly. In addition, they appear able to use auditory cues to assist in locating obstacles in space (Ashmead et al., 1989).

Vision is critical to many complex walking tasks, including obstacle avoidance, since visual inputs regarding upcoming obstacles are used to alter gait patterns in an anticipatory manner. For example, loss of the visual field on one side (hemianopsia) can have an impact on the person's ability to perceive potential threats to stability on the impaired side. This is shown in Figure 15.16, which illustrates a bus coming from the left that would be invisible to a person with left hemianopsia (Tobis & Lowenthal, 1960). Thus, loss of visual inputs will affect both route finding and obstacle avoidance.

Vestibular Deficits

The functional consequence of the loss of vestibular inputs appears to depend on the age of the individual at the time of the sensory loss. For example, individuals who lost vestibular function as infants had near-normal posture and gait control (Horak et al., 1994). However, this depends on the level of damage. In children with bilateral, moderate to profound sensorineural hearing loss since or shortly after birth, there is a delay in overall motor development, which either persists or is progressive depending on the task (Rine and Cornwall, 2000). Loss of vestibular function in adulthood can produce gait ataxia and difficulty in stabilizing the head in space.

Adult patients with vestibular deficits may walk more slowly than do individuals without impairment. Other changes include a prolonged double-support phase and a 6.5% longer cycle time than in normal subjects (Takahashi et al., 1988). Interestingly, when individuals with vestibular deficits were asked to walk at a normal velocity, using a metronome to establish the pace, the duration of their double-support phase became more normal. It is not clear why individuals

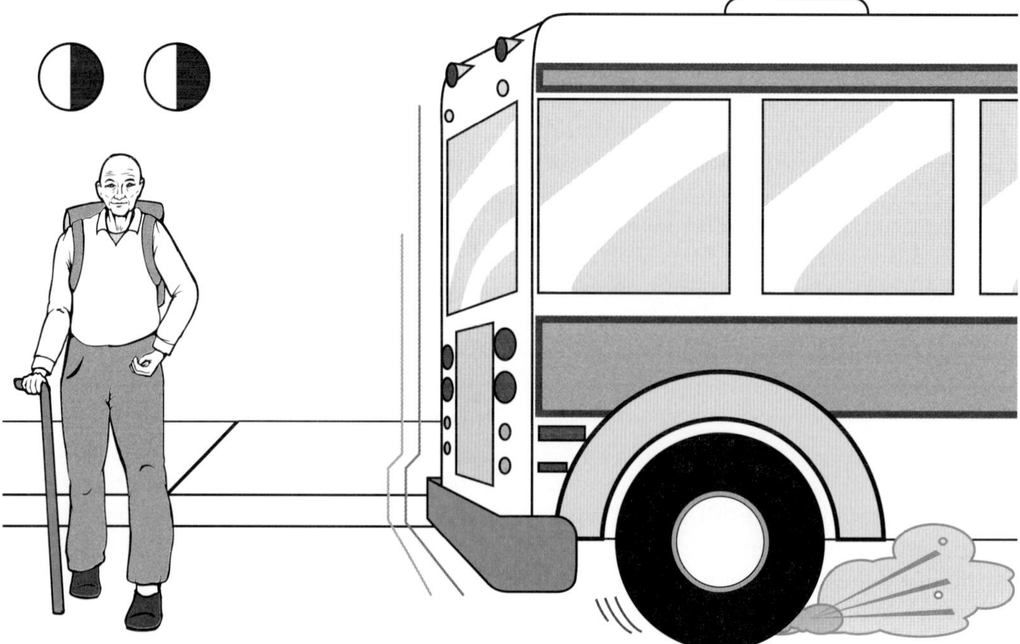

Figure 15.16 Functional effects of visual hemianopsia. A patient with a left hemianopsia would not perceive a bus coming from the left. (Adapted from Tobis JS, Lowenthal M. *Evaluation and management of the brain damaged patient*. Springfield, IL: Charles C Thomas, 1960:78, with permission.)

with vestibular deficits seem to prefer a slower gait speed and whether practicing at faster speeds would improve the kinematics of their gait cycle.

It has been reported that persons with vestibular deficits may also show impairments in head stabilization during gait, especially when walking in the dark (Pozzo et al., 1991; Takahashi et al., 1988). Gaze is equally stable for individuals with vestibular deficits and normal subjects during sitting and standing. However, when walking, the ability to stabilize gaze is impaired; thus, persons with vestibular deficits report impaired vision and oscillopsia. In addition, eye movements compensate for head movements more effectively during active head rotations than during similar movements made while walking. It has been suggested that this may be due to the predictable nature of active voluntary head movements versus the passive head movements that happen during locomotion (Grossman & Leigh, 1990).

When normal subjects walk or run in the dark, the amplitude and velocity of head rotations are decreased as compared with head movements during normal walking. However, these parameters increase for subjects with bilateral vestibular deficits when they walk in the dark (Pozzo et al., 1991).

Perceptual Problems Affecting Gait

As discussed in Chapter 5, perceptual problems are a common consequence of CNS pathology and make significant contributions to abnormal gait.

Body Image or Scheme Disorders

Body image deficits can result in a number of gait deviations, including ipsilateral trunk lean toward the stance leg, resulting in loss of stability. Impaired body image can also result in inappropriate foot placement and difficulty in controlling the COM relative to the changing base of support of the feet (Perry, 1992). Individuals with unilateral spatial neglect (USN, defined as the inability to perceive and integrate stimuli on one side of the body), affecting the left side, tend to veer to the right when walking, or bump into objects on the left side when walking or propelling a wheelchair.

Suzuki et al. (1997) used a dual-task method to examine the relationship between USN and gait in 31 individuals who had had a stroke, 12 with left hemiplegia (right hemisphere damage) and 19 with right hemiplegia (left hemisphere damage). They created a video face test involving use of a video monitor, placed in front of the patient, which showed a video of scenery associated with walking along a corridor. Faces appeared on the video periodically, positioned to the right or left of midline. The ability to perceive faces presented on the right versus the left side was examined while individuals were sitting, standing, or stepping continuously. Results from this study are summarized in Table 15.1. They found that many of the individuals with USN (see, for example, subjects 1, 5, and 6) were able to observe all 15 faces presented on the side contralateral to the lesion when sitting or standing; however, they were unable to perceive faces

TABLE 15.1 Scores on the Video Face Test in Patients with Unilateral Spatial Neglect: Number of Correct Identifications of Faces Presented on the Right or Left Side in Sitting, Standing, and Walking

		Sitting		Standing		Stepping	
Subject number	**Hemisphere >Lesion side**	**RT**	**LT**	**RT**	**LT**	**RT**	**LT**
1	Right	15	15	15	15	14	0
2	Right	15	15	15	15	15	7
3	Right	14	15	15	15	13	7
4	Right	14	13	15	15	15	0
5	Right	15	15	15	15	15	0
6	Right	15	15	15	15	15	0
7	Right	15	15	15	15	15	9
8	Right	15	0	15	0	15	0
9	Right	15	15	15	15	15	15
10	Right	14	15	15	15	15	15
11	Left	14	15	15	15	10	15
12	Left	0	15	0	15	0	15

Total possible, 15. *RT*, right; *LT*, left.

Source: Reprinted from Suzuki E, Chen W, Kondo T. Measuring unilateral spatial neglect during stepping. *Arch Phys Med Rehabil.* 1997;78:176, with permission.

(score of 0) while stepping. In contrast, subjects 8 and 12 show USN (as indicated by 0 scores) in sitting, standing, and stepping. These findings indicate that in some individuals, USN is context specific.

Interestingly, two of the individuals with USN (subjects 9 and 10) who performed normally on the video face test in stepping (score of 15) required more assistance to step during the test, suggesting that they allocated attention to the video task rather than to the stepping task. Other subjects were able to keep stepping with minimal or no assistance (Suzuki et al., 1997).

Spatial Relation Disorders

Purposeful locomotion toward a goal that is not visible from the start requires navigational strategies that depend on stored spatial knowledge (Patla, 2003). The impact of deficits in spatial cognition on mobility is considerable and particularly affects the ability to navigate safely through the environment, avoiding collisions with obstacles that are not readily perceived. Inability to remember the relationship of one place to another, called "topographic disorientation," can significantly affect route-finding aspects of locomotion (Patla, 2003).

Pain

Pain can also cause an alteration of movement patterns used for gait. An antalgic gait is defined as a gait pattern that results from pain of the lower back or lower extremity. Compensatory strategies used in the presence of pain are movements that (a) reduce weight-bearing time on the painful limb (e.g., shortening stance phase of gait), (b) avoid impact loads, (c) reduce joint excursion (e.g., limiting knee flexion during the stance phase of gait), and (d) decrease joint compressive forces by minimizing activity in muscles that cross the joint (e.g., side bending over a painful hip to bring the COM closer to the joint's center of rotation, reducing the need for hip abductor activity and concomitant joint compressive forces) (Eyring & Murray, 1964). Antalgic gait is often characterized by decreased gait velocity, shortened stance phase on the painful limb, a tendency to stiffen the limb in order to minimize joint motion, and a reduction in forceful foot contact or push-off.

COGNITIVE SYSTEMS AND IMPAIRED GAIT

Cognitive impairments also have an impact on mobility function, specifically, the ability to initiate gait, to adapt gait patterns to changing environmental demands, and to navigate in both familiar and unfamiliar locations. Cognitive impairments, as discussed in Chapter 5, include deficits affecting memory, attention, and executive function. A more complete discussion of higher-order gait disorders resulting from impaired cognitive function can be found elsewhere (Nutt et al., 1993; 1997).

Many studies have found that dementia is a major risk factor for falls (Alexander et al., 1995; Tinetti et al., 1988). Alexander and colleagues (1995) studied 17 subjects with Alzheimer's disease (AD). They found that the individuals with AD walked at half the speed of healthy older adults, had a higher obstacle contact rate, and tended to land more closely to the obstacle. These factors could contribute to falls, particularly trips, in persons with AD. In addition, falls during gait may be the result of impaired judgment, resulting in attempts to perform tasks that are beyond a person's physical capabilities.

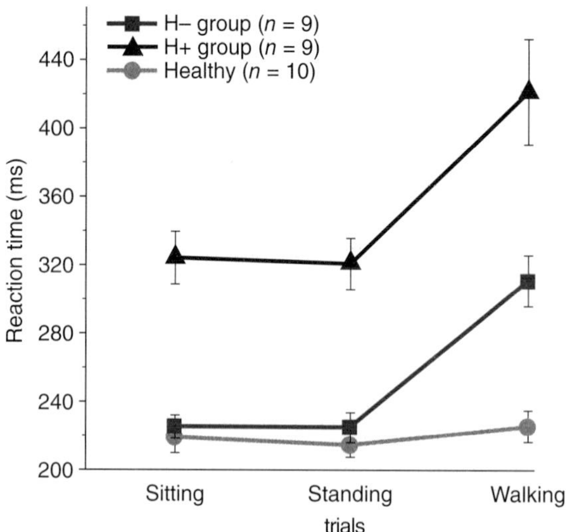

Figure 15.17 Changes of the mean reaction time across three different trials (sitting, standing, and walking on a treadmill at preferred speed) in healthy subjects, and in two groups of individuals with poststroke hemiparesis, those whose RT in sitting were the same as healthy controls (labeled *H–*) and those with a longer RT (labeled *H+*). *Error bars* indicate the standard deviation. (Adapted from Regnaux JP, David D, Daniel O, et al. Evidence for Cognitive Processes Involved in the Control of Steady State of Walking in Healthy Subjects and after Cerebral Damage. *Neurorehabil Neural Repair*. 2005;19:128, Fig. 2.)

Impaired Dual-Task Walking

Researchers have shown that posture, balance, and gait, although considered "automatic," require attentional resources (Lajoie et al., 1993; Teasdale et al., 1993; Woollacott & Shumway-Cook, 2002). Attentional demands associated with postural control in stance and gait are greater in individuals with impaired balance as compared with individuals without impairment. Regnaux et al. (2005) used a dual-task paradigm to compare the attentional demands associated with sitting, standing, and walking in participants with and without a history of stroke. Participants walked on a treadmill at their preferred speed; reaction time to a 10 ms shock to the neck was recorded using a pressure-sensitive sensor located in the mouth. Results, shown in Figure 15.17, found that attentional demands associated with sitting, standing, and walking were greater in persons with stroke as compared with nonimpaired controls. In addition, walking required more attentional resources, as indicated by the much slower reaction times during dual-task walking compared to dual-task sitting or standing, for all participants with stroke. This included both groups of individuals with stroke, those whose reactions in sitting were comparable to age-matched controls (labeled H group), as well as those whose reaction times in sitting were significantly slower than the controls (labeled H+). In this study, there were no effects of the secondary task on gait parameters, probably because treadmill speed was kept constant under both single- and dual-task conditions.

Performance of a secondary task while walking can impair stability in patients with various types of neurologic pathology, including stroke, PD, and traumatic brain injury. Bowen and colleagues (2001) compared the effects of a secondary task on gait speed in 12 persons with hemiparesis following a stroke (average time since stroke, 4 months) with a group of nonimpaired control subjects. Their results, shown in Figure 15.18, showed that performance of a secondary task decreased gait velocity in some but not all persons with stroke. We have added the BBS scores listed for each patient to this figure to illustrate that performance on the Berg test (a

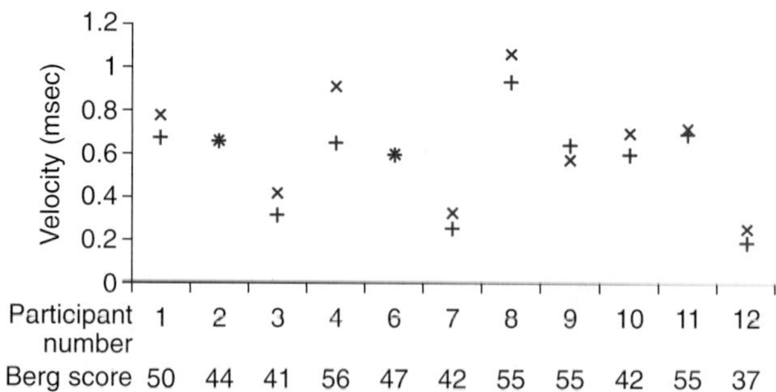

Figure 15.18 Effect of a secondary task on gait speed after stroke. Gait speed (m/s) in 12 persons with stroke under single- (x) and dual-task (+) conditions. Also shown are the scores on the BBS for each individual subject, illustrating the relationship between the Berg test and gait performance in single- and dual-task conditions. Note that not all participants with stroke demonstrate dual-task interference. In addition, extent of dual-task interference is not correlated with BBS. (Adapted with permission from Bowen A, Wenman R, Mickelborough J, et al. Dual-task effects of talking while walking on velocity and balance following a stroke. *Age Ageing*. 2001;30:319–323.)

nongait balance measure) did not predict who would have difficulty in the dual-task gait conditions.

Plummer-D'Amato and Altmann (2012) and Plummer-D'Amato et al. (2008) also examined dual-task interference during gait in individuals with stroke using three cognitive tasks that varied with respect to level of difficulty: a memory task (1-back test), a visuospatial task (clock), and a speech task (narrative). Dual-task interference was greatest during the single-limb stance phase of gait; as cognitive task demands increased, dual-task costs developed in other parts of the gait cycle as well. Dual-task costs affecting gait were greatest among participants with slow gait speed and significant lower-extremity motor impairment (as indicated by Fugl-Meyer scores). Following stroke, dual-task interference in gait was greatest among persons who walk the slowest; however, impaired dual-task gait performance was present even among individuals who were considered full community ambulators (Yang et al., 2007).

The addition of a secondary task also significantly affected turning strategies among individuals with stroke (Hollands et al., 2014). Persons with stroke, similar to age-matched older adults, turned more slowly and were more variable under dual-task conditions compared to single-task conditions. In addition, single-support phase of gait was prolonged when performing a secondary task in both groups. Since single-limb support is an unstable phase of gait, increasing the duration of the phase during turns under cognitively demanding conditions may be one reason why there is a high incidence of falls during turns in these two populations (Hollands et al., 2014).

A number of researchers have reported the effects of attentional demands on walking in individuals with PD (Bloem et al., 2006; Campbell et al., 2003; Galletly & Brauer, 2005; O'Shea et al., 2002; Plotnik et al., 2009; Rochester et al., 2004; Yogev et al., 2007). Campbell and colleagues (2003) tested the effect of two types of cognitive tasks (a low-attention task, repeating the same phrase over and over, and a high-attention task, saying the days of the week backward) on gait using the Timed Up and Go (TUG) test. Their results are shown in Figure 15.19, which compares times on the TUG test in the 10 healthy older adults and 9 individual subjects with PD in the three conditions (no task and the two secondary tasks). While the low-attention task did not interfere with TUG performance, the high-attention task did, with the greatest dual-task costs found in persons with the most disease progression.

Rochester et al. (2004) examined the effects of various types of secondary tasks: motor (carrying a tray), cognitive (answering questions), and multiple (both tasks together) on gait (speed, step length) in 20 subjects with idiopathic PD and 10 controls. Performance of both the cognitive task and the multiple tasks (but

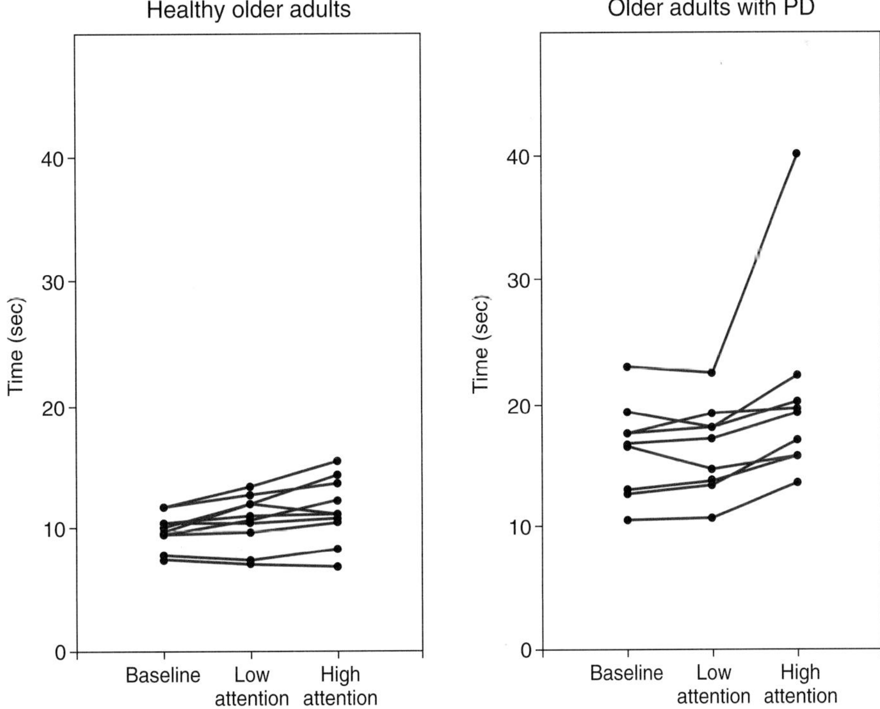

Figure 15.19 Effect of two types of secondary tasks on performance of the TUG test. Change in time on the TUG in three conditions, single task (baseline), low-attention task, and high-attention task, is compared in healthy older adults and subjects with PD. While the low-attention task did not interfere with TUG performance, the high-attention task did. Data from individual participants are shown. (Reprinted from Campbell C, Rowse J, Ciol MA, et al. The Effect of Cognitive Demand on Timed Up and Go Performance in Older Adults With and Without Parkinson Disease. *Neurol* Rep. 2003;27:2–7, Figure 1, with permission.)

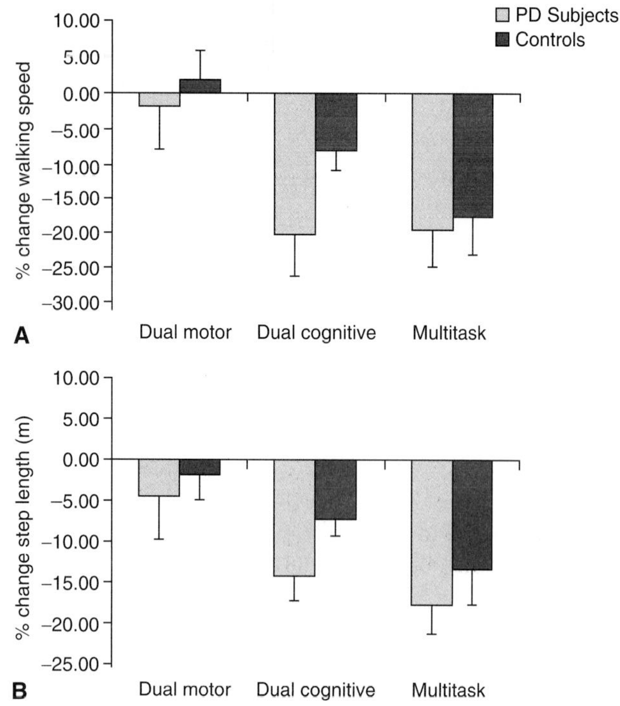

Figure 15.20 Effect of motor, cognitive, and combined tasks on gait speed (percent change) **(A)** and step length (percent change) **(B)** in persons with PD and age-matched controls. (Modified from Rochester L, Hetherington V, Jones B, et al. Attending to the task: interference effects of functional tasks on walking in Parkinson's disease and the roles of cognition, depression, fatigue and balance. *Arch Phys Med Rehabil.* 2004;85:1581, Figure 2, with permission.)

not motor alone) decreased both gait speed and step length in both groups (results shown in Fig.15.20); however, the greatest effect was in the group with PD. A secondary task influences many aspects of gait in persons with PD, including velocity, gait variability, bilateral coordination, and rhythmicity (Hausdorff et al., 1998; O'Shea et al., 2002; Plotnik et al., 2009; Yogev et al., 2005).

A number of researchers have reported that performance of a secondary task can impair stance and gait in persons with traumatic brain injury, even those with a relatively mild concussion (Brauer et al., 2004; Catena et al., 2007; Fait et al., 2009; Kern & Mateer, 1996; McCulloch, 2007; Pare et al., 2009; Parker et al., 2005; Rasmussen et al., 2008). Parker et al. (2005) studied the effects of a secondary task on gait 48 hours after a concussion injury. For subjects who had had a concussion, walking while performing a concurrent cognitive task resulted in significant changes in gait variables (decreased gait speed and step length, increased stride time) and an increase in mediolateral displacement and velocity of the COM as compared with age-matched controls. Thus, following concussive injury, there is a decrease in stability in gait that can be observed during dual-task conditions. Dual-task gait assessment was more sensitive in detecting instability following concussion than was single-task level walking (Catena et al., 2007). Following traumatic brain injury, measures of cognitive function, specifically executive function, can predict locomotor behavior, particularly in complex environments (Cantin et al., 2007).

Finally, children with CP show decreased foot clearance during dual tasking, which consequently may increase fall risk. Also, in children with CP, walking speed is slower during dual-task conditions compared to single-task conditions, and walking speed decreases more in children with CP during dual-task conditions compared with typical developing children (Roostaei et al., 2020). Moreover, other gait parameters (e.g., increased step width and step time or decreased stride length) occur in cognitive dual walking tasks more than during just walking conditions for children with CP. These changes in spatiotemporal gait parameters are related to children's ability to maintain gait stability.

All of these studies suggest the potential importance of evaluating walking function under more complex conditions in persons with neurologic pathology.

WHAT FACTORS LIMIT PARTICIPATION IN THE MOBILITY DOMAIN?

Limited participation in the mobility domain (referred to as mobility disability and defined by a limited ability to walk in a home and community environment) has been identified as one of the most debilitating aspects of neurologic pathology, including stroke (Lord et al., 2004; Robinson et al., 2007) and PD (Schenkman et al., 2002). The prevalence of mobility disability is high. For example, only 50% of survivors of stroke regain the ability to walk in the community, and 30% of individuals are unable to walk without the assistance of another person (Lord et al., 2004). Walking in the community, with its complex task demands, is particularly difficult. In one study on community walking following stroke, 4% of survivors of stroke reported moderate difficulty walking at home; however, 72% reported moderate difficulty when walking in the community (Robinson et al., 2010). In addition, as difficulty with walking increased, satisfaction with community walking skills decreased (Robinson et al., 2010).

The ability to manage complex environmental challenges is necessary to achieving successful participation in community walking (Lord et al., 2006), and an inability to manage specific environmental challenges is a critical determinant of impaired mobility function (Hirvensalo et al., 2000; Jette et al., 1998). Understanding the factors that limit participation in the mobility domain and contribute to mobility disability is critical to developing effective strategies for the rehabilitation of gait disorders.

Research suggests that outcomes such as gait speed and distance (referred to as "capacity" measures of mobility in the ICF framework) do not reliably predict the ability to walk in the community ("performance" in the ICF framework) (Kollen et al., 2006; Lord et al., 2004). In addition, other clinical measures of functional ambulation skills, including balance, paretic leg strength (Kollen et al., 2005; Patterson et al., 2007), and cardiovascular fitness (Michael et al., 2005; Patterson et al., 2007), have not been shown to predict participation in community walking following stroke. Robinson et al. (2007; 2010) examined the factors associated with participation in community ambulation among participants with chronic (>6 months) stroke. Following stroke, participation in community ambulation was reduced, as indicated by both a decrease in the number of trips made into the community and the number of walking-related activities performed on each trip (on average, 1) as compared with controls, who performed, on average, 2 or more walking-related activities per trip in the community.

The following factors were significantly correlated with participation in community ambulation: balance, usual gait velocity as well as velocity on complex walking tasks, and strength in the hemiparetic limb. However, regression modeling found that these factors, while significant, explained only a small portion of the variance in participation in community walking (Robinson et al., 2007). In a follow-up study, Robinson et al. (2010) found that personal factors, specifically balance and falls self-efficacy, depression, and fatigue, were also significantly associated with participation in community walking following stroke and that they explained a much larger portion of the variance in participation in the mobility domain.

Poor balance self-efficacy and fear of falling, resulting in avoidance of physical activity, including walking in the community, have been reported in a number of studies (Basler et al., 2008; Bertera & Bertera, 2008; Deshpande et al., 2008; Hellstrom et al., 2003; Pound et al., 1998; Salbach et al., 2006). In addition, depression has also been associated with reduced walking participation and function in activities of daily living in patients with neurologic dysfunction (Chemerinski et al., 2001; Goodwin & Devanand, 2008).

This research confirms that among persons with neurologic impairments, the ability to participate in community walking is perceived as very important. In addition, the prevalence of reduced participation (mobility disability) is very high among persons with neurologic pathology. It also suggests that poor participation results from a combination of factors including physical, psychological, and environmental factors. Impaired gait, while important, is only one of many factors influencing the recovery of mobility. Other factors, such as self-efficacy, fear, depression, and fatigue, may have a greater influence on long-term recovery of mobility in the home and community.

For children with CP, social and community participation most likely involves physical and skill-based activities instead of recreational activities. Moreover, children with the mildest forms of CP do the highest percentage of activities with friends and other nonfamily members because they have the ability to run and jump, which may enable social participation in games and sport activities. Conversely, children with more severe forms of CP (those who use a wheelchair for mobility purposes) are more likely to not have practiced any activities with friends and others in the past 4 months (Palisano et al., 2009).

Understanding the constellation of factors influencing participation is important to the development of treatment strategies effective in ensuring recovery of participation in persons with neurologic pathology.

DISORDERS OF MOBILITY OTHER THAN GAIT

Gait Initiation

Gait initiation is a critical part of mobility function and presents a challenge for many patients with CNS pathology. As discussed in Chapter 12, when initiating gait, the goal is to maintain dynamic balance while the body's COM first moves posteriorly and laterally toward the swing limb and then shifts toward the stance limb and forward outside the base of support and a step is taken. Anticipatory muscle activity, consisting of soleus muscle inhibition coupled with activation of the anterior tibialis muscle in the swing or leading limb, produces the forward momentum necessary for a safe and effective first step. Thus, anticipatory postural adjustments that control dynamic stability are critical to the complex process of gait initiation.

Widely distributed pathology in the CNS can interfere with gait initiation. Children with cerebral palsy (both hemiplegic and diplegic) demonstrate impaired gait initiation when compared to children who are typically developing. Children with hemiplegic CP demonstrate a preference for taking a first step with their more affected side, though this is associated with a reduced lateral shifting of the COP toward the stance (less affected) limb (Stackhouse et al., 2007). Similar findings have been reported in individuals with hemiparesis due to stroke. Several studies have reported that following stroke, initiation of gait is done primarily with the paretic limb as the leading limb. Onset of the TA muscle was delayed significantly with less amplitude when initiating gait with the paretic limb; this was associated with decreased generation of forward momentum (Brunt et al., 1995; Hesse et al., 1997; Ko et al., 2011; Sousa et al., 2015). This tendency to initiate gait with the paretic limb may be due in part to the fact that both children and adults with hemiplegia have a COP that is already biased toward their stance or trailing limb at the time of gait initiation (Stackhouse et al., 2007).

Individuals with PD also have difficulty with gait initiation, largely due to disruption of anticipatory postural control, including delayed and hypokinetic anticipatory postural adjustments (reduced scaling) (Mancini et al., 2009) and bradykinetic anticipatory postural adjustments (abnormal timing) (Delval et al., 2014). Alternatively, gait initiation can be characterized by multiple anticipatory postural adjustments, sometimes referred to as "knee trembling" (Jacobs et al., 2009), and a tendency to have greater interlimb weight shifts and associated increased COP shifts in the mediolateral and anterior directions (Elble et al., 1996).

Stair Walking

Like level walking, stair walking involves reciprocal movements of the legs through alternating stance and swing phases. Climbing stairs requires the generation of concentric forces at the knee and ankle (mostly the knee) for forward and vertical progression. Stability demands are greatest during the single-limb stance phase, when the swing leg is advancing to the next step (McFadyen & Winter, 1988).

In contrast to stair ascent, descent is achieved largely through eccentric contractions of the hip, knee, and ankle extensors, which control body position in response to the accelerating force of gravity. Energy absorption and a controlled landing are ensured through anticipatory activation of the gastrocnemius prior to foot contact with the step (McFadyen & Winter, 1988).

This means that in a person with a neurologic deficit, decreased concentric control will primarily affect stair ascent, while decreased eccentric control will primarily affect stair descent. Persons with a CNS lesion tend to walk stairs slowly, require the use of rails for support and progression, and, in severe cases of dyscontrol, are unable to use a reciprocal pattern for stair walking. Instead, they bring both feet to the same step prior to progressing to the next step.

Impaired visual sensation affects anticipatory aspects of this task. For example, gastrocnemius activity, which precedes foot contact, is lower when visual cues are reduced (Simoneau et al., 1991).

Transfers and Bed Mobility

During the performance of transfer activities such as sit-to-stand (STS), rolling, and rising from a bed, healthy young adults tend to use momentum to move the body smoothly and efficiently from one position to another. An alternative strategy that can be used when performing transfer tasks is the zero-momentum or force-control strategy (refer to Chapter 12 to review this material).

There are many reasons why persons with neurologic impairments might use a force-control strategy during transfers. Postural-control problems limiting stability, cardiovascular problems such as orthostatic hypotension, and episodes of dizziness may require a person to move slowly and make interim stops during the task. For example, when rising from a bed, a person with orthostatic hypotension would need to sit for a moment on the side of the bed before standing up or risk a sudden drop in blood pressure and loss of balance. The over reliance on a force-control strategy and upper-extremity control during transfer tasks, however, can limit persons' ability to adapt to changing environmental conditions. For example, they may find it difficult to stand up independently from a chair without arms (Carr & Shepherd, 1998; Schenkman et al., 1990).

There have been many studies examining pathologic gait in neurologic populations. In contrast, few studies have systematically explored problems constraining other mobility skills in this population.

Sit-to-Stand

Many persons with neurologic pathology report difficulty rising from a chair. In a survey of 379 older adults with varying neurologic diagnoses, 42% reported difficulty with rising from a chair at home (Munton et al., 1981). In a survey of persons with PD, 81% reported difficulty standing up (Brod et al., 1998). There are many impairments that potentially constrain the ability to perform STS behaviors effectively and efficiently. However, the majority of research has focused on the impact of neuromuscular impairments on STS in stroke, PD, and CP.

A number of studies have identified reduced force production as a major factor in difficulty with rising to stand. Lomaglio and Eng (2005) studied the relationship of lower-extremity joint torques and weight-bearing symmetry to STS performance in individuals with chronic stroke. A motion analysis system (kinematics) and two force plates (GRFs) were used to quantify characteristics of STS under self-paced and fast-paced conditions. An isokinetic dynamometer measured maximum concentric joint torques of the paretic and nonparetic ankle, knee, and hip (normalized to body mass).

The study found that paretic ankle dorsiflexion and knee extension torques were significantly correlated to the time taken to complete the self-paced STS condition, while paretic ankle dorsiflexion, plantarflexion, and knee extension torques were related to the time taken to complete fast-paced STS condition. Faster performance on STS was associated with greater weight-bearing symmetry.

Cameron et al. (2003) compared kinetic energy and duration of the task during STS and curb climbing in 15 individuals with hemiparetic stroke and age-matched controls. In addition, they compared performance on STS to standing balance, maximum weight-bearing ability of the paretic extremity, and knee extension strength. They reported that as compared with controls, STS in subjects with stroke was characterized by reduced kinetic energy and prolonged duration, with a significant correlation between STS kinetic energy and knee extension strength, standing balance, and maximum weight bearing.

Cheng et al. (2004) examined leg–muscle activation patterns (TA and soleus) and GRFs during self-paced STS from an armless chair in individuals with hemiparesis due to stroke (with and without a history of falls). They found that in 70% of the individuals with stroke who had a history of falls, TA activity was either absent or delayed in activation, with low amplitude. In addition, for half the subjects with poststroke hemiparesis and a history of falls, the soleus muscle exhibited early or excessive activity. This pattern of activity in the affected limb during STS was associated with compensatory excessive TA and quadriceps muscle activation in the unaffected limbs.

In an earlier study, Cheng et al. (1998) reported that the rate of rise in force production was significantly slower in persons who had a stroke and a positive history of falls than in those with no history of falls and healthy subjects. In addition, the COP movement in the mediolateral direction during rising and sitting down was much greater in persons with a history of falls than in those with no history of falls or healthy subjects. Patients with stroke exhibited an asymmetric body weight distribution, with significantly more body weight on their sound side (Cheng et al., 1998).

In contrast to these studies, Ng (2010) reported that following stroke, the ability to perform STS tasks (as indicated by performance on the five times STS test) was correlated with balance (BBS) but not muscle strength (Ng, 2010).

In a study with persons with MS, the authors found that thigh angular velocity in the pitch direction during the STS task was particularly high for HC compared to persons with MS (Witchel et al., 2018). The authors associated this finding with quadriceps weakness. Moreover, they found that spine angular velocity in the roll direction during an STS task was high for persons with MS compared to controls and related this finding to diminished postural control. Thus, the temporal features of the STS and stand to sit tasks can distinguish persons with MS from healthy individuals.

Impaired rate of force production has been reported in persons with PD. Bishop and colleagues (2005) examined lower-extremity muscle activation patterns in 41 people with PD (grouped according to time taken to complete the task) asked to stand up from a bench. Dual force plates were used to quantify GRFs, including peak acceleration and vertical GRF, the slopes of peaks, and the timing of events, while surface EMG was used to measure activity of the soleus and TA.

Results showed that in subjects with PD, increased duration of STS was due to a longer time for the seat-off phase. In addition, slower subjects demonstrated a slower rate of force production, took longer to complete the flexion-momentum phase (64% vs. 56% in faster subjects), and used more cocontraction. The authors noted that deficits recruiting the TA may contribute to the decreased rate of production of the acceleration forces and the longer time required for the seat-off phase and suggest that treatment strategies designed to facilitate TA activation may improve the functional performance of this task.

Inkster and colleagues (2003) reported lower hip and knee extensor torques in subjects with PD, with greater deficits found at the hip. Greater hip strength was related to better STS ability in subjects with PD; in contrast, greater knee strength was related to better STS ability in controls. The authors conclude that reduced strength, particularly at the hip, may be one factor that contributes to difficulty rising from a chair in persons with PD. These findings are supported by Mak et al. (2003), who reported smaller hip flexion torque and a slower torque buildup rate in seven subjects with PD, as compared with age-matched controls. The PD group demonstrated joint kinematic patterns similar to those of controls but slower angular displacement. The authors conclude that slowness of STS in people with PD could be due to reduced hip flexion joint torque and a prolonged rate of torque production. In addition to smaller hip flexion and ankle dorsiflexion joint torques, and prolonged time to peak torque, subjects with PD appear to have difficulty switching from flexion to extension during STS (Mak & Hui-Chan, 2002).

Force production has also been implicated in impaired STS in children with CP. Park et al. (2003) compared the kinetic and kinematic characteristics of STS in 27 children with spastic CP (15 with spastic diplegia, 12 with spastic hemiplegia) and 21 typically developing children. All children with CP performed the task more slowly than did typically developing children. In addition, STS in the children with CP was characterized by increased anterior pelvic tilt and hip flexion, an early abrupt knee extension (in diplegia only), decreased maximal knee extensor moment, and decreased extensor power generation of the hip and knee joints.

Finally, while impaired anticipatory postural control has been hypothesized to contribute to impaired STS in persons with PD, a study by Inkster and Eng (2004) did not support this hypothesis in subjects with mild PD. Their study found that subjects with PD used an exaggerated hip flexion strategy and moved their COM further forward during the preparation stage than did controls. The authors speculate that an exaggerated hip flexion strategy used in preparation for rising from a chair may have been compensatory to increased stiffness and reduced flexibility of the trunk. It could also be a strategy to reduce balance demands in the task by increasing the time the COM stays within the base of support. The authors caution that their study included only subjects with mild PD (9 of 10 scored normally on the STS item on the Unified Parkinson Disease Rating Scale [UPDRS]); hence, it may not apply to persons with more advanced disease.

Rise-to-Walk Task

Are similar impairments described in the STS task also found when the task required is to rise and walk? Biomechanical studies have shown that different motor strategies are used when healthy subjects rise to stand versus rise to walk. During STS, forward momentum of the body COM must be stopped on rising, whereas during rise to walking, forward momentum is maintained and stepping is initiated before reaching a full standing position (Dion et al., 2003). Thus, nonneurologically impaired subjects use a fluid motor strategy when performing the rise-to-walk (RTW) task. In contrast, after stroke, RTW is characterized by a nonfluid strategy, with the majority of individuals with stroke arresting forward motion before initiating stepping (Dion et al., 2003).

A scale to measure difficulty in the RTW task has been developed and is shown in Table 15.2 (Malouin et al., 2003). The relationship between scores on the RTW and patterns of forward momentum during the RTW task in subjects with hemiparetic stroke are shown in Figure 15.21. COM horizontal momentum mean curves are shown for controls (heavy line) and patient subgroups in each of the four categories of RTW scores. Note that horizontal momentum of the COM increases, peaking just before the seat-off phase, and then rises again as subjects rise to walk. Lowest scores on the RTW scale (0 category subgroup) are associated with a stop on rising (arresting forward momentum) (Malouin et al., 2003).

TABLE 15.2 Fluidity Scale for the Rise-to-Walk Task

Score	Descriptors
3	The foot (heel and toes)[a] is lifted off the ground while the subject's body is still moving forward; the trunk remains slightly flexed forward even when the subject stands up.[b]
2	The forward movement of the body stops, and as soon as the subject stands up with his body fully vertical, he lifts his foot.
1	The forward movement of the body stops; the subject stands up with his body fully vertical and then stops momentarily before he lifts his foot.
0	The forward movement of the body stops; the subject stands up with his body fully vertical, then stops momentarily before reaching for his cane, stops and then lifts his foot.

[a]The stepping limb is the affected limb.
[b]Stands up: is the maximal vertical position of the shoulder.

Description of the rise-to-walk task

Starting position
Subjects are seated on a chair without backrest and armrest, with the feet on the floor and two-thirds of the thighs in contact with the seat; they are asked to keep their arms folded in front of them during the task.

Instructions
Subjects are instructed to look ahead, to distribute their weight evenly, and, upon an auditory signal, to stand up, without using their hands, and walk, at a natural pace, toward the target (a table placed about 2 m in front of the subject), but are not required to cover the full distance.

Conditions
Patients are allowed to use a walking aid (cane) and wear their orthosis but are not provided external support. The stepping limb is the affected limb.

Source: Reprinted from Malouin F, McFadyen B, Dion L, et al. A fluidity scale for evaluating the motor strategy of the rise to walk task after stroke. *Clin Rehabil.* 2003;17:674–684 (appendix), with permission.

Bed Mobility Skills

Bed mobility skills include changing position while in bed (rolling supine to side lying or prone) and getting out of bed, either to a chair or standing up. Researchers have found that normal young adults use a variety of momentum-related strategies when performing bed mobility skills. There is incredible variety in how people move; in fact, none of the young adults tested used exactly the same strategy twice.

In contrast, force-control movement strategies are frequently used by patients with neurologic impairments and are characterized by frequent starts and stops. As mentioned previously, there are many reasons why a force-control strategy may be more appropriate than a momentum strategy in a patient with neurologic impairments (Richter et al., 1989).

The most common approach to rolling shown by normal young adults involves reaching and lifting with the upper extremity, flexing the head and upper trunk, and lifting the leg to roll onto the side and then over to prone. Most healthy young adults did not show rotation between the shoulders and pelvis, assumed by many clinicians to be an invariant feature of rolling (Richter et al., 1989). Because bed mobility skills are primarily initiated by movement of the head, upper trunk, and shoulders, impairments that affect these structures (such as weakness and or range-of-motion limitations) will limit performance of these skills.

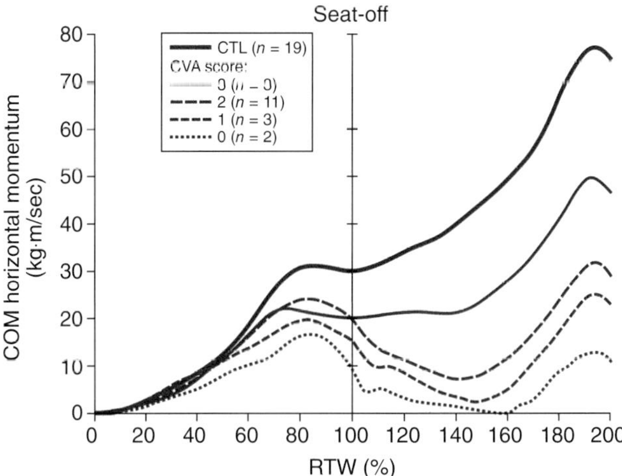

Figure 15.21 Relationship between scores on the rise-to-walk (RTW) scale (0–3) and patterns of forward body momentum in persons with stroke and controls during RTW. Shown are COM horizontal momentum mean curves in the control group and in patient subgroups in each category of the RTW scale. In contrast to controls, who maintain forward momentum on rising (seat-off), subjects with the lowest score (0) arrest forward momentum on rising (momentum closer to 0), then initiate gait. In contrast, participants with the highest RTW score (3) perform more like healthy controls. *CTL*, control subject; *CVA*, cerebral vascular accident. (Reprinted from Malouin F, McFadyen B, Dion L, et al. A fluidity scale for evaluating the motor strategy of the rise to walk task after stroke. *Clin Rehabil.* 2003;17:679, Figure 2, with permission.)

A CASE STUDY APPROACH TO UNDERSTANDING MOBILITY DISORDERS

We now turn to summarizing mobility disorders by diagnosis, using our case studies as examples. Again, as in the abnormal postural control chapter, it is important to remember that there is a great deal of heterogeneity among patients even with the same diagnosis. Thus, not all patients who have had a stroke will have a gait disorder similar to that observed in our case examples.

 Jean J and Genise T: Stroke

Stroke is the fifthleading cause of death in the United States and is considered to be a major cause of serious disability for adults (Kochaneck et al., 2014; Mozzafarian et al., 2016). The ability to walk is often a prime factor in determining residential status and level of productivity following a stroke. Loss of independent ambulation, particularly outdoors, is reported as one of the most debilitating consequences of stroke (Pound et al., 1998). A study of 115 stroke survivors reported that despite good mobility outcomes on standardized measures of balance and gait, nearly one-third of those studied reported that they were unable to go into the community without assistance (Lord et al., 2004).

Jean, our patient with right hemiparesis, is 5 years poststroke and continues to have significant balance and gait impairments. She has had numerous falls, particularly during walking-related activities. With her walker, she walks at 0.5 meters per second, which is 50% slower than individuals her age who have no neurologic impairment. With her cane, her gait velocity is further slowed to 0.3 meters persecond. Her slow gait velocity is the result of a number of factors, including her extensive muscle weakness, moderate spasticity, and presence of abnormal synergy patterns of movement. Because she is unable to achieve a walking speed of at least 48 meters per minute and has difficulty managing curbs and stairs, she relies on a wheelchair for community mobility and is not a community ambulator.

Genise is our 53-year-old woman who at the time of her initial video evaluation was 3 days poststroke. At this time, her paresis was profound, and she was unable to stand or walk without maximum assistance of two people. At 1 month poststroke, she is able to stand independently, though demonstrates significant weight-bearing asymmetry. She is able to walk with assistance using a walker and an AFO with a posterior plantarflexion stop to control her knee hyperextension. Her gait velocity is quite slow (0.08 m/s), suggesting she is still a nonfunctional ambulator.

Both Jean and Genise demonstrate abnormal spatiotemporal parameters associated with hemiparetic gait, including increased double-support time, decreased stance time by the involved leg, and a shortened step by the noninvolved leg. This results in a significant step asymmetry. A kinematic analysis of hemiparetic gait is significant for the following abnormalities in the stance phase: (a) equinovarus foot position, leading to a forefoot or flatfoot strike during loading; (b) knee hyperextension in midstance, with a forward lean of the trunk; and (c) limited hip extension during stance phase, resulting in an inability to place the hemiparetic leg in a trailing position during terminal stance. The pelvis is retracted on the stance leg and drops on the swing side, probably due to abductor weakness. In the swing phase of gait, we observe (a) toe drag, impeding progression because of inadequate flexion at the hip, knee, and ankle; (b) delayed hip flexion until after toe-off; (c) reduced knee flexion during preswing and swing; and (d) inappropriate foot placement because of incomplete knee extension and ankle dorsiflexion at the end of the swing phase.

An EMG analysis of gait in Jean and Genise would help determine some of the underlying causes of their abnormal gait patterns. By analyzing the activation of muscles during gait, we may be able to place Jean and Genise into one or more of the following categories of gait disorders: (a) "spastic pattern," characterized by exaggerated stretch response; (b) "paretic pattern," characterized by decreased (or absent) centrally generated patterned muscle activation; or (c) "coactivation pattern," produced by abnormal coactivation of multiple muscle groups (Knutsson, 1981; 1994; Knutsson & Richards, 1979). These patterns were described in more detail in early sections of this chapter.

For both Genise and Jean, a kinetic analysis of work and power may well indicate a reduction in the ability to generate a plantarflexion moment for push-off during stance, because of paresis. An increased use of hip flexor moment at pull-off in swing is used to compensate for a reduction in plantarflexion push-off (Nadeau et al., 1997; Olney et al., 1991).

We may be surprised to find that the oxygen cost for walking in both Jean and Genise is quite low, despite the abnormal appearance of their gait. The inefficiency associated with abnormal gait patterns appears to be offset by slow gait speed and muscular weakness. But these impairments might lead to diminished cardiovascular fitness. For example, research has shown that oxygen consumption in persons with stroke is strongly associated with their knee muscle strength (Baert et al., 2012). Research suggests that ambulation is not physiologically stressful for the typical stroke patient unless there are cardiovascular problems as well (Waters & Mulroy, 1999; Waters et al., 1988). But these studies examined energy costs in persons with stroke based on time walked. When distance walked is considered, energy expenditure associated with hemiparetic gait is twice as much as that of normal gait, because it takes persons with stroke, who walk at half the velocity of normal adults, twice as long to cover the same distance (Montgomery, 1987).

Both Jean and Genise have significant problems with dynamic gait activities, indicating a reduced ability to adapt locomotor patterns to changing task and environmental demands. They have difficulty traversing uneven terrains due to a reduced ability to modify both step height and length to step over obstacles. Control of posture and gait is less automatic and requires more attentional resources. Stability while walking is further compromised when they perform other attentionally demanding tasks. Jean performs the TUG test under single-task conditions in 32 seconds, and this increased to 42 seconds when performing the TUG under dual-task conditions. At 1 month poststroke, Genise requires 56 seconds to complete the TUG under single-task conditions and 69 seconds under dual-task conditions. In addition, both Genise and Jean make multiple errors on the secondary task while walking, which are not present when sitting.

Both Genise and Jean demonstrate asymmetry in gait initiation. Patients with hemiparesis demonstrate significant differences in timing, step length, mediolateral displacement of the COP, and COM movement velocity when starting with the affected versus the nonaffected leg.

Finally, both Jean and Genise have difficulty with other mobility tasks, including transfers such as STS and RTW. Reduced ability to develop symmetric torques results in an asymmetric STS pattern, with the majority of work being done by the nonparetic leg.

 Mike M: Parkinson's Disease

Mike has significant gait problems, which increase his probability for falls. The degree of his gait abnormality depends on both the progression of his disease and his medication state. Blin et al. (1990; 1991) studied 21 patients at various stages in the clinical progression of the disease (Hoehn and Yahr, stages I through IV [Hoehn & Yahr, 1967]). Compared with normal elderly controls, patients with PD showed a slower walking velocity, a shorter and more variable stride length, and longer stride duration. In addition, patients with PD showed an increased duration of stance and double-support phase and a concomitant decrease in the swing phase. Table 15.3 compares selected gait characteristics in patients with PD with those of healthy age-matched controls. Researchers have found a significant relationship between walking velocity in patients with PD and the stages of disability as described by the Schwab Classification of Progression (Schwab, 1960) or the Hoehn and Yahr Classification (Hoehn & Yahr, 1967).

Kinematic analysis of Mike's gait, especially when walking while in the off-medication state, indicates a reduction in the speed and amplitude of leg movements (resulting in characteristic short, shuffling steps) and arm movements (resulting in diminution of arm swing). Specific alterations in the stance phase of gait include (a) lack of heel strike; instead, he makes contact with the foot flat or with the forefoot; (b) incomplete knee extension during midstance; (c) inability to extend the knee and plantarflex the ankle in terminal stance, resulting in decreased forward thrust of the body; (d) forward trunk lean; (e) diminished trunk motion; and (f) reduced or absent arm swing. Decreased motion of the joints is apparent in swing phase as well, with decreased hip and knee flexion resulting in diminished toe clearance. In addition, reduced speed and amplitude of motion of the swing leg affect forward thrust of the body (Knutsson, 1972; Sofuwa et al., 2005; Stern et al., 1983).

An EMG study of Mike's gait may allow us to categorize him into one of three types of muscle activation patterns: (a) continuous EMG activity instead of cyclical activity, (b) reduced amplitude of muscle activation, and (c) abnormal coactivation of muscles (Knutsson, 1972). A kinetic analysis will likely show a reduction in ankle push-off power generation and a reduced hip flexion pull-off power even in the "on" phase of medication (Sofuwa et al., 2005).

When he is in the off-medication state, Mike demonstrates problems with freezing while walking, particularly when he is turning or trying to step over obstacles or when he is moving through doorways. Gait in patients with PD has been characterized by an

TABLE 15.3 Comparison of Selected Gait Characteristics in Patients with Parkinson's Disease and Healthy Age-Matched Controls

	Patients with PD ($N = 21$)	Controls ($N = 58$)	Patients with PD versus controls	
	Mean ± SD	**Mean ± SD**	***z* value**	***p* value**
Velocity (m/s)	0.44 ± 0.20	0.83 ± 0.23	5.25	<0.01
Stride length (m)	0.57 ± 0.26	0.97 ± 0.22	4.95	<0.01
Stride duration (sec)	1.29 ± 0.16	1.19 ± 0.15	2.17	<0.05
Swing duration (s)	0.40 ± 0.08	0.46 ± 0.05	2.88	<0.01
Stance duration (s)	0.88 ± 0.16	0.74 ± 0.12	3.50	<0.01
Swing velocity (m/s)	1.36 ± 0.44	2.12 ± 0.46	5.03	<0.01
Peak velocity (m/s)	2.00 ± 0.66	3.28 ± 0.72	5.31	<0.01
Double-support duration (s)	0.23 ± 0.08	0.13 ± 0.05	5.21	<0.01
Relative double-support duration (s)	35.8 ± 9.80	21.8 ± 6.80	5.24	<0.01
Stride duration variability	5.51 ± 5.10	4.75 ± 2.30	0.12	NS
Stride length variability	6.68 ± 4.27	5.17 ± 3.80	1.92	<0.05

Source: Reprinted from Blin O, Ferrandez AM, Serratrice G. Quantitative analysis of gait in Parkinson patients: increased variability of stride length. *J Neurosci.* 1990;98:95, with permission.

inability to control momentum. If a patient is unable to generate sufficient momentum, forward progression is arrested. This is often referred to as "freezing" (or "gait ignition failure"). Freezing episodes are transient, lasting from seconds to minutes. Freezing most often affects gait initiation (start hesitation) during turns, in narrow spaces, or when approaching obstacles (Fahn, 1995; Giladi et al., 1997). We may be able to help Mike reduce his freezing episodes using maneuvers such as counting or stepping over lines or visual targets displayed on a screen (Frazzitta et al., 2009; Stern et al., 1980).

In addition to freezing, Mike's gait is characterized by unrestrained momentum that leads to uncontrolled progression, called a "propulsive gait pattern." Propulsive gait disorders may be due to an exaggerated forward inclination of the body, resulting in an anterior displacement of the COM beyond the supporting foot. In some instances, however, propulsive gait is seen in patients who have normal vertical posture but seem unable to oppose forward momentum (Knutsson, 1972).

Mike, like many patients with PD, has problems with gait initiation, leading to akinesia (defined as loss of willed movement). Gait initiation has been cinematically studied in 31 patients with PD (Rosin et al., 1997). Gait initiation was divided into two phases, movement preparation time and movement execution. Patients with PD had significantly longer movement preparation time but not execution time. In addition, while initiation of ankle, knee, hip, arm, and trunk movements was delayed, the sequencing and timing of submovements was comparable between groups. The authors suggest that gait initiation problems in PD were not the result of dyscoordinated movements but rather were due to a deficit within the basal ganglia's internal cueing for movement sequences (Rosin et al., 1997).

Mike is taking medication to help control the symptoms of his PD; however, he shows considerable fluctuations in his motor performance, both throughout the course of the day as well as from one day to the next. Contributions to motor fluctuations include variation in levels of anti-PD medications, time of day, fatigue, stress, diet, and change in responsiveness to the medication (Nutt et al., 1984). A number of studies have examined the effect of medication (L-DOPA) on various gait parameters (Blin et al., 1991; MacKay-Lyons, 1998; Morris et al., 1996). Gait parameters particularly sensitive to changes in drug levels are walking velocity and stride length (Blin et al., 1991; MacKay-Lyons, 1998; Morris et al., 1996). In contrast, other variables, such as cadence, stride time, and swing duration, did not vary as a function of medication cycle (Blin et al., 1991;

Pedersen et al., 1991). Morris et al. (1996) concluded that characteristics of gait in patients with mild PD are reproducible during the "on" phase of medication (both across 30 minutes of peak dosage or at 24-hour intervals) but are more variable during the "off" phase. In contrast, MacKay-Lyons (1998) found extensive variability throughout the entire l-DOPA cycle in patients with moderately severe PD. Not all fluctuations in motor performance are predictable, however. Poewe (1994) found that approximately 15% of patients with PD have random fluctuations in motor performance that are not related to L-DOPA doses. This led Poewe to categorize fluctuations in motor performance in patients with PD as either predictable or random.

Mike relies heavily on visual cues during walking. Prokop and Berger (1996) found that when an optical flow pattern was imposed during stepping on a treadmill, patients with PD continuously modulated their speed in response to changing visual flow patterns, while HC did not. It has been hypothesized that increased reliance on visual cues to regulate gait is the result of impaired proprioceptive reflexes (Bronstein & Guerraz, 1999). In contrast to patients with spasticity, patients with PD show a reduced reflex sensitivity (Berardelli et al., 1983; Tatton et al., 1984).

Finally, Mike, like Jean and Genise, has difficulty with other mobility tasks, such as transfers, sitting to standing, and bed mobility. He takes longer to stand up, particularly off medication, because of a reduced rate of force production.

John C: Degenerative Cerebellar Injury

John, our 33-year-old with spinocerebellar degeneration, has significant gait problems. His walking, particularly without his shoes on, is characterized by staggering, irregular stepping, veering from side to side, and excessively high lifting of the feet above the ground (Gilman, 2000; Palliyath et al., 1998). John walks more slowly than do his age-matched peers and has a reduced step and stride length and longer stride durations (Earhart & Bastian, 2001). Palliyath et al. (1998) quantified gait in 10 patients with cerebellar ataxia, 6 with hereditary cerebellar cortical atrophy, and 4 with olivopontocerebellar atrophy. Mean quantitative differences in gait characteristics between patients and normal controls are shown in Table 15.4. Patients were, on average, slower than normal controls and showed more variability across all measures. Patients showed reduced step and stride length and motion at the ankle, knee, and hip. Interestingly, despite current clinical assumptions that cerebellar ataxic gait is characterized by increased step width and high steppage, in this study there was not a significant difference in step width or toe clearance between the two groups. Seidel and Krebs (2002) also found no increase in step width in persons with chronic ataxia.

A kinematic analysis of John's ataxic gait demonstrates poor intersegmental coordination with abnormal rates of motion between ankle and knee. Problems with intersegmental coordination are associated with increased frontal-plane instability, as indicated by increased displacement and velocity of the COM in the mediolateral direction during stepping tasks (Hudson & Krebbs, 2000).

John has problems adapting his gait to changes in external demands (Earhart & Bastian, 2001; Morton & Bastian, 2003; 2007). Researchers have reported that individuals with cerebellar pathology have difficulty adapting locomotor patterns to changing external constraints, including wedges in the walking path (Earhart & Bastian, 2001) and stepping over obstacles (Morton et al., 2004), because of reduced ability to coordinate the relative movement of multiple joints.

Sue: Multiple Sclerosis

Sue, our 66-year-old woman with MS, has significantly impaired mobility function. MS is a degenerative neurological disease affecting approximately 350,000 people in the United States and as many as 2 million worldwide (Noseworthy et al., 2000). MS is an immune-mediated disease that causes demyelination and degeneration within the brain and spinal cord. Symptoms depend on the location and severity of demyelination, are highly variable, but typically include sensory, cognitive, and motor impairment. MS is a progressive disease resulting in progressive disability, which is measured clinically by the Expanded Disability Status Scale (EDSS) (Kurtzke, 1983), a 0–10 scale in which 0.0 represents no impairment due to MS, 4.0 indicates the onset of significant walking impairment, 7.5 indicates wheelchair dependence, and 10.0 represents death due to MS.

Sue reports that impaired mobility, including gait abnormalities, is a major factor impacting her daily life. She uses a power scooter for community mobility and a seated four-wheeled walker for ambulating at home and for short distances in the community. Her EDSS score is 6.5 (or 7), since she requires constant bilateral assistance (4WW) when walking 20 m. She is independent in other mobility skills including transfers and bed mobility.

Sue, like other people with MS, reports impaired mobility as one of the most debilitating aspects of the disease (LaRocca, 2011). Research shows this is the case even among people with minimal disability (Nogueira et al., 2013). Sue has experienced multiple falls in the past 6 months. Impaired mobility is associated with increased risk for falls, with the highest risk for recurrent falls found among persons with impaired gait, who are not yet using assistive devices (Coote et al., 2014).

Sue walks slower, takes shorter steps, and has longer periods of double-support compared to age-matched HC walking at comparable speeds. Among

TABLE 15.4 Comparison of Selected Gait Characteristics in Patients with Cerebellar Ataxia and Healthy Age-Matched Controls

Descriptor	Control (mean ± SD)	Patient (Mean ± SD)	P From *t test*
Cadence (steps/min)	111.00 ± 7.60	102.20 ± 15.90	0.14
Step length (% height)	0.48 ± 0.20	0.29 ± 0.07	0.02[a]
Stride length (% height)	0.96 ± 0.40	0.59 ± 0.14	0.02[a]
Step width (% height)	0.16 ± 0.08	0.14 ± 0.03	0.68
Step length symmetry	1.00 ± 0.06	0.97 ± 0.17	0.64
Stride length symmetry	1.02 ± 0.02	1.00 ± 0.04	0.35
Step width symmetry	0.98 ± 0.06	1.02 ± 0.12	0.31
Stance time (sec)	0.66 ± 0.12	0.79 ± 0.17	0.07
Swing time (sec)	0.39 ± 0.05	0.43 ± 0.06	0.18
Step time (sec)	0.54 ± 0.04	0.61 ± 0.11	0.13
Stride time or gait cycle (sec)	1.08 ± 0.08	1.21 ± 0.22	0.11
Gait velocity (mm/sec)	0.90 ± 0.39	0.47 ± 0.17	0.01[a]
Ankle angle range of motion, degrees	31.50 ± 6.20	23.20 ± 5.10	0.004[a]
Ankle angle at heel strike	102.50 ± 5.90	103.00 ± 8.50	0.90
Heel-off time (% of gait cycle)	44.00 ± 4.00	50.00 ± 8.00	0.04[a]
Toe-off time (% of gait cycle)	66.00 ± 1.00	68.00 ± 3.00	0.04[a]
Knee angle range of motion	58.50 ± 2.10	53.90 ± 7.70	0.10
Knee angle range of motion during stance	11.50 ± 4.90	7.50 ± 3.80	0.07
Time of peak flexion of knee during swing (% of gait cycle)	2.70 ± 1.90	75.50 ± 3.20	0.02[a]
Hip angle range of motion	34.30 ± 5.90	31.30 ± 4.70	0.23
Foot height (cm)	11.90 ± 1.20	11.50 ± 1.90	0.62

[a]Seidel B, Krebs DE. Base of support is not wider in chronic ataxic and unsteady patients. *J Rehabil Med.* 2002;34:288–292.

Source: Reprinted from Palliyath S, Hallett M, Thomas SL, et al. Gait in patients with cerebellar ataxia. *Mov Disord.* 1998;13:962, with permission.

persons with MS, spatiotemporal gait impairments increase with increasing disability (Remelius et al., 2012; Sosnoff et al., 2011a). Consistent with research on persons with MS with greater disability, she demonstrates increased variability of step length and step time, though step width variability is smaller (Socie & Sosnoff, 2013). Many factors are thought to contribute to changes in gait variability in persons like Sue with MS, including fatigue (Huisinga et al., 2011; Socie et al., 2011), decreased muscle strength (Broekmans et al., 2013), and spasticity (Sosnoff et al., 2011b). Interestingly, unlike the findings from older adults, increased gait variability among persons with MS was not associated with increased risk for falls (Motl et al., 2011).

Sue's gait is notable for a flatfoot initial contact, reduced hip flexion and dorsiflexion during the swing phase of gait, resulting in bilateral decreased toe clearance. She has reduced plantarflexion in terminal stance. These characteristics are consistent with research on gait kinematics in persons with MS (van der Linden et al., 2014). Research has demonstrated that individuals with MS, like Sue, demonstrate less joint torque and reduced joint power compared to age-matched controls. In addition, research shows a strong correlation between biomechanical gait parameters of gait and EDSS score (Husinga et al., 2013). Impaired somatosensation in her lower extremities is a significant factor impacting Sue's gait, and she reports that she needs to see her feet to be able to maintain her balance during gait.

In addition to impairments in her steady-state gait, Sue, like other persons with MS, demonstrates reduced ability to adapt gait; this compromises her ability to perform complex walking tasks, such as stepping over obstacles or changing directions. When changing directions while walking, persons with MS reduce gait speed and cadence and have a smaller lateral stability margin (i.e., COM remains close to lateral edge of BOS) compared to age-matched individuals without impairment. Gait kinematics and stability margins in persons with MS are similar to balance-impaired older adults, suggesting that both groups use similar strategies to adapt locomotion as a result of impaired balance (Denommé et al., 2014).

Thomas: Spastic Diplegic Cerebral Palsy

Thomas, our 7-year-old with a spastic diplegic form of cerebral palsy, began walking much later than did his age-matched peers. He walks much more slowly than do his typically developing peers, averaging 0.5 meters per second without his assistive device. He is much faster when walking with his walker. At home and at school, Thomas walks with a walker or no assistive device, but he uses a scooter for community mobility. His gait is characterized by a reduced stride length and step width. He walks with a characteristic crouched-gait pattern, with excessive hip and knee flexion, in conjunction with excessive ankle plantarflexion, and anterior pelvic tilt during the stance and swing phases of gait. Foot strike is abnormal, with an equinovarus foot posture and often forefoot contact. This foot position is continued through the stance phase of gait. Excessive plantarflexion and knee and hip flexion are seen during loading and continue through the stance phase of gait. Excessive flexion persists into the terminal stance, and the preswing phase is minimal or absent because of an inability to extend the hip and knee. The swing phase of gait also shows excessive knee and hip flexion.

If Thomas had spastic hemiplegic, instead of spastic diplegic, cerebral palsy, he would likely present with a genu recurvatum gait pattern instead of a crouched-gait pattern. The former gait pattern is characterized by knee hyperextension during stance and excessive ankle plantarflexion. Hip flexion and forward lean of the trunk may occur as the patient leans forward to balance over a plantarflexed foot. Loading is onto the forefoot because of inadequate knee extension and excessive plantarflexion during swing. During swing, toe drag constrains progression, requiring contralateral trunk lean to free the foot and advance the thigh. The genu recurvatum gait pattern is more common in unilateral motor impairments such as spastic hemiplegia (Crenna, 1998; Gage, 1993).

An EMG analysis of Thomas's gait might allow us to separate his problems into one of four categories: (a) defective recruitment of motor units, referred to as a "paresis" or "weakness pattern;" (b) abnormal velocity-dependent recruitment during muscle stretch, the so-called spasticity pattern; (c) nonselective activation of antagonist muscles with a loss of a normal reciprocal inhibitory pattern, called the "cocontraction pattern;" and (d) problems associated with musculoskeletal restraint due to changes in mechanical properties of muscles, the nonneural problem pattern (Crenna, 1998).

Interestingly, in children with spastic hemiplegic cerebral palsy, a cocontraction pattern of muscle activity was found in both the hemiplegic leg and the noninvolved leg. Thus, researchers are now considering the possibility that cocontraction represents a compensatory strategy aimed at stiffening a joint to compensate for postural instability or paresis (Berger et al., 1984b; Crenna, 1998; Leonard et al., 2006). The particular gait profile seen in an individual will reflect a combination of the factors just listed. Thus, each individual with CP will present with a slightly different gait pattern.

When walking, Thomas's heart rate and oxygen rates are higher than are those of his age-matched peers. Researchers believe that this is because the flexed posture, which is typical of the crouched-gait pattern, requires additional muscle activity for stability. Interestingly, the physiological costs of walking decrease in typically developing children as they get older. In contrast, the physiological costs of walking increase as children with CP get older. Why does this happen? Increased physiological costs of walking are not due to an increase in motor abnormalities in CP, since it is a nonprogressive disease. Instead, researchers believe that oxygen rates associated with walking increase as children with CP get older because changes in body morphology, including increased body weight and size, interact with impaired motor control. This results in an increase in the physiological cost of gait in older children. As a result, the older child with CP may walk less and increasingly rely on a wheelchair (Palisano et al., 2009).

Finally, Thomas has difficulty with other mobility tasks, including standing up, because of neuromuscular impairments affecting his ability to generate and time the forces needed for the sitting-to-standing task.

SUMMARY

1. While abnormal gait is a common characteristic of many neurologic pathologies, the constellation of underlying problems that produce disordered gait will vary from patient to patient depending on (a)

primary impairments, such as inadequate activation of a muscle; (b) secondary impairments, such as contractures; and (c) compensatory strategies developed to meet the requirements of mobility in the face of persisting impairments. Neuromuscular impairments affecting gait include paresis or weakness, abnormalities of muscle tone, impaired selective control, and impaired intra- and intersegmental coordination. Impaired coordination includes (a) the inability to recruit a muscle during an automatic task such as posture or gait; (b) inappropriate activation of a muscle during gait, which is not related to stretch of the muscle; (c) coactivation of agonist and antagonist muscles around a joint, which increases stiffness and decreases motion; (d) desynchronization between the upper and lower limbs; and (e) problems related to scaling the amplitude of muscle activity during gait.

2. Musculoskeletal impairments constrain movement and increase the workload on the muscles, affecting a patient's ability to meet the requirements of gait. Decreased joint mobility during stance restricts forward motion of the body over the supporting foot, affecting progression. In swing, decreased joint mobility reduces foot clearance, affecting progression, and appropriate foot placement for weight acceptance, affecting stability.
3. Sensory disorders can lead to problems in the following areas of locomotor control: (a) signaling terminal stance and thus triggering the initiation of swing, (b) signaling unanticipated disruptions to gait, and (c) detecting upcoming obstacles important for modifying gait to changes in task and environmental conditions.
4. Impairments in cognitive systems, particularly the increased attentional demands associated with walking, can result in dual-task interference in many patients with CNS pathology. Dual-task interference during walking tasks such as turning or clearing obstacles can contribute to an increased risk for falls.
5. During the performance of transfer activities such as sitting to standing, rolling, and rising from a bed, healthy young adults tend to use a momentum strategy, which requires the generation of concentric and eccentric contractions to control motion, and ensures stability. In contrast, a force-control strategy, characterized by frequent starts and stops, is frequently used by patients with neurological impairments. This is related to impairments affecting both stability and progression aspects of the movement. This is also the strategy most commonly taught by clinicians when retraining transfer tasks.

CHAPTER 16

Clinical Management of the Patient with a Mobility Disorder

Learning Objectives

Following completion of this chapter, the reader will be able to:

1. Describe a task-oriented approach to evaluating mobility function in geriatric and neurologic populations.
2. Review functional tests and measures used to quantify functional mobility skills, including limited ability to participate in mobility functions in the context of a home and community environment ("performance" in the ICF framework) as well as clinical measures of functional mobility skills ("capacity" in the ICF framework).
3. Compare and contrast clinical methods for evaluating strategies for gait and other mobility skills, including measures used to assist the process of observational gait analysis.
4. Discuss a task-oriented approach to treating functional mobility limitations, including locomotion and transfers.
5. Define and give examples of part and whole mobility training.
6. Review the research evidence for locomotor training, including the evidence related to task-oriented training, treadmill training with and without body weight support, robotic-assisted locomotor training, and virtual reality.

INTRODUCTION

Management of mobility problems is often a key to return of functional independence in patients with neurologic pathology. Consider Genise T, our 53-year-old woman with poststroke hemiparesis. Prior to her stroke, she was living independently in her own home. At 4 days poststroke, Genise was dependent in most mobility functions, requiring assistance in moving about her bed, transferring to her wheelchair or commode, and standing up. At that point, she was unable to walk, requiring the assistance of two people to step. Since mobility is essential to many basic activities of daily living (BADLs), such as toileting, transfers, and dressing, as well as many instrumental activities of daily living (IADLs), such as shopping, cleaning, and cooking, regaining mobility function is a critical determinant of Genise's ability to recover functional independence and return to living in her own home. Given the importance of mobility to recovery of functional independence, a critical issue for her therapist is to determine the most effective way to examine and retrain mobility skills.

This chapter presents a task-oriented approach to examining and treating individuals with mobility dysfunction, with a main focus on examination and treatment of walking. As is true throughout this book, our task-oriented approach is based on both the International

Classification of Functioning, Disability and Health (ICF) and the systems framework. We begin with examination, reviewing some of the tests and measures that can be used to document functional abilities related to mobility, including the following: (1) level of mobility disability, defined as a restriction in participation of mobility-related activities in the person's home and community environment (referred to as "performance" in the ICF framework), and (2) functional mobility skills within a standard setting (referred to as "capacity" in the ICF framework). Including tests and measures at both these levels is important since it enables the distinction between what a person *actually* does during daily life (performance) and what a person *can* do in a daily environment (capability) (Holsbeeke et al., 2009). It is important to remember that the specific constellation of tests and measures chosen to evaluate function will vary according to practice setting, level of function of the patient, and in many cases the specific diagnosis. More detailed information on the specific tests and measures recommended for different practice settings and diagnoses may be found on the Academy of Neurologic Physical Therapy Edge task force website from the American Physical Therapy Association (APTA).

As part of our task-oriented examination, we discuss the process of observational gait analysis (OGA), an approach to assessing strategies used to accomplish the main tasks of gait, including progression, stability, and adaptation.

The second half of the chapter addresses issues related to describing a task-oriented approach to retraining mobility skills in the person with neurologic pathology, with a primary focus on walking. We begin with a discussion of clinical strategies used to improve underlying impairments constraining mobility function and review some of the research to determine whether treatment of underlying impairments alone is sufficient to change mobility (locomotion) function. We then discuss clinical strategies used to modify the underlying gait pattern (GP) and review the evidence that supports these strategies. We move on to a review of functional task training, including strategies for improving the performance of complex walking tasks essential to ambulation in a home and community environment. The research evidence in support of a task-oriented approach to mobility training is reviewed. Finally, we consider strategies for training mobility skills other than walking and review the evidence in support of these strategies.

A TASK-ORIENTED APPROACH TO EXAMINATION

In a task-oriented approach, examination of mobility analyzes performance at three levels: (1) the functional-task level, (2) the essential strategies used to accomplish the requirements of mobility, and (3) the underlying sensory, motor, and cognitive impairments that constrain mobility. The three-level examination attempts to answer the following questions:

1. To what degree can the patient perform functional mobility tasks? What is the effect of impaired mobility on the ability of the patient to be engaged in daily life activities and social roles?
2. What strategies does the person use to accomplish mobility tasks? In the case of walking, is the GP effective in meeting the progression and stability requirements of walking? Is the person able to adapt gait to changing task and environmental conditions?
3. What are the sensory, motor, and cognitive impairments that constrain mobility? Can these impairments be altered through intervention, thereby enhancing the person's capabilities?

The following section reviews a wide range of tests used to measure mobility function, with a specific focus on gait. Within the ICF, mobility is considered both an activity (e.g., a task performed by an individual) and a domain of *Participation* (e.g., the societal level of functioning). This can make it difficult to classify tests of mobility function. In this chapter, a mobility test performed in a standardized clinical environment is classified as an activity measure designed to capture the ICF's concept of *capacity* (i.e., the extent of activity limitation that is inherent to the patient's health status). A test is classified as a measure of participation, or performance, when it gathers information about the person's mobility behavior (self-reported or observed) in his or her current environment (i.e., the extent of participation restriction that represents the person's involvement in a life situation) (WHO, 2003). It is important to remember that outcomes on activities measures (such as gait speed on the 10-meter walk clinical test) may or may not predict mobility participation, that is, behavior in the person's own environment (ICF concept of performance). We recognize that not everyone will agree with our approach to classifying tests and measures, and many may disagree with the way a specific test or measure is classified. Though subject to interpretation and error, we feel that it is important to create a consistent framework across research areas and health disciplines for the presentation of these materials.

Measuring Participation: Mobility Performance in the Home and Community Contexts

For many people with neurologic pathology, reintegration into community life marks a significant, if not the most important, goal in rehabilitation. For example, in older adults with or without disability, low mobility is strongly associated with low engagement in social life inside and outside their homes (e.g., participation in organizations and use of senior centers) (Rosso et al., 2013). Among older adults, even concerns about falling may significantly reduce social participation (Choi et al., 2020).

Therefore, ambulation in home and community contexts is an important part of the community reintegration process. As discussed in Chapter 12, mobility in daily life requires the ability to walk in diverse environments. Because of this, mobility measured in a controlled context, like the clinic, may not capture the complexity of walking in natural environments; thus, it may not predict participation in the mobility domain (e.g., mobility behavior and restrictions in the person's real-life context). Most measures of participation rely on self-report (by the individual or their proxy) to determine the degree to which the person is mobile during the performance of social roles and daily life activities. Alternatively, technology such as pedometers and activity monitors can be used to objectively measure mobility, specifically walking behavior, directly. Activity-based monitors and self-report mobility measurements offer different but significant complementary information. Thus, clinicians and researchers should consider both types of evaluations in order to achieve a complete description of mobility deficits.

Self-Report Measures

A number of self-report instruments designed to examine participation in multiple domains including mobility are available. In a review of the literature, Andrews (2012) listed the most commonly cited mobility-related measures; these included the Medical Outcomes Study Short Form-36 (physical function subscale), the National Health and Nutrition Examination Survey (Physical Functioning Questionnaire), the Barthel Index (self-report), the Lower Extremity Functional Scale, and the Craig Handicap Assessment and Reporting Technique (mobility subscale) (Andrews, 2012). Other examples of self-report mobility measures include the Mobility and Self-Care (MOSES) Questionnaire, which measures perceived difficulty with mobility and self-care activities performed in the home and community (Farin et al., 2007), and the Participation Survey/Mobility (PARTS/M), which measures perceived choice, importance, and satisfaction related to components of participation (Gray et al., 2006). The Craig Handicap Assessment and Reporting Technique (CHART) measures participation (handicap) in multiple dimensions, including physical independence, mobility, occupation, social integration, and economic self-sufficiency (Hall et al., 2001; Walker et al., 2003; Whiteneck et al., 1992). The Assessment of Life Habits (LIFE-H) measures the level of difficulty, the type of assistance, and satisfaction in several domains, including mobility. It also documents the impact of assistive technology on participation (Noreau et al., 2004).

Another approach to examining mobility participation is through the use of life space, defined as the size of the spatial area a person purposely moves through in his or her daily life, as well as the frequency and duration of travel within a specific time frame (Baker et al., 2003; Johnson et al., 2020; May et al., 1985). The Life Space Questionnaire (LSQ) is an example of a measure used to document a person's mobility within their home and community (Peel et al., 2005; Stalvey et al., 1999).

Activity Monitors

Activity monitoring has been used to gain insight into locomotor activity in a person's own environment. The pedometer is a simple device often used to measure locomotor activity by counting the number of steps taken. Simple physical activity monitors can also be used to measure walking activity during inpatient stroke rehabilitation (Klassen et al., 2017). However, as mentioned earlier, locomotor activities in daily life consist of walking in complex environments while performing other activities, and this illustrates one of the limitations of the pedometer. Another limitation is that output from pedometers (and some actigraphs—that is, accelerometers to measure activity of the body) is confounded by gait speed and pattern (Cyarto et al., 2004).

Orendurff and colleagues (2008) used step activity monitors (SAMs) to examine walking patterns in healthy young adults employed and living in a typical urban environment. They found that walking in daily living for this sample of people, similar to infant walking (Lee et al., 2018), overwhelmingly comprised short-duration walking bouts. Forty percent of all walking bouts were less than 12 steps in a row, and 60% of all walking bouts lasted 30 seconds or less. The authors suggest that walking in daily living is predominantly short duration with lots of initiation, termination, speed modulation, corner negotiation, and maneuvering. This has implications for locomotor training in geriatric and neurologic populations, as it suggests that restricting training to long bouts of walking practice in a constant context (such as a single speed) may be insufficient preparation for walking in daily life.

SAMs and pedometers have been used to examine walking behavior in various environments following a stroke. Studies using a SAM have reported that among healthy young adults, average step count per day was 5,951. Step counts in persons with neurologic pathology are considerably lower; for example, for persons with stroke, step counts ranged from 2,500 to 4,700 (Michael et al., 2005; Mudge & Stott, 2009; Robinson, 2010; Shaughnessy et al., 2005).

Activity monitors, including pedometers, are not routinely used in therapy to either evaluate or treat locomotor function (as a source of feedback to patients). While there are many technical limitations to work out, they may prove to be a useful way to encourage locomotor activity outside the context of a clinical setting and thus could be useful in facilitating increased participation in mobility. In addition, ambulatory monitoring may prove to be a useful outcome measure for patients involved in mobility training programs and may provide insight into participation in the mobility domain.

Standardized Measures of Walking Capacity

Examination of walking function often focuses on determining the distance a patient can walk, the time it takes to traverse this distance, and the level of assistance (LOA) needed (Katz et al., 1970; Keith et al., 1987; Lawton, 1971). The individual being tested can be asked to walk a specified distance (e.g., 150 ft), and the time taken to walk that distance can be recorded. Alternatively, the person can be asked to walk for a specified time period, and the distance walked can be recorded.

Measuring Gait Velocity

A number of researchers have suggested that gait velocity is the single best measure of gait function as it is simple and quick and appears to be a composite measure of temporal and distance variables (Brandstater et al., 1983; Murray et al., 1970; Richards et al., 1995). For example, a study of ambulatory children and adolescents with cerebral palsy (CP) has shown that there is clinical value in examining self-paced walking compared to fast-paced walking in gait parameters such as velocity and stride length (Chakraborty et al., 2020). You can gain experience in calculating self-paced and fast-paced gait velocity in Lab Activity 16.1. Converting a person's self-selected gait velocity to a percentage of normal can be an effective way to communicate locomotor abilities to the individual, families, and insurers (Bohannon, 1997; Montgomery, 1987). In order to find the percentage of normal gait velocity, reference values for non-neurologically impaired individuals are needed. In some cases, a standard reference value of 80 m/min is used. Bohannon (1997) published normative values for comfortable and maximum gait speed based on data from 230 healthy non-neurologically impaired individuals. Reference values are both gender and age (by decades) specific and include both actual gait speed (cm/sec) and gait speed normalized to height (actual gait speed [cm/sec]/height [cm]). Norms from this study (converted to meters per minute) are shown in Table 16.1.

TABLE 16.1 Reference Values for Gait Speed: Comfortable versus Maximum Velocity by Decade of Age and Gender

	Comfortable (m/min)		Maximum (m/min)	
Decade	**Men**	**Women**	**Men**	**Women**
20s	83.6	84.4	151.9	148.0
30s	87.5	84.9	147.4	140.5
40s	88.1	83.5	147.7	127.4
50s	83.6	83.7	124.1	120.6
60s	81.5	77.8	115.9	106.4
70s	79.8	76.3	124.7	104.9

Source: Adapted from Bohannon RW. Comfortable and maximum walking speed of adults aged 20 to 79 years: reference values and determinants. *Age Ageing.* 1997;26:15–19, with permission.

LAB ACTIVITY 16.1

Objective: To determine gait velocity under self-paced and fast-paced conditions.

Procedure: Measure a 10-m (33-ft) walking course. You will be calculating a steady-state gait velocity, so you want to be walking at a constant speed, not speeding up or slowing down. Starting at about 3 feet before the first mark, begin walking at a comfortable pace, and keep walking for at least 3 feet after the second mark. Using a stopwatch, calculate the time it takes to walk the middle (marked) 10 m. Repeat this 3 times, recording the time for each trial. Now, repeat the test walking the 10 m as fast as you can, and record the time. You may also wish to try this test using a distance of 5 m, as recommended by Salbach et al. (2001), to determine differences in gait velocity that occur with distance. In addition, you can repeat the test using various types of assistive devices, such as a single-point cane or a pickup or front-wheeled walker to determine the effect of an assistive device on gait speed.

Assignment

Question 1. Average the three trials for each condition and calculate gait velocity (divide the total walking distance of 10 m [or 5 m] by the elapsed time in seconds, multiply by 60 to get meters per minute) for both the self-paced and fast-paced conditions. Convert self-selected gait velocity to a percentage of normal. Compare self-selected gait velocity to fast-paced velocity, and calculate the percentage increase in gait speed. How does using an assistive device change your gait velocity?

What is the best distance to use when calculating gait velocity? One common method calculates gait speed measured over 10 m (33 ft) indoors (Collen et al., 1990). Guralnik and colleagues (1994) reported that 4 m (13 ft) was the distance of choice because it is feasible in both a home and clinical setting; however, the longer distance improved measurement accuracy (Guralnik et al., 1994). An important assumption in the measurement of any gait variable, including gait velocity, is that measures taken in the clinic are ecologically valid—that is, reflecting the person's capabilities in the real world. This may not be true. Gait speeds observed in natural environments were slower than those observed in the clinic (Dean et al., 2001; Moseley et al., 2004). It is possible that slower gait speed in more complex environments, such as in a shopping mall and a busy hospital corridor, was due to additional demands on mobility in these environments.

For any measure to be useful as an outcome measure, the minimal amount of change that is clinically meaningful and associated with an important difference in function needs to be determined. Tilson and colleagues (2010) estimated that the minimally clinical important difference (MCID) for usual gait speed was 0.16 m/s in persons between 20 and 60 days after stroke.

MCID may vary as a function of baseline gait speed and diagnosis. Both Palombaro et al. (2006) and Perera et al. (2006) reported that the MCID for gait speed was 0.10 m/s. This estimate was derived from data from a range of participants including older adults with mobility disability (e.g., hip fracture), poststroke survivors, and community-dwelling older adults. Among older adults, a change in gait speed of 0.10 m/s was associated with reduced disability and better survival rates (Hardy et al., 2007). Bohannon and Glenney (2014) showed that in groups of people with stroke, hip fracture, multiple sclerosis, or mixed conditions, a MCID of .10 to .20 m/s for gait speed can be used across multiple patient groups.

Being able to calculate an individual's self-selected gait velocity is important, as it represents a cumulative score of both ability and confidence in walking (Brandstater et al., 1983; Richards et al., 1995). It can also be used to infer the level of disability related to mobility, since an individual whose gait speed is less than 30% of normal does not usually become a community ambulator (Perry et al., 1995). However, clinicians need to be careful when assuming that gait speed measured during short distances under relatively ideal clinical conditions reflects walking ability for longer distances and in more natural (and often less than ideal) contexts.

Measuring Walking Endurance: 2-, 6-, or 12-Minute Walk Tests

Independent mobility in the community requires not just sufficient speed but walking endurance as well (Hesse et al., 1994). Thus, measuring the distance a patient can walk is an important outcome when retraining gait. Activities of daily living (ADL) scales, such as the Functional Independence Measure (FIM), evaluate independence in walking based on distance measures (Keith et al., 1987).

The 12-minute walk test was designed to examine exercise tolerance in patients with chronic respiratory disease (McGavin et al., 1976). However, researchers have determined that both the 2- and 6-minute walk tests are equally reliable, although slightly less sensitive in discriminating a patient's level of exercise tolerance compared to the 12-minute walk test (Butland et al., 1982). The 6-minute walk test is among the recommended measures identified by the majority of the APTA's Academy of Neurologic Physical Therapy Edge task forces.

Age- (community-dwelling older adults 65 years of age or older) and gender-specific normative values for the 6-minute walk test have been published as part of the Functional Fitness Test (Rikli & Jones, 2001). In addition, in a study examining mobility measures in subjects with chronic stroke, Ng and Hui-Chan (2005) reported that the average distance walked in the 6-minute walk test was 202 ± 88 ft in subjects with stroke, as compared with 416.5 ± 95.7 ft in age-matched controls.

Wise and Brown (2005) estimated that the MCID for the 6-minute walk test is 54 to 80 m. However, clinical meaningful differences in walking measures vary based on the distance walked (e.g., 2 vs. 6 minutes), the diagnosis, and the severity of walking impairment (Baert et al., 2014). Bohannon and Crouch (2017) determined a MCID in the 6-minute walk test of 14.0 to 30.5 m for people with chronic obstructive pulmonary disease, lung cancer, coronary artery disease, diffuse parenchymal lung disease, and non-cystic fibrosis bronchiectasis, and adults with fear of falling.

Technological Devices for the Clinic. The use of laboratory methods (e.g., motion analysis, electromyography [EMG], and force plates) for analyzing gait is expensive and time consuming and requires specialized expertise; as a result, it is not realistic in clinical settings. However, there are a growing number of simple devices being developed that can quantify spatial and temporal aspects of gait and can be used in the clinic. These devices vary in their complexity and cost but can improve the therapist's ability to measure specific gait parameters within the clinical setting.

For example, portable stride analyzers (i.e., insoles that contain four compression closing foot switches that connect to a lightweight mobile data collection box worn on a belt) and gait analyzers based on instrumented walkways or wearable sensors can be used to objectively evaluate walking abilities in clinical settings and during real life situations. Some studies are currently incorporating novel wearable sensors during walking activities or even when people with different conditions perform validated clinical tests, such as the Dynamic Gait Index or Timed Up and Go (Anastasi et al., 2019; Carpinella et al., 2018). Shah and colleagues (2020) measured objectively the quantity and quality of ambulation in people with MS and Parkinson's disease (PD) and age-matched controls. The participants wore 3 inertial sensors on the top of their feet and the lumbar area. They found that the quantity of mobility (e.g., median number of strides) best discriminated walking deficits in people with MS from controls; whereas quality of movement, measured as turn angles, best discriminated mobility deficits in people with PD from controls.

Measures of Complex Walking Tasks

Measurement of spatial and temporal aspects of gait, while important, is limited to examining gait under rather static conditions (walking in a straight path, at a comfortable speed over level ground, in ideal ambient conditions). A number of mobility scales have been developed to examine a broader range of walking skills that are more characteristic of mobility in community environments, including starts and stops, changes in direction and speed, stepping over and around obstacles, and the integration of multiple tasks such as talking, turning to look at something, or carrying objects during gait. Thus, these tests include not only the examination of unimpeded gait, defined as a closed-skill task, but also the ability to modify and adapt gait to both expected and unexpected disturbances to locomotion. When selecting a test, clinicians should keep in mind the severity of mobility impairment in the patient being tested and choose a scale that is appropriate, in order to avoid either a ceiling (a test that is too easy) or floor (a test that is too difficult) effect.

Timed Up and Go Test. The Get Up and Go (TUG) test (Mathias et al., 1986) was developed as a quick screening tool for detecting balance problems affecting daily mobility skills in older adults. The test requires that subjects stand up from a chair, walk 3 m, turn around, and return. Performance is scored according to the following scale: 1 = normal; 2 = very slightly abnormal, 3 = mildly abnormal; 4 = moderately abnormal; and 5 = severely abnormal. An increased risk for falls was found among older adults who scored 3 or higher on this test.

The TUG test modifies the original test by adding a timing component to performance (Podsiadlo & Richardson, 1991). You can see the TUG test being performed in the mobility segment of the following video case studies: Jean, Mike, John, Sue, and Thomas. The TUG is among the core measures recommended by the APTA's Academy of Neurologic Physical Therapy Edge task forces.

Neurologically intact adults who are independent in balance and mobility skills are able to perform the test in less than 10 seconds. This test correlates well with functional capacity as measured by the Barthel index. Adults with neurologic pathology who took longer than 30 seconds to complete the test were dependent in most activities of daily living and mobility skills. Isles et al. (2004) published normal values for a variety of balance tests, including the TUG, in 456 community-dwelling, independently ambulatory women, 20 to 80 years of age with no known neurologic or musculoskeletal diagnoses. Age-related changes in time(s) taken to complete the TUG are summarized in Table 16.2. Also shown in this table is a comparison of data from the two oldest age groups, with data from other published studies. There are also age- (65 years and older) and gender-based norms for an 8-foot version of the TUG (an individual walks 8 ft rather than 10 ft as is used in the original test), developed as part of the Functional Fitness Test for neurologically intact older adults (Rikli & Jones, 2001).

Adding a secondary task to the TUG allows clinicians to examine the effect of cognitive demand on gait. The dual-task TUG (TUG_{DT}) was originally created to

TABLE 16.2 Comparison of Timed Up and Go Values

	Age					
	20–29 (*n* = 40)	**30–39 (*n* = 47)**	**40–49 (*n* = 95)**	**50–59 (*n* = 93)**	**60–69 (*n* = 90)**	**70–79 (*n* = 91)**
Mean ± SE	5.31 ± 0.25	5.39 ± 0.23	6.24 ± 0.67	6.44 ± 0.17	7.24 ± 0.17	8.54 ± 0.17
Published normative value	NA	NA	NA	NA	8 (60–88) Steffen 8.42 (65–85) Shumway-Cook 13.05 (65–86) Hughes	8.5 (70–84) Podsiadlo 8 (60–88) Steffen 8.42 (65–85) Shumway-Cook

Source: Adapted from Isles RC, Chow NL, Stur M, et al. Normed values of balance tests in women 20–80. *J Am Geriatr Soc.* 2004;53:1370 (Table 1), with permission.

see whether adding a secondary task would increase the sensitivity and specificity of the TUG as a measure of fall risk in community-living older adults (Shumway-Cook et al., 2000). Because so many older adults have difficulty maintaining stability while performing multiple tasks, it was hypothesized that performing the TUG under dual-task conditions would be a more sensitive way to identify fall-prone older adults. Results indicate that while the time taken to complete the TUG was significantly longer in the dual-task conditions, the TUG alone was a sensitive and specific indicator of fall status in community-dwelling older adults. Thus, the TUG, a relatively simple screening test, which takes only minutes to complete, appears to be a valid method for screening both level of functional mobility and risk for falls in community-dwelling older adults.

The TUG has also been shown to be a reliable and valid test for examining mobility following stroke (Faria et al., 2009; Ng & Hui-Chan, 2005) and PD (Campbell et al., 2003; Dibble & Lange, 2006; Morris et al., 2001). Following stroke, the time to complete the TUG was significantly associated with strength in the hemiparetic plantarflexors (but not spasticity), gait parameters (e.g., gait velocity and step length), and walking endurance (distance covered on the 6-minute walk test) (Ng & Hui-Chan, 2005). Researchers have also found that performing the TUG simultaneously with another motor task (holding a glass of water) is reliable and valid for assessment of functional mobility in people with stroke, correlating with the Fugl-Meyer Assessment for the Lower Extremities, Berg Balance Scale scores, and performance time of the 5-Times Sit-to-Stand (STS) (Chan et al., 2017). The authors reported that for persons with chronic stroke, the minimum detectable change in TUG_{motor} time was 3.53 seconds.

The TUG is also a valid and reliable test of mobility function in children with and without physical disabilities (Gan et al., 2008; Williams et al., 2005). Minor modifications to testing procedures (e.g., beginning to time when the child starts to move rather than with the instruction to go) have allowed the test to be used in children as young as 3 years of age (Williams et al., 2005). In typically developing children 3 to 5 years of age, the mean (±SD) time to complete the TUG was 6.7 ± 1.2 seconds but decreased to 5.1 ± 0.08 seconds in children 5 to 9 years of age. A systematic review from Himuro et al. (2017) showed that the TUG can be easily performed within 5 minutes to measure the capacity of children and adolescents with CP in functional ambulatory mobility and dynamic balance. However, the authors note a number of limitations in the current research, including small number of participants and limited evidence on measurement error and responsiveness (i.e., the ability to detect a clinical change).

The TUG has been used to evaluate mobility in those case studies in which the patient can walk unassisted (Jean, Mike, John, Sue, Thomas, and Bonnie). To see the TUG being performed, refer to the mobility section of the video case studies.

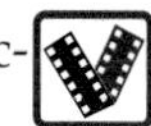

Dynamic Gait Index. The Dynamic Gait Index (DGI) was developed by Shumway-Cook et al. (1997a) to evaluate and document a patient's ability to modify gait in response to changing task demands. The original scoring system used two factors, GP and LOA, to rate walking performance on an ordinal scale of 0 to 3. A score of 19 out of 24 is considered an indicator of increased risk for falls among older adults (Shumway-Cook et al., 1997a). A study of community-dwelling older adults established a MCID of 1.90 for the DGI (Pardasaney et al., 2012). The authors of this study proposed two MCID values for two subgroups based on their DGI baseline values—older adults with DGI < 21/24 had a MCID of 1.80 and older adults with DGI ≥ 21/24 had a MCID of 0.60.

A modified version of the DGI (the mDGI) was developed by Shumway-Cook and colleagues (2013) and tested on a population of 995 persons (855 patients with neurologic pathology and mobility impairments and 140 non-neurologically impaired controls) (Matsuda et al., 2014, 2015; Shumway-Cook et al., 2013, 2015). The mDGI retains the original eight tasks but uses a new scoring system, which rates three aspects of performance: LOA, GP, and time. The mDGI is shown in Assessment Tool 16.1. A number of researchers have demonstrated good reliability (interrater and test–retest) and validity of the DGI (Hall & Herdman, 2006; Herman et al., 2009; Jonsdottir & Cattaneo, 2007; Marchetti et al., 2008; McConvey & Bennett, 2005; Whitney et al., 2000, 2003; Wrisley et al., 2003) and mDGI (Shumway-Cook et al., 2013; 2014; Matsuda et al., 2014a; 2014b). The MCID for the DGI appears to be 4 points (Wrisley et al., 2002). The DGI is an excellent outcome measure for patients who are community ambulators. However, it is not appropriate for patients such as Genise and Malachi, who are unable to walk unassisted.

Functional Gait Assessment. The Functional Gait Assessment (FGA) tool is a 10-item assessment of complex walking tasks based on the DGI (Wrisley et al., 2004); it is shown in Assessment Tool 16.2. Wrisley and colleagues examined the psychometric properties of the FGA within a population of persons with vestibular disorders. Interrater reliability was good (ICC = 0.86), as was intrarater reliability (ICC = 0.74). The FGA has good concurrent validity with other balance measures, including the TUG, DGI, Activities-specific Balance Confidence (ABC) Scale, and Dizziness Handicap Index. A cutoff score of ≤22/30 was effective in classifying fall risk in older adults and predicting unexplained falls in community-dwelling older adults (Wrisley & Kumar, 2010). The FGA has been validated as a measure of fall risk in people with PD, with a cut point of 18/30. The FGA is among the core measures recommended by the APTA's Academy of Neurologic Physical Therapy Edge task forces.

Assessment Tool 16.1

Modified Dynamic Gait Index

1. Gait Level Surface

Equipment: Measuring tape, masking tape for floor, stop watch

Setup: A 23 ft distance is needed for this test. Mark the beginning of the walking course with a piece of tape. Place a piece of tape at the 10 and 20 ft distance; participant should be instructed to continue walking past the 20-ft point another 3 ft.

Instructions to Participant: Begin with your toes on this line. When I tell you "Begin," start walking at your normal pace from here to *past* this line (Point out the 20-ft line to the participant). Make sure you continue to walk past this line. Do you understand what I want you to do? Are you ready? Begin.

Examiner Instructions and Grading: Timing begins when the tester says "Begin." Stop timing when *the first foot* crosses the 20-ft line. Circle ordinal score for level of assistance and gait pattern. Mark the *lowest* category that applies.

Time: _______________ seconds

Ordinal Time Level: __________

- **(3) <6.0 seconds**
- **(2) 7.6 to 6.0 seconds**
- **(1) 15.2 to 7.7 seconds**
- **(0) >15.2 seconds or unable**

Gait Pattern:

- (3) **NORMAL:** Walks 20 ft, normal gait pattern, no evidence for imbalance
- (2) **MILD IMPAIRMENT:** Walks 20 ft, mild gait deviations or mild imbalance
- (1) **MODERATE IMPAIRMENT:** Walks 20 ft, moderate gait deviations, clear evidence for imbalance, but recovers independently
- (0) **SEVERE IMPAIRMENT:** Cannot walk 20 ft or walks with severe gait deviations or cannot maintain balance independently

Level of Assistance

- (2) No assistance
- (1) Used an assistive device (excludes orthosis or brace)
- (0) Required the physical assistance of another (includes contact guard)

2. Change in Gait Speed:

Setup: Same as for 1

Instructions to Participant: Begin with your toes on this line. When I tell you *"Begin,"* start walking at your normal pace. When I say *"Go Fast,"* I want you to walk as quickly and safely as you can until I tell you *to stop*. Do you understand what I want you to do? Are you ready? *Begin*.

Examiner Instructions and Grading: Timing begins when the tester says *"Begin."* Stop timing when *the first foot* crosses the 20-ft line. At 10 ft, tell the participant to *"go fast."* Observe whether the participant is able to significantly change speed, evidence for gait, or balance problems. Circle the score for level of assistance and gait pattern. Mark the *lowest* category that applies.

Time: _____________seconds

Ordinal Time Level: __________

- **(3) <4.9 seconds**
- **(2) 6.8 to 4.9 seconds**
- **(1) 11.7 to 6.9 seconds**
- **(0) >11.7 seconds or unable**

Gait Pattern:

- (3) **NORMAL:** Able to smoothly change walking speed without loss of balance or gait deviation. Shows a significant difference in walking speeds between normal and fast speeds
- (2) **MILD IMPAIRMENT:** Is able to change speed but demonstrates mild gait deviations or mild imbalance, **or** no gait deviations but unable to achieve a significant change in velocity
- (1) **MODERATE IMPAIRMENT:** Makes only minor adjustments to walking speed, or accomplishes a change in speed with significant gait deviations, or loses balance but is able to recover and continue walking
- (0) **SEVERE IMPAIRMENT:** Cannot change speeds, or loses balance and is unable to recover independently.

Level of Assistance

- (2) No assistance
- (1) Used an assistive device (excludes orthosis or brace)
- (0) Required the physical assistance of another (includes contact guard)

3. Gait with Horizontal Head Turns

Setup: Same

Instructions to Participant: Begin with your toes on this line. When I say *"Begin,"* start walking at your normal pace. When I tell you *"Look Right,"* keep walking straight but turn your head to the right. Keep looking right until I tell you *"Look left,"* then keep walking straight and turn your head to the left until I tell you *"Look Straight,"* then keep walking straight but return your head to the center. Do you understand what I want you to do? Are you ready? *Begin*.

Examiner Instructions and Grading: Timing begins when the tester says *"Begin."* Stop timing when *the first foot* crosses the 20-ft line. After the participant has walked about 3 steps, ask them to *look right*; after about 3 more steps, ask them to *look left*; and after about 3 steps, ask them to *look straight*. Circle ordinal score for level of assistance and gait pattern. Mark the *lowest* category that applies.

Time: ____________seconds

Ordinal Time Level: __________

- **(3) <6.2 seconds**
- **(2) 8.5 to 6.2 seconds**
- **(1) 14.5 to 8.6 seconds**
- **(0) >14.5 seconds or unable**

(continued)

Assessment Tool 16.1

Modified Dynamic Gait Index (*continued*)

Gait Pattern:

(3) **NORMAL:** Performs head turns smoothly with no change in gait pattern or evidence of imbalance

(2) **MILD IMPAIRMENT:** Mild reduction in head motion **or** performs head turns with mild changes in gait pattern **or** minor disruption to gait path **or** mild imbalance

(1) **MODERATE IMPAIRMENT:** Moderate reduction in head motion **or** performs head turns with moderate change in gait pattern, or moderate imbalance but recovers independently

(0) **SEVERE IMPAIRMENT:** Unable to turn head **or** performs head turns with severe disruption of gait, that is, staggers outside 15-in. path, **or** stops, **or** loses balance and is unable to recover independently

Level of Assistance

(2) No assistance

(1) Used an assistive device (excludes orthosis or brace)

(0) Required the physical assistance of another (includes contact guard)

4. Gait with Vertical Head Turns

Setup: Same

Instructions: Begin with your toes on this line. When I tell you *"Begin,"* start walking at your normal pace. When I tell you *"look up,"* keep walking straight but tilt your head and look up to the ceiling. Keep looking up until I tell you *"Look down,"* then keep walking straight and tilt your head down, and look at the floor until I tell you *"Look Straight,"* then keep walking straight but return your head to the center. Do you understand what I want you to do? Are you ready? *Begin.*

Examiner Instructions and Grading: Timing begins when the tester says *"Begin."* After the participant has walked about 3 steps, ask them to *look up*; after about 3 more steps, ask them to *look down*; and after about 3 steps, ask them to *look straight*. Stop timing when *the first foot* crosses the 20-ft line. Circle ordinal score for level of assistance and gait pattern. Mark the *lowest* category that applies.

Time: ___________ seconds

Ordinal Time Level: _________

(3) <6.0 seconds

(2) 8.2 to 6.0 seconds

(1) 13.9 to 8.3 seconds

(0) >13.9 seconds or unable

Gait Pattern:

(3) **NORMAL:** Performs head turns smoothly with no change in gait pattern or evidence of imbalance

(2) **MILD IMPAIRMENT:** Mild reduction in head motion **or** performs head turns with mild changes in gait pattern **or** minor disruption to gait path **or** mild imbalance

(1) **MODERATE IMPAIRMENT:** Moderate reduction in head motion **or** performs head turns with moderate change in gait pattern, or moderate imbalance but recovers independently

(0) **SEVERE IMPAIRMENT:** Unable to turn head **or** performs head turns with severe disruption of gait, that is, staggers outside 15-in. path, **or** stops, **or** loses balance and is unable to recover independently

Level of Assistance

(2) No assistance

(1) Used an assistive device (excludes orthosis or brace)

(0) Required the physical assistance of another (includes contact guard)

5. Gait and Pivot Turn: ______

Setup: Place a piece of tape at the end of the 10 ft. Participant will be asked to turn around at the 10-ft point.

Instructions to participant: Begin with your toes on this line. When I tell you *"Begin,"* start walking at your normal pace. When I tell you *"turn around,"* turn around as quickly and SAFELY as you can and walk back to the starting point. Do you understand what I want you to do? Are you ready? Begin.

Examiner Instructions and Grading: Timing begins when the tester says *"Begin."* Ask the participant to *turn around* at the 10-ft mark. Stop timing when *the first foot* crosses the line at the start of the course. Circle ordinal score for level of assistance and gait pattern. Mark the *lowest* category that applies.

Time: ____________seconds

Ordinal Time Level: _________

(3) <6.9 seconds

(2) 9.4 to 6.9 seconds

(1) 16.9 to 9.5 seconds

(0) >16.9 seconds or unable

Gait Pattern:

(3) **NORMAL:** Pivot turns safely using 3 steps or less and continues walking in opposite direction with no gait deviations and no imbalance.

(2) **MILD IMPAIRMENT:** Turns using 3 to 5 steps **or** with mild gait deviations or imbalance before, during, or after turning

(1) **MODERATE IMPAIRMENT:** Turns using multiple steps (>5 steps), or has moderate gait deviation or imbalance before, during, or after turning but is able to recover independently

(0) **SEVERE IMPAIRMENT:** Cannot turn safely, loses balance, and is unable to recover independently

Level of Assistance

(2) No assistance

(1) Used an assistive device (excludes orthosis or brace)

(0) Required the physical assistance of another (includes contact guard)

6. Step Over Obstacle: ______

Equipment: Measuring tape, masking tape for floor, stopwatch, two semirigid pieces of foam rectangles, dimensions are 76 cm long, 12 cm wide, 5 cm thick.

Assessment Tool 16.1

Modified Dynamic Gait Index (*continued*)

Setup: A 23 ft distance is needed for this test. Mark the beginning of the walking course with a piece of tape. Place the first obstacle with the 12-cm side flat on the floor at 8 ft from start. Place the second obstacle with the 12-cm side up 8 ft past the first obstacle (about 16 ft from the start). Place a piece of tape at the end of the 20 ft distance.

Instructions to participant: Begin with your toes on this line. When I tell you *"Begin,"* start walking at your normal pace. When you come to each obstacle, step over and keep walking to past this line (point out the 20-ft line on the floor). Do you understand what I want you to do? Are you ready? *Begin.*

Examiner Instructions and Grading: Timing begins when the tester says *"Begin."* Stop timing when the first foot crosses the 20-ft line but make sure the participant keeps walking 3 ft past the 20-ft mark. Make sure to observe whether the participant clears both obstacles completely without touching them with either the lead or trailing foot. Circle an ordinal score for level of assistance and gait pattern. Mark the *lowest* category that applies.

Time: ____________ seconds

Ordinal Time Level: __________

- **(3) <6.0 seconds**
- **(2) 8.5 to 6.0 seconds**
- **(1) 17.4 to 8.6 seconds**
- **(0) >17.4 seconds or unable**

Gait Pattern:

- (3) **NORMAL:** Is able to step over and clear both obstacles without changing gait speed, no evidence for gait deviations or imbalance
- (2) **MILD IMPAIRMENT:** Is able to step over and clear both obstacles, but with mild gait deviations (e.g., slowing down and adjusting steps to clear obstacles) or mild imbalance
- (1) **MODERATE IMPAIRMENT:** Is able to step over the obstacles but must stop, then step over, **or** strikes an obstacle **or** is significantly unsteady when crossing, but able to recover without assistance
- (0) **SEVERE IMPAIRMENT:** Cannot step over one or both obstacles or loses balance and is unable to recover independently

Level of Assistance

- (2) No assistance
- (1) Used an assistive device (excludes orthosis or brace)
- (0) Required the physical assistance of another (includes contact guard)

7. Steps Around Obstacles:______

Equipment: Measuring tape, masking tape for floor, stopwatch, two semirigid foam cylinders, and dimensions are 76 cm long and 12 cm diameter

Setup: A 23 ft distance is needed for this test. Mark the beginning of the walking course with a piece of tape. Place the first foam cylinder upright 8 ft from start. Place the second foam cylinder upright 8 ft past the first cylinder (about 16 ft from the start). Place a piece of tape at the end of the 20ft distance, but make sure there is another 3 ft walking distance past this line.

Instructions to participant: Begin with your toes on this line. When I tell you *"Begin,"* start walking at your normal pace. When you come to the first obstacle, walk around it to the left. When you come to the second obstacle, walk around it to the right and keep walking till I tell you to *stop*. Do you understand what I want you to do? Are you ready? *Begin.*

Examiner Instructions and Grading: Timing begins when the tester says *"Begin."* Stop timing when the first foot crosses the 20-ft line but make sure the participant keeps walking 3 ft past the 20-ft mark. Make sure to observe whether the participant touches or brushes the foam cylinders as they walk by. Circle an ordinal score for level of assistance and gait pattern. Mark the *lowest* category that applies.

Time: ____________ seconds

Ordinal Time Level: __________

- **(3) <6.0 seconds**
- **(2) 8.2 to 6.0 seconds**
- **(1) 14.5 to 8.2 seconds**
- **(0) >14.5 seconds or unable**

Gait Pattern:

- (3) **NORMAL:** Is able to walk around both cylinders with normal gait pattern and no evidence of imbalance
- (2) **MILD IMPAIRMENT:** Is able to walk around both cylinders but shows mild gait deviations (i.e., may need to slow down and adjust steps) **or** shows mild imbalance
- (1) **MODERATE IMPAIRMENT:** Is able to walk around both cylinders but shows moderate gait deviations (i.e., must stop, then step around) **or** touches one or both cylinders **or** has moderate imbalance but is able to recover independently
- (0) **SEVERE IMPAIRMENT:** Cannot step around one or both cylinders, or loses balance and is unable to recover independently

Level of Assistance

- (2) No assistance
- (1) Used an assistive device (excludes orthosis or brace)
- (0) Required the physical assistance of another (includes contact guard)

8. Up Stairs: ______

Equipment: 10 steps with railing and stopwatch

Setup: Position participant at the bottom of the stairs.

Instructions to participant: When I tell you *"Begin,"* start walking up the stairs as you would at home or in the community. If you normally use a rail, do so. Walk to the top of the stairs and stop. Do you understand what I want you to do? Are you ready? *Begin.*

(*continued*)

Assessment Tool 16.1

Modified Dynamic Gait Index (*continued*)

Examiner Instructions and Grading: Timing begins when the tester says *"Begin."* Stop timing when *both* of the participant's feet are on the 10th step (or landing). Circle an ordinal score for level of assistance and gait pattern. Mark the *lowest* category that applies.

Time:____________ seconds

Ordinal Time Level: __________

(3) <6.1 seconds
(2) 9.0 to 6.1 seconds
(1) 19.7 to 9.1 seconds
(0) >19.7 seconds or unable

Gait Pattern:

(3) **NORMAL:** Alternating feet, no rail
(2) **MILD IMPAIRMENT:** Alternating feet, must use rail
(1) **MODERATE IMPAIRMENT:** Two feet to a stair, must use rail
(0) **SEVERE IMPAIRMENT:** Cannot do safely

Level of Assistance

(2) No assistance
(1) Used an assistive device (excludes orthosis or brace)
(0) Required the physical assistance of another (includes contact guard)

Dynamic Gait Index Score Sheet

Task Scores	**Time (0–3)**	**Gait Pattern (0–3)**	**Level of Assistance (0–2)**	**Total Task Score (0–8)**
Usual Pace Task				
Change Pace Task				
Horizontal Head Task				
Vertical Head Task				
Pivot Turn Task				
Over Obstacles Task				
Around Obstacles Task				
Stairs Task				
Performance Scores	**Time (0–24)**	**Gait Pattern (0–24)**	**Level of Assistance (0–16)**	
DGI Total Score (0–64)				

Adapted from Shumway-Cook A, Taylor C, Matsuda PN, et al. Expanding the scoring system of the Dynamic Gait Index. *Phys Ther.* 2013;93:1493–1506, with permission.

Assessment Tool 16.2

Functional Gait Assessment

Requirements: A marked 6-m (20-ft) walkway that is marked with a 30.48 cm (12 in.) width.

1. Gait level surface____

Instructions: Walk at your normal speed from here to the next mark (6 m [20 ft]).

Grading: Mark the highest category that applies.

(3) Normal—Walks 6 m (20 ft) in less than 5.5 seconds, no assistive devices, good speed, no evidence for imbalance, normal gait pattern, deviates no more than 15.24 cm (6 in.) outside the 30.48-cm (12-in.) walkway width.

(2) Mild impairment—Walks 6 m (20 ft) in less than 7 seconds but more than 5.5 seconds, uses assistive device, slower speed, mild gait deviations, or

Assessment Tool 16.2

Functional Gait Assessment (*continued*)

deviates 15.24 to 25.4 cm (6 to 10 in.) outside the 30.48-cm (12-in.) walkway width.
- (1) Moderate impairment—Walks 6 m (20 ft), slow speed, abnormal gait pattern, evidence for imbalance, or deviates 25.4 to 38.1 cm (10 to 15 in.) outside the 30.48-cm (12-in.) walkway width. Requires more than 7 seconds to ambulate 6 m (20 ft).
- (0) Severe impairment—Cannot walk 6 m (20 ft) without assistance, severe gait deviations or imbalance, deviates more than 38.1 cm (15 in.) outside the 30.48-cm (12-in.) walkway width or reaches and touches the wall.

2. Change in gait speed_____

Instructions: Begin walking at your normal pace (for 1.5 m [5 ft]). When I tell you "go," walk as fast as you can (for 1.5 m [5 ft]). When I tell you "slow," walk as slowly as you can (for 1.5 m [5 ft]).

Grading: Mark the highest category that applies.
- (3) Normal—Able to smoothly change walking speed without loss of balance or gait deviation. Shows a significant difference in walking speeds between normal, fast, and slow speeds. Deviates no more than 15.24 cm (6 in.) outside the 30.48-cm (12-in.) walkway width.
- (2) Mild impairment—Is able to change speed but demonstrates mild gait deviations, deviates 15.24 to 25.4 cm (6 to 10 in.) outside the 30.48-cm (12-in.) walkway width, or no gait deviations but unable to achieve a significant change in velocity, or uses an assistive device.
- (1) Moderate impairment—Makes only minor adjustments to walking speed, or accomplishes a change in speed with significant gait deviations, deviates 25.4 to 38.1 cm (10 to 15 in.) outside the 30.48-cm (12-in.) walkway width, or changes speed but loses balance but is able to recover and continue walking.
- (0) Severe impairment—Cannot change speeds, deviates more than 38.1 cm (15 in.) outside 30.48-cm (12-in.) walkway width, or loses balance and has to reach for wall or be caught.

3. Gait with horizontal head turns_____

Instructions: Walk from here to the next mark 6 m (20 ft) away. Begin walking at your normal pace. Keep walking straight; after three steps, turn your head to the right and keep walking straight while looking to the right. After three more steps, turn your head to the left and keep walking straight while looking left. Continue alternating looking right and left every three steps until you have completed two repetitions in each direction.

Grading: Mark the highest category that applies.
- (3) Normal—Performs head turns smoothly with no change in gait. Deviates no more than 15.24 cm (6 in.) outside the 30.48-cm (12-in.) walkway width.
- (2) Mild impairment—Performs head turns smoothly, with slight change in gait velocity (e.g., minor disruption to smooth gait path), deviates 15.24 to 25.4 cm (6 to 10 in.) outside the 30.48-cm (12-in.) walkway width, or uses an assistive device.
- (1) Moderate impairment—Performs head turns with moderate change in gait velocity, slows down, deviates 25.4 to 38.1 cm (10 to 15 in.) outside the 30.48-cm (12-in.) walkway width but recovers, and can continue to walk.
- (0) Severe impairment—Performs task with severe disruption of gait (e.g., staggers 38.1 cm [15 in.] outside the 30.48-cm [12-in.] walkway width, loses balance, stops, or reaches for wall).

4. Gait with vertical head turns_____

Instructions: Walk from here to the next mark (6 m [20 ft]). Begin walking at your normal pace. Keep walking straight; after three steps, tip your head up and keep walking straight while looking up. After three more steps, tip your head down, keep walking straight while looking down. Continue alternating looking up and down every three steps until you have completed two repetitions in each direction.

Grading: Mark the highest category that applies.
- (3) Normal—Performs head turns with no change in gait. Deviates no more than 15.24 cm (6 in.) outside the 30.48-cm (12-in.) walkway width.
- (2) Mild impairment—Performs task with slight change in gait velocity (e.g., minor disruption to smooth gait path), deviates 15.2 to 25.4 cm (6 to 10 in.) outside the 30.5-cm (12-in.) walkway width, or uses assistive device.
- (1) Moderate impairment—Performs task with moderate change in gait velocity, slows down, deviates 25.4 to 38.1 cm (10 to 15 in.) outside the 30.5-cm (12-in.) walkway width but recovers, and can continue to walk.
- (0) Severe impairment—Performs task with severe disruption of gait (e.g., staggers 38.1 cm [15 in.] outside the 30.5-cm [12-in.] walkway width, loses balance, stops, reaches for wall).

5. Gait and pivot turn_____

Instructions: Begin walking at your normal pace. When I tell you to turn and stop, turn as quickly as you can to face the opposite direction and stop.

Grading: Mark the highest category that applies.
- (3) Normal—Pivot turns safely within 3 seconds and stops quickly with no loss of balance.
- (2) Mild impairment—Pivot turns safely in <3 seconds and stops with no loss of balance, or pivot turns safely within 3 seconds and stops with mild imbalance and requires small steps to catch balance.
- (1) Moderate impairment—Turns slowly, requires verbal cueing, or requires several small steps to catch balance following turn and stop.
- (0) Severe impairment—Cannot turn safely, requires assistance to turn and stop.

(*continued*)

Assessment Tool 16.2

Functional Gait Assessment (*continued*)

6. Step over obstacle____

Instructions: Begin walking at your normal speed. When you come to the shoe box, step over it, not around it, and keep walking.

Grading: Mark the highest category that applies.

(3) Normal—Is able to step over two stacked shoe boxes taped together (22.9 cm [9 in.] total height) without changing gait speed; no evidence of imbalance.

(2) Mild impairment—Is able to step over one shoe box (11.4 cm [4.5 in.] total height) without changing gait speed; no evidence of imbalance.

(1) Moderate impairment—Is able to step over one shoe box (11.4 cm [4.5 in.] total height), but must slow down and adjust steps to clear box safely. May require verbal cueing.

(0) Severe impairment—Cannot perform without assistance.

7. Gait with narrow base of support____

Instructions: Walk on the floor with arms folded across the chest, feet aligned heel to toe in tandem for a distance of 3.6 m [12 ft]. The number of steps taken in a straight line is counted, for a maximum of 10 steps.

Grading: Mark the highest category that applies.

(3) Normal—Is able to walk for 10 steps heel to toe with no staggering

(2) Mild impairment—Walks 7 to 9 steps

(1) Moderate impairment—Walks 4 to 7 steps

(0) Severe impairment—Walks less than 4 steps heel to toe or cannot perform without assistance

8. Gait with eyes closed____

Instructions: Walk at your normal speed from here to the next mark (6 m [20 ft]) with your eyes closed.

Grading: Mark the highest category that applies.

(3) Normal—Walks 6 m (20 ft), no assistive devices, good speed, no evidence of imbalance, normal gait pattern, deviates no more than 15.2 cm (6 in.) outside the 30.5-cm (12-in.) walkway width. Walks 6 m (20 ft) in less than 7 seconds

(2) Mild impairment—Walks 6 m (20 ft), uses assistive device, slower speed, mild gait deviations, deviates 15.2 to 25.4 cm (6 to 10 in.) outside the 30.5 cm (12-in.) walkway width. Ambulates 6 m (20 ft) in less than 9 seconds but more than 7 seconds

(1) Moderate impairment—Walks 6 m (20 ft), slow speed, abnormal gait pattern, evidence for imbalance, deviates 25.4 to 38.1 cm (10 to 15 in.) outside the 30.5-cm (12-in.) walkway width. Requires more than 9 seconds to walk 6 m (20 ft)

(0) Severe impairment—Cannot walk 6 m (20 ft) without assistance, severe gait deviations or imbalance, deviates more than 38.1 cm (15 in.) outside the 30.5-cm (12-in.) walkway width or will not attempt task

9. Ambulating backward____

Instructions: Walk backward until I tell you to stop.

Grading: Mark the highest category that applies.

(3) Normal—Walks 6 m (20 ft), no assistive devices, good speed, no evidence for imbalance, normal gait pattern, deviates no more than 15.2 cm (6 in.) outside the 30.5-cm (12-in.) walkway width

(2) Mild impairment—Walks 6 m (20 ft), uses assistive device, slower speed, mild gait deviations, deviates 15.2 to 25.4 cm (6 to 10 in.) outside the 30.5-cm (12-in.) walkway width

(1) Moderate impairment—Walks 6 m (20 ft), slow speed, abnormal gait pattern, evidence for imbalance, deviates 25.4 to 38.1 cm (10 to 15 in.) outside the 30.5-cm (12-in) walkway width.

(0) Severe impairment—Cannot walk 6 m (20 ft) without assistance, severe gait deviations or imbalance, deviates more than 38.1 cm (15 in.) outside the 30.5-cm (12-in.) walkway width or will not attempt task

10. Steps____

Instructions: Walk up these stairs as you would at home (i.e., using the rail if necessary). At the top, turn around and walk down.

Grading: Mark the highest category that applies.

(3) Normal—Alternating feet, no rail

(2) Mild impairment—Alternating feet, must use rail

(1) Moderate impairment—Two feet to a stair, must use rail

(0) Severe impairment—Cannot do safely

Total score: _____ *(Maximum score: 30)*

Adapted from Wrisley DM, Marchett GF, Kuharsky DK, et al. Reliability, internal consistency, and validity of data obtained with the functional gait assessment. *Phys Ther.* 2004;84:906–918, with permission of the American Physical Therapy Association.

Stops Walking When Talking. The Stops Walking When Talking (SWWT) test examines the effect of a secondary task, talking, on walking. In this test, the examiner begins a conversation with an individual who is walking; the individual who stops walking in order to talk defines a positive response. The SWWT test was a good predictor of falls among frail, institutionalized, older adults (Lundin-Olsson et al., 1997), with 95% specificity but only 48% sensitivity. The SWWT test did not predict falls in persons with PD (Bloem et al., 2000). Hyndman and Ashburn (2004) examined the predictive ability of the SWWT test following stroke.

Of the 63 subjects tested, 26 stopped walking when talking and 16 of them fell during the 6-month follow-up period. Thus, in persons with stroke, the SWWT test had a specificity of 70% (23 of 33) and a sensitivity of 53% (16 of 30). The SWWT test is limited because a positive outcome is defined relative to whether an individual SWWT. Thus, a person who slows but does not stop walking, or alternatively, maintains speed but is unsteady, will not be identified as at risk by the SWWT test. In an effort to capture individuals who slow but do not stop walking when talking, clinicians have examined the effect of a secondary task on usual gait speed measured during a 4-, 8-, or 10-Meter Walk test. A reduction in gait speed during performance of a secondary task has been shown in a variety of persons with neurologic pathology, including those with stroke (Bowen et al., 2001), PD (Rochester et al., 2004), and older adults at risk for falls (Shumway-Cook et al., 2000). Li and colleagues (2014) investigated in a group of healthy older adults the cost of two types of dual-task talking while walking paradigms: walking while reciting alternate letters of the alphabet and walking while counting backward by sevens. Their findings show that both dual-task paradigms compromise gait performance, with slower gait velocity in the dual-task that involved counting backward. They also found that faster gait velocity was associated with higher cognitive accuracy; which may suggest that older adults with greater attention resources are more capable of coping with the concurrent cognitive and motor demands.

Measuring Mobility in Low-Functioning Persons

Several measures are available to examine a variety of mobility tasks in low-functioning individuals.

Physical Performance and Mobility Examination. The Physical Performance and Mobility Examination (PPME) was developed to measure performance of physical function and mobility in hospitalized and frail older adults (Winograd et al., 1994). The PPME was designed to assess function without overtaxing frail or acutely ill subjects. Six mobility tasks integral to everyday life were chosen for the test, which does not examine constituent abilities such as strength and range of motion (ROM). This test includes both high-level tasks, such as standing up 5 times from a chair, and lower-level tasks, such as bed mobility and transfer skills. The PPME has been shown to be responsive in older adults undergoing rehabilitation after hip fracture (Farag et al., 2012). The test is summarized in Assessment Tool 16.3. Shown are the list of tasks, a description of how the task is to be performed, and the response dimensions.

Assessment Tool 16.3

Physical Performance and Mobility Examination

Tasks	Description	Response Dimension
1. Bed mobility	Sit up in bed from lying down	Need for assistance, time to complete
2. Transfers	Stand up from bed (from sitting) move to chair, sit down, stand up from chair once	Need for assistance, use of arms
3. Multiple chair stands	Stand up from chair 5 times	Need for assistance, use of arms, time to complete
4. Standing balance	Ability to hold 4 positions for 10 seconds, feet apart, feet together, semitandem, tandem	Need for assistance, time
5. Step up	Step up one step with handrail	Need for assistance, use of handrail
6. Ambulation	Walk 5 m, 2 trials	Time at usual pace, number of steps

Reprinted from Winograd CH, Lemsky CM, Nevitt MC, et al. Development of a physical performance and mobility examination. *J Am Geriatr Soc.* 1994;42:743–749, with permission.

The Boston University Activity Measure for Post Acute Care "6-Clicks," Basic Mobility Short Form. Boston University has created the Activity Measure for Post Acute Care (AM-PAC), to measure activity limitations in three functional domains: basic mobility, daily activities, and applied cognitive. The Basic Mobility Test (or "6-Clicks") evaluates the difficulty a person has and the assistance a person requires when performing six basic mobility tasks. The AM-PAC has a predictive use to determine the physical activity status of hospitalized patients. In an observational retrospective study, Johnson and colleagues (2020) used the AM-PAC to investigate the relationship of physical function in the acute hospital setting and physical outcomes during inpatient rehabilitation in 1,323 patients. Compared to patients with very low physical function, those with moderately low, moderately high, or high physical function at hospital discharge were more likely to improve their physical outcomes during inpatient rehabilitation and be discharged from the inpatient facility to the community; they also had shorter length of stay at inpatient rehabilitation.

This test is shown in Assessment Tool 16.4. This tool was used to evaluate Genise's function immediately following her stroke and again on admission to the inpatient rehabilitation unit.

Assessment Tool 16.4

Activity Measure for Post Acute Care Mobility Short Form

AM-PAC Inpatient Basic Mobility Short Form

Boston University AM-PAC™ "6 Clicks"
Basic Mobility Inpatient Short Form

Please check the box that reflects your (the patient's) best answer to each question.

How much difficulty does the patient currently have...	Unable	A Lot	A Little	None
1. Turning over in bed (including adjusting bedclothes, sheets and blankets)?	☐1	☐2	☐3	☐4
2. Sitting down on and standing up from a chair with arms (e.g., wheelchair, bedside commode, etc.)	☐1	☐2	☐3	☐4
3. Moving from lying on back to sitting on the side of the bed?	☐1	☐2	☐3	☐4

How much help from another person does the patient currently need...	Unable		A Little	
4. Moving to and from a bed to a chair (including a wheelchair)?	☐1	☐2	☐3	☐4
5. Need to walk in hospital room?	☐1	☐2	☐3	☐4
6. Climbing 3-5 steps with a railing?	☐1	☐2	☐3	☐4

Raw Score: ____________ CMS 0-100% Score: ____________

Standardized Score: ____________ CMS Modifier: ____________

Note: Use the AM-PAC Basic Mobility Inpatient Short Form Conversion Table to convert raw scores.

AM-PAC Short Form Manual (v. 3)

Predicting Participation from Functional Activity and Impairment Measures

An important part of rehabilitation of persons with gait disorders is predicting the ability to participate in mobility-related activities within his or her own environment (level of mobility disability). However, there are few guidelines to assist the clinician in the prediction process. The relationships among impairments (body functions and structures), limitations in functional abilities (capacity), and restricted level of participation (mobility disability) are not clear. Gait velocity measured in the clinic has been shown to relate to strength (an impairment measure), but neither measure has been shown to correlate well with home versus community independence (a disability measure) (Lord & Rochester, 2005; Robinson et al., 2007, 2011a).

Hoffer et al. (1973) suggested a classification of walking disability including the following: nonambulator (a person who cannot meet the requirements of ambulating within the home or community), nonfunctional ambulator (an individual who walks for therapeutic but not functional purposes), household ambulator (an individual who can safely perform the tasks that define mobility within the home environment), and community ambulator (no limitations to the individual's ability to meet the demands of moving within the community). This classification system was expanded and modified by Perry and colleagues (1995), and it is summarized in Table 16.3. They studied 147 patients who had had a stroke in order to identify the best combination of measures that predicted mobility status. Measures used to predict level of ambulation included a self-report questionnaire regarding walking abilities, calculation of stride characteristics using a footswitch stride analyzer, a test of proprioception, and the upright motor control test (a test that examines the ability to extend the knee in the paretic limb during single-limb stance).

Gait velocity was one of several variables important in predicting walking classification. A velocity of at least 0.42 m/s predicted community ambulation. The mean walking velocity of the highest category of community walkers among the stroke subjects was 0.8 m/s, significantly slower than the normal population value of 1.33 m/s, and not fast enough to cross a street safely (Perry et al., 1995).

Perry's findings were consistent with a study by Lerner-Frankiel and colleagues (1990), who reported that the requirements for being a community ambulator included the ability to (1) walk at greater than 33% of a normal adult's velocity (0.45 m/s), or about 1.0 mph; (2) walk 80 m/min for 13 to 27 meters in order to cross a street safely in the normal time allotted by stoplights; and (3) negotiate 7- to 8-inch curbs independently (with assistive devices as needed). The study also found that, in general, clinicians underestimated the distance and speed needed to function independently within a community environment (Lerner-Frankiel et al., 1990). This may be because tests of normal ADL

TABLE 16.3 Perry's Proposed Scheme for Classifying Mobility Function

Discriminant functions	Functional walking category: Physiological	Limited household	Unlimited household	Most-limited community	Least-limited community	Community
Bathroom	4.32[a]	11.78[a]	16.93[b]	16.96[b]	16.60[b]	17.09
Bedroom	3.39[a]	8.35[a]	12.68[b]	11.83[b]	11.25[b]	10.83
Enter/exit	1.80[c]	3.67[c]	5.47[a]	7.83[b]	7.24[b]	7.05
Curb	−0.14[c]	1.94[c]	4.77[a]	7.04[b]	7.94[b]	8.40
Grocery	−0.06[b]	−0.37[b]	−0.01[b]	−0.03[a]	1.61[b]	1.58
Shopping center, uncrowded	0.21[b]	0.74[b]	1.54[b]	1.34[a]	3.79[b]	2.98
Shopping center, crowded	0.30[c]	0.02[c]	0.05[c]	−0.22[b]	−2.10[a]	1.19
Constant	−6.70	−33.51	−76.24	−88.13	−92.45	−101.47

[a]Questionnaire item had a strong influence on placement between the two adjacent walking groups.
[b]Questionnaire item had minimal or no influence on placement between the two adjacent walking groups.
[c]Questionnaire item had moderate influence on placement between the two adjacent walking groups.

TABLE 16.4 Functional Ambulation Classification Scale

Score	Description
0	(Nonambulation): Absolute walking incapacity, even with external help.
1	(Nonfunctional ambulation): Dependent walking that requires permanent help of others. The patient must be firmly supported by one or two people, and/or walking is possible only within a therapy session at home or at the hospital between parallel bars.
2	(Household ambulation): Walking is only possible indoors, on flat, horizontal surfaces, usually within a known and controlled area, such as in the home.
3	(Neighborhood ambulation): Patients are able to walk indoors and outdoors on uneven surfaces, and they are able to climb an occasional step or stair. Therefore, the patient is able to walk in the street, albeit within a limited and restricted walking distance.
4	(Independent community ambulation): Patients are able to walk on all types of irregular surfaces. They can ascend and descend steps, or stairs, ramps, curbs, etc. They have a considerable, even unrestricted, walking distance so that they are capable of shopping for food and accomplishing other basic chores. However, they are not considered normal walkers because they have aesthetic anomalies, such as an obvious limp.
5	(Normal ambulation): Walking is completely normal in both distance and appearance, both at home and outside and with an unlimited distance. There is no aesthetic anomaly or limp. They can tiptoe, walk on their heels, and in tandem.

Source: Reprinted from Viosca E, Martinez JL, Almagro PL, et al. Proposal and validation of a new functional ambulation classification scale for clinical use. *Arch Phys Med Rehabil.* 2005;86:1234–1238, with permission.

skills, for example, the FIM, often define complete independence in locomotor skills as being able to walk 150 ft safely (Keith et al., 1987). However, this standard may underestimate the requirements for being truly independent within the community.

Similar results were found in a more recent study examining factors that predicted ambulation in home and community settings following stroke (Fulk et al., 2017). Four ambulation categories were identified: home (100–2,499 steps/day), most limited community (2,500–4,499 steps/day), least limited community (5,000–74,999 steps/day), and full community (≥7,500 steps/day). The 6-minute walk test (endurance), Berg Balance Scale (functional balance), and Fugle-Meyer (motor function) were the strongest predictors of home versus community and limited versus unlimited community ambulators. Performance on the 6-minute walk test was the single best predictor. The authors observed that a comfortable gait speed of 0.49 m/s discriminated between home and community ambulators, while 0.93 m/s discriminated between limited and full community ambulators. Moreover, a 6-minute walking test distance ≥205 m discriminated between home and community ambulators, and a distance ≥288 m discriminated limited from unlimited community ambulators. However, while gait speed discriminated between home and community walkers, it overestimated actual walking activity (Fulk et al., 2017).

The Functional Ambulation Classification (FAC) scale includes six functional levels ranging from 0 (absence of walking capacity) to 5 (recovery of normal ambulation) (Viosca et al., 2005). This scale is shown in Table 16.4. This scale was tested on 31 patients with poststroke hemiplegia and a control group of five healthy adults. The test was found to have good interrater reliability (kappa = 0.74) and a strong correlation to walking velocity (Spearman correlation = 0.84).

A functional walking classification scale for children was developed by researchers at Gillette Hospital (Novacheck et al., 2000). The Gillette Functional Assessment Questionnaire (FAQ)-Walking Scale, shown in Assessment Tool 16.5, is a parent report, 10 level walking scale, encompassing a wide range of walking abilities from nonambulatory to community ambulation. In a study with 41 children with neurologic pathology (83% of the children had a diagnosis of CP) resulting in a range of ambulation skills, the test was found to have good test–retest reliability among parents and good interrater reliability between parents and community caregivers. The test had good content and construct validity, as indicated by a significant correlation with the pediatric version of the Functional Independence Measure (Wee FIM), and a significant inverse correlation to laboratory measures of oxygen consumption (Novacheck et al., 2000).

Assessment Tool 16.5

Gillette Functional Walking Scale

Choose one answer in the following that best describes your child's typical walking ability (with the use of any needed assistive devices).

1. Cannot take any steps at all
2. Can do some stepping on their own with the help of another person. Does not take full weight on feet: does not walk on a routine basis
3. Walks for exercise in therapy and less than typical household distances. Usually requires assistance from another person
4. Walks for household distances, but makes slow progress. Does not use walking at home as preferred mobility (primarily walks in therapy)
5. Walks more than 15 to 50 ft but only inside at home or school (walks for household distances)
6. Walks more than 15 to 50 ft outside the home, but usually uses a wheelchair or stroller for community distances or in congested areas
7. Walks outside the home for community distances, but only on level surfaces (cannot perform on curbs, uneven terrain, or stairs without the assistance of another person)
8. Walks outside the home for community distances, is able to perform on curbs and uneven terrain in addition to level surfaces, but usually requires minimal assistance or supervision for safety
9. Walks outside home for community distances, easily gets around on level ground, curbs, and uneven terrain but has difficulty or requires minimal assistance with running, climbing, and/or stairs
10. Walk, runs, and climbs on level and uneven terrain without difficulty or assistance

Reprinted from Novacheck TF, Stout JS, Tervo R. Reliability and validity of the Gillette Functional Assessment Questionnaire as an outcome measure in children with walking disabilities. *J Pediatr Orthop*. 2000;20:76 (Table 1), with permission.

A MCID of a 2-point increase in the Gillette FAQ walking scale has been determined in children with neuromotor disorders, including CP, traumatic brain injury, and stroke in the inpatient setting (Ammann-Reiffer et al., 2019).

Limitations of Functional Gait Measures

All functional measures, whether of mobility, balance, or general motor control, are indicators of the end product only and do not provide information about the way performance is achieved. Thus, these measures do not provide insight into underlying impairments that require treatment. However, functional measures are good indicators of overall function and, therefore, are important indices of change.

Examining the Gait Pattern

Quantitative measures such as gait speed provide an objective measure of function but do not describe the quality of performance (e.g., the ways in which gait patterns deviate from normal). Therefore, examination of gait must include a systematic description of the GP and its ability to meet the requirements inherent in locomotion. In the ICF classification system, evaluating the underlying GP is part of measuring the Body Structures and Functions component of mobility.

Observational Gait Analysis

OGA is a common method for examining the GP in clinical practice (Krebs et al., 1985). OGA is the observation of kinematic patterns of movement used for gait. Observation of atypical kinematic patterns of movement is used to identify major gait deficits; however, nonobservable deficits, such as weakness, coordination, and spasticity, can be inferred only from observation and require confirmation with appropriate testing. OGA is used as both an evaluative tool (e.g., to monitor change over time) and a diagnostic tool (e.g., to determine the causal factors producing atypical gait) (Lord et al., 1998; Winter, 1993). In OGA, the observer describes characteristics of gait without the aid of electronic devices.

There are many standardized forms available to help clinicians structure their approach to visual gait analysis. One example is the gait assessment portion of the Performance-Oriented Mobility Assessment described in Chapter 11. Other examples of visual gait analysis forms that are helpful in guiding a clinical examination of gait patterns in the patient with neurologic impairments follow.

Rancho Los Amigos Gait Analysis Form. The Gait Analysis Form, developed at Rancho Los Amigos Hospital and shown in Assessment Tool 16.6, is a comprehensive approach to gait analysis (Perry, 1992; Perry & Burnfield, 2010). It is based on Perry's classification system, shown in Figure 16.1 (Perry, 1992). Gait is broken down into component parts. The observer focuses on one period of gait at a time (e.g., stance vs. swing), considers the functional tasks to be performed during those periods (e.g., weight acceptance, single-limb support, and limb advancement), and observes motion at each of the major joints (e.g., ankle, knee, hip, pelvis, and trunk) in each of the phases of gait (initial contact, loading response, midstance, etc.).

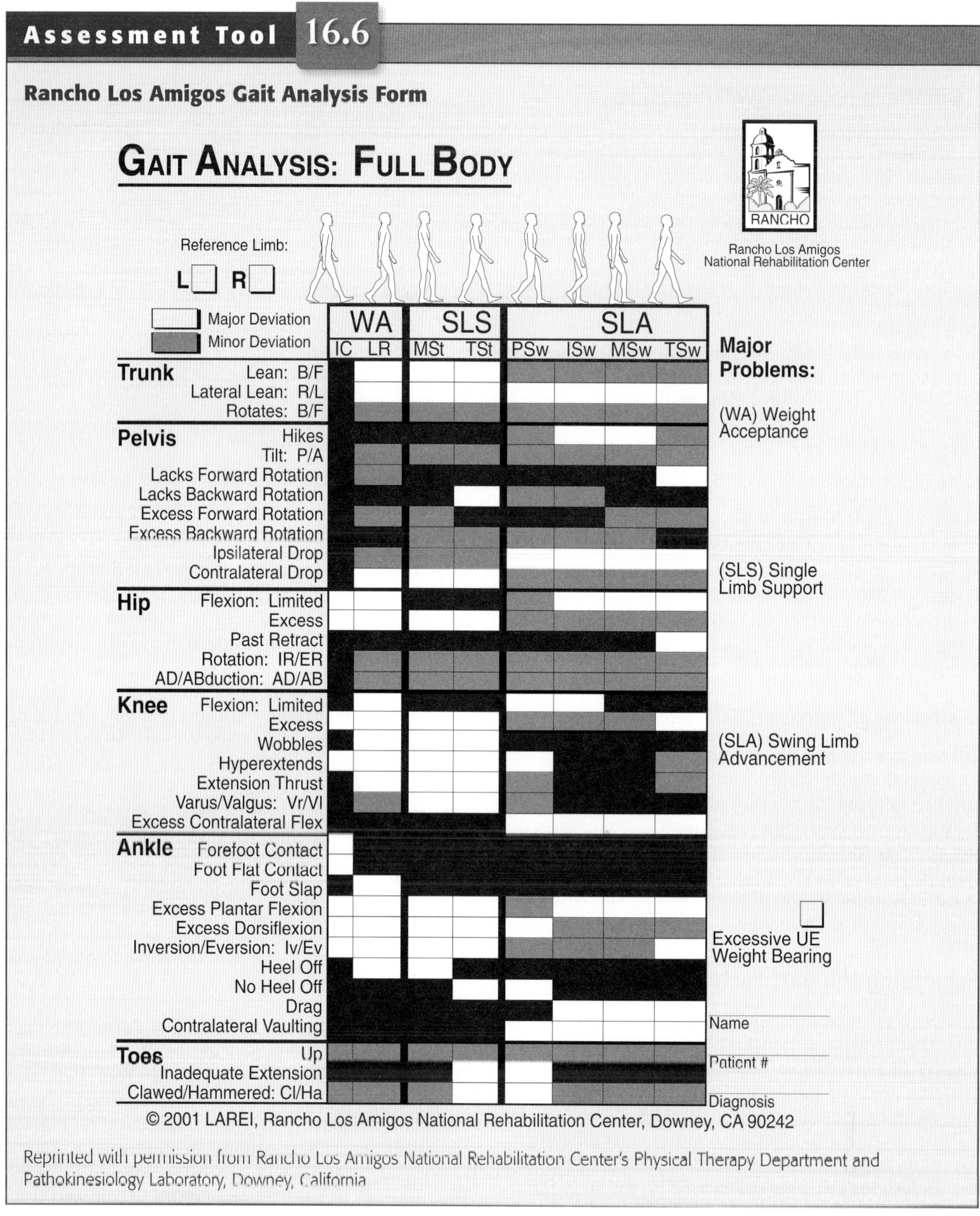

Assessment Tool 16.6

Rancho Los Amigos Gait Analysis Form

GAIT ANALYSIS: FULL BODY

RANCHO

Rancho Los Amigos National Rehabilitation Center

Reference Limb: L☐ R☐

☐ Major Deviation

■ Minor Deviation

		WA		SLS		SLA			
		IC	LR	MSt	TSt	PSw	ISw	MSw	TSw
Trunk	Lean: B/F								
	Lateral Lean: R/L								
	Rotates: B/F								
Pelvis	Hikes								
	Tilt: P/A								
	Lacks Forward Rotation								
	Lacks Backward Rotation								
	Excess Forward Rotation								
	Excess Backward Rotation								
	Ipsilateral Drop								
	Contralateral Drop								
Hip	Flexion: Limited								
	Excess								
	Past Retract								
	Rotation: IR/ER								
	AD/ABduction: AD/AB								
Knee	Flexion: Limited								
	Excess								
	Wobbles								
	Hyperextends								
	Extension Thrust								
	Varus/Valgus: Vr/Vl								
	Excess Contralateral Flex								
Ankle	Forefoot Contact								
	Foot Flat Contact								
	Foot Slap								
	Excess Plantar Flexion								
	Excess Dorsiflexion								
	Inversion/Eversion: Iv/Ev								
	Heel Off								
	No Heel Off								
	Drag								
	Contralateral Vaulting								
Toes	Up								
	Inadequate Extension								
	Clawed/Hammered: Cl/Ha								

Major Problems:

(WA) Weight Acceptance

(SLS) Single Limb Support

(SLA) Swing Limb Advancement

☐ Excessive UE Weight Bearing

Name

Patient #

Diagnosis

Gait Assessment Rating Scale. The Gait Abnormality Rating Scale (GARS), developed by Wolfson and colleagues (1990), is shown in Assessment Tool 16.7. The scale also allows the quantification and documentation of three categories of gait abnormalities, a general category, a lower-extremity category, and a trunk, head, and upper-extremity (UE) category. The scale is sensitive to change and has high interrater reliability. A modified 7-item version of the GARS including (1) variability, (2) guardedness, (3) staggering, (4) foot

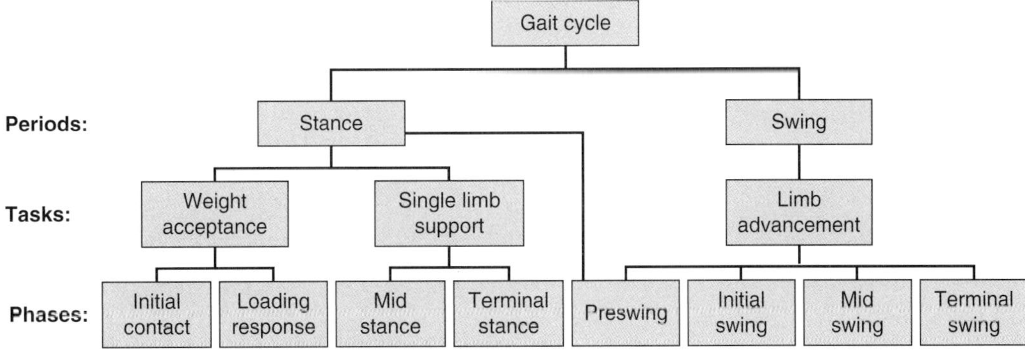

Figure 16.1 Conceptual framework for analyzing gait suggested by Perry (1992).

Assessment Tool 16.7

Gait Assessment Rating Scale

General Categories

1. Variability—a measure of inconsistency and arrhythmicity of stepping and of arm movements
- 0 = Fluid and predictably paced limb movements
- 1 = Occasional interruptions (changes in velocity), approximately <25% of time
- 2 = Unpredictability of rhythm approximately 25% to 75% of time
- 3 = Random timing of limb movements

2. Guardedness—Hesitancy, slowness, diminished propulsion, and lack of commitment in stepping and arm swing
- 0 = Good forward momentum and lack of apprehension in propulsion
- 1 = Center of gravity of HAT projects only slightly in front of push-off, but still good arm–leg coordination
- 2 = HAT held over anterior aspect of foot and some moderate loss of smooth reciprocation
- 3 = HAT held over rear aspect of stance phase foot and great tentativeness in stepping

3. Weaving—An irregular and wavering line of progression
- 0 = Straight line of progression on frontal viewing
- 1 = A single deviation from straight (line of best fit) line of progression
- 2 = Two to three deviations from line of progression
- 3 = Four or more deviations from line of progression

4. Waddling—A broad-based gait characterized by excessive truncal crossing of the midline and side bending
- 0 = Narrow base of support and body held nearly vertically over feet
- 1 = Slight separation of medial aspects of feet and just perceptible lateral movement of head and trunk
- 2 = 3 to 4 in. of separation between feet and obvious bending of trunk to side so that COG of head lies well over ipsilateral stance foot
- 3 = Extreme pendular deviations of head and trunk (head passes lateral to ipsilateral stance foot) and further widening of base of support

5. Staggering—Sudden and unexpected lateral partial losses of balance
- 0 = No losses of balance to side
- 1 = A single lurch to side
- 2 = Two lurches to side
- 3 = Three or more lurches to side

Lower-Extremity Categories

1. Percent Time in Swing—A loss in the percentage of the gait cycle constituted by the swing phase
- 0 = Approximately 3:2 ratio of duration of stance to swing phase
- 1 = A 1:1 or slightly less ratio of stance to swing
- 2 = Markedly prolonged stance phase but with some obvious swing time remaining
- 3 = Barely perceptible portion of cycle spent in swing

2. Foot Contact—The degree to which heel strikes the ground before the forefoot
- 0 = Very obvious angle of impact of heel on ground
- 1 = Barely visible contact of heel before forefoot
- 2 = Entire foot lands flat on ground
- 3 = Anterior aspect of foot strikes ground before heel

3. Hip ROM—The degree of loss of hip range of motion seen during a gait cycle
- 0 = Obvious angulation of thigh backward during double-support (10 degrees)
- 1 = Just barely visible angulation backward from vertical
- 2 = Thigh in line with vertical projection from ground
- 3 = Thigh angled forward from vertical at maximum posterior excursion

4. Knee ROM—The degree of loss of knee range of motion seen during a gait cycle
- 0 = Knee moves from complete extension at heel strike (and late stance) to almost 90 degrees (70 degrees) during swing phase.
- 1 = Slight bend in knee seen at heel strike and late stance and maximal flexion at midswing is closer to 45 degrees than 90 degrees.

(continued)

Assessment Tool 16.7

Gait Assessment Rating Scale (*continued*)

2 = Knee flexion at late stance more obvious than at heel strike; very little clearance seen for toe during swing
3 = Toe appears to touch ground during swing, knee flexion appears constant during stance, and knee angle during swing appears 45 degrees or less.

Trunk, Head, and Upper-Extremity Categories

1. Elbow Extension—A measure of the decrease of elbow range of motion
0 = Large peak-to-peak excursion of forearm (~20 degrees), with distinct maximal flexion at the end of anterior trajectory
1 = 25% decrement of extension during maximal posterior excursion of upper extremity
2 = Almost no change in elbow angle
3 = No apparent change in elbow angle (held in flexion)

2. Shoulder Extension—A measure of the decrease of shoulder range of motion
0 = Clearly seen movement of upper arm anterior (15 degrees) and posterior (20 degrees) to vertical axis of trunk
1 = Shoulder flexes slightly anterior to vertical axis.
2 = Shoulder comes only to vertical axis, or slightly posterior to it during flexion.
3 = Shoulder stays well behind vertical axis during entire excursion.

3. Shoulder Abduction—A measure of pathological increase in shoulder range of motion laterally
0 = Shoulders held almost parallel to trunk
1 = Shoulders held 5 to 10 degrees to side
2 = Shoulders held 10 to 20 degrees to side
3 = Shoulders held greater than 20 degrees to side

4. Arm–Heel Strike Synchrony—The extent to which the contralateral movements of an arm and leg are out of phase
0 = Good temporal conjunction of arm and contralateral leg at apex of shoulder and hip excursions all of the time
1 = Arm and leg slightly out of phase 25% of the time
2 = Arm and leg moderately out of phase 25% to 50% of time
3 = Little or no temporal coherence of arm and leg

5. Head Held Forward—A measure of the pathological forward projection of the head relative to the trunk
0 = Earlobe vertically aligned with shoulder tip
1 = Earlobe vertical projection falls 1 inch anterior to shoulder tip
2 = Earlobe vertical projection falls 2 inches anterior to shoulder tip
3 = Earlobe vertical projection falls 3 inches or more anterior to shoulder tip

6. Shoulders Held Elevated—The degree to which the scapular girdle is held higher than normal
0 = Tip of shoulder (acromion) markedly below the level of chin 1 to 2 inches
1 = Tip of shoulder slightly below the level of chin
2 = Tip of shoulder at the level of chin
3 = Tip of shoulder above the level of chin

7. Upper Trunk Flexed Forward—A measure of kyphotic involvement of the trunk
0 = Very gentle thoracic convexity, cervical spine flat, or almost flat
1 = Emerging cervical curve, more distant thoracic convexity
2 = Anterior concavity at midchest level apparent
3 = Anterior concavity at midchest level very obvious

COG, center of gravity; HAT, head, arms, trunk; ROM, range of motion.

Reprinted from Wolfson L, Whipple R, Amerman P, et al. Gait assessment in the elderly: a gait abnormality rating scale and its relation to falls. *J Gerontol.* 1990;45:M12–M19, with permission.

contact, (5) hip ROM, (6) shoulder extension, and (7) arm–heel–strike synchrony has been developed for use with frail older community-dwelling individuals. The modified GARS is valid and reliable to report gait changes associated with an increased risk of falls (VanSwearingen et al., 1996).

Interpreting Observational Gait Analysis: Framework for Determining Causes of Atypical Gait

Systematically observing and documenting gait abnormalities is the first step in generating hypotheses regarding the possible causes for these deviations. Table 16.5 illustrates a gait diagnostic chart developed by Winter (1993) to serve as a framework for understanding possible causes of gait abnormalities observed during a visual gait analysis. The chart has three columns: the first lists the observed abnormalities, the second column lists the possible causes of the abnormality, and the third column describes the type of biomechanical or neuromuscular evidence that might be gathered to determine which of the possible causes is likely to be producing the observed abnormality. Thus, results from a visual gait analysis are tied to hypotheses regarding possible underlying causes and the types of diagnostic tests needed to confirm

TABLE 16.5 Winter's Framework for Understanding Atypical Gait Patterns

Observed abnormality	Possible causes	Biomechanical and neuromuscular diagnostic evidence
Foot slap at heel contact Forefoot or flatfoot initial contact	Below-normal dorsiflexor activity at heel contact a. Hyperactive plantarflexor activity in late swing b. Structural limitation in ankle range c. Short step length	Below-normal TA EMG or dorsiflexor moment at heel contact a. Above-normal plantarflexor EMG in late swing b. Decreased dorsiflexion ROM c. See (a), (b), (c), and (d) immediately following
Short step length	a. Weak push-off prior to swing b. Weak hip flexors at toe-off and early swing c. Above-normal knee extensor activity during push-off d. Excessive deceleration of leg in late swing	a. Below-normal plantarflexor moment or power generation or EMG during push-off b. Below-normal hip flexor power or power or EMG during late push-off and early swing c. Above-normal quadriceps EMG or knee extensor moment or power absorption in late stance d. Above-normal hamstrings EMG or knee flexor moment or power absorption late in swing
Stiff-legged weight bearing	a. Above-normal extensor activity at the ankle, knee, or hip early in stance	a. Above-normal EMG activity or moments in hip extensors, knee extensors, or plantarflexors early in stance
Stance phase with flexed but rigid knee	a. Above-normal extensor activity during weight acceptance at the ankle and hip with reduced knee extensor activity b. Excessive ankle dorsiflexion	a. Above-normal EMG activity or moments in hip extensors and plantarflexors in early and middle stance b. Hyperactivity of dorsiflexors or excessive dorsiflexion of ankle orthosis
Weak push-off accompanied by observable pull-off	a. Weak plantarflexor activity at push-off b. Normal or above-normal hip flexor EMG activity during late push-off and early swing	a. Below-normal plantarflexor EMG, moment, or power during push-off b. Normal or above-normal hip flexor EMG, moment, or power during late push off and early swing
Hip hiking in swing with or without circumduction of lower limb	a. Weak hip, knee, or ankle flexor activity during swing b. Overactive extensor synergy during swing	a. Below-normal TA EMG or hip or knee flexors during swing b. Above-normal hip or knee extensor EMG or moment during swing
Trendelenburg gait	a. Weak hip abductors b. Overactive hip adductors	a. Below-normal EMG in hip abductors: gluteus medius and minimus, tensor fasciae latae b. Above-normal EMG in hip adductors, adductor longus, magnus and brevis, and gracilis

Source: Reprinted from Winter DA. Knowledge base for diagnostic gait assessments. *Med Prog Technol.* 1993;19:72, with permission.

LAB ACTIVITY 16.2

Objective: To perform a visual gait analysis.

Procedure: Get a partner. Choose one or more of the visual gait analysis forms presented in this chapter. Observe your partner walking at his or her comfortable gait speed, first from the sagittal plane, then from the frontal plane. You may wish to videotape several cycles of gait from both the sagittal plane and frontal plane. If you have access to a patient with an atypical gait pattern, you may wish to repeat this assignment with them.

Assignment

Question 1. Complete the gait analysis form you have chosen. If you use several different forms, consider the ease of using each form. How long did it take you to complete a visual gait analysis?

the cause. This information is used when determining appropriate interventions for retraining gait.

To practice your skills in OGA, perform Lab Activity 16.2.

Limitations to Observational Gait Analysis

Studies have shown that a major limitation of most OGA is poor reliability even among highly trained and experienced clinicians (Krebs et al., 1985). In addition, a detailed qualitative gait analysis is very time consuming and often unrealistic in a busy clinical environment. Finally, strong evidence does not support that OGA forms are sensitive to changes in gait patterns in response to therapy. This is the reason why technological systems are gaining support as methods to quantify movement patterns, muscle activation patterns, and forces used in gait. However, this technology is usually beyond the reach of most clinicians, and is extremely expensive, is time consuming, and requires considerable technical expertise to use.

Examination at the Impairment Level

A complete examination includes identifying underlying impairments that are potentially constraining mobility function and participation. The physical examination of underlying systems important to gait is often referred to as a "static evaluation," since it evaluates factors such as strength, ROM, and tone in passive situations such as while the patient is sitting or lying down. In contrast, a "dynamic evaluation" examines these systems while the patient is performing functional movements such as gait. Examination of underlying impairments was discussed in Chapter 5 and will not be repeated in this chapter.

Do Impairments Predict Gait Performance?

Static examination of factors such as strength, ROM, and spasticity is important; however, these factors do not always predict gait performance in patients with neurologic lesions. Nadeau et al. (1997) studied the relationship between plantarflexor strength and gait speed in subjects with hemiplegia. Results showed that subjects with hemiparesis were significantly weaker and slower compared to controls; however, strength in the plantarflexors was not significantly related to gait performance. Some patients with good plantarflexor strength walked at relatively slower speeds; in contrast, some patients with decreased plantarflexor strength could walk at relatively fast velocities (over 60 m/min). These individuals produced the faster gait velocity using alternative movement strategies, such as increased use of hip flexors for "pull-off" during swing as a substitute for decreased push-off in terminal stance (Nadeau et al., 1997).

While ankle strength may not predict gait performance, knee strength might. Perry and colleagues (1995) found that a combination of gait velocity and knee extension control was highly predictive of mobility function in individuals who had a stroke. Strong knee extension and a gait velocity of 16 m/min predicted community ambulation. Moderate and weak knee extension required at least 24 m/min and 32 m/min, respectively, to achieve community-level ambulation. In these patients, the loss of knee control required the substitution of other mechanisms to achieve the required gait speed.

While strength may not always correlate with gait parameters, sensation appears to. In the study by Nadeau et al. (1997), the patients with the lowest sensory scores tended to be the slowest walkers, supporting the findings of others (Brandstater et al., 1983; Lord et al., 1996; Perry et al., 1995).

Among persons with poststroke hemiparesis, perceived balance ability also has a significant effect on gait speed. Liphart and colleagues (2015) reported that gait speed was strongly related to perceived balance self-efficacy. Interestingly, there was a significant difference between perceived ability (as reported on the ABC test) and actual balance (as determined by performance on the BBS) in 35% of the 352 participants (Liphart et al., 2015).

Thus, the relationship between impairment and gait parameters is very complex and depends on many factors, including the type and extent of impairment, the functional level and perceived abilities of the individual, and the capacity for compensation by other systems.

Measuring Mobility: Do We Really Need All These Tests and Measures?

As you can see, examination of mobility using a task-oriented approach is very complex. It uses a range of tests and measures to quantify functional status (capacity in the ICF framework) and level of disability (performance in the ICF framework), describe gait strategies, and document underlying impairments. In this time of health care reform, when the amount of time available to examine and treat a patient is shrinking rapidly, do we really need all these measures? Is it really necessary to measure functional mobility, perform a visual gait analysis, and examine underlying impairments? We would argue that each provides essential information when establishing a plan of care for the person with mobility limitations.

For example, a static examination of underlying impairments determines the resources and constraints affecting gait and other aspects of mobility function. A dynamic evaluation using visual gait analysis can help a clinician determine the extent to which current strategies meet the requirements of gait in the face of underlying impairments. Functional measures, whether a single measure such as gait velocity or multiple measures available through mobility scales, document level of function and may help to predict disability. These measures are important for justifying the need for therapy and serve as outcome measures, quantifying change over time and in response to intervention. Thus, a clinician can use information from all levels of assessment to develop a comprehensive plan of care designed to maximize functional mobility status.

Before moving on to treatment, the reader is encouraged to review the case study presented in Figure 16.2 and complete Lab Activity 16.3, applying a task-oriented approach to examination.

Genise T is a 53-year-old woman, admitted to the hospital with right-sided weakness. An MRI indicated an ischemic stroke affecting the left periventricular corona radiata, extending into the posterior limb of the internal capsule with some extension in the external capsule. She is currently *1 month* poststroke. To see a video of Genise, refer to her video case study, which examines her underlying impairments and functional skills at 1 month poststroke.

Reason for referral: Outpatient therapy for continued impairments and functional limitations related to her stroke.

Medical history: She has a history of type II diabetes, hypertension, and hyperlipidemia, for which she takes medication. Following her 4-day stay in acute care, she spent 2 weeks in rehabilitation and was discharged to her home.

Social and work history: Genise lives with her husband in a single-level home. Prior to her stroke she was independent in all ADLs and IADLs. Prior to her stroke she worked as a worship leader in her church, composing and performing music.

ON EXAMINATION

I. Self-report participation and fall/balance history

Genise relies primarily on her wheelchair for mobility in her home and community. She reports walking in her own home with her cane and posterior stop AFO. She is independent in self-care activities (grooming, dressing, toileting, etc.), but requires assistance for all IADLs. Her primary social support is her husband; however, her mother and sister live nearby and are available to provide assistance as needed. She has had several falls since her return home; several while standing and leaning over to pick something up, or while walking.

II. Impairments in Body Structure and Function

A. Motor System Impairments

1. Voluntary, isolated movement: When asked to move her right arm, she has partial flexion at the elbow and shoulder, performed within a flexor synergy. With her arm supported to minimize the effect of gravity, she still has no active extension in her paretic arm. When she tries to extend her hand and wrist, instead of recruiting the extensors, a flexor synergy is recruited, resulting in flexion of the arm. When asked to flex her paretic leg, she flexes at the hip and knee and is now beginning to recruit ankle dorsiflexors within a flexor synergy pattern. Similarly, when extending her leg, plantarflexors are now recruited within an extensor synergy pattern. When asked to move only her ankle, she is not able to isolate ankle movement and instead recruits both the ankle dorsiflexors and plantarflexors within a total synergy pattern.

2. Range of motion: She has full range of motion at the shoulder and elbow but is beginning to develop tightness in her wrist and fingers flexors. She has limited range of motion in her right dorsiflexors.

3. Spasticity: Quick stretch of the biceps, wrist flexors, and ankle plantarflexors indicates the presence of spasticity. Her Ashworth score is 3.

B. Sensation

Genise has impaired light touch, two-point discrimination, and proprioception in both her paretic arm and leg; distal loss is greater than proximal loss. She has no visual problems.

C. Cognition

She has no cognitive impairments.

III. Postural Control

Impaired postural control is a significant factor contributing to Genise's limited functional abilities. She has had several falls since her return home; several while standing and leaning over to pick something up, or while walking.

Figure 16.2 Case Study of Genise T, at 1 month poststroke. *(continued)*

A. Sitting

Steady-state balance: Steady-state sitting balance is fairly good; her weight is slightly displaced to her left but she shows minimal sway. However, when her attention shifts to respond to questions, sway increases. She is able to maintain independent steady-state sitting balance with eyes closed. When displaced off vertical, with her eyes closed, she is not able to return to a symmetrical vertical position, suggesting verticality perceptions may be impaired.

Reactive balance: She is able to recover independently from small perturbations in all directions while sitting. However, in response to a large displacement to her paretic side, she is unable to reach for support with her paretic arm and has to be caught to prevent a fall.

Proactive balance: She has good proactive balance in sitting, and is able to reach forward > 10″, pick things up from the floor, and turn her head and trunk without loss of balance.

B. Standing

Steady-state balance: At 1 month, her steady-state balance in standing is better than it was at 4 days, but is still significantly impaired. She maintains stability but only for a few minutes, and stands asymmetrically with her weight shifted to the left. Note that when distracted, she sways back and to the right requiring assistance to prevent a fall. Steady-state balance does not change when she closes her eyes, suggesting that she is not overly reliant on vision, and is able to use somatosensory and vestibular inputs for postural control.

Reactive balance: She is unable to recover from loss of balance in either the forward or backward direction using an inplace strategy, and requires assistance to prevent a fall. In response to the lean and release test, Genise does step with her nonparetic leg, but requires assistance with recovery. Note that when she loads the paretic leg in order to step with the nonparetic leg, the knee snaps back into hyperextension to prevent collapse of the paretic leg.

Proactive balance: She has difficulty maintaining her balance during forward reach, and requires assistance to perform the task. She reports several falls when leaning over to pull up her pant legs when standing.

IV· Mobility

Bed mobility: She is independent in bed mobility skills, including rolling, and moving to the edge of bed.

Locomotion: At 1 month, Genise is able to walk without assistance using a quad cane and an ankle–foot orthosis. She is considered a nonfunctional, physiological walker, since her gait speed on the 10-Meter Walk test is 0.08 m/sec.Without an AFO, her gait pattern is characterized by an equinovarus foot position at initial contact, knee hyperextension at loading and throughout stance, and limited hip extension at terminal stance. She is unable to generate a push-off force with her paretic plantarflexors and uses hip flexion (pull off) to advance her paretic limb. During swing, she has reduced knee flexion and persistent plantarflexion, resulting in poor foot clearance. Using an AFO with a plantarflexion stop reduces knee hyperextension in stance and foot clearance in swing. Her gait speed does not change with an AFO. She completes the Timed Up and Go in single task conditions in 56 sec, indicating her increased risk for falls. When the TUG is performed with a secondary task, her time increases to 69 sec, and she makes multiple errors on the secondary task.

Figure 16.2 (*continued*)

LAB ACTIVITY 16.3

Objective: To apply a task-oriented approach to examining mobility function in a patient with hemiplegia and to establish goals and a plan of care for walking based on assessment information.

Procedures: Read the case study of Genise T in Figure 16.2. (or use a real case study if you have access to a patient with a neurologic diagnosis).

Assignment

Based on the information you have, answer the following questions

1. How would you classify Genise using the Perry ambulation classification system?
2. Which aspects of gait are affected in Genise, progression, stability, or adaptation?
3. What impairments are contributing to her hemiparetic gait pattern?

TRANSITION TO TREATMENT

Setting Goals

As is true for goal setting related to other physical skills, clinicians need to establish both long- and short-term goals during mobility retraining that are objective, measurable, and meaningful to the patient.

Long-Term Goals (Outcomes)

Long-term goals, or functional outcomes, are often stated in terms of functional performance and level of disability. They usually reflect ambulation outcomes with respect to level of independence and/or the context or conditions under which a patient will be able to walk. Examples of long-term goals might be the following: the patient will be able to walk independently a minimum of 1,000 ft in the community with the use of a cane and orthosis; the patient will be able to walk independently with a quad cane, 50 ft in her home environment; the patient will be able to walk independently using a single-point cane up and down curbs, on inclines and uneven surfaces; and the patient will be able to sustain a walking speed of 32 m/min with the use of a cane and orthosis for a distance of 1/4 mile.

Short-Term Goals

Short-term goals for mobility retraining can be expressed in terms of the following:

1. Changing underlying impairments. One example would be to decrease flexion contractures at the hip by 20 degrees, at the knee by 15 degrees, and at the ankle by 20 degrees.
2. Improving gait patterns. One example would be to decrease forward trunk flexion by 20 degrees and thereby improve upright posture during the stance and swing phases of gait.
3. Accomplishing interim steps toward long-term goals. Examples include the following: (a) increasing distance walked, with only standby assist, from 10 to 25 ft; (b) to increase speed, patient will be able to walk 200 ft, standby assist only, in 45 seconds; and (c) to become independent in the use of a front-wheeled walker.

Short-term goals usually lead to treatment strategies aimed at resolving underlying impairments and improving the quality of gait strategies. Long-term goals often lead to treatment strategies related to improving the overall performance of ambulation, such as increasing the distance walked or the speed of ambulation. Often, the two are interrelated, as when the goal is to improve a particular aspect of the locomotor pattern to increase the velocity of gait.

With comprehensive and realistic goals established, based on the patient's desires and problems, the clinician can move ahead to planning treatments designed to meet these goals.

TASK-ORIENTED APPROACH TO LOCOMOTOR TRAINING

The remaining portion of this chapter discusses a task-oriented approach to retraining mobility function, with an emphasis on locomotor training. While there is considerable evidence to support the importance of task specificity when retraining motor skills like walking, there is no consensus as to what constitutes a task-oriented approach to locomotor training. Task-specific locomotor training has been described as walking on a treadmill with (or without) body weight support (BWSTT) or alternatively using robotic devices used to assist or retrain stepping patterns. In their review, Winstein and Wolf (2009) suggest that in order for a training program to be considered task oriented, that is, focused on improving the performance of functional tasks, it must be as follows:

1. **Challenging** enough to induce variability and errors, require new learning, and to engage attention to solve the motor problem.
2. **Progressive and optimally adapted** to the patient's capability and the environmental context. Training must not be so simple or repetitive that the patient is not challenged, but neither can it be so challenging that the patient is unable to learn and to develop a sense of competence.
3. Interesting enough to invoke **active participation.**

A task-oriented approach (as defined in this book) to locomotor training includes a range of therapeutic interventions that are progressively challenging and organized around the goal of improving locomotor function. Our approach includes treatments aimed at (1) reducing underlying impairments of body structure and function that constrain gait, (2) modifying the GP to effectively and efficiently meet the progression and stability requirements of gait, and (3) developing the ability to adapt gait to changing task and environmental demands in order to maximize participation and minimize mobility disability. While this approach does not use preambulation skill training, it does use both part and whole practice to retrain mobility skills, including locomotion.

As discussed in Chapter 2, part practice refers to the process of breaking a skill such as walking down into component parts and practicing them in isolation. Part practice is always combined with whole-task practice, for example, using strategies such as BWSTT and overground walking to maximize stepping practice. Finally, our approach to task-oriented training places considerable emphasis on practicing locomotion (and other mobility skills) under varied task and environmental conditions in order to facilitate the ability to adapt functional skills to varying situations.

Interventions at the Impairment Level

The goal of treatment aimed at the impairment level is to maximize the sensory–motor resources available for the performance of functional mobility skills. As shown in Table 16.5, special emphasis can be given to musculoskeletal and other biomechanical impairments that constrain the use of gait strategies that are effective in meeting the essential requirements of progression, stability, and adaptation. For example, impairments that have a specific impact on the goal of progression include weakness of the ankle plantarflexors, which limits a forceful push-off in terminal stance, and shortened hip flexors and/or ankle plantarflexors, which limits the ability to advance the body over the stance foot. Weakness of the hip flexors will also impact the ability to advance the swing limb using a pull-off strategy. Impairments that have an impact on the goal of stability include weakness of the ankle, knee, and hip extensors, limiting the generation of an extensor support moment, and weakness of the hip abductors, which has an impact on mediolateral stability. Examples of treatment strategies aimed to improve impairments include stretching, sensory stimulation, voluntary movements with active-assistance, and strength training.

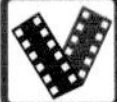

In the treatment case study of Genise, you can see examples of treatments aimed at her underlying impairments, including paresis or weakness and limited ROM. Prior to working on gait retraining, the therapist works on reducing musculoskeletal tightness in the foot and ankle through slow stretch of the intrinsic foot muscles and ankle plantarflexors. Slow stretching is done with the knee flexed as well as extended. In addition, by placing Genise's foot on her thigh, the therapist provides plantar stimulation and increased pressure through the joints to simulate weight-bearing through the limb. To improve recruitment of active movement in the paretic limb, the therapist uses a combination of quick stretch to the ankle dorsiflexors, combined with bilateral voluntary flexion at the hip, knee, and ankle. A second therapist is providing resistance to flexion on the nonparetic side, using overflow to assist flexion in the paretic limb. Treatments at the impairment level are immediately followed by task-specific practice of components of the GP, including use of a pull-off strategy to advance the paretic limb, as well as a push-off strategy.

Research Evidence

Does changing impairments improve gait function? Although most clinicians use treatment strategies to remediate underlying impairments, research summarized in the following suggests that improving underlying impairments alone may not be enough to ensure recovery of functional ambulation skills. For example, researchers have found that, while therapeutic strategies were effective in significantly increasing hip flexion ROM and improving trunk strength, improvements in these areas did not significantly improve gait speed (Godges et al., 1993). Judge and colleagues (1993) reported that gait measures did not change significantly in older adults following strengthening exercises. Krebs et al. (1998) examined the effect of moderate-intensity strength training on gait in 132 functionally limited older adults. Following 6 months of progressive resistive exercises, strength improved by 17.6%. While gait velocity did not significantly change, mediolateral stability (as measured by mediolateral center-of-mass [COM] excursion and velocity) significantly improved (Krebs et al., 1998).

Ouellette and colleagues (2004) used a program of high-intensity resistance training in long-term stroke survivors (average time since stroke, 32 months) and found significant improvements in muscle strength and peak power but no change in capacity-based measures of walking distance (6-minute walk) or speed (habitual or maximal gait velocity). Flansbjer et al. (2008) also reported that among persons with chronic stroke, progressive resistance training improved lower-extremity strength but did not affect scores on the TUG or the Stroke Impact Scale (their measure of participation). In contrast, Dragert and Zehr (2013) reported that high-intensity unilateral strength training of the **nonparetic** anterior tibialis (TA) in persons with chronic stroke produced significant improvement in strength and muscle activation in the paretic TA, which was more active in gait. The authors suggest that even when strength training of a paretic limb is not possible, high-intensity training of the nonparetic limb may be an effective strategy for both improving recruitment of muscles in the paretic limb and improving gait (Dragert & Zehr, 2013).

DeBolt and McCubbin (2004) examined the effects of a home-based resistance exercise program on power, balance, and mobility in adults with multiple sclerosis (see Chapter 11 for a more detailed description of the study) and found that resistance strength training resulted in increased lower-extremity power, but no changes in mobility as assessed by the TUG test.

Damiano and colleagues (2010) (Daminao and Abel, 1998) in a series of studies examined the effect of strength training on physical function in children with CP. These studies showed that children with CP had significantly improved strength in the targeted muscles. The effect of improved strength on gait parameters was variable, however. While in some children gait patterns improved, in others, gait patterns either did not change or were slightly worse. The authors suggest that given the variability of outcomes in strengthening studies in CP, methods are needed to better identify the individuals who are most likely to benefit from strengthening (Damiano et al., 2010).

Dibble and colleagues (2006, 2015) reported that among persons with PD, progressive resistance strength training in combination with flexibility exercises and static and dynamic balance exercises performed 3 times per week for 19 weeks significantly improved muscle strength and locomotor function (as measures on the FGA and 6-minute walk test) but did not impact measures of participation (Parkinson's Disease Questionnaire-39). While improvements were found in both on- and off-medication states, the largest effect size was found when exercise and medication were combined. In their systematic review and meta-analysis Li and colleagues (2020) reported that among persons with PD, lower limb resistance training has a positive effect on strength, quality of life, and can improve some aspects of gait performance.

Why are there conflicting research results on the effects of strength training on gait velocity? Research has shown that there is a nonlinear relationship between strength and gait speed in the lower-extremity muscles (Buchner et al., 1996). This is shown in Figure 16.3A, which plots leg strength versus usual gait speed in a group of older adult (average age 76 years) participants (Buchner et al., 1996). The hypothesized relationship between leg strength and gait speed is shown in Figure 16.3B. Since walking does not require maximum strength, normal walking

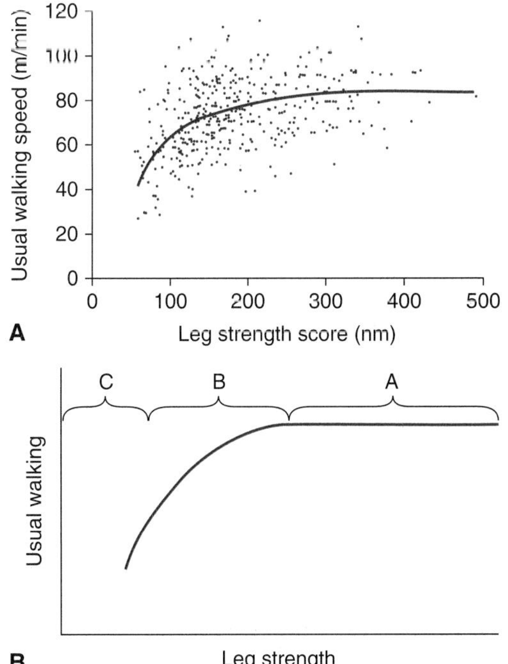

Figure 16.3 Relationship between strength and walking speed. **(A)** Plot of leg strength scores versus usual gait speed in older adult subjects. Shown also is the regression curve plotting strength versus speed for the average age of 76 and average body weight of 71 kg. **(B)** The hypothesized nonlinear relationship between gait speed and strength predicting the effect of changes in strength on gait speed. See text for further explanation. (Redrawn from Buchner DM, Larson EB, Wagner EH, et al. Evidence for a non-linear relationship between leg strength and gait speed. *Age Ageing*. 1996;25:387, with permission.)

speed could be maintained in the presence of a range of strength abilities (this is shown as a range of strength marked with an A in Fig. 16.3B). Thus, it is proposed that a patient who is already walking at this speed will not show further changes in gait speed in response to changes in strength. In contrast, the strength range marked by area B corresponds to the range in which decrements in strength will affect walking speed; thus, changes in strength will have an impact on gait speed. Finally, the strength range marked C illustrates the range of strength deficits in which walking is no longer possible.

A number of studies have shown that among persons with poststroke hemiplegic gait, augmenting conventional gait rehabilitation programs with visual mirror feedback and movement training in the nonparetic limb resulted in greater improvements in gait than conventional therapy alone (Ji & Kim, 2015; Sütbeyaz et al., 2007; see Thieme et al., 2012 for a review). Mirror therapy involves performing movements of the unimpaired limb while watching its mirror reflection superimposed over the (unseen) impaired limb, thus creating a visual illusion of enhanced movement capability of the impaired limb. This type of therapy is considered a special form of bilateral training and thought to exploit similar mechanisms (see Cauraugh & Summers, 2005; Thieme et al., 2012 for a review). Because there are very few studies on the use of mirror therapy in persons with stroke, there is no widely accepted agreement on the duration, timing, and frequency needed to achieve optimal outcomes.

In summary, current research suggests that treatments aimed at the resolution of impairments alone may not be enough to ensure recovery of ambulation skills. To optimize the recovery of locomotion, interventions aimed at improving gait strategies and functional performance are required as well.

Intervention at the Strategy Level: Improving the Gait Pattern

The goal of retraining at the strategy level is to assist the individual in developing a GP that is effective and efficient in meeting the essential requirements of progression, stability, and adaptation. While much of gait retraining strives to assist individuals in the recovery of previously used "normal" gait patterns, this may not be a realistic goal in the face of permanent sensory and motor impairments. Thus, a better standard for judging the efficacy of a person's GP is to ask, "Is he or she effective in meeting the demands of the task in the face of current impairments? Are current impairments potentially modifiable, and how will this change the strategies used for gait?"

Whole versus Part Practice Locomotor Training

Should gait training focus on practice of the whole pattern of walking, or can components of the gait cycle be practiced in isolation, so-called part practice? There is no consensus on the relative merits of part versus whole practice when retraining gait. As reviewed in Chapter 2, motor learning research suggests that breaking a motor skill down and practicing component parts (part practice) is effective when it is combined with whole-task practice. Whole GP practice can be performed overground without the use of additional equipment. Alternatively, whole practice gait training can involve use of technology such as BWSTT or robotic devices.

A number of researchers have proposed that whole practice alone, with its focus on achieving a high repetition of steps, is the most important aspect of locomotion training (see Hornby et al., 2011 for a review). However, other research has shown that an equally intense program of strength training combined with stance balance activities (including part practice gait strategies discussed in the following) was as effective in improving gait as whole practice using BWSTT in persons with stroke (Duncan et al., 2011). Thus, the approach to gait training presented here includes strategies for improving components of the GP (part-task practice) as well as whole-task practice.

Part Practice to Improve Components of the Gait Pattern

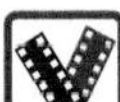

Postural Alignment and Stability. Treatments aimed at improving postural control include improving postural alignment of the HAT (head–arms–trunk) segment, effective generation of an extensor support moment in the stance limb, control of mediolateral stability (including placement of the foot at initial contact of stance), and improving balance in the single- and double-support phases of gait. Some stroke studies show that paresis of trunk muscles (flexors and extensors) interferes with balance, stability, and functional disability, and that postural alignment influences body control during walking and foot pressure (Karatas et al. 2004; Yang et al., 2015). Thus, many of the activities used in part practice gait training are designed to improve the stability component (controlled movement of the center of mass). This type of practice is often referred to as dynamic balance training.

Examples of part practice gait training activities may be seen in the treatment of stroke case study. Finally, assistive devices that broaden the base of support are another approach to managing stability problems during gait. To improve vertical alignment and stability in the HAT, manual cues can be given to the patient at the shoulders (shown in Fig. 16.4) combined with verbal cues to "look up." Assistive devices such as long poles (shown in Fig. 16.5) can be used to facilitate extension of the trunk and hips during walking.

Postural stability requires the ability to load the stance limb without collapsing. In patients who do not have sufficient knee control to prevent collapse during loading, the therapist can use manual cues and assistance to prevent collapse, while the patient works on weight-bearing activities in stance and gait. This activity can be seen in Genise's treatment video. Because Genise has difficulty loading her paretic limb without hyperextending the knee, the therapist uses both manual cues and physical assistance to control her knee position during activities such as STS, standing weight shifts, and during gait training. Other activities that can help a patient learn to load the paretic limb and practice controlling the center of mass relative to the changing base of support include stepping up onto a higher surface, such as a stool or taped newspapers (shown in Fig. 16.6), and weight shifting from side to side (Fig. 16.7A) and diagonally forward and backward (Fig. 16.7B).

In many persons with hemiparesis, such as Genise, hyperextension of the knee during loading and midstance is a frequent occurrence and can be controlled with an ankle–foot orthosis (AFO) with a plantarflexion stop (Montgomery, 1987; Mulroy et al., 2003; Perry & Burnfield, 2010; Rosenthal et al., 1975). A systematic review and meta-analysis study of randomized

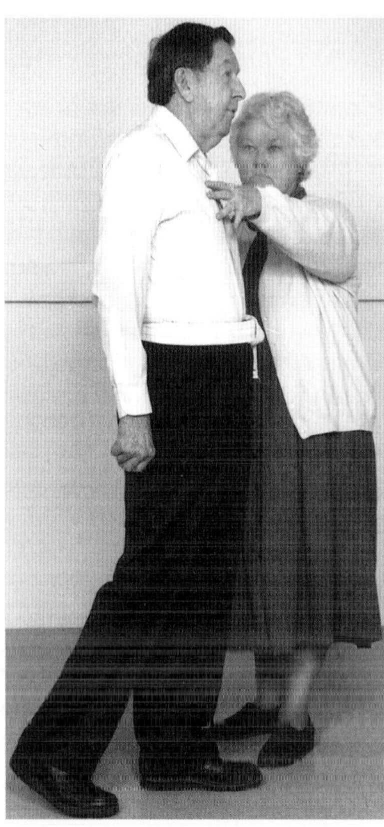

Figure 16.4 Assisting a patient learning to maintain a vertical trunk posture during gait with manual cues.

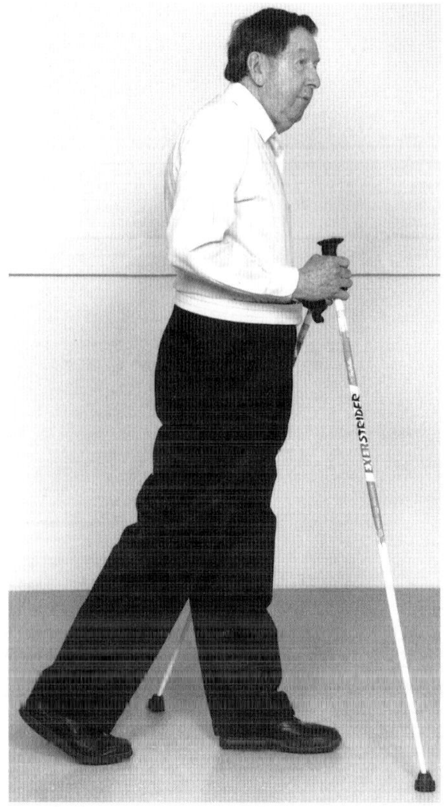

Figure 16.5 During gait retraining, long poles can be used to facilitate extension of the HAT segment.

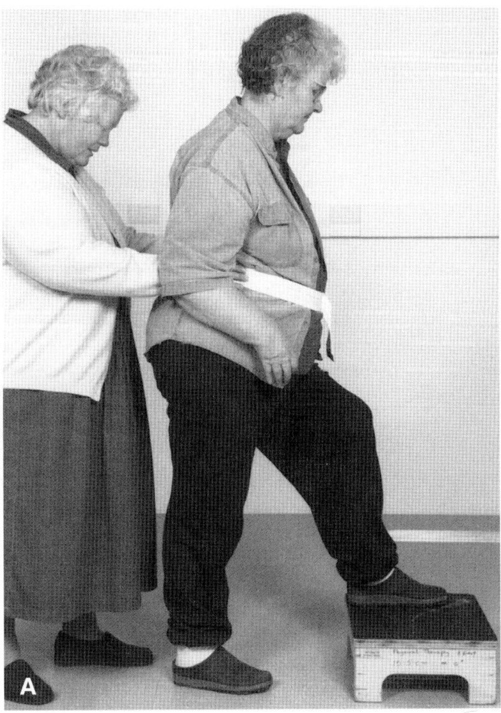
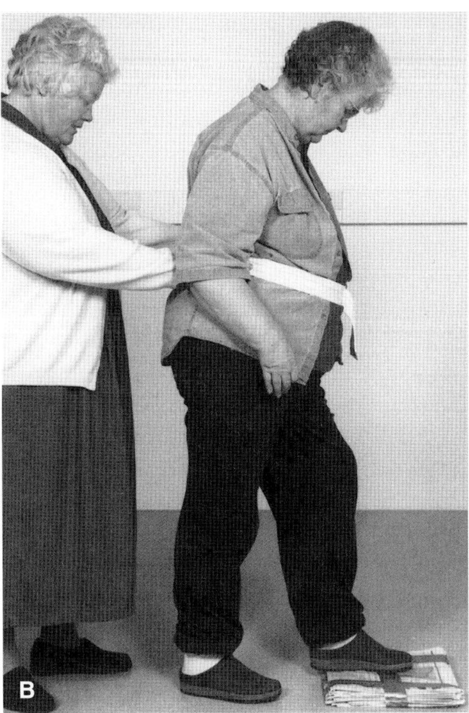

Figure 16.6 Activities that increase weight bearing in a single-limb stance include stepping up to a low stool **(A)** or to a taped stack of newspapers **(B)**.

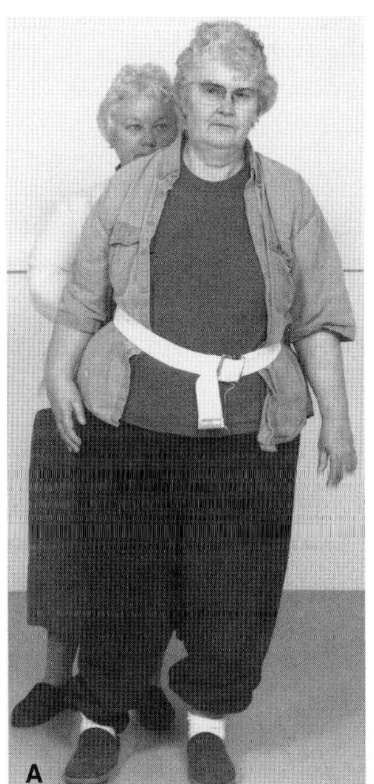
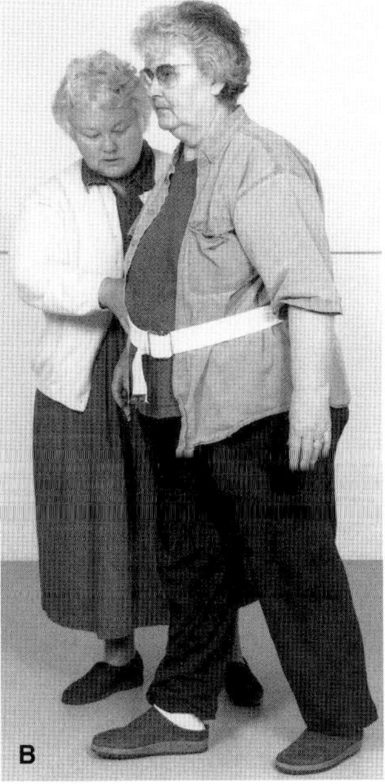

Figure 16.7 To improve stability, patients practice controlled movement of the COM in the lateral direction **(A)**, in the antero-posterior direction **(B)**, and in the diagonal direction (not shown).

controlled trials showed that an AFO implemented to control foot drop secondary to stroke can improve walking speed (Nascimento et al., 2020). The effect of this type of AFO on hyperextension during walking can be seen in the mobility section of Genise's case study video. Compare her gait as she walks with and without an AFO with a posterior stop to limit plantarflexion and control knee hyperextension. When plantarflexor spasticity is a primary contributor to knee hyperextension, techniques to decrease muscle tone in the plantarflexors have been recommended, including having the individual practice weight bearing with the ankle dorsiflexed, thus providing a slow stretch to the triceps surae (Carr & Shepherd, 1998; Montgomery, 1987).

Foot placement during initial contact and throughout the stance phase of gait is a major factor in determining stability; thus, improving movement and control of the ankle and foot at initial contact and during loading can significantly improve stability. Heel-strike foot contact with a smooth transition to a stable flatfoot position will facilitate both forward progression and a stable base of support important for stability. The treatment of problems impairing heel strike depends on the underlying cause.

Reducing musculoskeletal impairments that constrain a dorsiflexed position of the foot at initial contact is important. This includes stretching tight plantarflexors and hamstrings muscles to allow knee extension and ankle dorsiflexion. The use of myofascial release techniques to reduce tightness in the intrinsic muscles and fascia of the foot can be helpful in preparing the foot to accept weight and allowing motion at the foot as the shank moves forward over the stance foot. In Genise's treatment video, the therapist uses these treatments to prepare the paretic leg for task-specific part and whole practice of gait.

Inability to activate the TA muscle is a common cause of impaired heel strike in the patient with neurologic impairments. Strengthening exercises to increase force production of the TA are important in making sure the TA is capable of generating force in response to descending commands. Unfortunately, the capacity to generate force during a voluntary contraction of the muscle does not ensure that the muscle will be recruited automatically during gait. Nonetheless, strengthening is necessary to ensure that the capability for force generation is at least present.

Biofeedback and/or electrical stimulation of the TA in conjunction with a foot switch placed inside the patient's shoe has been used effectively to increase activation of the TA at heel strike and retrain the temporal activation of TA (Basmajian et al., 1975; Damiano et al., 2013; Pilkar et al., 2014; Takebe et al., 1975; Waters et al., 1975). Other studies have confirmed the positive effects of Functional Electric Stimulation (FES), timed to the gait cycle, on gait patterns in persons with stroke (Kim et al., 2012a; Lee et al., 2014; Tan et al., 2014; see Kafri & Laufer, 2015 for a review) and in children with CP (Damiano et al., 2013).

Manual cues to facilitate hip flexion, knee extension, and ankle dorsiflexion at terminal swing in order to ensure a heel-first foot-strike pattern can be used; this is shown in Figure 16.8. Use of manual cues to improve swing limb trajectory and initial foot placement can also be seen in Genise's treatment video. During her overground walking practice, the therapist uses verbal and manual cues to help Genise with flexion of the paretic limb as she moves into the swing phase of gait. In addition, manual guidance is used to help her achieve a smoother swing limb trajectory and improve her foot placement at initial contact.

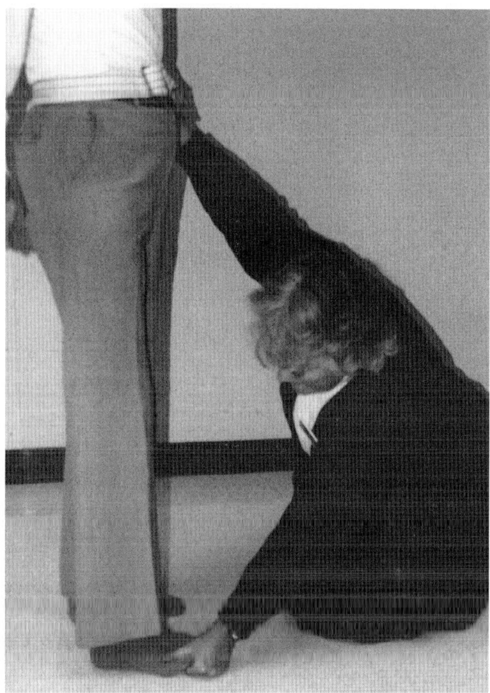

Figure 16.8 Helping the patient to accomplish a heel-first foot-strike pattern. This position will allow the body to move smoothly over the foot with good weight-bearing surface, enhancing both postural control and progression.

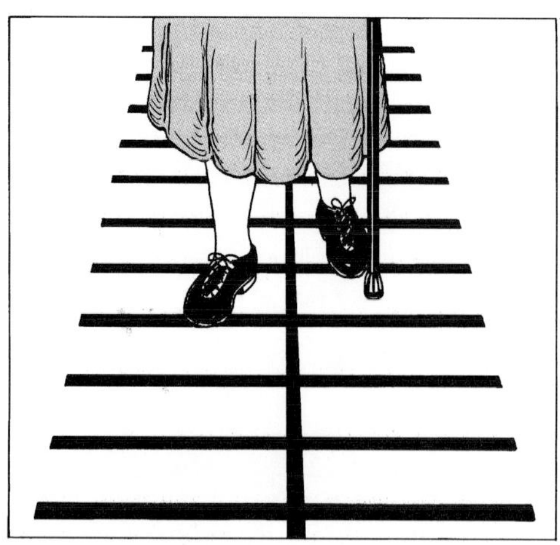

Figure 16.9 An example of a floor grid that can be used to visually guide patients toward better foot placement during gait. (Redrawn from Jims C. Foot placement pattern, an aid in gait training: suggestions from the field. *Phys Ther.* 1977;57:286, with permission of the American Physical Therapy Association. This material is copyrighted, and any further reproduction or distribution requires written permission from APTA.)

Improving foot placement by increasing step length can be assisted by making a grid on the floor, which helps to visually guide patients in establishing a better foot placement pattern. This is shown in Figure 16.9. The distance between horizontal stripes can be individualized to the patient's desired stride length (Jims, 1977).

Use of Assistive Devices. Assistive devices contribute to postural stability by widening the base of support and providing additional support against gravity. A variety of assistive devices are available to provide support, including walkers (standard and rolling), canes (quad, tripod, and single point), and various types of crutches (see Bateni & Maki, 2005, for a review). A progression of assistive devices is often prescribed based on changing stability requirements of the patient and the amount of support provided by the device (e.g., walker, quad or tripod cane, single-point cane). A number of factors are considered when prescribing an assistive device for a patient with neurologic impairments, including extent of physical disability, cognitive impairment, and the patient's personal motivations and desires (Allet et al., 2009; Schmitz, 1998). In addition, it is important to consider the effects of using various assistive devices on factors other than gait skills, such as attentional resources and their potential interference with balance in certain situations.

Wright and Kemp (1992) reported that attentional costs varied depending on the type of assistive device used and the person's familiarity with the device; for example, a rolling walker was less attention demanding than a standard pickup walker (Wright & Kemp, 1992). Since there is some evidence that competing demands for attentional resources by postural and cognitive systems contribute to instability in older adults (Shumway-Cook et al., 1997b), understanding the attentional requirements of the assistive devices we give patients is an important consideration during gait training.

In addition, while assistive devices do improve balance and mobility in many patients, they may also increase the risk of falling by causing trips or disruption of balance. A number of studies have reported that inappropriate device use, inadequate training, and use of nonprescribed assistive devices contribute to falls (Bateni et al., 2004a, 2004b; Milczarek et al., 1993).

Progression. The progression requirement of gait depends on both the generation of energy through concentric contractions and the absorption of energy through eccentric contractions. Impairments such as paresis and weakness will limit the generation of forces necessary for progression, while impairments such as spasticity and muscle shortening may result in inefficient gait through excessive energy absorption.

Strategies used to improve the progression component of gait, which can be seen in Genise's treatment video, are based on the research that energy generated for gait comes from a combination of the gastrocnemius contributing to push-off in terminal stance and the hip flexors, which pull off during initial swing. Patients practice a forceful push-off (concentric contraction of the plantarflexors) while maintaining an extended leg posture (e.g., hip extension coupled with plantarflexion of the ankle), as shown in Figure 16.10 and in Genise's treatment video. Genise stands in a trailing limb position and practices pushing off with her paretic leg, lifting the heel while the hip is extended and the knee flexes. This movement is associated with shifting her body weight diagonally over the nonparetic limb. Manual cues and assistance are given by her therapist as needed to facilitate this component of gait.

Functional electrical stimulation could be used to facilitate activation of paretic plantarflexors during walking (Awad et al., 2015). Since walking at faster speeds increases the posterior position of the paretic limb during double-support phase of gait, combining FES of the plantarflexors while walking on a treadmill at the patient's fastest speed has been shown to be effective in improving activation of paretic plantarflexors during gait (Awad et al., 2013, 2014). A randomized controlled trial investigated the additive effects of neuromuscular electrical stimulation (NMES) on walking (Yang et al., 2018). The experimental group received 20 minutes of NMES on either ankle dorsiflexors (TA) or ankle plantarflexors (medial gastrocnemius); the control group received 20 minutes of ROM and stretching exercises. After treatment, all received 15 minutes of ambulation training. The training program was 3 times per week for 7 weeks. The authors found that static and dynamic spasticity of ankle plantarflexors were significantly decreased after training, and the

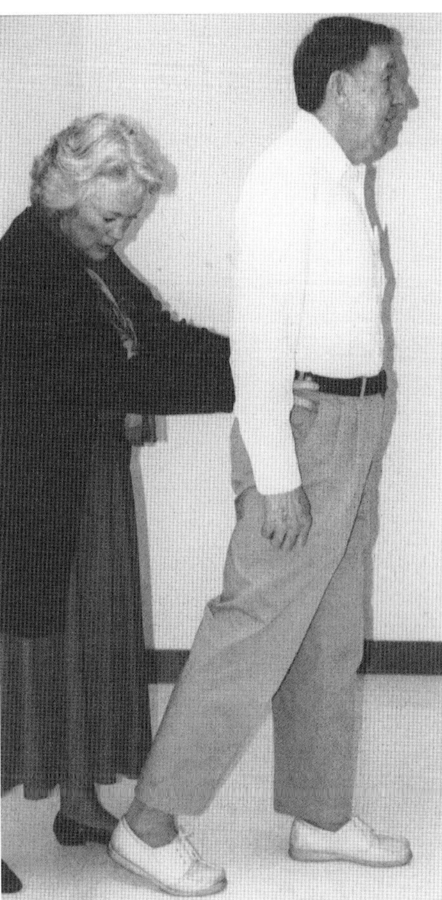

Figure 16.10 The patient practices a forceful push-off (concentric contraction) of the gastrocnemius, in an extended leg posture.

reduction in dynamic spasticity of ankle plantarflexors was significantly greater in the group that received NMES on TA compared to medial gastrocnemius. The authors also found that the group that received ankle dorsiflexors-NMES had greater improvements in spatial asymmetry, ankle plantarflexion during push-off, and muscle strength (ankle dorsiflexors) compared to control subjects (Yang et al., 2018).

To improve the ability of the hip flexors to participate in generation of power for progression, Genise also practices pull-off (exaggerating hip flexion) during the initiation of swing. Manual cues and support of the leg are provided by the therapist as needed. Other activities to facilitate hip flexion during swing have been used, including marching in place and practicing a high-step gait—that is, bringing the knee up into an exaggerated flexed position (Fig. 16.11). Finally, as shown by Olney et al. (1991, 1994), increasing the speed of walking will have a tendency to increase the speed and amplitude of hip flexion during the initiation of the swing phase of gait, and this will facilitate passive knee flexion for toe clearance.

To advance the swing limb, clearing the supporting surface with the foot requires activation of the plantarflexors at push-off in conjunction with hip flexors at

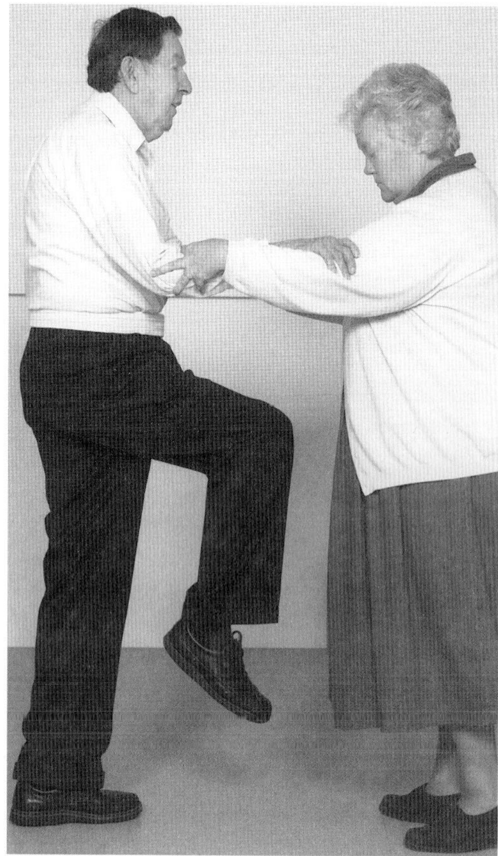

Figure 16.11 Improving the use of the hip flexors to pull off the swing limb through practice of a high-step gait pattern.

the initiation of swing, to draw the thigh segment forward with sufficient force to passively flex the knee. In addition, activation of the TA to dorsiflex the ankle is also important to the achievement of foot clearance. Thus, loss of foot clearance can be caused by (1) weakness of the plantarflexors, hip flexors, and/or TA, (2) spasticity of the ankle plantarflexors and/or hamstrings, or (3) neural control problems affecting the appropriate activation of muscles such as the TA muscle during swing. Thus, treatments aimed at each of these problems combined with task-specific practice of the swing phase of gait are indicated. Additional suggestions to improve flexion of the swing limb were described in earlier sections on postural support and stability.

Improving Arm Swing. Evidence indicates that upper and lower limb movements influence each other during locomotor-like tasks (Hong et al., 2020; Meyns et al., 2012a; Stephenson et al., 2010). Thus, including arm movements in rehabilitation of gait in order to affect interlimb coordination has been shown to improve gait in a number of patient populations, including PD (Behrman et al., 1998), stroke (Dietz, 2011), and children with CP (Meyns et al., 2012b). Improved coordination of the upper and lower extremities normalized angular momentum and decreased energy expenditure during gait (Bruijn et al., 2008), thus impacting the progression component of gait. In addition, improved arm swing had an impact on mediolateral stability, thus impacting the stability component of gait. Instructions to actively increase arm swing amplitude resulted in improved gait in persons with stroke (Ford et al., 2007a, 2007b; Wagenaar et al., 1994) and PD (Behrman et al., 1998; Bruijn et al., 2008).

Sliding handles on a handrail have also been used to enhance arm swing during gait training on a treadmill. Additionally, compared to fixed handrails, sliding handrails resulted in increased lower limb muscle activation and reduced weight bearing through the upper limbs (Stephenson et al., 2009). Similarly, the rhythmic swing of upper limbs during a robot-assisted walking training in patients with subacute stroke is associated with greater improvements in the Berg Balance Scale, Fugl-Meyer, and modified Barthel index score (Kang et al., 2018).

Research Evidence. Does locomotor training alter underlying gait patterns in persons with stroke? The evidence for this is mixed. Mulroy and colleagues (2010) characterized changes in gait parameters in participants with post-stroke hemiparetic gait who had completed 6 weeks of locomotor training. Gait characteristics were compared among a high-response group (participants who showed an increase in gait speed of greater than 0.08 m/s) versus a low-response group (those with less than a 0.08 m/s improvement). After the intervention, the high-response group had greater improvements in kinematic, kinetic, and muscle activity patterns as compared with the low-response group. These changes—including increased terminal stance hip extension, hip flexion power, and intensity of soleus muscle EMG activity—were associated with increases in gait speed. The results of this study suggest that in persons with stroke, training that results in improved gait velocity is associated with concomitant changes in the underlying GP.

In contrast, Den Otter et al. (2006) found that improvements in gait speed were not associated with a change in the temporal pattern of muscle activity in the lower extremities in persons with stroke participating in 10 weeks of locomotor rehabilitation. Despite improved gait speed and function, duration of muscle coactivity, abnormal muscle timing, and gait asymmetry persisted. The authors conclude that recovery of walking ability following stroke is not dependent on normalization of the temporal coordination of muscle activity. Thus, the degree to which training affects underlying characteristics of abnormal gait is uncertain.

Whole Practice Gait Training

As mentioned earlier, motor learning research suggests that part practice of the components of gait must be combined with whole-task practice, that is, practice of the entire gait cycle itself, in order to be effective. Whole-task gait training over level ground is at the heart of most locomotor training programs (LTPs).

Whole practice gait training can also involve the use of technology such as BWSTT and robotic devices. A large percentage of Genise's LTP both in the clinic and at home includes practice walking overground using an assistive device. Gait training is done with her AFO and also without her AFO to facilitate the use of ankle muscles during gait. Practice is done both with and without manual and verbal feedback cues. In the clinic, BWSTT with therapist provided manual assistance is also used to increase step practice.

Unfortunately, research suggests that the amount of walking practice within a therapy session may be insufficient to optimize learning. While gait training was the most practiced activity performed in physical therapy (~40% of time of PT sessions), patients averaged only 300 to 800 steps per PT session (Lang et al., 2007, 2009; Moore et al., 2010). This is far below animal models of locomotion training, where the number of repetitions of steps ranged from 1,000 to 2,000 steps per session (Cha et al., 2007; De Leon et al., 1998). In light of this research, many researchers have recommended the use of technology such as BWSTT or robotic-assisted stepping to enhance walking practice.

Research Evidence. How important is the use of this technology to locomotor recovery? What evidence do we have that technology-assisted locomotor training improves walking function? Is technology-assisted locomotor training superior to other forms of training?

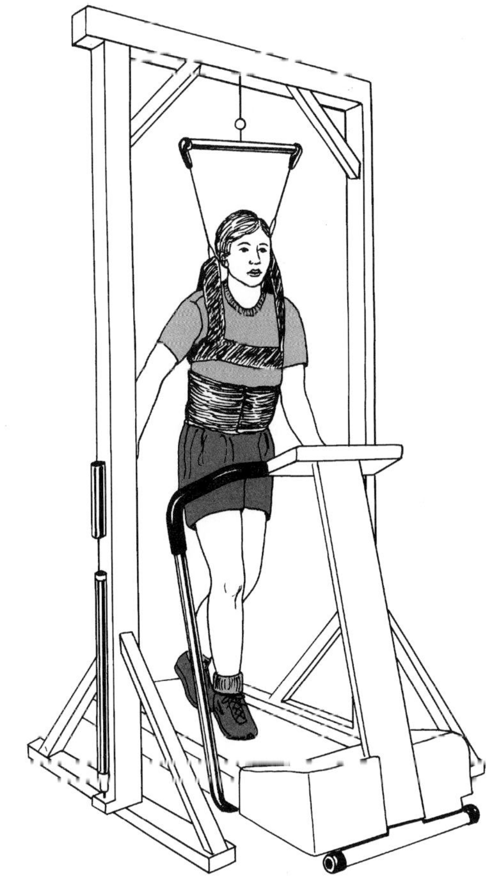

Figure 16.12 Gait retraining using a treadmill and harness system for partial support of body weight.

Treadmill training with and without body weight support. BWSTT uses a harness to provide partial body weight support in conjunction with a motorized treadmill to facilitate extended practice of the entire GP. An example of a BWSTT system is shown in Figure 16.12.

Some of the earliest training studies supporting the effectiveness of BWSTT were by Hesse and colleagues (1994, 1995, 1999). Since then, a number of studies have confirmed the positive effects of BWSTT on gait function in persons with stroke (Ada et al., 2003; Richards et al., 2004; Sullivan et al., 2002) and other patient populations, including those with PD (Cakit et al., 2007; Miyai et al., 2002), children with CP (Gates et al., 2012; Johnston et al., 2011; Richards et al., 1997), and young children with Down syndrome (Ulrich et al., 2001).

Research is beginning to identify the specific dosage required to impact gait in various populations. While in the Sullivan study, 4 weeks of treadmill training significantly improved gait in persons with stroke, a 2-week program of treadmill training was not effective in modifying ataxic gait in 12 patients with acute cerebellar stroke (Bultmann et al., 2014). Given the nature of motor learning deficits in persons with cerebellar pathology, a longer period of training may be needed to improve function. In a single case study, a 6-month program of almost daily (5 days/week) locomotor training using BWS on a treadmill in conjunction with overground gait training was an effective way to improve ambulatory function in a 13-year-old child with severe cerebellar ataxia (Cernak et al., 2008). Further research is needed to determine the dose of locomotor training needed to improve locomotor function in persons with cerebellar ataxia and patients with other neurologic diagnoses.

Is BWSTT superior to other approaches to balance and gait training? Several studies suggest that this is not the case (Duncan et al., 2011; Middleton et al., 2014; Richards et al., 2004). The Locomotor Experience Applied Post-Stroke (LEAPS) trial was a single-blinded, randomized rehabilitation trial to determine if, in addition to usual care, a specialized LTP that included BWSTT was superior to a physical therapy program of progressive strength and balance exercises delivered in a home environment. In this study, 408 participants (mean age 62 years), stratified according to severity of walking impairment (moderate 0.4 to >8 m/s vs. severe <0.4 msec), were randomly assigned to one of three groups: early LTP involving BWSTT begun at 2 months poststroke, late LTP involving usual care from 2 to 6 months followed by BWSTT begun at 6 months poststroke, or a home exercise program involving a physical therapist–directed program of progressive strength and balance exercises begun at 2 months poststroke. Interventions involved 36 sessions, 90 minutes each, over 12 to 16 weeks. At 1 year poststroke, outcomes were comparable across all three groups; 52% of all participants had significantly improved their functional walking. At 6 months, the two groups receiving augmented therapy (either BWSTT or home exercise program) in addition to usual care had better outcomes than the group receiving just usual care alone (Duncan et al., 2011).

A Cochrane systematic review compared no walking or overground walking to mechanically assisted walking training with or without body weight support in children with CP. The authors concluded that compared with no walking, mechanically assisted walking training (with or without body weight support), may result in small increases in walking speed and may improve gross motor function (when combined with body weight support). It appears that dose-matched overground walking and mechanically assisted walking training with body weight support result in comparable improvements in walking speed and gross motor function. The authors cautioned that robust conclusions could not be made from the reviewed papers because for the most part results were not clinically significant, sample sizes were small, and the risk of bias and intervention intensity were highly variable across studies (Chiu et al., 2020)

Results from these studies suggest that BWSTT may be an effective approach to improving gait in a wide variety of patient populations, though not necessarily superior to other forms of training given at equal intensity. Helbostad (2003) suggested that while not superior to other forms of therapy, BWSTT may be the only alternative for walking training in persons who are not able to walk, even with support from walking aids or other persons.

Robot-aided gait training. Robotic devices, such as the Lokomat (Hocoma, Inc., Zurich, Switzerland), have been developed to automate locomotor training in neurorehabilitation (Westlake & Patten, 2009). A number of randomized clinical trials have demonstrated that robot-aided locomotor training is effective in improving gait in stroke (Hidler et al., 2009; Hornby et al., 2008; Schwartz et al., 2009; Westlake & Patten; 2009), PD (Picelli et al., 2012a, 2012b), MS (Lo & Triche, 2008; Schwartz et al., 2012; Vaney et al., 2012), and CP (Carvalho et al., 2017; Meyer-Heim et al., 2009; Wu et al., 2014). Kang and colleagues (2017) used a motorized-cable driven robot called the Tethered Pelvic Assist Device (TPAD) to retrain crouch gait in children with spastic diplegic CP (GMFCS II). TPAD consists of a lightweight belt placed on the waist with four wires connecting it to motors connected to an external rigid frame. The cables are controlled in real time to generate a constant downward pull while the child walks on a treadmill. The robotic gait intervention included fifteen training sessions (16 minutes each) for 6 weeks. Results showed a significant increase in the activation and improved timing of the soleus muscle, a straighter positioning of lower limbs during the mid-stance phase, and improved overground walking as measured by the 6-minute walking test.

A number of studies have reported that robot-aided training is not superior to (1) therapist-assisted gait training in persons with stroke (Hornby et al., 2008) and CP (Drużbicki et al., 2013), (2) equal-intensity treadmill training or therapist-directed balance training in persons with PD (Picelli et al., 2013, 2015), or (3) other forms of therapy in persons with MS (Lo & Triche, 2008; Schwartz et al., 2012; Vaney et al., 2012). Therefore, the appropriateness of using complex and highly expensive technology in locomotor training in persons with neurologic pathology is being questioned. In their review, Dobkin and Duncan (2012) suggest that because research has not shown the superiority of BWSTT and robotic-assisted step training over a comparable dose of progressive overground training, these technologies should not replace overground walking training in routine clinical practice.

Training Adaptation: Complex Walking Tasks

A comprehensive LTP includes having patients practice walking under a variety of tasks and environments in order to learn to adapt gait to functional demands likely to be encountered in the home and community environment. As patients learn to develop strategies effective in meeting the task requirement of locomotion in relatively nondemanding environments, such as on a level surface, training is broadened to include achieving functional walking skills under more complex and challenging conditions. As discussed earlier, these activities are often referred to as dynamic gait or complex walking activities.

Complex walking activities are designed to improve both anticipatory and reactive components of postural control during ambulation. In addition, tasks are used to improve the ability to walk under altered sensory contexts or while performing other tasks (e.g., varying the cognitive load). In Table 16.6, we summarize a framework for organizing dynamic gait activities based on the eight environmental dimensions identified in the work by Shumway-Cook and colleagues (Patla & Shumway-Cook, 1999; Shumway-Cook et al., 2002, 2003, 2005b). This table lists the eight dimensions, the goal for gait training in each dimension, and examples of some of the activities that could be used to train each dimension of locomotor adaptation. Examples of activities for training in the density dimension (avoidance of static and dynamic obstacles) include practicing stepping over

TABLE 16.6 Summary of Environmental Dimensions and Associated Activities to Promote Locomotor Adaptation, Based on a Proposed Framework by Patla and Shumway-Cook (1999)

Dimension	Items
Distance	**Goal:** Increase distance walked at comfortable speed, community ambulation goal 1,200 ft. **Activities:** • Practice continuous walking while gradually increasing distance walked.
Temporal	**Goal:** Increase comfortable and fast walking speeds, ability to change speeds safely. Community ambulation goal: comfortable walking speed of ≥0.45 m/s, with ability to walk ≥0.8 m/s for distances of 40 ft (to cross streets). **Activities:** • Practice continuous walking at comfortable speed, gradually increasing gait velocity. • Practice fast walking, gradually increasing gait velocity. • Practice increasing and decreasing speed safely, with short bursts of fast walking for distances of 40 to 60 ft.
Ambient	**Goal:** Walk safely under different light and weather conditions. **Activities:** • Practice walking under different light-level conditions and during transitions in light (e.g., light to dark, dark to light). • Practice walking outside in different light and weather conditions.
Terrain	**Goal:** Ability to walk safely under changing terrain characteristics. **Activities:** • Practice walking on uneven surfaces, up and down curbs, ramps. • Practice walking up- and downstairs.
Physical load	**Goal:** Ability to walk safely while interacting with physical loads, including carrying/pushing/pulling loads. **Activities:** • Practice walking while carrying weights, gradually increasing the weight of objects carried. • Practice carrying weight distributed over one or two packages carried in the arms (e.g., grocery bag) or held by hand (e.g., plastic bag with handles). • Practice carrying loads of varying fragility and predictability (e.g., paper cup vs. water glass [filled to various levels], tray with rolling ball or egg). • Practice opening/closing manual doors of varying weights. • Practice walking while pushing/pulling loads of varying weights.
Postural transitions	**Goal:** Ability to walk safely while making postural transitions **Activities:** • Practice static stance tasks—standing reach above, below, and forward; stepping forward, sideways, backward; stepping up (forward, sideways).

(*continued*)

TABLE 16.6 Summary of Environmental Dimensions and Associated Activities to Promote Locomotor Adaptation, Based on a Proposed Framework by Patla and Shumway-Cook (1999) (*continued*)

Dimension	Items
	• Practice dynamic tasks that require proactive balance control, such as walking with postural transitions, including walking with head turns; change in direction; pivot turns; walking forward, sideways, and backward; walking with wide/narrow base of support; walking with long/short steps, stops, and starts; sit-to-stand and walk. • Practice recovery of balance while walking: walking on treadmill with varying speeds, walking against unpredictable and variable resistance from elastic tubing, walking while recovering from small external perturbations given manually.
Attentional demands	**Goal:** Maintain safe ambulation while concurrently performing a secondary manual or cognitive task. Also includes ability to walk in noisy distracting environments and to navigate in novel environments. **Activities:** • Practice walking while simultaneously performing secondary cognitive tasks (see Table 11.11 for examples of tasks used in training). • Practice walking in noisy, crowded, and distracting environments (busy hallways, hospital dining room, therapy rooms with loud distracting music playing, malls). • Practice walking and navigating to familiar and unfamiliar places.
Density and collision avoidance	**Goal:** Ability to walk safely while avoiding contact with obstacles in the environment. **Activities:** • Practice walking over, around, and under static objects that vary in height/width and fragility. • Practice walking over and around dynamic (moving) obstacles. • Collision avoidance should be practiced with objects presented on the floor as well as overhead, requiring persons to duck under an object.

obstacles of various heights (Fig. 16.13A) or walking around obstacles (Fig. 16.13B). Training activities in the postural dimension include walking a straight path while turning the head (Fig. 16.14); training in the physical load dimension includes walking while interacting with an external physical load, such as carrying an object (Fig. 16.15A) or opening a heavy door (Fig. 16.15B). What is the evidence that task-oriented practice of functional gait tasks improves locomotor function in different patient populations?

Research Supporting Locomotor Training in Specific Patient Populations

There is a broad and extensive body of research examining the effect of training on locomotor function in patients with specific neurologic pathology, including stroke, MS, PD, CP, and traumatic brain injury. A review of some of these studies may be found in Extended Knowledge Box 16.1.

Virtual Reality

Recognizing the importance of incorporating changing tasks and contexts into locomotor retraining in order to facilitate gait adaptation, researchers are combining treadmill training with virtual reality (VR) or augmented reality (AR) systems that simulate obstacles and other tasks that require modifying step characteristics (van Ooijen et al., 2013, 2015). These systems can be used to project visual images down onto a treadmill or onto a screen in front of a treadmill to add contextual variability. A systematic review and meta-analysis identified that the addition of virtual reality and biofeedback during functional gait training can increase engagement and magnify the therapeutic effects in children and young adults with CP (Booth et al., 2018).

Examples of visual tasks projected onto a treadmill are shown in Figure 16.16 and include visually guided stepping (practice of foot positioning relative to a projected sequence of irregularly spaced stepping

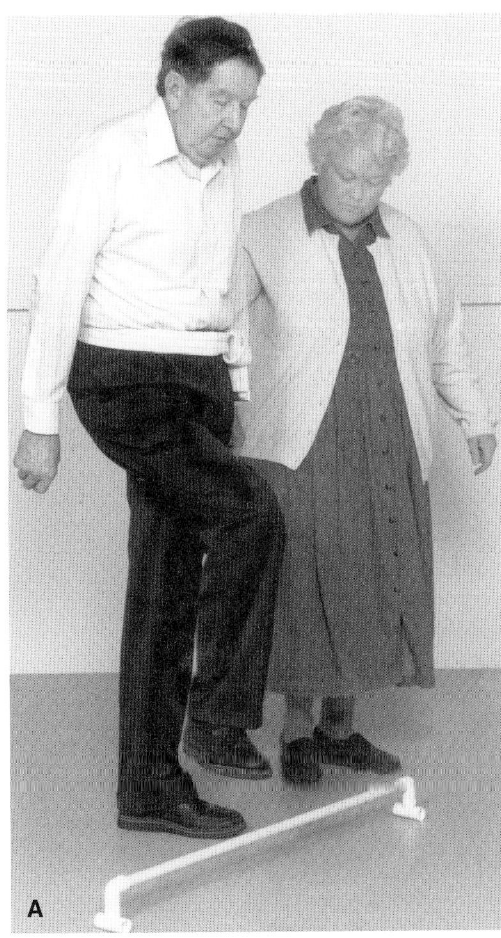

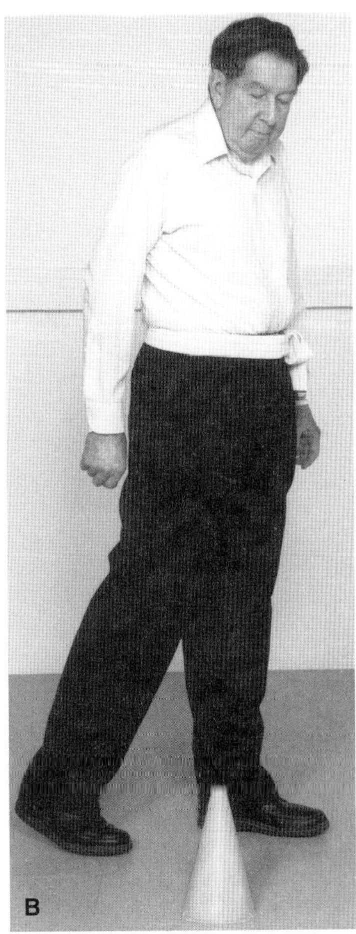

Figure 16.13 Retraining complex walking tasks. Practicing collision avoidance by stepping over **(A)** and around **(B)** obstacles.

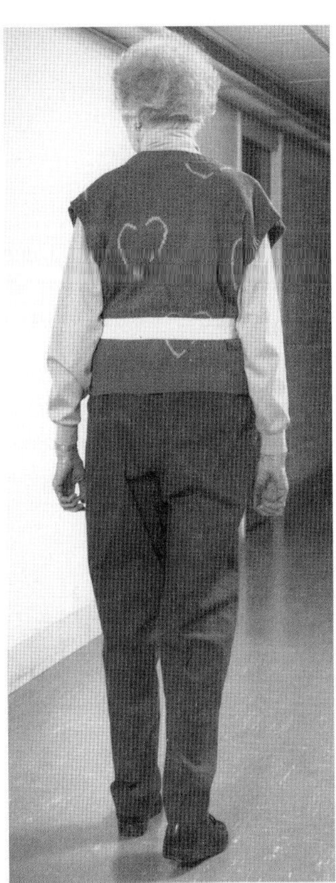

Figure 16.14 Retraining complex walking tasks. Walking a straight path while practicing head turns.

targets) (Fig. 16.16A), obstacle avoidance (practice of avoidance of visual obstacles projected onto the belt's surface) (Fig. 16.16B and C), speeding up and slowing down, tight-rope walking, and other functional gait adaptability games (kicking interactive targets, such as balls [Fig. 16.16D], or avoiding stepping onto obstacles). What is the evidence to support the use of VR systems such as the one described previously in locomotor training?

Research Evidence. VR exercise programs use computer-simulated interactive environments to promote movement. Researchers have examined the use of VR with and without treadmill training and have shown it to improve clinical measures of functional mobility in adolescents with CP (Brien & Sveistrup, 2011; van der Krogt et al., 2014), persons with traumatic brain injury (Thornton et al., 2005), community-living older adults (Bisson et al., 2007), and persons with stroke (Cho & Lee, 2014; Lloréns et al., 2015; Navarro et al., 2013). Mirelman and colleagues (2011) developed a VR system that incorporates treadmill training with virtual obstacle negotiation and investigated its effects among patients with PD. Twenty patients (mean age 67 years) received 18 sessions (3 per week) of progressive intensive treadmill training with virtual obstacles. Training resulted in significant improvements in gait speed under

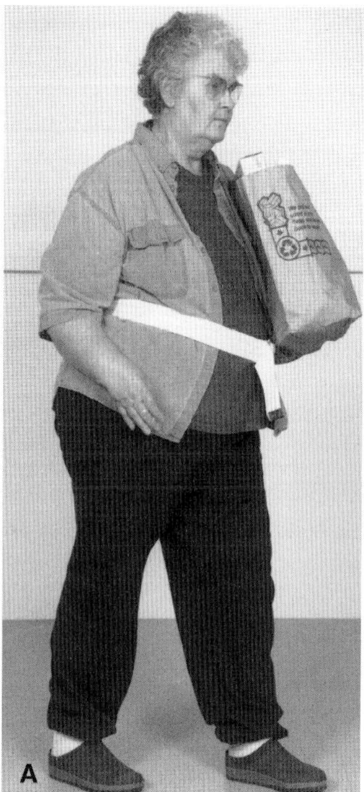

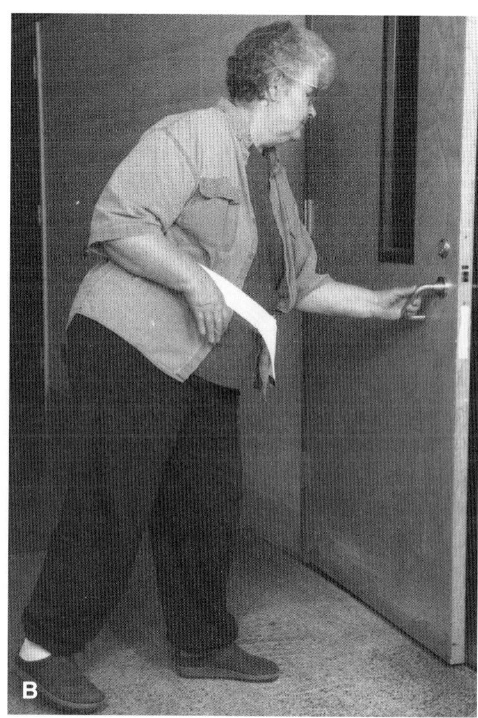

Figure 16.15 Retraining complex walking tasks. Practicing gait while interacting with external physical loads such as carrying an object **(A)** or opening a heavy door **(B)**.

Extended Knowledge 16.1

Research Supporting Locomotor Training in Specific Patient Populations

Stroke

There is considerable research examining task-oriented locomotor training in persons with stroke. In the study by Salbach et al. (2004), 91 individuals less than 1 year poststroke were randomly assigned to receive a 6-week intervention (60 minutes, 3 times a week) that targeted walking or UE function. Locomotor training included a progressive program of 10 functional tasks, including walking on a treadmill, standing up and walking to and sitting down on a chair, kicking a soccer ball against a wall, walking a balance beam, performing step-ups, walking an obstacle course, walking while carrying an object, walking at maximal speed, walking backward, and walking up and downstairs. A control group practiced UE tasks while sitting. Results found that compared to those in the UE training, participants in the walking intervention improved on all measures of gait, with the greatest improvements found in the subjects with moderately severe gait problems.

Circuit based-exercises (or circuit training) include diverse task oriented locomotor activities. According to the terms defined by Medical Subject Headings, circuit training is defined as "an alternate set of exercises that works out different muscle groups and that also alternates between aerobic and anaerobic exercises, which, when combined together, offer an overall program to improve strength, stamina, balance, or functioning." Mudge and colleagues (2009) reported that following 12 sessions of circuit-based locomotor training participants with stroke walked significantly further on the 6-minute walk test, though improvements were not retained at 3 months. Dean and colleagues (2000) also reported improvements in gait function following 12 sessions (3 times a week for 4 weeks) of circuit training in persons with chronic stroke.

Pang and colleagues (2005) reported that a multidimensional group-based community fitness and mobility exercise program performed 1 hour, 3 times a week for 19 weeks significantly improved VO_2max, 6-minute walk test distance, paretic leg muscle strength, and hip bone density in persons with chronic stroke compared to controls receiving a seated exercise program.

Multiple Sclerosis

A multidimensional exercise program incorporating task-oriented practice has been shown to improve mobility in persons with MS with a range of disability (Chisari et al., 2014; Kalron et al., 2015; Motl et al., 2012). Motl and colleagues (2012) examined the effect of a multidimensional exercise program on mobility in persons with MS and moderate disability (EDSS 4 to 6). The program was delivered by a trained professional, 60 minutes, 3 times a week for 8 weeks, and included aerobic exercise (i.e., leg cycle ergometry, treadmill walking, elliptical, or seated rowing exercise), resistance exercise (i.e., squats, knee flexion/extension, and ankle dorsiflexion/plantarflexion using resistance bands), and task-oriented balance and activities (i.e., single-leg stands, figure eights, stair stepping, and heel-to-toe line walk). Exercise was associated with significant improvements in mobility measures including TUG, timed 25-foot walk test, and Multiple Sclerosis Walking Scale-12 (Motl et al., 2012). Similarly, Kalron et al. (2015) reported that in persons with relapsing–remitting MS, a 3-week multidimensional exercise program resulted in significant improvements in walking measures (10-meter walk test, TUG, and 2 minute walk test); the greatest improvements were in the moderate and severe groups compared to the mild gait disability group. In a single-blinded randomized controlled trial, Özkul and colleagues (2020) investigated the effects of a task-oriented circuit training on motor and cognitive performance in people with MS. The authors found that the investigated

Extended Knowledge 16.1 *(continued)*

training program substantially improved balance as well as walking abilities in patients with MS. However, they did not find a significant effect on cognitive performance, except for verbal memory.

Parkinson's Disease

A number of studies have demonstrated the positive effects of different training strategies on locomotor function in persons with PD. The evidence for BWSTT and robotic-assisted training in persons with PD were reviewed earlier and so will not be discussed here. Morris (2006) has provided an overview of training at different stages of progression in PD. Consistent across all stages is the repetitive practice of walking under varying task (straight line walking, turns, obstacles, etc.) and environmental conditions (e.g., varying distances and surfaces).

Task-oriented locomotor training combined with verbal instructions to focus on different aspects of gait has been shown to improve gait in persons with PD (Behrman et al., 1998; Lehman et al., 2005; Werner & Gentile, 2010). For example, walking practice with instructions to increase step length (e.g., "think big" or "take a big step") or stride length ("long strides") improved gait function in persons with PD (Farley & Koshland, 2005; Morris et al., 1996; Werner & Gentile, 2010), with improvements retained up to 1 month (Sidaway et al., 2006; Werner & Gentile, 2010). Combining walking practice with performance of a secondary task has also been shown in improve gait function in persons with PD (Bilney et al., 2003; Brauer & Morris, 2004). These studies all suggest that repetitive practice of locomotor tasks can significantly improve gait function in persons with PD and that improvements may be retained following completion of training.

In summary, this research examining the effects of repetitive practice of walking-related tasks shows significant improvements in locomotor function in a wide range of persons with neurologic pathology.

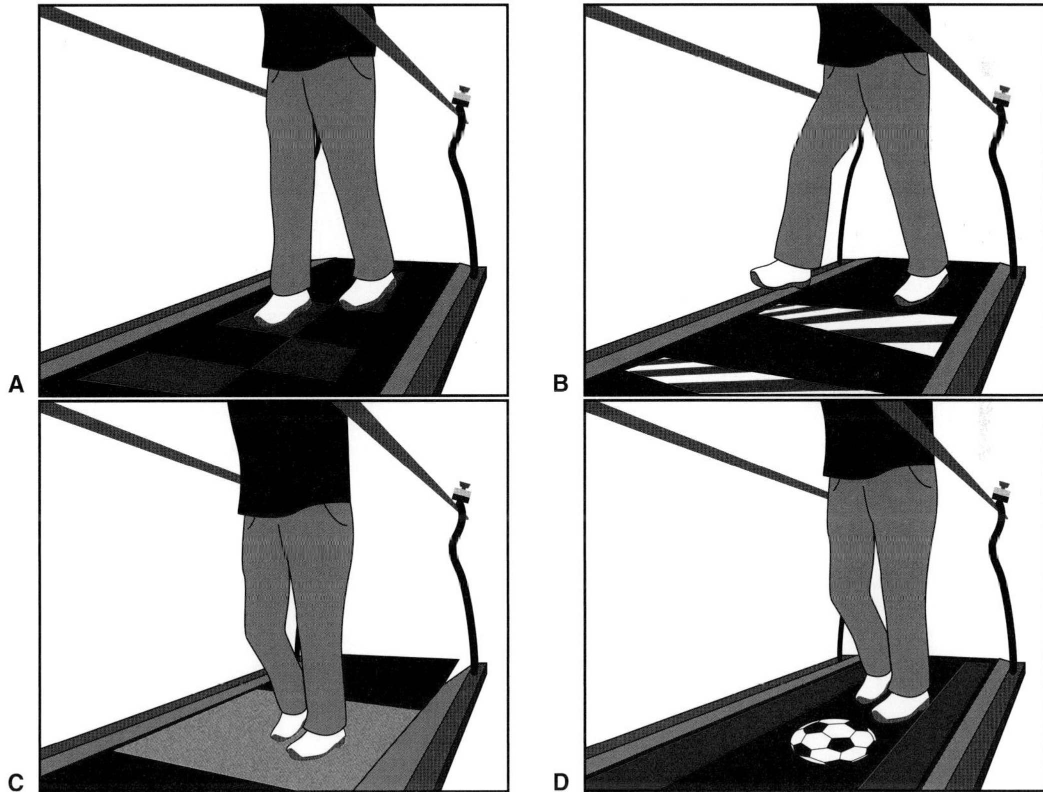

Figure 16.16 A method for training gait adaptability using a treadmill and a system for projecting virtual objects. Tasks used to train gait adaptation include visually guided stepping to a sequence of irregularly spaced stepping targets **(A)**, obstacle avoidance **(B)**, speeding up and slowing down by maintaining position in an anteriorly–posteriorly moving walking zone **(C)**, and all of the above in a functional and interactive gait adaptability game **(D)**. (Adapted from van Ooijen MW, Heeren A, Smulders K, et al. Improved gait adjustments after gait adaptability training are associated with reduced attentional demands in persons with stroke. *Exp Brain Res*. 2015;233:1008, Fig. 1.)

single- and dual-task conditions. In addition, training-related improvements transferred to improved ability to negotiate obstacles during overground walking.

The integration of VR into clinical services, including both inpatient rehabilitation and outpatient ambulatory services, is just the beginning. McEwen and colleagues (2014) examined the effects of augmenting conventional inpatient stroke rehabilitation with a VR-based exercise program. Participants included 59 inpatients receiving stroke rehabilitation services; half were randomized to a VR-based balance training in standing (e.g., soccer goaltending, snowboarding performed in a standing position, challenging balance, and requiring weight shifting), while half (n = 29) received non–balance-related VR exercises performed in sitting. Participants in both groups improved and reached the minimal clinical important difference on the 2-minute walk test and TUG test, with the group receiving VR in standing showing the greatest improvement.

Shema et al. (2014) examined the effects of VR training in a heterogeneous group of patients referred for treatment of gait instability in an ambulatory care setting. Sixty individuals received 15 one-hour sessions of VR gait training (3 times per week for 5 weeks). VR gait training consisted of walking on a treadmill while negotiating virtual obstacles (see Fig. 16.17). The virtual environment (VE) simulated an obstacle course situated along different pathways in an outdoor scene. Feedback was provided by the simulation and consisted of knowledge of performance (allowing the participants to see their steps), symmetry, and obstacle clearance using immediate visual and auditory cues. After 5 weeks of training, time to complete the TUG decreased by 10.3%, the distance walked during the 2-minute walk test increased by 9.5%, and performance on the Four Square Step Test improved by 13%.

In summary, this research review suggests that VR done alone or in conjunction with treadmill training may be an effective way to train complex walking skills, such as obstacle negotiation. Training appears to transfer to improved obstacle negotiation in non-trained conditions (e.g., during overground walking). Whether it is superior to other forms of training is not yet established (see Laver et al., 2015 for a Cochrane Review of VR in stroke rehabilitation).

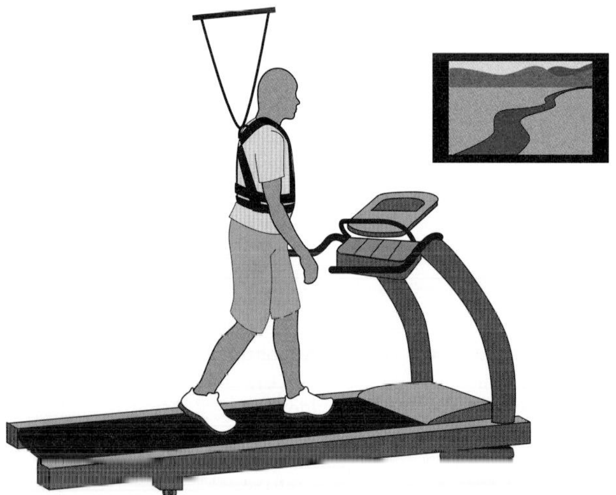

Figure 16.17 A VR gait training system utilizes a treadmill with a safety harness and a computer that generates the virtual reality simulation presented on the screen. (From Shema SR, Brozgol M, Dorfman M, et al. Clinical experience using a 5-week treadmill training program with virtual reality to enhance gait in an ambulatory physical therapy service. *Phys Ther.* 2014;94:1322: Fig. 2.)

Dual-Task Locomotor Training

Improving performance on complex walking tasks also involves locomotor training under both single- and dual-task conditions. Dual-task gait training involves practicing walking while simultaneously practicing additional motor and cognitive tasks. Dual-task gait training can be done with instructions to focus on the gait task, the secondary task, or to alternate between tasks. What evidence do we have that training is effective in improving dual-task gait?

Research Evidence. As discussed in Chapter 11, Silsupadol et al. (2006, 2009a, 2009b) described the outcomes of a 4-week training of balance and gait under three conditions—single task, dual task with fixed-priority instructions, and dual task with variable-priority instructions—in older adults with balance impairment. All three forms of training improved balance (BBS) and gait speed (10-meter walk test); however, only participants who received dual-task training improved gait speed under dual-task conditions (Silsupadol et al., 2009a). In addition, variable-priority instructional set was more effective than the fixed-priority instructional set in improving dual-task gait measures.

Does attentional focus influence the effect of a training program in persons with PD? Landers et al. (2015) randomly assigned 49 participants with PD to 4 weeks of dual-task balance and gait training, under three instructional focus conditions (balance training + external focus instructions, balance training + internal focus instructions, and balance training + no attentional focus instructions). A control group received no training. Training included 10 minutes of treadmill training without holding onto the railing so as to challenge balance, 10 minutes of obstacle course negotiation, and 10 minutes of balance training on a compliant surface in a harness (tandem stance, narrow support stance, single leg stance, eyes closed, and external perturbations). All four groups (including the nontrained controls) improved performance on measures of balance, though gait speed did not change. The authors suggest that 4 weeks of training, regardless of instructional focus, was not sufficient to improve balance in persons with PD.

Gait-related dual-task deficits are present among many persons who have had a stroke even after conventional rehabilitation and may persist for months following discharge from rehabilitation (Cockburn et al., 2003; Dennis et al., 2009; Hyndman et al., 2006; Plummer et al., 2013; Plummer-D'Amato et al., 2008, 2010). Because of these sustained deficits, a number of researchers are beginning to explore the effects of dual-task training in persons with stroke.

Yang and colleagues (2007b) provided dual-task motor training (walked while manipulating either one or two balls of various sizes) to persons with chronic stroke. Training was 30 minutes, 3 times per week for 4 weeks. Compared to 12 patients who did not receive any intervention, the 13 patients who received dual-task training significantly improved their gait speed, cadence, stride duration, and stride length in single- and dual-task (tray carrying) walking. A blind randomized controlled trial investigated the preliminary effects of dual-task training on walking and balance in people with chronic stroke (Fishbein et al., 2019). The dual-task training consisted of walking while performing virtual reality activities (ball and reaching games). In the control group, participants just practiced single-task treadmill walking. The authors measured the 10-minute walking test, Timed Up and Go, Functional Reach Test, Lateral Reach Test, Activities-specific Balance Confidence scale, and Berg Balance Scale. Those participants allocated to the dual-task training group achieved greater balance and gait ability than controls.

In a case series study, Plummer et al. (2014) examined the feasibility of dual-task gait training in 7 persons with stroke. Gait training sessions were 30 minutes, 3 times a week, for 4 weeks. The gait activities used for this training were organized according to Gentile's taxonomy and are shown in Table 16.7; the cognitive tasks used are also shown in this table. Following training, five of the seven participants had improved gait speed under dual-task conditions, providing preliminary evidence that training can improve dual-task gait in some persons with stroke. An interesting finding from this case series is that most participants did not demonstrate improvements in single-task walking speed after the training. The authors note that this may be due to the fact that there was no single-task practice during the dual-task gait training sessions (Plummer et al., 2014).

Training Reactive Balance during Gait

Strategies to retrain compensatory responses to unexpected perturbations to gait (reactive balance training) include unexpectedly changing the speed of a treadmill while the patient is walking on it. It is also possible to ask the individual to walk against resistance (using elastic tubing) and to unexpectedly release the resistance to give an unexpected perturbation to forward progression. It is very important to have the patient wear a gait belt (or harness system) and to guard them carefully during dynamic gait tasks in order to prevent a fall.

Research Evidence. A number of researchers have developed methods for training reactive balance during gait in order to reduce slip-related falls (Bhat & Pai, 2008; Bhatt et al., 2006; Grabiner et al., 2012; Lockhart et al., 2005; Mansfield et al., 2010; Pai et al., 2003, 2010; Parijat et al., 2012; Wang et al., 2011). A variety of methods have been used to deliver forward-directed perturbations, including steel rollers or low-friction movable platforms integrated in overground walkways (Bhatt et al., 2006; Marigold & Patla, 2002) or low-friction material surface such as a vinyl tile covered with oil (Brady et al., 2000). This research is encouraging in demonstrating the feasibility and efficacy of training recovery from an unexpected slip or trip in young and older adults (Pai et al., 2010; Parijat et al., 2012). Training using technology such as a treadmill or low-friction moveable platforms appears to transfer to improved ability to recover from an unexpected slip or trip under different conditions (such as during overground walking) (Bhatt & Pai, 2009; Yang et al., 2013). Most encouraging slip-related training in a group of older adults reduced frequency of falls in daily life by half (Pai et al., 2014). The effects of slip-resistant gait training can be retained for up to 6 months (Bhatt et al., 2012). Allin and colleagues (2020) investigated a perturbation-based balance training for fall prevention secondary to slips and trips in older adults. The authors found that specifically targeting slipping and tripping can improve reactive balance and fall incidence during lab-induced slips but not lab-induced trips. They proposed that a difference in dosage and training specificity could explain this discrepancy in the outcomes.

In summary, this research provides evidence to support a task-oriented exercise program in improving gait function in a variety of patient populations. Studies vary as to the duration and intensity of intervention. Some include treatment at the impairment level (e.g., strength training), but all include progressively challenging task-oriented practice of functional locomotor skills.

Improving Participation and Reducing Mobility Disability

The ultimate goal of any form of locomotor training is to improve participation. In the ICF, *Participation* refers to a person's involvement in a life situation. Reduced participation as indicated by reduced involvement in social, recreational, and purposeful activity is reported in over half of all persons living at home 6 months after stroke (Ashe et al., 2009, Mayo et al., 2002). Can locomotor training improve participation in the mobility domain? How can we improve a person's ability to walk more in their daily life?

Unfortunately, little is known about the effects of interventions aimed at impairments and functional mobility skills (capacity) on performance of mobility tasks in the person's daily life (participation). This is because of the paucity of measures related to participation in the mobility domain and the fact that few studies use measures of participation as outcomes in intervention studies. Often, locomotor interventions use change in gait velocity as a primary outcome measure, but this does not necessarily mean improved function in the context of daily life. Mudge et al. (2009) found that among chronic stroke patients, circuit training improved distance walked on the 6-minute walk test but found no change in average steps per day as measured by an SAM. In contrast, a study by Moore and colleagues (2010) found improvements in daily steps outside of therapy in participants 6 months poststroke with high-intensity

TABLE 16.7 Overview of Gait and Cognitive Activities Used for Dual-Task Gait Training

A

	Predictable	**Unpredictable**
Stationary	Closed tasks: i. Walking in flat, wide space ii. Walking over/around obstacles, all of the same height and equally spaced iii. Walking with a narrow base of support	Variable motionless tasks: i. Walking around obstacles with variable spacing ii. Walking over obstacles of variable height iii. Walking over changing floor surfaces
Moving	Consistent motion tasks: i. Walk toward/beside/behind a person moving at a consistent speed and direction ii. Walk under different lighting conditions	Open tasks: i. Walking in a crowded corridor ii. Walking outdoors in the car park iii. Walking and negotiating a moving obstacle

B

Task	**Description**
Random number/ letter generation	i. Randomly naming numbers between 100 and 500 (without repetition or consecutively ii. Randomly naming odd (or even) numbers between 1 and 100 (without repetition or consecutively) iii. Randomly naming consonants of the alphabet (without repetition or consecutively)
Word association	Easy: i. Naming as many words as possible in a category (e.g., animals, fruits) ii. Naming opposites of words Hard: i. Naming as many words as possible beginning with a particular letter ii. Naming as many words as possible in a category (e.g., European cities)
Working memory	Easy: i. Reciting a sequence of numbers (3 or 4 number sequence) ii. Reciting a grocery list (3 or 4 items) Hard: i. Reciting a sequence of numbers (5 numbers per sequence) ii. Reciting a grocery list (5 items)
Calculating a time	Easy: Adding or subtracting minutes to a given time within the hour (e.g., 3:15 + 5 minutes; 1:30–15 min) Hard: Adding or subtracting minutes to a given time into the next hour (e.g., 4:40 = 25 min; 1:15–30 min)
Backward recitation	i. Reciting number sequences backward ii. Months of the year iii. Days of the week iv. Backward spelling (4- or 5-letter words) v. Counting backward (by 2, 3, 6, 7, 8; starting between 75 and 100)

Source: Adapted from Plummer P, Villalobos RM, Vayda MS, et al. Feasibility of dual-task gait training for community-dwelling adults after stroke: a case series. *Stroke Res Treat.* 2014;2014:538602, Tables 1 & 2, with permission.

locomotor training (15 minutes of treadmill training with an average of 4,000 steps per session).

Mayo and colleagues (2015) used a randomized clinical trial to investigate the extent to which participation in personal, family, social, and community life could be enhanced in persons with chronic stroke, through the provision of a community-based structured program. The Getting on with the Rest of Your Life: Mission Possible© program was a group-based intervention provided in a community setting that included exercise- and project-based activities to promote learning, leisure, and social activities. After the 9-month intervention, 45% of the participants increased their participation in meaningful activity (not necessarily defined by increased walking) by 3 hours per week, while 39% increased by 4 to 5 hours. Increased hours in meaningful activity was associated with reports of a higher degree of satisfaction with meaningful roles and also by improvements in gait speed. The authors conclude that it is possible to improve participation among persons with chronic stroke, but an extended period of participation in community-based programs may be required.

In summary, preliminary research suggests that locomotor training may improve participation in mobility and other domains; however, the intensity and duration of training needed to impact participation may be extensive.

RETRAINING OTHER MOBILITY SKILLS

Stair Walking

The ability to safely manage stairs is of particular concern since many falls occur during stair descent. Locomotion on stairs is associated with high musculoskeletal, balance, and cardiovascular demands (Jacobs, 2016; Startzell et al., 2000); thus a wide variety of patients with neurologic disorders will have problems negotiating stairs. Several clinical strategies for retraining stair walking have been proposed for patients with stroke and are shown in Figures 16.18 and 16.19 (Bobath, 1978; Voss et al., 1985).

During stair ascent, the patient is taught to advance the nonhemiplegic leg first. As shown in Figure 16.18, manual assistance is given as needed to guide and control the involved leg.

During stair descent, shown in Figure 16.19, the patient with stroke is taught to advance the hemiplegic leg first. The therapist assists with foot placement as needed and in knee control, to prevent collapse of the leg when the noninvolved leg is advanced during swing.

Research has shown that certain stair features are critical in establishing effective movement strategies for stair walking. Thus, it is possible that accentuating stair features, such as the edge of the step or the height of the step and drawing the patient's attention to these features may enhance the ability to develop effective stair walking strategies.

Research Evidence

Is there evidence available on the efficacy of locomotion training while ascending and descending stairs in patients with neuromotor disorders? As with any other motor task, we should always consider the task, the individual, and the environmental constraints. In a systematic review, Jacobs (2016) focused on studies examining these constraints in healthy young and old people. Specifically, older adults negotiated stairs with less stability and at greater risk to tripping. Older adults showed the following performance deficits: a slow GP on stairs,

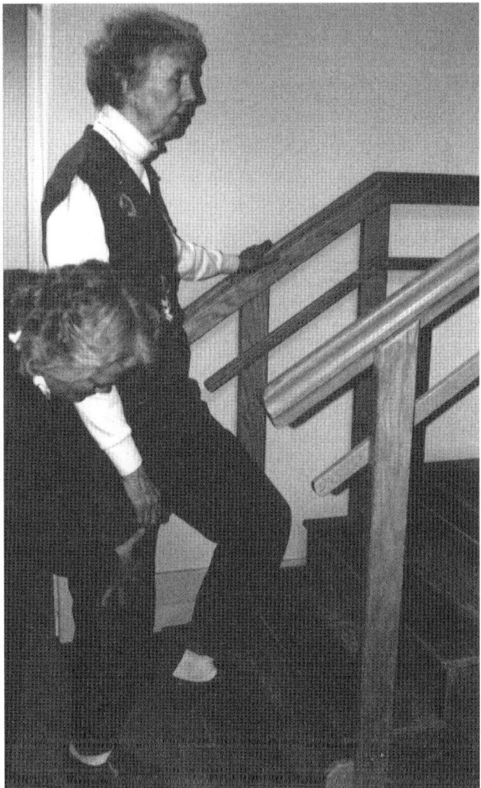

Figure 16.18 Assisting stair walking, controlling the involved leg for single-limb stance in stair ascent.

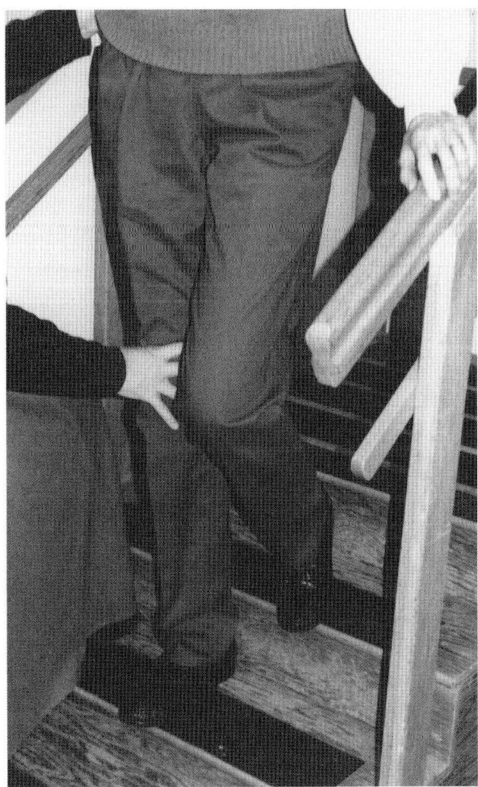

Figure 16.19 Manually assisting control of the knee during stair descent.

greater double-support time, diminished vertical forces while accepting weight and pushing off, increased force at midstance, less motion or force at ankle and knee but increased motion or force at the hip, impaired coordination, decreased strength, small and variable foot clearance, large and fast horizontal displacements of the body's COM, less capacity to control fast vertical COM displacements, and potential increased fear of falling with cautious motor strategies. Regarding environmental factors, stair architecture and ambient lightning seem to be critical. High stair heights and decreased tread length can reduce COM stability. Even with regular stairs, older adults perform close to their maximum joint ROM and force production capacity. Well-lit stairwells may increase step speed, and visual cues on stair edges or handrails can enhance foot clearance, COM stability and promote and improve handrail grasping performance. Finally, negotiating stairs with a handrail can improve cadence and balance. Older adults also show dual-task costs and thus attention-to-task should be emphasized. Stair mobility in some other pathological populations such as stroke or PD can be found in this review as well.

Sit-to-Stand

Standing up is critical to mobility function; thus, learning to transfer from a bed or a seated position to standing (and walking) is an important part of mobility training. A task-oriented approach to training transfers, including STS, focuses on having patients practice this functional task in a variety of contexts. Remember from Chapter 12 that there are two basic strategies that can be used separately or in combination to stand up: a momentum strategy and a force control strategy. A patient should be allowed to explore the possibilities for using momentum when performing a transfer task, since this strategy is most efficient and requires the least amount of muscular activity.

Essential elements of teaching a momentum strategy include encouraging the patient to move quickly, but safely, and avoid breaks in the motion. The clinician can verbally instruct the patient to move quickly, with no stops. An appropriate prompt might be, "Now we are going to try standing up again, but this time I want you to move quickly, with no stops." Manual cues can be used at the shoulders to set the pace. Patients who have trouble generating force quickly with the trunk can try swinging their arms freely while standing up, to increase momentum generated in upper body segments.

When teaching a momentum strategy, clinicians should be aware of the stringent stability requirements of this strategy and adequately safeguard a patient with poor postural control to prevent a fall. The risk for a backward fall will be greatest at the beginning of the movement if the patient tries to transfer momentum from the trunk to the legs for a vertical lift before the COM is sufficiently forward over the feet. This is often characteristic of STS in a patient who is hemiparetic. In contrast, the risk for a forward fall will be greatest at the end of the movement in patients who are unable to control horizontal forces affecting the COM. When this occurs, the COM continues to accelerate forward of the base of support of the feet after the patient reaches a vertical position, resulting in a fall forward. This is often characteristic of STS in patients with cerebellar pathology, who have difficulty scaling forces for movement.

In contrast to the momentum strategy, a force control strategy is characterized by frequent stops. In using a force control strategy, patients are taught to bring the buttocks forward toward the edge of the chair. The trunk is brought forward, bringing the "nose over the toes." This is shown in Figure 16.20. This brings the COM over the base of support of the feet. The patient is then cued to stand up. Patients with weakness, making it difficult to achieve a vertical position from a normal-height chair, can begin learning STS from a raised chair, reducing the strength requirement for lifting the body (Fig. 16.21). As the patient improves, the seat height can be lowered.

In patients with asymmetrical force-production problems, facilitating symmetry is important when possible, since symmetrical weight bearing enhances both progression and stability during the task. A symmetrical weight-bearing posture is possible only in patients who can generate sufficient force to control the knee and prevent collapse of the body when the impaired limb is loaded. When this is not the case, the clinician will have to manually control the knee—for

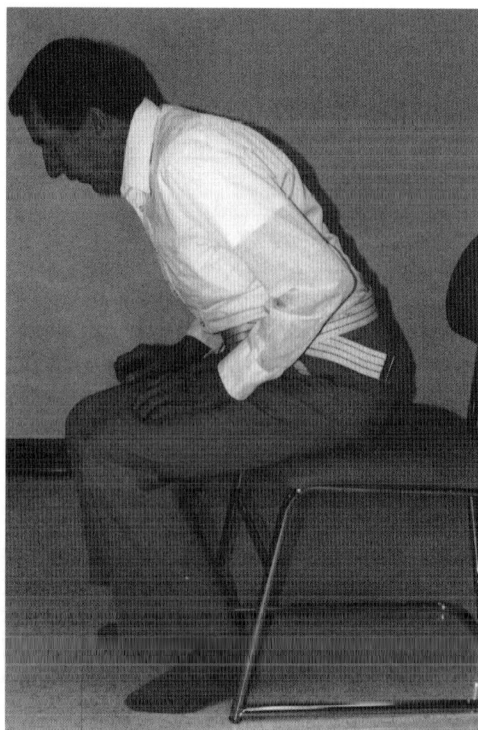

Figure 16.20 Teaching a force control strategy for accomplishing STS involves asking the patient to move forward to the edge of the chair, incline the trunk forward until the "nose is over the toes," and then stand up.

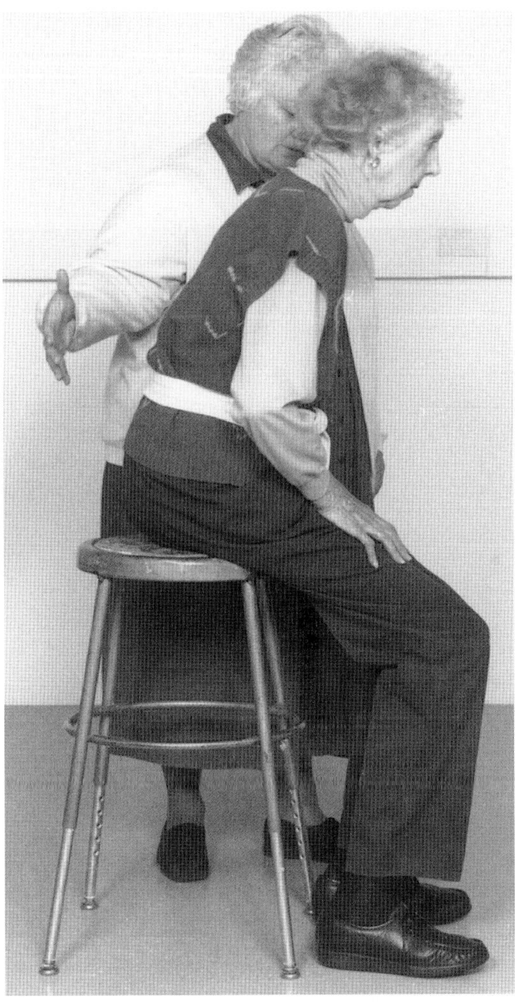

Figure 16.21 Teaching STS from a raised chair reduces the strength requirement for lifting the body and allows a weak patient to accomplish the task.

example, as illustrated in Figure 16.22 and demonstrated in Genise's treatment video. It is important that when manually assisting knee control, forward motion of the knee is not blocked as the patient stands up.

It is often easier for a patient to learn to sit down than to stand up because eccentric force control is often gained prior to concentric force control (Carr & Shepherd, 1998; Duncan & Badke, 1987). When teaching a patient to sit down, the therapist asks the patient to practice flexing the knees in preparation for sitting. This requires eccentric contraction of the quadriceps to control premature collapse of the knee.

Research Evidence

What evidence do we have that training improves STS performance in patients with neurologic pathology? Monger and colleagues (2002) examined the effect of a 3-week home-based task-oriented exercise program (activities summarized in Table 16.8) on STS performance in individuals with chronic stroke (mean time since stroke, 2.6 years). Exercises were performed daily for 20 minutes; in addition, a researcher worked with

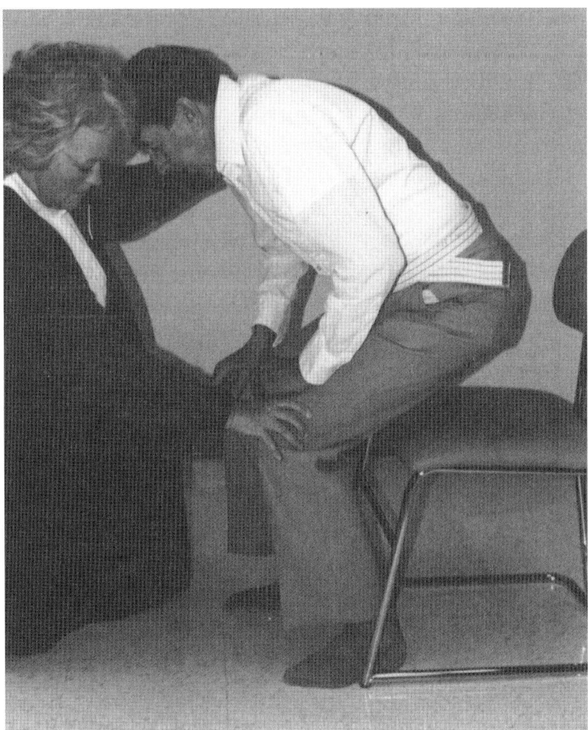

Figure 16.22 Manually controlling the knee when assisting a patient who is moving from a sitting to a standing position.

each person 3 times a week in order to progress activities (decreasing seat height, increasing step height, and increasing the number and speed of repetitions). Verbal feedback about weight distribution and encouragement were provided. Five of six subjects improved their score on the standing up item from the Movement Assessment Scale, while all six improved self-selected walking speed (10-meter walk test). In addition, laboratory measures showed improved timing (but not magnitude) of the peak vertical ground reaction force during STS. Grip strength, which was not trained, did not change.

Importance of Varying Task and Environmental Demands

Just as in gait, patients must learn to perform functional tasks, such as STS and transfers, under varying task and environmental demands. To assist in the process of exploring movement strategies that are effective in meeting changing task and environmental demands, conditions of training are varied. For example, as shown in Figure 16.23, during the process of learning to move from a sitting to a standing position, the patient may practice standing up from a wheelchair (Fig. 16.23A), from the bed (Fig. 16.23B), from a chair without arms (Fig. 16.23C), and from a low soft chair (Fig. 16.23D). In addition, patients may learn to embed STS in a variety of other tasks, such as stand up and stop, stand up and walk, or stand up and lean over. This type of variability encourages the patient to modify strategies used to stand up in response to changes in task and environmental demands.

Often, as therapists, we are quick to guide patients toward the use of strategies that we know will be effective in meeting the demands of the task. Patients rarely have the time to experiment with a variety of solutions that are effective in meeting task demands. This concept of trial-and-error exploration in the learning of strategies that are effective in meeting task goals has a number of important implications for clinicians. Initial performance may be quite poor as patients learn to explore and to find their own

TABLE 16.8 Task-Specific Activities for Training Sit-to-Stand

Sit–stand–sit	• 10 times (or maximum number up to 10 that can be performed without a rest). • Repeat 3 times (30 repetitions in total). • Move feet backward, look straight ahead, swing trunk forward at the hips, and stand up with weight evenly distributed through both feet. • Do not use your arms.
Step-ups	• Standing, affected foot on 8-cm block, step up and down with other leg: a. to shift body mass forward on to affected leg b. to shift body mass sideways on to affected leg • Exercise near furniture to steady yourself if necessary. • Do three sets of 10 repetitions (or a maximum number up to 10 that you can perform without a rest).
Calf stretch	• Standing with affected knee straight and extended arm(s) resting on wall: • Keeping body straight, pivot the body forward at the ankles, keeping heel on the floor until you feel that the calf muscle is stretched. • Hold for 2 min, relax, and repeat 10 times.

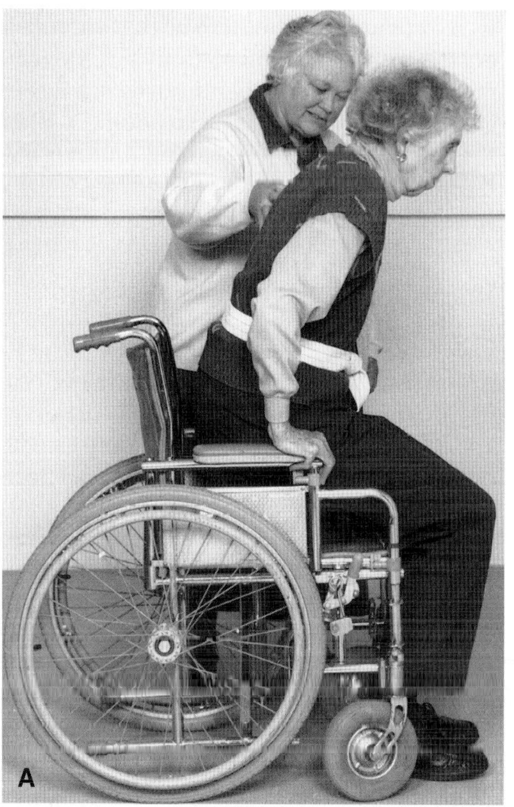
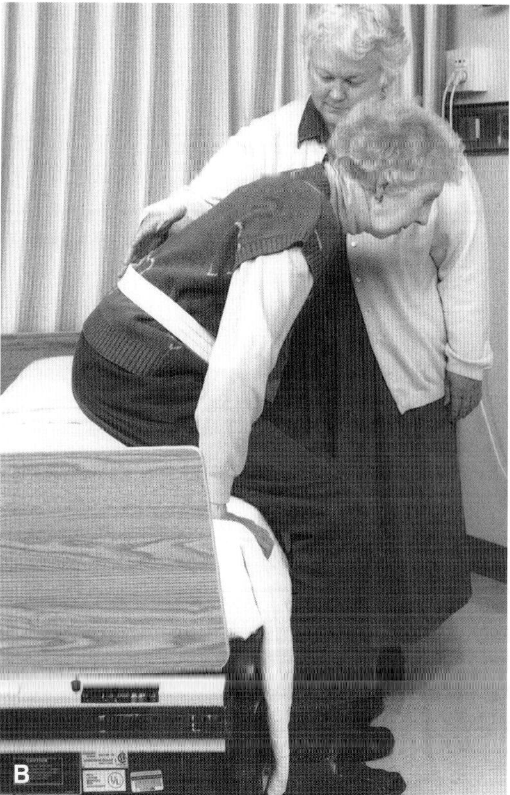

Figure 16.23 Varying the environmental conditions while learning the STS task. Practice conditions involve standing up from a wheelchair **(A)**, from the bed **(B)**, from a chair without arms **(C)**, and from a low soft chair **(D)**.

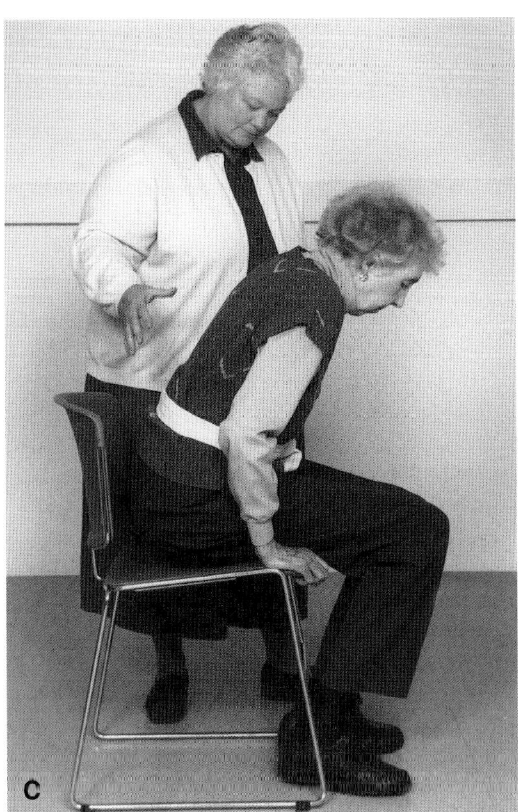

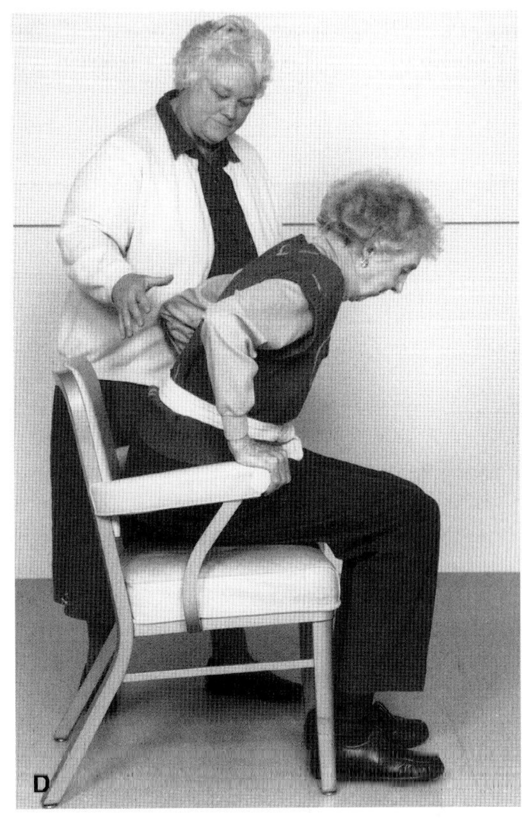

Figure 16.23 *(continued)*

solutions. Patients may not progress as quickly as if they were taught a single solution to the task being learned. If we value the importance of multiple solutions to task demands, short- and long-term therapy goals may need to include the ability to perform a functional task under multiple conditions.

Lab Activity 16.4 provides a framework for developing a treatment program for retraining locomotor function in our patient Genise T Review our case study in Figure 16.2 and the information gained through Lab Activity 16.3. Complete the table proposed in Lab Activity 16.4, identifying the specific individual system to be targeted (column 1), the task or activity to be practiced (column 2), the environmental conditions under which practice will occur (column 3), and the research evidence that supports this aspect of treatment (column 4).

LAB ACTIVITY 16.4

Objective: Apply a task-oriented approach to locomotor training in Genise (or a patient of your own choice). Identify the research evidence to support clinical decisions regarding specific treatment interventions.

Procedure: Reread the case study presented in Figure 16.2 and your assignment from Lab Activity 16.3.

Assignment

1. Create a table identifying the various treatments you will use to improve mobility function in Genise. List the specific individual system to be targeted (column 1), the task or activity to be practiced (column 2), the environmental conditions under which practice will occur (column 3), and the research evidence that supports this aspect of treatment. For example, you may decide to do progressive resistance strength training with Genise because paresis or weakness is an underlying impairment contributing to her impaired gait. The individual component listed in the table is motor: strength, the task is strength training, and the specific environmental condition you choose may be free weights at 60% 1 RM. Several research studies support your decision to incorporate progressive resistive strength training with Genise, including the meta-analysis by Ada et al. (2006). Is strength training alone enough to insure recovery of gait? What other aspects of mobility will you train? What research supports your decision?

(continued)

LAB ACTIVITY 16.4 *(continued)*

Individual component of balance	Task or activity	Environmental conditions	Research evidence
Motor: Strength	Progressive resistance strength training	Free weights, 60% of 1 RM	Ada et al. (2006); Duncan et al. (2003); Ouelette et al. (2004)
Motor: Gait Pattern: Progression	Walking—part practice	Hip pull-off while standing in a diagonal leg position Push-off while standing with hemiparetic limb in a trailing limb position	Milot et al. (2008); Olney et al. (1991, 1994)
Motor: Gait pattern	Walking—whole-task practice	Treadmill and body weight support Manual and verbal cues related to gait pattern	Ada et al. (2003); Hesse et al. (1994, 1995, 1999); Sullivan et al. (2002)
Motor: Gait pattern	Walking—whole-task practice	FES to the plantarflexors and dorsiflexor	Kesar et al. (2009)
Motor: Velocity and distance	Walking for progressively longer distances	Treadmill and overground Vary distance and speed	Sullivan et al. (2002)
Motor: Gait pattern, velocity	Walking	Lateral wedge insole	Chen et al. (2010)
Motor: Complex walking tasks	Walking under varying task and environmental conditions	Task-oriented training of complex walking tasks using the eight environmental dimensions Circuit training	Bassile et al. (2003); Dean et al. (2000); Duncan et al. (2003); Mudge et al. (2009); Salbach et al. (2004)
Sensory: Organization of Sensory Inputs for Balance	Walking	Eyes open, closed, while wearing opaque glasses Firm, foam surface Carpeted surfaces	Bayouk et al. (2006); Bonan et al. (2004); Smania et al. (2008)
Cognitive: Dual-Task Balance Training	Walking Sit-to-stand	Practice tasks under dual-task conditions, adding secondary cognitive tasks	Silsupadol et al. (2009a and b); Yang et al. (2007b)

RM, Repetition maximum.

SUMMARY

1. The key to recovery of mobility skills following neurologic injury is learning to meet the task requirements of progression, stability, and adaptation, despite persisting sensory, motor, and cognitive impairments. Research examining mobility strategies in neurologically intact individuals suggests that there is no one right strategy that can, or should, be used to meet these requirements.
2. Retraining the person with impaired mobility skills begins with an examination of the following: (a) mobility skills in daily life (performance in the ICF framework), (b) functional mobility skills (capacity in the ICF framework), (c) strategies used to accomplish the progression and stability requirements of gait, and (d) underlying sensory, motor, and cognitive impairments that constrain the performance of functional mobility skills.
3. Visual gait analysis is the clinical tool most commonly used to aid therapists in systematically analyzing a person's gait pattern.
4. A task-oriented approach to treatment (as defined in this book) focuses on helping patients to resolve

specific impairments constraining a functional task, to develop strategies effective in meeting essential task requirements, and to learn how to adapt and modify these strategies so performance can be sustained under a wide variety of conditions.

5. There is considerable evidence to support effectiveness of task-specific locomotor training on improving functional mobility skills in persons with neurologic disorders.
6. The use of technology such as BWSTT and robotic-assisted gait training, while effective in improving mobility function, has not been shown to be superior to other forms of therapy provided with comparable intensity.

ANSWERS TO LAB ACTIVITY ASSIGNMENTS

Lab Activity 16.1

1. Compare the data from this lab to the norms listed in Table 16.1.

Lab Activity 16.2

1. If you have analyzed an atypical gait pattern, refer back to Table 16.5 and examine the possible causes of the gait abnormalities you observed.

Lab Activity 16.3

1. At 1 month poststroke, Genise walks at less than 0.4 m/s and requires stand by assistance to ensure her safety. She is unable to walk 500 m, a distance considered critical to community mobility. This information suggests that at this point in her recovery, she is a nonfunctional (physiological) ambulator.
2. Her paresis limits Genise's ability to meet the stability and progression requirements of steady-state gait. She has reduced ability to generate forces for progression; this results in slowed gait speed. In addition, she is unable to adapt gait to changing task and environmental demands, including an inability to recover stability following an unexpected challenge to balance (impaired reactive balance) and to modify gait in advance of a potentially destabilizing challenge to gait (impaired anticipatory balance). She cannot modify her step height or length, so has difficulty crossing obstacles. Because she must use a walker for balance, she is unable to carry packages and thus requires assistance on all shopping trips.
3. Refer to Table 16.5 to determine the relationship between her underlying impairments and her gait pattern. For example, her hyperextension in midstance could be the result of one or more of the following: spasticity in her plantarflexors (or quads), reduced ROM in her ankle, weakness in her knee extensors (compensatory passive locking of the knee), extensor mass synergy pattern, and/or poor recruitment and selective control.

Lab Activity 16.4

1. It is important to remember that there is no single correct way to train walking in Genise. It is essential that all aspects of gait be included in her rehabilitation program (e.g., progression, stability, and adaptation) and that a range of tasks and conditions be used to help her develop a variety of gait strategies so that she is able walk safely in a wide diversity of tasks and conditions. The specific order, duration, and timing of each activity may vary from therapist to therapist.

   We begin by determining Genise's main concern and goals related to her walking. She wants to increase the speed and distance that she is able to walk so that she can walk in her home and community. She wants to improve her stability when she walks, particularly when faced with environmental challenges to gait (such as stepping over obstacles).

   Therefore, our approach to training walking will focus on improving underlying impairments (her paresis or weakness and reduced ROM); improving movement patterns effective in achieving progression, stability, and adaptation; and practicing functional mobility tasks under a variety of conditions.

   Activities will be goal directed, and progressively challenging, beginning with relatively simple challenges (e.g., walking on a firm flat surface with good lighting or standing up from a 17-inch chair with arms) to more complex (e.g., changing speeds, irregular terrains, with manual loads, increased attentional demands, or standing up from a lower-height chair, a chair without arms, or a rocking chair). In order to facilitate extended practice, we will perform locomotor training with body weight support on a treadmill system. We may also include circuit training, setting up stations in which she can practice complex walking tasks under single- and dual-task conditions (see Table 16.7 for treatment ideas for these stations).

   We will incorporate motor learning principles into her training. Initially, we will have her practice functional tasks in a blocked manner (practicing each task for a time, before switching to a different task). As she improves, we will shift to a more random practice pattern (alternating the types of tasks she practices) and modify the conditions under which she practices as well (variable practice). As she is reacquiring balance ability, we will vary the timing and extent of the external feedback she is given.

   There is considerable research to support our clinical decision-making regarding a task-oriented approach to treatment. What research can you find to support your evidence-based mobility rehabilitation program?

PART IV

Reach, Grasp, and Manipulation

"Upper-extremity function is the basis for both fine motor skills, such as grasping and manipulating objects, and gross motor skills, such as crawling, walking, and recovering balance."

CHAPTER 17

Normal Reach, Grasp, and Manipulation

Learning Objectives

Following completion of this chapter, the reader will be able to:

1. Discuss upper-extremity function, including reach, grasp, and manipulation, within the context of the International Classification of Functioning, Disability and Health (ICF).
2. Describe the principal components of eye–head–trunk–hand coordination during reach and grasp skills.
3. Discuss the contributions of neural and musculoskeletal systems to reach and grasp skills and predict the skill deficits that would occur with lesions to these systems.
4. Discuss the general principles of motor control of reach and grasp, including the way the nervous system plans movements, and different theories of the control of reach and grasp.

INTRODUCTION

How important is upper-extremity function to successfully moving through the activities of our day? Take a moment to scan the activities you completed within the first hour after waking up this morning. They probably included brushing your teeth, combing your hair, buttoning your clothes as you dressed, and using your spoon as you stirred your coffee or ate your breakfast. In reviewing the typical activities of our day, it becomes apparent that upper-extremity function is the basis for the fine motor skills important to activities such as feeding, dressing, and grooming. In addition, upper-extremity function plays an important role in gross motor skills such as crawling, walking, the ability to recover balance, and the ability to protect the body from injury when balance recovery is not possible.

Because of this interweaving of upper-extremity control with both fine and gross motor skills, recovery of upper-extremity function is an important aspect of retraining motor control and thus falls within the purview of most areas of rehabilitation, including both occupational and physical therapies.

Where does upper-extremity function fit into the International Classification of Functioning, Disability and Health (ICF) framework? As you can see in Figure 17.1, upper-extremity function, including reach, grasp, and manipulation, fits into the ICF framework in a number of ways. "Carrying, Moving, and Handling Objects" is a subcomponent of the domain of *Mobility*, in the component *Activity and Participation*. Upper-extremity function is also important in other domains of *Activity and Participation*, including *Self-Care and Domestic Life* (specifically the ability to do household tasks).

The ICF has classified many of the underlying movements contributing to functional upper-extremity activities within the component of *Body Structure and Function*. Movements, such as *visually directed movements* and *eye–hand coordination*, are considered part of *Control of Voluntary Movement*, which is in the category of *Neuromusculoskeletal and Movement-Related Function*. Finally, contextual factors also impact upper-extremity function, including environmental factors, such as characteristics of objects to be lifted or carried.

In upper-extremity control, as in postural control and mobility, three factors contribute to sensorimotor

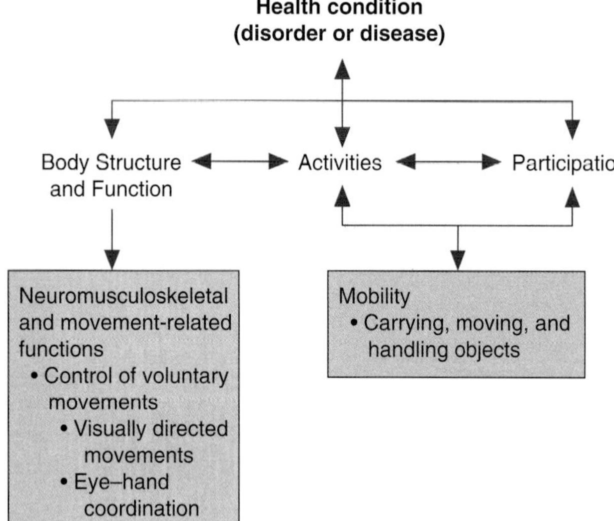

Figure 17.1 Upper-extremity function in the ICF framework.

processing: (1) the constraints of the individual, including age, experience with the task, and presence or absence of pathology; (2) the type of task (e.g., to point at an object, to grasp and manipulate an object, or to grasp and throw an object); and (3) the specific environmental constraints, including the properties of the objects to be grasped.

How does the nervous system accomplish the complex process of upper-extremity control? Before we can answer this question, we need to understand the basic requirements of reach, grasp, and manipulation. This will provide a framework for discussing both normal control (covered in this chapter) and the effect of neurologic pathology on functional grasp and manipulatory skills (covered in Chapter 19). In addition, it will provide the structure for clinical management of upper-extremity dysfunction in patients with neurologic impairments, presented in Chapter 20.

The following components are key elements of upper-extremity reach, grasp, and manipulation skills: (a) locating a target, also called "visual regard," which requires the coordination of eye–head movements and is essential in guiding movements of the hand; (b) reaching, involving transportation of the arm and hand in space as well as postural support; (c) grasping, including grip formation, grasp, and release; and (d) in-hand manipulation skills.

As we mentioned in earlier chapters, the systems theory of motor control predicts that there are specific neural and musculoskeletal subsystems that contribute to the control of the components of reach, grasp, and manipulation. Musculoskeletal components include joint range of motion, spinal flexibility, muscle properties, and biomechanical relationships among linked body segments. Neural components encompass the following: (a) motor processes, including the coordination of the eye, head, trunk, and arm movements and coordination of both the transport and grasp phases of the reach; (b) sensory processes, including the coordination of visual, vestibular, and somatosensory systems; (c) internal representations important for the mapping of sensation to action; and (d) higher-level processes essential for adaptive and anticipatory aspects of manipulatory functions.

In addition, control of manipulation involves both reflexive and voluntary movements and both feedback and feedforward processing. Voluntary movements also obey specific psychophysical principles (e.g., motor programs have invariant features, and movements show a lengthening of reaction time [RT] with increasing information to be processed) (Ghez & Krakauer, 2000).

We begin our discussion with a review of some general principles of movement control that apply equally to eye, head, and hand coordination during reaching. We then move to a discussion of components of reach, grasp, and manipulation, beginning with visual regard, which describes the manner in which the eyes and head are coupled during target location. We then discuss the components of reach and grasp, describing the role of the motor and sensory systems, and higher-level adaptive abilities. Finally, we review some of the theories of the control of reaching movements.

MOVEMENT CONTROL PRINCIPLES

Feedforward versus Feedback Control of Movement

In Chapters 7 and 12, on the control of posture and locomotion, we emphasized the importance of both feedback and feedforward (anticipatory) processes in movement control. Efficient reaching also involves both feedback and feedforward control processes. We learn to improve our reaching efficiency and accuracy with practice, as we both *anticipate* the requirements of the task and obstacles that might perturb the arm movement trajectory and *correct* for the effects of perturbations. An example of feedback control is shown in Figure 17.2A. Feedback control involves input from the sensory systems (typically visual or somatosensory) being compared to a reference signal, representing a desired state of the system (e.g., a position of the arm). The difference between the sensory input and the reference signal (error signal) is used to update the output of the system (e.g., the muscles controlling the arm, called "actuators"). For example, the goal may be to maintain the position of the arm while catching a ball. The reference signal would indicate the muscle contraction required to do this. Sensory information from the somatosensory or visual system would provide feedback on the current position of the arm, and the difference between the current arm position and the

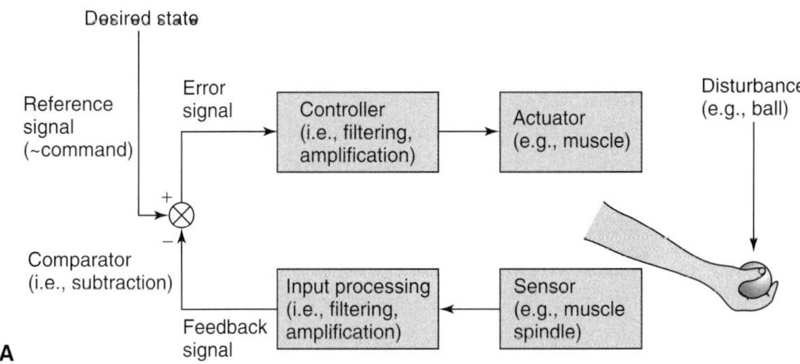

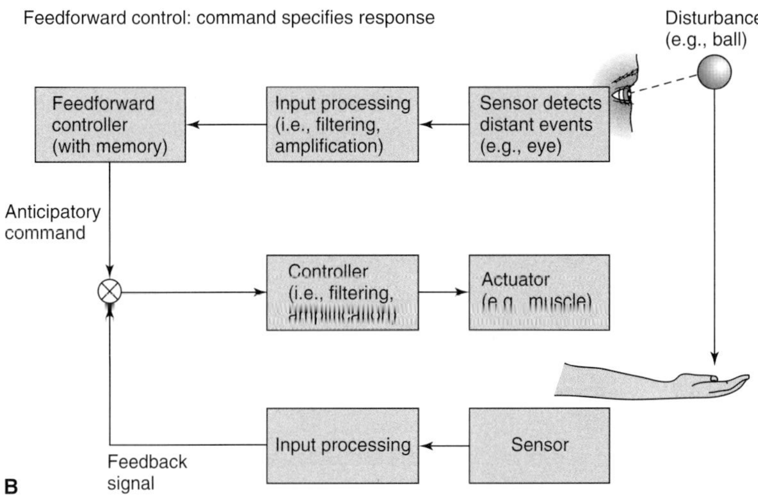

Figure 17.2 **(A)** A feedback control circuit. In feedback control, a signal from the sensory systems (marked "sensor" and typically visual or somatosensory sensors) is processed by higher centers (input processing) and then compared with a reference signal, representing a desired state of the system (e.g., a position of the arm). The difference between the sensory input and the reference signal (error signal) is used to update the output of the system, including the controller (e.g., motor cortex) and the actuator (e.g., the muscles controlling the arm). **(B)** A feedforward control circuit for catching a ball. Information from a distance sensor (e.g., the eye) is processed (input processing) and then sent to the feedforward controller (with memory access to paths of previously thrown balls) to anticipate the path of the ball and the best response. The anticipatory command is sent to the controller and actuator (as in the feedback condition in panel **A**). Feedback control is then used once the ball hits the hand and activates cutaneous and muscle receptors. (Reprinted from Ghez C, Krakauer J. The organization of movement. In: Kandel E, Schwartz J, Jessel T, eds. *Principles of neural science*, 4th ed. New York, NY: McGraw-Hill, 2000:655, with permission.)

desired position would be used to activate arm muscles to maintain that position (Ghez & Krakauer, 2000).

Feedforward, or anticipatory, control takes advantage of previous experience to predict the consequences of sensory information that is received. This occurs before the feedback sensors are stimulated and thus reduces the reliance on feedback control. For example, when catching a ball (Fig. 17.2B), we use visual information about the trajectory of the ball's movement to anticipate where to move the hand to catch it. This activates a feedforward controller (continuously updated through information from prior experience), and the controller activates the muscles at the correct level to catch the ball. After the ball hits the hand, feedback processes will also be used to react to the perturbation of hand position by the ball (Ghez & Krakauer, 2000).

These two mechanisms can be seen to contribute to the muscle activation patterns involved in catching a ball, as shown in Figure 17.3. The feedforward or anticipatory responses are indicated by the arrows and occur in the biceps, triceps, and flexor and extensor carpi radialis (ECR). After the ball hits the hand, feedback control consists of a short-latency reflex at about 50 msec after impact, in both flexor and extensor muscles. These same processes underlie the accurate movement of the eye, head, and hand toward a target, topics to be discussed in the following (Ghez & Krakauer, 2000).

LOCATING A TARGET

Eye–Head–Trunk Coordination

In order to reach for an object successfully, we must first locate the object in space, and this requires the control of rapid eye movements (smooth pursuit or saccades). Normally, vision is used for object location and to guide the movements of the hand (for reach, grasp, and manipulation). Object location typically involves movement of the eyes alone, when the target is in our central visual field, or the eyes and head, when the target is in our peripheral visual field.

How are reaching movements of the arm coordinated with the movements of the eye and head? Do we move our eyes first to a target, then our head, and finally our hand? Kinematic studies have shown that when an object to be grasped appears in the peripheral visual field, there is normally the following sequence of movements. The eye movement onset has the shortest latency, so it begins first, even before the head. The eyes

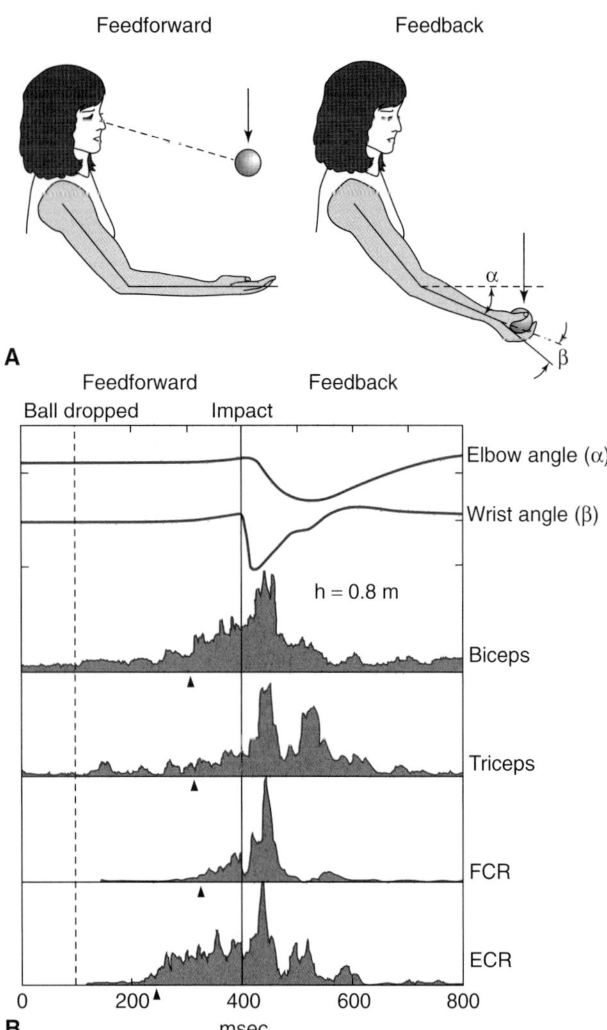

Figure 17.3 (A) Experimental conditions for feedforward/feedback control experiments. Initial input is feedforward (using vision), while final input is feedback (using somatosensory inputs from the arm/hand). The ball is dropped from different heights. **(B)** Angular changes in the elbow and wrist and muscle responses (rectified surface electromyograms) from the biceps, triceps, flexor carpi radialis (*FCR*), and extensor carpi radialis (*ECR*). Anticipatory (feedforward) responses are indicated by the *arrowheads*. Feedback responses occur after impact. (Reprinted from Ghez C, Krakauer J. The organization of movement. In: Kandel E, Schwartz J, Jessel T, eds. *Principles of neural science,* 4th ed. New York, NY: McGraw-Hill, 2000:655, with permission.)

reach the target first because they move very quickly, so they focus on the target before the head stops moving (Jeannerod, 1990). Electromyographic (EMG) studies have shown that activation of neck muscles usually occurs 20 to 40 msec prior to activation of the muscles controlling eye movements. However, because the eyes have less inertia than the head, the eyes move first, even though the neural signal occurs first in the neck muscles.

When head movement is needed to look at an object, the amplitude of head movement is usually only about 60% to 75% of the distance to the target (Biguer et al., 1984; Gresty, 1974). However, when arm movements requiring great accuracy are performed, this behavior may be modified. It has been shown that people trained to throw with great accuracy make combined eye and head movements that go most of the distance to the target (Roll et al., 1986).

Reaching to objects located in the far visual field requires a combination of eye, head, and trunk movements. Because of this heterogeneity of movement requirements, researchers have argued that eye–head coordination is not controlled by a unitary mechanism but rather emerges from an interaction of several different neural mechanisms. These could include one neural mechanism that subserves the ability to locate objects in the near periphery, requiring primarily eye movements; a second mechanism to locate objects in the further periphery, controlling combined eye–head movements; and a third mechanism to locate objects in the far periphery, controlling the movements of eye, head, and trunk together (Jeannerod, 1990).

What is the functional significance of this information to understanding and retraining a patient who has problems with functional grasp? Part of the patient's problems may relate to the coordination of eye–head movements needed for visual regard. Thus, when retraining impaired upper-extremity function, the clinician might focus on training the different control systems separately. For example, the clinician might begin by retraining eye movements to targets located within the central visual field, then progress to retraining eye–head movements to targets located in the peripheral visual field. Finally, movements involving eye, head, and trunk motions could be practiced as patients learn to locate targets oriented in the far periphery.

Interactions between Eye Movements and Hand Movements

There is evidence that eye and hand movements both interact with and influence each other. For example, when accompanied by eye movement, hand movements are more accurate. In addition, during smooth pursuit eye movements, there is an increase in gain if the hand is also following the target (Gauthier et al., 1988). Vercher and colleagues (1996) found that even in deafferented subjects, there was an increase in gain and reduction in latency for smooth pursuit when the hand was used to follow the target. Thus, they suggest it is the efference copy or corollary discharge about limb movement that helps the smooth pursuit system, rather than proprioceptive feedback from the hand movement.

Other research has shown that proprioceptive signals from the eye muscles do contribute to our ability to localize targets in extrapersonal space. Gauthier and colleagues (1988) performed an experiment in which they perturbed the movement of one eye, so it was deviated 30 degrees to the left while the subject was asked to point at a target located straight ahead. They found that the subjects were not accurate when localizing the targets, with shifts in the leftward direction of 3 to 4 degrees.

REACH AND GRASP

It is interesting to note that the control of arm movements changes depending on the goal of the task. For example, when the arm is used to point to an object, all the segments of the arm are controlled as a unit. But when the arm is used to reach for and grasp an object, the hand appears to be controlled independently of the other arm segments, with the arm carrying out movements related to transport and the hand carrying out movements related to grasping the object. In this case, reaching for an object can be divided into two subcomponents—the reach component versus the grasp component—which appear to be controlled by separate areas of the brain.

In this section, we first examine the kinematic characteristics of reaching movements and the way kinematics change depending on the task and the environment. We then discuss the contributions of specific neural and musculoskeletal subsystems to the control of visual regard, reach, and grasp.

Kinematics of Reach and Grasp

Studies have been performed to better understand the way that reach-and-grasp movements are affected by both task and environment. As you will see, this research suggests that the ability to adapt how we reach is a critical part of upper-extremity function, since reaching movements vary according to the goals and constraints of the task.

Researchers have shown that the velocity profiles and movement durations of a reach vary depending on the goal of the task. If the subject was asked to grasp the object, the movement duration of the reach was much longer than if the subject was asked to point and hit the target. Also, when preparing to grasp an object, the acceleration phase of the reaching movement was much shorter than the deceleration phase, but if the subject was asked to hit the target with the index finger, the acceleration phase was longer than the deceleration phase, with the subject hitting the target at a relatively high velocity (Marteniuk et al., 1987). This is shown in Figure 17.4, which shows the different velocity profiles for the arm over time for grasping versus pointing movements.

In addition, if the subject grasped the object, then either fit it in a small box or, alternatively, threw it; movement times and velocity profiles were also different. Movement times were shorter for grasp and throw versus grasp and fit. In addition, the acceleration phase of the movement was longer for grasp and throw than for grasp and fit. Clearly, the task constraints and goals affect the reaching phase of the movement. This finding has implications for the clinician engaged in retraining

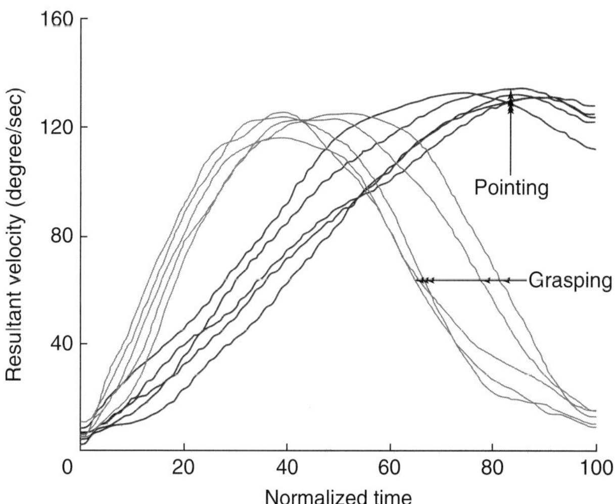

Figure 17.4 Velocity of the arm versus time (velocity profile) for a number of individual trials of both pointing and grasping movements. Note that in the grasp, the acceleration phase is shorter than the deceleration phase, while in the point, the reverse is true. (Reprinted from Jeannerod M. *The neural and behavioral organization of goal-directed movements,* Oxford, UK: Clarendon Press, 1990:19, with permission.)

the patient with problems related to reach and grasp. Since movements used during reaching for an object vary depending on the nature of the task, reaching movements need to be practiced within a variety of tasks. For example, these tasks might include practicing reach during reach and point; reach and grasp; reach, grasp, and throw; and reach, grasp, and manipulate.

NEURAL CONTROL OF REACH AND GRASP

Research on both monkeys and humans has shown that many systems are critical to the control of reach and grasp, including sensory systems and three areas of the cerebral cortex. These include the primary motor cortex, premotor cortex, and areas of the posterior parietal lobe. In addition, the cerebellum is important for the control of both feedforward and feedback control of these skills. In the following sections, we discuss the contributions of each of these areas to reach and grasp.

Sensory Systems

What is the role of sensory information in controlling reach and grasp? You may recall that in Chapter 3, to better understand the function of the different levels of the nervous system, we took a specific upper-extremity function task and walked through the pathways of the nervous system that contributed to its planning and execution. We gave the example of you being thirsty and wanting to pour some milk from the milk carton in front of you into a glass.

Sensory inputs come in from the periphery to tell you what is happening around you, where you are in space, and where your joints are relative to each other: they give you a map of your body in space. Sensory inputs from the visual system go through two parallel pathways involved in goal-directed reaching: one related to what is being reached for (perception and object recognition) and the other related to where the object is in extrapersonal space (localization) and the action systems involved in object manipulation. The perceptual pathway goes from visual cortex to temporal cortex, while the localization and action pathway goes from visual cortex to parietal lobe.

Higher centers in the cortex take this information (using, e.g., the parietal lobes and premotor cortex) and make a plan to act on it in relation to the goal: reaching for the carton of milk. You make a specific movement plan: you're going to reach over the box of cornflakes in front of you. This plan is sent to the motor cortex, and muscle groups are specified. The plan is also sent to the cerebellum and basal ganglia, and they modify it to refine the movement.

The cerebellum sends an update of the movement output plan to the motor cortex and brainstem. Descending pathways from the motor cortex and brainstem then activate spinal cord networks, spinal motor neurons activate the muscles, and you reach for the milk. If the milk carton is full, when you thought it was almost empty, spinal reflex pathways will compensate for the extra weight that you did not expect and activate more motor neurons. Then, the sensory consequences of your reach will be evaluated, and the cerebellum will update the movement—in this case, to accommodate a heavier milk carton.

From this description, you can see that sensory information plays many roles during the control of reaching. Sensory information is used to correct errors during the execution of the movement itself, ensuring accuracy during the final portions of the movement. In addition, sensory information is used proactively (feedforward) in helping to make the movement plan.

In the following section, we will discuss research exploring the role of specific visual pathways involved in reach and grasp.

Visual Pathways Related to Visual Regard, Reach, and Grasp

Researchers have identified four major brain areas, in addition to the superior colliculus, that are involved in the voluntary and reflexive control of eye movements: the frontal eye field, the supplementary eye field, the parietal eye field, and the cingulate eye field (Rizzo et al., 2017). When we move our eyes to locate a stationary target we want to grasp, that object excites successive locations on the retina during the movement. In spite of this continual shift in input across the retina, we perceive a stable visual environment. How does the brain deal with the problem of transforming a sensory stimulus coded at the level of the retina into a motor output code for controlling reach and grasp motions? The relationships between eye, head, and hand movements can be best understood in relationship to the role of optimizing vision for the guidance of hand motion (Crawford et al., 2004). Research has shown that neurons in the parietal cortex use information about the intended eye movement to update the brain's representation of visual space. The neurons anticipate the retinal consequences of the intended eye movement and shift the cortical representation first. Then, the eye catches up.

These neurons thus send a corollary discharge of the output to the eye muscles to other areas of the brain, allowing the visual world to be remapped with each eye movement into the coordinates of the current gaze location. Research (Duhamel et al., 1992a, 1992b) has shown that these corollary discharge visual cells in the lateral intraparietal area (LIP) start to increase their firing rate about 80 msec before a saccade occurs.

The two visual pathways involved in reach and grasp include the dorsal stream pathway, going from the visual to the parietal cortex, and the ventral stream pathway, going from visual cortex to the temporal lobe. Research (Goodale & Milner, 1992; Goodale et al., 1991) suggests that the dorsal stream projection to the parietal cortex provides action-relevant information about all phases of the reaching movement, including object position, structure, and orientation, while ventral stream projections to the temporal lobe provide our conscious visual perceptual experience.

Goodale and Milner (1992) note that the dorsal and ventral stream visual pathways are different with respect to their access to consciousness. For example, a patient with "ventral stream" lesions had no conscious perception of the orientation or dimension of objects, but she could pick them up with great adeptness. Thus, it may be that information in the dorsal system can be processed without reaching conscious perception (Goodale & Milner, 1992).

Evidence supporting the concept of separate visual pathways for perception (ventral stream) and action (dorsal stream) in normal subjects comes from the work by Haffenden and Goodale (1998). In this experiment, they used a visual illusion to separate perceptual judgments about an object's size and the ability to reach for it accurately. They used the Ebbinghaus illusion, in which two target circles of equal size are surrounded by an array of either smaller or larger circles. Subjects typically report that the circle surrounded by the smaller circles is larger than the one surrounded by larger circles. If the same pathway controlled perception and action, one would expect that both perception and grasp would be equally affected by the illusion.

In this experiment, subjects were asked to either reach for a disk placed in the center of one of the two sets of circles (hypothesized dorsal stream) (Fig. 17.5A) or manually estimate the size of the center disk (hypothesized ventral stream), as shown in Figure 17.5B. Participants were tested under two conditions. In the first, the size of the two center targets was the same, though they were perceived as different due to differences in the size of the surrounding circles. In the second condition (shown in C), the two disks were different in size; however, the surrounding circles gave the illusion that the two target disks were the same size. As shown in Figure 17.5C, which presents the data from the second condition, grip size was scaled to actual target size rather than apparent size. Note that maximum grip aperture was significantly greater for the larger disk compared to the smaller disk (see histograms on the left). However, when asked to estimate the size of the two target disks, the subjects reported that the different-sized disks were identical in size (see histograms of manual estimation of target size on the right) (Haffenden & Goodale, 1998).

Thus, it appears that the ventral stream projections to the temporal cortex play a major role in the perceptual identification of objects, while the dorsal stream projections to the parietal cortex mediate the required sensorimotor transformations for visually guided actions directed at those objects (Goodale & Milner, 1992).

There are a number of clinical implications of this research. It suggests that clinicians should assess both perceptual and action components of visually guided reaching, because they are subserved by different neural components. Understanding the essential perceptual features of an object to be grasped is as important as the ability to modify grasp to accommodate those features. In addition, treatment should focus on training both perceptual and action components of the movement.

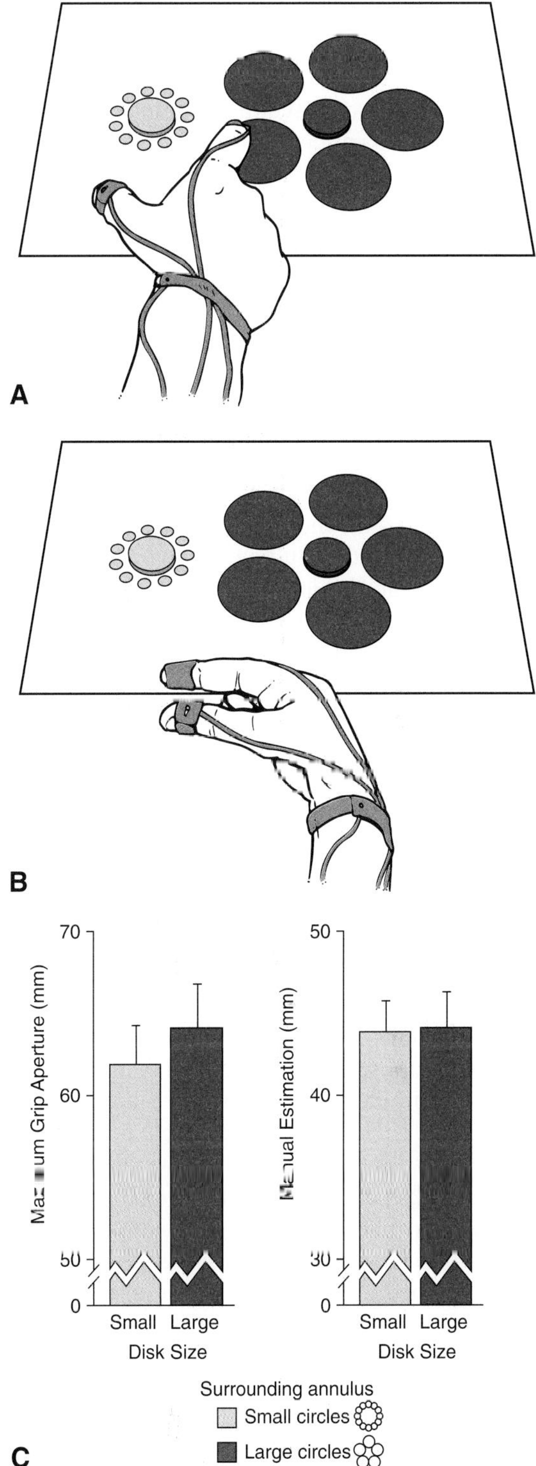

Figure 17.5 Reaching and manual estimation tasks. Shown are both the subject's hand in the grasping task on the way to the target **(A)** and in the manual estimation task **(B)**. Also shown are graphs of mean maximum grip aperture (histograms on the left) on trials in which participants are reaching for disks of two different sizes, though they were perceived as the same size **(C)**. Note that the grip aperture is correctly scaled to target size. Histograms on the right show their manual estimation of the two target disks, indicating the illusion that the two targets were the same size. (Adapted from Haffenden AM, Goodale MA. The effect of pictorial illusion on prehension and perception. *J Cogn Neurosci.* 1998;10:127, 128, with permission.)

Posterior Parietal Cortex and Sensorimotor Transformations

Ongoing research suggests that the control of eye and hand movements emerges from a gradient of sensory and motor neuronal connections across the parietal and frontal areas of the cortex (see Battaglia-Mayer et al., 2016 for a review). This network processes sensory information and transforms it into motor outputs according to abstract rules. This enables the construction of appropriate action goals and strategies to plan, execute, and coordinate eyes and hands during simple reaches, movement sequences, and higher-order complex actions such as tool use and constructions tasks.

It is interesting to note that most neurons in the dorsal stream area (in the posterior parietal cortex, or PPC) show both sensory-related and movement-related activity and thus may be involved in sensorimotor transformation processes involved in both eye movements toward the object to be grasped and subsequent reach and grasp movements of the object as well. For example, the LIP serves as a sensorimotor processing area or interface for the production of saccadic eye movements toward an object. As is found in other sensory processing areas, the LIP governs both sensory attention (required for reaching for a specific object within the sensorimotor map) and eye movements. This interface is a shared boundary between the sensory and motor systems involved in reaching. The strongest eye movement related activity is typically found in the inferior parietal lobule, which includes Brodmann's area 7a and the LIP (Buneo & Andersen, 2006).

There is also evidence that the PPC carries the sensory-motor transformations for planning and controlling intentional high-level cognitive reaching movements (Andersen & Bruneo, 2002). The parietal activity seems to be strongest in the superior parietal lobule, which includes Brodmann's area 5 and the parietal reach region (PRR)—which is composed of the intraparietal sulcus (IPS), medial bank of the intraparietal sulcus (MIP), and V6A (Budisavljevic & Castiello 2017). Moreover, specific visuomotor cortical brain areas have a different degree of involvement depending on the nature of the visuomotor action. A region that corresponds to the posterior portion of the superior parietal lobe (V6A) and the dorsal premotor cortex is mainly active during grasping of large objects, whereas the grasping of small objects would mainly recruit the inferior parietal lobe and the ventral premotor cortex (Battaglia-Mayer et al., 2016).

What computations does the brain need to make in order to make an accurate reach? First of all, it needs to determine both the hand position and the target position. As shown in Figure 17.6, the target in this case is the doorknob used to open the door. The brain can define these positions either in terms of an eye-centered coordinate system (represented by the red lines in Fig. 17.6) or with respect to a body-centered coordinate system (in Fig. 17.6, the gray lines show the coordinates involving the right shoulder, for a right-handed person). Then, it can compute the motor error (M), which is the difference between the hand position (H) and the target position (T) (Buneo & Andersen, 2006).

Research has shown that some neurons in the PPC (those in the PRR) encode target position and current hand position in eye-centered coordinates, while other PPC neurons encode reach-related variables in limb-centered coordinates. A third group of neurons encodes these variables in both eye- and limb-centered coordinates; this suggests that they may play a crucial role in transforming spatial information between the two reference frames (Buneo & Andersen, 2006).

In fact, the PPC is involved in a number of different types of sensorimotor transformations, including the following: (1) movement planning or what could be called "intention" for the movement (the goal of the movement and the type of movement; for example, "I wish to pick up my glass of milk"), which also includes decision-making (a competition between different intentions) and the specifics of how to reach for and grasp the glass; (2) the formation of internal models; and (3) coordinate transformations as part of the process of carrying out the movement plan (Andersen & Cui, 2009).

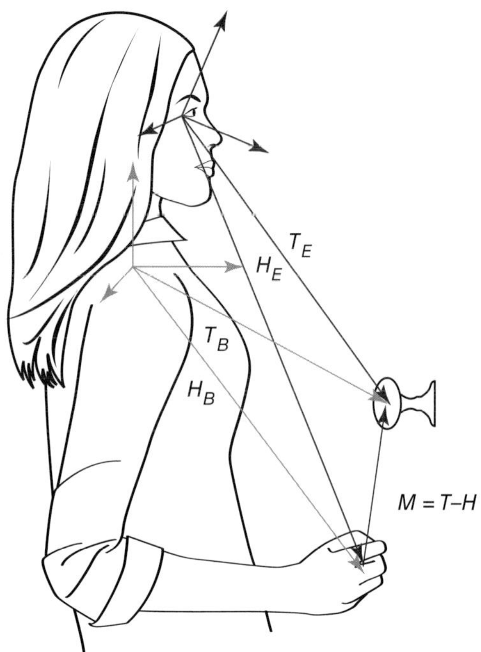

Figure 17.6 Drawing illustrating both an eye-centered representation for reaching to a doorknob (target and hand are shown as *red lines* and coded with respect to the current point of visual fixation) and a body-centered representation (target and hand are shown as *gray lines* and coded with respect to a fixed position on the trunk). The motor error (*M*) is the difference between the hand position (*H*) and the target position (*T*) and is shown by the *black arrow*. *B*, body-centered coordinates; *E*, eye-centered coordinates. (Reprinted from Buneo CA, Andersen RA. The posterior parietal cortex: sensorimotor interface for the planning and online control of visually guided movements. *Neuropsychologia.* 2006;44:2594–2606, with permission.)

Movement Planning and Intentional Maps

Research using functional magnetic resonance imaging (fMRI) in humans and single-unit recording in nonhuman primates suggests that there is a map related to movement planning or intention in the PPC. As shown in Figure 17.7, area LIP (lateral intraparietal cortex) is specialized for saccade planning; area MIP (medial intraparietal), also called the PRR, is specialized for planning of a reach; area AIP (anterior intraparietal) is specialized for planning of a grasp; and area MST (medial superior temporal) is for planning smooth pursuit eye movements. If area AIP, the grasp area, is reversibly inactivated in monkeys, there is a deficit in the shaping of the hand prior to grasping. This is similar to what is found in humans who have PPC damage (Andersen & Buneo, 2002).

For example, it has been shown that patients with lesions in the PPC, resulting in optic ataxia, have problems not only with reaching in the right direction but also with positioning their fingers or adjusting the orientation

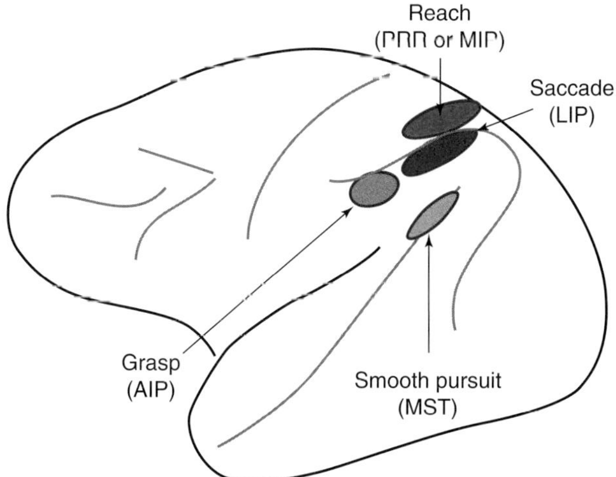

Figure 17.7 Map of intentional areas (involved in early plans for movement) in the posterior parietal cortex of a nonhuman primate. Area LIP (lateral intraparietal area) is specialized for saccade planning; area MIP (medial intraparietal area), also called the parietal reach region (PRR) for reaching; area AIP (anterior intraparietal area) for grasping; and area MST (medial superior temporal) for smooth pursuit eye movements. (Reprinted from Andersen RA, Buneo CA. Intentional maps in posterior parietal cortex. *Annu Rev Neurosci.* 2002;25:199, with permission.)

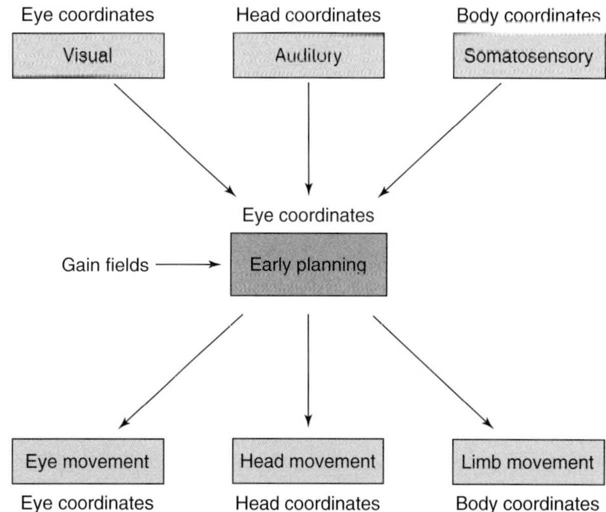

Figure 17.8 Model for multisensory integration and eye, head, and body coordinate transformations occurring within the posterior parietal cortex (PPC). See text for details. (Reprinted from Andersen RA, Buneo CA. Intentional maps in posterior parietal cortex. *Annu Rev Neurosci.* 2002;25:207, with permission.)

of their hand when reaching toward an object. They also have trouble adjusting their grasp to reflect the size of the object they are picking up. Researchers have found that damage to the parietal lobe can impair the ability of patients to use information about the size, shape, and orientation of an object to control the hand and fingers during a grasping movement, even though this same information can be used to identify and describe objects. In particular, patients with superior parietal lesions have problems with scaling maximum grip aperture to the size of the object to be grasped. In addition, fMRI studies in humans have shown that the AIP along with premotor cortex, sensorimotor cortex, and other areas of the PPC are active during a precision grip in humans (Binkofski et al., 1998; Castiello, 2005; Goodale & Milner, 1992).

Coordinate Transformations. Making a movement in response to a sensory stimulus is an amazingly complex task, requiring that our brain solve a large number of difficult computational tasks. The first task requires sensing current hand- and eye-position and using this sensory information to fine-tune movement-related activity neurons (e.g., directional tuning motor neurons) (Battaglia-Mayer, 2019). This task is complex since different types of sensory inputs (e.g., visual, auditory, touch) use different reference frames when coding where the body and the object are in space. As shown in Figure 17.8, visual information is coded in eye-centered coordinates, auditory information in head-centered coordinates, and somatosensory information (e.g., touch) in body-centered coordinates (Andersen & Buneo, 2002). Therefore, the central nervous system (CNS) needs to resolve the discrepancies among the reference coordinate systems in some way, as all three systems may be needed to guide the movement in different contexts. All of the coordinate frames must then be transformed into motor coordinates to command muscles during eye, head, and arm movements, which are the final execution systems to carry the movements.

As shown in Figure 17.8, the nervous system can solve this problem during the early planning of the movement by using the eye-centered coordinate system as a common coordinate system. Using a common coordinate frame facilitates eye–hand coordination, and as vision is the most accurate of all the senses, it also improves movement accuracy (Andersen & Buneo, 2002).

The next problem to be solved is to convert the information into limb-centered coordinates for the reach itself. There is evidence to suggest that, at least in some contexts, this is solved by using a direct transformation scheme, using eye coordinates to subtract the current hand position from the current target position (seen in Fig. 17.6), and creating a motor vector in limb coordinates. Researchers have found that cells in Brodmann's area 5, a somatosensory–motor cortical area within the PPC, code the locations of targets in both eye-centered and limb-centered coordinates. The transformation process appears to involve simple gain changes in neuron responses (Andersen & Buneo, 2002).

Bernier and Grafton (2010) have shown that within the multiplicity of coordinate systems, the sensory modality used in perception of a target can determine the coordinate frame of reference to be used for the sensorimotor transformations that are required for making the reach toward the target. For example, when the target is defined visually, the motor goal is encoded in a gaze-centered system by the anterior precuneus, while the parieto-occipital junction, Broadman's area 5, and the dorsal premotor cortex combine gaze- and body-centered coordinates. On the other hand, when proprioception is used to identify the target, these brain areas use a body-centered frame (Bernier & Grafton, 2010).

Role of Visual Feedback in Reach and Grasp

The primary function of visual feedback in reaching appears to be related to the attainment of final accuracy. It has been hypothesized that the constancy of thumb position with relation to the wrist during reaching may be part of a strategy of providing clear visual feedback information regarding the end point of the limb (Wing & Frazer, 1983).

To determine the function of visual feedback in reaching, studies have been performed to compare reaches made with and without vision. Reaches with visual feedback showed a longer duration than those performed without feedback. Absence of visual feedback did not alter the grasp component of the reach (Jeannerod, 1990).

Can reaching still occur in the absence of visual cortex function? It is usually accepted that destruction of the visual cortex in humans produces total blindness, except for very poor visual perception of illumination changes. However, research on monkeys with visual cortex lesions has shown some very interesting results related to visual–motor control. Although these monkeys appeared to be blind when their visual behavior was tested, they could still reach for objects that appeared in or moved across the visual field. It has been hypothesized that the superior colliculus in the midbrain contributes to this residual reaching behavior (Humphrey & Weiskrantz, 1969).

Since the studies in monkeys were performed, studies in humans have verified these results. In extending the studies in monkeys to humans, these researchers used a new experimental paradigm that had not been used before in humans. Instead of asking humans with visual cortex lesions if they could see an object, they asked them to try to point to where they "guessed" the target would be. It was shown that subjects did not point randomly; there was a significant correlation between pointing and target position. However, subjects did show larger constant errors when reaching within their blind visual fields. They typically overshot targets when they were within 30 degrees of midline and undershot them when they were beyond 30 degrees (Perenin & Jeannerod, 1975; Weiskrantz et al., 1974).

Visually Controlled Reaches across the Midline

Is visual processing more complex when reaching to the contralateral side of the body? Yes. Researchers have consistently found that reaching movements across the midline (toward targets in the visual hemifield of the opposite arm) are slower and less accurate than movements to targets on the same side as the arm. Ipsilateral (uncrossed) reaches in these studies were shorter in latency, made with higher maximum velocity, completed more quickly, and made significantly more accurately than contralateral (crossed) reaches (Fisk & Goodale, 1985).

Thus, even normal adults show decrements when reaching to the contralateral side of the body. This must be remembered when evaluating patients with reaching problems. In addition, when structuring a training program, one may wish to begin with reaching to objects placed on the ipsilateral side prior to progressing to objects placed on the contralateral side.

Somatosensory Contributions to Reach

Is somatosensory input essential for the production of reaching movements? Taub and Berman (1968) have shown that within 2 weeks of deafferentation, monkeys were able to perform adequate reach-and-grasp movements as long as vision was available. They noted that the monkeys' movements were awkward at first, with animals only sweeping objects along the floor. Monkeys then developed a primitive grasp with four fingers together and no thumb and finally redeveloped a crude pincer grasp a few months after the lesion was made.

Other experiments discussed later in this chapter have shown that deafferented monkeys can still make reasonably accurate single-joint pointing movements, even when vision of the arm is occluded, when the pointing task was learned before deafferentation (Polit & Bizzi, 1979). In this case, even displacing the arm before the movement did not substantially affect terminal accuracy, even though the monkeys could not see or feel their arm positions. Thus, it was concluded that monkeys are capable of using a central motor program to perform previously learned reaching movements and that kinesthetic feedback is not required for achieving reasonable accuracy when performing well-learned movements.

Experiments performed with humans with severe peripheral sensory neuropathy in all four limbs have shown similar results. One person was able to perform a wide variety of hand movements, such as tapping movements and drawing figures in the air, even with the eyes closed. However, when he was asked to repeat the movement many times with the eyes closed, his performance deteriorated quickly. Thus, it appears that somatosensory information is not required for arm movement initiation or execution, as long as the movements are simple or nonrepetitive. However, if individuals have to make complex movements requiring coordination of many joints, or repeat movements, without visual feedback, they are unable to update their central representations of body space and show considerable movement "drift" and problems with coordination (Rothwell et al., 1982).

Research suggests that in individuals with an intact CNS, proprioceptive information is used to update the internal representation of limb movement dynamics. However, in those with impaired proprioception, there exist disrupted reaching paths and interactive joint torque coordination problems in the upper limb. In this case, the use of vision can partly compensate for these errors (Ghez & Sainburg, 1995). Furthermore, Lefumat and colleagues (2016) investigated how two proprioceptively deafferented individuals with specific damage of sensory Aβ axons (i.e., selective loss of kinesthesia, tendon reflexes, touch, vibration, pressure, position and movement sense) controlled upper limb dynamics during perturbed reaches with the dominant arm and whether there was transfer learning of the reaching task in the opposite arm. Vision of the reaching arm was allowed in their experiment. Their results showed that the two participants not only adjusted reaching control to the imposed perturbative external force fields but also demonstrated interlimb transfer of the sensorimotor adaptation to the non-adapted limb, which is critical for motor learning generalization across limbs and movement directions.

All these experiments suggest that certain movements may be carried out without somatosensory feedback or learned with visual compensation. Nevertheless, considerable work has also shown the important contributions of sensory feedback to the fine regulation of movement.

Researchers originally thought that it was mainly joint receptors that controlled position sense during reaching. However, more recent research suggests that joint receptors are active mainly at the extremes of joint motion, but not at midposition. This would thus make it impossible for these receptors to signal limb position in the mid–working range of joints (Jeannerod, 1990).

Other research has begun to build evidence for a strong role for muscle spindles in position sense. Experiments have been performed in which tendons were vibrated, specifically activating muscle spindle Ia afferents. Subjects consistently had the illusion that the joint was moving in the direction that it would have been moving if the muscle were being stretched. For example, when the biceps tendon was vibrated, it produced the illusion of elbow extension (Goodwin et al., 1972).

Cutaneous afferents are also important contributors to position sense. Mechanoreceptors in the glabrous area of the hand are strongly activated by isotonic movements of the fingers (Hulliger et al., 1979).

Interestingly, individuals who are recovering from paralysis report that when the muscle is still completely paralyzed, they have no feeling of heaviness in the limb. But as they begin to regain movement ability, they feel as if the limb is being held down by weights. These sensations of heaviness are reduced as movements become easier and strength increases. This could be due to an internal perception of the intensity of motor commands (Jeannerod, 1990).

Somatosensory Contributions to Grasp

Cutaneous afferent input is essential for the control of grip forces. If objects are slippery, cutaneous afferents will detect the slip and activate pathways to increase activity in finger muscles to increase the grip force and in shoulder and elbow muscles to slow the acceleration of the hand. When experiments were performed in which fingers were anesthetized to prevent cutaneous feedback, subjects used the strategy of increasing grip forces to compensate for lack of information, but coordination between grip and load forces was lost, even if the person had previous experience lifting the object (Witney et al., 2004).

In addition, the grip force declined significantly over a 20- to 30-second hold period, and 7 of 10 subjects dropped the object at least once. Adaptation to this loss of information did not occur, even with vision of the grasping hand. Individuals with polysensory neuropathy (complete loss of primary afferent sensory inputs) also have similar difficulty with the control of grip forces and show little to no ability to adapt with time. However, those with moderately impaired sensation have shown no problems of this type (Augurelle et al., 2003; Monzee et al., 2003; Nowak et al., 2003; Witney et al., 2004).

Elegant studies have shown that the CNS areas critical for this control include the somatosensory cortex (SI). Studies inactivating the finger area of SI showed that this was correlated with uncoordinated grip and load forces and an increase in grip force (Brochier et al., 1999). Single-cell recording in SI during lift-and-hold tasks in primates has shown that rapidly adapting cells are briefly active at grip onset, slowly adapting cells show continuous activity during the holding phase, and both cell types respond strongly to slip. They also receive input from movement-related areas of the brain and may play a role in the activation of responses when afferent input suddenly changes from its normal pattern (Salimi et al., 1999a, 1999b).

Visual and Somatosensory Contributions to Anticipatory (Feedforward) Control of Reach and Grasp

An essential component of all reaching movements is proactive visual and somatosensory control, which is responsible for the correct initial direction of the limb toward the target and the initial coordination between limb segments. In addition, visual information about the characteristics of the object to be grasped is used proactively to preprogram the forces used in precision grip.

It has been hypothesized that visual and somatosensory information is also used to update proprioceptive and visual body maps that allow the accurate programming of reaching movements. To determine the influence of updated maps of the body workspace on the accuracy of a reaching movement, experiments were performed to manipulate visual information regarding hand and target positions prior to movement. It was shown that when a person could not see the hand prior to movement, there were large errors in reaching the target. It was thus concluded that a proprioceptive map of the hand, by itself, was not adequate to appropriately code the hand position in the reaching workspace. This suggests that somatosensory inputs must be calibrated by vision in order for the proprioceptive map and the visual map to be matched (Jeannerod, 1990).

Research has shown that individuals with a healthy CNS can smooth hand paths that undergo external perturbative forces using either visual or proprioceptive feedback. This is because the two types of sensory information are encoded within different coordinate systems. Proprioception is mainly encoded as muscle length and rate of length change, whereas the spatial location of the object is visually registered within egocentric coordinates. Because they use different coordinate systems, researchers propose that proprioception and vision control different segments of the reaching task. Vision is proposed to regulate hand path direction and spatial trajectory, while proprioception facilitates the terminal hand position and limb status (Scheidt et al., 2005; Sober & Sabes 2003). When the object is in motion, visual feedback from the moving object is of critical importance to predict synchronous grip and load forces in a timely manner in order to control the grasp of the object. Furthermore, research suggests that grip force regulation is facilitated when visual attention is directed toward the moving object (inverse dynamics computations) and not toward the hand for the estimation of hand position errors (forward computations) (Takamuku & Gomi, 2019).

Motor Systems

Premotor and Primary Motor Cortex Involvement

As noted previously, in the section on visual contributions to reach and grasp, the PPC is involved in encoding goals for movement, such as the intended hand formation and orientation toward the object. Information is then sent to the premotor and primary motor cortex (Castiello, 2005; Crawford et al., 2004). Though we think of the parietal cortex as "sensory" and the premotor and motor cortexes as being involved with movement execution, there are both interesting similarities and differences related to activity in the PPC and in the premotor cortex. For example, neurons in both the AIP grasp area and the motor areas code for grasping actions that relate to the type of object that will be grasped (e.g., precision vs. power grip), but the AIP neurons represent the entire action, while the premotor neurons are concerned with a particular part of the action. In addition, the AIP codes objects in visual coordinates, while premotor cortex codes in body coordinates (as noted in the lower part of Fig. 17.8, under eye movement, head movement, and limb movement) (Andersen & Buneo, 2002; Castiello, 2005).

Two separate descending pathways are also involved in reach and grasp, as described in the following.

Two Separate Descending Pathways for Reach and Grasp

During reaching, the arm movement carrying the hand to the target is performed in parallel with the preshaping of the fingers for grasping the object. There are many experiments that suggest that the respective motor systems contributing to reach and grasp involve separate descending motor pathways.

For example, reaching is observed in newborn infants, although grip formation develops later. Research has shown that 1-week-old infants may reach for and intercept moving objects and come into contact with them, but this is done with a hand that is wide open, with no grip formation. Grip formation appears to develop at about 10 to 22 weeks of age (Bruner & Koslowski, 1972).

This is also the case in monkeys. It has been shown that the appearance of the grasp component, at 8 months of age, is correlated with the maturation of connections between the corticospinal tract and the motor neurons (Kuypers, 1962). Thus, a successful grasp requires an intact primary motor cortex and corticospinal tract: if either of these areas has lesions, there is a clear problem with individual finger control for grasping. However, lesions here do not affect synergistic control of fingers for power grips. Interestingly, it has also been shown that motor cortex neurons that are active during fine movements, like a precision grip, become inactive during a power grip (Castiello, 2005; Muir & Lemon, 1983).

Children with pyramidal lesions show problems with the grasp component of reaching, although the transport component may be normal (Jeannerod, 1990). This suggests that midbrain and brainstem pathways such as the red nucleus and reticular nuclei may control the more proximal muscles involved in reaching movements, while pyramidal pathways are required for the fine control of grasping movements.

Information from primary motor cortex to the spinal cord is also sent to the cerebellum (intermediate lobe), since the cerebellum is also important for the control of hand movements during grasping; [illegible]% of output neurons from the cerebellum were more active during reaching out and grasping than during simply gripping an object (Castiello, 2005; Gibson et al., 1994).

Experiments on monkeys performing a precision grip versus a power grip task (Fig. 17.9) have shown that there are neurons in the primary motor cortex that

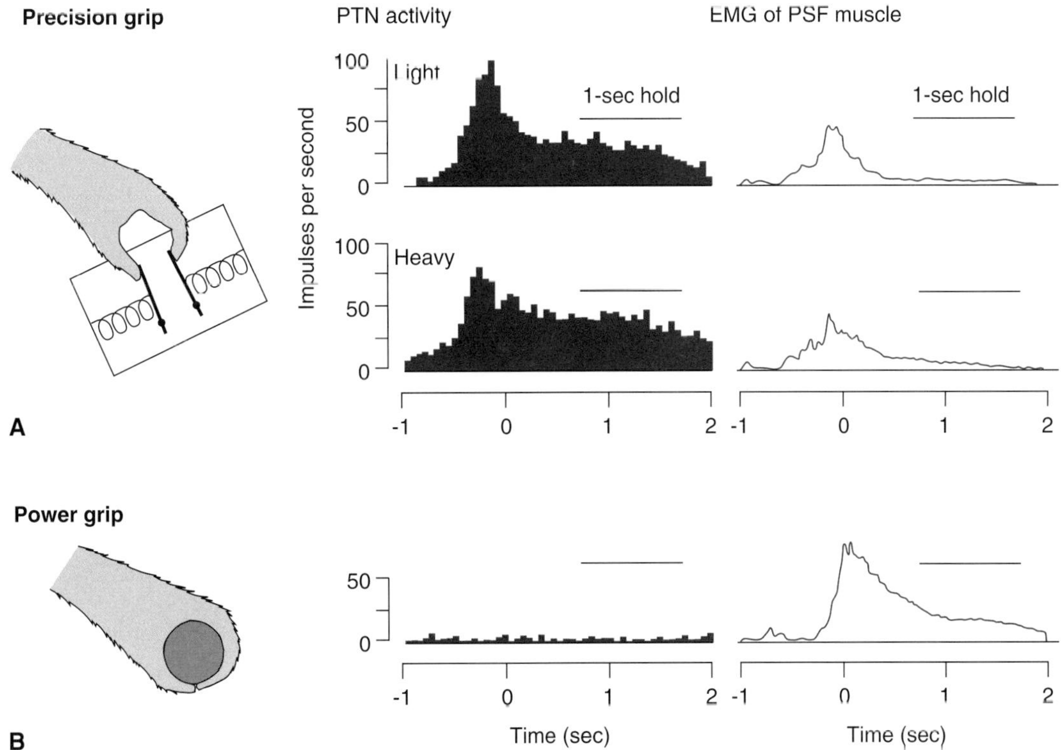

Figure 17.9 Graph of activity (impulses/second) of a pyramidal tract neuron (*PTN*) and an interosseus muscle (*PSF*) during two different tasks: **(A)** a precision grip task executed with light versus heavy force (top two traces) and **(B)** a power grip task (bottom trace). Note that these neurons are active during a precision grip but not a power grip. (Redrawn from Muir RB, Lemon RM. Corticospinal neurons with a special role in precision grip. *Brain Res.* 1983;261:312–316, with permission.)

fire during the execution of a precision but not a power grip. This indicates that their connections are with intrinsic hand muscles rather than with forearm muscles. These neurons show a short-latency burst onset (~11 msec) prior to muscle activation, which suggests they are monosynaptically connected to the motor neuron pools (Lemon et al., 1986; Muir & Lemon, 1983). Figure 17.9 shows the activity of a pyramidal tract neuron (PTN) and an interosseus muscle during a precision grip task with light versus heavy force and during a power grip task (grasping a cylinder). Note that the PTN is activated only during the precision grip task at both force levels, but is not activated during the power grip task. However, the interosseus muscle showed activity in all three tasks.

Musculoskeletal Contributions

Reaching also involves a complex interaction of musculoskeletal and neural systems. Musculoskeletal components include joint range of motion, spinal flexibility, muscle properties, and biomechanical relationships among linked body segments. In particular, it has been suggested that the following types of joint motion are essential to the ability to move the arm normally: scapular rotation; appropriate movement of the humeral head; the ability to supinate the forearm, shoulder, and elbow flexion to approximately 100 to 120 degrees; the ability to extend the wrist to slightly beyond neutral; and sufficient mobility in the hand to allow grasp and release (Charness, 1994).

Motor aspects of reaching include appropriate muscle tone, muscle strength, and coordination. More specifically, this involves appropriate activation of muscles to stabilize the scapula, rib cage, and humeral head during upper-extremity reaching movements and activation of muscles at the shoulder, elbow, and wrist joint for transport of the arm.

The work of Kaminski et al. (1995) provides evidence for coupling between the trunk, scapula, and arm when one reaches toward targets. The authors found motion of the trunk to make a significant contribution during arm transport, which affected both the velocity and the path of the hand. Specific evidence of coupling was documented during reaches for anteriorly placed targets; in that trunk, rotation was countered by glenohumeral horizontal abduction and scapular retraction in order to keep the hand moving in a straight path.

In a patient with neurologic deficits, it is often not easy to determine the relative contribution of neural versus musculoskeletal problems to abnormal reaching. Motor control problems that affect the inertial characteristics of the system will give rise to coordination problems, even when the patterns of activation are normal. For example, an increase in stiffness will change the inertial characteristics of the head, arm, and/or trunk, making the initiation of motion more difficult. Thus, we see the important interaction between the biomechanics of movement and the neural control mechanisms.

Postural Support of Reaching

As was discussed in Chapter 7, postural control, defined as the ability to control the body's position in space for the purpose of stability and orientation, has a strong influence on upper-extremity function. The ability to control the body's position in space is essential to being able to move one part of the body, in this case one or both arms, without destabilizing the rest of the body.

Research has shown that a key brain structure involved in the learning of anticipatory postural adjustments during a bimanual task (e.g., holding an object in one hand and lifting it with the other) is the cerebellum. Studies of task efficiency in individuals with cerebellar lesions showed that although well-learned anticipatory postural adjustments in this task were mainly intact, short-term adaptation of the adjustment was not possible. In addition, individuals with cerebellar abnormalities were not able to learn to make an anticipatory postural adjustment for a task for which they had previously not been trained. The authors conclude that adaptation of these responses and the acquisition of novel anticipatory adjustments require the cerebellum. They also found that individuals with cerebellar damage showed poorly timed anticipatory adjustments, with responses beginning earlier than in normal adults (Diedrichsen et al., 2005).

Just as manipulatory control is task dependent, postural requirements also vary according to the task. For example, postural requirements involved in a seated reaching task will be less stringent than those in a standing task and thus may require only muscles in the trunk. In contrast, postural demands during reaching while standing are greater, requiring more extensive activation of muscles in both the legs and the trunk to prevent instability. Postural demands can affect the speed and accuracy of an upper-extremity movement. When postural demands are decreased by providing external support, upper-extremity movements are faster, since prior postural stabilization is not necessary (Cordo & Nashner, 1982).

For healthy young adults, additional postural support of the trunk while seated (e.g., at the midribs) did not change arm and trunk kinematics of the reach. However, as we will see in the next chapters, on both development and impaired reach and grasp, external trunk support improves reaching kinematics for children and individuals with neurologic pathology (Rachwani et al., 2015; Santamaria, 2016). Therefore, helping patients with upper-extremity dysfunction to regain sufficient postural control to meet the postural requirements inherent in a reaching task is essential to retraining. The reader is urged to review Chapters 7 to 11, which discuss postural control, its relationship to reaching, and issues related to retraining the patient with postural disorders.

GRASPING

Classification of Grasping Patterns

Grasping patterns vary as a function of location, size, and shape of the object to be grasped (Johansson, 1996). In 1956, Napier classified human grasping movements as either power or precision grips. He found that precision and power grips could be used alternatively or in combination for almost every type of object. He also believed that it was not solely the shape or size of the object that determined the grip pattern but also the intended activity, since a cylindrical object could be used for writing (precision grip) or hammering (power grip) (Castiello, 2005; Jeannerod, 1996; Napier, 1956).

The anatomical difference between the two grips involves the posture both of the thumb and that of the fingers. In a power grip, the finger and thumb pads are directed toward the palm to transmit a force to an object. Power grips include a hook grasp (holding a handle of a suitcase), a spherical grasp (holding a softball), and a cylindrical grasp (holding a bottle). In contrast, during a precision grip, the forces are directed between the thumb and fingers. The two grips are used very differently in manipulative skills: the precision grip allows movements of the object relative to the hand and within the hand, while the power grip does not.

In addition to the power versus precision distinction, researchers have shown that subjects tend to classify objects into four broad categories according to prior knowledge about the object. These categories are the four hand shapes: poke, pinch, clench, and palm. The boundaries between categories are determined by the pattern of hand movements used with these objects when they are grasped and manipulated. This differentiation of hand shape also appears during actual reaching in the preshaping of the grasp (Castiello, 2005; Jeannerod, 1996; Klatzky et al., 1987).

Two important requirements are necessary for successfully grasping an object. First, the hand must be adapted to the shape, size, and use of the object. Second, the finger movements must be timed appropriately in relation to transport so that they close on the object just at the appropriate moment. If they close too early or too late, the grasp will be inappropriate (Jeannerod, 1990). Most of the research related to grip formation has been on precision grip, and this will be discussed in the following section.

Anticipatory Control of Grasping Patterns: Precision Grip Formation

When reaching forward to grasp an object, the shaping of the hand for grasping occurs during the

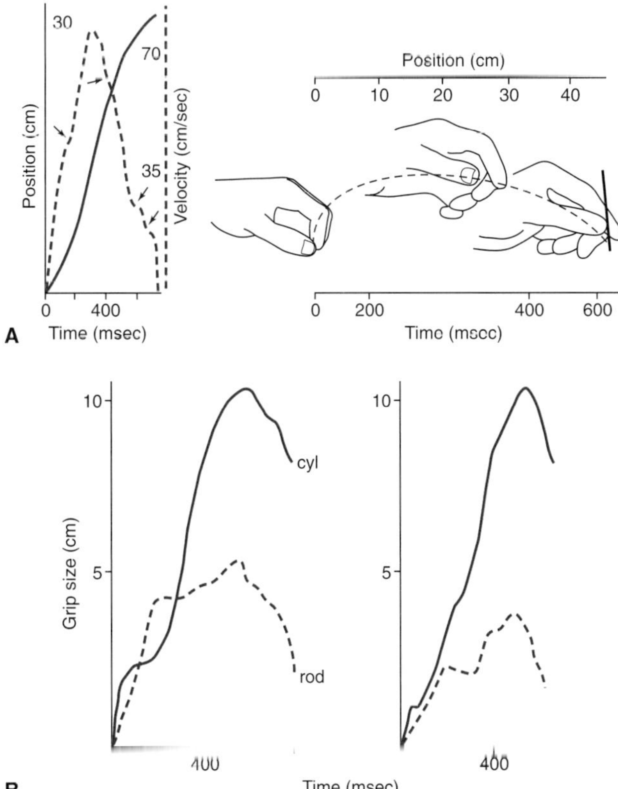

Figure 17.10 Characteristics of the transport phase of reaching. **(A)** *left*. Changes in hand movement velocity (*dotted line*) and position (*solid line*) as a function of time during a reach. **(A)** *right*. Drawing of hand movement changes, including grip opening, during reach. (Adapted from Brooks VB. *The neural basis of motor control*. New York, NY: Oxford University Press, 1986:133.) **(B)** Changes in grip size over time for two different subjects reaching for a 2-mm-diameter, 10-cm-long rod (*dashed lines*) versus a 55-mm-diameter, 10-cm-long cylinder (cyl) (*solid lines*). Note that there are different grip sizes but similar curve shapes. (Reprinted from Jeannerod M. *The neural and behavioral organization of goal-directed movements*. Oxford: Clarendon Press, 1990:61, with permission.)

transportation component of the reach. Figure 17.10 shows changes in both hand movement velocity (Fig. 17.10A, left) and grip size (Fig. 17.10A, right) during a reach. This pregrasp hand shaping appears to be under visual control. What are the properties of an object that affect anticipatory hand shaping? Lab Activity 17.1 will help answer this question.

As you can see from Lab Activity 17.1, there are two different categories of properties of objects that affect pregrasp hand shaping: intrinsic properties, such as the object's size, shape, and texture, and extrinsic or contextual properties, such as the object's orientation, distance from the body, and location with respect to the body (Jeannerod, 1984).

Remember that grip formation takes place during the transportation phase and is anticipatory of the characteristics of the object to be grasped. The size of the maximum grip opening is proportional to the size of the object. This relationship is shown in Figure 17.10B,

LAB ACTIVITY 17.1

Objective: To examine how properties of the task affect reach-and-grasp movements.

Procedures: You will be working in pairs for this lab. You will need the following items: a pitcher of water, a glass, a quarter, a pencil, a block, and a plastic glass covered with oil. In the first part of the lab, observe the arm and hand movements of your partner while they pick up and set down the glass, quarter, pencil, block, and plastic glass coated with oil. Next, set the glass upright next to the water pitcher. Observe your partner while they reach for and pour a glass of water. Now, pour the water back in the pitcher and invert the glass next to the pitcher. Again, observe your partner while they reach for and pour a glass of water.

Assignment

1. Describe the properties of the objects that affected how you reach for and grasp the various objects.
2. During the pouring task, how did changing the orientation of the glass affect the movement strategy used to pick up the glass?
3. During the reach for an object, did the hand begin to shape in preparation for grasp?
4. How did characteristics of the object affect anticipatory hand shaping?

with a subject reaching for a 2-mm rod versus a 55-mm cylinder. Each increase of 1 cm in object size is associated with a maximum grip size increase of 0.77 cm (Marteniuk et al., 1990). When subjects change the grip opening, they do it almost entirely with finger movements, while the thumb stays in one place. When reaching for an object, as the arm is transported forward, the fingers begin to stretch, and the grip size increases rapidly to a maximum and then is reduced to match the size of the object (Castiello, 2005; Jeannerod, 1990).

Subjects show differential hand shaping for different shapes of objects as well. The distance between the thumb and index finger is usually largest during the final-slow-approach phase. It has been shown that adults with prosthetic hands show this same relationship between grasp and transport phases (Fraser & Wing, 1981). Apparently, this relationship is not due to neural constraints but may be the most efficient way to reach. Furthermore, the probability of being successful while grasping relies upon the level of sensorimotor uncertainty (e.g., visual constraints such as blurred or monocular vision). This means that the brain needs to account for and estimate the margin of error in order to adjust the hand configuration to the object's features (Keefe et al., 2019).

Aging has been shown to contribute to reduced control of precision hand movements. A study investigated age-related reductions in hand control with the Simple Test for Evaluating Hand Functions (STEF) and kinematics in healthy older and young adult groups. They found that motor performance was lower in older adults than controls, independent of the use of the non-dominant or dominant hand. In addition, older adults showed compensatory kinematic grasping patterns during the hand actions. Older adults grasped with an earlier peak tangential velocity of the wrist and with greater inter-fingertip distances that followed arch-like fingertip trajectories, for all objects regardless of their size. The authors concluded that this compensatory kinematic pattern allowed a longer adjustment time for the reach and grasp components and reduced errors prehension (Tamaru et al., 2017).

Grasp and Lift Tasks

The types of objects that are picked up during a given day may vary from a light pen to a heavy slick bottle of oil. The nervous system is capable of adapting precision grip so that it accommodates objects of many different weights and surface characteristics. The control mechanisms underlying these abilities have been carefully investigated. It has been shown that there are discrete phases to any lifting task. These phases are associated with responses in sensory receptors of the hand.

The first phase of, for example, lifting an object off a table starts with contact between the fingers and the object to be lifted, as you see in Figure 17.11A. When contact has been established, the second phase begins, with the grip force and the load force (load on the fingers) starting to increase. This is shown by the dotted line on the load and grip force graphs in Figure 17.11B. The third phase begins when the load force has overcome the weight of the object and it starts to move. This is shown in the position graph (lowest trace in black) in Figure 17.11B, when the position begins to move upward from 0. The fourth phase occurs at the end of the lifting task, when there is a decrease in the grip and load force shortly after the object again makes contact with the table (not shown) (Johansson & Edin, 1992). The figure shows force and position measurements for three different known weights of objects, 200, 400, and 800 g. Note that the grip force increases proportionately, as the weight of the object increases.

This type of an organizational control scheme has many advantages. For example, it allows great flexibility in lifting objects of different weights. Thus, the duration of the loading phase depends on the object's weight: heavier objects require higher load forces before they move. This also ensures that proper grip forces are used during the load phase. This scheme also requires limited sensory processing, since the end of one phase serves as the trigger for the next.

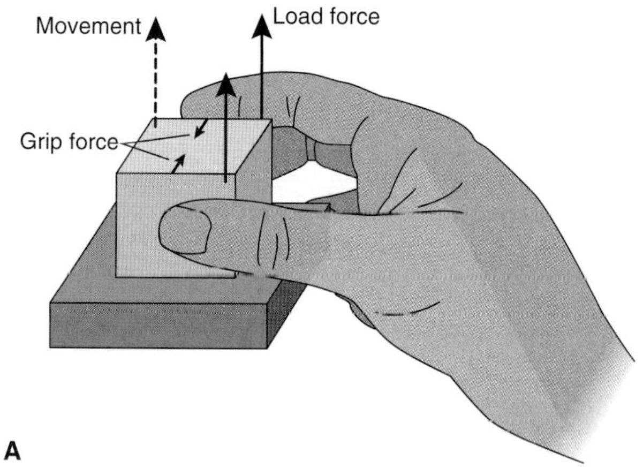

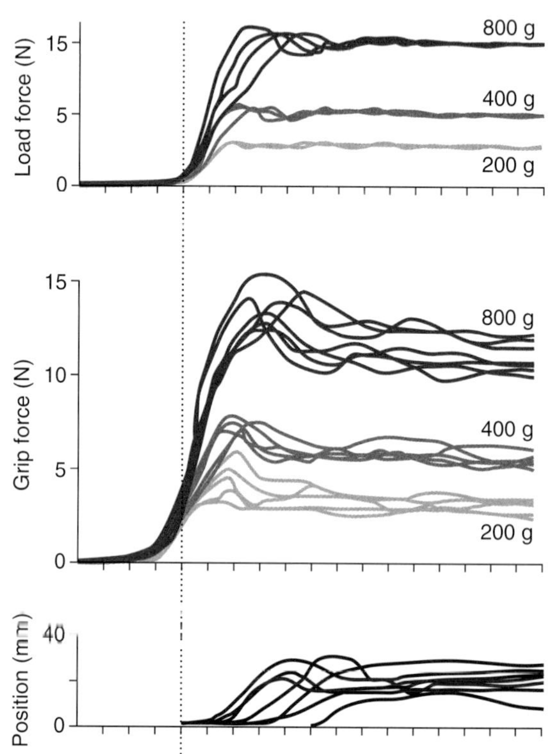

Figure 17.11 **(A)** A subject lifts an object from a table that is instrumented with both grip force and load force detectors. **(B)** The person knows the object's weight (200, 400, or 800 g) in advance, and thus, the forces used are appropriate for lifting the object, as you see in the three sets of traces (load force, grip force, and position) from multiple trials. Note that the grip force is scaled in proportion to the weight of the object so that the object doesn't slip. (Reprinted from Kandel ER, et al. *Principles of neural science.* 5th ed. New York, NY: McGraw Hill, 2013. Fig. 33-14, p. 758, with permission.)

Once the object is grasped, the grip-to-load force ratio has to be above a certain level to ensure a safe grip; otherwise, slipping will occur. How does the nervous system choose the correct parameters for grip and load force? Two objects of the same weight will not necessarily require the same grip force, since one may be much more slippery than the other. The CNS appears to use both previous experience and afferent information during the task to choose correct grip parameters. If there is a mismatch between the expected and actual properties of an object, then receptors in the finger pads are activated. Pacinian corpuscles are very sensitive and capable of easily detecting that an object has started to move earlier than expected. In addition, visual and other types of cutaneous cues are important in determining the choice of grip parameters (Johansson & Edin, 1992).

This research suggests the importance of haptic feedback for the precise control of grip tasks that involve the thumb and the index finger or multiple digits, as well as for discriminating other object properties such as a change in weight in the absence of visual cues (Miall et al., 2000, 2019). A study by Miall et al. (2019) has shown that individuals with damage to large-fiber sensory axons have both functional deficits and altered hand control strategies during reach-grasp-lift tasks. In the reach-to-grasp component, these individuals show slowed movement, larger grip aperture, and less dynamic modulation of grip aperture. In the lifting phase, they showed greater variability in hand postures, mainly while grasping small objects, and they adopted hand postures that facilitated visual guidance and a reduction of complexity in the control of the hand.

The cerebellum appears to be a key system contributing to predictive control of grip forces. In studies in which monkeys were required to maintain their grip on an object during perturbations that simulated object slip, it was found that cerebellar interpositus nucleus and cortical neurons with inputs from cutaneous receptors were activated about 45 msec after the perturbation. The cerebellar neurons also showed anticipatory increases in activation along with grip force increases over repeated trials (Monzee & Smith, 2004). This indicates that the cerebellum plays a role in organizing predictive responses. Research indicates that primary, premotor, and supplementary motor areas do not show predictive responses of this type. This research is supported by work with patients with cerebellar lesions, who have poor predictive control of grip forces, especially related to timing of these forces. On the contrary, patients with hemiparesis have normal timing of predictive grip forces but with reduced response amplitudes (Babin-Ratte et al., 1999; Boudreau & Smith, 2001; Wiesendanger & Serrien, 2001; Witney et al., 2004).

COORDINATION OF REACH AND GRASP

Although the neurophysiological and developmental research discussed previously indicates that the two components, reach and grasp, are controlled by different motor systems, to be functionally effective, they must be coordinated with each other. Thus, transport of the hand must be coordinated with the shaping of the fingers to ensure that reaching ends when the fingers come in contact with the object.

Researchers have used kinematics to determine whether there are invariant relationships between reach components and grasp components. It has been shown that there is a fixed ratio of maximum grip aperture to total movement time, such that it occurs at about 75% to 80% of movement time (Jeannerod, 1984; Wallace et al., 1990). This ratio was invariant across variations in movement time and speed and different initial finger postures and was preserved even in pathological conditions. This is a strong indication of functional coupling of the two components (Jeannerod, 1996).

Invariance related to the coordination of reach and grasp has also been studied by examining the effect of a perturbation of one component on the second component. For example, in order to perturb the transport (reach) component, researchers displaced the object to be grasped and found that this perturbation of reach also affected grasp, since there was a brief interruption in grip aperture formation. In addition, when object size was changed in order to perturb the grip component, it affected the transport component. Thus, the two components were kinematically coupled during corrections for these perturbations (Paulignan et al., 1990). Although the two components are correlated, they appear to be only loosely coupled in time. Thus, they appear to be functionally linked, without stereotyped structural relationships (Jeannerod, 1996).

Based on this research, we could hypothesize that in the case of Genise, our patient with upper-extremity paresis complicated by spasticity, both reach (transport) and grasp will be affected. We might predict, based on the neurophysiological research, that Genise will recover the reach phase earlier and more completely than the grasp phase (De Souza et al., 1980). While the two components are controlled separately, they require coordination to be functionally effective; thus, Genise will need to train reach and grasp both separately and together (i.e., part- and whole-task training). For example, as shown in Genise's treatment video, Genise begins practicing the reach component by moving her arm on the sliding board toward an object but not actually grasping it. Because even the reach phase is task dependent, it is important to practice reaching within the context of many different types of functional tasks, such as reach and point, reach in preparation for a grasp, reach in preparation for a grasp and lift, or grasp and move.

Using a mirror for visual feedback training, Genise also practices grasp and release bimanually, alleviating the need for controlling reach. At this stage in her recovery, she has very little capacity to grasp and release with her paretic arm and requires assistance. Eventually, as she improves, she may work on combining reach components and grasp components.

GENERAL PRINCIPLES OF NEURAL CONTROL OF REACH AND GRASP

Until now, we have described the biomechanical and neural contributions to the different components of reach and grasp. However, another approach to studying the control of reaching has come from the field of psychology, where researchers have focused on describing basic characteristics of reaching and formulated principles and theories about the neural control of reaching based on these characteristics.

Invariant Features of Movement: Motor Programs

In Chapter 1, we mentioned that most movements are performed with similar characteristics even when made with different body segments or limbs. Thus, you can write a word with your fingers, with your left or right arm, or with the pen in your mouth, and the word will have similar characteristics. This feature has been called "motor equivalence," and it predicts that most movements are represented in the brain in terms of abstract rules that can be used to activate any set of muscles and are not represented solely at the level of muscle contractions or joint motions.

Reaction Times for Reach and Grasp

RT is defined as the period between a stimulus and the beginning of a voluntary response (measured as the activation of muscle responses or movement). Voluntary movements require significantly more processing time than reflexes, with the fastest RTs being about 80 to 120 msec for a voluntary response to a somatosensory cue. In contrast, monosynaptic reflex responses are about 40 msec in response to similar cues. Visually initiated RTs are even longer, on the order of 150 to 180 msec, because of increased synaptic processing in the visual system (Ghez & Krakauer, 2000).

RT also varies according to the amount of information to be processed in making the decision to move. RT is fastest if the subject knows in advance the response that is required and is increasingly slowed by adding choices (different cues indicating different movements to be made) or more complex tasks. Figure 17.12A shows how RT increases with the addition of response alternatives. This is called the "choice effect." It has led researchers to hypothesize that movement processing involves three general stages: stimulus identification, response selection (varying with the number of choices to be made), and response programming (Fig. 17.12B). Although it has been hypothesized that movement processing involves three stages, it has also been shown that parallel processing of movement characteristics, such as movement direction and movement extent, can occur, thus speeding movement processing. RT also becomes faster with learning, as shown in Figure 17.12C. If one group of subjects is given 10 blocks of 10 trials (pressing a key under one of four lights when it is illuminated) each with a repeated sequence and a second group is given a completely random set of responses, there is a substantial drop in RT in the first case but not in the second (Ghez & Krakauer, 2000).

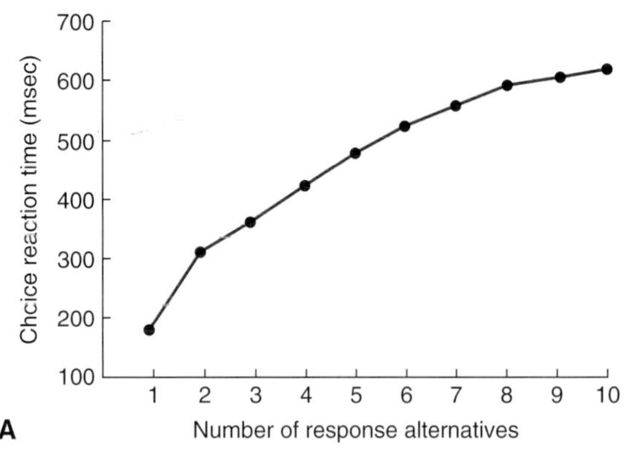

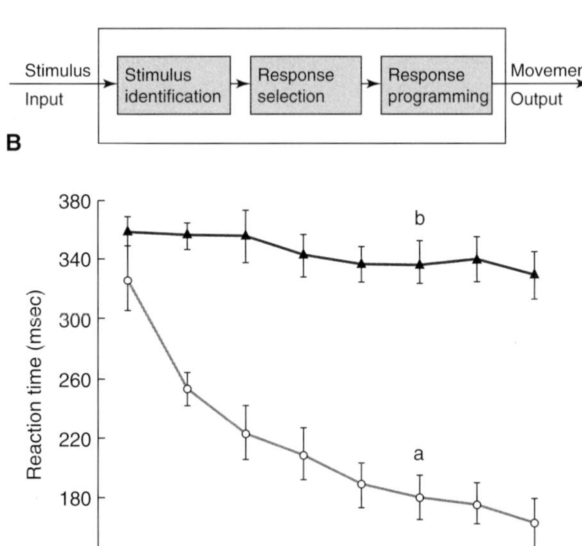

Figure 17.12 (A) A comparison of reaction time (RT) and the number of response alternatives available. Note that RT increases nonlinearly with the number of response alternatives. **(B)** Information-processing model with three stages between stimulus input and movement output. **(C)** Comparison of RT during successive blocks of trials (10 trials/block) when responding to a predictable (*a*) versus a nonpredictable (*b*) stimulus. On each trial, one of four lights flashed and participants pressed the key under the light. The same 10-trial sequence was given for each block in the predictable condition. Note that RT decreases with predictable stimuli (*a*) but does not change with successive blocks of nonpredictable (random) stimuli (*b*). (Reprinted from Ghez C, Krakauer J. The organization of movement. In: Kandel E, Schwartz J, Jessel T, eds. *Principles of neural science,* 4th ed. New York, NY: McGraw-Hill, 2000:662, with permission.)

Fitts's Law

Some basic characteristics of arm movements that you may find intuitively obvious are that whenever arm movement precision is increased or movement distance is increased, movement time becomes longer. In the 1950s, Fitts quantified these characteristics in the following experiments. He asked subjects to move a pointer back and forth between an initial position and a target position as quickly as possible, as you see in Figure 17.13. In the set of experiments, he systematically varied the movement distance (signified by the distance A in the figure) and the width of the target (signified by the W in the figure). For a particular distance, A, Fitts varied the width of the target on consecutive trials. The graph in Figure 17.13 shows the movement time for a different target width (from narrow to broad) for four different movement distances, when subjects were asked to move as fast as possible. He found that he could create a simple equation relating movement time to the distance moved and the target width. This equation, which has become known as Fitts's law, is shown in the following equation:

$$MT = a + b\log_2 2D/W$$

where a and b are empirically determined constants, MT is movement time, D is distance moved, and W is the width of the target. The term $\log_2 2D/W$, which is the label of the x-axis in the graph, has been called the "index of difficulty." Thus, narrower target widths and longer distances contribute to slowing the speed of the task. Movement time increases linearly with the index of difficulty; that is, the more difficult the task, the longer it takes to make the movement (Fitts, 1954; Keele, 1981).

Fitts's law relates movement time to movement accuracy and distance and applies to many different kinds of tasks, including discrete aiming movements, moving objects to insert them in a hole, moving a cursor on a screen, small finger movements under a microscope, and even throwing darts. Fitts's law has proven accurate in describing movements made by subjects of all ages, from infants to older adults (Keele, 1981; Rosenbaum, 1991).

What are the constraints of the individual and the task that lead to this particular law regarding movement? It has been suggested that movement time increases with distance and accuracy, due in part to the constraints of our visual system. It is difficult to translate our visual perception of the distance to be covered precisely into an actual movement; thus, as the hand approaches the target, time is needed to further update the movement trajectory (Keele, 1981). Lab Activity 17.2 gives you the opportunity to explore Fitts's law and the relationship between task difficulty and movement time.

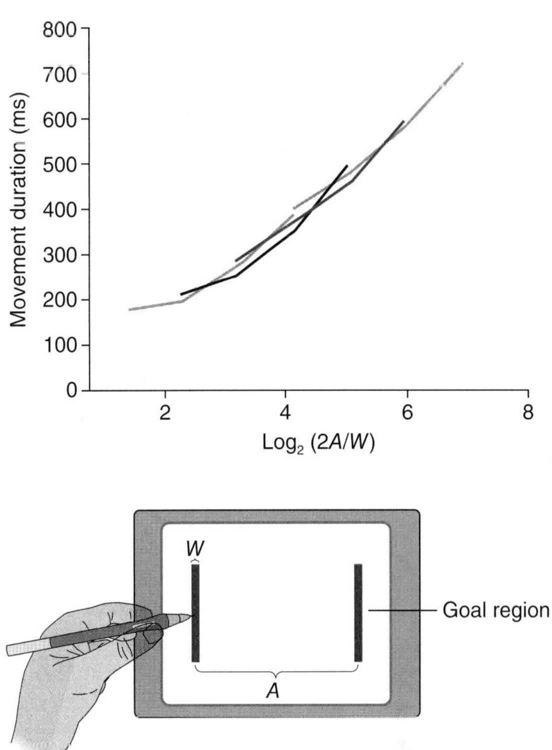

Figure 17.13 An example of a subject performing the Fitts's law task. The person moves the stylus between two targets of changing widths (W) and separated by different distances (A). The graph shows duration of movements for different target widths over four different distances. It shows that over many movement widths and distances, movement time is linearly dependent on the formula $\log_2 (2A/W)$, which is known as the index of difficulty. (Adapted from Jeannerod M. *The neural and behavioural organization of goal-directed movements.* Oxford, UK: Clarendon Press, 1988.)

How Does the Nervous System Plan Movements? Muscle Coordinate, Joint Angle Coordinate, and End Point Coordinate Strategies

In Chapter 1, when we discussed theories of motor control, we mentioned Bernstein's contributions to systems theory. Remember that Bernstein proposed that a given nervous system program will produce different outcomes in different situations because the response of the body will depend on the initial position of the limbs and on outside forces such as gravity and inertia. When body segments act together, the nervous system must also take into account the forces they generate with respect to each other. Bernstein hypothesized that the nervous system possessed a central representation of the movement that was in the form of a "motor image," representing the form of the movement to be achieved, not the impulses needed to achieve it. He believed that proprioception was important to the final achievement of the movement, not in a reflex-triggering sense, but as it contributed to the central representation of the

LAB ACTIVITY 17.2

Objective: To examine the effect of task difficulty on reaching (Fitts's law). Remember, Fitts defined task difficulty in terms of target size (*W*, which is the width of the target) and the distance to move (*D*, which is the distance between targets). He thus quantified task difficulty (which he called "index of difficulty" or simply *ID*) by using the following equation: $ID = \log_2 2D/W$.

Procedure: For this lab, you will work in pairs. With a pencil, tap quickly and accurately between two targets that vary in width and distance. The objective is to make as many *accurate* tapping movements as possible in a 10-second period. Accuracy is important. Remember that there should be no more errors made in the most difficult task than in the easiest tasks. If the number of errors exceeds 5% of the pencil dots, the trial should be done again.

Two combinations of task difficulty will be used. The first and easiest task has $D = 2$ cm and $W = 2$ cm. Solving the equation for *ID*, that would be log (base 2) of $(2 \times 2)/2$. This works out to the $\log_2$ of 2, which is 1. The most difficult task has $D = 16$ cm and $W = 1$ cm—that is, the $\log_2$ of $(2 \times 16)/1$, which is 5.

Each person will perform three trials (10 seconds each) for the two task conditions. When you are the subject, your partner will time each trial and count and record the number of dots in each target. Your partner should tell you to "start" and "stop" on each 10-second trial. The rest interval between trials should be the amount of time needed to count and record the taps. After the three trials, you can switch jobs with your partner.

Make a table and record the number of taps on each of the three trials for both the easy and the difficult tasks. Calculate the mean and standard deviation as well. For each task, calculate the average movement time (in milliseconds) for a single movement of the tapping task. Do this by dividing each number of taps by 10, which will give you the number of taps per second during the 10-second trial. Record this value in the table as well. Next, take the inverse of this number ($1/x$, where x is the average number of taps). Then, multiply this number by 1,000 to obtain the average movement time in milliseconds. Record this average movement time in the table.

Assignment

1. What impact did the difficulty of the task have on movement time?
2. If you tried to maintain the same speed on the difficult task as you used on the easy task, how would this affect your accuracy?
3. Describe a functional task that has relatively low demands for accuracy and distance versus a functional task that has relatively high demands for accuracy.
4. What impact will these differences in task difficulty have on your patient's performance?

movement. He also suggested that one way to control the high number of degrees of freedom involved in any complex movement was to organize the actions in terms of synergies or groups of muscles or joints that were constrained to act as a unit (Bernstein, 1967).

In fact, many researchers have now shown that hand movements are organized synergically or through coordinative structures. For example, it was shown that when subjects were asked to use their two hands to point at two separate targets, they moved their hands simultaneously, even if the pointing tasks were very different in difficulty (e.g., one was near and large and the other one was far away and small). Other researchers have noted this same tight bimanual coordination when subjects reached forward to manipulate an object with two hands. Thus, it has been suggested that independent body segments become functionally linked for the execution of a common task (Jeannerod, 1990; Kelso et al., 1979).

How does the nervous system control complex arm movements to reach targets with speed and elegant precision? This is an intricate problem that could be solved in different ways. For example, the nervous system could plan reaching movements with respect to the activation sequences of individual muscles; this has been referred to as a "muscle coordinate strategy." Alternatively, reaching could be planned in relationship to joint angle coordinates—that is, planning the movements of shoulder, elbow, and wrist joints to arrive at the target. This would mean that the nervous system was planning the movement around a set of intrinsic coordinates of the body, expressed in terms of the joint angles. Finally, the nervous system could plan arm movements in terms of the final end point coordinates, using extrinsic coordinates in space (Hollerbach, 1990).

Levels of planning could also be considered in terms of a hierarchy, with, for example, both kinematic and kinetic levels of planning. Kinematic levels of planning would be organized around geometry, such as joint angle variables and end point variables. Kinetic levels of planning would be organized around forces such as those of muscle activation and joint torques.

On the one hand, it seems intuitively obvious that we would need to use some variation of end point coordinate planning in order to do something like picking up a glass of water. If we plan a movement using intrinsic coordinates alone, without regard to the actual position of the object in space, the accuracy of the movement with respect to the end position needed is likely to be decreased. But when the nervous system plans according to end point coordinates, it needs to make a complex mathematical transformation called an "inverse kinematics transformation," which would transform end point coordinates into joint angle coordinates. Then, it has to create this trajectory by producing the appropriate muscle activation patterns (Hollerbach, 1990).

It has also been proposed that movements are planned in terms of joint angle coordinates, which has the advantage of not requiring an inverse kinematics transformation. This would mean that the organization of movement by the nervous system would be simplified. However, the nervous system would still have to do an inverse dynamics transformation that would transform joint angle coordinates into muscle torques and muscle activation patterns required to make the movement.

If trajectories were planned in terms of the muscle activation pattern, this planning would have the advantage of simplifying the inverse kinematics and inverse dynamics problems. But as we have also mentioned, muscle activation patterns are only indirectly related to final joint positions. Thus, programming movements in this manner could cause large inaccuracies (Hollerbach, 1990).

How does one go about answering the question of how the nervous system plans movements? In Hollerbach's (1990) excellent review of the research on arm movement planning, he mentions that Bernstein (1967) actually made the following statement, which has guided modern physiologists in their experiments exploring the control of reaching movements:

If the spatial shape of a trajectory is invariant irrespective of the muscle scheme or the joint scheme, then the motor plan must be closely related to the topology of the trajectory and considerably removed from joints and muscles.

Thus, experimenters have begun to look for invariant characteristics in different variables related to the reach. If invariances are found across different conditions, this could be considered evidence that the nervous system uses this variable to plan movements.

It has been shown that the path of the wrist in an arm movement is unaffected by movement speed or by load (weights held in the hand). In addition, the velocity profiles of a movement are also unaffected by movement speed or load. These findings support the concept that the nervous system uses kinematic variables for planning (Atkeson & Hollerbach, 1985).

Remember that there are two types of kinematic variables that could be used for movement planning: joint angle coordinates and end point coordinates. If the nervous system controls movements in joint angle coordinates, the hand should move in a curved line, because the movements will be about the axis of a joint, as shown in Figure 17.14A. However, if it plans movements with respect to extrapersonal space or end point coordinates, the hand would be expected to move in a straight line (Fig. 17.14B) (Hollerbach, 1990; Rosenbaum, 1991).

To answer this question, researchers (Morasso, 1981) asked subjects to point to different targets (see Fig. 17.15A, T1–T6) in two-dimensional space (on a surface) and recorded their hand trajectories (see Fig. 17.15B). They found that subjects tended to move the hand in straight lines, with hand velocity characteristics having the same shape and scale in relation to the distance the hand moved. However, elbow and shoulder joints went through complex angular changes (see Fig. 17.15C). Even when they were asked to draw curved lines, the subjects tended to draw a series of straight-line subunits. These results (straight hand path and similar velocity characteristics) support the concept that the CNS programs movements according to hand and movement end point coordinates (Ghez & Krakauer, 2000).

Other researchers have explored arm movement control further and have shown that the nervous system can directly control the joints and still produce straight-line movements. This is done by varying the onset times for the joint movements, with all joints stopping at the same time. This method of control gives movements with almost straight-line paths. This

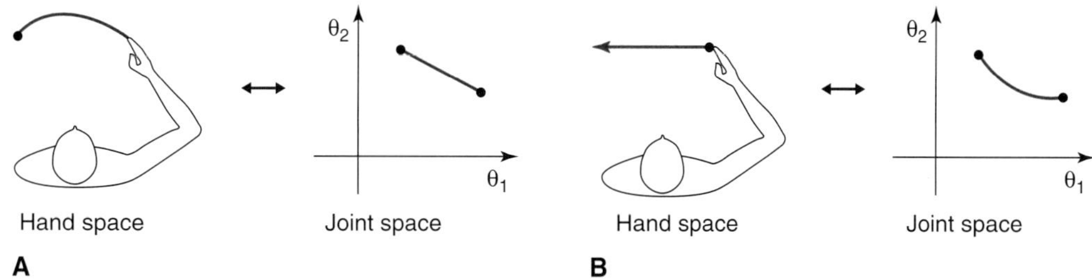

Figure 17.14 Different variables that can be used for planning arm movements. **(A)** If movements are controlled in joint angle coordinates, hand trajectories are curved. **(B)** If movements are controlled in end point coordinates, joint space is curved (a complex elbow and shoulder movement is required). (Adapted from Hollerbach JM. Planning of arm movements. In: Osherson DN, Kosslyn SM, Hollerbach JM, eds. *Visual cognition and action: an invitation to cognitive science,* vol. 2. Cambridge, MA: MIT Press, 1990:187.)

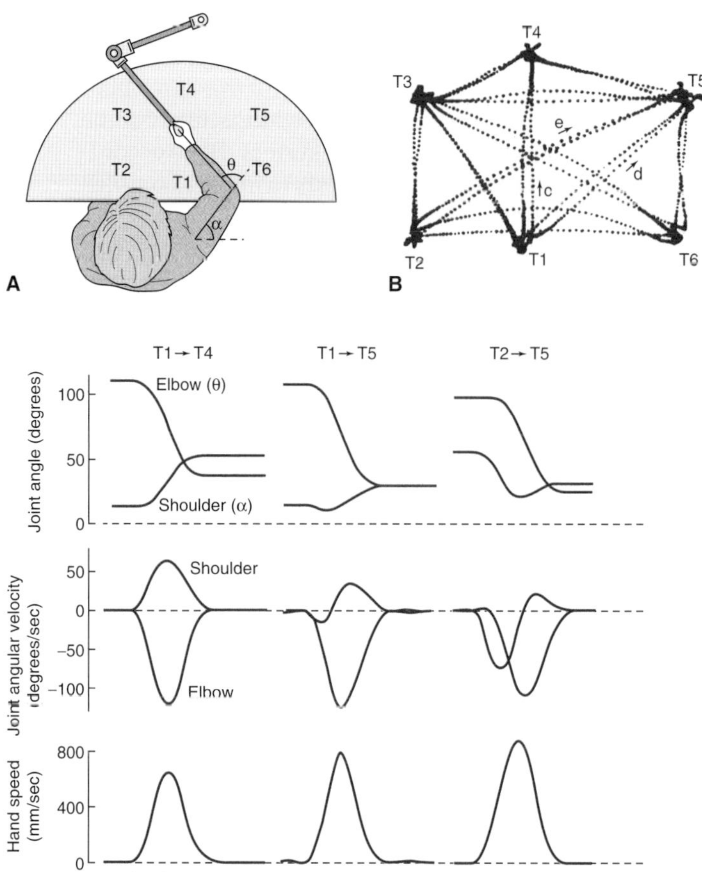

Figure 17.15 (A) Subject sitting in front of a plate, grasping a handle, which can be moved to one of six positions. The two-jointed handle system records hand position. **(B)** Hand position paths of one participant when moving to different targets. **(C)** Elbow and shoulder joint angle and joint angular velocity, in addition to hand speed when moving among three different targets. Elbow and shoulder angles differ for the three paths. Hand paths are approximately straight, and hand speed curves have similar shapes in proportion to distance between targets, suggesting that movement planning is made with reference to the hand. (Reprinted from Ghez C, Krakauer J. The organization of movement. In: Kandel E, Schwartz J, Jessel T, eds. *Principles of neural science,* 4th ed. New York, NY: McGraw-Hill, 2000:658, with permission.)

suggests that straight-line trajectories can occur even when the CNS is using joint angle coordinates to program movements. Thus, it is not clear whether the CNS programs movements exclusively by one method or the other (Hollerbach, 1990).

Russian researchers have shown that the elbow and wrist joints are controlled as a synergic unit. When subjects were asked to move the elbow and wrist joint congruently (flexing both together), the subjects could perform this task with ease, with joint motions starting and stopping as a unit. When asked to move the joints incongruently (flexing one and extending the other), they performed the task with considerable difficulty, moving the joints much less smoothly. This is additional evidence for joint-based planning (Kots & Syrovegin, 1966).

A number of additional theories on the control of reaching will be described in the following section. The first group of theories tends to assume that the nervous system is programming distance in making movements, while the second group of theories suggests that final location is the parameter being programmed.

Distance versus Location Programming Theories

What do we mean by programming distance versus location? According to the distance programming theory, when making an arm movement toward a target, people visually perceive the distance to be covered. Then, they activate a particular set of agonist muscles to propel the arm the proper distance to the target. At a particular point, they turn off the agonist muscles and activate antagonist muscles at the joint in order to provide a braking force to stop the movement (Keele, 1986).

According to the location programming theory, the nervous system programs the relative balance of tensions (or stiffness) of two opposing (agonist and antagonist) muscle sets. According to this theory, every location in space corresponds to a family of stiffness relations between opposing muscles, as we explain later in the chapter. Let's first look at distance programming theories.

Distance Theories

Multiple-Corrections Theory. It has been shown repeatedly that accuracy of arm movements decreases when vision is absent. For example, when subjects were asked to make arm movements of different durations to a target, movements of 190 msec or less were unaffected by loss of vision, while movements of 260 msec or more were affected by loss of visual feedback (Keele & Posner, 1968). Thus, it appears that movement trajectories are corrected based on visual feedback and that it takes about 200 to 250 msec for vision to be able to update a movement trajectory. Considering that some movement time must occur before the limb is close enough to the target to use visual feedback, one realizes that the visual processing time is slightly shorter. It has been shown (Carlton, 1981) that subjects need to see their hand for at least 135 msec during a movement to use vision to improve movement accuracy.

In the 1960s, researchers (Crossman & Goodeve, 1983; Keele, 1968) proposed that aiming movements consisted of a series of submovements, each responding to and reducing visual error. Thus, an initial movement, before any visual correction takes place, covers most of the distance to a target and is independent of final precision. This model predicts a constant b for Fitts's law, which is almost identical to the one that Fitts and Peterson calculated originally (Keele, 1981).

There are, however, some problems with this model. Typically, aiming movements to a target have only one correction, if any, and when corrections are made, they do not have constant durations or proportions of the distance to the target (Rosenbaum, 1991).

How might this theory be used to explain problems related to inaccurate reaching movements commonly found in patients with neurologic deficits? The multiple-corrections theory stresses the importance of visual feedback when making corrections during a movement to increase accuracy. Thus, inaccurate movements could be the result of loss of visual feedback. When retraining a patient using a multiple-corrections theory, the clinician could have the patient practice slow movements, requiring a high degree of accuracy, drawing the patient's attention to visual cues relating hand movement to target location.

Schmidt's Impulse Variability Model. Another way of explaining the characteristics of arm movement seen in Fitts's equation is to hypothesize that the initial phase of the movement, involving the generation of a force impulse, is more important than later phases of the movement dealing with ongoing control. This would be particularly true in cases in which the movement is too fast to use visual feedback to aid in accuracy.

Schmidt performed research in which subjects were asked to make fast movements over a fixed distance. These movements required large amounts of force, since high-velocity movements require large forces to generate the movement. He showed that the size of the subject's error increased in proportion to the magnitude of the force used. Thus, when he asked subjects to make a fast but accurate movement, the large forces required caused increased force variability. This increased variability resulted in decreased movement accuracy (Schmidt et al., 1989). These movement characteristics were described in the following equation:

$$W_e = a + bD/MT$$

where W_e is variation in movement end point expressed in standard deviation units, D is distance moved, and MT is movement time. This equation is similar to Fitts's law. It indicates that simply taking into account the fact that faster movement requires more force can explain Fitts's law, without having to factor in a need for visual feedback for movement accuracy (Keele, 1981).

This theory alone cannot be used to explain aiming movements, since as we have seen previously, many movements, particularly those lasting longer than 250 msec, do use visual feedback for accuracy.

Nonetheless, this theory does have relevance for the clinician involved in retraining upper-extremity control. It suggests the importance of practicing fast movements of varying amplitudes during therapy sessions. In this way, patients learn to program forces appropriately for quick and accurate movements.

Hybrid Model: Optimized Initial Impulse Model. The previous two models deal with two extremes of movement control: (a) the use of visual feedback to improve accuracy during ongoing portions of slower movements and (b) very fast movements that cannot easily use visual feedback and thus are controlled only through the amplitude of the initial impulse. In an attempt to create a model to explain the entire range of possible aiming movements, a hybrid model has been proposed that combines elements of both of these models (Meyer et al., 1988). This hybrid model is referred to as the "optimized initial impulse model."

Researchers involved in studying this model hypothesized that a subject makes a first movement toward a target, which, if successful, is the sole movement. However, if it is inaccurate (e.g., if it undershoots or overshoots the target), another movement will be required involving visual feedback during ongoing movement control. Clearly, the subject needs to find a balance between moving quickly, which requires a large initial force, and moving slowly enough to allow for corrections to the ongoing movement, thereby ensuring accuracy.

It was found that an equation taking these issues into account was similar to Fitts's law:

$$T = a + b(n(D/W)^{1/n})$$

where T is movement time, D is distance, W is width of the target, and n is the number of submovements used to reach the target (Rosenbaum, 1991).

Since functional activities require a variety of movements, both fast and slow, with varying degrees of accuracy, it is important to retrain a patient's ability to perform a continuum of movements that vary in both speed and accuracy.

Location Programming Theories

As we mentioned previously, the nervous system could program arm movements in one of two ways: distance programming or programming the end point location of the movement (Feldman, 1974; Keele, 1981). The example of a café door swinging on springs has sometimes been used to explain the location programming model (Keele, 1986). Figure 17.16A shows the door in a closed position. The movement of the café door is described as occurring when there is a reduction in the length of one spring and the lengthening of the other spring. When the door is released, the imbalance between the springs causes the door to return to its closed position, in which the springs are at their resting length. If you want to keep the door open, you can simply change one spring for another of a different stiffness, and then, it will have a new resting position (Fig. 17.16B).

It has been suggested that the agonist–antagonist muscle pairs at the joints are like the springs of the café door. We can change the position of the joint simply by changing the relative stiffness of the two muscles, through higher or lower relative activation levels. Although this may sound like an unusual way for the nervous system to program reaching movements, experiments have shown that this occurs in many circumstances.

For example, experiments performed on monkeys (Polit & Bizzi, 1979) suggest that many movements may be controlled through location rather than distance programming. In these experiments, the monkeys were trained to make elbow movements to different targets whenever lights above those targets were turned on, as shown in Figure 17.17D. The monkeys wore a large collar that blocked sight of the arm, eliminating visual feedback. In addition, in certain experiments, the dorsal roots of the spinal cord were severed, eliminating kinesthetic feedback from the arm. The accuracy of the monkeys' arm movements was measured with and without visual and kinesthetic feedback. Researchers found that the monkeys' reaching was normal, despite a loss of visual and kinesthetic feedback (Fig. 17.17A).

The investigators then gave a perturbation to the deafferented monkey's arm, moving it from its original position, just after the target light was turned on but before the monkey began to move. Remember that the monkeys could not feel or see the arm position when it was perturbed. Nevertheless, the monkeys reached for the target with reasonable accuracy (Fig. 17.17B and C). If the monkeys were using distance programming for reaching, this would have been impossible, because they would have applied a fixed force pulse

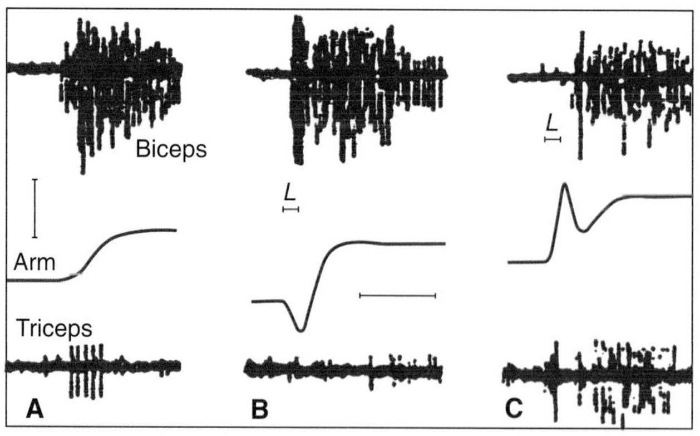

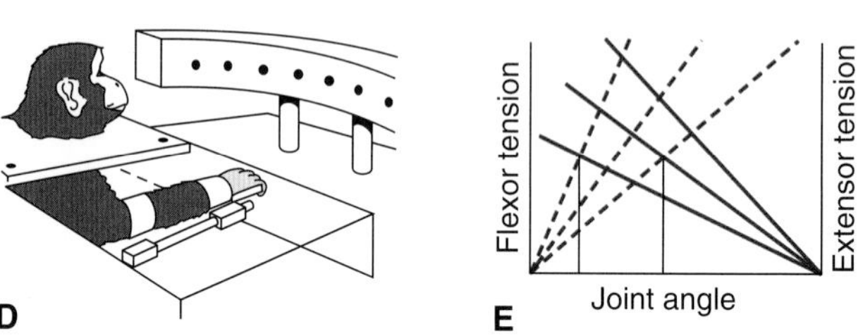

Figure 17.17 Experimental setup to test the mass–spring model of control. The deafferented monkey is pointing to a target but is unable to see its hand (see part **D**). **(A)** The monkey flexes the arm at the elbow to move to the target in a control trial. Biceps, triceps, and arm position traces are shown. Note that the biceps muscle is predominantly active, with little activity in the triceps. **(B)** The hand is moved by a torque motor to a new position further from the target after the target is illuminated but before the hand starts to move. Note that the biceps muscle is active and the triceps silent. **(C)** The hand is moved by a torque motor to a new position past the target after the target is illuminated but before the hand starts to move. Note that now the triceps muscle also shows considerable activity, since the monkey must extend the arm slightly. As shown in the movement traces, the monkey was able to successfully point to the target, even when the unseen deafferented hand was perturbed. For **A**, **B**, **C**. Time calibration, 1 second, vertical bar, 15 degrees. L indicates timing and duration of load application. Target light is on during actual pointing. Initial forearm position was different from trial to trial. **(E)** A graph showing different flexor (*dotted lines*) and extensor (*solid lines*) muscle tension levels that would move the arm to different joint angles. The intersection of two curves on the *x*-axis shows the resultant joint angle produced by two combined tensions (left vertical line = greater angle of flexion, next line to right = great extension). (Reprinted from Brooks VB. *The neural basis of motor control.* New York, NY: Oxford University Press, 1986:138, with permission.)

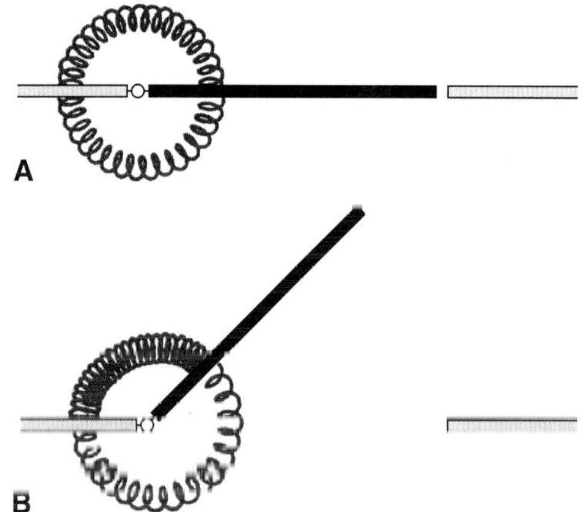

Figure 17.16 The café door model. Simplified explanation of the mass–spring model of motor control. **(A)** When a café door is at rest, it resembles a joint at midpoint, with both muscles at midlength. **(B)** When one spring of a café door is shortened and the other is lengthened, the door is open, analogous to one muscle contracting and the other relaxing to allow the joint to flex.

in the elbow muscles to move the arm to the new position. Since the arm had already been perturbed, they should have ended up in the wrong place.

The only way these results can be explained is through the use of end point location programming. In this case, what the nervous system would program is the stiffness (or background activity level) settings on the agonist and antagonist muscles of the arm. For example, if the arm were originally in a flexed position, there would be high background activity levels in the elbow flexors and low levels in the extensors. To move the arm precisely to the new location (increased extension angle), the background activity (stiffness) levels would simply change so that the spring constant of the elbow flexors was at a lower level and that of the extensors was at a higher level. This is shown graphically in Figure 17.17E. Once this new spring setting was made, it would not matter where the limb was perturbed, because, just like the café door, the limb would swing to its new spring setting. Thus, the monkey did not have to know its starting point in order to go to the correct end point.

It is interesting that in these experiments, the monkeys were not able to continue to make accurate movements when the shoulder position was changed. It appears that without visual or somatosensory feedback from the arm, they could not update a central reference concerning shoulder position changes. These changes then threw off the elbow location programming (Polit & Bizzi, 1979).

Work by Kelso and Holt (1980) with humans produced similar results. In this study, subjects were blindfolded, and their fingers were anesthetized by using a pressure cuff. Before testing began, they were trained to move their fingers to a specific position in space. They were then given brief finger perturbations during the course of their finger movement. With complete loss of finger sensation, there was very little difference in terminal error between the perturbed and unperturbed movements.

These results suggest that the nervous system is able to encode the location of body segments in space, in relation to a base body position as varying activation levels of agonist and antagonist muscles. What does this mean? It has been suggested that this could explain why we can perform a skill (such as reaching for a cup or throwing a ball) hundreds of times without repeating exactly the same movement. According to classic programming theory, one would have to make a new program for each movement variation, but according to the mass–spring model, one would have to program the appropriate muscle activity ratios, and the limb would move appropriately to its final position (Keele, 1986).

Do these results suggest that distance programming is wrong? No. Most likely, both strategies are used for arm movements, depending on the task and the context. For example, it has been shown that when humans make rapid elbow flexion movements (Hallett et al., 1975), they show a triphasic burst of contraction: first, the biceps are activated, followed by the triceps (braking the movement), and then the biceps again. This same pattern was found in patients with loss of kinesthetic sensation. However, when subjects were asked to move more slowly and smoothly, they showed continuous biceps activity and no triceps activity. This has led some researchers to argue that the subjects are using mass–spring or location programming for slow movements and a combination of distance programming and location programming for faster movements. There are also limitations to the mass–spring model. The model holds only with single-joint, one-plane movements. Most movements involve many joints, are carried out in three-dimensional space, and have to take gravity into account (Keele, 1981).

Ghez (1979) has also proposed a pulse-step model for arm movement control, in which an initial pulse of force is followed by a step change in force levels. He states that the initial pulse component is required to overcome the constraints imposed by mechanical properties of the muscle and limb. This again could be considered a combined distance/location type of movement control.

In summary, research appears to indicate that single-joint movements that are shorter than 0.25 second are too short to take advantage of visual feedback, while those longer than 0.25 second involve visual feedback in the homing-in phase. Slower movements may involve location programming, while faster movements may involve a combination of distance and location programming.

This model would suggest that the capacity to modulate stiffness levels between the agonist and antagonist muscles is an important part of retraining accurate upper-extremity movements.

INTERFERENCE BETWEEN REACHING AND THE PERFORMANCE OF SECONDARY COGNITIVE TASKS

In previous chapters, we have discussed interference that occurs in the performance of both postural and gait tasks when they are performed simultaneously with a cognitive task, when attentional resources are not sufficient for the efficient execution of both tasks. This phenomenon has also been documented for reaching tasks (Ghillery et al., 2013). This is of relevance since reaching tasks and the manipulation of objects are typically performed at the same time as other cognitive tasks.

One study examined the extent to which a precision grip task required cognitive resources, using a dual-task paradigm. The secondary task was a complex visual search task, which was accompanied by counting. The results showed that the cognitive task interfered with the initial force scaling that occurred during the preload phase as the person began to grasp the object and in the fine-tuning of the grip force as the person held the object, suggesting that these parts of the task require attentional resources. The authors suggest that this type of dual-task paradigm may be useful for examining changes in task performance in patients undergoing neurologic rehabilitation, as increased automaticity with retraining should improve dual-task performance (Ghillery et al., 2013).

A second study examined the performance of goal-directed reaching movements when attention was divided between the reaching task and competing stimuli (Long & Wyatt, 2014). The two tasks included a pointing task to a target in the periphery and a visual letter search task in central vision (participants needed to count the number of times they saw a specific letter flash on the screen during a trial). The authors found that performance on both the central visual search task (increased percentage of errors) and peripheral pointing tasks was impaired under dual-task conditions. Movement onset of the pointing task, but not movement time, was slowed under the dual-task conditions. This suggests that in this reaching task, dual-task costs were associated with movement planning rather than execution.

These results suggest that reaching performance, like postural and gait control, requires attentional resources, and the complexity of both the motor and the secondary task contributes to the extent of dual-task interference in young adults.

SUMMARY

1. From a kinematic perspective, coordination in reaching is characterized by the sequential activation of eye, head, and then hand movements. However, muscle responses in these segments tend to be activated synchronously, not sequentially. Thus, inertial characteristics play an important part in the final movement characteristics.
2. Reach and grasp represent two distinct components that appear to be controlled by different neural mechanisms. Thus, patients with motor control problems can have difficulties in one or both aspects. This has implications for retraining.
3. Certain aspects of the grasp component, such as force of the grasp, are based on the person's perception of the characteristics of the object to be grasped and thus are programmed in advance.
4. Visual and somatosensory information are also used reactively for error correction during reach and grasp.
5. Fitts's law expresses the relationship between movement time, distance, and accuracy, stating that when the demands for accuracy increase, movement time will also increase.
6. There are two theories regarding the neural control of reaching: distance programming and location theories.
7. According to the distance programming theory, when people make an arm movement toward a target, they visually perceive the distance to be covered, and then they activate a particular set of agonist muscles to propel the arm the proper distance to the target. At a particular point, they turn off the agonist muscles and activate antagonist muscles at the joint to provide a braking force to stop the movement.
8. According to the location programming theory, the nervous system programs the relative balance of tensions (or stiffness) of two opposing (agonist and antagonist) muscle sets. According to this theory, every location in space corresponds to a family of stiffness relations between opposing muscles.
9. It is probably the case that both strategies are used for arm movements, depending on the task and the context.
10. Dual-task research suggests that even among young adults, reach and grasp is attentionally demanding. As was true for posture and gait, attentional demands vary with task complexity, including both the primary reach and grasp task and the secondary cognitive task.

ANSWERS TO LAB ACTIVITY ASSIGNMENTS

Lab Activity 17.1

1. The properties that affect reach and grasp include the object's size, shape, and surface texture (including its slipperiness) as well as the object's orientation, distance from the body, and location with respect to the body.
2. The orientation of the hand was opposite for the two glass orientations (glass right side up: thumb up; glass upside down: thumb down, so that the hand or glass orientation would be the same for the final upright position of the glass).
3. Almost from the beginning of the reach.
4. It was wider for larger objects.

Lab Activity 17.2

1. Movement time was longer.
2. Accuracy would decrease.
3. Functional task with low demands for accuracy/distance: Placing a coffee cup on a nearby shelf. High demands: Fitting a screwdriver in a small screw head at arm's length.
4. Either accuracy or movement time will go down in the task with high distance/accuracy demands.

CHAPTER 18

Reach, Grasp, and Manipulation: Changes across the Life Span

Learning Objectives

Following completion of this chapter, the reader will be able to:

1. Discuss the developmental changes in neural and musculoskeletal systems involved in reach-and-grasp skills across the life span.
2. Describe the changes in reach and manipulation skills that occur with each stage of development up to adulthood and any decrements that occur as part of the aging process, and discuss the underlying subsystem changes contributing to these changes in skill.

INTRODUCTION

The development of reach, grasp, and manipulation skills is complex and actually involves the development of many behaviors, each of which emerges progressively over time in association with maturation of different parts of the nervous and musculoskeletal systems and with experience. For example, the infant's ability to transport the arm toward an object precedes the ability to grasp. The ability to grasp emerges at 4 to 5 months of age, preceding the infant's ability to use the hands to explore objects, which does not emerge until about the first year of life. Thus, the development of mature upper-extremity function, including reach, grasp, and manipulation, occurs gradually over the first few years of life.

This chapter explores research on the development of reaching abilities in infants and children, as well as the changes in reaching abilities that occur in older adults. We first discuss some of the early hypotheses concerning the development of reaching, which propose that reaching results either from the inhibition of primitive reflexes or from the integration of those reflexes into voluntary movement (Twitchell, 1970). We also discuss the relative contributions of genetics versus experience to the emergence of reaching in the neonate. We then review more recent studies that come from newer theories of motor control, such as the ecological and systems approaches.

PRINCIPLES UNDERLYING THE DEVELOPMENT OF REACHING BEHAVIORS

Role of Reflexes in the Development of Reaching Behaviors

Is early reaching controlled reflexly? This is a question that has been debated in the developmental literature for many years. Early theories of the development of reaching argued that reflexes provide the physiological substrate for complex voluntary movements, such as reaching (Twitchell, 1970). According to these theories, the transition from reflexes to voluntary reaching is a continuous process, with newborn reflexes gradually being incorporated into a hierarchy of complex coordinated actions (McDonnell, 1979). A review of eye–hand coordination development mentions that early developmental theoreticians may have overlooked another possibility regarding the development of reaching: that eye–hand coordination may emerge concurrently with the maturation of reflex function rather than emerging from the modification of reflex function (McDonnell, 1979). Thus, reflexes such as the grasp reflex may develop separately from the eye–hand coordination system and may underlie different functions.

Reaching Behaviors: Innate or Learned?

Another question that has intrigued researchers concerns the extent to which the integration of sensory and motor systems underlying eye–hand coordination is genetically predetermined and/or experientially determined.

If the integration of eye–hand coordination was completely genetically predetermined, it would imply that the nervous system has a ready-made map of visual space and one of manipulative space laid out in a one-to-one correspondence. Thus, just by seeing an object, an infant would know exactly where to reach. In contrast, if eye–hand coordination was completely experientially determined, experience would be required to "map" visual space onto motor space or to learn to adjust arm spatial coordinates with coordinates of the object.

The first hypothesis implies that once the nervous system's sensory and motor pathways for visually guided reaching have matured, the infant will be able to reach accurately for an object, with little or no prior experience. The second hypothesis predicts that a learning period is required in development, during which the infant creates, through trial and error, the visual map or perceptual rules that overlay the motor map or actions required for reaching.

In the 1950s, Piaget's research on child development led him to believe that although nervous system maturation is a requirement for the appearance of a behavior, experience is responsible for its coordination with the senses. He believed that only through repeatedly and simultaneously looking at and touching an object would the visual and manipulative impressions be associated (Piaget, 1954).

Other researchers gave further support to this concept when they noted that neonates showed both visual and manual activities in the first few weeks after birth, but these movements were apparently unrelated (White et al., 1964). Thus, in the 1960s, many researchers in developmental science supported the theory that visual and hand control systems are unrelated at birth.

In the 1970s, a group of scientists (Bower et al., 1970a, 1970b) presented interesting evidence that they believed supported the opposite concept: that there was clear coordination of eye and hand in the newborn. They reported that infants between 7 and 14 days of age showed arm movements that were clearly directed toward an object in the visual field. They said a significant proportion of reaches were within 5 to 10 degrees of the object and that in 30% to 40% of the reaches, the hand closed around the object. They also observed that infants differentiated between objects that could be grasped (small objects) from those that could not (large objects at large distances): they reached for the first but not the second.

Many researchers initially had difficulty replicating these experiments, and thus, the results were questioned (Dodwell et al., 1976). However, later studies indicated that an early form of eye–hand coordination does exist in the neonate, although reaching does not seem to be as accurate or as coordinated as originally indicated (Vinter, 1990; von Hofsten, 1982).

In 1980, Amiel-Tison and Grenier wrote a surprising article on neonatal abilities. They reported that when the heads of neonates were stabilized, giving them postural support, amazing coordination of other behaviors was seen. For example, they reported that chaotic movements of the arms became still, and the infants appeared to be able to reach forward toward objects, as shown in Figure 18.1. Their article is one example of research that supports the hypothesis that infants are born with certain innate abilities or behaviors, which have sometimes been termed "prereaching behaviors." It also suggests that, as was true in the development of independent mobility function, postural control is a rate-limiting factor in the development of coordinated reaching.

In the late 1970s and 1980s, von Hofsten (1984, 1993) began exploring the development of eye–hand coordination in the neonate. He placed infants in an infant

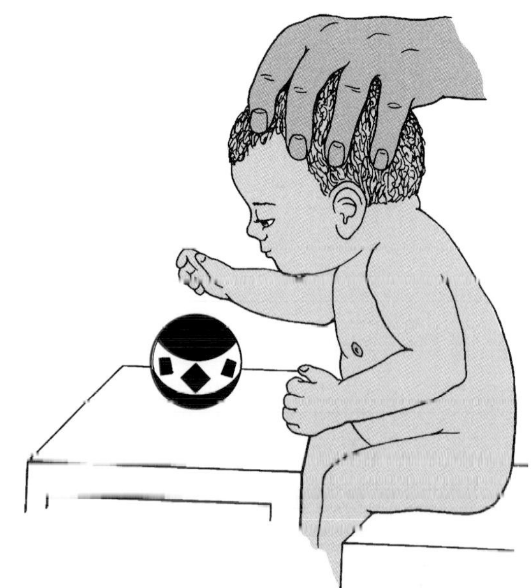

Figure 18.1 The release of reaching movements in a neonate by stabilizing the head. (Modified from Amiel-Tison C, Grenier A. *Evaluation neurologique du nuveau-ne et du nourrisson*. Paris, France: Masson, 1980:95.)

seat and moved an object in front of them, as shown in Figure 18.2, and carefully documented the number and accuracy of reaches. He showed that the number of extended movements performed when the infants were visually fixating on the object was twice as high as when the infants did not fixate on the object. The reaching movements were not very accurate. However, those that were made while the infants fixated on the target were aimed within an average of 32 degrees laterally and 25 degrees vertically toward the target, while those that were made without fixation were only within 52 degrees laterally and 37 degrees vertically. Although these reaching movements were not as accurate as had previously been postulated, they were clearly aimed at the target, since they were significantly more accurate than the nonvisually fixated movements. Other researchers have corroborated these findings showing that in the month or two before infants can successfully reach for and contact toys, their arm movements are faster, smoother, and closer toward toys that are visually present as opposed to toys that are out of view (Bhat & Galloway, 2006). All these results thus show a clear effect of vision on reaching movements. Von Hofsten also noted that the system works from hand to eye as well. Several times, the infant accidentally touched the object and immediately turned the eyes toward it. Neonates also have proprioceptive control of hand movements: they reach toward their mouth or body without vision, in a goal-directed way. Indeed, these general exploratory behaviors, also known as spontaneous movements because they seem to not be elicited by external triggers, can be found as early as in 8-week fetuses, and they continue to develop even after visually guided reaching has emerged (Einspieler & Prechtl, 2005; von Hofsten, 1984).

A subset of spontaneous behaviors involves waving or flapping, which have also been referred to as "prereaching" movements. Van der Meer et al. (1995) recorded the arm-waving movements of newborn infants as they lay supine, with the head facing to the side. They were given vision of the arm they were facing, vision of the opposite arm through a monitor,

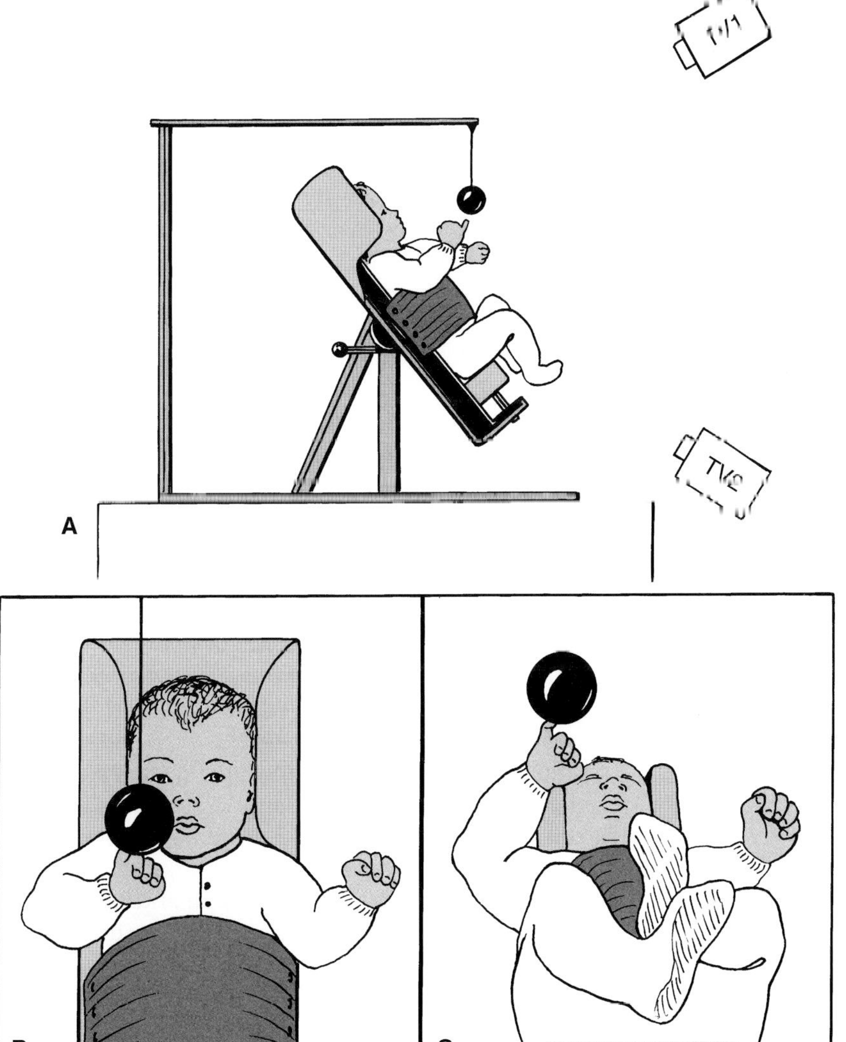

Figure 18.2 (A) Experimental setup used to study reaching in neonates. The infant is placed in an infant seat (50-degree angle) that has head support on the back and sides but allows the arms freedom to move. **(B and C)** Diagram of the outline of the infant as it touched the object, taken from single frames from the two video cameras seen in part **A.** (Adapted from von Hofsten C. Eye–hand coordination in the newborn. *Dev Psychol.* 1982;18:452, with permission.)

or vision of neither arm. They found that the infants would counteract small forces applied to the wrist in order to keep the limb up and moving if they could see it but did not do this if they could not see it. This also suggests that infants have visual control of arm movements shortly after birth (Gordon, 2001).

Thus, this research suggests that some aspects of reaching, in particular the ability to locate objects in space and transport the arm, may be present in rudimentary form (prereaching behaviors) at birth, while other components, such as grasp, develop later in the first year of life. In addition, the emergence of reaching is constrained by the development of postural control. These findings suggest support for the hypothesis that at least some aspects of reaching are innate.

In the next sections, we follow the progression of the development of reaching and manipulation skills through infancy and childhood, exploring the emergence of various aspects of reaching and manipulation behaviors. We have already seen that location of an object in space is possible in the neonate and that the ability to transport the arm toward the object in a rudimentary way is also available at birth. However, as you will see, more accurate reaching and the grasp component of reaching do not develop until 4 to 5 months of age, with pincer grasp developing at 9 to 13 months. Higher cognitive aspects of reaching begin to emerge at about 1 year of age. Throughout development, there appears to be a repetitive shift between visually triggered (or proactively guided reaching) and visually guided (or feedback-controlled) reaching.

LOCATING A TARGET: EYE–HEAD COORDINATION

In order to reach for a target, the infant must first locate the target in space. If the target is moving, this requires that the infant stabilize the gaze on the moving target and move the gaze at the same speed as the image of the target. This may involve eye movements alone or eye and head movements in combination, and control of these movements involves visual, vestibular, and proprioceptive information. How do infants develop the coordination of head and eye movements for gaze control? To do this, they need to master two tasks: moving the eyes to specific targets and stabilizing gaze on the targets. This is done using a combination of saccadic eye movements (moving the eye to the target) and smooth-pursuit movements (stabilizing the eye on the target) (von Hofsten, 2003, 2007).

Shifting Gaze

The control of saccadic eye movements develops before that of smooth pursuit. In fact, saccadic movements are present in the neonate. Tracking targets is done with saccadic eye movements at this age. To shift gaze, the infant needs to shift attention from the current object of fixation to a new object. This ability is also present at birth. However, as attention matures, it goes through a period in which the infant has difficulty looking away from a target (called "obligatory attention"). At about 4 months of age, infants become able to disengage attention and examine new objects at will (von Hofsten, 2003).

Tracking Object Movements

Limited smooth-pursuit tracking ability is present in the neonate. Researchers have shown that neonates can follow visually observed objects, which are large, covering a wide angle of visual space (about 16 degrees or more) and moving slowly (10 degrees per second or less) with smooth eye movements, but eye movements become jerky for small targets (Aslin, 1981). Rosander and von Hofsten (2002) also observed that 1-month-old infants followed large moving vertical gratings more smoothly than small objects. But they found that when the saccades were subtracted from the recordings, the remaining smooth tracking was not different for the two targets. This suggests that the reason the pursuit of the small objects appears jerky is because the infants are making many catch-up saccades to stay with the small target, which they do not need to do for the larger target. Von Hofsten (2003) proposes that this is because a wide-angle pattern of vertical stripes allows the eyes to always be on the target, however they move. Nevertheless, as with the size of the object, researchers have shown that if the target moves quickly, the duration of smooth pursuit decreases and the saccadic frequency needs to increase to catch up with the target (Pieh et al., 2012).

By about 6 weeks of age, smooth pursuit of objects begins to improve quickly (Shea & Aslin, 1990). In addition, 1-month-olds show a substantial lag (180 msec) in following a moving stimulus that follows a sinusoidal trajectory, although this lag decreases with age. By about 3 months of age, infants can keep the eyes on target most of the time, and by 5 months of age, they show predictive abilities and thus are able to lead the sinusoidal motion of a visual target (von Hofsten, 2003, 2007; von Hofsten & Rosander, 1996, 1997).

Is head motion involved in the early use of smooth pursuit? Yes, it is present even in 1-month-olds and increases with age through at least 5 months. However, its lag is always large (250 msec). In spite of this lag, the infants are able to finely coordinate head and eye movements to track moving targets accurately. Figure 18.3 shows the eye and head tracking ability in two infants, tested between the ages of 2 and 5 months. Note that head involvement is not substantial until 5 months. As head movement increases, the contribution of eye movement naturally goes down. Note that gaze, which is the combination of head and

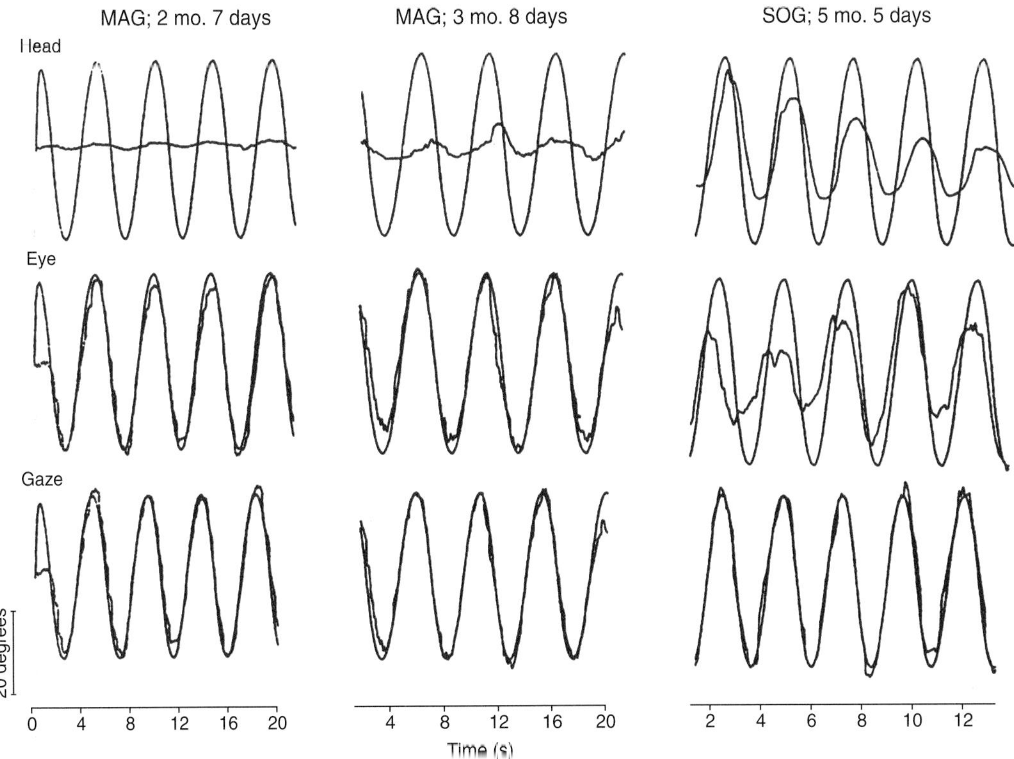

Figure 18.3 Examples of pursuit tracking of a sinusoidal motion by infants of two **(left)**, three **(middle)**, and five **(right)** months of age. Movement of the head (upper trace), eye (middle trace), and gaze (lower trace) is shown. Note that head involvement is not substantial until 5 months of age. As its involvement increases, the contribution of eye movement naturally goes down. Note that gaze, which is the combination of head and eye movements, tracks the target almost perfectly, taking into account head movement lag as well as the relative contribution of eye and head to total gaze. MAG, SOG, codes for individual subjects. (Reprinted from von Hofsten C, Rosander K. Development of smooth-pursuit tracking in young infants. *Vision Res.* 1997;13:1803, with permission.)

eye movements, tracks the target almost perfectly, taking into account head movement lag, as well as the relative contribution of eye and head movements to total gaze (Rosander & von Hofsten, 2000; von Hofsten & Rosander, 1997).

Von Hofsten and Rosander's results support the concept that one system is responsible for smooth tracking both large and small objects. They note that both the visual areas of MT (medial temporal cortex) and MST (medial superior temporal cortex) are involved in smooth tracking and that their function improves quickly after 6.5 weeks. Research suggests that the gain of the smooth-pursuit system is set in the frontal cortex, which develops rapidly during this period. The smooth-pursuit gain improves gradually from 6.5 to 15 weeks, in agreement with this research (Rosander & von Hofsten, 2002; von Hofsten, 2003, 2007; von Hofsten & Rosander, 1997).

Development of Visual Pathways for Reaching

In Chapter 17, we discussed the Ebbinghaus illusion, in which adults typically misjudge the physical size of a central disk when it is surrounded by smaller disks, yet, despite this misperception, scale their hand aperture to the actual size of the disc. We suggested that separate processing in the ventral versus the dorsal stream visual pathways for perception and action underlies this phenomenon. In a study of the development of this dissociation between perception and action, Hanisch et al. (2001) asked children between the ages of 5 and 12 years to both estimate the size of the central disk in the Ebbinghaus test and grasp the disk. They found that when children of all ages were asked to estimate the size of the object without grasping it, they experienced the same illusion as adults. However, when asked to estimate the size and then grasp the disk, the younger (5–7 years) children's perceptual judgments were unreliable, although adults still showed the effect of the illusion for 80% of the trials. In addition, the younger children were more affected by the illusion created by the surround when making their grasp opening. They grasped disks of the same size with a smaller grasp opening when the disks were surrounded by smaller disks, although they perceived the central disks as being larger. The younger children also had the largest safety margin during grasping, with a larger grasp opening than required. The researchers conclude that ventral and dorsal stream pathways may not be functionally segregated in early and middle childhood, with children using both of the visual processing streams during perceptual and visuomotor tasks.

Eye–Head–Hand Coordination Development

In Chapter 17, we mentioned that the eye, head, and hand are coordinated when adults reach, such that the eyes move first, followed by the head, and then the arm. How does eye, head, and hand coordination develop in children?

At 2 months, head–arm movements become coupled very strongly as the infant gains control over the neck muscles (von Hofsten, 1984, 1993). Over the next 2 months, there is an increased uncoupling of head and arm movements, which allows more flexibility in eye–head–hand coordination. At about 4 months, infants begin to gain trunk postural stability, so they have a more stable base for reaching movements. As infants gain increased trunk postural stability and more experience in upright sitting, infants' postural–visual–manual coordination improves. This relation is shown by a study from Rachwani and colleagues (2019). They tested 6- to 12-month-old infants on a motorized chair that rotated them past a toy (Fig. 18.4A). All infants were independent sitters at the time of testing, but their independent sitting experience ranged from 0 to 174 days. Infants wore a head-mounted eye tracker to record when the toy appeared in the infant's field of view and when infants fixated their eyes on the toy (Fig. 18.4B). Results showed that the infant's quick reaches toward the toy played out in a coordinated sequence of actions. Infants started turning their head and trunk to bring the toy into view, which in turn instigated the start of the reach. Visually fixating the toy to locate its position in space guided the hand to contact the toy and retrieve it. Infants with more independent sitting experience displayed better performance—they quickly implemented all coordinated actions to retrieve the toy during the midst of a spin.

A significant number of developmental changes thus converge after 4 months of age, all of which are essential for the emergence of successful reaching. This supports the concept that the emergence of successful reaching is not due to the maturation of a single system but to contributions and coordination of multiple maturing systems (Bertenthal & von Hofsten, 1998; von Hofsten, 1984, 1993).

REACH AND GRASP

Motor Components

Early Development

During the first year of life, there are a number of clear transitions in the infant's reach-and-grasp motor abilities. As mentioned earlier, rudimentary "prereaching" movements can be observed in infants at birth. Until about 2 months of age, whenever the infant extends the arm, the hand opens in extension at the same time, so that it is difficult to grasp an object. At about 2 months of age, the first motor transformation in reaching occurs (von Hofsten, 1984). At this age (about 7 weeks), the amount of reaching is substantially reduced, and the hand becomes fisted instead of remaining open during arm extension toward the object. Von Hofsten (1984) has hypothesized that the reduction in reaching at this age is due to an inhibition that is associated with the development of the corticospinal pathway; he proposed that

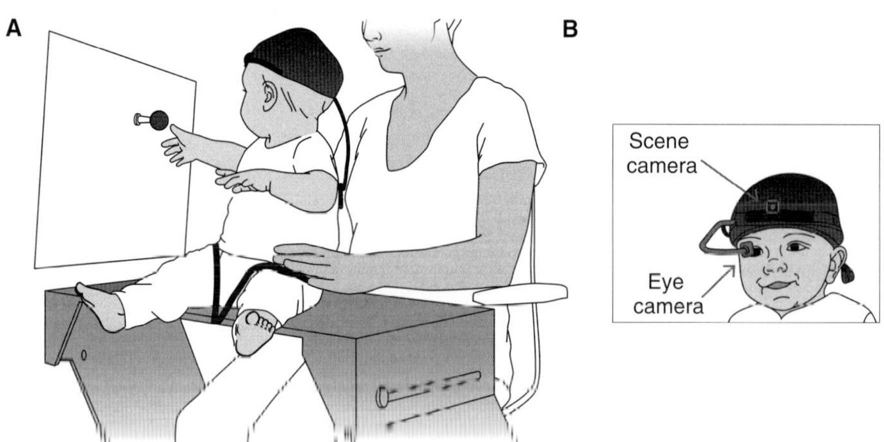

Figure 18.4 (A) A typical infant sitting on a bench attached to the motorized rotating chair with the caregiver seated behind. Infants had to reach toward a toy placed at different locations on the reaching board as the motorized chair rotated the infant past the toy. **(B)** Line drawing shows infant wearing a head-mounted eye tracker. The scene camera records the view of the infant. The eye camera records the movements of the infant's eye. The software calculates the infant's point of gaze in the scene. (Adapted with permission from Rachwani J, Herzberg O, Golenia L, Adolph, KE. Postural, visual, and manual coordination in the development of prehension. *Child Dev.* 2019;90:1559–1568.)

it is not yet synchronized with the brainstem pathways, involving whole arm extension and flexion synergies.

After this short period of about 1 to 2 weeks, the proportion of fisted reaches decreases again, and the arm becomes controlled in a more functional fashion so that only when the infant fixates on an object does the hand open in preparation for intentionally grasping and manipulating the object. Thus, an intentional reach begins to emerge, with the extension synergy being broken up, so that the fingers flex as the arm extends toward the desired object (von Hofsten, 1984, 1993).

At about 4 months, infants enter a new developmental phase, involving integration of the newly developed skill of reaching. The movement of reaches of 4-month-olds typically consists of several subunits (often called "movement units"), and the final approach toward the object is crooked and awkward. In the next 2 months, the approach path straightens and the number of movement units in the reach is reduced in number, with the first part of the reach getting longer and more powerful. The largest movement units in a reach move closer to the beginning of the reach with age. Studies show that at the age of 2 years, 75% of trials show a velocity profile with a single peak (von Hofsten, 1984, 1991, 1993).

More recently, researchers have performed longitudinal studies examining reaching in infants from 2 months to 3 years of age. Figure 18.5 shows examples of sagittal hand paths of one infant reaching at four different developmental times. As you see, infant reaches are curved at early ages and become much straighter by 2 years of age. This has been defined by the "straightness ratio," which is about 2 at reach onset and decreases to 1.3 to 1.4 by 2 to 3 years of age, still less straight than for adults, who have a ratio of about 1. This is accompanied by an increase in smoothness (or decrease in jerk) of the movements. In addition, maximum hand speed during the reach occurs closer to the beginning of the reach with development, being at 0.35 to 0.5 of the reach in the earliest ages and moving to 0.2 to 0.4 of the reach by 2 to 3 years of age. However, average reaching speed does not increase during this time period.

Laboratories have begun using a dynamic systems approach to explore the development of reaching. In one set of studies, the transition to the development of reaching was explored in infants from the age of 3 weeks through 1 year (Thelen et al., 1993, 1996). Thelen and colleagues noted that the four infants studied entered the transition to reaching at different ages and with different activity levels and preferred movement patterns. They suggest that the process of learning to reach is one of discovering the match between intrinsic dynamics (the opportunities and constraints of their bodies) and their intention to move the hand (using proprioceptive and/or visual cues) to the toy (using visual cues). They found that infants chose the patterns for executing a reach in a flexible way, in relation to their dynamic resources and the demands of the task, rather than from a preexisting motor program.

For example, at the time of reach onset, each infant had characteristic intrinsic dynamics, including preferred postures, movements, and energy levels. They noted that two of the infants had higher energy levels and energized their muscles with large coactive phasic bursts, often rhythmically. Movements looked like bilateral flapping (described as similar to limit cycle oscillators). When they reached for the toy, they converted these oscillations into a task-specific movement (described as a point attractor) by damping down their oscillations and stiffening the arm with cocontraction of the muscles.

The second two infants were quieter and thus needed to lift their arms against gravity and move them forward. These movements were slow and sustained,

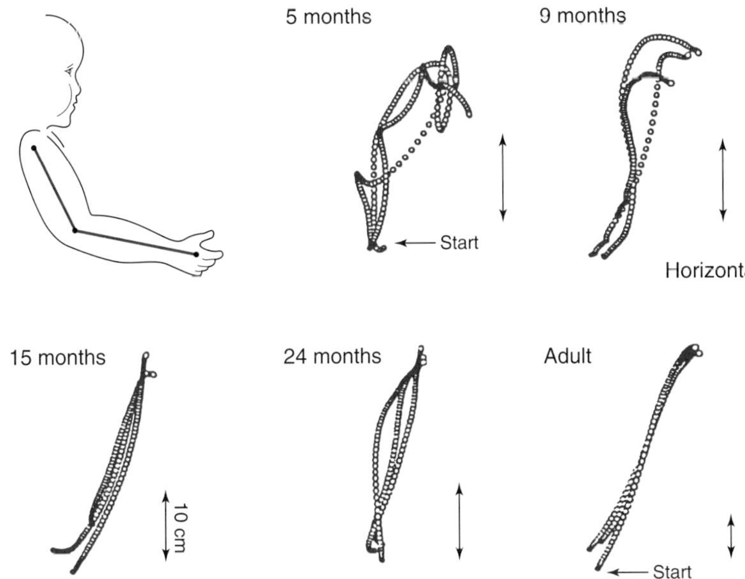

Figure 18.5 Example of hand paths used by one infant at four different ages, recorded in the sagittal plane. Three different reaches are shown for each age. Note the progression toward the smoothing of the end point motion. The time interval between successive points is 10 msec. (Reprinted from Konczak J, Dichgans J. The development toward stereotypic arm kinematics during reaching in the first 3 years of life. *Exp Brain Res.* 1997;117:348, with permission.)

with limbs relatively compliant instead of stiff, and without perturbations from motion-dependent forces from connected segments. The authors conclude that smooth trajectories and coupling of joints were a byproduct of particular levels of force and arm stiffness or compliance (Thelen et al., 1993).

They also noted that infants acquired stable head control several weeks before reaching onset. Reaching onset involved a reorganization of muscle patterns in trapezius and deltoid muscles, serving to stabilize the head and shoulders and provide a stable base for reaching (Thelen & Spencer, 1998).

The authors state that their results support mass-spring (or equilibrium-point) models of motor control in which the trajectory of the hand, joint angles, and muscle patterns is not explicitly planned in advance. Instead, the central nervous system (CNS) sets up new spring constants for the muscles at the involved joints that bring the joint to the desired position (Hogan et al., 1987).

Additional research by Konczak and colleagues (1995, 1997), studying nine infants longitudinally from 4 to 15 months of age, has shown that there are two developmental phases in hand trajectory formation: a first phase between 16 and 24 weeks involved rapid improvements, including reductions in movement time and number of movement units. This was followed by a second phase (28–64 weeks) involving fine-tuning of the sensorimotor system, in which there were more gradual changes in end point kinematics. They noted that early reaching was not limited by lack of ability to generate adequate levels of muscle torques. This suggests that, as for postural and locomotion development, muscle strength is not the rate-limiting factor for the onset of reaching. However, there were significant increases in the production of muscle flexor torque with time, with early reachers using a combination of flexion and extension torque and mature reachers using only adult-like flexor torques. Thus, mature reachers, like adults, took advantage of motion-dependent and gravitational forces to extend the arm.

In addition, relative timing of muscle- and motion-dependent torque peaks showed a systematic development toward adult profiles with increasing age. They suggested that control problems of proximal joint torque generation could account for the segmented hand paths seen in early reaching. They concluded that the development of stable patterns of interjoint coordination does not only occur simply by regulating torque amplitude but also by modulating the correct timing of force production and by the system's use of reactive forces (Konczak et al., 1995, 1997). Like Thelen and colleagues, they also noted variability in the longitudinal profiles of each infant, indicating that each child followed his or her own strategy to explore the internal and external forces that are the basis of coordinated movements.

In a longitudinal study of reaching development in 12 infants during varying periods from reaching onset to 20 months of age, Berthier and Keen (2006) found a gradual slowing of reach speed and a more rapid reduction in movement jerk with development (probably similar to the second phase of reaching development described by Konczak and colleagues, 1997 [see earlier discussions]). Infants first learning to reach primarily used the shoulder muscles to extend the hand to the target. The use of the elbow gradually increased after the onset of reaching and reached a plateau at about 6 months of age. The increase in use of the elbow coincides with the rapid or active phase of learning, observed by Konczak et al. (1995) and Thelen et al. (1996). These developmental changes in reaching support Bernstein's (1967) hypothesis that early in skill development, there is a fixing of the degrees of freedom of a limb, with a gradual release of these degrees of freedom with skill acquisition (Berthier & Keen, 2006; Konczak & Dichgans, 1997; Thelen et al., 1996). Thus, there are probably a number of developmental changes that contribute to this improvement, including development of trunk postural control.

Early reaches are often bimanual, with both mirror movements and nondifferentiated movements of both limbs being typical of the infant's early reaching behavior. By 6 months of age, unilateral reaching begins to dominate. However, mirror movements persist during some unilateral reaching, and become less frequent during upright sitting and when infants watch their acting hand (Soska et al., 2012). It has been suggested that the early mirror movements could be due to crossed corticospinal projections from the right and left hemispheres, which are reduced during development (Gordon, 2001).

Researchers believe that the development of the corticospinal tract contributes to the emergence of independent finger movements. However, it is also possible that the maturation of the tract depends on the use of the hands and fingers. In fact, animal studies have shown that the formation of normal patterns of corticospinal tract development depends on neural activity in the sensorimotor cortex in early postnatal development and that blocking this activity results in the inability to create normal reaching movements (Martin, 1999, 2000). This suggests that there may be an early critical period for the development of reaching, in which practice in manipulative activity shapes the development of corticospinal circuits (Gordon, 2001).

Von Hofsten (2007) emphasizes this issue, noting that the neural starting point of development in the neonate is not a set of reflexes that are triggered by sensory stimuli but a set of action systems activated by the infant. This creates a dynamic system in which the development of the nervous system and the development of action each influence the other through activity and the infant's experience. He notes that infants have a number of endogenous skills present at birth, including visually controlling their arms in space and that these skills give activity-dependent input to the sensorimotor and cognitive systems. This allows the infant to explore the relationship between commands and movements and between the different sensory modalities (vision, somatosensation, etc.) and to discover all the possibilities of their actions and the ways their actions are constrained by the environment. We must remember that a key driving force for all these actions is exploration and social interaction.

Indeed, experimental studies in healthy infants have highlighted the importance of active experience in the performance of infant reaching. For example, three sessions of reach training led 3.5-month-old infants to contact toys more frequently, with shorter and smoother arm movements, compared to same-aged infants who were only exposed to social interactions (Cunha et al., 2015). Moreover, just 2 hours of toy contact training over a 2-week period in 3-month-old infants, with the help of sticky mittens, led to higher attempts of infants contacting and grasping toys barehanded, and to more sophisticated object exploration, than infants who observed objects being moved and touched by their parents (Libertus & Needham, 2010).

Clinical implications for this research are that it is important to help children with developmental disabilities to actively explore their environment as well as to initiate social interactions with others. These are key factors in habilitation of the nervous system.

Development of Postural Support of Reaching. As you may remember from Chapters 7 and 8, a critical element that contributes to the accuracy of reaching is postural control. Research on the development of postural control and its relationship to reaching in seated infants has been performed in a longitudinal study on infants from 2.5 to 8 months of age (Rachwani et al., 2015). As shown in Figure 18.6A, infants were seated and provided either thoracic or pelvic support, and a toy was dropped in front of the child at arm's length. As the child reached for the toy, kinematics of trunk motion and arm reach trajectory and success rate were recorded. Table 18.1 shows the rate of reaching success for the infants, while Figures 18.6B and C show the changes in both the variability of trunk angle during the reach and the straightness of the reach trajectory for infants from 3 to 4 months prior to sitting onset through 2 months after onset of independent sitting. Note in the table that the success rate for reaching was substantially higher with thoracic compared to pelvic support in the months prior to sitting onset (i.e., within the interval from −4 to −1 months before independent sitting). At this point, success rate became equivalent at 100%. Figure 18.6B shows that with only pelvic support (red lines and circles), infants showed a high variability of trunk angle during the reach, which was gradually reduced in the months prior to sitting onset, while with thoracic support trunk angle, variability remained minimal through sitting onset. Figure 18.6C shows that straightness of arm trajectory also was significantly reduced in the months prior to independent sitting with thoracic compared to pelvic support, with no change between straightness score for the two levels of support after sitting onset. These results support earlier research indicating that postural control, specifically control of the trunk, is a key rate-limiting factor in success and performance efficiency of reaching in young infants. These results also support the concept that development of trunk control underlying sitting balance involves the sequential development of control over successive segments of the trunk in a top-down order (Rachwani et al., 2015; Saavedra et al., 2012).

Development in Childhood

A study by Schneiberg et al. (2002) further examined the development of coordination during reaching in children from 4 to 11 years of age. They asked children to reach from the seated position with the dominant arm and to grasp a cone placed in front of them. Kinematic data from markers placed on the arm, head, and trunk showed that younger children used immature patterns of reaching, characterized by increased variability. With increasing age, hand trajectories became smoother and less variable, while interjoint coordination became more consistent. Finally, trunk displacement and variability also decreased with age. By 8 to 10 years of age, children showed variability similar to that in adults.

A second study (Kuhtz-Buschbeck et al., 1998) examined the kinematics and coordination of reaching and grasping for a cylindrical target in children 4 to 12 years of age. Across this age range, movement duration and normalized peak spatial velocity of the reaching hand did not change significantly. However, the authors found that the hand path became straighter and the coordination between hand path and grip formation improved, creating smooth predictable kinematic trajectories by the age of 12 years. They noted that younger children opened their grip relatively wider than older children, using a higher safety margin. In addition, the children showed a decrease in the use of visual control with development. Thus, only the oldest children were able to scale the grip opening appropriately to object size, when vision of the object was not available during the reach. The authors concluded that the development of control of manipulation skills continues through about 10 to 12 years of age.

Another study aimed to look at age-related differences in reach planning (Domellöf et al., 2020). Young (6 years) and older (10 years) children, and a group of adults, were asked to transport a vertical cylindrical peg with either a circular or semicircular base from a start-holder to a goal-holder. For the round peg, the start- and goal-holder were identical; however, for the semicircular peg, the goal-holder was presented in four different orientations (0°, 90°, 180°, or −90°). Thus, participants had to rotate the semicircular peg various

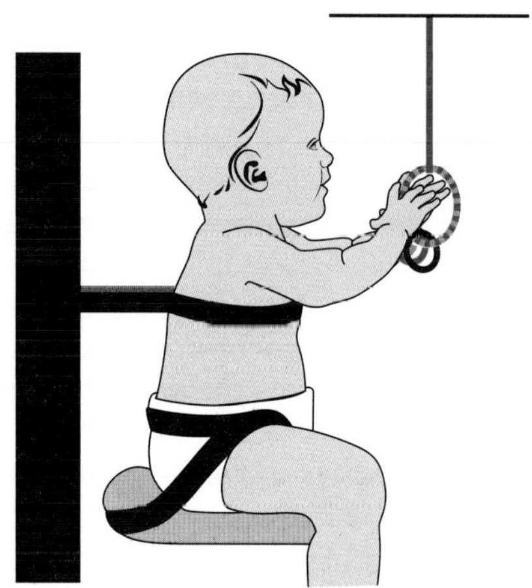

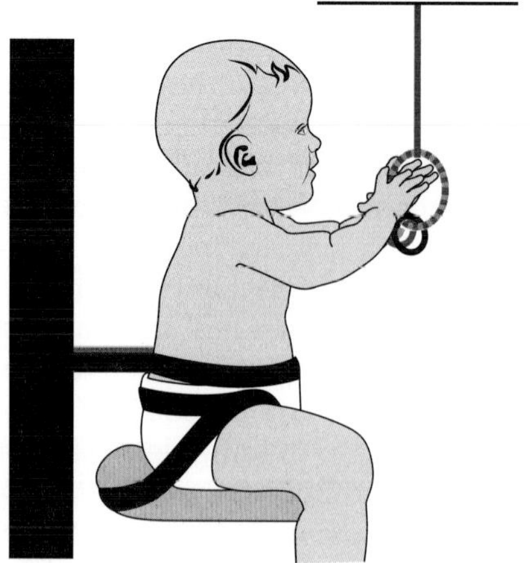

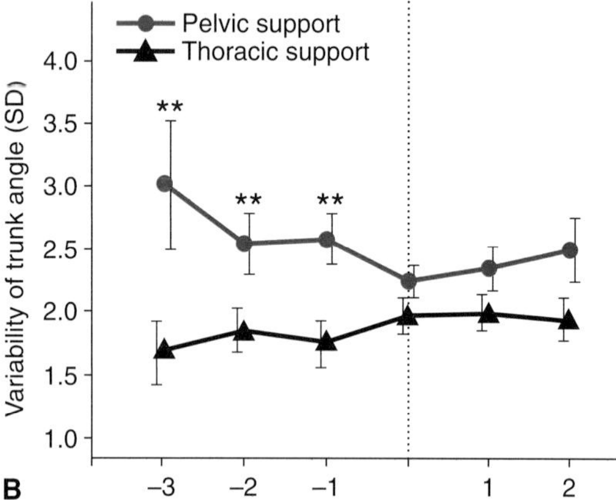

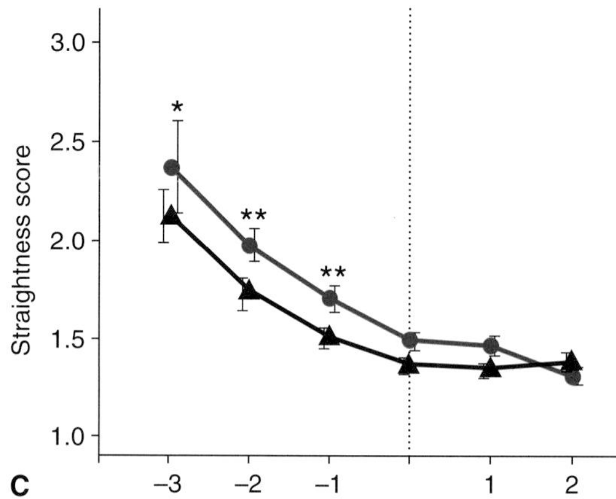

Figure 18.6 (A) Image of infant supported at either the thoracic level or the pelvic level of the trunk in a reaching task. **(B and C)** Changes in both the variability of trunk angle **(B)** during the reach and the straightness of the reach **(C)** for infants from 3 to 4 months prior to sitting onset (–3 to –1) through 2 months after onset of independent sitting *(1, 2)*. *Vertical dotted lines* indicate onset of independent sitting. (* $p < 0.05$, ** $p < 0.01$). Pelvic support: *circles* and *red lines*. Thoracic support: triangles and black lines. Note the improvement in both trunk variability and reaching straightness score in the months prior to sitting onset, when thoracic support is provided. (Adapted from Rachwani J, Santamaria V, Saavedra S, et al. The development of trunk control and its relation to reaching in infancy: a longitudinal study. *Front Hum Neurosci.* 2015;9:94. doi: 10.3389/fnhum.2015.00094. Ecollection 2015, Fig. 4, p. 8.)

TABLE 18.1 Success Rate for Infant Reaching with Either Thoracic or Pelvic Support

	–4 Months	–3 Months	–2 Months	–1 Month	Sitting onset	1 Month	2 Months
Success rate/ infant: Thoracic support	40% (N = 7)	67% (N = 9)	96% (N = 10)	100% (N = 10)	100% (N = 10)	100% (N = 9)	100% (N = 7)
Success rate/ infant: Pelvic support	18% (N = 3)	47% (N = 8)	86% (N = 10)	100% (N = 10)	100% (N = 10)	100% (N = 9)	100% (N = 7)

Adapted from Rachwani J, Santamaria V, Saavedra S, et al. The development of trunk control and its relation to reaching in infancy: a longitudinal study. Front Hum Neurosci 2015;9:94. doi:10.3389/fnhum.2015.00094. Ecollection 2015, Table 2.

amounts horizontally before fitting it into its final position. In line with previous research, 6 year olds in this study had less efficient reaching movements—they displayed shorter reach onset latencies, higher reaching velocities and shorter time to peak velocities, and longer grasping durations than adults. Most importantly, adults rotated the peg during the transport phase of the reach while children made the corrective rotations once the hand had arrived at the goal. Thus, the authors conclude that while children and adults are capable of grasping, transporting, and rotating the target, they do so at different skill levels.

Development of Force Adaptation during Reaching

In order to be able to reach accurately in many different contexts, children need to learn to adapt to the forces used during reaching to task and environmental demands. It has been hypothesized that humans learn to make reaching movements in a variety of contexts by creating an internal motor model of their limb dynamics. In order to determine the gradual time course of development of inverse dynamics models for reaching in children, Konczak et al. (2003) examined the movement characteristics of children (4–11 years of age) as they adapted to changes in arm dynamics.

The children sat, and their forearm was secured in a device attached to a torque motor. They made goal-directed forearm movements, while the torque motor applied different external damping forces. The researchers found that all children showed aftereffects from the previous condition in response to changes in damping, which suggests that their neural control systems did not rapidly adapt to changes in damping forces. However, they found that with increasing age, there was a reduction in the number of trials required for adaptation, although it did not reach adult levels by 11 years of age. The youngest children showed the most difficulty compensating for damping forces, with the path of the forearm most perturbed and most variable when making reaches under these conditions. These findings suggest that the neural representations of limb dynamics are less precise and less stable in young children. The researchers propose that this instability might be a cause of the high kinematic variability seen in children during many motor tasks.

Sensory Components

Visually Guided versus Visually Triggered Reaching

Early Development. It has been long-hypothesized that infants initially need to alternate their look between their hand and a target to guide the hand progressively and finally aim at the target. This is known as visually guided reaching. It was assumed to be a precursory step for the development of a more direct arm movement toward the target. A vast number of studies performed between the 60s and 80s support the visually guided reaching hypothesis for learning to reach. To study the development of visually guided reaching in infants, researchers have fitted infants with prism lenses to visually provide a lateral shift of the target position as the infants reach for small toys (McDonnell & Abraham, 1979). Authors showed that by 5-1/2 months of age, when the hand comes into view, the infant is able to perceive the discrepancy between the hand and target positions in order to correct the reaching trajectory. However, McDonnell and Abraham noticed that after 7 months of age, infants' adaptation to the displacing prism decreased. They concluded that infants over 7 months relied less on vision to guide their reaching movements. After 7 months, visually guided reaching is gradually replaced by visually triggered reaching, where infants look at the target (not the hand) to make contact with the target. During visually triggered reaching, infants integrate object properties and its location into their reach and pre-shape their hand movement in anticipation of grasping the object (Lockman et al., 1984).

The visually guided hypothesis for learning to reach was corroborated by other studies that also used displacement prisms or mirrors to examine infants' reliance on the sight of their hand to contact the target. However, many other discoveries have proved that the emergence and development of infant reaching do not occur primarily under the control of vision. One of the most convincing studies was performed by Clifton and colleagues (1993), who looked at seven infants between 6 and 25 weeks of age. Each session consisted of a condition where objects were presented in the light and another condition where glowing or sounding objects were presented in the dark. Authors found that infants began contacting and grasping the objects in both conditions at comparable ages. They concluded that proprioceptive cues—not the sight of the hand—guided early reaching, and thus, very young infants perform visually triggered reaching instead of visually guided ones. Many researchers nowadays agree that the visually guided hypothesis does not hold; however, there still exists a continuous debate about this matter. For example, Pogetti and colleagues (2013) assessed the movement kinematics during reaching in 5-month-old infants and compared their movements performed under full vision versus visual occlusion. They found that visual occlusion led to decreased straightness of the arm displacement toward the toy compared to full vision. Thus, Pogetti and colleagues proposed a "flexibility" in the use of sensory information during early reaching (similar to the multisensory reweighting model for balance control). They proposed that infants use visual feedback to guide their hands when available, but when not available, infants would rely on proprioceptive feedback rather than visual feedback for movement control.

Development in Childhood. To determine whether there are continued developmental changes in children's use of visual feedback in making reaching movements, studies were performed in which children from 4 to 11 years of age were asked to make movements with or without visual feedback. Hay (1978) has shown that there are interesting changes in the use of visual information by children between 4 and 11 years of age. Children between 4 and 6 years of age can make movements without visual feedback with reasonable accuracy, as shown in Figure 18.7, which displays the magnitude of error when reaching without feedback in children ages 4 to 11 and in adults. (Note that although 5-year-olds may appear to be more accurate than adults, there are no significant differences between these groups.) However, as the figure illustrates, at age 7, there is an abrupt reduction in this ability, as seen in the increased errors made in reaching without visual feedback. The accuracy then begins to increase again, reaching adult levels by 10 to 11 years of age. As we describe in the next section, this reduction in accuracy is reflected in an increased dependence on visual feedback at the age of 7 years. This is one piece of research that supports the hypothesis that the age of 7 is a transition time in the development of reaching (Dellen & Kalverboer, 1984; Hay, 1990).

Other studies analyzing the kinematics of reaching movements without visual feedback in children ages 5 to 11 also support this hypothesis. Figure 18.8 shows that 5-year-olds produce mainly ballistic movements, with sharp decelerations at the end of the movement (labeled 1 in the top rectangle and shown by the dark orange bars below). This pattern shows a sharp decrease in children aged 7. At this age, a ramp-and-step movement pattern increases (labeled 3 in the top rectangle and shown as light bars below). At the same time, ballistic patterns with a smooth deceleration at the end of the movement increase and continue to increase through 9 years of age (labeled 2 and shown by the striped bars). It has been hypothesized that this could be due to the increased use of proprioceptive feedback control in 7-year-olds and the progressive restriction of feedback control to the final homing-in phase in older children, possibly the result of increased efficiency of the movement braking system (Hay, 1979).

For a closer look at developmental changes in the use of visual feedback in reaching movements in children, experiments were performed in which children ages 5 to 11 were asked to make reaches while wearing prismatic lenses, which make an illusory shift in the image of the object. These experiments are similar to those described earlier, examining the use of visual feedback in reaching in neonates and infants. As shown in the upper part of Figure 18.9, as the children made a reach, the kinematics of the hand movement showed a

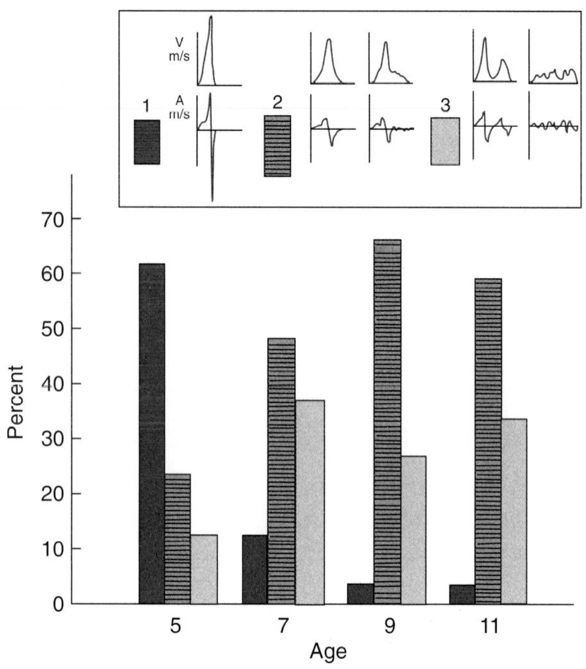

Figure 18.8 Percentage of time three different reaching movement patterns were seen in children from 5 to 11 years of age. *1*, ballistic pattern with sharp accelerations/decelerations; *2*, ballistic patterns with smooth decelerations; *3*, step-and-ramp patterns. Note that the 5-year-olds used the highest levels of ballistic patterns, while the 7-year-olds used high levels of step-and-ramp patterns, indicating increased reliance on vision. Children 9 to 11 years old used the highest levels of ballistic patterns, with smooth decelerations, indicating primary use of visual feedback at the end of the movement. *V*, velocity; *A*, acceleration. (Adapted from Hay L. Developmental changes in eye-hand coordination behaviors: preprogramming versus feedback control. In: Bard C, Fleury M, Hay L, eds. *Development of eye–hand coordination across the lifespan*. Columbia, SC: University of South Carolina Press, 1990:231, with permission.)

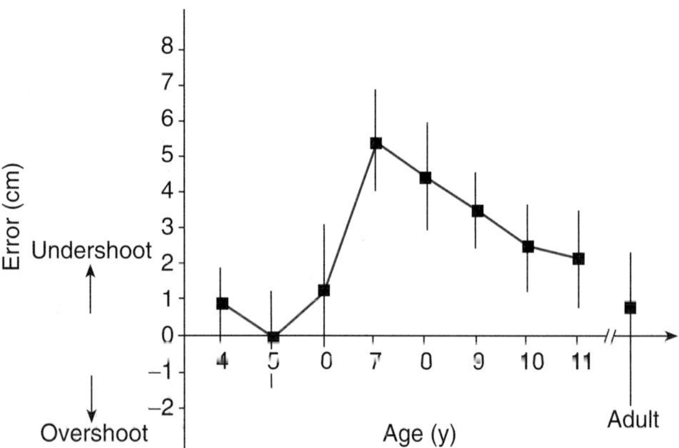

Figure 18.7 Graph showing pointing errors when visual feedback is not present for children from 4 to 11 years of age, as compared with adults. Note that large errors appear at 7 years of age, indicating reliance on visual feedback for reaching. These gradually are reduced in subsequent years, as children restrict feedback to the homing-in phase of the reach. (Adapted from Hay L. Developmental changes in eye–hand coordination behaviors: preprogramming versus feedback control. In: Bard C, Fleury M, Hay L, eds. *Development of eye–hand coordination across the lifespan*. Columbia, SC: University of South Carolina Press, 1990:228, with permission.)

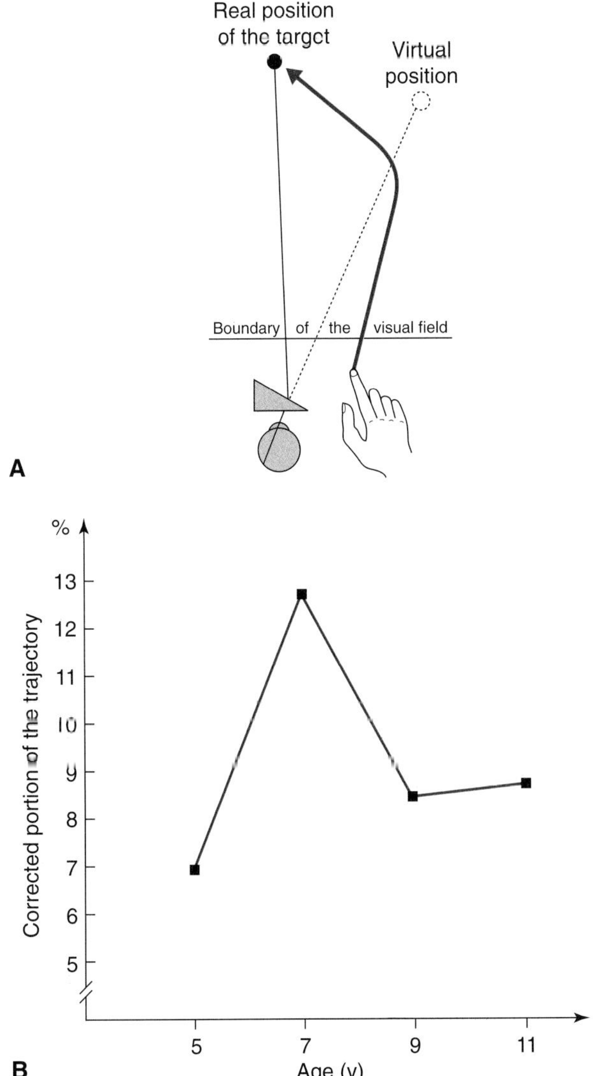

Figure 18.9 (A) Diagram of reaching movements of children who wore prismatic lenses, displacing the apparent position of the target in the visual field. **(B)** Corrected portion of the reaching trajectory for 5-, 7-, 9-, and 11-year-olds. Note that 7-year-olds correct the reaching movement much earlier than the other age groups, indicating increased use of visual feedback. (Adapted from Hay L. Spatial-temporal analysis of movements in children: motor programs versus feedback in the development of reaching *J Mot Behav.* 1979;11:196, 198.)

curved, rather than a straight-line trajectory toward the object. This occurred as the hand shifted from an initially incorrect path, due to the shift in the visual image caused by the prismatic lenses, to a correct path when the hand came into view, based on visual information of the relative hand and target positions. The length of the visually corrected path indicates the amount of visual feedback used in the movement (Hay, 1979).

As evident in the bottom half of Figure 18.9, 5-year-old children corrected the movement late in its trajectory, and in fact, the majority of these children did not make a correction until they reached the virtual target, indicating minimal use of visual feedback. Thus, in this age group, visual control occurs mainly after, rather than during, reaching movements. This is correlated with highly stereotyped movement times seen in this age group.

The 7-year-old children corrected the movements earlier than any other group, indicating a strong use of visual feedback. While this gives rise to an increased flexibility in reaching behavior, it is coupled with increased variability in movement times and decreased accuracy when visual feedback is not present.

The 9- and 11-year-olds showed an intermediate level of trajectory correction, indicating a shift in the use of visual control toward the final phase of the movement trajectory. Thus, between 5 and 9 years of age, there appears to be a reorganization in the programming of reaching movements from mainly feedforward or anticipatory activation of reaching, to predominantly feedback control, and finally to an integration of the feedforward and feedback control, resulting in fast, accurate movements by 9 years of age.

Grasp Development

Emergence of Hand Orientation

In the neonatal period, infants show reflexive grasping patterns. What transitional changes occur as these patterns are transformed into effective grasping patterns? In order to answer this question, researchers made video recordings of the spontaneous hand and finger movements made by infants during their first 5 months. They found that during this period, spontaneous hand and digit movements gradually changed from the predominant occurrence of fist postures to nearly continuous random movements and finally to self-directed grasping movements. They noted that voluntary grasp movements can be observed at about 2 to 3 months of age (Wallace & Whishaw, 2003).

Researchers found four grasping patterns during the first 5 months of life, defined as fists, preprecision grasps associated with numerous digit postures, precision grips including the pincer grasp, and self-directed grasps. They proposed that the wide range of independent digit movements and grasp patterns during this time suggests that some direct connections of the pyramidal tract may be functional relatively early in infancy. They also suggest that "hand babbling," defined as first random and then self-directed movements, is part of the preparatory process for the emergence of accurate reaching (Wallace & Whishaw, 2003).

When do infants first begin to orient their hands to the position and shape of the object? To answer this question, researchers placed brightly colored rods either horizontally or vertically in front of the infant and recorded the characteristics of their reaching movements, as shown in Figure 18.10. Preparatory adjustments of hand orientation (vertical vs. horizontal, depending on object orientation) occurred when infants

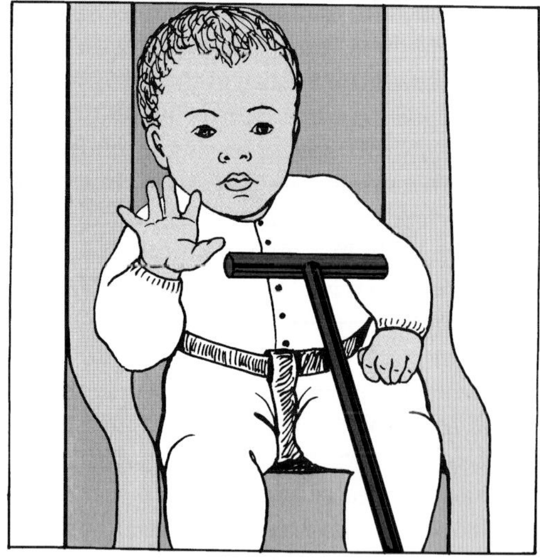

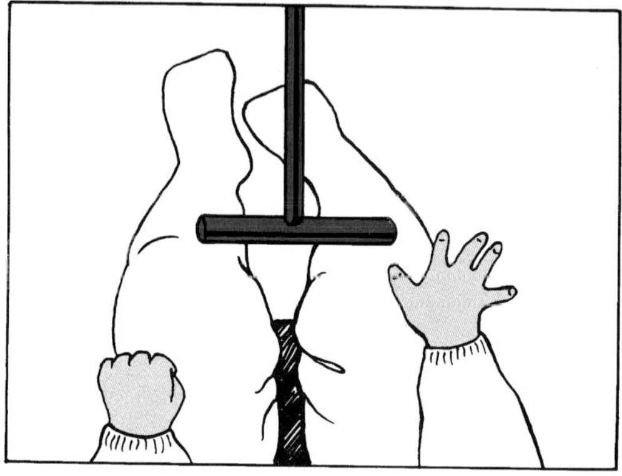

Figure 18.10 Two video camera views of an infant reaching for a horizontally oriented bar. Note that the infant uses correct hand orientation for grasping the bar. (Adapted from von Hofsten C, Fazel-Zandy S. Development of visually guided hand orientation in reaching. *J Exp Child Psychol.* 1984;38:210.)

first began to grasp objects, as early as 4-1/2 to 5 months of age (von Hofsten & Fazel-Zandy, 1984). However, the adjustments of the hand to the orientation of the object became more precise with age. Adjustments of the hand were often made before or during the early part of the reach, although they could also be seen during the approach phase. Infants are also able to use predictive control to reach for a rotating rod; they prepare to grasp it by creating a hand orientation that is aligned with the future orientation of the rod (von Hofsten, 2007).

To reach smoothly for an object, the infant must time the grasp appropriately with relation to encountering the object. If the hand closes too late, the object will bounce off the palm, and if the hand closes too early, the object will hit the knuckles. This type of planning requires visual control, since tactile control would not allow the hand to close until after touching the object (von Hofsten & Fazel-Zandy, 1984).

In experiments in which the kinematics of reaching in 5-, 6-, 9-, and 13-month-olds were compared with those of adults, it was shown that infant grasping was visually controlled as early as 5 to 6 months of age, with the hand starting to close in anticipation of reaching the object. Also, the opening of the hand was related to the size of the object for the 9- and 13-month-olds, but not in the younger group. Finally, the 13-month-olds initiated the grasp farther away from the target than the younger groups, with timing of the grasp similar to that seen in adults. The grasp component of the reach is still not mature in 13-month-olds, however, since, unlike adults, they do not yet correlate the onset of closing of the hand with the size of the object to be grasped (von Hofsten & Ronnqvist, 1988).

Development of the Pincer Grasp

There are two different ways that objects can be grasped—in a power grip, using the palm and palmar surface of the fingers, with the thumb reinforcing this grip, or in a precision grip, between the terminal pads of the finger and the thumb. The precision grip requires that the fingers be moved independently and is a prerequisite for accurate and skilled manipulation of objects (Forssberg et al., 1991; Napier, 1956).

In the first months after birth, infant grasping movements are controlled by tactile and proprioceptive reflexes. Thus, when an object contacts the palm, the fingers close. Also, when the arm flexes, the hand closes, as part of a flexor synergy. At about 4 months of age, with the onset of functional reaching, the infant uses the palmer grasp exclusively. With subsequent development, first the thumb and then the fingers begin to operate independently, and at about 10 months of age, pincer grasp (with opposition of the thumb) develops (Forssberg et al., 1991).

Developmental changes related to reaching and grasping skills correlate well with research performed on the anatomic development of the primate motor system. In primates, it has been shown that neural pathways controlling movements of the arm are different from those that control the fine movements of the fingers and hand. The two systems develop at different times. Arm control, which appears to be coordinated mainly at the brainstem level, develops earlier than hand and finger control, which appears to be coordinated at the cortical level (Kuypers, 1962, 1964).

Researchers found that infant monkeys show arm movements toward objects early in development but do not show independent finger and hand movements until they are 3 months old (Lawrence & Hopkins, 1972). It has also been shown that at about 9 to 13 months of age, with the development of the pyramidal tract, infants are able to control fractionated finger movements and thus develop more difficult grasping skills, such as the pincer grasp (von Hofsten, 1984, 2007).

Experiments have followed the development and refinement of precision grasp in human infants and children ranging in age from 8 months to 15 years. Remember from Chapter 17 that when an adult is asked to lift an object, as soon as his or her fingers touch the object, cutaneous receptors activate a centrally programmed response that consists of an increase in grip forces and load forces, designed to lift the object without letting it slip through the fingers. In adults, these two forces are always programmed in parallel, to prevent slips and to avoid squeezing the object too hard (Forssberg et al., 1991).

This parallel programming of grip and load forces was not found in human infants. In fact, until 5 years of age, the children pushed the object into the table as they increased the grip force, showing a reversed coordination between the two forces. In these children, the grip force had to be very high before the load force increase occurred. In addition, the timing and sequencing of the different phases of lifting were much longer in the infants. For example, the time between first and second finger contact was three times as long in 10-month-olds and two times as long in children up to 3 years of age, as compared with adults. It was common in the younger children to have several touches by the thumb and index finger before the object was properly gripped. Also, any finger could be the first to contact the object (Forssberg et al., 1991).

In a similar study (Pare & Dugas, 1999), distinct developmental milestones were found for the maturation of precision grip from 2 to 9 years of age. For the grasps of 2-year-old children, the peak vertical acceleration of the object during lifting was negatively correlated with peak grip force. By 3 years of age, peak acceleration and peak grip force during lifting became positively correlated, and the correlation continued to strengthen up to 9 years of age. By 4 years of age, children controlled both the acceleration and deceleration of the lifting movement in a symmetrical pattern and used a single burst of grip force to grasp the object, suggesting that they had begun to use an anticipatory control strategy for grasping. To explore for yourself the ages at which children refine control in the grasping of different types of objects, complete Lab Activity 18.1.

When Do Children Start Using Anticipatory Control in Grasping and Lifting Objects?

In the study by Pare and Dugas (1999), it was noted that children younger than 2 years of age did not increase grip and load forces in parallel but used a sequential force activation with grip force increases occurring prior to load force increases. They also showed force increases in steps, indicating a feedback strategy, since the forces were not scaled in one force rate pulse. In a second study, Forssberg and colleagues (1992) further examined the development of this anticipatory control of precision grip, exploring how weight from the previous lift is used to scale current forces. They found that anticipatory control of isometric force output during lifts with precision grip emerges during the 2nd year. The youngest children, those younger than 18 months of age, showed no or very small differences in force rates for lifts using different weights, while children older than 18 months showed this ability. This anticipatory control develops gradually, with large changes occurring between 1 and 4 years of age and more gradual changes occurring from 4 to 11 years, with adult levels being reached at about 11 years of age.

Forssberg and colleagues (1995) also noted that the younger children used a high grip-to-load-force ratio,

LAB ACTIVITY 18.1

Objective: To examine how properties of the task affect reach-and-grasp movements in children of different ages.

Procedures: For this lab, you will find one child from at least two of the following age groups—8 to 12 months, 12 to 18 months, 2 to 3 years, and 4 to 6 years—in your community and observe them performing the following tasks. Bring the following items with you when you work with the children (you can vary the size of the items so they are appropriate to the size of the child): two small plastic glasses (one with water in it and one without), a small block (small square shape), a crayon (something long and narrow), and a second small plastic glass or cylinder that you have coated with oil. In the first part of the lab, observe the arm and hand movements of the children while they pick up the empty plastic glass, block, crayon, plastic glass with water, and plastic glass coated with oil. For the older children, place the two cups (one with water and one without) next to each other. Ask the child to pour you a cup of water. Then, try it again, but invert the empty glass and place it near the glass with water.

Assignment

1. Describe how the children of the different age groups reached for and grasped the various objects.
2. When during the reach for an object, did the hand begin to shape in preparation for grasp? How did characteristics of the object affect anticipatory hand shaping?
3. For the older children, how did changing the orientation of the glass affect hand orientation? Were they able to modify the orientation of the hand so they did not have to pour the water in multiple steps?
4. Compare the data from the children to your own or other adult reach/grasp characteristics from Lab Activity 17.1. Do your results agree with those of von Hofsten and Forssberg et al. on developmental changes in anticipatory hand shaping and in lifting objects?

particularly in trials with nonslippery objects (sandpaper). This showed their use of a large safety margin against slips, indicating an immature capacity to adapt to the frictional condition. The safety margin decreased during the first 5 years of life, along with a lower variability in the grip force and a better adaptation to the current condition.

They found that by 18 months of age, children could adapt grip forces to a surface condition when the same surface was presented in blocks of trials but failed when the surface was unexpectedly changed. They suggest that this may indicate a poor capacity to form a sensorimotor memory representation of the friction. These memory abilities increased gradually with age, with older children requiring only a few lifts and adults, only one lift to update their force coordination to a new surface friction.

Adaptation of Grip Forces

One aspect of adaptation of grasping is the ability to increase or decrease grip forces smoothly depending on external sensory information. In order to study the development of grip force adaptation, Blank et al. (2000) asked children from 3 to 6 years of age, and adults, to use visual feedback to increase or decrease isometric forces on a small cylindrical sensor using a pinch grip. Participants could see their actual applied grip force as a red bar on the computer screen and had to reach the target force, shown as a blue bar. After they reached the target force level, they had to maintain the grip force continuously for 5 sec. Visual feedback was then withdrawn after 10 sec, and participants had to hold the requested force level without visual control. There were clear developmental changes in the precision of force tracking. For children up to 4 years of age, there was a tendency to overshoot the target force change by "jumping and waiting." The older children overshot the target only when there was a slow target force decrease. In contrast, adults used small amounts of undershooting as they followed the target change in all conditions, suggesting that they used a continuous "following" strategy. The time to establish the target force level also decreased with age. Notably, in contrast to older children and adults, most of the 3-year-olds and some 4-year-olds were not able to sustain the force level without visual feedback. However, the older children and adults were better under the condition of visual feedback versus after withdrawing visual feedback, suggesting their reliance on visual versus internal proprioceptive control for pinch grip force regulation. These results suggest that there is a developmental strategy change for the adaptation of grip forces from a feedforward strategy with intermittent use of sensorimotor feedback toward parallel and integrated feedback and feedforward processing, with a critical transition period at 5 to 6 years of age.

Learning to Reach for and Grasp Moving Objects (Catching)

Studies have also been performed to determine the emergence of the ability of infants to reach for and grasp a moving object; this could be considered a rudimentary form of catching behavior. Researchers have shown that by the time infants could reach successfully for nonmoving objects, they were also successful at reaching for moving objects. Infants as young as 18 weeks could catch objects moving at 30 cm/s. Fifteen-week-olds could intercept the object but were not yet able to grasp it. These results suggest that infants are able to predict where the object will be at a future point in time because they must start reaching early to intercept it in its path. It was noted that the infants did not automatically reach toward every object that passed by. Rather, they seemed to be able to detect in advance whether they had a reasonable chance to reach it (von Hofsten & Lindhagen, 1979).

Cognitive Components

Emergence of Object Exploration

When do infants first begin to change their manipulative activities in relation to the characteristics of the objects grasped? During the first year, the actions infants perform with objects tend to be mouthing, waving, shaking, or banging. Rigid objects tend to be banged, while spongy objects are squeezed or rubbed (Gibson & Walker, 1984). In studies on 6-, 9-, and 12-month-olds, it was noted that mouthing activity decreased with age and that object rotation, transferring the object between hands, and looking at and fingering the object increased (Corbetta & Mounoud, 1990; Ruff, 1984).

At about 1 year of age, infants begin to acquire the understanding of how to use objects, but even before this age, they can discover simple, functional relationships if these require little precision. Thus, an infant first uses a spoon for banging or shaking before using it for eating. The infant establishes the relationships between spoon and hand, spoon and mouth, and spoon and plate as subroutines before putting them together for the act of eating, in which the spoon is filled at the plate and transported to the mouth with an anticipatory opening of the mouth (Connolly, 1979).

If infants are given a spoon to grasp when they are young (in the first year), they tend to ignore the handle orientation and grasp it with the preferred hand even if this creates an awkward grasp. However, in their 2nd year, they begin to understand the task and grasp the handle of the spoon with the appropriate hand using an efficient grip (McCarty et al., 1999).

At about 14 to 16 months of age, the infant develops the ability to adapt reaching to the weight of objects, using shape and size as indicators of weight. At about 16 to 19 months of age, infants begin to understand that certain objects go together culturally, such as a cup in a saucer. Finally, at the end of the 2nd year, they begin to perform symbolic actions like pretending to eat or drink (Corbetta & Mounoud, 1990).

After 1 year of age, infants begin to develop skills requiring more precision of movement and closer relationships between objects, such as fitting one object into another. At 13 to 15 months, infants begin piling two cubes on top of each other; at 18 months, three cubes; at 21 months, five cubes; and at 23 to 24 months, six cubes. This shows that the infant is gradually developing coordinated reaching and manipulation, so that objects can be placed and released carefully (Bayley, 1969; Corbetta & Mounoud, 1990). One of the most complex hand skills—in-hand manipulation of objects—develops over a number of years. This allows the development of activities of daily living such as eating, handwriting, buttoning clothes, and brushing the teeth (Gordon, 2001).

A study to examine the onset of manipulation abilities encouraged infants to insert elongated objects of various shapes into snuggly fitting holes. Infants who were younger than 18 months understood the task, tried hard, but had little concept of how to do it. They simply pressed the object against the hole without regard to orientation. Children who were 22 months old, however, systematically raised the horizontally placed objects when transporting them to the hole, and the 26-month-old children turned the objects before arriving at the hole so that they were oriented appropriately. The authors state that a pure feedback strategy (used by the 18-month-olds) would not work for this task and that infants needed to acquire and master a variety of skills, including motor competence, perception of the spatial relationship between the object and the hole it fit into, and mental rotation of the object (Örnkloo & von Hofsten, 2007; von Hofsten, 2007).

Thus, to functionally operate cultural artifacts (e.g., opening a container lid, unzipping a jacket), children must know what to do and have the perceptual-motor skills to implement the required actions as the designers intended successfully. Kachwani and colleagues (2020) documented a three-step developmental progression in learning the designed actions—from non-designed exploratory actions at younger ages (e.g., banging and mouthing), to display of the designed actions at intermediate ages (e.g., twisting a container lid or pulling the tab of a zipper), to successful implementation of the designed actions at older ages (continuous left-twisting of a container lid or pulling the tab toward the teeth of the zipper). The authors showed that children's display of the designed actions does not guarantee successful implementation because many artifacts involve complex, motorically challenging operations. Children must know the detailed biomechanical requirements to operate each artifact and possess the bimanual coordination, dexterity, and strength to successfully implement them.

Attentional Demands: Upper-Extremity Function in Dual-Task Contexts

In previous chapters on development, we have discussed how the interference that occurs in the performance of both postural and gait tasks when they are performed simultaneously with a cognitive task changes as children mature. This phenomenon has also been documented for the development of reaching tasks and is of relevance since reaching tasks and the manipulation of objects are typically performed at the same time as other cognitive tasks.

One study examined the ability of 570 children from 5 to 17 years of age to perform a tracking task and a cognitive task (the digit sequence recall task), both in single-task and dual-task contexts. It has been shown previously that older children have increased cognitive capacity (associated with front lobe maturation), so it would be expected that they would have reduced dual-task costs in dual-task procedures. Results showed that all participants showed decreased performance in the tracking task in the dual-task condition, and older children performed better in the tracking task than younger children. However, the younger age groups showed a larger dual task cost for tracking and for the digit recall task than the older groups. Figure 18.11 shows the overall results of their study.

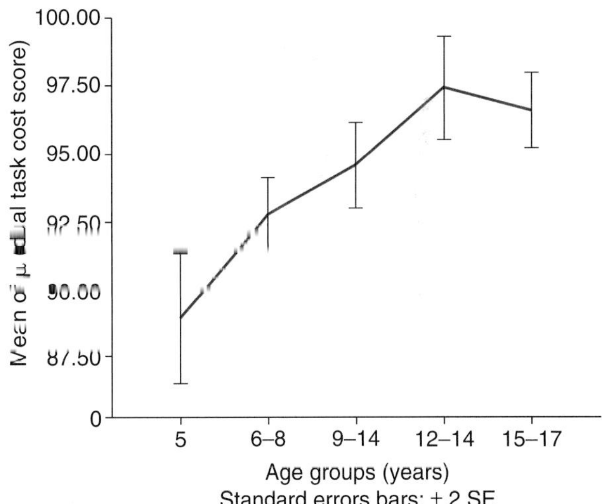

Figure 18.11 Graph showing dual-task costs for children from 5 to 17 years of age when performing a manual tracking and a digit recall task simultaneously. The *y*-axis shows a combined dual-task cost score, μ, created by taking the proportional reduction in performance of each task in the dual- versus single-task condition and combining them (called "dual-task coordination"). This score μ is shown for each of the age groups, with scores near 100 indicating very little dual-task costs. Note that the youngest age groups showed higher dual-task costs, which gradually diminished, with increased age, reaching a plateau at about 15 years of age. (Adapted from Sebastian MV, Hernandez-Gil L. Do 5-year-old children perform dual-task coordination better than AD patients? *J Atten Disord*. 2013, Nov 14. doi: 10.1177/1087054713510738. [Epub ahead of print], Figure 2, P.6, with permission.)

The y-axis shows a combined dual-task cost score, μ, created by taking the proportional reduction in performance of each task in the dual- versus single-task condition and combining them (called "dual-task coordination"). This score μ is shown for each of the age groups, with scores near 100 indicating very little dual-task costs. Note that the youngest age groups showed higher dual-task costs, which gradually diminished, with increased age, reaching a plateau at about 15 years of age. This suggests that dual-task costs for tracking skills are highest in young children and reach adult levels at 15 years of age.

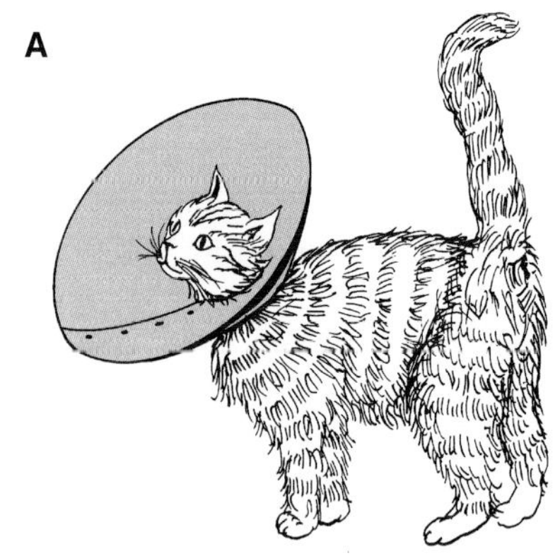

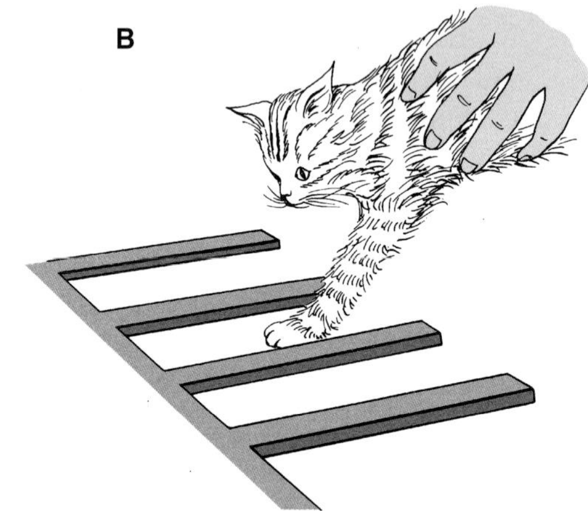

Figure 18.12 (A) Experimental collar worn by kittens to block the view of their paws during early development. **(B)** Pronged apparatus for testing visually guided reaching. (Adapted from Hein A, Held R. Dissociation of the visual placing response into elicited and guided components. *Science.* 1967;158:391, with permission.)

THE ROLE OF EXPERIENCE IN THE DEVELOPMENT OF EYE–HAND COORDINATION

Remember that in humans, reaching behavior has two aspects, a visually triggered portion and a visually guided portion. These two aspects of eye–limb coordination are also found in cats. Elegant studies on the development of these two aspects of eye–limb coordination have shown that movement-produced visual feedback experience is essential for the visually guided portion to develop (Hein & Held, 1967).

In these experiments, kittens were raised in the dark until 4 weeks of age and then allowed to move freely for 6 hours each day in a normal environment. But during this time, they wore lightweight opaque collars that kept them from seeing their limbs and torso. This is shown in Figure 18.12A. For the rest of the day, they remained in the dark. After 12 days of this treatment, the animals were tested for the presence of visually triggered versus visually guided placing reactions. This was accomplished by lowering the kitten toward a continuous surface (requires only visually triggered placing, since accuracy is not required) versus a discontinuous surface, made up of prongs (requires visually guided placing to hit the prong). All animals showed a visually triggered placing reaction, in which they automatically extended the forelimb toward a continuous surface. But they showed no greater than chance hits for a placing reaction to a pronged surface (Fig. 18.12B). However, after removal of the collar, the animals needed only 18 hours in a normal environment to show visually guided placing. It was thus concluded that visually triggered paw extension develops without sight, but visually guided paw placing requires prolonged viewing of the limbs (Hein & Held, 1967).

The researchers then asked: What kind of contact with the environment is important for visually guided behavior? Is passive contact sufficient, or must it be active? To answer this question, they tested 10 pairs of kittens. One kitten of each pair was able to walk freely in a circular room, pulling a gondola, and the other kitten was placed in the gondola and was passively pulled around the room. This is shown in Figure 18.13. Thus, both kittens had similar visual feedback and motion cues, but for the kittens who walked, the cues were active, and for the kittens who rode, they were passive.

The kittens had experience with the apparatus for 3 hours a day. At the end of the experiment, the active animals showed normal visually guided placing reactions and responses to a visual cliff test (in which a normal animal does not walk out over an illusory cliff), but the passive animals did not. Thus, the researchers concluded that self-produced movement is necessary for the development of visually guided behavior. However, once again, after 48 hours in a normal environment, the passive group of animals showed normal visually guided paw placement (Held & Hein, 1963).

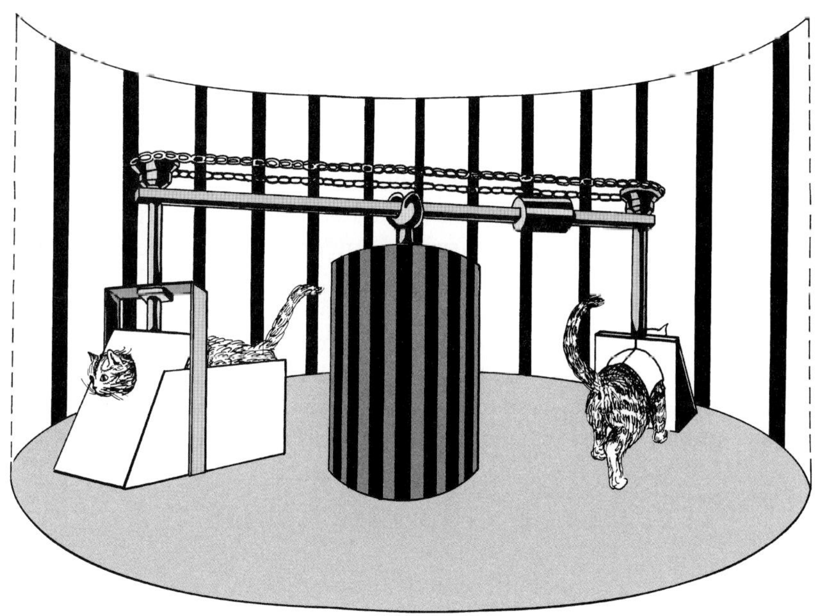

Figure 18.13 Experimental apparatus in which one kitten actively pulls a second kitten, which is passively pulled, in the gondola. (Adapted from Held R, Hein A. Movement-produced stimulation in the development of visually guided behavior. *J Comp Physiol Psychol.* 1963;56:873.)

REACTION TIME REACHING TASKS

A great deal of research has been performed on developmental changes in reaction time (RT) tasks. In general, it has been shown that for simple RT tasks, RTs times become faster as children mature. The greatest changes occur until about 8 to 9 years of age, with slower changes occurring subsequently, until RTs reach adult levels at 16 to 17 years. However, when children are asked to perform more complex movements as part of the RT task, these developmental changes vary according to the task. For example, in a study in which 2- to 8-year-old children were asked to make target-aiming movements, a decrease in RT was observed from 2 to 5 years of age, followed by a stabilization in RT (Brown et al., 1986; Favilla, 2005; Hay, 1990).

Movement time in most RT tasks also changes as a function of age. Remember from Chapter 17 that movement time depends on the accuracy and distance requirements of a task. Strategies for programming movements also vary, depending on whether the movement requires an accurate stop. If an accurate stop is required, the individual must use a braking action controlled by antagonist muscles. Alternatively, if the movement can be stopped automatically by hitting a target, antagonist muscle activation is not required.

Studies analyzing movement time in children from 6 to 10 years of age, for either type of movement, have shown a reduction in movement time with increased age. As might be expected, movements that require an accurate stop are slower at all ages. However, the difference between the speed of the two types of movements is about three times higher at 6 years of age than at 8 to 10 years of age. It has been hypothesized that this could be due to a difficulty experienced by the 6-year-olds in modulating the braking action of the antagonist muscle system (Hay et al., 1986).

In a slightly different cross-sectional study of children 6 to 9 years of age (in addition to a single child tested longitudinally across this period), participants were asked to reach as quickly and accurately as possible to a visual target, thus minimizing visual feedback corrections after the movement began. Results showed that RTs decreased between 6 and 7 years of age. Accuracy decreased temporarily at 7 years of age, followed by an increase at age 8. By age 9, both accuracy and RT reached approximately adult levels. Movement times were similar in all age groups. It is possible that the differences in this study as compared with earlier studies (lack of change in movement time with age and RTs being approximately at adult levels by age 9) relate to the conditions used, involving minimizing visual feedback corrections (Favilla, 2005).

Fitts' Law

Remember from Chapter 17 that Fitts' law shows a specific relationship between the time to make a movement and the amplitude and accuracy of that movement (see Fig. 17.12 for diagram of the task). The difficulty of the task is related both to the accuracy and the amplitude requirements and is represented by the following equation:

$$ID = \frac{\text{Log}_2\, 2D}{W}$$

where *D*, distance of the movement; *W*, width of the target; and *ID*, index of difficulty (Fitts, 1954).

Studies testing the extent to which Fitts' law applies to children have found that movement time decreases with age. This decrease is in general a linear change, except for a regression, which appears to occur at about 7 years of age (recall from our visual control of reaching section that this is a time when visually guided reaching is predominant). Remember also that in the development of postural control, there is a similar regression, as indicated by an increase in postural response latencies, between 4 and 6 years of age. A study examining 5- to 9-year-olds has shown that these developmental decreases and regressions in movement time are not related to any changes in biomechanical factors, such as growth of the bones of the arm (Kerr, 1975; Rey, 1968; Shumway-Cook & Woollacott, 1985a).

Using Fitts' law, one can plot movement time as a function of index of difficulty for different age groups. This relationship is shown in Figure 18.14. The intercept of the line with the *y*-axis reflects the general efficiency of the motor system, while the slope of the line reflects the amount of information that can be processed per second by the motor system. Almost all studies have shown that the *y*-intercept decreases with age, indicating increased efficiency (note, e.g., in Fig. 18.14, the difference in the *y*-intercept in a 5-year-old vs. an 11-year-old). However, age-related improvements in slope appear to depend on the task involved and appear to be more evident in discrete rather than serial movements (Hay, 1990; Sugden, 1980). To examine the effect of age on the ability of children to perform a reciprocal tapping task and how Fitts' law applies to these movements in children, complete Lab Activity 18.2.

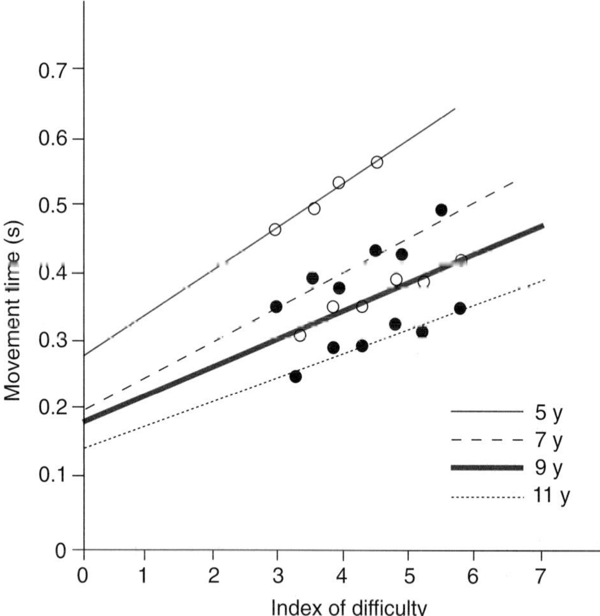

Figure 18.14 Graph showing the relationship between movement time and the index of difficulty of a task, for four age groups of children. The intercept of the line with the *y*-axis reflects the general efficiency of the motor system, while the slope of the line reflects the amount of information that can be processed per second by the motor system. Almost all studies have shown that the *y*-intercept decreases with age, indicating increased efficiency. (Data adapted from Hay L. Developmental changes in eye–hand coordination behaviors: preprogramming versus feedback control. In: Bard C, Fleury M, Hay L, eds. *Development of eye–hand coordination across the lifespan.* Columbia, SC: University of South Carolina Press, 1990:227, with permission.)

In summary, the emergence of reach, grasp, and manipulation occurs gradually during development and is characterized by changes in many systems. With the emergence and refinement of these skills, one sees changes in timing, coordination, and modulation of forces used for reach and grasp. We now turn to examine age-related changes in reach, grasp, and manipulation.

CHANGES IN OLDER ADULTS

As we have noted in our previous chapters on age-related changes in postural control and mobility skills, there are specific changes in these skills with age. These can be divided into (a) time-related changes, such as slowing of onset latencies for postural response or decreased movement speed in locomotion; (b) coordination factors, related to changes in movement or muscle activation patterns; and (c) changes in the use of feedback and feedforward control of both postural and mobility skills. We will find that these same factors are important to consider in examining age-related changes in reaching and grasping skills.

Reaching: Changes with Age

Changes in Reaching Movement Time with Age

A review of studies examining changes in the speed of reaching movements with age has shown that discrete reaching movements show a range of 30% to 90% reduction in velocity with aging, depending on the ages compared and the task performed. For example, one study examining changes in the speed of discrete arm movements showed a 32% reduction between the ages of 50 and 90 years, while another showed a reduction in movement speed of 90% when comparing subjects from 20 to 69 years performing a repetitive tapping task (Welford, 1982; Williams, 1990).

What are some of the age-related changes in different systems of the body that might contribute to this slowing in reaching movements? Different systems that could contribute to the slowing include (a) sensory and perceptual systems, such as the visual system's ability to detect the target, (b) central processing systems, (c) motor systems, and (d) arousal and motivational systems (Welford, 1982). For a review of changes in individual sensory, motor, and cognitive subsystems that could contribute to these changes, see Chapter 9.

Welford performed an experiment to determine whether changes in central mechanisms contribute to

LAB ACTIVITY 18.2

Objective: To examine the effect of age on the ability of children to perform a reciprocal tapping task. Remember, Fitts defined task difficulty in terms of target size (*W*, which is the width of the target) and the distance to move (*D*, which is the distance between targets). He thus quantified task difficulty (which he called "index of difficulty" or simply *ID*) by using the following equation: $ID = \log_2 2D/W$.

Procedure: For this lab, find children from at least two of the following age groups—5, 7, 9, and 11 years—in your community and observe them performing the following task. When you work with each child, bring with you a pencil and six pieces of paper, one for each of the three trials in each task. They should be already marked with appropriate target sizes and distances (see subsequent discussion). Ask the children to tap quickly and accurately between two targets that vary in width and distance. The objective is to make as many *accurate* tapping movements as possible in a 10-sec period. Accuracy is important. Remind the children that there should be no more errors made in the most difficult task than in the easiest tasks. If the number of errors exceeds more than 5% of the pencil dots, the trial should be done again.

Two combinations of task difficulty will be used. The first and easiest task has $D = 2$ cm and $W = 2$ cm. Solving the equation for *ID*, that would be log (base 2) of $(2 \times 2)/2$. This works out to the $\log_2$ of 2, which is 1. The most difficult task has $D = 16$ cm and $W = 1$ cm. That is, the $\log_2$ of $(2 \times 16)/1$, which is 5.

Each child will perform three trials (10 sec each) for the two task conditions. You will time each trial and count and record the number of dots in each target. You should verbally tell the child when to start and stop each 10-sec trial (use a watch with a second hand). The rest interval between trials should be the amount of time needed to count and record the taps.

Assignment

1. Make a table with a record of the number of taps on each of the three trials for both the easy and difficult tasks for each child. Calculate the mean and standard deviation as well. For each task, calculate the average movement time (in milliseconds) for a single movement of the tapping task. Do this by dividing each number of taps by 10, which will give you the number of taps per second during the 10-s trial. Record this value in the table as well. Next, take the inverse of this number (1/*x*, where *x* is the average number of taps). Then, multiply this number by 1,000 to obtain the average movement time in milliseconds. Record this average movement time in the table for each child. What impact did the difficulty of the task have on movement time for children in the different age groups? How did the children's performance change with increasing age? Compare your results with those of others in the class. Did you find a regression (slowing) in movement time for 7-year-olds as compared with the younger and older children?

the slowing in reaching speed in older adults. In these experiments, subjects were asked to keep a pointer (which they could move with a handle) in line with a target that continuously moved from side to side, in an irregular sinusoidal fashion, with the movement varying in both speed and extent. He found that as the speed of the target movement was increased, the subjects could follow it less easily, until at some point it was impossible to follow.

However, there was a difference between the older and younger subjects. As shown in Figure 18.15, the ability to follow the movements dropped off sooner in the older adults than in the young adults. Welford (1977) hypothesized that the limitation in the performance of the older adults was not due to problems with the motor system because they could move faster if they were not following the target. He theorized that the limitation was not sensory because the older adults could easily see the target. Therefore, he concluded that the limitation was in central processing abilities—that is, in the older adults' ability to match the target and pointer and react quickly to changes in target direction. This implies that the time spent in actual movement itself slows little as compared with the time taken to make decisions about the next part of the movement sequence.

Changes in Reaching Coordination with Age

Motion analysis of the trajectories of older adults performing rapid aiming movements has indicated that they spend more time in the target approach, or deceleration, phase than do young adults (Fradet et al., 2008). This is the period of sensory processing that ensures accuracy in reaching the target. A number of studies have explored possible contributing factors to this slowing in the target approach phase. A study by Pohl et al. (1996) compared the movements of young (mean age, 25 years) and older (mean age, 71 years)

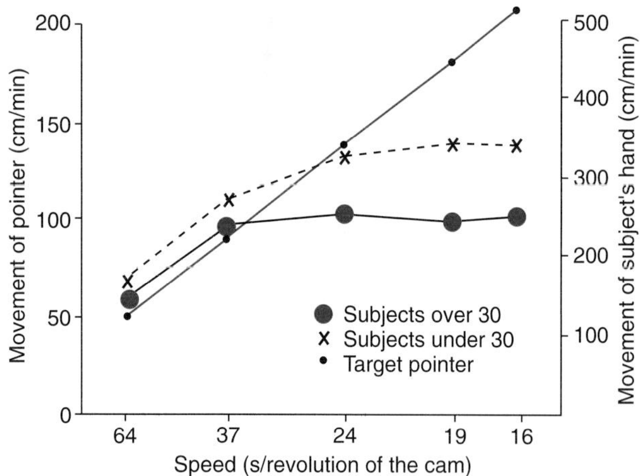

Figure 18.15 The ability of young versus older adults to follow unpredictable target movements of different speeds. Note that older adults have more problems following the target movements at higher speeds. (Adapted from Welford AT. Motor skills and aging. In: Mortimer JA, Pirozzolo FJ, Maletta GJ, eds. *The aging motor system*. New York, NY: Praeger, 1982:159, with permission.)

adults in a reciprocal tapping task with different accuracy requirements (8-cm-wide vs. 2-cm-wide targets, 37 cm apart). They noted that the older adults showed significantly more movement adjustments, coupled with a longer absolute adjustment time and a longer reversal time when moving between the two targets. The authors suggest that the young adults used more online and feedforward processes in achieving the goals of speed and accuracy in movement, while the older adults relied more on slower feedback processes.

Other researchers have suggested that the increased submovements during the deceleration phase of the reach are not necessarily related to corrective adjustments but may also be due to velocity fluctuations caused by the lower movement speed at the end of the reach observed with aging. Young adults also have increased submovements at lower movement speeds; however, the velocity fluctuations in older adults are even greater than those seen in young adults. This may be attributed to a reduction in motor units in older adults, which results in a reduced ability to generate smooth muscle forces, especially at low force levels (Fradet et al., 2008).

Additional studies of movement kinematics in young versus older adults used a task that required drawing a line to 5-, 10-, and 20-mm targets (a digitizing tablet was used) and compared subjects at similar movement speeds (Morgan et al., 1994). Older adults showed comparable overall accuracy on the tasks but again showed more hesitancy and submovements, implying possible increased reliance on visual guidance. The authors concluded that this indicates a central deficit in motor coordination. Other research has examined changes in force production during reaching movements in older adults and shown similar discontinuities in their movement trajectories (Vrtunski & Patterson, 1985). It is interesting to remember that increased submovements were characteristic of early reaching patterns in normal infants (von Hofsten, 1993). Like older adults, these submovements in infants are often associated with higher reliance on visual feedback during reaching (Hay, 1979).

It has also been shown that hand steadiness decreases with age during reaching tasks (Williams, 1990). When older adults were asked to insert a small stylus in slots of different diameters (1/2–1/8 inch), steadiness dropped by 77%, from 50 to 90 years of age. Steadiness deteriorated faster in the nonpreferred hand than in the preferred hand.

Based on the literature, there appears to be little change in performance speed for reaching movements with age, if subjects are asked to repeat the same simple action, like tapping a pencil between two targets or performing a simple RT task (Welford, 1977, 1982). In this case, the slowing may be as little as 16%. But if the complexity of the task is increased, by making the target smaller, using successive targets, or using a choice RT task, then slowing can range from 86% to 276%. To observe changes in reciprocal movement patterns found in old adults under a variety of conditions and how Fitts' law applies to their movement patterns, perform Lab Activity 18.3.

Table 18.2 gives examples of differences in the slowing of the performance of reaching movements in older adults with the complexity of the task. The largest slowing in performance was in tasks involving symbolic translations (using a code to relate a stimulus to a response) or spatial transpositions (e.g., a light cue

LAB ACTIVITY 18.3

Objective: To examine the effect of aging on the ability to perform a reciprocal tapping task.

Procedure: Repeat the procedure from Lab Activity 18.2, but with an older adult (70 years or older) from your community.

Assignment

1. Repeat the assignment from Lab Activity 18.2, with the following changes in questions. What impact did the difficulty of the task have on movement time for the older adult, as compared with your own or other young adult times, from Lab Activity 18.2?
2. Did you notice any additional movement or hesitancy in making the movements? Do you think that the fitness level of the older adult would affect performance on the task?

TABLE 18.2 Age-Related Slowing in the Performance of Reaching Movements as a Function of Task Complexity

Task	Age groups compared	Percentage increase[a]
Simple key press or release to light or sound	20s with 60s	
Average of 11 studies listed by Welford		16
Ten-choice (Birren et al., 1962)	18–33 with 65–72	
a. Straightforward relationship		27
b. With numerical code, mean of five studies	25–34 with 65–72	50
c. With verbal code, mean of two studies		45
d. With color code		94
e. With part color and part letter code		86
Ten-choice (Kay, 1954, 1955)		
a. Signal lights immediately above response keys		−13 (no error made)
b. Signal lights 3 ft from keys		26 (−43)
c. As b, but signal lights arranged so that leftmost responded to with		46 (−19)
rightmost key, and so forth		56 (+138)
d. With numerical code		299 (+464)
e. The difficulties of d and b combined		

[a]Adapted from Welford AT. Motor skills and aging. In: Mortimer JA, Pirozzolo FJ, Maletta GJ, eds. *The aging motor system.* New York, NY: Praeger, 1982:163.

on the left requiring a reach to the right). Although decrements have been found in performance on many RT tasks, one study has also shown that when older adults are not instructed to worry about accuracy on such a task, they demonstrate no decrease in reaching speed (Williamson et al., 1993).

The primary source of the slowing in complex RT tasks is in the first phase of performance, the time to observe the signals and relate them to action, rather than in the second phase, the time to execute the movement (Welford, 1977, 1982). When performing more continuous tasks, the second phase, that of movement execution, can overlap to some extent with the first. For example, a person may process the information relating to the next signal while making the first response. This type of task appears to be more difficult for older adults, possibly because they need more time to monitor their responses, and thus have difficulty processing other signals simultaneously (Welford, 1982).

For example, older adults (63–76 years) were compared with younger adults (19–29 years) on a task in which they moved as quickly as possible to one of two end points, with one farther away than the other, in the same direction (Rabbitt & Rogers, 1965). The younger subjects could overlap the time required to choose the end point with the initial stages of the movement itself, while the older subjects were less able to do this. Although there is no evidence that the time taken for monitoring increases with age, older adults seem less able to suppress monitoring.

What reasons might there be for this lack of suppression? It has been hypothesized that suppression of monitoring occurs when the outcome of a task is certain; thus, if there is a possibility of error, monitoring will be more probable. In addition, suppression of monitoring may be possible when movement sub units are coordinated into higher units of performance (Welford, 1982). However, to do this often requires that the subject hold the movement subunits together in working memory while performing the task.

A study tested this ability in older (60–81 years) versus young (17–28 years) adults. Subjects were asked to perform two serial key pressing tasks, one that had few subunits (12, 12, 12, etc.) and one that was more complex (1234, 32, 1234, etc.). The investigators found that the older adults were slower than the young adults, particularly with the second series (Rabbitt & Birren, 1967).

Grasping: Changes with Age

One of the problems faced by older adults is a decrease in manual dexterity. Researchers have shown that older people have decreased coordination of individual digit forces and difficulties producing high and accurate forces with their fingers compared to young adults (Shim et al., 2004). These impairments become apparent in tasks such as tying shoelaces and fastening buttons. For example, the time required to manipulate a small object increases 25% to 40% by 70 years of age. These age-related changes have been explored by measuring the fingertip forces used to grip and lift objects, in experiments similar to those performed with young children, described earlier. Figure 18.16 shows the experimental apparatus often used to measure grip forces in older adults. It is known that tactile sensation is reduced in older adults, and this may affect their ability to detect how strongly they are holding an object (Agnew et al., 1982; Cole, 1991; Keogh et al., 2006).

Studies by Cole and colleagues have shown that older adults (mean age, 81 years) used grasp forces that were, on average, twice as large as those of young adults, with some older adults producing forces that were many times larger than the young adult mean. Figure 18.17 shows examples of grasp force records for a young versus an older adult for the third trial picking up a nonslippery object (covered with sandpaper) and the first and third trials picking up a slippery object (covered with rayon). Note that the older subject shows much larger grasp forces and takes longer to adapt to the final grasp force for the rayon object than the young adult. A portion of the increased force was due to increased skin slipperiness. In addition, the older adults simply produced a higher margin of safety against object slippage. Variability of grip forces was also much higher across trials, and the direction of fingertip forces was not aligned with vertical in the older as compared with the young adults. It is hypothesized that this may contribute to clumsiness in older adults during fine manipulation (Cole, 1991, 2006; Cole et al., 1999).

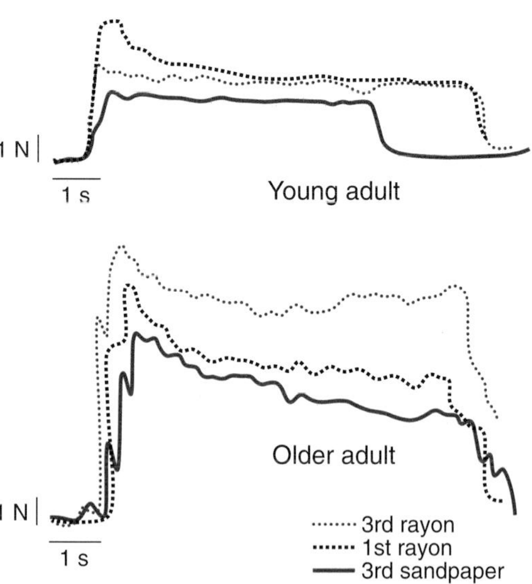

Figure 18.17 Grasp force traces from a young subject and an older adult showing typical grasp force patterns when lifting an object with a nonslippery (sandpaper) versus a slippery (rayon) surface. Traces represent the third lift with sandpaper followed by the first and third rayon trials. N, Newtons. (Reprinted from Cole KJ. Grasp force control in older adults. *J Motor Behav.* 1991;23:255, with permission.)

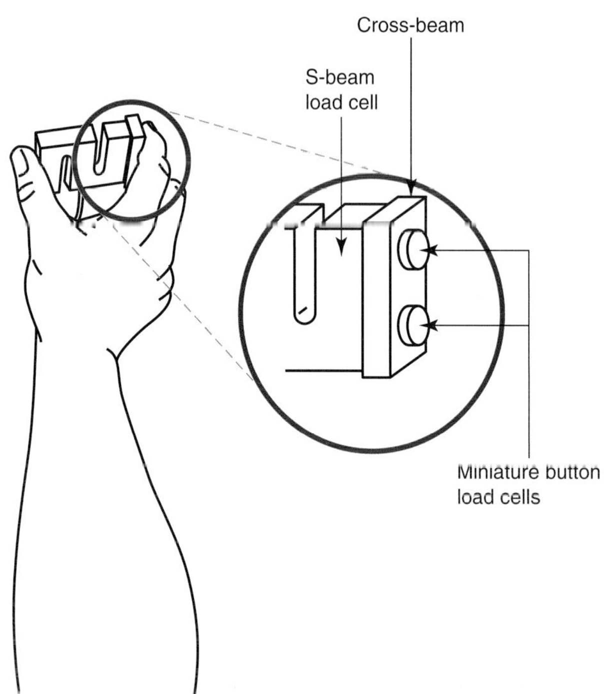

Figure 18.16 Experimental apparatus used for the recording of digit forces during finger pinch tasks. The magnified area shows the positions of the load cells for measuring finger forces. (Reprinted from Keogh J, Morrison S, Barrett R. Age related differences in inter-digit coupling during finger pinching. *Eur J Appl Physol.* 2006;97:79, with permission.)

Sensory and Motor Contributions to Impaired Grasp

What are the relative contributions of sensory and motor systems to impaired grasp in older adults? Experiments have examined whether this increased safety margin is due to decreased tactile sensation or decreased ability to encode skin–object frictional properties (Cole & Rotella, 2001; Cole et al., 1998, 1999). Results suggest that declining cutaneous afferent function contributes to safety margin increases after about 60 years of age. Researchers noted that grip force adjustments to new surfaces were delayed about 100 msec in older adults as compared with young adults. They also found that when a grasped handle was pulled unexpectedly, older adults (mean age, 78 years) showed a twofold increase in the force required to evoke a response, showed delays in response onsets, and showed significantly larger resulting fingertip forces than young adults. Previous research has shown that friction is signaled locally by fast-adapting afferents, which decrease in number with age; thus, this could account for the delays in force adjustments.

In a separate set of experiments, Cole et al. (1998) hypothesized that if age-related tactile changes were the cause of decreased manual dexterity, then performing a grip-and-lift task in the dark would cause a disproportionate increase in the duration of the grip-and-lift task in older as compared with younger adults. Their results showed that the grip–lift duration in the no-vision condition was equally increased for the young (mean age, 45 years) and older (mean age, 74 years) adult groups, with ratios of 2.1 and 2.3 for the duration in the vision and no-vision conditions for the respective groups. The authors conclude that these results fail to support the hypothesis that age-related declines in dexterity were due predominantly to changes in availability of tactile information.

In additional experiments, Kinoshita and Francis (1996) attempted to determine whether there are age-related changes in the control of precision grip force during the lifting and holding of objects with different surface textures (slippery [silk] and nonslippery [sandpaper]). They compared the performance of two groups of active older adults (69–79 years and 80–93 years) and a group of young adults (18–32 years) in a grasp-and-lift task. They found that the older adults (especially the 81-to-93-year-old group) had increased fluctuations in the grip force rate curve and longer force application time than the younger subjects during lifting. They also noted that prior experience with one surface had less effect on the performance with the next surface in the older adults. The authors conclude that this indicates a decrease in the capacity to program force production with aging. As noted previously, they found that the fingers of the older subjects were more slippery, and they used a larger grip force safety margin than younger adults. The overall results demonstrated that the capacity for precision grip force control declines with advancing age.

The age-associated decrease in force control during lifting is believed to be related to decreased motor unit control. For example, older adults show increases in average motor unit force, motor unit force variability, and modulation of motor unit firing rate. In addition, older adults show a reduced coupling between the force output of the fingers of the hand when grasping (Keogh et al., 2006).

One possible reason that older adults have difficulty lifting objects efficiently is that aging impairs the ability to learn the visual–motor associations needed to set appropriate fingertip forces for handling familiar objects. Cole and Rotella (2002) tested the ability of young (mean age, 22 years) versus older (mean age, 77 years) adults to use visual color cues about the texture (sandpaper vs. acetate) or weight (200 g vs. 400 g) of an object to control fingertip forces during a grasp-and-lift task. Objects to be lifted were color coded according to the weight or slipperiness in the "visual cue" condition, and these properties changed unpredictably across trials in the "no visual cue" condition. When object texture was visually cued, grip forces of young adults were 24% smaller; however, grip forces for older adults did not vary in response to the visual cues, although they accurately reported the surface colors prior to lifts. Similar results were found for prior cueing concerning object weights to be lifted (older adults did not use cueing information), although old and young adults each used approximately a 2-N grip force when lifting the 200-g object.

The researchers concluded that the older adults' inability to adjust grip force to object properties when the color cue was present was not due to a general inability or unwillingness to use a low grip force when handling objects but that aging affects the associative learning linking visual identification of objects with fingertip forces required to efficiently lift the object. In contrast to these results, the grip force of older and young adults was affected by the prior lifting, suggesting that more than one internal representation contributes to predictive control of forces during grasp-and-lift tasks (Cole & Rotella, 2002).

Reach–Grasp Adaptation: Changes with Age

Do older adults have more difficulty adapting to unexpected changes in object size? In order to answer this question, Bennett and Castiello (1995) compared the movement trajectories of older (60–70 years) and younger (20–26 years) adults in response to a perturbation of object size during a reach-to-grasp movement. In most trials (80 of 100), participants reached for and grasped an illuminated cylinder of small (0.7 cm) or large (8.0 cm) diameter. In 20 trials, a visual perturbation (switching from one to the other cylinder) occurred at the onset of the reach, requiring a switch from precision to power grip or vice versa.

Although the older group successfully adapted to these changes, they used a more conservative strategy, involving a longer approach time to the object and the use of the standard coordination pattern between transport and manipulation components. Younger adults, instead, used a new pattern, with a decrease of temporal coordination between the components. The authors suggest that the more rigid movement pattern of older adults with regard to the unexpected changes in grip requirements could contribute to a higher incidence of accidents during manipulation tasks. To examine how properties of a task affect reach-and-grasp movements in older adults, perform Lab Activity 18.4.

Compensation and Reversibility of Decrements in Reaching Performance

Although decrements in reaching performance may be found in older adults under experimental conditions, they are often not observed in the workplace or in activities of daily living. It has been suggested that performance is preserved because many

LAB ACTIVITY 18.4

Objective: To examine how properties of a task affect reach-and-grasp movements in older adults.

Procedures: For this lab, you will repeat Lab Activity 18.1, but now, you will find an older adult (70 years or older) in your community and observe him or her performing the same tasks as described in Lab Activity 18.1.

Assignment

1. Describe how the older adult reached for and grasped the various objects.
2. When during the reach for an object, did the hand begin to shape in preparation for grasp? How did characteristics of the object affect anticipatory hand shaping?
3. Compare the data from the older adult to young adult reach-and-grasp characteristics from Lab Activity 18.1. Do your results agree with those of Cole's (1991) regarding ability to change lift forces easily with changing object surface characteristics?

compensatory strategies are used to improve reach-and-grasp skills. Many of these compensatory strategies used by older adults appear to be unconscious, automatic processes. For example, older adults may increase the effort they put into the movement. In the workplace, they may work more continuously with fewer brief pauses. They may also prepare for movements that require speed and accuracy in advance, thus allowing anticipatory processes to aid in performance. In many tasks, they may also make a trade-off between speed and accuracy. Finally, it has also been shown that older adults set higher criteria for responding to RT signals in sensory discrimination tasks (Welford, 1982).

Can the changes in reaching skills that occur with aging be counteracted by practice or training? Yes. This can occur with training at both the impairment level (muscle strength training) and at the functional level (eye–hand coordination skill training). Keogh et al. (2007) compared the performance of a group of older adults (70–80 years) who underwent upper limb strength training (2 times per week for 6 weeks) with that of a control group of older adults (70–80 years) on finger pinch force control. They found that the strength training group showed significantly greater reductions in force variability and target error as well as greater increases in finger pinch force than did the control group. This suggests the importance of upper limb strength to high-level performance on precision grip tasks.

In addition, clear improvement with practice has been reported for eye–hand coordination skills in older adults (Falduto & Baron, 1986). The greatest improvement is seen in more complex tasks. Interestingly, older adults show more improvement with practice than do younger adults on performance of RT tasks (Jordan & Rabbitt, 1977). This may occur because young adults are closer to their ceiling of performance when starting to learn the task. However, practice does not eliminate the age differences in the performance of these tasks.

Practice also improves performance in older adults with regard to the perceptual processes involved in eye–hand coordination tasks, such as visual acuity, signal detection, and auditory discrimination. In addition, the effects of practice remain high, even 1 month after practice on eye–hand coordination tasks had ended. One study compared the performance of young (19–27 years) and older (62–73 years) adults on a task that involved fine movements of the hands, signal detection, memory scanning, visual discrimination, and anticipation timing, called "space trek." Subjects were given 1-hour practice sessions, 51 over a period of 2 to 5 months. One month after training ended, there was only a small decrease in performance levels (Welford, 1982).

In another study, older adults (57–83 years) were given practice in eye–hand coordination skills by playing video games. These games involved making fast decisions about changes in the speed and direction of hand movements. Over a 7-week period, scores tripled on the task. In addition, practice on the video games transferred over to other RT tasks that required subjects to select a motor response quickly (Clark et al., 1987).

Improving Cognitive Impairments with Aging and Manipulation: Dual-Task Costs

Many older adults have additional slowing or error production as compared with young adults when asked to perform two tasks simultaneously because attentional resources must be shared between the two tasks. Can motor practice improve this decrease in performance under dual-task conditions? To answer this question, researchers asked young and older adults to perform a precision grip sine wave force tracking and a working memory task simultaneously before and after 100 motor training trials. Results showed that motor practice improved force tracking in both groups. Younger adults showed higher performance at both pretraining and posttraining than older adults, but older adults reached the younger adult pretraining performance levels after extended practice. Interestingly, this training did not prevent the decline in motor performance in the older adult group when going from the single- to the dual-task condition. After training, however, the cognitive task performance was improved in older adults (Voelcker-Rehage & Alberts, 2005, 2007).

Most of these studies suggest that older adults learn as much as if not more than young adults with practice and that they retain the learned skills as well as young adults do. However, it appears that motor training does not eliminate the decrements in dual-task performance seen in older as compared with younger adults. In addition, the way subjects improved with practice was similar for the young and older adults; however, the older adults simply learned more slowly. This slower rate of learning of eye–hand coordination skills in older subjects may be due to material taking longer to register in long-term memory (Welford, 1982).

What does this mean in terms of determining the best strategies for teaching eye–hand coordination skills to older adults? Since the time required for registering information in long-term memory lengthens with age, learning needs to be unhurried. Otherwise, extra information to be processed during the time required to register information in longer-term memory will simply disrupt the memory process.

In teaching eye–hand coordination skills, there are sometimes problems in translating verbal instruction into motor performance. To avoid this, one can use demonstrations. However, in this case, the pace of the demonstration should be under the learner's control. Thus, using slow-motion, self-paced videos in training may help (Welford, 1982).

Active decision making is also an important factor in learning at any age. In a maze study with adults, it was shown that learning took place much faster if the correct pathway was marked, but the subject had to make an active choice. This helped subjects of all ages, but it especially helped older adults (Wright, 1957).

It was also shown that using a mixture of mental practice and physical practice when learning a pursuit rotor task was as good as physical practice alone for 65- to 69- and 80- to 100-year-olds (Surberg, 1976).

Thus, learning of eye–hand coordination tasks by older adults can be facilitated by using a type of discovery learning, which involves demonstrations that can be self-paced, active learning, and a combination of physical and mental practice (Welford, 1982).

During development, the emergence of mature reach-and-grasp behavior is characterized by a reduction in RT, a decrease in safety margins during grip and lift, and a reduction in the number of subunits during the reaching movement, resulting in a smoother trajectory. Similarly, a decline in reach and grasp with aging is characterized by an increase in RT, an increase in safety margins, and an increase in the number of subunits contributing to a reaching movement. Multiple factors may be contributing to these characteristic changes across the life span. These include both primary deficits in the nervous and musculoskeletal systems and secondary strategies used to compensate for these deficits.

A CASE STUDY APPROACH TO UNDERSTANDING AGE-RELATED CHANGES IN REACH, GRASP, AND MANIPULATION

Bonnie B is a 90-year-old woman with impaired balance and gait resulting in multiple falls. Like many older adults, Bonnie has impaired upper limb function resulting from age-related changes in reach, grasp, and manipulation. With respect to her participation, Bonnie is limited in her activities of daily living and has a home health aide 3 days per week to help with shopping, cooking, cleaning, and laundry. Bonnie cannot stand and walk without the use of a walker, limiting her ability to carry objects; thus, she requires assistance when shopping as well.

Bonnie's functional movements are slowed, and she has reduced end point accuracy when reaching for targets or picking up small objects. Reach-and-grasp problems are often worse when Bonnie is performing multiple tasks simultaneously. Researchers have found that age-related changes in reach, grasp, and manipulation include time-related changes, such as slowed reaction and movement times, coordination factors related to changes in multijoint movements and muscle activation patterns, and changes in the use of feedback and feedforward control. In addition, older adults like Bonnie demonstrate velocity fluctuations resulting from a reduction in motor units that affect the ability to generate and coordinate muscle forces, particularly those used in precision grip. Among older adults, reduced ability to allocate attention appropriately can reduce upper limb function under dual-task conditions. Researchers have found that many older adults like Bonnie have a reduced ability to adapt reach-and-grasp forces to unexpected changes in task and environmental demands, which contributes to a higher incidence of accidents during manipulation tasks (Bennett & Castiello, 1995).

Bonnie demonstrates age-related decreases in manual dexterity affecting her ability to perform tasks such as writing, tying shoelaces, and fastening buttons. Her movements are slow, and accuracy is reduced, increasing the time required to perform common daily tasks.

Like many older adults, Bonnie has age-related changes in motor, sensory, and cognitive systems; thus, many impairments contribute to her functional limitations and restricted participation. Motor impairments include reduced range of motion and strength in her upper extremities. She has reduced multijoint coordination affecting the coordination of reach and grasp.

Bonnie has deficits in multiple sensory systems. She has age-related changes to vision, including reduced contrast sensitivity, problems with depth perception, and reduced visual acuity. She also has somatosensory changes including reduced vibratory sense, proprioception, and light touch sensation. Reduced somatosensation in her hands contributes to a reduced ability to regulate fingertip forces during grip-and-lift tasks. Bonnie also has reduced vestibular function associated with a history of Ménière disease. Finally, Bonnie has some cognitive deficits, including problems with short-term memory and mildly impaired executive function, which contribute to impaired upper limb functions.

Bonnie's impaired balance plays a significant role in her reduced upper limb function. In addition to reduced steady-state postural control in standing, Bonnie has significantly impaired anticipatory postural control, which makes it difficult for her to maintain stability during the performance of many upper limb tasks, such as reaching, lifting, and leaning over to pick up objects from the floor. In addition, impairments in reactive balance control limit her ability to recover stability and avoid a fall when she performs these tasks.

Practice would most likely improve Bonnie's upper limb function. Researchers have found that practice can reduce, though not eliminate, many age-related changes in reach-and-grasp skills (Clark et al., 1987; Falduto & Baron, 1986; Keogh et al., 2007; Voelcker-Rehage & Alberts, 2007).

SUMMARY

1. Infants as young as a week old show prereaching behaviors, in which they reach toward objects that are in front of them. These reaches are not accurate, and the infants do not grasp the object, as an extension synergy controls the arm and hand movements. When the arm is extended, the hand is open. But the reaches are clearly aimed at the object, since they are significantly more accurate than arm movements in which the eyes are not fixated on the object.
2. At about 2 months, the extension synergy is broken up so that the fingers flex as the arm extends. At this time, head–arm movements become coupled as the infant gains control over the neck muscles.
3. At about 4 months, infants begin to gain trunk stability, along with a progressive uncoupling of head–arm–hand synergies. These changes allow the emergence of functional reach-and-grasp behavior.
4. The progressive development of trunk stability is an essential factor contributing to both success and accuracy in infant reaching.
5. From 4 months onward, reaching becomes more refined, with the approach path straightening and the number of segments of the reach being reduced.
6. Visually triggered reaching is dominant in the newborn, changing to visually guided reaching at about 5 months of age and returning to visually triggered reaching by 1 year of age, although guided reaching is still available.
7. The development of hand orientation begins to occur at the onset of successful reaching, at about 5 months of age.
8. The pincer grasp develops at about 9 to 10 months of age, along with the development of the pyramidal tract.
9. Reaction time shows a progressive reduction with age, with sharper changes occurring up to 8 to 9 years, followed by slower changes up to 16 to 17 years.
10. Children from 4 to 6 years of age make predominantly visually triggered (feedforward) movements, using little visual feedback. At 7 to 8 years, visual feedback is dominant, leading to poor reaching in the dark but more accurate reaching with vision present. By 9 to 11 years, there is an integration between feedforward and feedback movements.
11. Children gradually improve their ability to perform manipulation tasks effectively within dual-task contexts between the ages of 5 and 15 years.
12. Older adults show a slowing in reaching movements, with much of this due to central processing slowing. The slowing in performance on reaching movements is greater for more complex tasks.
13. Part of the slowing may result from an inability to suppress monitoring of movements, due to either uncertainty concerning the accuracy of the movement or an inability to integrate movement subunits into larger chunks in working memory.
14. Older adults are less efficient than young adults when performing grip-and-lift tasks, using higher grip forces (a larger safety margin), and showing more variability in grip-and-lift forces and a longer time to attain the final grip force.
15. Most age-related decrements in reaching performance can be improved with training. Training effects remain high for at least a month after training has ended and also transfer to other reaching tasks.

ANSWERS TO LAB ACTIVITY ASSIGNMENTS

Lab Activity 18.1

1. Hand closes in anticipation of reaching object.
2. Hand shaping and orientation:

8 to 12 months: Child may use palmer grasp for everything if about 8 months but will shift to pincer grasp at about 9 to 10 months for block (if small enough) and crayon. Opening of hand is related to size of object from 9 months of age. Cannot adapt to sudden changes in friction of object (slippery glass).

12 to 18 months: Use pincer grasp for block and crayon and palmer grasp for glass. Opening of hand is related to size of object. They initiate the grasp farther from the target than 8- to 12-month-olds. Cannot adapt to change in friction of object.

2 to 3 years: Like 12- to 18-month-olds, with the addition that arm movements are smoother than in the younger age groups. Can adapt to unexpected changes in friction when given in blocks of trials but not when suddenly changed (slippery glass).

4 to 6 years: Use pincer grasp, smooth arm movement, adapt to changes in friction (slippery glass) with just a few practice trials. May be able to orient hand to glass when upside down, to make single smooth movement.

3. To be determined by student's observed data.
4. To be determined by student's observed data.

Lab Activity 18.2

1. With increased age, there will be a decrease in movement time for the tasks. Increased difficulty of the task should increase movement time more in the younger children than in the older children. There may be a slight slowing in movement in the 7-year-olds as compared with the other children.

Lab Activity 18.3

1. Depending on the age and health of the older adult, you may find that increasing the difficulty of the task increases movement time more than for a young adult.
2. Again, you may find that a very old adult or one who has low fitness levels will have lower performance levels than a fit older adult or a young adult.

Lab Activity 18.4

1. Healthy older adults would be expected to grasp objects like young adults. The very old or unfit older adults would possibly show slowing and hesitation in reaching, causing increased movement units in the reach and decreased smoothness of the trajectory.
2. To be determined by student's observed data.
3. Most healthy and fit older adults would show results similar to young adults.
4. To be determined by student's observed data.

CHAPTER 19

Abnormal Reach, Grasp, and Manipulation

Learning Objectives

Following completion of this chapter, the reader will be able to:

1. Describe problems with reach, grasp, and manipulation within the ICF framework.
2. Discuss the effect of central nervous system (CNS) pathology on reach and grasp.
3. Discuss the role of sensory deficits on reach and grasp.
4. Compare and contrast deficits in reach and grasp in persons with poststroke hemiparesis, Parkinson's disease, cerebellar pathology, multiple sclerosis, and cerebral palsy.

INTRODUCTION

Normal upper-extremity function, including the ability to reach for, grasp, and manipulate objects, is the basis for fine-motor skills important to activities such as feeding, dressing, grooming, and handwriting. Limitations in upper-extremity function significantly impact independence in daily life activities and contribute to increased health and other related costs. For example, impaired upper-extremity function may be associated with increased costs for health care providers, long-term care expenditures as well as home and car modifications. More specifically, in persons with multiple sclerosis (MS), upper-extremity function is the best predictor of disease related expenses (Koch et al., 2014).

In addition to fine-motor skills, upper-extremity function plays an important role in gross motor skills such as crawling, walking, the ability to recover balance, and the ability to protect the body from injury when postural recovery is not possible. Because upper-extremity control is intertwined with both fine and gross motor skills, development and recovery of upper-extremity function are important aspects of training and retraining the patient with impaired motor control and fall within the purview of most areas of rehabilitation, including both occupational and physical therapy.

The importance of upper limb function in balance recovery was discussed in the postural control chapters of this book. The current chapter focuses on understanding problems related to reach, grasp, and manipulation in persons with neurologic pathology. In Chapter 17, we examined normal upper-extremity function within the context of the International Classification of Functioning, Disability, and Health (ICF) framework. In this chapter, we also use the ICF framework to understand impaired reach, grasp, and manipulation resulting from central nervous system (CNS) pathology. Restrictions in upper-extremity function, specifically the ability to carry, move, and handle objects, are considered limitations or restrictions in the *Activities and Participation* component of the ICF. However, problems in the key elements of upper-extremity control, such as eye–hand coordination and visually directed arm and hand movements, are considered impairments in body function, thus classified in the *Body Structure and Function* component.

In this chapter, we first review problems related to the key components of upper-extremity control, incorporating a discussion of sensory, motor, and cognitive problems that affect the key components, including (a) locating a target, involving the coordinated movement of the eyes, head, and trunk; (b) reaching, involving transportation of the arm and hand in space as well as postural support; (c) grasp, including grip formation, grasp, and release; and (d) in-hand manipulation skills. We then use a case study approach to explore the types of upper-extremity problems found in patients with specific types of neurologic diagnoses.

TARGET LOCATION PROBLEMS

A critical aspect of manipulatory function is the ability to locate a target and maintain gaze on that target preceding a reach. Depending on the task, target localization requires some combination of eye, head, and trunk motion, depending on how far from midline the target is located. Thus, neural pathology affecting the ability to coordinate eye, head, trunk, and hand movements can affect the ability to locate targets or objects in space. In addition, gaze stabilization problems can result from (a) oculomotor system pathology disrupting visually driven eye movements; (b) damage to the vestibular system, which disrupts vestibuloocular reflex control of eye movements in response to head movements; and (c) inability to adapt the vestibuloocular reflex to changes in task demands because of cerebellar damage (Martin et al., 1993). All of these types of problems affect the patient's ability to stabilize gaze on an object when moving the head. However, in this chapter, we focus primarily on problems related to visually driven eye movements that affect the ability to locate targets or objects to be reached. In addition, we review research on problems affecting the ability to coordinate and integrate eye movements with head and hand movements for tasks such as pointing to a target or reaching for an object.

Visual Deficits and Object Localization

CNS lesions affecting the processing of visual signals will impair the ability to locate a target or object in space. Visual field deficits following a stroke, such as homonymous hemianopsia, restrict a person's ability to visually locate objects in half the visual field, affecting reach and grasp in the contralesional hemifield (Jeannerod, 1990). More than 50% of children with spastic hemiplegic cerebral palsy (CP) have homonymous hemianopsia and many compensate with atypical head postures in order to improve visual acuity and binocular vision (Porro et al., 2005; Prayson & Hanahoe, 2004).

Can localization of a target in the affected hemifield improve with practice? The answer may be yes. Individuals with hemianopsia (due to hemispherectomy) were asked to point to a target when it appeared in either the normal visual field or the affected field. Because participants said they could not see an object when it was in the affected field, they were asked to "guess" where it was. Although participants were initially very poor at reaching for objects in this manner, with practice, they showed a clear and rapid improvement in their abilities, suggesting that in this population, target localization improved with practice (Zihl & Werth, 1984).

Visual neglect and visual extinction, now often referred to as hemi-inattention, are often the consequence of damage to the right cerebral hemisphere. Individuals with visual neglect show a profound lack of awareness of the contralesional side of personal and external space. In the case of visual extinction, patients can detect a stimulus presented in either hemifield, but will report only the ipsilesional stimulus when two visual stimuli are simultaneously and bilaterally presented in both visual fields, or even within the same visual hemifield (Rapcsak et al., 1987; Rorden et al., 2009). Research studies have shown that the level of visual extinction is more related to the spatial location of the stimuli than to any potential temporal mismatch during the presentation of the visual stimuli (Rorden et al., 2009). However, it is unclear whether visual neglect and extinction are related to sensory, attentional, or other factors. Current emphasis on labeling these deficits as hemi-inattention suggests a focus on attentional processes as a primary contributor to neglect, which may not be the case in all patients with the problem.

In both visual neglect and visual extinction, the relative location of the target appears to influence the patient's ability to detect an object or a target in space. Smania et al. (1998) examined the spatial distribution of visual attention in subjects with right hemispheric damage and either hemineglect or extinction. Subjects were required to press the space bar of a computer keyboard after the appearance of a light flash in one of four positions (10, 20, 30, or 40 degrees along the horizontal meridian) presented in either the left or right visual field. Both the neglect and the extinction groups were less able to detect targets presented in their left hemifield. In addition, impairments in detecting targets increased with target eccentricity. This study reminds us that patients with right hemisphere damage who also have left unilateral neglect will have difficulty reaching for objects presented on the left side of the body because of difficulty in locating objects presented in the left visual field. In addition, the more eccentric the target, the more difficulty the patient will have in reaching.

Individuals with parietal lesions also show problems with eye movements when these movements are a part of exploratory visual searches or reaching behaviors. They may have problems breaking visual fixation (Balint's syndrome) or in optic ataxia; they also may have slowed reaction times for saccades, with the saccades subdivided into staircase patterns (Balint, 1909; Waters et al., 1978). Patients with Balint's syndrome also show oculomotor apraxia (i.e., inability to shift gaze but without lesion of extraocular muscles) and simultagnosia, defined as an inability to perceive more than one object, or all the details and items of a complex visual image at a time (Parvathaneni & Das, 2020). Visual deficits also impact the planning and execution of reach and grasp. Experiments with healthy young adults, in which the field of view was reduced to 11 degrees, showed that reducing peripheral vision affected the planning and execution of both reach and grasp (González-Alvarez et al., 2007). In persons with reduced binocular vision, the reach phase of movement was significantly slower as compared with individuals with intact vision, particularly during the end phase of reaching, which was characterized by a prolonged final approach, more velocity corrections, and poorer coordination during object contact. In addition, during the grasp phase, reduced visual information resulted in increased reliance on somatosensory inputs, with a subsequent increase in the number of grip adjustments after contact had been made with the object to be grasped (Melmoth et al., 2009).

Finally, problems in the visual system can affect perceptual aspects of object identification and localization. In Chapter 17, we discussed the two visual pathways involved in reach and grasp, including the dorsal stream pathway going from the visual to the parietal cortex, which provides critical information for all phases of a reach, and the ventral stream pathway, going from visual cortex to the temporal lobe, which provides conscious visual perceptions (Goodale & Milner, 1992; Goodale et al., 1991). Thus, a person with ventral stream lesions will have no conscious perception of the orientation or dimension of objects but will show great skill in picking them up, while the opposite may be true for a person with a dorsal stream lesion.

PROBLEMS WITH EYE–HEAD–HAND COORDINATION

Remember from Chapters 17 and 18 that some target location tasks require eye movements alone, while others require a combination of eye and head movement, and still others require a combination of eye, head, and trunk movements, depending on the eccentricity of the target in space. This has led researchers to suggest that eye–head coordination is not controlled by a single mechanism but, rather, emerges from an interaction of several different neural mechanisms (Jeannerod, 1990).

Problems coordinating eye, head, and hand movements contributing to impaired reaching abilities have been reported in a number of neurologic populations, including CP (Saavedra et al., 2009), developmental coordination deficits (Wilmut et al., 2006), stroke, and cerebellar pathology (van Donkelaar & Lee, 1994). Saavedra and colleagues (2009) compared the coordination of eye, head, and hand movements during seated reaches in 10 children with CP, 6 to 16 years of age, with that in typically developing children. The children made eye and hand movements either together or in isolation with different levels of external postural support. Children with CP had a reduced ability to isolate eye, head, and hand movements, suggesting that inappropriate coupling of eye, head, and hands contributes to impaired reach and grasp in children with CP. Interestingly, providing external postural support to the children with CP did not affect eye or head movements but did affect the initiation and execution of hand movements. This is consistent with other research demonstrating the effect of providing additional postural support at the trunk on reach and grasp, which will be discussed in more detail in the postural control section of this chapter. In addition to deficits in the control of gaze and hand during reaching and grasping, children with hemiplegic CP show deficits in anticipatory visual control, defined as the ability to scan the visual scene and identify task-relevant landmarks in advance of an action. Anticipatory visual deficits may secondarily affect the planning and execution of goal-directed actions (Surkar et al., 2018).

Van Donkelaar and Lee (1994) examined the interaction between eye and hand movements in individuals with cerebellar pathology. They compared kinematic output of the eye and hand motor systems in both nonimpaired participants and participants with cerebellar pathology during the performance of two tasks: (a) tracking a moving target with the hand and (b) performing a pointing movement to intercept a target. As one might expect, individuals with cerebellar damage were slower to begin tracking the visual target and had more inaccurate and variable hand movements as compared with the nonimpaired participants. A large amount of the increased variability in hand movements occurred just prior to and after each corrective eye movement (ocular saccade) made to track the object. Interestingly, the increased variability in hand movements could be decreased when vision of the hand was restricted. Figure 19.1A shows that in a nonimpaired participant, variability of hand velocity did not change in the three visual conditions: normal, visual fixation, and restricted vision (e.g., the individual cannot see his or her hand). In contrast, Figure 19.1B indicates that hand velocity in a person with cerebellar damage is greatest under unrestricted visual conditions (normal) and is reduced when vision is either fixed or restricted. The authors conclude that there is a reciprocal interaction between the eye and hand motor systems.

In addition, among persons with cerebellar pathology, problems affecting the output of one system adversely affect the other, so that inaccuracies in hand movements are influenced by inaccuracies in eye movements, and vice versa. This is supported by a case study that assessed eye–hand coordination in two patients with stroke—one case with cerebellar stroke and another one with cortical stroke (Rizzo et al., 2020). The authors found that in the patient with cerebellar stroke, the timing control of eye and hand movements was decoupled and highly variable. The decoupling variance was attributed to inadequate timing in the control of saccades (i.e., short and long saccade latencies). In contrast, the temporal

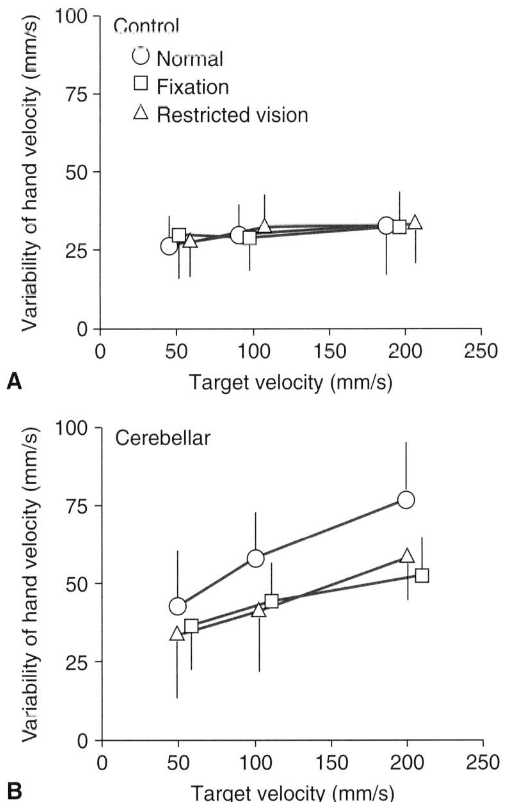

Figure 19.1 A comparison of hand velocity variability produced in a tracking task during normal visual conditions (Normal), when eye motion is restricted (Fixation), or when vision of the hand is restricted (Restricted vision) in a nonimpaired individual **(A)** and a subject with cerebellar pathology **(B)**. (Redrawn from van Donkelaar P, Lee RG. Interactions between the eye and hand motor systems: disruptions due to cerebellar dysfunction. *J Neurophysiol.* 1994;72:1679, with permission.)

eye–hand decoupling was less variable in the patient with cortical stroke. This was surprising in light of the fact that this patient demonstrated a greater degree of spatial variability in hand paths during the reach compared to the patient with cerebellar stroke. These data highlight the role of the cerebellum in the temporal and spatial prediction of eye and hand movements. Difficulties with eye–hand–head coordination during reach and grasp can be seen in the upper-extremity portion of the video of John, our case study on cerebellar pathology.

PROBLEMS WITH REACH AND GRASP

As we mentioned earlier, reaching is controlled by a different neural mechanism from that for grasping; hence, individuals with CNS pathology can have impaired reach but intact grasp or vice versa. For most individuals who are neurologically impaired, however, both reach and grasp are affected, reflecting dysfunction in the multiple systems controlling upper-extremity function. Separating the two, while artificial, makes it easier to analyze problems in each. However, it is important to remember that because of their close coordination and synchronization, pathology affecting reach most often disrupts grasp as well.

Impairments of Reach

Remember that during normal reaching, movement trajectories involving more than one joint tend to be straight and smooth and to have bell-shaped velocity profiles (Hogan et al., 1987). In contrast, movement trajectories in persons with neurologic pathology are often characterized by poor synergistic muscle control and loss of joint coordination. Disruptions in the coordination of movements can affect the timing and trajectory of movements. Many types of impairment can disrupt the timing and accuracy of reaching movements including motor impairments such as changes in muscle tone, weakness, decreased range of motion, and impaired multijoint coordination. In addition to motor impairments, sensory problems, including both peripheral and central processing problems, can disrupt reaching and are discussed in later sections of this chapter. Finally, postural control problems can disrupt the timing and sequencing of reaching movements.

Motor Problems

Timing Problems. Studies on reach and grasp have consistently shown delayed movement times (MT) in most types of neural pathology. For example, a number of researchers have reported that after stroke, reaching movements are slower, less accurate, and not as well coordinated as those made by nonimpaired individuals (Beer et al., 2000; Cirstea et al., 2003; Dewald & Beer, 2001; Levin, 1996; Reisman & Scholz, 2003). In addition, the ability to adapt reach to changing task demands is also impaired after stroke; individuals poststroke have difficulty adjusting reach extent and tend to overshoot closer targets and undershoot the more distant targets (van Vliet & Sheridan, 2009). Due to a combination of spasticity and paresis, Jean, our patient with chronic stroke, has great difficulty extending her arm and reaching for objects, as can be seen in the upper-extremity portion of her video case study.

Similarly, children with CP also have difficulty making coordinated reaching movements to point at or grasp objects (Mackey et al., 2006; Petrarca et al., 2009; Ronnqvist & Rosblad, 2007; Saavedra et al., 2009; Verrel et al., 2008). Reaches in children with CP are characterized by slower reaction times (Petrarca et al., 2009; Saavedra et al., 2009; van Thiel et al., 2000; Utley & Sugden, 1998), slower MT, and increased submovements (Chang et al., 2005; Mutsaarts et al., 2006; Saavedra et al., 2009; van der Heide et al., 2005). In addition, underlying patterns of muscle activity used for reaching are more variable in children with CP as compared with children who are typically developing (Zaino & McCoy, 2008). Differences are more apparent in the affected versus the unaffected arms in children with hemiplegia (Hung et al., 2004; Mackey et al., 2006; Ronnqvist & Rosblad, 2007; Steenbergen et al., 1998). For example, children with spastic hemiparetic CP use more trunk movement when reaching with the impaired arm as compared with the nonimpaired arm (Ricken et al., 2005). This is similar to research in adults with poststroke hemiplegia who, when compared to nonimpaired adults, tend to use increased trunk movement when reaching (van der Heide et al., 2004; Van Thiel & Steenbergen, 2001).

Interestingly, several researchers have shown that despite their motor impairments, children with CP were able to accurately reach for and grasp even quickly moving targets. These researchers found that the children aimed their reaches well ahead of the moving targets, suggesting that when planning a reaching movement, the children were able to compensate for the movement deficits that resulted in their slowed MT (Forsstrom & von Hofsten, 1982; Ricken et al., 2005).

Reaching in individuals with cerebellar dysfunction is also characterized by delayed MT (Rand et al., 2000; van Donkelaar & Lee, 1994). Van Donkelaar and Lee (1994) found that both response onset and MT were prolonged when reaching to moving targets. They suggest that delays in timing may be due to the person's need for more time to determine target velocity. Impaired reaching in a person with cerebellar pathology can be seen in the upper-extremity portion of the video case study on John, our patient with spinocerebellar degeneration.

Delayed reaching times have been shown in persons with Parkinson's disease (PD) (Bertram et al., 2005; Kelly et al., 2002; Negrotti et al., 2005; Wang et al., 2006). Kelly et al. (2002) examined the effect of medication (levodopa) and external cueing on voluntary reaching in nine people with PD (tested on and off medication) and nine age-matched controls. Participants were asked to reach to a target under speed constraints versus accuracy constraints and in one of two cue conditions: noncued (self-initiated) versus cued (triggered by a light). Results showed that persons with PD had slower reaching times under all conditions as compared with nonimpaired adults. Both levodopa and cueing increased the velocity of reaching movements of participants with PD; however, these factors were not additive. Levodopa increased movement speed more when reaches were self-initiated as compared with cued, and it improved self-paced reaches more than fast reaches. In a related study, these researchers also examined the effect of levodopa on the modulation of muscle activity (e.g., the ability to activate agonist muscles and inhibit antagonist muscles) during reaching movements (Kelly & Bastian, 2005). As had been reported previously, medication improved the speed of reaches in persons with PD and improved the ability to activate agonist muscle activity, but it did not improve the ability to inhibit antagonist muscle activity. Instead, the activity of both agonist and antagonist muscles increased with levodopa; thus, the medication, while improving the speed of movement, did not improve muscle modulation during voluntary reaching. The effects of medication on upper-extremity function can be observed in the upper-extremity section of Mike's video case study.

Thus, impaired timing, including delayed reaction and MT, is a common feature of reaching in persons with a wide variety of CNS pathology. One factor implicated in prolonged MT is a disruption to the coordination of multijoint movements.

Problems with Interjoint Coordination. Normally, elbow and shoulder joint angles change smoothly and at synchronized rates related to one another to produce a smooth reaching movement with a fairly straight trajectory. Children develop this coordination gradually during the first years of reaching (Konczak et al., 1995, 1997). In contrast, many studies have reported that in persons with CNS pathology, reaching movements are characterized by multijoint incoordination, leading to abnormal movement trajectories.

For example, Bastian and colleagues (1996, 2000; Bastian, 2002) studied movement trajectories in adults with cerebellar pathology. Movement trajectories were characterized by either undershooting or overshooting the target (dysmetria) and decomposition (moving one joint at a time). Figure 19.2 compares movement trajectories in a nonimpaired adult and a person with cerebellar pathology. In Figure 19.2A and B, wrist trajectories in a nonimpaired adult are smooth and straight during both slow accurate (A) and fast accurate (B) reaches. In addition, the movements are quite accurate; this can be seen by comparing the position of the fingertip (shown as an open circle) to the target (shown as a shaded circle). In contrast, the wrist trajectories and finger-point accuracy for a person with cerebellar pathology are shown in Figure 19.2C (slow accurate conditions) and 19.2D (fast accurate conditions). For both the slow and the fast movements, wrist trajectories show a fragmented trajectory (i.e., movement decomposition)—this can be seen by an initial vertical movement (primarily related to shoulder flexion), followed by a horizontal movement (related to elbow extension) during the latter half of the reach. While nonimpaired participants initiated shoulder and elbow motion within 73 msec of one another, participants with cerebellar pathology initiated shoulder flexion approximately 296 msec before the onset of elbow extension. In addition, the slow reaching movements were hypometric (undershooting) while the fast movements were hypermetric (overshooting) (Bastian et al., 1996).

Bastian and colleagues hypothesized that impaired multijoint coordination reflects the role of the cerebellum in anticipating and controlling interaction torques generated during multijoint movements. An interaction

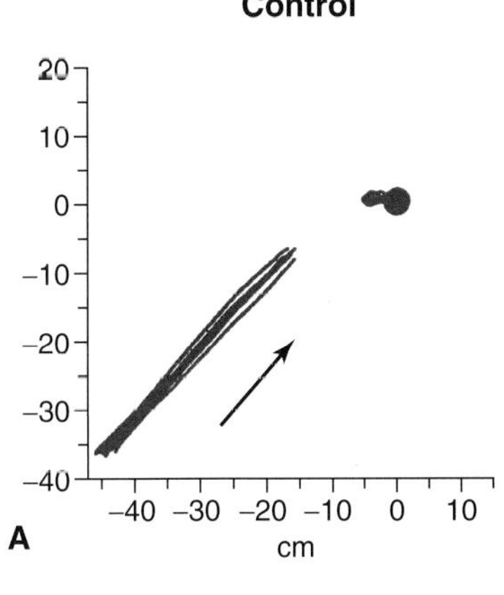

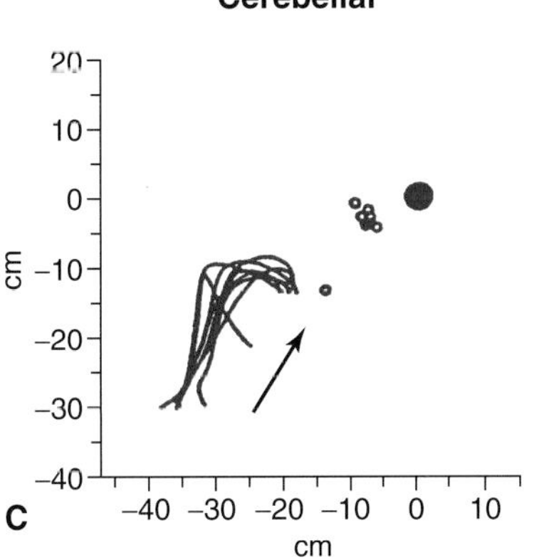

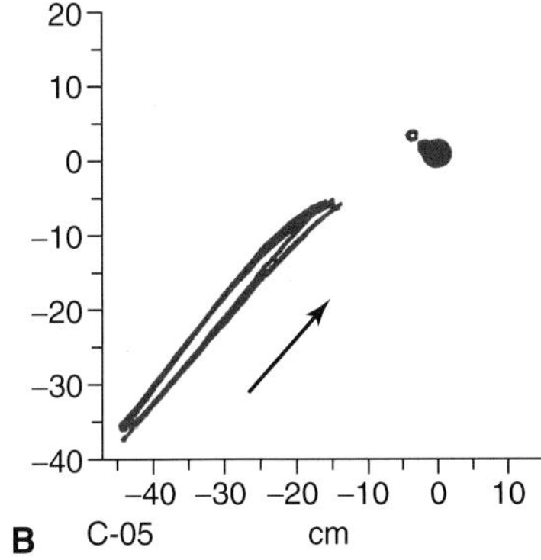

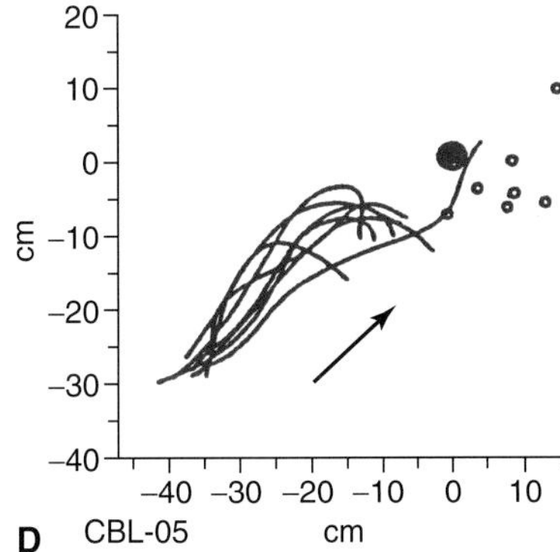

Figure 19.2 A comparison of wrist path in a nonimpaired individual **(A and B)** versus a subject with cerebellar pathology **(C and D)** moving in slow accurate **(A and C)** and fast accurate **(B and D)** conditions. *Arrows* indicate the direction of movement. The *shaded circle* indicates the location of the target. *Open circles* indicate the position of the tip of the index finger at the end of the movement. (Redrawn from Bastian AJ, Martin TA, Keating JG, et al. Cerebellar ataxia: abnormal control of interaction torques across multiple joints. *J Neurophysiol.* 1996;76:497, with permission.)

torque reflects the effect of movement at one joint (e.g., the elbow) on another joint (e.g., the shoulder). They examined multijoint coordination between the shoulder and elbow during a pointing task requiring elbow flexion (Fig. 19.3) when the shoulder was free to move (Fig. 19.3A) versus constrained (Fig. 19.3D). Eight individuals with cerebellar pathology and eight age-matched controls were tested. Control subjects (Fig. 19.3B and E) made few end point errors in either condition. In contrast, persons with cerebellar pathology made large end point errors in the free condition (data from trials for each person are shown as numbers in Fig. 19.3C) but not in the constrained condition (Fig. 19.3F). Elbow movements were near normal in the constrained condition (when the movement was performed at a single joint). In contrast, multijoint movements were associated with excessive shoulder flexion and an inability to control interactive torques, and this resulted in large end point errors (Bastian, 2002). The effect of cerebellar pathology on segmental coordination during reach can be observed in the video case study of John, our patient with spinocerebellar degeneration.

Impaired multijoint coordination has also been reported in several studies examining upper-extremity movements in individuals with PD (Bertram et al., 2005; Teulings et al., 2002; Wang et al., 2006; Wiesendanger & Serrien, 2001). Tuelings et al. (2002) used handwriting-like tasks to study upper-extremity control

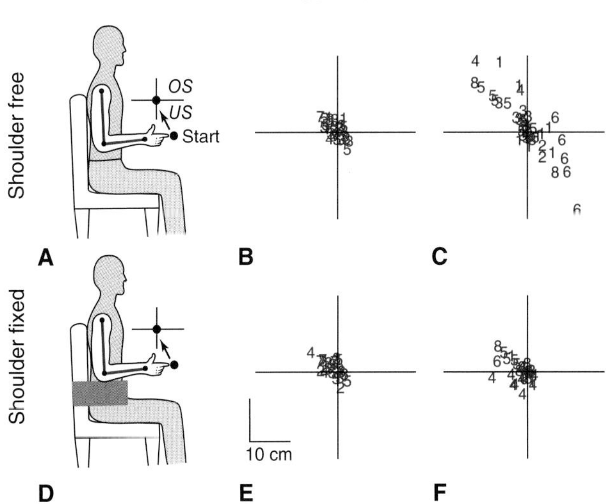

Figure 19.3 Experimental method used to study multijoint coordination between the shoulder and elbow during a pointing task requiring elbow flexion under two conditions: when the shoulder was free to move **(A)** and when it was constrained **(D)**. Nonimpaired individuals **(B and E)** made few end point errors in either condition. Individuals with cerebellar pathology made large end point errors in the free condition **(C)** but not in the constrained condition **(F)**. For all plots, numbers represent data from multiple trials in individual participants. *OS*, overshoot; *US*, undershoot. (Reprinted from Bastian AJ. Cerebellar limb ataxia: abnormal control of self-generated and external forces. *Ann NY Acad Sci.* 2002;978:18, with permission.)

in individuals with PD. They found that many of the fine-motor control problems in persons with PD (as shown by their handwriting-like tasks) were caused by a reduced ability to coordinate wrist and finger movements and by a reduced ability to control wrist flexion. Researchers have also reported that individuals with PD have difficulty coordinating arm, hand, and trunk motion during tasks that require trunk-assisted reaching (Bertram et al., 2005; Wang et al., 2006).

Bertram et al. (2005) examined multisegmental coordination in persons with PD and healthy aged-matched controls during a prehension task that involved reaching for a glass of water with and without a cover, placed beyond the reach of the outstretched arm. The task required coordinated movement of the arm and trunk. MT in persons with PD were comparable to those in healthy controls when reaching for a covered glass of water but were significantly slower when reaching for an uncovered glass. In addition, there was a difference in the strategy used when reaching for the uncovered cup, with individuals with PD using less trunk motion during forward reaches than did age-matched controls. Results suggest the presence of task-specific changes in strategies used for reach and grasp in persons with PD. The effects of task and medication on reach and grasp in a person with PD can be seen in the upper-extremity section of Mike's video case study.

Various researchers have documented deficits in interjoint coordination in children with hemiplegic CP. In their study of reaching toward a stationary and a moving ball, Ricken and colleagues (2005) found greater variability and joint segmentation in the coordination patterns between the elbow, shoulder, and trunk of the more-affected side. The children tended to show increased trunk motion, perhaps in an effort to compensate for the reduction in shoulder and elbow excursion.

Other studies have also provided evidence of greater joint segmentation in children with CP, describing the reaching pattern of the affected limb as one with increased movement units (Chang et al., 2005; van der Heide et al., 2005). A biomechanical analysis of a forward reaching task in standing children with unilateral and bilateral CP and typically developing children (6–14 years) showed that children with CP demonstrated decreased active range of motion of shoulder and trunk (dos Santos Soares et al., 2019). Children with spastic hemiplegic CP also showed deficits during dynamic control of neuromuscular interlimb patterns when two body segments (e.g., both arms or an arm and a leg) were involved in a continuous motor task. These children showed impaired continuous interlimb coordination (i.e., movement relationship between limbs) and low motor stability (i.e., inconsistent motor patterns) while performing continuous *in-phase* upper limb movements (i.e., the arms move in the same direction at the same time) during *in-place* marching (i.e., flexion-extension of lower extremities). However, when children practiced the continuous upper limb movements in a standing position, and the lower limbs were eliminated from the task (i.e., less degrees of freedom to control and coordinate), they did not show interlimb coordination deficits (Sidiropoulos et al., 2020).

Problems with coordination during reach and grasp have also been reported in children with developmental coordination disorder (DCD). Astill and Utley (2008) studied the kinematics of reach and grasp during a catching task in 10 children with DCD and found that during reach, initiation and MT were slower and the grasp phase of the movement occurred earlier and was more variable as well. The authors suggest that during reach and grasp, children with DCD use a decomposition strategy to simplify the movement control of the transport and grasp phases of a catch (Astill & Utley, 2008).

Loss of Movement Individuation, Synergies, and Global Synkinesis. Atypical movement patterns, specifically the presence of abnormal synergies and difficulty with selective movement, are commonly observed in individuals who have had a stroke. Pathological synergies have been defined as fixed patterns of movement involving an entire extremity, with an inability to isolate movements outside the synergy pattern (Twitchell, 1951). Historically, clinicians have characterized recovery from stroke relative to movements both within and outside synergy patterns, with the highest level of recovery associated with the ability to make isolated movements in individual joints (Brunnstrom, 1966; Twitchell, 1951). However, research has shown that in individuals without neural pathology, the CNS spatially and temporally constrains complex muscle activations into synergies in order to simplify the control of reaching and postural movements. This suggests that the CNS applies muscle synergies as heuristic solutions to transform task-level motor intentions into detailed spatiotemporal muscle patterns in order to reduce the complexity of control (D'Avella & Lacquaniti, 2013; Profeta & Turvey, 2018; Ting & McKay, 2007).

Micera and colleagues (2005) examined interjoint arm synergies during 12 different reaching movements in persons with hemiparesis and healthy controls. Motion analysis was used to examine upper-extremity kinematics, specifically the synergistic relationship between shoulder and elbow angular velocity profiles during different reaching movements. While angular trajectories for the shoulder and elbow were very consistent in the healthy control subjects (strong synergistic coupling), they varied significantly in the group with hemiparesis. Among individuals with poststroke hemiparesis, there was a disruption to the normal synergistic coupling between shoulder and elbow motion during reaching movements. Pan and collaborators (2018) investigated an upward reaching task with a 2-second holding component at the end of the reach in stroke survivors and age-matched controls.

They found that for most participants in both groups, a total of three muscle synergy structures were used to control the reaching task. Overall, participants with stroke displayed a characteristic co-activation of trapezius and deltoids, increased activation of pectoralis major, and decreased activation of triceps. However, the participants with stroke at the recovery stages III–IV (increased and decreased spasticity, respectively, according to the Brunnstrom Motor Recovery Stage Levels) significantly differed with respect to controls. Moreover, those subjects at stage III showed the largest elbow joint angles and the greatest motor difficulties to withhold the reaching arm. Thus, deficits in muscle synergies during reaching are more prominent in severely impaired stroke survivors, and lesser in mild-to-moderately impaired patients.

Levin (1996) used pointing movements to study upper-extremity control in 10 persons with poststroke hemiplegia and 6 nonimpaired participants to determine the relationship between functional upper-extremity limitations and underlying impairments such as abnormal synergies and spasticity. Participants were seated in front of a horizontal surface and made reaching movements to four targets located in front of them (200 and 400 mm) and in the ipsilateral and contralateral workspace (Fig. 19.4). The targets were arranged as follows: (a) moving toward the ipsilateral target required an out-of-synergy movement (e.g., a combination of shoulder horizontal abduction and elbow extension), (b) moving toward a contralateral target could be performed with an extensor synergy (e.g., shoulder adduction and elbow extension), and (c) movement to near and far targets required a combination of flexor and extensor synergies in order to move the arm forward. Kinematic data were used to study coordination of finger, wrist, elbow, and shoulder joints to the four targets. In addition, subjects underwent clinical evaluation to assess spasticity (modified Ashworth scale) and sensorimotor function (Fugl–Meyer scale).

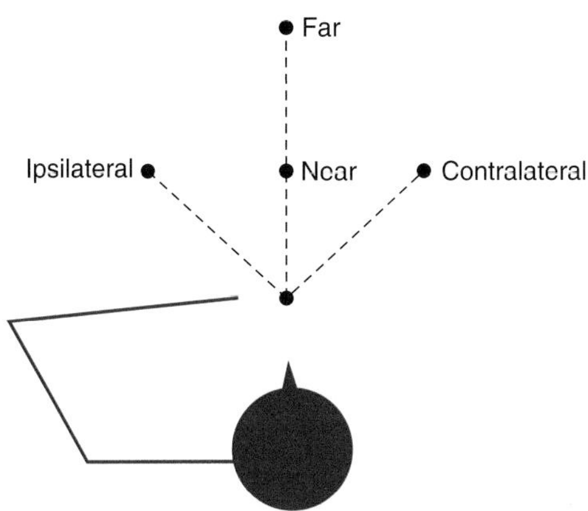

Figure 19.4 A diagram of the target positions (*black circles*) for reaching movements made on a horizontal surface, by patients with poststroke hemiplegia. (Reprinted from Levin MF. Interjoint coordination during pointing movements is disrupted in spastic hemiparesis. *Brain.* 1996;119:283, with permission.)

For all participants with hemiparesis, MT were significantly longer and movement amplitudes smaller in the affected arm as compared with the less affected arm (see Fig. 19.5A). In the affected arm, trajectories were characterized by segmented movements, increased variability, and disrupted interjoint coordination. This can be seen in Figure 19.5B, which compares interjoint coordination to all four targets in the less affected arm and the affected arm of one of the participants with hemiparesis. As can be seen in Figure 19.5B, right panels, in the less affected arm, the trajectories were smooth

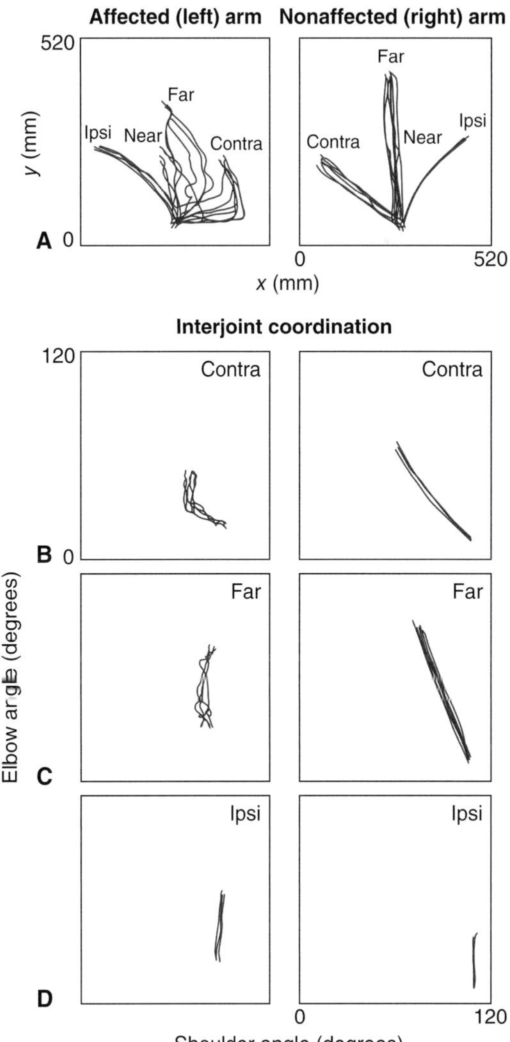

Figure 19.5 A comparison of trajectories to contralateral (*Contra*), far, near, and ipsilateral (*Ipsi*) targets in spatial coordinates **(A)** and interjoint coordination (elbow and shoulder) **(B–D)** in angular coordinates for the affected left arm **(left panels)** and the nonaffected arm **(right panels)** for a subject with hemiparesis and severe spasticity. (Redrawn from Levin MF. Interjoint coordination during pointing movements is disrupted in spastic hemiparesis. *Brain.* 1996;119:285, with permission.)

and continuous, with good coordination of movement in the elbow and shoulder joints.

In contrast, the participant could not produce smooth end point trajectories in the affected arm (left panels), and movement to the contralateral target was segmented and poorly coordinated. Movement segmentation resulted from a lack of coordination between shoulder and elbow joint movements, reminiscent of the findings from studies on reaching in persons with cerebellar pathology. This disruption of interjoint coordination led to a limitation in active range of elbow and shoulder joint motion, resulting in hypometric movements that undershot the target.

Poor coordination was obvious for both movements made within the extensor synergy (to the contralateral target) and those requiring out-of-synergy movements (to near and far targets). Thus, the disruption to movements was not solely due to the presence of pathologic movement synergies. Finally, severity of spasticity was correlated with both movement time and amplitude, but not with interjoint coordination measures. The author suggests that regardless of the location of the lesion, following a stroke, the CNS may not be able to determine the optimal set of relationships between muscles and segments to perform smooth coordinated reaching movements (Levin, 1996).

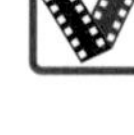

In the case studies of both Jean and Genise, individuals who have had a stroke, we observe the presence of a flexor synergy as a predominant movement pattern in the upper extremity. Both have profound paresis and spasticity as well, constraining their capacity to make voluntary movements of the upper extremity outside the flexor synergy pattern.

While many researchers have examined the role of upper extremity synergistic relationships to reaching, others have focused on examining the ability to make isolated motions of individual joints or body segments, referred to as "individuation" (Zackowski et al., 2004). Poor individuation results in excessive and unintended motion at linked body segments (Beer et al., 2000; Lang & Schieber, 2004). Studies have shown abnormal coupling between elbow and shoulder torques in the paretic limbs of individuals with hemiparetic stroke that closely parallel abnormal movement synergies characteristic of upper-extremity movement following stroke (Dewald et al., 1999). Abnormal torque coupling makes it difficult for a person with stroke to extend the elbow while simultaneously flexing the shoulder. The video case study of Genise, which tracks upper-extremity function in a patient recovering from an acute stroke, provides an example of abnormal coupling of upper extremity joints during shoulder flexion.

Zackowski et al. (2004) studied the impact of impaired joint individuation during reaching in people with chronic hemiparesis. In this study, 18 subjects with chronic hemiparesis and 18 age- and gender-matched controls were evaluated while either reaching up (requiring flexion at both the shoulder and elbow) or reaching out (flexion at the shoulder and extension at the elbow). In addition, subjects performed three upper-extremity individuation movements, shoulder individuation (shoulder flexion with the remaining limb segments in extension), elbow individuation (elbow flexion with no associated movement at the shoulder or wrist), and wrist individuation (wrist extension without associated movement at the elbow and shoulder). Other impairments tested in this study included strength (using a handheld dynamometer), spasticity (response to passive movements using the modified Ashworth scale), and fine touch sensation using a monofilament test.

Results indicated that while both types of reaches were abnormal in the group with hemiparesis, performance was worse on the reach-out versus the reach-up task. In addition, the ability to individuate movement at shoulder, elbow, and wrist was significantly impaired. Abnormal individuation is shown in Figure 19.6, which compares individuation at the shoulder (top traces), elbow (middle traces), and wrist (lower traces) in a nonimpaired participant (A) compared with two persons with hemiparesis (B and C). The nonimpaired individual was able to flex the shoulder 73 degrees, with less than 8 degrees of combined motion at the wrist and elbow, resulting in an individuation index of 0.97. Individuation was similarly good at both the elbow and the wrist. In contrast, both persons with hemiparesis had difficulty making individuated movements, with participant labeled 04 (Fig. 19.6B) showing mild deficits as compared with participant labeled 08 (Fig. 19.6C). For the participant with mild hemiparesis (labeled 04), shoulder flexion to 70 degrees was associated with 15 degrees of elbow flexion and 20 degrees of wrist extension, for an individuation index of 0.79. Similar patterns were also present in the elbow and wrist individuation tasks (middle and lower traces). For the participant with severe hemiparesis, shoulder flexion of 40 degrees was associated with 65 degrees of elbow motion and 20 degrees of wrist motion, resulting in a 0.29 individuation index.

Finally, these researchers used regression analysis to determine which combination of impairments best explained deficits in reaching, including reach trajectories and end point error, and found that individuation explained most of the variance. Sensation also contributed, while strength and spasticity did not. Strength did explain variance in reaching velocity. They conclude that deficits in joint individuation are the primary problem affecting impaired reaching in persons who have had a stroke.

In contrast to Zackowski et al., who did not find strength a major factor in reaching trajectories and end point error, McCrea and colleagues (2005) argue that insufficient force generation in paretic arm muscles results in the compensatory activation of additional arm muscles,

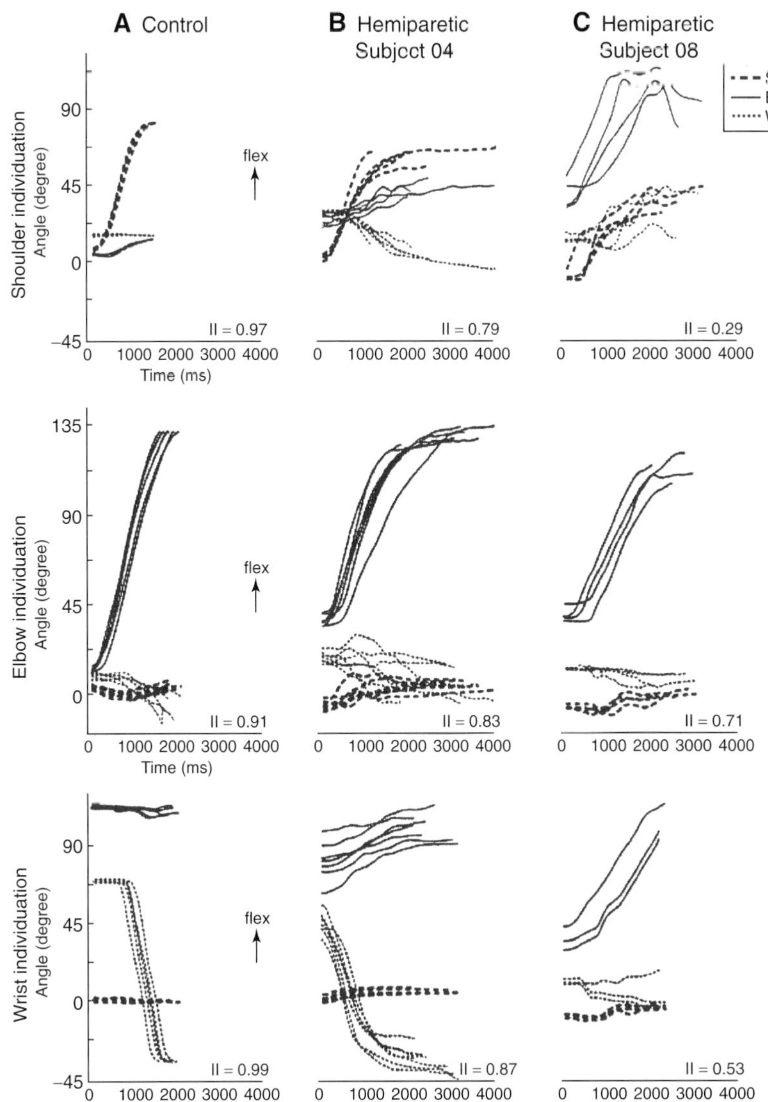

Figure 19.6 Abnormal individuation at the shoulder **(top traces)**, elbow **(middle traces)**, and wrist **(lower traces)** in a nonimpaired individual **(A)** and two individuals with hemiparesis **(B and C)**. Bold dashed lines are shoulder angular excursion, narrow solid lines are elbow angular excursion, and narrow dashed lines are wrist angular excursion. Note that in the nonimpaired individual, individuated motion at the shoulder **(top trace)** is associated with minimal motion at the elbow and wrist. This is also true for elbow and wrist motion **(middle and bottom panels)**. In contrast, in both individuals with hemiparesis **(B and C)**, motion at the shoulder is associated with significant motion at the elbow and wrist. This is also true when the primary movement is at the elbow **(middle panels)** and wrist **(lower panels)**. *II*, individuation index. (Reprinted from Zackowski KM, Dromerick AW, Sahrmann SA, et al. How do strength, sensation, spasticity and joint individuation relate to the reaching deficits of people with chronic hemiparesis? *Brain.* 2004;127:1041, with permission.)

which contributes to atypical movement trajectories during reaching movements following stroke. McCrea and colleagues (2005) compared patterns of muscle recruitment in paretic and nonparetic limbs during a forward reaching movement in 20 individuals who had a stroke and 10 healthy age-matched controls. They hypothesized that paretic arm muscles would be maximally activated (i.e., saturated) during a sagittal plane reach, thus requiring compensatory recruitment of other muscles, and this would result in out-of-plane movement trajectories.

Results indicated that muscle recruitment and arm trajectories in the nonparetic arm of the persons with stroke were similar to those in nonimpaired participants; however, in the paretic limb, there was increased activation of all muscles, especially the lateral deltoid and anterior deltoid. This pattern of muscle activation resulted in shoulder abduction, segmented interjoint movement, and indirect hand motion. They suggest that the inability to generate sufficient force in paretic arm muscles involved in a forward reach task results in the recruitment of additional muscles in order to successfully complete the task (McCrea et al., 2005).

The studies by McCrea and Zackowski and their colleagues have examined excessive and atypical recruitment of muscles within a paretic limb during a reaching task. Another characteristic of movement following stroke is referred to as global synkinesis or motor irradiation, described as the involuntary and unintentional movement of one limb when the opposite limb is active. Neuroimaging has suggested that global synkinesis results from the bilateral excitation of the motor cortex and a loss of inhibitory influence on the opposite hemisphere via transcallosal fibers (Meyer et al., 1995; Schnitzler et al., 1996).

Hwang and colleagues (2005) used surface electromyography (EMG) to characterize motor irradiation in the paretic upper extremity during flexion movements of the nonparetic contralateral limb in 20 persons with poststroke hemiparesis, classified into one of two groups according to severity of involvement, and 20 nonimpaired individuals. In subjects with poststroke hemiparesis, muscle activation in the nonparetic limb was associated with widespread activation of muscles in the paretic limb—global synkinesis. Interestingly, increased levels of global synkinesis were associated with better motor recovery. While nonimpaired participants showed some level of global synkinesis (primarily in the elbow flexors), the pattern of muscle recruitment was significantly different in the two groups of participants with poststroke hemiparesis (primary recruitment of shoulder adductors) as compared with the nonimpaired group. Improved recruitment of muscle activity in the paretic limb associated with activity in the nonparetic limb is often exploited in rehabilitation of upper-extremity function in persons with poststroke hemiparesis. As 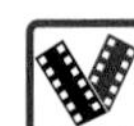 discussed in Chapter 20, and shown in the treatment video of Genise our patient with an acute stroke, practicing voluntary movements of the nonimpaired hand combined with mirror visual feedback is used to facilitate recruitment of muscle activity in the paretic limb.

Impairments in Postural Support of Reaching. As discussed in Chapters 17 and 18, a critical element that contributes to the speed and accuracy of reaching is postural control. Hung and Spingarn (2018) investigated a bimanual pickup task that involved the whole body to retrieve an object from the floor in children with spastic hemiplegic CP and compared their performance to children with typical development. The aim of this study was to investigate how both groups organized their upper extremities as well as their whole-body movements during the pickup task. Children with CP had longer overall MT, slower times when reaching down and when grasping, and demonstrated impaired spatial and temporal bimanual coordination. Additionally, the group of children with CP demonstrated uneven weight bearing and postural control deficits during the whole-body pickup task compared to typically developing children. Deficits in postural control were evidenced by greater asymmetric bilateral ground reaction forces and larger lateral and anterior excursion of the center of mass (COM).

Tsang and colleagues (2013) examined the effect of postural stability on eye–hand coordination in 15 participants with poststroke hemiplegia (average age 58 years, average time since stroke 7 years). Participants used their index finger to touch a moving target presented on a visual screen at shoulder height. The fast finger-pointing task was done in sitting and in standing, both paretic and nonparetic limbs were tested and participants were asked to move as quickly as they could. They found that reaction and MT were slower in the paretic compared to the nonparetic arm, though accuracy was similar for the two arms. In addition, when the task was performed with the paretic limb, reaction time (but not accuracy) was slower in standing compared to sitting, though MT were slightly faster in standing. Finally, in standing, postural sway (total sway path and anteroposterior sway path) was significantly greater when the task was performed with the paretic arm compared to the nonparetic arm. Faster MT were associated with increased forward reaching, suggesting that in the standing position, participants with stroke used a strategy of forward lean toward the target to compensate for upper-extremity limitations.

Trunk control is key to independent sitting as well as to reaching performance. Previous research has shown that restraining trunk motion in participants with stroke who were sitting and reaching resulted in increased motion at the shoulder, elbow, and wrist (Michaelsen et al., 2001). Research in children with CP has also explored the relationship between postural control and reaching, specifically the effects of external support at different trunk segments on seated postural control and reaching (Santamaria et al., 2016). In this study, the Segmental Assessment of Trunk Control (SATCo) was used to categorize children from 2 to 15 years (classified as GMFCS III–V) into three groups (mild, moderate, and severe). All children were instructed to perform a self-paced reach toward a toy placed at midline. The level of trunk support did not have an impact on seated postural or reaching control in children classified with mild trunk control deficits. However, children classified with moderate deficits were able to improve their reaching and seated postural control when the external support was placed at the most-impaired trunk segment or above (midribs or axillae support in comparison to pelvic support). Children in the severest group were unable to sit independently even with pelvic support. In addition, while they showed improved postural head and trunk control when the trunk support was placed at axillae compared to midrib level, reaching performance did not improve. Results, shown in Figure 19.7, compare the straightness of the reaching path at the three different levels of support, in the three groups of children. Note that children with moderate trunk control deficits showed significant improvements in straightness score (in which a value closer to 1 indicates better straightness) when support was at either axillae or midribs compared to pelvic level. Moreover, children in the moderate group showed improvements in movement time, path length, and in the number of movement units with higher trunk supports. However, reaching performance did not differ between axillae and midribs support. Hence, the researchers concluded that providing trunk support at the specific level at which trunk stability is compromised for a child with moderate-to-severe CP improves seated postural and reaching performance. The effect of providing external support to the trunk on 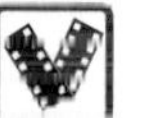 upper-extremity function is shown in the case study of Malachi, our child with severe CP.

In a similar fashion, systematically lowering the external support from least to most-impaired segmental trunk control has been used when training upper-extremity control in children with CP. Santamaria and

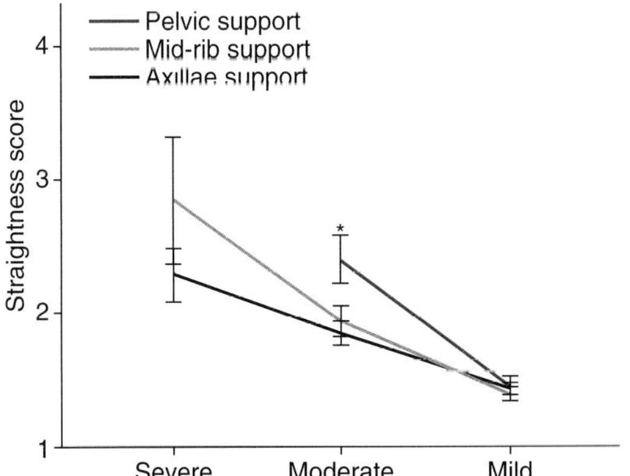

Figure 19.7 A comparison of the straightness of the reach, with support at three different levels in three groups of children with cerebral palsy. Note that the moderately involved group showed significant improvements in straightness score (lower numbers, closer to 1, indicate better straightness) when support was at the axillae (*black line*) or midrib level (*light orange line*) compared to the pelvis (*dark orange line*). More severely involved children showed improvements with support at the axillae. (Adapted with permission from Santamaria V, Rachwani J, Saavedra S, Woollacott MH. Effect of segmental trunk support on posture and reaching in children with cerebral palsy. *Ped Phys Ther.* 2016;285–293.)

colleagues (2020) developed a novel robotic-aided therapeutic method to dynamically support the trunk, at the most-impaired region, while applying a seated postural and reaching control training, based on motor learning and control principles. They used a robotic platform, called the Trunk-Support-Trainer (TruST), that delivered "assist-as-needed" circular force fields corresponding to the individual stability boundaries in sitting. Based on the child's level of trunk control, the authors systematically increased the diameter of the postural assistance during practice. With this progressive training, all four children improved their reaching control, stability limits, and independent sitting ability. Figure 19.8 shows data from three children.

In summary, this research underscores the critical importance of postural control as a constraint on upper-extremity function in both adults and children with CNS pathology. It also reminds us that constraints in upper-extremity function, such as reduced ability to reach, can impact strategies used to maintain postural stability in both sitting and standing.

Sensory Problems

The ability to adapt reaching movements to changes in task and environmental demands is an essential component of normal upper-extremity control. Multisensory integration is critical to adapting movements and is used to correct errors during the execution of upper-extremity movement, ensuring accuracy during the final portions of the movement. Thus, disruption to peripheral and central sensory systems can disrupt the timing and accuracy of reaching movements and limit the capacity to adapt movements to changing task and environmental demands.

Effect of Visual Deficits on Visually Guided Reach. The primary function of visual feedback in reaching appears to be related to the attainment of final accuracy. It has been hypothesized that the constancy of thumb position with relation to the wrist during reaching may be part of

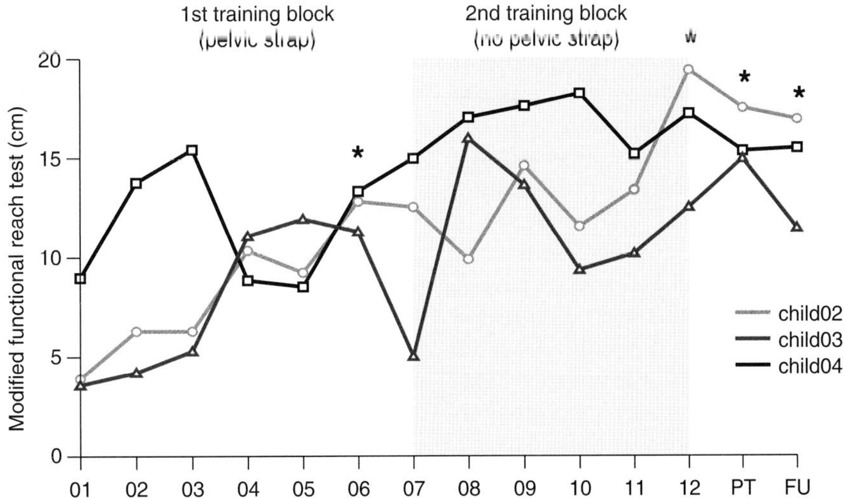

Figure 19.8 The modified functional reach test (forward direction) was measured with pelvic strapping (1st training block) and without pelvic straps (2nd training block). Overall, the graph shows a steady increase in the modified functional reach test in the three children with training. Most importantly, the children showed short-term and long-term improvements in reaching control during independent sitting at 1 week post training and at the 3 months follow-up. *$P < 0.05$ compared to session 01. (Adapted with permission from Santamaria et al., 2020. *Promoting Functional and Independent Sitting in Children with Cerebral Palsy Using the Robotic Trunk Support Trainer. TNSRE,* doi: 10.1109/TNSRE.2020.3031580.)

a strategy of providing clear visual feedback information regarding the end point of the limb (Wing & Frazer, 1983). However, one might ask which type of visual information is most helpful to the CNS during the planning and control of reaching accuracy (knowledge of limb position prior to reaching, online tracking of the moving arm, or target location)? Research has shown that knowledge of the starting hand position increases reaching accuracy when visual information of the moving limb is absent. Still, some studies show that proprioceptive inputs are critical to register the position of limb configuration at the start of the reach (Sarlegna & Sainburg, 2009). Lesions on either side of the posterior parietal area in humans can cause marked eye–hand coordination impairment, or optic ataxia. Optic ataxia is defined as the inability to reach for objects in extrapersonal space, in the absence of extensive motor, visual, or somatosensory deficits (Jeannerod, 1990). Patients with optic ataxia are impaired in their ability to reach and grasp, although they retain the ability to describe objects. In contrast, patients with bilateral occipitotemporal cortex lesions have impaired shape perception (visual form agnosia) but retain the ability to reach and grasp for objects, although they cannot describe them (Rossetti et al., 2005).

Optic ataxia was first described by Balint in 1909, using the term *visual disorientation*. He noted that the patient could reach normally with his left hand, but when asked to reach with his right hand, he made mistakes in all directions, until he eventually bumped into the object with his hand. He found that the problem was related to visual control of that hand, because if he asked the patient to first point to the object with his left hand, then he could reach accurately with his right hand. On autopsy, it was found that the patient had a lesion in the posterior parietal areas, including the angular gyrus and the anterior occipital lobe on both sides of the brain (Jeannerod, 1990).

There are specific motor disorganization problems in these individuals as well. It has been hypothesized that their problems relate to programming visually guided goal-directed movements. It has been shown that the deceleration phase of reaching is much longer than that in the normal hand, with many small peaks. In addition, these patients have problems with grasp formation. Figure 19.9 shows a reach of a person with optic ataxia with his normal hand (A), and with his affected hand, with visual feedback (B), and (C) without vision. Note that even with visual feedback, the affected hand did not begin to close until the last moment and the terminal grip size was too big. Without visual feedback, grasp formation did not occur (Jeannerod, 1990). Thus, it has been suggested that optic ataxia results from a specific problem with eye–hand coordination mechanisms responsible for adjusting finger posture to the shape of the object (Jeannerod, 1990).

Visual motor problems in reaching to a target in individuals with optic ataxia were also described by Rossetti et al. (2005). In this experiment, persons with optic ataxia reached for a target under congruent and incongruent conditions. In the congruent condition, the target was presented at the same location prior to and after a delay during which the target was not visible. In the incongruent task condition, the target was displayed at one location, and then, after a delay, participants reached for a target that was presented at a different location. Results are shown in Figure 19.10. The nonimpaired participant (Fig. 19.10A) demonstrated smooth and efficient reaching trajectories to point B under both congruent (target placement at point B both before and after the delay) and incongruent (before delay, target at point A, after delay, target at point B) conditions. Both participants with optic ataxia (B and C) showed impaired trajectories in both conditions. During the incongruent condition trials, participants with optic ataxia reached initially toward the remembered target (located at position A) rather than the actual target (located at position B). The authors suggest that individuals with optic ataxia rely more on remembered information (slow cognitive control) rather than on online visual information (fast visuomotor control) when reaching (Rossetti et al., 2005).

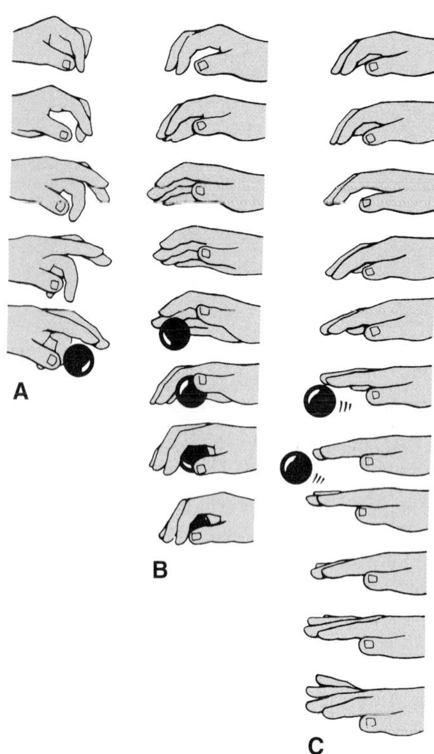

Figure 19.9 Grip patterns of an individual with optic ataxia. **(A)** Normal hand. **(B)** Affected hand, visual feedback. **(C)** Affected hand, no visual feedback. (Reprinted from Jeannerod M. *The neural and behavioral organization of goal-directed movements.* Oxford, UK: Oxford University Press, 1990:225, with permission.)

Effect of Somatosensory Deficits on Reach. Is somatosensory input essential for the production of reaching

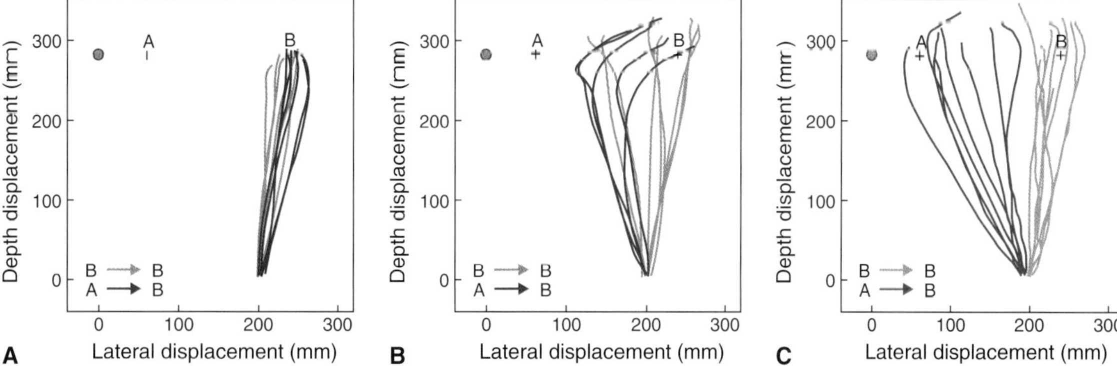

Figure 19.10 Reaching trajectories made in congruent (*dark lines*) and incongruent (*light lines*) conditions in a nonimpaired individual **(A)** and two individuals with optic ataxia **(B and C)**. The nonimpaired control **(A)** demonstrates smooth and efficient reaching trajectories to point *B* under both congruent (target placement at point *B* both before and after the delay) and incongruent (before delay target at point *A*, after delay target at point *B*) conditions. Both individuals with optic ataxia **(B and C)** show impaired trajectories in both conditions. During the incongruent trials, individuals with optic ataxia initially reach toward the remembered target (located at position *A*) rather than the actual target (located at position *B*). (Reprinted from Rossetti Y, Revol P, McIntosh R, et al. Visually guided reaching: bilateral posterior parietal lesions cause a switch from fast visuomotor to slow cognitive control. *Neuropsychologia*. 2005;43:171, with permission.)

movements? As noted in earlier chapters, experiments by Sherrington in the late 1800s showed that monkeys that were deafferented on one side of the spinal cord stopped using the affected limb. He concluded that sensory feedback was critical to movement control. In contrast, researchers who deafferented both limbs of animals showed that the animals recovered motor function. Movements were initially awkward but improved within as little as 2 weeks, as long as visual feedback was available (Taub & Berman, 1968).

Interestingly, recovery starts with the animals being able to only sweep the object across the floor. Then, a coarse grasp with all four fingers develops, and then, a pincer grasp reappears (Taub, 1976). It has been suggested that when unilateral deafferentation occurs, the animals may learn not to use the deafferented limb or may even develop inhibition of the deafferented arm (Taub, 1976). This learned disuse hypothesis is supported by the fact that unilaterally deafferented animals recover movement coordination as well as bilaterally deafferented animals if their nonaffected limb remains immobilized so that they have to use the deafferented limb (Jeannerod, 1990). Results from these studies form the basis of constraint-induced treatment of upper-extremity function discussed in Chapter 20.

Also, remember from Chapter 17 that experiments on deafferented monkeys showed that, when making single-joint movements, they could reach targets with relative accuracy, even when they could not see the hand. Displacing the forearm just prior to movement onset during a reach also did not significantly disturb pointing accuracy in these deafferented animals. It was thus concluded that single-joint movements depend on changes in muscle activation levels that are programmed prior to movement onset and that no feedback is required for reasonably accurate execution of these movements (Polit & Bizzi, 1979).

In addition, experiments on humans after pathological deafferentation have confirmed the results from experiments on monkeys (Rothwell et al., 1982). One individual had suffered a severe peripheral sensory neuropathy, with a significant loss of sensation in both the arms and the legs. Light touch, vibration, and temperature sensation were impaired or totally absent in both hands. Tests showed that in spite of these problems, this individual could perform many motor tasks, even without vision. For example, it was possible to tap, do fast alternating flexion and extension movements, and draw figures in the air, using only the wrist and fingers (Jeannerod, 1990; Rothwell et al., 1982).

It was also noted that EMG activity during flexion and extension of the thumb was similar to that seen in a nonimpaired individual. Finally, the individual with sensory loss could learn new thumb positions with vision and then reproduce those positions without vision suggesting that motor learning was also possible. However, performance declined rapidly when it was necessary to repeat the movement many times with the eyes closed.

In a second study, individuals with peripheral sensory neuropathy could perform repetitive flexion and extension movements of the wrist, with normal EMG activity, as long as the movements were not too fast. At a certain point, however, the intervals between the EMG bursts tended to disappear. It was hypothesized that this was due to high levels of co-contraction of agonist and antagonist muscles (Sanes et al., 1985). In addition, individuals with sensory neuropathy could hold a steady posture with their deafferented limb as long as they had visual feedback. However, without visual feedback, large errors were made, and the limb drifted back to its initial

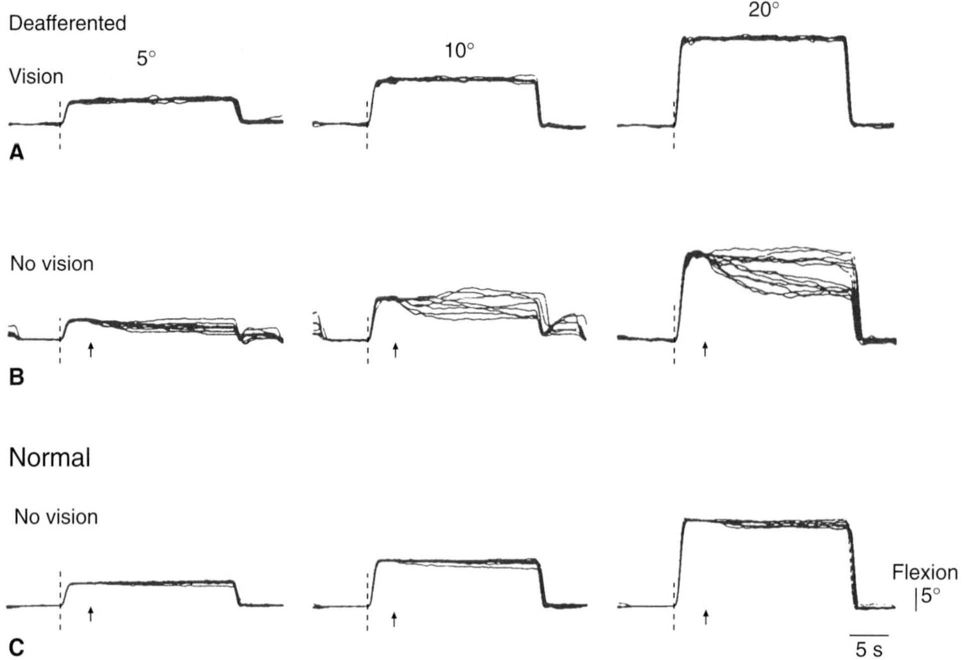

Figure 19.11 Recordings of wrist position of an individual with peripheral sensory neuropathy. The individual was asked to rotate the wrist to reach positions of 5, 10, and 20 degrees against an elastic load. **(A)** With vision, the individual had no problems. **(B)** When the visual cue related to the position to be maintained was removed (shown by the up-pointing *arrow*), the position drifted back in the direction of the load. **(C)** A nonimpaired individual's performance, showing that even when the visual position cue is removed, wrist position is fairly well maintained. (Redrawn from Sanes JN, Mauritz KH, Dalakas MC, et al. Motor control in humans with large-fiber sensory neuropathy. *Hum Neurobiol.* 1985;4:101, with permission.)

position, as shown in Figure 19.11 (Sanes et al., 1985). These findings were supported in work by Sainburg and colleagues (1993, 1995), who compared individuals with proprioceptive deafferentation and nonimpaired controls during a pantomimed task of slicing bread. This task required sharp joint reversals in movement direction. They found that without visual feedback, nonimpaired individuals exhibited synchronous movements of the shoulder and elbow at the reversal, exploiting the interaction torques. However, individuals with proprioceptive deafferentation showed timing errors at shoulder and elbow joint reversals, resulting in large trajectory errors. The authors concluded that without proprioception, there is a reduced ability to control the interaction torques necessary for smooth interjoint coordination. Performance improved significantly with vision.

What does this information tell us about the role of kinesthetic feedback in reaching? It appears that it is not required for movement initiation and execution. However, it is still important for accurate reaching involving multiple joints. Individuals with peripheral sensory neuropathy are able to make accurate movements if they involve single joints or if they were able to compensate using vision; however, they show great problems in performing natural movements used in everyday life (Sanes et al., 1985).

Cognitive Contributions

Many types of cognitive problems can contribute to impaired reach and grasp in persons with neural pathology. The following section focuses on attentional contributions, specifically the effects of dual-task demands, on reach and grasp in persons with neural pathology.

Houwink and colleagues (2013) used a dual-task paradigm to assess automaticity of upper limb motor control in persons with mild to moderate stroke and nonimpaired controls. Participants made circular hand movements alone or in combination with an auditory Stroop task with the arm either unsupported or supported at the elbow and wrist. Dual-task interference was not present in either the participants with mild stroke or in the nonimpaired group in either condition of support. In contrast, in the unsupported condition, participants with moderate stroke showed significant dual-task interference when they used their affected compared to their nonaffected arm, suggesting reduced automaticity. Interestingly, when the paretic limb was supported at the elbow and wrist, dual-task interference was eliminated. The authors suggest that following moderate stroke, arm movements made with the paretic limb are less automatic and thus require more attentional resources than movements made with the nonparetic limb, which may contribute to learned disuse of the paretic limb. In addition, providing antigravity support reduces the attentional load associated with moving the paretic limb. In a similar fashion, cognitive-motor interference (i.e., limited capacity to engage cognitive and motor resources during a task) has also been reported during practice of robotic-aided reaching tasks performed simultaneously with numerical or speech-related tasks in participants with stroke. This finding suggests that following a stroke, target-directed reaches require greater cognitive resources (Shin et al., 2017).

Pohl and colleagues (2011) also examined the effects of secondary tasks on hand movements in 19 persons with poststroke hemiparesis. Participants performed a rhythmic hand movement (either pressing a small clicker between thumb and fingers or holding a music shaker in the palm of their hand) with the paretic and nonparetic hand under single- and two dual-task conditions (while walking and during a conversational speech task). In contrast to results by Houwink et al., Pohl did not find increased dual-task costs when participants moved with their paretic arm. As shown in Figure 19.12A, the rate of hand movement was the same in all three conditions when participants used their affected limb (Fig. 19.12A histograms on the left); thus, there was no dual task cost for hand movements made with the paretic limb and combined with either walking or speech. In contrast, there was a dual-task cost in the nonparetic limb (Fig. 19.12A histograms on the right and labeled less affected hand); the rate of hand movement in the nonparetic arm movement was increased during the walking (but not the speech) task. As shown in Figure 19.12B, when walking was combined with paretic hand movements, cadence decreased (middle histogram); there was no change in cadence when walking was combined with nonparetic hand movements (dark pink histogram on the far right). Hand movements, whether performed by the affected or nonaffected hand, did not affect speech rate (data not shown) (Pohl et al., 2011).

Results from these studies suggest that following stroke, dual-task effects on upper-extremity function depend on a number of factors including the severity of stroke, the specific combination of tasks being performed, whether the upper-extremity task is being performed with the paretic versus nonparetic arm, and the degree of support provided.

Among persons with PD, dual-task interference has been shown to affect a number of upper-extremity tasks including handwriting (Broeder et al., 2014), dexterity (Proud & Morris, 2010), and the control of grip forces (Pradhan et al., 2010, 2011). Pradhan and colleagues (2011) examined the effects of medication on attentional demands of precision and power grip tasks in persons with PD. An instrumented twist cap device was used to examine force control during precision and power grip trials performed alone or in combination with an auditory Stroop task. Participants were tested on and off medication. Participants with PD were significantly less accurate in controlling grip forces (both power and precision) under dual- compared

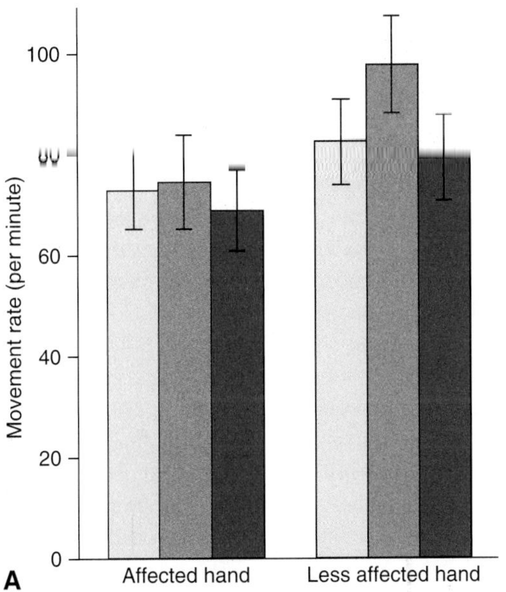

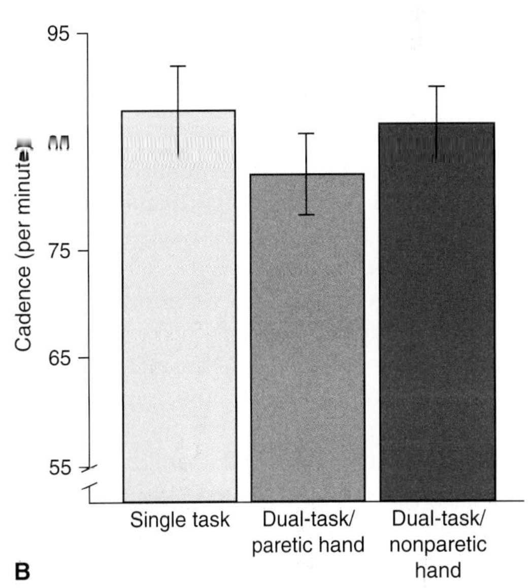

Figure 19.12 The effects of secondary tasks on hand movements in persons with poststroke hemiparesis. **(A)** Dual-task costs, as shown by change in rate of hand movements, are present when hand movements are made with the nonparetic hand (shown on right and labeled less affected hand) but not the paretic hand (shown on the left and labeled affected hand), where hand movement rate is the same across all three conditions. **(B)** Compared to the single task condition (left histogram), there was a dual-task cost to walking (decreased cadence) when hand movements were made with the paretic limb (middle histogram) but no change in cadence when movements were made with the nonparetic hand (histogram on the far right). (Adapted from Pohl PS, Kemper S, Siengsukon CF, et al. Dual-task demands of hand movements for adults with stroke: A Pilot Study. *Top Stroke Rehabil.* 2011;18: Fig. 1, page 242, Fig. 2, page 243.)

to single-task conditions. In addition, dual-task costs for response latency on the auditory Stroop task were greater for both grips when participants were on- compared to off medication, suggesting that even on medication, the control of forces for both power and precision grip tasks is attentionally demanding.

In order to understand the neural correlates of dual-task performance in PD, Wu and Hallett (2008) obtained fMRIs in 15 persons with PD and 14 nonimpaired controls, before and after practicing a simple and complex dual task. While 12 of the 15 participants with PD learned to perform the simpler dual task correctly, only 3 could perform the more complex task correctly. Functional MRIs indicated that both groups activated similar brain regions for all tasks, with an increased activation of bilateral precuneus during dual-task performance. Though brain regions were similar, persons with PD had greater activity in all brain regions compared to nonimpaired controls. Importantly, practice decreased dual-task costs and improved performance in persons with PD.

Lang and Bastian (2002) used a dual-task paradigm to examine the effect of practice on automaticity (attentional demands) in persons with cerebellar damage and nonimpaired controls. Participants stood and performed a figure 8 movement using their arm, under single- and dual-task (while performing an auditory vigilance task) conditions. Errors were recorded while participants practiced the movement task alone or in combination with the auditory task. Results demonstrated that practice resulted in only limited amounts of improvement in persons with cerebellar pathology compared to nonimpaired controls. In addition, under dual-task conditions, performance on the upper-extremity task declined to prepractice levels in persons with cerebellar damage while the nonimpaired controls showed no decline in the practiced tasks under dual-task conditions. The authors conclude that practicing upper-extremity motor tasks results in a reduction in attentional demands, and the cerebellum is critical to this practice-related shift toward automaticity (Lang & Bastian, 2002).

Interestingly, several studies reported that during the performance of upper-extremity tasks, persons with MS demonstrated significant impairments in motor control (greater force variability and motor overflow [involuntary movements]); however, the ability to perform upper-extremity motor tasks while concurrently performing a cognitive task appeared to be preserved (Stoquart-Elsankari et al., 2010; Ternes et al., 2014). In the study by Ternes and colleagues (2014), while performance on the motor task was preserved, persons with MS showed a decline in cognitive task performance (digit span test) under dual-task conditions, suggesting they may have prioritized the motor task at the expense of performance on the cognitive task.

In summary, these studies suggest that upper-extremity function is more attentionally demanding in persons with CNS pathology. Dual-task interference when upper-extremity tasks are performed concurrently with other tasks is present in some but not all persons with CNS pathology compared to nonimpaired individuals. Among persons with stroke, increased attentional demands associated with using the paretic limb may contribute to learned disuse. In addition, medication and practice may have only a limited effect on dual-task interference in some persons with CNS pathology.

Problems with Grasp

Appropriate regulation of grip force is essential in performance of various activities of daily living such as drinking, eating, and buttoning a shirt. For example, a number of researchers have described deficits in grasp following stroke, including slower and less accurate finger and hand movements, poorly modulated fingertip forces, and a reduced ability to control individual fingers (Hermsdörfer et al., 2003; Lang & Schieber, 2004; van Vliet & Sheridan, 2007). Not surprisingly, the degree of deficit shown is highly dependent on the severity of stroke. For example, among individuals with less severe paresis, the ability to scale grip aperture to object size for different grasp types is retained; however, timing deficits—including slowed MT, prolonged deceleration times, and earlier time to maximal grip aperture—remain (Michaelsen et al., 2009).

Because the greatest proportion of inputs from the corticospinal tract is to motor neuron pools of the distal upper segments, it has been reported that the severity of hemiparesis following stroke is most often greatest in the distal as compared with the proximal muscles (Colebatch & Gandevia, 1989). This has led to the hypothesis that after stroke, deficits in grasp, which rely on distal limb segments, are greater than those in reach, which rely on proximal segment motion. In contrast with this hypothesis, Lang et al. (2005) found that among persons with acute hemiparesis, the ability to perform a purposeful movement with the distal segments was not more disrupted than movements made with the proximal segments.

In examining the recovery of reach and grasp following stroke, these researchers reported that the majority of recovery in both reach and grasp occurred by the 90-day time point, with little change occurring between the 90-day and 1-year time points. Movement speed improved over time for both reach and grasp, as did deficits in accuracy in both components. In contrast, deficits in efficiency did not improve, and they were greater in grasp than reach (Lang et al., 2006).

Reach-and-grasp deficits may vary as a function of the side of the lesion, since hemispheric specialization appears to contribute to differential reach-and-grasp impairments following stroke. Tretriluxana and colleagues (2008, 2009) investigated the role of hemispheric specialization in visuomotor transformation of grasp preshaping and the coordination between transport and grasp in individuals after stroke. Components of grasp preshaping, including changes in aperture velocity and peak aperture relative to three different object dimensions, were measured in persons with right versus left hemiparesis. There were significant differences between the groups. MT were prolonged for the right- but not the left-stroke group. In addition, for the group with right-sided stroke, grasp preshaping began earlier but was less coordinated as compared with the group with left-sided stroke, whose primary deficit was in scaling grasp preshaping. The authors suggest that the left hemisphere is specialized for the visuomotor transformation of grasp preshaping while the right hemisphere specialization is related to transport–grasp coordination (Tretriluxana et al., 2009).

Bradykinesia contributes to slowing in both the reach-and-grasp components in individuals with PD, though the degree of slowing may be task dependent (Majsak et al., 2008; Rand et al., 2006, 2009). Majsak et al. (2008) reported that among persons with PD, slowing was present when reaching for a stationary object, but MT were comparable to those of controls when reaching for moving objects (Majsak et al., 2008). In addition, disease progression appears to affect grasp components more than reach components. Grasp was characterized by slower velocity of hand opening and closing, a smaller maximal aperture, a longer time to maximal aperture (Majsak et al., 2008), and increased variability in aperture timing and scaling as compared with nonimpaired individuals (Alberts et al., 2000).

Interestingly, even in a relatively advanced stage of the disease, persons with PD retain the ability to modify reach and grasp in response to object properties (Negrotti et al., 2005; Weiss et al., 2009). Medications, such as L-dopa, appear to improve the kinematics of reach more than grasp (Negrotti et al., 2005; Schettino et al., 2006), leading to the hypothesis that slowed reach in PD is in part a strategy used to compensate for deficiencies in the grasp component of the task (Negrotti et al., 2005). Aside from bradykinesia, limb-kinetic apraxia—defined as a loss of the ability to make precise, independent, and coordinated finger and hand movements—impairs activities of daily living that require dexterity (e.g., buttoning and unbuttoning). A study by Foki and colleagues (2016) investigated the relationship between limb-kinetic apraxia and bradykinesia with a coin rotation task versus a typical tapping task, in order to determine which task was the best predictor of movement dexterity during buttoning and unbuttoning. Results indicated that a tapping task revealed deficits in agonist-antagonist activations associated with bradykinesia. In contrast, a coin rotation task revealed deficits in limb-kinetic apraxia. In addition, the coin rotation task performed with the dominant hand was the only significant predictor of movement dexterity during a buttoning and unbuttoning task (Foki et al., 2016).

Studies have examined the reach-and-grasp behavior of children with CP and with other developmental delays (Cole et al., 1998, Eliasson et al., 1991; Jeannerod, 1986; Kearney & Gentile, 2003; Mackey et al., 2006; Petrarca et al., 2009; Ronnqvist & Rosblad, 2007; Saavedra et al., 2009; Verrel et al., 2008). These children show muscle weakness of both the more and less affected upper extremities (Dekkers et al., 2020). In some cases of mild impairment, hemiplegia is not readily identified until about 40 weeks, when the infant first begins to use the pincer grasp and manipulate objects (Jeannerod, 1990). In a 23-month-old child, the hand with hemiplegia was used only when the normal hand was immobilized, and even then, it was with great difficulty that the child grasped objects. Figure 19.13, adapted from film records, illustrates the child reaching for a prong from a pegboard with the nonparetic hand (Fig. 19.13A) and the hemiparetic hand (Fig. 19.13B), with visual feedback. Note that the nonparetic hand did not anticipate the shape of the object; a finger extension/flexion pattern was used instead. In addition, contact of the hand with the object caused the fingers to close around the object. The hemiplegic hand (Fig. 19.13B) also showed an exaggerated opening during the entire movement, with no anticipatory grasp formation. There was a very slight closing of the hand after contact with the object, giving a very clumsy

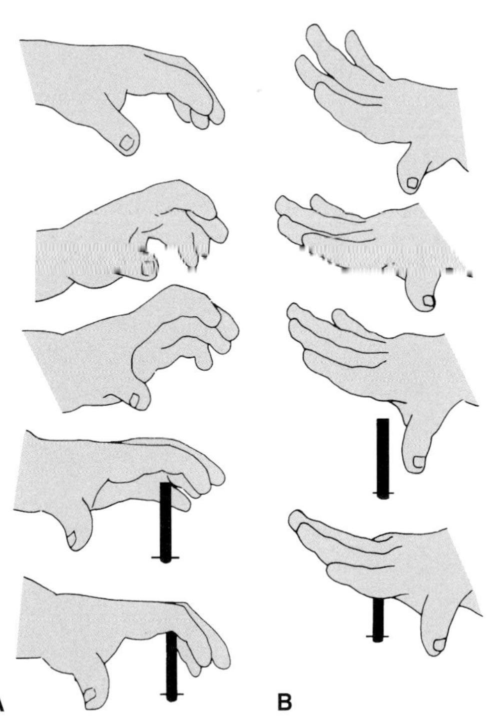

Figure 19.13 Drawing from film records of the reaches of a 23-month-old child with hemiplegia reaching for a prong from a pegboard with the nonparetic hand **(A)** and the paretic hand **(B)**. (Redrawn from Jeannerod M. *The neural and behavioral organization of goal-directed movements.* Oxford: Oxford University Press, 1990:72, with permission.)

grasp (Jeannerod, 1990). This type of impaired grasp can be seen in the upper-extremity section of the video case study of Malachi, our child with severe CP.

In a second child, 5 years of age, the hemiplegic hand showed more normal reach-and-grasp movements. The authors suggest that more normal movement patterns may be the result of many years of rehabilitation training (Jeannerod, 1990). Figure 19.14 depicts film records of her reaching movements with her normal hand (A) and her hemiplegic hand (B, C, and D). Note that reaching with the hemiplegic hand was affected only in relation to the pattern of grip formation. Finger shaping was abnormal, with the index finger extended in an exaggerated manner, and then flexing only slightly, if at all, before contacting the object. Because of these problems, the objects were sometimes dropped during the grasp (Jeannerod, 1990).

Hanna and colleagues (2003) also examined changes in hand function (Peabody fine-motor scores) and upper-extremity movement using the Quality of Upper Extremity Skills Test (QUEST; DeMatteo et al., 1992) in 51 children with CP (29 boys and 22 girls, mean age 36 months) studied prospectively four times over 10 months. Results indicated that hand function developed differently from overall upper-extremity function. Figure 19.15 compares Peabody fine-motor scores in

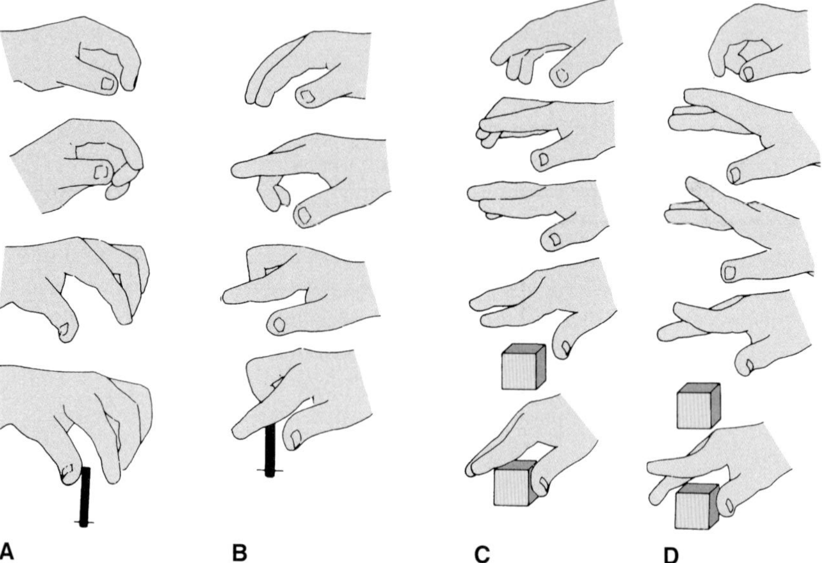

Figure 19.14 Drawing from film records of the reaches of a 5-year-old child with hemiplegia after many years of rehabilitation reaching with the nonaffected hand **(A)** and the affected hand **(B–D)**. (Redrawn from Jeannerod M. *The neural and behavioral organization of goal-directed movements.* Oxford, UK: Oxford University Press, 1990:73, with permission.)

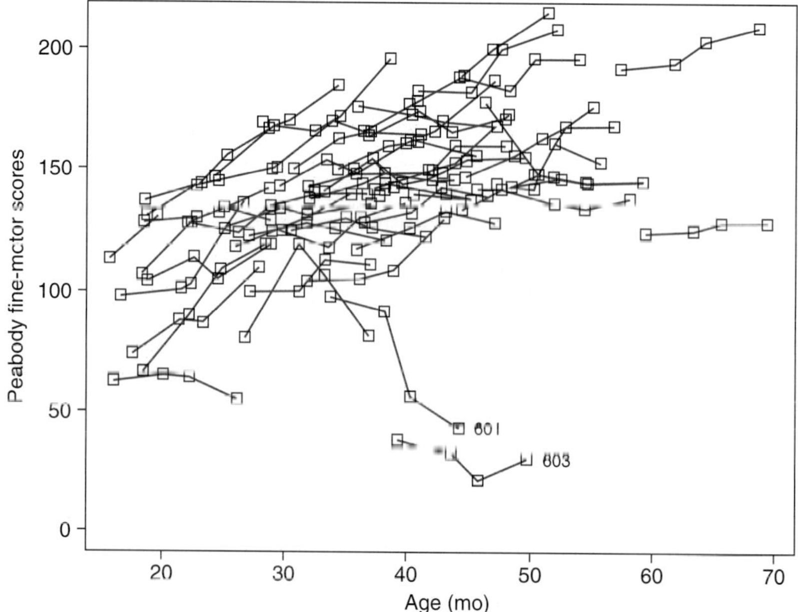

Figure 19.15 Changes in hand function in children with cerebral palsy studied four times over a 10-month period. Shown are observed Peabody fine-motor scores as a function of children's ages. Numbers 601 and 603 indicate the study numbers of children with atypical patterns of change. (Reprinted from Hanna SL, Law MC, Rosenbaum PL, et al. Development of hand function among children with cerebral palsy: growth curve analysis for ages 16 to 70 months. *Dev Med Child Neurol.* 2003;45:449, with permission.)

children with CP as a function of children's ages. At 16 months of age, children had a mean hand function score of 101.9 points and showed a positive improvement, on average, of 2.36 points per month. This average rate of improvement was slower in the older children while interindividual variation increased. In contrast to the hand function measures, measures of upper-extremity movement using QUEST scores demonstrated significant interindividual variability across all ages.

Experiments have been performed in which the reach-and-grasp skills of persons with lesions in the somatosensory pathways at brainstem levels and at parietal cortex levels were examined. In the individual with a lesion at the brainstem level, the hand ipsilateral to the lesion was affected. When vision was present, grasp formation was normal, as shown in Figure 19.16A, except that it was longer in duration than it was in the normal hand. However, without vision, the grasping movements were critically changed (Fig. 19.16B and C). Finger grip was either absent altogether or incomplete. In the first reach the person made with no visual feedback, there was no grip formation at all, while in the second reach, there was incomplete grip formation (Jeannerod, 1990).

Individuals with lesions to the parietal lobe, particularly the postcentral gyrus and the supramarginal gyrus, show patterns for reach and grasp that are similar to persons with peripheral sensory problems. In a detailed study on the recovery of reach and grasp in an individual with a parietal lobe lesion, researchers found that the she did not use her right hand spontaneously immediately following her lesion but later used it in many actions, as long as she had visual feedback. Without visual control, her movements were very awkward. For example, she could not sustain repetitive tapping movements unless she could see or hear her fingers moving (Jeannerod, 1990).

In contrast to individuals with peripheral deafferentation, who could grip normally as long as visual feedback was present, grip formation was impaired in an individual with a parietal lesion, even with visual feedback present (Jeannerod, 1990). Figure 19.17A shows the grasp component of a reach with the nonimpaired hand, while B and C show the grasp of the affected hand both with and without visual feedback. When this individual had visual feedback while reaching with the affected hand, she made grasps using the whole palm of the hand. Without visual feedback, only the initial part of the transportation phase was normal. Then, the hand seemed to "wander above the object, without a grasp" (Jeannerod, 1990, p. 207). Thus, loss of sensory information results in abnormal grip-and-lift forces and problems in the control of fine movements of the hand.

Problems with Precision Grip and Lift

As discussed in Chapter 17, the ability to produce and regulate force is an important aspect of tasks in which an object has to be grasped and lifted. Tactile sensation from the fingertips is particularly important when lifting objects with a precision grip in order to adjust the amplitude of forces used to grip and lift. If grip force is too tight, the object cannot be manipulated; if it is too loose, the object will be dropped. In a precision grip, forces for gripping and lifting are generated simultaneously and appear to be very dependent on cutaneous input.

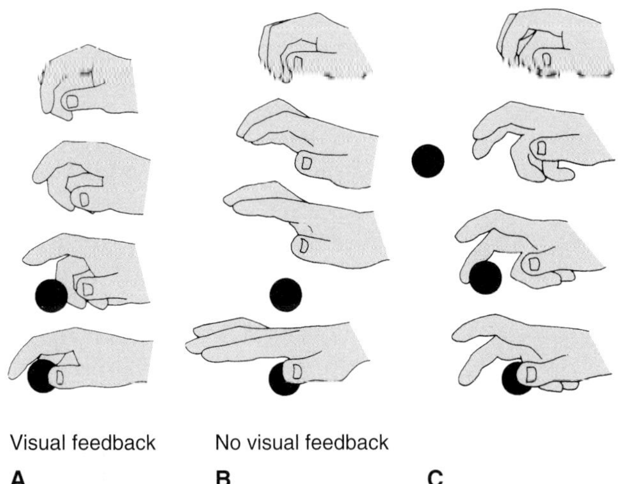

Figure 19.16 Drawing from film records of the grip patterns of an individual with a lesion of the somatosensory pathway at the brainstem level. **(A)** With vision, grasp was normal. **(B and C)** Without vision, grasp was absent or incomplete. (Redrawn from Jeannerod M. *The neural and behavioral organization of goal-directed movements.* Oxford, UK: Oxford University Press, 1990:205, with permission.)

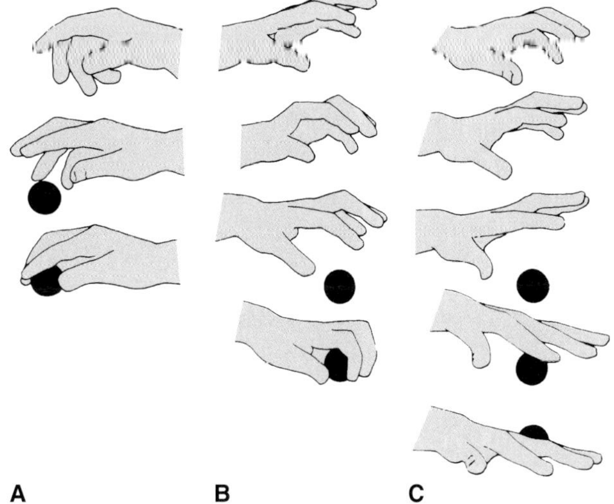

Figure 19.17 Drawing of the grip patterns of an individual with a parietal lobe lesion. **(A)** Normal hand, visual feedback. **(B)** Affected hand, visual feedback. **(C)** Affected hand, no visual feedback. (Redrawn from Jeannerod M. *The neural and behavioral organization of goal-directed movements.* Oxford, UK: Oxford University Press, 1990:208, with permission.)

Many studies have reported deficits in the control of grip-and-lift forces in a wide variety of persons with CNS pathology (see Weisendanger & Serrien, 2004 for a review). For example, disruptions to the initiation and sequencing of grip-and-lift forces have been reported in individuals with PD. Grip forces in persons with PD are much greater than those of nonimpaired individuals, and force development is slower (Rand et al., 2009; Weiss et al., 2009). Despite these deficits, individuals with PD were able to adapt grip force to load conditions (Weiss et al., 2009). Ingvarsson and colleagues (1997) reported frequent oscillations and fluctuations in the force profiles associated with grip-and-lift movements in participants with PD while off medication. The amplitude of oscillations decreased when participants were on medication, suggesting the oscillations were due to action tremor superimposed on the force trajectories.

Fellows et al. (1998) investigated force development in 16 individuals with PD and 12 age-matched controls. Subjects performed a grip-and-lift task under conditions in which the weight of the object was altered both with and without warning. Results for the grip-and-lift task under the four conditions (expecting and lifting a light load [labeled Light in Fig. 19.18], expecting and lifting a heavy load [labeled Heavy], expecting a heavy load and lifting a light load [labeled Unload], and expecting a light load and lifting a heavy load [labeled Load]) are shown in Figure 9.18. Participants with PD, like the nonimpaired participants, lifted the unpredictable load using grip force parameters they had used in the preceding lift. Both groups were able to modulate grip forces to the new load during the lift. However, participants with PD required a significantly longer time to develop grip force as compared with nonimpaired participants in all conditions. In addition, they showed significantly higher levels of grip force during the lift phase of the movement, indicating a higher safety margin, but were capable of modulating grip forces to match changes in the object weight.

Impaired control of forces during precision grip has also been reported following stroke (Buckingham et al., 2015; Dispa et al., 2014; Eidenmüller et al., 2014; Raghavan et al., 2006). Seo and colleagues reported significantly impaired grip force development in the paretic hand in individuals with hemiparesis. Impaired force control was observed regardless of grip size, grip force level, and object stability and resulted in slips in 55% of all trials (Seo et al., 2010).

Children with CP also show excessive and oscillatory grip forces (Eliasson et al., 1991). Eliasson et al. also found that in contrast to children who were typically developing, children with CP did not coordinate grip-and-lift forces simultaneously, but sequentially. The authors suggested that these excessive grip forces, establishing a high safety margin against slips, may be compensatory to unstable motor output. This type of safety margin has been reported in older adults and in typically developing children under the age of 5, who also show oscillations in force control.

In PD, and other brain-related disorders like Olivo-Ponto-Cerebellar degeneration, studies have shown that people demonstrate reduced stability of multifinger force-stabilizing synergies, decreased finger individuation (i.e., enslaving), and delayed and reduced

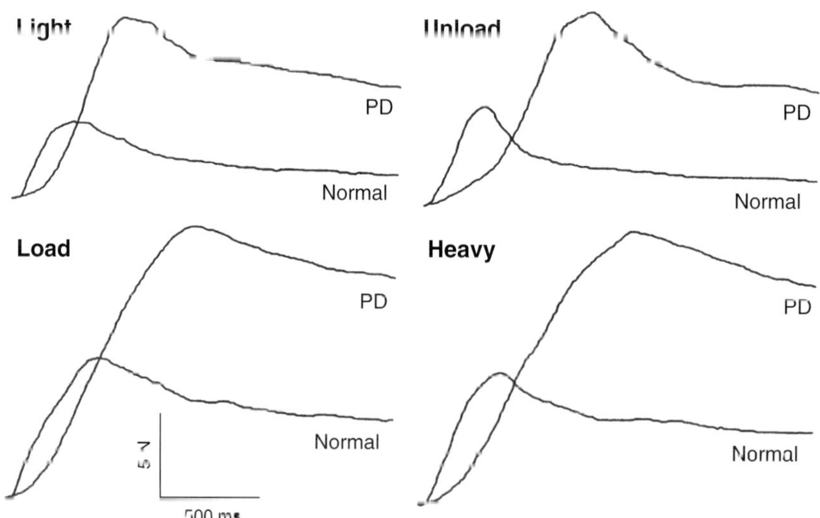

Figure 19.18 Mean grip force curves for an individual with PD and an age matched nonimpaired individual, obtained from five lifts performed under four conditions (expecting and lifting a light load [Light], expecting and lifting a heavy load [Heavy], expecting a heavy load and lifting a light load [Unload], and expecting a light load and lifting a heavy load [Load]). As expected, for both individuals with Parkinson's disease and nonimpaired controls, peak grip force values were higher for the heavier loads as compared with values for lighter loads (compare "Heavy" traces with "Light"). Individuals with Parkinson's disease tended to produce inappropriately high grip forces compared with nonimpaired controls in all conditions. *5 N*, 5 Newtons. (Redrawn from Fellows SJ, Noth J, Schwarz M. Precision grip and Parkinson's disease. *Brain*. 1998;121:1776, with permission.)

anticipatory adjustments of synergies prior to rapid finger force generation (de Freitas et al., 2020; Park et al., 2012, 2013). Neuromotor disorders characterized mainly by cortical damage such as stroke or CP also show decreased maximal finger force production and enslaving; but interestingly, these individuals do not show impaired multifinger synergies for stable force production (Jo et al., 2016; Kong et al., 2019).

Iyengar and colleagues (2009) examined the regulation of grip-and-lift forces in persons with MS as they performed two tasks: lifting and placing an instrumented object on a shelf and lifting the object and bringing it close to the mouth to mimic drinking. Results demonstrated that persons with MS used significantly larger peak grip force than nonimpaired control subjects while performing both tasks and for both hands. The authors suggest that the use of excessive grip force could contribute to fatigue and musculoskeletal overuse trauma in persons with MS.

Several studies have reported impaired control of load and grip forces in persons with mild MS (Expanded Disability Status Scale scores of < 5), resulting in overgripping objects (Krishnan et al., 2008; Marwaha et al., 2006). Persons with mild MS displayed poorer task performance (as assessed by the ability to produce appropriate task-specific load forces) and impaired force coordination (indicated by impaired coupling of grip and load forces) compared to nonimpaired individuals (Krishnan & Jaric, 2008).

What are some of the other factors that contribute to impairments in force regulation during grip-and-lift tasks? A number of studies suggest sensory deficits as a primary cause.

Sensory Deficits and Precision Grip. How does loss of somatosensation affect precision grip? It appears that, in addition to impaired force production, impaired somatosensation and large-fiber sensory loss contribute to reduced hand function and positioning following stroke (Blennerhassett et al., 2007; Miall et al., 2019; Robertson & Jones, 1994). In individuals with poststroke hemiparesis, reduced somatosensation, specifically impaired friction discrimination ability, contributed to altered timing and force adjustment during tasks that required a precision pinch grip (Blennerhassett et al., 2007). A study compared object manipulation in the more-impaired hand in people with right versus left hemispheric stroke (Cunha et al., 2019). Regardless of the brain hemisphere damaged (right or left), people with stroke showed similar capability for generating gripping forces and coordinating grip and load forces. Interestingly, participants with left-brain stroke presented a delayed onset in lifting the object. Hence, the authors suggested that people with left-sided stroke might require more time to register somatosensory information from the time of contact with the object. In addition, reduced somatosensation (pressure sensitivity and two-point discrimination) significantly affected the regulation of grip-and-lift forces. While the ability to adapt forces correlated with poor performance on object recognition tests, it did not predict performance on functional hand tests, such as the Jebsen–Taylor test (Robertson & Jones, 1994).

Lesions of the anterior parietal lobe result in somatosensory deficits that limit precision grip and in-hand manipulation skills (Jeannerod, 1996). Pause et al. (1989) referred to these motor impairments due to central sensory deficits as tactile apraxia. In contrast, lesions of the posterior parietal area produce spatial disorientation and impaired reach, specifically the ability to shape the hand according to object size and configuration. Deficits are more severe in the absence of visual feedback from the limb (Jeannerod, 1996). Damage to posterior parietal areas produces a disconnection between visual and proprioceptive inputs, so that limb and object positions in space are no longer matched with each other. Thus, the importance of the posterior parietal lobe is in organizing object-oriented action. Sakata et al. (1985) suggest that neurons in this area are able to integrate visual and motor signals related to object-oriented action, thus linking sensory information on object properties with corresponding motor commands. Detailed information on the neural basis for object-oriented action is provided in Chapters 3 and 17.

Impaired Anticipatory Control of Precision Grip. As discussed in Chapters 17 and 18, the development of precision grip and manipulation depends on the availability of both tactile information (from both slow- and fast-adapting afferents, which convey information on texture) and weight-related information (from muscle spindles and tactile afferents) (Johansson, 1996). During an ongoing lift, small slips between the skin and the object result in activation of cutaneous receptors, which causes the grip force to be increased. Activity in the dorsolateral pathway (ventral premotor area and anterior intraparietal area) is critical to the coordination of grasp-and-lift actions (Marneweck & Grafton, 2020b). When controlling grip-and-lift forces, the CNS does not rely only on reactive hand adjustments to the object's dynamics. Sensorimotor information is used in the development of internal representations about the object's physical characteristics to generate accurate motor predictions. In a series of object lifts, expectations based on internal representations of the object are used to preprogram grip-and-lift forces. Among the different neural substrates that may take part in this anticipatory process, the cerebellum seems to be crucial to form an internal model to further create and update effective predictive grip force control for subsequent lifts (Marneweck & Grafton, 2020a). Thus, scaling of forces is also performed prior to the lift and is dependent on both sensorimotor memory (internal representations) and current sensory (visual and tactile) information (Gordon et al., 1997). As discussed in

Chapter 18, anticipatory control emerges with development. By 6 to 8 years of age, anticipatory control of fingertip forces (both pinch and vertical lift) is adult-like (Forssberg et al., 1992; Gordon et al., 1992).

Gordon and Duff (1999a) studied anticipatory grip-and-lift forces in 15 children, ages 8 to 14 years, with spastic hemiplegic CP. They found that children with CP were initially impaired in their ability to scale forces during the first few trials of a grip-and-lift task. However, they eventually learned to use anticipatory control of load forces based on the texture and weight of an object, but only after extended practice with the object.

Duff and Gordon (2003) also investigated the effects of practice on anticipatory aspects of grasp in children with hemiparetic CP who were learning to grasp novel objects. In this study, 18 children with hemiparetic CP practiced lifting three novel objects of varying weight but constant volume 27 times using either a blocked or random practice schedule. Children with CP were able to form and retain internal representation of novel objects for anticipatory control of grasp, but anticipatory control was not as well differentiated in the children with CP as compared with age-matched typically developing children. They also reported that while blocked practice was superior during the acquisition of novel grasp tasks, retention was comparable in both practice types, leading the authors to conclude that for children with hemiparetic CP, the amount of practice is more important than the type of practice when learning to grasp novel objects.

What is the basis for the deficits found in children with CP in initial ability to scale the rate of force to the weight of the object to be lifted? Gordon and Duff (1999a) report no clear relationship between degree of spasticity and anticipatory control of grip and lift in children with CP suggesting that spasticity while present was not the major factor related to impaired grip and lift. In addition, they found that sensory information from the less affected hand could transfer to improved anticipatory scaling of forces by the contralateral (affected) hand in subsequent manipulations (Gordon and Duff 1999a). These two findings suggest that sensory deficits account for many problems related to precision grip and lift.

The assumption that sensory deficits are a major factor in impaired precision grip in children with CP is supported by results from a study by Eliasson and Gordon (2000), who found impaired tactile regulation of isometric fingertip forces during grasping in these children. They suggest that children with CP who have sensory impairments may not be able to extract enough information during initial manipulatory experiences to form internal representations of the object's properties. Instead, they appear to require considerable practice to form accurate internal representations of objects.

Impaired anticipatory control of precision grip is also present in persons with poststroke hemiparesis (Buckingham et al., 2015; Dispa et al., 2014; Eidenmüller et al., 2014; Raghavan et al., 2006). Eidenmüller and colleagues (2014) compared anticipatory grip force scaling when lifting everyday objects in persons with right versus left hemiparesis and age-matched controls and reported that impaired grip force scaling was present in persons with left-brain damage (right hemiparesis) but not in those with right-brain damage (left hemiparesis), suggesting that the left hemisphere is engaged in anticipatory grip force scaling for lifting everyday objects. In contrast, Buckingham and colleagues (2015) reported that impaired anticipatory grip forces were present in both groups of participants, those with right-brain damage and those with left-brain damage. Raghavan et al. (2006) reported impaired anticipatory grip force control in the paretic hand in persons with right hemiparesis (left-brain damage). Interestingly, when participants practiced precision grip with the nonparetic hand, control of anticipatory grip forces was better in the paretic hand. The authors suggest that during rehabilitation, practice with the left (nonaffected) hand prior to practice with the right (affected) hand may improve planning of grasping behavior in patients with right hemiparesis.

Impaired Adaptation. Daily life activities require us to continually modify and adapt how we reach and grasp to changing task conditions. Vision modulates how the CNS enhances object-related tactile sensitivity before grasping objects. The disruption of visual information impairs both the ability to scale forces and the perception of an object's weight (Juravle et al. 2018; van Polanen et al., 2019). Objects to be picked up and manipulated vary in size, shape, and weight. This necessitates the ability to adjust to uncertain and changing conditions, and this is done through practice. During trial–error practice, the CNS creates implicit sensorimotor memories. A study compared young and elderly participants during performance of an object lifting task in which the object's COM was randomly varied between trials to bias the tilting point of the object (Schneider et al., 2019). After each lift, the participants had to indicate the perceived COM location and weight of the object. The authors found that sensorimotor torque memories associated with lifting errors significantly impaired not only the perception of torques and weight but also the planning of the torque in the subsequent lifting task. This suggests that impairments that alter the ability to create, adjust, and update the sensorimotor plan controlling the interactive torques between the object's surface and our fingers will hamper object manipulation during activities of daily living.

Cerebellar pathology reduces a person's ability to adjust to novel loads through trial-and-error practice (Bastian, 2002; Lang & Bastian, 1999, 2001). Bastian and colleagues used a catching task to examine adaptation to a novel load (light vs. heavy ball). The experimental setup is shown in Figure 19.19A. Participants caught a ball dropped vertically. Adaptation was determined from measures of impact displacement, and the rate of adaptation was defined by how quickly impact

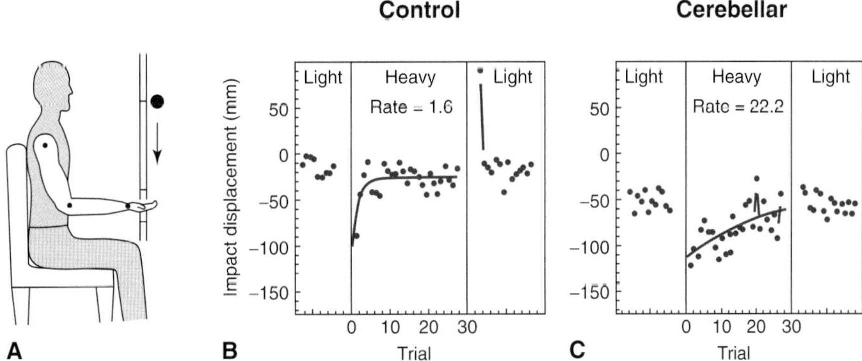

Figure 19.19 Experimental setup for adaptation of a catching task. Participants sit and catch a ball, which is dropped vertically **(A)**. Impact displacement values are plotted as a function of trials. A nonimpaired individual **(B)** catches a light ball initially **(left panel)** and then adapts within two trials to catching a heavy ball **(middle panel)**. When the light ball is reintroduced **(right panel)**, the person shows a large negative impact displacement on the first trial. In contrast, the individual with cerebellar pathology **(C)** requires 22 trials to adapt to the heavy ball **(middle panel)** and has no negative impact displacement on the first trial when the light ball is reintroduced **(right panel)**. (Adapted from Bastian AJ. Cerebellar limb ataxia: abnormal control of self-generated and external forces. *Ann NY Acad Sci.* 2002;978:23, 24.)

displacement changed after exposure to a new ball. Figure 19.19 compares impact displacement in a nonimpaired participant (B) and a person with cerebellar pathology (C) as participants initially caught a light ball (left panel), adapted to a heavy ball (middle), and then were reintroduced to the light ball (right). As can be seen in the middle panel, when learning to catch a heavy ball after exposure to a light ball, the participant with cerebellar pathology adapted much more slowly as compared with the nonimpaired person. Nonimpaired participants adapted rapidly (average 1.6 trials) as compared with participants with cerebellar pathology (average 24.6 trials). In addition, when the light ball was reintroduced, the nonimpaired participants showed a large aftereffect (large impact displacement in the first trial of the right panel) while individuals with cerebellar pathology did not. These results support the hypothesis that the cerebellum is important in the ability to adapt movements to changing task demands through practice.

PROBLEMS WITH IN-HAND MANIPULATION

In nonimpaired individuals, prehension and in-hand manipulation are associated with a complex interaction between the fingers in order to isolate motion (Hager-Ross & Schieber, 2000; Schieber, 1995) and coordinate forces (Scholz et al., 2002). While mechanical coupling may be responsible for limitations in finger independence in typical individuals (Lang & Schieber, 2004), after a subcortical stroke, adults show greater deficits in finger individuation (Raghavan, 2007), perhaps stemming from disruptions in corticomotoneuronal loops. In contrast, persons with Down syndrome (DS) show a less complex pattern of interfinger coordination in which forces within individual fingers are not independently modifiable; rather, force control among the fingers is linked but can be modified with practice (Latash et al., 2002).

Carpinella and colleagues (2014) used inertial sensors to compare task performance and subphases of movements (reaching, manipulation, transport, release, and return) in 21 persons with MS and 12 nonimpaired volunteers while performing the Arm Research Action Test (a clinical measure of upper-extremity function discussed in Chapter 20). Compared to nonimpaired controls, persons with MS were significantly slower (on average 70% increase in task duration) and less smooth when performing all tasks. Poor task performance was primarily due to problems in the manipulation phase of movements (Carpinella et al., 2014).

Problems with Release

Gordon and colleagues (1997) studied task-dependent problems during release of an object in persons with PD, both on and off medication. Results showed that impairments in grasping and releasing objects were dependent on the task condition. Coordination of grip and load forces in persons with PD approximated those of nonimpaired adults during object replacement and release at preferred speeds. In contrast, when instructed to move as quickly as possible, release was significantly slower as compared with nonimpaired adults. These findings were consistent with those of Kunesch and colleagues (1995), who also found that release of an isotonic force was impaired in persons with PD. Impaired release is apparent in the upper-extremity section of the video case study on Mike, our individual with PD. 

Eliasson and Gordon (2000) examined object release in children between 8 and 14 years of age who had hemiplegic CP. They found that these children tended to replace objects abruptly as compared with controls, and they took a longer time to release objects from finger contact. In a follow-up study (Gordon et al., 2003), the speed (self-paced and as fast as possible) and accuracy requirements (stable and unstable release surface) of the task were altered. The authors found that the impairments in temporal coordination of replacement and release of the novel object were greater and significantly different from those of typically developing children when the speed and accuracy requirements were higher. Interestingly, impairments in release were also found in the less affected hand. Impaired release of objects can be seen in the upper-extremity section of Malachi's video case study.

INTERLIMB COUPLING AND BIMANUAL TASKS

Bimanual coordination is required in many activities of daily living, such as when someone needs to tie their shoe laces. This type of activity requires dexterous string-pulling behaviors (Singh et al., 2019). In normal conditions, bimanual control requires coordination between upper limb motion and vision. Thus, the CNS allocates and switches the attentional focus between intrinsic muscle coordinates for movement performance and extrinsic visual coordinates for the goal-directed bimanual task (Sakurada & Kansaku, 2020; Sakurada et al., 2016). In addition, movement preparation takes more time when a bimanual reaching task requires asymmetric compared to symmetric reaching movements (Blinch et al., 2018). Impaired performance on bimanual tasks has been reported in a number of neurologic populations including stroke, CP, and MS. For instance, impaired control of grip-load forces during the performance of bimanual tasks has been reported in persons with MS (Gorniak et al., 2014).

Researchers have studied the effect of coupling the paretic and nonparetic limbs during bimanual reaching in individuals with hemiparesis in order to determine whether paretic arm reaching improves under the bilateral condition as compared with the unilateral condition (Gosser & Rice, 2015; Harris et al., 2005; Rose & Winstein, 2004; Utley & Sugden, 1998; Wu et al., 2008). Rose and Winstein (2004) compared unimanual to bimanual aiming in individuals with hemiparesis secondary to a cerebrovascular accident (CVA) and found that during bimanual reaches, the less affected limb extended its movement time to allow nearly simultaneous target contact. When the bimanual condition was compared with the unimanual condition, peak velocity decreased for the less affected limb and increased for the affected limb.

Similar results were recorded by Gosser and Rice (2015) who showed that among participants with stroke, the unimpaired limb accommodated its movements to that of the less efficient paretic limb during bimanual conditions. While there was no difference in paretic limb movement parameters in unimanual and bimanual tasks, the nonimpaired limb was less efficient in the bimanual task compared to the unimanual task. The authors suggest that following stroke, motor efficiency in the unimpaired upper extremity may be adversely influenced when yoked with the impaired limb during symmetrical bimanual tasks. Thus, subtle task-dependent motor impairments may be apparent in the nonimpaired limb (Gosser & Rice, 2015).

The authors of studies using animal stroke models propose the training of dexterous bimanual tasks to prevent movement disuse and to encourage functional improvements with the paretic hand (Dutcher et al., 2021). Metrot et al. (2013) investigated the recovery of unimanual and bimanual reaching tasks over the first 3 months of standard rehabilitation treatment following a stroke. Beginning about 3 weeks poststroke, 12 participants receiving a standard rehabilitation program for mild to moderate hemiparesis (9 men, age 65.6 ± 9.7 years) underwent eight kinematic assessments of reach-to-grasp movements (once a week for 6 weeks [week 0 to week 6] with a follow-up assessment at 3 months). The experimental setup is shown in Figure 19.20A. Participants grasped a 5-cm diameter ball and moved it at a self-selected speed, 20 cm to a target under three conditions: unimanual with the nonparetic limb (UN), unimanual with the paretic limb (UP), and bimanual movement (BN/BP). During bimanual reaching, participants were asked to simultaneously initiate the movement of both upper limbs and to hold the ball with both hands. A belt prevented compensatory trunk movements. Kinematic analysis measured MT and segmental characteristics of the movement including the number of velocity peaks (NVPs), the maximal reaching velocity (Vmax), and the directness of the trajectory (DT).

Results (shown in Fig. 19.20B) demonstrated that bimanual reaches were performed more slowly, with more segmented movements, compared to unimanual reaches. With respect to the recovery, on average over the eight sessions, reaching movements in both arms became smoother, faster, and more stable. In addition, movement characteristics were similar in both paretic and nonparetic hands in both the uni- and bimanual conditions. However, initially (first 3 weeks of rehabilitation), the paretic and nonparetic limbs operated asymmetrically during bimanual reaching, after which the kinematics of the two hands became similar. The authors suggest that improvements in reaching were likely a combination of both spontaneous recovery (which is maximum during the first 4 weeks of recovery) (Krakauer, 2006) and practice-dependent neural plasticity (Metrot et al., 2013).

Similar to the findings on adults with poststroke hemiparesis, Utley and Sugden (1998) reported that during bimanual reaches in children with CP, the affected

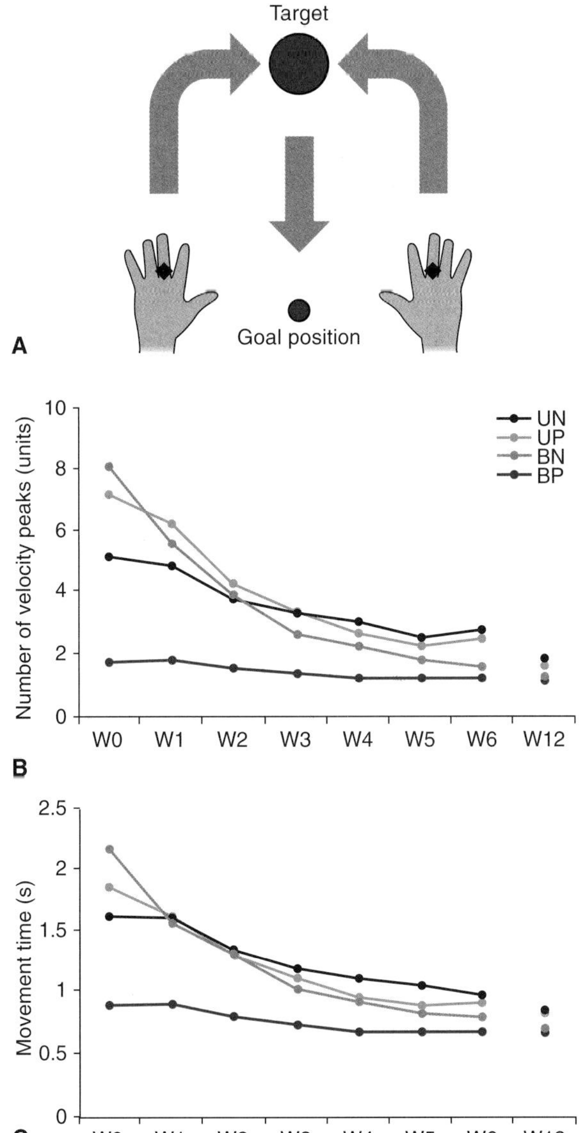

Figure 19.20 **(A)** The experimental setup used to examine the recovery of bimanual skills following stroke. **(B)** Number of velocity peaks for a unimanual task performed with the nonparetic hand (labeled *UN* and shown in *black*) and the paretic hand (labeled *UP* and shown in *gray*) and for a bimanual task for both the nonparetic (labeled *BN* and shown in *light orange*) and paretic hand (labeled *BP* and shown in *dark orange*). Number of velocity peaks **(B)** and movement time **(C)** plateau after 3 weeks of standard rehabilitation. (Adapted from Metrot J, Mottet D, Hauret I, et al. Changes in bimanual coordination during the first 6 weeks after moderate hemiparetic stroke. *Neurorehabil Neural Repair.* 2013;27:251–259.)

limb sped up and the less affected limb slowed down during bimanual reaching tasks, resulting in greater coupling between limbs. Interestingly, speed may improve coordination during bimanual tasks. Hung et al. (2004) examined the coordination of involved and noninvolved hands during a bimanual task in children with hemiplegic CP (mean age 13 years) and 10 age-matched typically developing children. Children were asked to reach forward and open a drawer with one hand and then activate a light switch inside the drawer with the contralateral hand. The children with hemiplegic CP were slower and less coordinated than the typically developing children. However, when asked to complete the task as fast as possible, the faster speed facilitated better bimanual coordination.

Finally, Klevberg and colleagues (2018) investigated the development of bimanual performance in children with unilateral or bilateral CP. They found that performance on tasks of bimanual hand function (Manual Ability Classification System [Mini-MACS/MACS], Assisting Hand Assessment [AHA], or Both Hands Assessment [BoHA]) at 19 months predicted the development of hand use in CP. In both unilateral and bilateral CP, children who were classified as level I in Mini-MACS/MACS and scored high in AHA or BoHA reached the highest limits of performance. Overall, children with bilateral CP were more impaired than those with unilateral CP, and children who showed symmetric hand use reached the highest developmental limits.

Reach and Grasp in the Ipsilesional Nonhemiparetic Limb

Traditionally, it was believed that impairments associated with unilateral cerebral lesions were limited to the limb contralateral to the lesion. However, as noted in many of the studies in this chapter, researchers are finding subtle deficits affecting the ability to reach on the nonhemiparetic side and the ipsilesional limb (Giulliani et al., 1993; Gordon et al., 1999; Haaland et al., 2004; Nowak et al., 2007; Quaney et al., 2005; Sunderland, 2000). For example, a study examining motor problems in the ipsilesional nonhemiparetic limb has suggested that weakness is a contributing factor in reaching problems in both the nonparetic and paretic limb (Giulliani et al., 1993). Other studies have found that problems in reaching in the ipsilesional nonparetic arm following unilateral hemispheric lesion may involve other factors as well.

The severity of a stroke is a major factor in determining the extent to which the more-impaired or less-impaired hand is used in real-life reaching situations. Demartino and colleagues (2019) found that people with mild or moderate stroke tend to use the paretic upper extremity more frequently for whole-hand stabilization (71.2%) compared to digital grasping (28.8%). This finding was shown for both the paretic and nonparetic limbs in the moderate group, but only in the paretic upper limb in the mild group. In addition, digital grasping with the nonparetic upper limb was more frequently observed during reach-to-grasp actions only in people with mild stroke. Finally, the study showed that the spontaneous use of the paretic hand in people with severe stroke is limited.

Gordon et al. (1999) studied the coordination of fingertip forces during object manipulation in both affected and nonaffected hands of children with hemiplegic CP. They found subtle deficits in sequencing of grip-and-lift movements in the nonaffected hand. Sunderland (2000) studied dexterity and apraxia in the ipsilesional hands of 24 persons following an acute stroke. All showed initial deficits in the ipsilesional hand on tests of dexterity and apraxia; however, most had recovered by 6 months after the stroke. Seven individuals, all of whom had left hemispheric damage, continued to show persistent problems related to dexterity and apraxia in the ipsilesional hand.

Bilateral impairments in hand function found in both children with CP and in adults who have had a unilateral stroke are not surprising, considering that 10% to 30% of fibers in the lateral corticospinal tract are uncrossed. These data support an anatomical substrate for bilateral impairment in hand function in individuals with lesions affecting one hemisphere.

APRAXIA

In the preceding sections, our discussion of abnormal reach and grasp has related to the examination of problems in each of the constituent components: visual regard, reach, grasp, manipulation, and release. However, the use of the upper extremity in the performance of simple everyday tasks is more than the simple summation of these components. It requires the integration of these components into an action plan. An action plan specifies the conceptual content of the action, along with its hierarchical and sequential organization (Poizner et al., 1990). The left cerebral cortex includes structures specialized for higher-order motor programming or the formation of action plans (Schwartz et al., 1991).

Researchers have studied the nature of these motor programs by analyzing the types of errors made by persons with left hemispheric damage. Disorders that result from dysfunction of this specialized left hemisphere have been termed apraxias. One type of apraxia that has been studied extensively is ideational apraxia, also referred to as frontal apraxia (Luria, 1966) or frontal lobe executive disorder (Wilkins et al., 1987). This is a disorder of the execution of movement that cannot be attributed to weakness, incoordination or sensory loss, or poor language comprehension or inattention to commands.

To understand this disorder, it is helpful to first appreciate what occurs when a nonimpaired adult decides to perform a task. The first step involves forming the intention to perform the task and then formulating an action plan. The essential requirement of an action plan is that it specifies the goal of the action along with the hierarchical and sequential organization of nested actions that are required to achieve the ultimate goal. Intentions, as defined by activated action plans, are an integral feature of all purposeful behavior. It has been hypothesized that the core of the intentional disorder of frontal apraxia is a weakening of the top-down formulation of action plans—that is, an inability to sustain the intent to the completion of the action plan (Schwartz et al., 1991).

Because intent to act cannot be sustained, irrelevant objects exert a strong influence on the action plan, and this leads to numerous performance errors. Researchers have begun to develop a system for coding performance errors based on this concept of hierarchically organized units of action within an action plan. These studies have enumerated examples of errors during the performance of common activities of daily living, including buttering hot coffee; putting clothes on backward or inside out; drinking from an empty cup; skipping key steps during activities such as shaving, toothbrushing, or hair brushing; using a fork to eat cereal; putting toothpaste on a razor; scrubbing the upper lip and chin with a toothbrush; eating toothpaste; and applying arm deodorant over a shirt (Schwartz et al., 1991). In a classic paper, Luria (1966) describes the behavior of an individual with frontal apraxia who would light a candle and put it in his mouth to perform the habitual movements of smoking a cigarette.

Haaland and colleagues (Wetter et al., 2005) compared dexterity using the Jebsen–Taylor hand function test in adults with left versus right hemispheric damage, with and without apraxia. Dexterity impairments were similar with damage to the right and left hemisphere; however, individuals with left hemispheric damage and apraxia exhibited greater impairments than those with left hemispheric damage but without apraxia.

Pizzamiglio and colleagues (2020) investigated perceptual and action-related factors in hand movements during a reach-to-grasp task in people with left-sided stroke, with and without apraxia. Participants were instructed to grasp the top or bottom of a cup and either lift it or turn it over, resulting in either a comfortable or uncomfortable hand position at the completion of the task (end-state comfort). The effect of compatibility between the initial hand-cup orientation and end-state comfort on action selection was examined. Individuals with stroke and apraxia showed increased errors and delayed responses when there was poor compatibility between initial orientation and end-state comfort compared to both participants with stroke but no apraxia and age-matched healthy participants.

A CASE STUDY APPROACH TO UNDERSTANDING UPPER-EXTREMITY DISORDERS

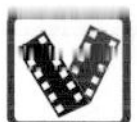 Jean J and Genise T: Reach-and-Grasp Problems Following Cerebrovascular Accident

Upper-extremity impairment is common following a stroke, with 85% of individuals in the acute phase showing functional deficits affecting the upper extremity, while 40% of persons with chronic stroke continue to have these impairments (Parker et al., 1986). However, the type of problem will depend on the location of the lesion. In the case of Jean J, our patient who is 5 years poststroke, reach-and-grasp movements in her right paretic arm are characterized by decreased movement speed and a lack of smoothness and coordination in movement trajectories due to abnormal patterns of muscle activity (Alt Murphy et al., 2011). Deficits in coordinated arm movements are most evident in the limb contralateral to her lesion and occur together with spasticity, muscle weakness, and stereotypic movement patterns. As can be seen in the upper-extremity section of her video case study, Jean has very limited function in her right upper extremity. When Jean reaches with her affected arm, the movement trajectory is segmented, with increased variability due to impaired interjoint coordination. She has very impaired grasp due to a limited ability to extend her fingers, and she shows fluctuations in force due to impairments in her ability to regulate forces.

Immediately following her stroke, Genise has total paralysis of her right upper extremity. As can be seen in her video case study, at 4 days poststroke, Genise is developing the ability to move, though movements are limited to partial elbow and finger flexion, made within the context of a flexor synergy. At 1 month poststroke, her paresis is still quite profound and spasticity has increased. While her ability to recruit muscles in the paretic arm has improved, movements are still confined to a flexor synergy pattern with no ability to recruit extensor muscles at the elbow, wrist, or fingers. At 6 months poststroke, voluntary movement in her upper extremity continues to improve, though the flexor synergy pattern is still predominant. Voluntary extension of her paretic limb at the elbow and wrist is just beginning to emerge.

Though it is not the case for either Jean or Genise, many patients with stroke have visual problems such as field deficits (homonymous hemianopsia) and hemi-inattention (visual neglect and extinction), which will affect the ability to reach and grasp objects presented in the contralesional hemifield. Both Jean and Genise do have other sensory impairments within the somatosensory system, which significantly impair reach, grasp, and manipulation.

Jean had several complications that interfered with her early recovery of upper-extremity function, including pain and swelling in her hemiparetic arm. Approximately 15% of patients who have had a stroke also have a shoulder–hand syndrome, which includes pain when moving and loss of range of motion in both the shoulder and the hand. In severe cases, there is pain at rest. If the shoulder–hand syndrome is prolonged, it can lead to a "frozen" shoulder. There is no agreement concerning the underlying cause of shoulder pain following stroke, nor is there agreement on methods for treatment (Cailliet, 1980; Partridge et al., 1990; Roy, 1988).

Mike M: Reach-and-Grasp Problems in Parkinson's Disease

Bradykinesia, or slowed movement, is a classic symptom of PD and has a significant impact on upper-extremity function in Mike. As can be seen in the upper-extremity section of his video case study, movements are slower than expected for someone his age. However, his impairments in reach and grasp are task dependent. For example, when he is performing fast, accurate movements, reaching impairments related to force regulation are most apparent. In contrast, in simple motor tasks, or during slow movements where speed and accuracy are not important, he shows much better control of both reach and grasp.

Mike is less impaired when performing a reach-and-grasp movement at his preferred speed, or when the movement amplitude is small. In addition, his ability to adjust to external perturbations during reach and grasp is less impaired than adjustments to self-generated perturbations. Across all tasks, however, he shows a reduced capability for coordinating multiple joints. In addition, tremor results in a disrupted force trajectory. Mike takes longer to develop grip force and uses excessive forces when lifting an object to ensure that it does not slip. However, surprisingly, Mike retains the ability to modulate forces to match changes in object weight. Finally, he has difficulty when releasing an object.

Medication has a strong impact on Mike's upper-extremity function. His video compares reach, grasp, and manipulation both on and off medication. The medication he takes improves his ability to reach, but not grasp. On medication, the speed of his movements increases, and this is most apparent in self-generated movements and movements that require increased accuracy. His tremor significantly interferes with his upper-extremity function, especially as his medication wears off.

John C: Reach-and-Grasp Problems Following Cerebellar Pathology

Cerebellar damage results in dysmetria, which is characterized by errors in the direction, amplitude, velocity, and force of movement. As can be seen in the upper-extremity section of his video case study, John has ataxia; thus, during reach-and-grasp tasks, his movements are slower and less accurate and there is increased variability in the movement trajectory. When reaching for an object, or pointing to a target, he either undershoots (if he is moving slowly) or overshoots (if he is moving quickly) the target. In addition, his movements are segmented (decomposition of movement), with movements at multiple joints occurring sequentially rather than synchronously. Both eye and hand movements are inaccurate when John is reaching for a stationary object. In addition, when reaching for moving objects, he is unable to match the target velocity and thus demonstrates inaccuracies when reaching or tracking.

Thomas: Reach-and-Grasp Problems in Cerebral Palsy

In addition to lower-extremity problems affecting postural control and mobility functions, Thomas, our 7-year-old child with spastic diplegia, has impairments in upper-extremity function. In children with CP, the level of hand function depends on a number of factors, including severity of motor impairments such as paresis, spasticity, and discoordination, as well as the extent of sensory loss (Ohata et al., 2008). Brændvik et al. (2010) reported that the combination of limited active supination range at the wrist and elbow in conjunction with reduced muscle strength in the elbow, forearm, and grip explained 74% of the variance in actual use of the hands in bimanual activities in children with hemiplegic or diplegic forms of CP.

What kinds of problems with reach and grasp do we see in Thomas? As can be seen in his video case study, his MT are delayed during reach and grasp. Thomas has particular difficulty reaching for a moving target, since when altering his trajectory of reach, he quickly loses his balance. He has poor anticipatory grasp formation during reaches. In addition, his grip and load forces are uncoordinated. He uses excessive grip forces when lifting an object to compensate for poor motor control. Thomas has difficulty when first learning to perform a task that requires precision grip. However, with practice, he improves significantly, as he develops better internal representations of the object.

Both sensory and motor impairments contribute to impaired reach, grasp, and manipulation in Thomas as in other children with CP. Neuromuscular impairments include weakness, spasticity, abnormal synergies, muscle imbalance, and incoordination. Sensory problems include impaired stereognosis, two-point discrimination, and position sense.

Malachi: Reach-and-Grasp Problems in Severe Dystonic/Spastic Cerebral Palsy

Both the postural control and upper-extremity segments of his video case study demonstrate that Malachi's ability to perform reach, grasp, and manipulation tasks varies greatly with the amount of external trunk support provided. With no support, Malachi has essentially no ability to reach for or grasp and manipulate objects. In addition, his ability to visually locate and track objects is limited due to poor head control. With support, head control and upper-extremity function improve dramatically. Because he is severely involved, upper-extremity function is best when full trunk support is provided (support at the shoulder level); however, even with this level of support, head control is intermittent.

Sue: Reach-and-Grasp Problems in Multiple Sclerosis

Sue is our 66-year-old woman with moderately severe relapsing–remitting MS affecting primarily her lower extremities. Sue is independent in all activities of daily living and reports she has very little difficulty with upper-extremity tasks. She has normal strength and range of motion in her upper extremities and demonstrates only mild problems with end point accuracy on her coordination tests. As can be seen in the upper-extremity portion of her video case study, her performance on the 9-Hole Peg test is only slightly slower than expected for a woman her age. Thus, upper-extremity function in Sue is largely intact.

SUMMARY

1. Problems with reach, grasp, and manipulation are a common finding in most individuals with neural pathology.
2. Understanding the causes of these problems is complex because of the many interactions between neural substrates affecting reach, grasp, and manipulation skills.
3. A critical aspect of reach and grasp is the ability to locate a target and maintain one's gaze on that target preceding a reach. Problems affecting target localization and gaze stabilization include (a) disruption of visually driven eye movements because of damage within the oculomotor system; (b) damage to the vestibular system, which disrupts vestibuloocular reflex control of eye movements in response to head movements; and (c) inability to adapt the vestibuloocular reflex to changes in task demands, because of cerebellar damage.
4. Visual deficits affecting target localization also appear to have an impact on hand motor function because of the reciprocal interaction between the eye and hand motor systems.
5. Impaired interjoint coordination is common in many types of neural pathology and affects both the timing and the trajectory of movements made during reach and grasp. In addition, most individuals with neural pathology show delayed MT.
6. Sensory impairments can also affect reach, grasp, and manipulation. Sensory impairments can affect the regulation of forces in response to the slip of a lifted object during an ongoing grip-and-lift task. In addition, sensory impairments can affect the formation of internal representations, which are important to regulating forces in subsequent lifts.

7. Cognitive impairments, specifically impairments in attentional resources, have been reported in most persons with CNS pathology. Upper-extremity tasks require increased attentional resources in persons with neural pathology compared to non-impaired individuals, resulting in dual-task interference when performed in combination with other attentionally demanding tasks. The degree of dual-task interference depends on the location and severity of CNS pathology, as well as the specific combination of tasks being performed. The effect of practice and medication on dual-task interference is variable across patient populations.
8. It appears that each hemisphere has a specialized role in the control of goal-directed voluntary movements. The right hemisphere appears to have a role in processing visual feedback for movement adjustments affecting control of aiming movements in tasks with high demands for accuracy. In contrast, the left hemisphere appears to have a role in some aspects of motor programming, including the timing and sequencing of movement phases specifically related to the ballistic components of the reaching movement.
9. Traditionally, researchers have maintained that unilateral cerebral lesions manifest in the limb contralateral to the lesions. Now, researchers are also finding subtle deficits affecting the ability to reach on the nonparetic side.
10. Damage to the left hemisphere may cause apraxia, a disorder of the execution of movement that cannot be accounted for by weakness, incoordination, sensory loss, poor language comprehension, or inattention to commands. The core of this disorder may be a weakening of the top-down formulation of action plans (i.e., an inability to sustain the intent to the completion of the action plan). As a result, irrelevant objects exert a strong influence on the action plan, leading to performance errors.

CHAPTER 20

Clinical Management of the Patient with Reach, Grasp, and Manipulation Disorders

Susan V. Duff
Jaya Rachwani
Victor Santamaria

Learning Objectives

Following completion of this chapter, the reader will be able to:

1. Discuss the clinical implications of both the ICF (International Classification of Functioning, Disability and Health) and systems framework on the assessment and treatment of prehensile disorders.
2. Discuss clinical tests and measures for assessing prehension and consider the evidence regarding the psychometric properties of these tests in neurologic populations.
3. Describe a task-oriented approach to improving functional prehension including reach, grasp, and manipulation skills.
4. Review the evidence for best practice related to prehensile training in neurologic populations.

INTRODUCTION

Reach, grasp, and manipulation disorders have an impact on participation in life roles and activities performed in daily life. As such, they are a major focus of intervention for clinicians involved in the rehabilitation of persons with neurologic pathology. However, time constraints in rehabilitation influence the number of assessments and intervention strategies employed. Therefore, the administration time and information gained from each assessment must be considered. It is also essential that the treatment be closely evaluated to identify the active ingredients responsible for change from baseline (Whyte & Hart, 2003). The intention of this chapter is to review research evidence that guides the reader in the process of choosing outcome measures and designing treatment strategies for persons with prehensile disorders stemming from neurologic pathology.

The conceptual framework of the task-oriented approach, described throughout this book, is based on the International Classification of Functioning, Disability and Health (ICF) and the systems framework. Prehension is multifaceted, therefore examination and intervention for reach, grasp, and manipulation disorders can incorporate all levels of the ICF. For example, strength, range of motion (ROM), and sensibility naturally fall into the category of *Body, Structure, and Function*. Assessment of dexterity and activities of daily living (ADLs) are often placed in the category of *Activity*. Finally, involvement in recreational activities that involve reach, grasp, and manipulation such as playing cards or golf is often placed in the category of *Participation*. The delivery of evidence-based practice based on the ICF and systems framework requires that clinicians choose sensitive outcome measures and employ effective treatment strategies at all levels of the ICF. Also, varying the environmental context (e.g., cognitive load) under which function is assessed and treated is an essential part of the both the ICF and systems framework.

In this chapter we refer to a few of the case studies introduced in other chapters to exemplify points made throughout. Jean is our client who sustained a stroke in the left hemisphere 6 years ago. She continues to deal with deficits in ADLs and insufficient use of her right arm. She has isolated, yet weak and uncoordinated arm movement. Genise is our client who also sustained a middle cerebral artery stroke, and is in the acute phase of recovery. The third case, Tim is a 4.5-year-old boy mainstreamed in a regular preschool who has been referred to therapy by his teacher because of her concerns about his fine motor skills. Tim was born preterm at 28 weeks of gestation. He prefers his right hand for prehension tasks and holds a crayon with a cross-thumb grasp. He has difficulty tracing shapes, and while he copies letters and numbers from a visual model, he reverses select letters and uses varying sizes. He also has difficulty securing fasteners, tying his shoes, and performing other manual tasks. Finally, we have Malachi who is a 3.7-year-old boy who presents with dyskinetic-spastic quadriplegia, mixed cerebral palsy (CP); athetoid and dystonic components) with trunk hypotonia and spasticity in both lower extremities. He has slight bilateral wrist hypertonia but has complete ROM. His primary goal is to improve trunk control to support upper-extremity (UE) function.

The first half of the chapter focuses on examination of UE function. We review psychometric properties of tests that are useful based on the entry point into rehabilitation. The second half of the chapter uses a task-oriented approach to review intervention options aimed at: (a) reducing impairments limiting UE function, (b) developing effective and efficient strategies and components of movement used to perform unimanual or bimanual tasks, and (c) improving functional abilities, including the ability to adapt to changing task and environmental demands in order to increase participation in daily activities and life roles.

EXAMINATION

A comprehensive assessment of UE function begins with the effect of impaired reach, grasp, and manipulation on the person's ability to participate in life roles. A functional assessment uses tests and measures to determine the person's abilities in his or her actual living environment (*Performance* in the ICF framework), and in a standard (clinical) environment (*Capacity* in the ICF framework). Examination also includes evaluation of strategies used to accomplish the underlying components of prehension, including visual regard, reach, grasp, manipulation, and release (Duff, 2012). Finally, underlying impairments in body structure and function that potentially constrain functional movement skills are examined.

The following section reviews a wide range of standardized tests available to clinicians when evaluating UE function in adults and children. The reader is also referred to web-based sources for information. In many instances, classifying a test within the ICF framework can be difficult and often controversial. Many tests include items considered an *Activity* within the ICF (e.g., task performed by an individual), as well as items related to *Participation* (e.g., societal level of functioning). When a test is performed in a standardized clinical environment it measures the ICF's concept of *Capacity*, and it may or may not predict actual performance in the person's own environment (ICF concept of *Performance*). In this book, a test is classified as a measure of participation (*Performance*) when it gathers information about the person's actual behavior (self-reported or observed) in his or her environment. We classify tests and measures performed in a clinical (standardized) environment as measures of activity (*Capacity*). We recognize that not everyone will agree with this approach and that many may disagree with the way a specific test or measure is classified. However, we believe that it is important to create a consistent framework for the presentation of these materials.

Examining the Effect of Prehension on Participation

Understanding the effect of prehensile limitations on elements of participation can be based on objective or subjective information obtained during the initial interview of the client and family. Difficulty with prehensile control can influence one's ability to take part in life roles (e.g., student or homemaker) and should be considered first in an examination because of the personal importance it holds (Trombly, 1993).

Along with medical and social information, the initial interview is directed toward gathering information on current symptoms and primary areas of concern.

Within the interview, information about any restrictions in tasks and activities that the individual has difficulty performing can be obtained, as well as perceptions on satisfaction with the ability to participate and beliefs regarding the underlying cause of the problem (e.g., weakness). Information on family and cultural values that influence task performance should also be investigated, as they may have an impact on treatment outcome. For example, a child who ties his or her shoes at school may not carry this over at home because of time constraints when getting ready for school or parental values related to functional independence. An interview allows clinicians to gain a general sense of an individual's cognitive status and can help them structure and establish priorities for the formal examination.

Measures of Participation

Most measures of participation rely on self-report (by individual or his or her proxy) to determine the degree to which UE function interferes with execution of everyday activities and social roles. Limits in participation can be verified through observation of the individual performing tasks in his or her home or community. Since observation outside the clinic is not easily done, simulated home and community environments may allow for this assessment.

Adult and Pediatric Measures. Scales that examine participation are not exclusive to UE function. A portion of those available to children and adults are discussed below.

Canadian Occupational Performance Measure. The Canadian Occupational Performance Measure (COPM; Carswell et al., 2004; Law et al., 2005) is an outcomes assessment based on a structured interview identifying client or caregiver-identified problem areas in self-care, productivity, and leisure (Law et al., 2005). The three to five most important problems are rated on a scale of 1 to 10 for performance and satisfaction. Upon reassessment, a change score over 2 is considered to be meaningful. The COPM is a valid and reliable way to identify key areas of concern and measure of improvement following intervention in adult neurologic (Karhula et al., 2013; Song et al., 2019) and pediatric populations (Brandão et al., 2014; Cusick et al., 2006, 2007; Ferre et al., 2015; Gillick et al., 2014). It is being used more frequently as an outcome measure for context-based training studies involving participation (Anaby et al., 2018; Law et al., 2015). This tool would be useful for most of the case studies presented.

Community Integration Questionnaire. The Community Integration Questionnaire (CIQ) is a 15-item, self-rated or interview-based measure used to assess the factors of home and social integration and productivity (Kaplan, 2001). It was designed for persons who sustained moderate-to-severe traumatic brain injury (TBI; Willer et al., 1993) and continues to be used to examine community integration with this population (Sandhaug et al., 2015). American Physical Therapy Association (APTA) StrokEDGE II Taskforce of the Academy of Neurologic Physical Therapy (PT) recommends that the CIQ be used for the TBI population during outpatient and community rehabilitation.

Goal-Attainment Scale. Goal-Attainment Scaling (GAS) was introduced for use in the field of mental health (Kiresuk & Sherman, 1968) and is now used to establish and monitor individualized goals during intervention in adult (Debreceni-Nagy et al., 2019; Quinn et al., 2014) and pediatric (Bloom et al., 2010; Cusick et al., 2006) populations. The procedure is as follows: (a) identify three to five goals; (b) weigh the goals for importance and difficulty. Expected outcomes are set on a 5-point scale: –2 = much less than expected; –1 = somewhat less than expected; 0 = expected level of attainment if the client receives the intended treatment program; +1 = somewhat better than expected; and +2 = much better than expected. Alternative rating and analysis methods exist (Krasny-Pacini et al., 2013; Turner-Stokes & Williams, 2010). The GAS could be useful in all of our case studies to examine one's perception of the impact of treatment on set goals.

Stroke Impact Scale. The Stroke Impact Scale (SIS; Duncan et al., 2002) is a 59-item scale measuring eight domains of self-reported function in adults: strength, hand function, ADLs, mobility, emotion, memory, communication, and social participation. Clients rate the impact of the stroke on a 5-point scale for each section. Lin et al. (2010) found the Minimally Clinically Important Difference (MCID) for hand function to be 17.8 and 5.9 points for ADL/IADL. An expert panel recommends the SIS as an UE outcome measure in clinical intervention trials with chronic stroke (Bushnell et al., 2015). The APTA StrokEDGE II Taskforce highly recommends the SIS for use in subacute and chronic stroke rehabilitation. Thus, the SIS would be a useful test for Jean.

Pediatric Measures. Two measures of participation for children 6 to 21 years of age are the Children's Assessment of Participation and Enjoyment (CAPE) and the Preferences for Activities of Children (PAC; King et al., 2004, 2006; Law et al., 2005). A combination of these two measures (CAPE/PAC) allows an examination of the dimensions of diversity, intensity, with whom, where, enjoyment, and preference. The Children's Leisure Assessment Scale (CLASS, Rosenblum et al., 2010) is another scale that has convergent validity with the CAPE/PAC (Brown & Thyer, 2020). The Child Engagement in Daily Life Measure (Chiarello et al., 2014) is a scale with acceptable to high validity and reliability for young children with CP. These measures would be fitting for Tim and Malachi.

Examining Prehension in Functional Activities

Many standardized tests designed to examine function include UE capability. Select tools have measures of participation. Some standardized assessment tools are discussed subsequently.

Adult and Pediatric Functional Scales

One of the most widely used basic scales is the Functional Independence Measure (FIM; Keith et al., 1987). The FIM is a motor and cognitive test using a 7-point scale to rate 18 items; with resultant scores from 18 to 126. A meta-analysis found reliability of the FIM to be acceptable (Ottenbacher et al., 1996). MCID scores for stroke were established as a total score of 22 points; motor score of 17 points; and cognitive score of 3 points (Beninato et al., 2006). The WeeFIM is adapted from the adult FIM for use with children via interview or observation (Braun & Granger, 1991) with norms available for infants and children 6 months to 7 years of age (Msall et al., 1994). It is reliable and valid for children with and without disabilities (Chen et al., 2005a; Park et al., 2013; Tur et al., 2009) and responsive to change (Ottenbacher et al., 2000). The WeeFIM 0–3 is available for children 0 to 3 years of age (Niewczyk & Granger, 2010). The FIM would be useful for Genise and Jean and the WeeFIM for Malachi.

Standardized instrumental ADL scales assess higher-level UE function by examining skills that require environmental interaction (e.g., shopping). For instance, the Assessment of Motor and Process Skills (AMPS; Fisher, 2003) identifies deficits in functional performance and underlying causes based on observation. This interval scale has good reliability and validity. The AMPS is also a valid measure for children 4 to 15 years of age with and without mild disabilities (Gantschnig et al., 2013). The AMPS would be useful for Jean and Tim.

Pediatric-Specific Measures of Function. The Pediatric Evaluation of Disability Inventory (PEDI; Haley et al., 1992) is standardized for children 6 months to 7.5 years of age. It evaluates skills a child can perform with assistance or independently in the areas of self-care, mobility, and social function on three separate scales (functional skills, caregiver assistance, and modifications required for function). The PEDI has established reliability and validity in standard form (Nichols & Case-Smith, 1996) and as a computer adaptive test (PEDI-CAT; Dumas et al., 2012). The PEDI-CAT includes the domains of daily activities, mobility, and social and cognitive function with selective assessment of UE function. It can be used from 0 to 20 years of age and has strong construct validity and reliability in children with CP (Shore et al., 2019). The PEDI or PEDI-CAT would be useful with Malachi.

The School Functional Assessment (Costner et al., 1998) is normed for children from kindergarten to sixth grade (Assessment Tool 20.1). It identifies strengths and limitations related to performance of school-related tasks in three separate parts: participation, task supports, and activity performance. Part 3 includes physical and cognitive/behavioral task performance, and rates execution on a 1 to 4 scale. Part 3 is a useful test of UE function. The School Function Assessment (SFA) is valid and reliable (Davies et al., 2004). The initial assessment time is 1½ to 2 hours (Sakzewski et al., 2007). Once Tim enters kindergarten this tool would be appropriate.

Amount and Quality of UE Use

The Motor Activity Log (MAL) was developed to determine the amount and quality paretic arm use poststroke during functional tasks (Taub & Wolf, 1997). It incorporates two separate Likert scales ranging from 0 to 5 measuring the amount and quality of use in the affected arm and hand based on observation or interview. The MAL documents baseline and progressive use for pertinent, individualized, everyday tasks in adults poststroke (Blanton & Wolf, 1999; Rand & Eng, 2015) and children with unilateral CP (Charles et al., 2001). The log is reliable and valid (Uswatte et al., 2006b) and recommended for use in subacute and chronic stroke rehabilitation by the APTA StrokEDGE II Task Force of the Academy of Neurologic PT. A revised MAL, the Rasch-based MAL-18, can be used in person with chronic stroke or multiple sclerosis (Van de Winckel & Gauthier, 2019).

The Pediatric MAL (PMAL) is a modification of the original MAL for children 7 months to 8 years of age (Taub et al., 2004). This parent-reported measure includes 22 tasks requiring fine- to gross-unilateral and bilateral UE movements. Based on Rasch analysis using a collapsed 3-point rating scale (Wallen et al., 2009) the PMAL has been found to have strong psychometric properties including construct validity and reliability (Assessment Tool 20.2). PMAL has been revised (PMAL-R) so it is now administered in a structured interview as originally designed (Uswatte et al., 2012). The MAL would be appropriate for Jean and Genise. The PMAL or PMAL-R would be useful for children with hemiplegia.

Inertial Measurement Units (IMUs), which capture acceleration, angular rate of change, and gravitational orientation, allow arm use to be quantified use during everyday tasks (Lang et al., 2007) without changing a person's daily routine. IMUs are reliable and valid measures of arm use in adults with acute or chronic stroke (Gebruers et al., 2014; Urbin et al., 2015; Uswatte et al., 2005, 2006a), multiple sclerosis (Carpinella et al., 2014), children with hemiparesis (Howcroft et al., 2011), and infants at risk for CP (Gravem et al., 2012; Heinz et al., 2010). IMUs have also been used to assess interlimb coordination in adults and children with hemiparesis during everyday tasks with early validation against clinical tools (Miller et al., 2018, 2020). Data from IMUs from Jean, Genise, and Malachi

Assessment Tool 20.1

School Functional Assessment

Three parts of assessment with adaptations checklist
1. Participation
2. Task supports
3. Activity performance
   a. Physical tasks
   b. Cognitive/behavioral tasks

Sample: activity performance–physical tasks
1. Travel
2. Maintaining and changing positions
3. Recreational movement
4. Using materials
5. Setup and cleanup
6. Eating and drinking
7. Hygiene
8. Clothing management
9. Up/down stairs
10. Written work
11. Computer and equipment use

Rating for activity performance
1. Does not perform
2. Partial performance
3. Inconsistent performance
4. Consistent performance

Tasks within "clothing management"

Task				
1. Removes hat	1	2	3	4
2. Removes front-opening garment top (e.g., coat)	1	2	3	4
3. Puts on hat	1	2	3	4
4. Puts on front-opening garment top (e.g., coat)	1	2	3	4
5. Lowers garment bottoms from waist to knees and pulls up from knees to waist (e.g., for toileting)	1	2	3	4
6. Zips and unzips, not including separating/hooking zipper	1	2	3	4
7. Removes pullover garment top (e.g., sweatshirt)	1	2	3	4
8. Removes shoes/boots	1	2	3	4
9. Hangs clothing on hook or hanger	1	2	3	4
10. Puts on pullover garment top (e.g., sweater)	1	2	3	4
11. Puts on and removes socks	1	2	3	4
12. Puts on shoes/boots (do not consider tying closures)	1	2	3	4
13. Secures shoes by tying or using Velcro	1	2	3	4
14. Separates and hooks zippers	1	2	3	4
15. Buttons a row of buttons with one-to-one correspondence	1	2	3	4
16. Fastens a belt buckle	1	2	3	4
17. Buttons small buttons (less than 1 in.)	1	2	3	4

would provide useful information on the amount of arm use and interlimb coordination after prehensile or segmental trunk training respectively. As issues relevant to sensor drift, cost, and data analysis are resolved, the clinical use of inertial sensors may be feasible.

Unimanual and Bimanual Function

The following tools are examples of those available for adults and/or children.

Action Research Arm Test. The Action Research Arm Test (ARAT), shown in Assessment Tool 20.3, was developed to examine UE function and activity limitations in adolescents and adults with neurologic dysfunction, including persons with cerebellar ataxia, poststroke, or TBI (Lyle, 1981; Reoli et al., 2020). The ARAT correlates with the UE portion of the Fugl-Meyer Assessment (FMA-UE; r = 0.94) (De Weerdt & Harrison, 1985). The ARAT was found to be more responsive than the FMA-UE with regard to increased UE function in persons with chronic stroke who participate in forced use paradigms (van der Lee et al., 2001). The ARAT has been used with inertial sensors to quantify arm function in persons with multiple sclerosis (Carpinella et al., 2014). The ARAT would be a useful test to use with Jean and for Genise as she recovers arm function, and is recommended by the APTA StrokEDGE II Task Force of the Academy of Neurologic PT.

Assisting Hand Assessment. Krumlinde-Sundholm and Eliasson (2003) introduced the standardized, criterion-referenced Assisting Hand Assessment (AHA). The AHA was intended to determine the degree to which the affected limb of a child with unilateral disability is engaged in bimanual tasks. All versions of the AHA are scored on a 3- to 4-point rating scale from videotape, yet, differ depending on the tool and age at administration.

Assessment Tool 20.2

Pediatric Motor Activity Log

This assessment is intended for use with the parents of children with hemiplegia.

Instruction: I am going to read a list of activities to you. After each activity, I would like you to use the scales in front of you to tell me about the use that your son/daughter (or you) has in his/her affected arm for each activity listed. We will go over the activities list twice. First, I will ask you to think about the amount of use of your son/daughter's affected arm 1 year ago and then we will go through the list again thinking about the quality of use in the affected arm 1 week ago.

How often scale

0 = Never or seldom uses the affected arm when the task is attempted.
1 = Sometimes uses the affected arm when the task is attempted.
2 = Uses affected arm on most or all of the occasions the task is attempted.

How well scale

0 = Movements were poor: The affected arm was not used; the affected arm was not helpful or was of some use (moving slowly or with difficulty) but needed some help from the other arm.
1 = Movements were fair. The affected arm was used for that activity, but movements were slow or were made with some effort.
2 = The movements made by the affected arm for that activity were almost typical for age but not quite as fast or as accurate (almost normal) or appeared normal.

Sample tasks

1. Open door/cabinet
2. Stops or rolls a ball
3. Carries an object from place to place
4. Push arm through sleeve of clothing
5. Pick-up and hold a large item while sitting in a chair
6. Eats finger food such as popcorn, potato chips, etc., with the affected hand
7. Takes off shoes or socks

Adapted with permission from Wallen M, Bundy A, Pont K, Ziviani J. Psychometric properties of the Pediatric Motor Activity Log for children with cerebral palsy. *Dev Med Child Neurol.* 2009;51:200–208.

The original AHA, designed for children with unilateral CP or brachial plexus birth palsy, 18 months to 12 years of age, was revised and renamed the Kids AHA 5.0 (Holmefur & Krumlinde-Sundholm, 2016). The Kids AHA 5.0 is now a 20-item scale with strong psychometric properties based on Rasch analysis and is more responsive to change over time (Holmefur & Krumlinde-Sundholm, 2016; Holmefur et al., 2009). The Mini-AHA is similar to the AHA yet is standardized for children with clinical signs of unilateral CP 8 to 18 months of age (Greaves et al., 2013). The Hand Assessment of Infants (HAI) is a unimanual and bimanual assessment for infants at risk for unilateral CP, 3 to 12 months corrected age (Krumlinde-Sundholm et al., 2017a). New versions of the AHA include: (a) the Adolescent AHA (Ad-AHA) Go with the Floe board Game, a 20-item scale for adolescents 13 to 18 years of age (Louwers et al., 2016, 2017); and (b) the Adult AHA Stroke, a 19-item scale for adults with hemiparesis poststroke, scored from one of two tasks: unwrapping and wrapping a present or making sandwich (Krumlinde-Sundholm et al., 2017b). The AHA has been expanded to include other conditions and teens with hemiparesis after acquired brain injury (Davis et al., 2019). The Kids AHA 5.0 would be useful with Malachi. The Ad-AHA Stroke would be useful for Jean and Genise.

Bimanual Fine Motor Function. The Bimanual Fine Motor Function (BFMF) test (Beckung & Hagberg, 2002) classifies a child's ability to grasp, hold, and manipulate objects in each hand separately. It rates the child's bimanual function on a five-level ordinal scale. At Level I they can manipulate objects without restriction in one hand and without limits in advanced fine motor skills with the other hand. At Level V they have severe limits holding objects with both hands and require total assistance even with adaptations. The BFMF has construct and content validity (Elvrum et al., 2016) when tested against the Manual Abilities Classification Scheme (MACS).

Both Hands Assessment. The Both Hands Assessment (BoHA; Elvrum et al., 2018) was designed for children with bilateral CP, 18 months to 12 years of age at MACS levels I-III. In this tool, each hand is assessed on 11 items and bimanually for 5 items. Performance is compared between hands creating an asymmetry index. Bimanual items are converted to an interval logit measure via Rasch analysis revealing bimanual performance. Children with asymmetric or symmetric disability can be assessed using two calibration scales. Construct validity and internal consistency are strong for both scales, yet, further research should examine response to change and reliability. The BoHA would be useful for Malachi.

Chedoke Upper Limb and Hand Activity Inventory. The Chedoke Upper Limb and Hand Activity Inventory (CAHAI) was designed to assess arm and hand recovery poststroke (Barreca et al., 2004, 2005). It contains 13 functional tasks that an individual performs while being timed. Scoring is as outlined in Assessment Tool 20.4.

Assessment Tool 20.3

Action Research Arm Test

Scoring: 0–3 points on 19 items in four subtests with 57 total possible points. If the subject passes the first item in a subtest, no more need be administered, and he or she scores top marks for that subtest. If the subject fails the first item and fails the second item in a subtest, he or she scores 0, and again no more tests need to be performed in that subtest. Otherwise, he or she needs to complete all tasks within the subtest.

Scale:

0 = Can perform no part of the test
1 = Performs test partially
2 = Completes test but takes an abnormally long time or has great difficulty
3 = Performs test normally

Subtests:

Grasp (6) Attempt to pick up the following per directions above:

1. 10-cm wood block (If score = 3, total = 18 and go to Grip)
2. 2.5-cm wood block (If score = 0, total = 0 and go to Grip)
3. 5-cm wood block
4. 7.5-cm wood block
5. Ball (cricket), 7.5 cm diameter
6. Stone, 10 × 2.5 × 1 cm

Grip (4) Attempt the following per directions above:

1. Pour water from glass to glass (If score = 3, total = 12 and go to Pinch)
2. Pick up 2.25-cm tube (If score = 0, total = 0 and go to Pinch)
3. Pick up tube, 1 × 16 cm
4. Place washer (3.5 cm diameter) over bolt

Pinch (6) Attempt to pick up the following per directions above:

1. Ball bearing, 6 mm, third finger and thumb (If score = 3, total = 18 and go to Gross Movements)
2. Marble, 1.5 cm, index finger and thumb (If score = 0, total = 0 and go to Gross Movements)
3. Ball bearing, second finger and thumb
4. Ball bearing, first finger and thumb
5. Marble, second finger and thumb
6. Marble, first finger and thumb

Gross Movements (3) Attempt the following:

1. Place hand behind head
2. Place hand on top of head
3. Hand to mouth

Reprinted with permission from Lyle RC. A performance test for assessment of upper limb function in physical rehabilitation treatment and research. *Int J Rehabil Res.* 1981;4:483–492.

Assessment Tool 20.4

Chedoke Arm and Hand Activity Inventory

This assessment tool was designed to measure response to change in hand and arm function in adults after a stroke.

Scale:

1. Total assist (weak upper limb <25%)
2. Maximal assist (weak upper limb = 25%–49%)
3. Moderate assist (upper limb = 50%–74%)
4. Minimal assist (weak >75%)
5. Supervision
6. Modified independence (device)
7. Complete independence (timely, safely)

Subtests affected limb score

1. Open jar of coffee ____holds jar ____holds lid ____
2. Call 911 ____holds receiver ____dials phone ____
3. Draw a line with a ruler ____holds ruler ____ holds pen ____
4. Put toothpaste on toothbrush ____holds toothpaste ____holds brush ____
5. Cut median consistency putty ____holds knife ____ holds fork ____
6. Pour a glass of water ____holds glass ____holds pitcher ____
7. Wring out washcloth ____
8. Clean a pair of eyeglasses ____holds glasses ____ wipes lenses ____
9. Zip up the zipper ____holds zipper ____ holds zipper pull ____
10. Do up five buttons
11. Dry back with towel ____reaches for towel ____grasps towel end ____
12. Place container on table ____
13. Carry bag up stairs

Reprinted with permission from Barreca S, Gowland CK, Stratford P, et al. Development of the Chedoke Arm and Hand Activity Inventory: theoretical constructs, item generation, and selection. *Top Stroke Rehabil.* 2004;11(4):31–42.

The CAHAI (CAHAI-9/CAHAI-13) correlated with the ARAT (r = 0.93, 1 month poststroke; and r = 0.95, 3 months poststroke) yet, was found to be more sensitive to clinical important change (Barreca et al., 2006). It also correlates with the Fugl–Meyer Scale (r = 0.95) and the FIM (r = 0.79) (Gowland et al., 1993). It is recommended by the APTA StrokEDGE II Taskforce. This tool would be useful with Jean and Genise.

Jebsen–Taylor Hand Function Test. The Jebsen–Taylor Hand Function test (JHFT) was designed to simulate hand function common to many ADL tasks (Jebsen et al., 1969). It contains seven timed subtests: writing, card turning, picking up small items, simulated feeding, stacking checkers, picking up light cans, and picking up heavy cans (Fig. 20.1), and requires that both hands be tested (nondominant first). The test takes 10 to 15 minutes to administer. It has established norms for adults (Jebsen et al., 1969) and children (Taylor et al., 1973). The JHFT generally has excellent test–retest reliability, with the exception of writing and feeding subtests, which tend to show practice effects (Stern, 1992). It has been found responsive to change with intervention in children with unilateral CP (Araneda et al., 2019) and within the first 6 months after stroke in adults (Beebe & Lang, 2009). The JHFT would be useful to assess unimanual hand function in all of our cases.

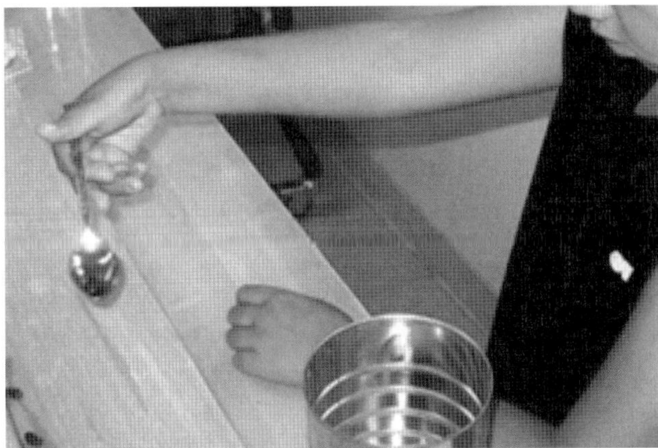

Figure 20.1 Jebsen–Taylor Hand Function Test. One item from this seven-item test includes use of a spoon to lift five beans to simulate feeding.

Manual Abilities Classification Scheme. The MACS was designed for children 4 to 18 years of age with CP, to quantify typical hand use in everyday activities (Eliasson et al., 2006). The MACS was adapted to create the Mini MACS for children with signs of CP 1 to 4 years of age (Eliasson et al., 2017). The MACS (Assessment Tool 20.5) and Mini MACS rate the child's manual ability on a five-level scale from handling objects easily at Level I to severe limits in the ability to handle objects at Level V. The MACS is reliable and valid (Eliasson et al., 2006) and the Mini MACS also has strong psychometric properties (Eliasson et al., 2017). The MACS can be used to identify service needs and assess longitudinal improvements as well to identify and classify research participants (Sakzewski et al., 2015). Function and participation have been found linked with MACS level (Lee et al., 2015). Malachi's hand use could be classified with the MACS.

Manual Ability Measure. The Manual Ability Measure (MAM) is a task-oriented, client-focused outcome measure (Chen et al., 2005b; Chen & Bode, 2010). This two-part tool uses self-reports to assess unimanual and

Assessment Tool 20.5

Manual Abilities Classification System (MACS)

This assessment tool is intended for use with children 4 to 18 years of age who have CP. The therapist observes the child performing everyday manual tasks. The child's typical manual ability is graded on a five-level scale:

Level I: Handles objects easily and successfully. Limitations only in speed and accuracy of manual performance, not ADLs.

Level II: Handles most objects but with somewhat reduced quality and/or speed of achievement. Performs tasks as in level I, but with reduced quality and speed. Certain tasks may be avoided, or achieved with difficulty. ADL independence is maintained.

Level III: Handles objects with difficulty: needs help to prepare and/or modify activities. Independent with setup or adaptations. Performance may be slow or achieved with limited success in terms of quality and quantity.

Level IV: Handles a limited selection of easily managed objects in adapted situations. Requires continuous support, partial assistance, or adaptive equipment in all activities just to achieve partial success.

Level V: Does not handle objects and has severely limited ability to perform even simple actions. Requires total assistance. Participates best if given simple tasks, such as pushing a button.

Reprinted with permission from Eliasson AC, Krumlinde-Sundholm L, Rosblad B, et al. The Manual Ability Classification System (MACS) for children with cerebral palsy: scale development and evidence of validity and reliability. *Dev Med Child Neurol.* 2006;48:549–554. See also Mini-MAC (Eliasson et al., 2017).

Assessment Tool 20.6

Manual Ability Measure (MAM-16)

Please choose one response from the scale, regarding how difficult it is for you to perform the following activities:

Scale:

(4) Easy
(3) A little hard
(2) Very hard
(1) Cannot do
(0) Almost never do

A little hard = Compared with the time before I had the disabilities (due to injuries or illness), it takes me more time, or causes me discomfort, or it tires me out to do the activity. However, I would usually do it. Very hard = Unless absolutely necessary, I prefer others to do it for me. Almost never do = I just never do the activity, because I cannot.

_____ **1.** Eat a sandwich.
_____ **2.** Pick up a half-full water pitcher.
_____ **3.** Use a spoon or fork.
_____ **4.** Cut meat on my plate with a knife.
_____ **5.** Squeeze toothpaste onto a toothbrush.
_____ **6.** Brush my teeth.
_____ **7.** Wring a towel.
_____ **8.** Zip my jacket.
_____ **9.** Button my shirt or clothes.
_____ **10.** Use a telephone.
_____ **11.** Turn a key to open a door.
_____ **12.** Open a wide-mouth jar (jam, pickle) previously opened.
_____ **13.** Open a medication bottle with child-proof cap.
_____ **14.** Count money (bills and coins).
_____ **15.** Take things out of my billfold (ID, credit card, bills).
_____ **16.** Write three to four sentences legibly.

Reprinted with permission from Chen CC, Granger CV, Peimer CA, et al. Manual Ability Measure (MAM-16): a preliminary report on a new patient-centered and task-oriented outcome measure of hand function. *J Hand Surg Br.* 2005;30:207–216. See also MAM-36 (Chen & Bode, 2010).

bimanual function. The first part documents demographics, and the second part evaluates function on 16 task items, MAM-16 (Assessment Tool 20.6), or 36 items, MAM-36. Using Rasch analysis, the MAM-16 and MAM-36 were found to have good validity and reliability (Chen et al., 2005b; Chen & Bode, 2010). It may be used as a screening tool to assess hand function or used in conjunction with other assessment (Rallon & Chen, 2008). This tool has the potential to be used with children, yet it currently would be most useful with Jean or Genise.

Wolf Motor Function Test. The Wolf Motor Function Test (WMFT; Wolf et al., 2001, 2006a) is a standardized UE assessment for adults poststroke. It quantifies performance on 15 timed tasks and two strength measures. Tasks are arranged from proximal to distal in order of complexity (Wolf et al., 2001) (see Assessment Tool 20.7). The WMFT-time has high interrater reliability, internal consistency, test–retest reliability, and adequate stability (Morris et al., 2001; Wolf et al., 2001). The WMFT-Functional Ability Scale (FAS) examines movement quality from video-capture on a 6-point rating scale; 0 (no use of the affected side attempted) to 5 (normal) with a peak rating of 75 points (15 tasks). The WMFT-FAS has been shown to have high interrater reliability (Duff et al., 2015; Morris et al., 2001). Together, the WMFT-FAS and WMFT-time may provide insight into neural recovery mechanisms. This tool would be useful for Jean as shown on the UE portion of her case study video.

Handwriting. Dysfunctional motor behaviors detected during handwriting in children and adults may include an unstable grip on the pen or pencil (see UE portion of Malachi's case study video), poor wrist stabilization, or failure to secure the paper when writing. Formal tests measure global legibility, writing speed, pencil management, and components such as near- and far-point copying. Adult handwriting can be assessed with the writing portion of the JHFT test (Jebsen et al., 1969) or the Handwriting Assessment Battery for Adults (Faddy et al., 2008). Tools available to assess handwriting in children include the JHFT (Taylor et al., 1973) or the Evaluation Tool of Children's Handwriting (ETCH) (Amundson, 1995). The ECTH-Manuscript and the ETCH-Cursive have good interrater reliability and content validity (Duff & Goyen, 2010; Feder & Majnemer, 2003). Computerized tools, instrumented pens, and tablets successfully assess visuomotor control of handwriting in children and adults (Cascarano et al., 2019; Guilbert et al., 2019; Israely & Carmeli, 2017; Lin et al., 2017). Features displayed by children with left unilateral CP correlate with speed and dexterity, bilateral coordination, visual–spatial perception, and visual–motor organization (Bumin & Kavak, 2010). A formal test should be coupled with analysis of motor strategies and resources such as attention, visual skills, or hand strength.

Some handwriting problems, such as difficulty copying from the blackboard or copying small text, may require referral to a specialist such as an optometrist. Due to potential discrepancies between formal testing and classroom performance (Sudsawad et al.,

Assessment Tool 20.7

Wolf Motor Function Test

The tasks listed below are performed as quickly as possible while being timed. Scoring is based on time maximal time recorded for task performance, for a maximum of 120 seconds (WMFT-time) and based on the Functional Ability Scale (WMFT-FAS) discussed subsequently.

Tasks:

1. Forearm to table (side): Subject attempts to place forearm on the table by abduction at shoulder.
2. Forearm to box (side): Subject attempts to place forearm on the box by abduction at shoulder.
3. Extend elbow (side): Subject attempts to reach across the table by extending the elbow (to side).
4. Extend elbow (to the side), with weight: Subject attempts to push the sandbag against outer wrist joint across the table by extending the elbow.
5. Hand to table (front): Subject attempts to place affected hand on the table.
6. Hand to box (front): Subject attempts to place hand on the box.
7. Reach and retrieve (front): Subject attempts to pull 1-lb weight across the table by using elbow flexion and cupped wrist.
8. Lift can (front): Subject attempts to lift can and bring it close to lips with a cylindrical grasp.
9. Lift pencil (front): Subject attempts to pick up pencil by using three-jaw chuck grasp.
10. Pick up paper clip (front): Subject attempts to pick up paper clip by using a pincer grasp.
11. Stack checkers (front): Subject attempts to stack checkers onto the center checker.
12. Flip cards (front): Using the pincer grasp, Subject attempts to flip each card over.
13. Turning the key in lock (front): Using pincer grasp, while maintaining contact, Subject turns key fully to the left and right.
14. Fold towel (front): Subject grasps towel, folds it lengthwise, and then uses the tested hand to fold the towel in half again.
15. Lift basket (standing): Subject picks up basket by grasping handles and placing it on bedside table.

WMFT-FAS 6-point ordinal rating scale

0. —Does not attempt with UE being tested.
1. —UE being tested does not participate functionally; however, attempt is made to use the UE. In unilateral tasks, the UE not being tested may be used to move the UE being tested.
2. —UE being tested participates functionally but requires assistance of the UE not being tested for minor readjustments or change of position, or requires more than two attempts to complete, or accomplishes very slowly. In bilateral tasks, the UE being tested may serve only as a helper.
3. —UE being tested participates functionally but movement is influenced to some degree by synergy or is performed slowly or with effort.
4. —UE being tested participates functionally; movement is close to normal[a] but slightly slower; may lack precision, fine coordination, or fluidity.
5. —UE being tested participates functionally; movement appears to be normal.[a]

[a]Here are guidelines when comparing performance in the affected to the less-affected arm:

- "Normal" for some may involve what appears to be a compensatory strategy.
- Try to discern what is compensatory versus alternate movement patterns that are "normal" for that person. The first would be downgraded, the latter would not.

Reprinted with permission from the supplement of: Duff SV, He J, Nelsen MA, et al. Inter-rater reliability of the wolf motor function test-Functional Ability Scale: why it matters. *Neurorehabil Neural Repair.* 2015;29(5):436–443. doi: 10.1177%2F1545968314553030

2001), it is important to obtain an opinion from the teacher in addition to reviewing results from formal testing. It may be useful to formally assess handwriting in persons who must transfer hand dominance due to a neurological condition (Yancosek & Mullineaux, 2011) as with Jean or Genise. Assessment of handwriting would also be beneficial for Tim.

Assessing Prehensile Strategies

Although an individual may perform a functional task successfully, his or her repertoire of movement strategies may be limited, restricting transfer of performance. Examination at the strategy level involves key elements of prehension, including (a) visual regard, (b) reach and grip formation, (c) grasp, (d) manipulation, and (e) release (Duff, 2012). Deficits in any element can limit function even if resources are sufficient (e.g., strength). For clients with unilateral neural pathology (e.g., stroke), assessment should include both limbs, since the limb on the same side as the lesion often exhibits control problems too (Poole et al., 2009; Schaefer et al., 2009; Tretriluxana et al., 2009). The client's ability to adapt to changes in the task and context should be assessed (Wu et al., 1994, 1998). It would be useful to assess prehensile strategy, in all of our cases.

Visual Coordination. Examination of eye–head coordination, which underlies localization of an object to be grasped, requires the assessment of three components (Herdman et al., 2001; Shumway-Cook & Horak, 1990). First, the client's ability to locate and maintain a stable gaze on a fixed or moving target, presented in the central and/or near peripheral visual field, is examined and graded on a 3-point scale: intact, impaired, or unable. The client is asked to keep the head still and move only the eyes. Saccadic eye movements to fixed targets and smooth pursuit movements used to track moving targets are tested. This type of testing can be seen in the impairment section of John's video case study. Figure 20.2 shows a client making saccadic eye movements to a still target in the near peripheral field. Subjective reports related to blurred or unstable vision, dizziness, or nausea are recorded. Following stroke, many clients, such as Genise, have difficulty making accurate eye movements to targets in their left visual field and tracking moving targets.

Next, the client's ability to locate and stabilize gaze on targets in the far peripheral visual field is examined (Fig. 20.3) and graded as previously described. Clients should be able to localize a target with the eyes and maintain a stable gaze on that target while the head is moving. Finally, the client's ability to make eye–head–trunk movements to locate targets in the far periphery is examined. Clients are tested initially while seated; then if they are capable, in standing and during walking (Shumway-Cook & Horak, 1990). An expanded method of measuring eye, head, and trunk coordination can be done during targeted tracking tasks using motion analysis and an eye-tracker (Gadotti et al., 2016, 2020).

Reach and Grasp. Reaching and reach-to-grasp behaviors have distinct features that may reveal underlying problems with planning and anticipatory control. Grip formation, or hand shaping, begins in the later part of the reach (transport) in anticipation of object size and shape incorporating finger opening and closure (Jeannerod, 1994, 1986) (Fig. 20.4). Reach-to-grasp kinematics provide excellent information, yet are not practical for the clinic. Yet, behaviors can be simply assessed by videotaping performance, using a stopwatch and/or inertial sensors. Videotaping allows the clinician to analyze components by repeated viewing segments of interest. A stopwatch allows for capture of temporal features, such as movement time. Inertial sensors allow monitoring of movement within or outside of the clinic by storing data within the sensors then calculating select reach parameters such as acceleration. Estimation of hand shaping is best done with motion capture and small sensors (Bańkosz & Winiarski, 2020; Chen, 2013; El-Gohary & McNames, 2015; Held et al., 2018).

Tasks that incorporate pointing or reach-to-grasp behaviors in different parts of the workspace demand that the individual use a range of movement strategies. To assess a client's repertoire, targets or objects could be placed ipsilateral and contralateral to the reaching arm, above or below shoulder height, within arm's reach, or at the extreme ends of the workspace. During testing, it is important to remember the speed–accuracy trade-off

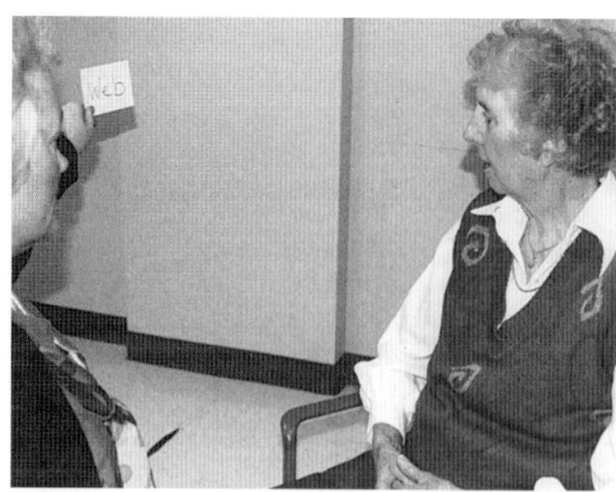

Figure 20.3 Testing eye–head coordination. The client's ability to make coordinated eye–head movements to locate a target in the far peripheral visual field is shown.

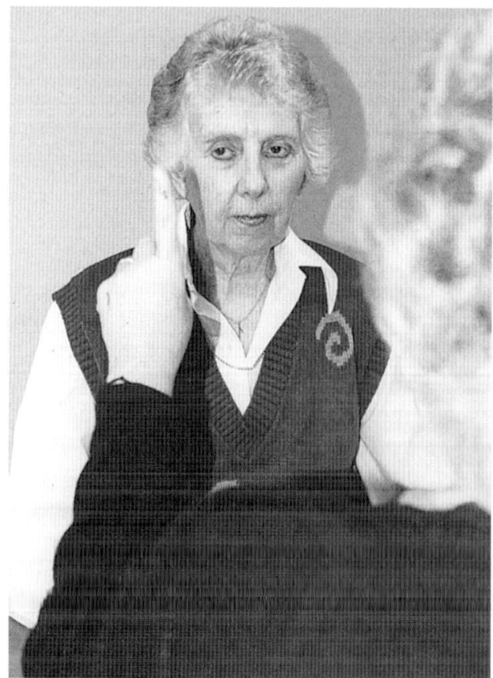

Figure 20.2 Testing eye–head coordination. Shown is the client's ability to make saccadic eye movements to locate and maintain gaze on a target in the near peripheral field.

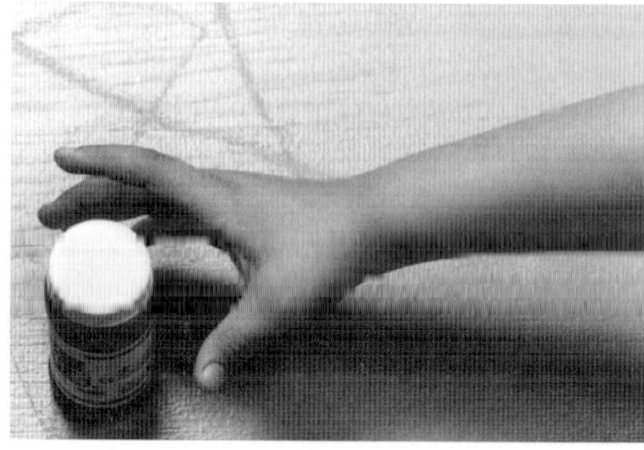

Figure 20.4 The development of grip formation during transport in anticipation of object size and contour.

or Fitts' law (Fitts, 1954). If accuracy demands are high (fragile or unstable target object), persons often slow down (decelerate) during the final phase of the reach.

Two problems you might expect to see in clients with underdeveloped, or impaired reach are increased movement time and an inefficient hand trajectory. Problems with grip formation include: (a) insufficient finger opening for wider objects due to weakness in finger/thumb extensors; and (b) premature finger closure, resulting in unstable grasp points on the object. During observations or video review, one could assess the path of the reach, hand orientation, and shape of the fingers relative to the thumb. One can determine the point in the reach when the hand opens maximally then begins to close to prepare for object contact, noting whether the thumb remains stable, thereby serving as a reference point.

The trunk should be analyzed for its role as a postural stabilizer during reach (Harbourne & Kamm, 2015; Massion, 1992) and in eye–hand–head coordination during object retrieval across the lifespan (Rachwani et al., 2019). As shown by Kaminski et al. (1995), when reaching for anteriorly placed targets, trunk rotation is countered by shoulder horizontal abduction and scapular retraction to keep the hand moving in a straight path (Fig. 20.5). Levin et al. (2002) examined trunk motion during forward reaching and found that it made a greater contribution and was used earlier in the reach in adults with hemiparesis than controls. During a lateral reaching task, Rachwani et al. (2019) found adults, initiated head–trunk turning and began to reach before objects came into view displaying anticipatory control. Yet, infants 6 to 12 months of age, first turned the head and trunk then began to reach once the toy was visually located displaying emerging anticipatory control. Based on its importance, trunk motion should be analyzed from lateral, posterior, and anterior views during reach-and-grasp tasks in various locations, particularly during reaches for objects placed at the terminal end of the workspace or initially out of view. Although an eye-tracker can capture eye–head coordination and visual fixation on targets it is often not available to clinicians. Thus, an overhead video camera could help to monitor trunk and arm coordination during reach-to-grasp movements during rehabilitation.

Anticipatory Control of Grasp. In preparation for grasp, relevant object features (e.g., texture, weight) are identified. We draw upon previously formed internal representations and body awareness to plan movements and forces in advance. If anticipatory scaling is impaired, one must use sensory feedback to modify fingertip forces, which is often too late and may result in object slips or crushes unless compensatory strategies are used.

Behavioral signs of impaired anticipatory control include: (a) repeatedly knocking over objects due to insufficient finger opening (underestimated aperture), (b) contacting objects with the web space first versus the fingertips (delay in finger closure), (c) denting or crushing lightweight objects during grasping (excess grip force), and (d) difficulty raising heavy but liftable objects off a table (underestimated load force rate). If one or more signs are evident, the clinician should determine the reason for the impaired anticipatory control (e.g., diminished sensibility distorting internal representations). Since anticipatory grip formation and object contact depend on accurate identification of object location and properties, remember to examine visual acuity and perception.

Grasp Stabilization. An individual's repertoire of grasp patterns can be ascertained easily using Sollerman's (1984) grasp-and-lift test during direct observation or video review. The nine test items require the use of various patterns such as a spherical grip to open a jar and a three-jaw chuck to open a tube of toothpaste. After each lift, the examiner rates the pattern on a scale of 1 to 4 to document baseline and progress.

Numerous tasks require a sustained grip on a utensil or tool. Weakness due to hemiplegia or dystonia may contribute to an awkward grip posture and limited endurance for sustained writing tasks and thus warrants close examination. Ten pencil and

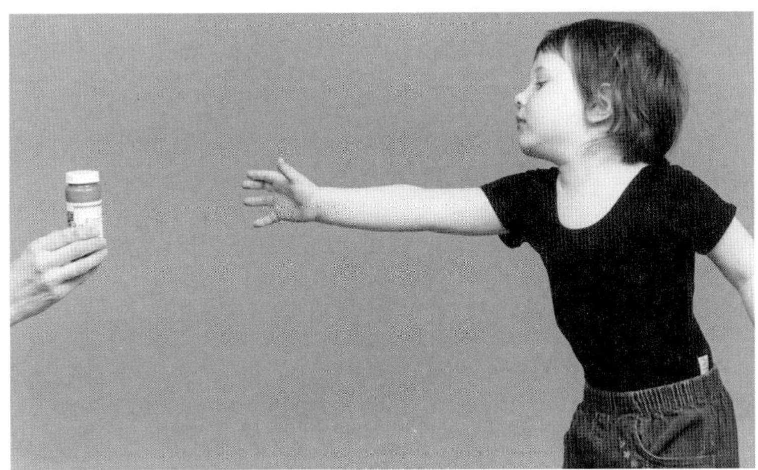

Figure 20.5 The importance of coupling movements between the trunk, glenohumeral joint, and scapula during reaching for anteriorly placed targets.

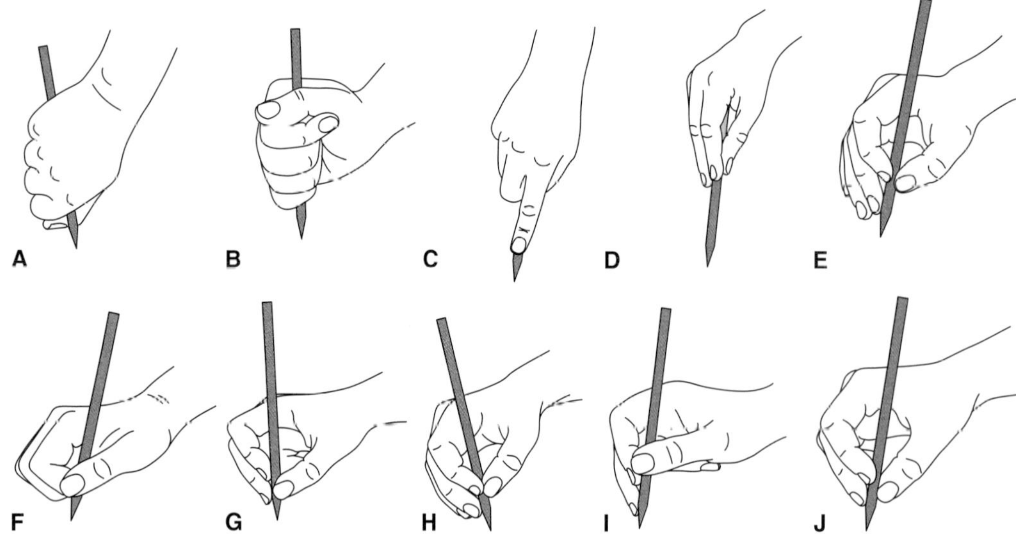

Figure 20.6 (A-J) Ten pencil and crayon grips observed during development. (Redrawn with permission from Schneck CM, Henderson A. Descriptive analysis of the developmental progression of grip position for pencil and crayon control in non-dysfunctional children. *Am J Occup Ther.* 1990;44:895.)

crayon grips often observed during development, compiled from various authors are shown in Figure 20.6 (Schneck & Henderson, 1990). These grip postures can be used as a guide when analyzing pencil grip in children and adults. Children younger than 4 years of age use a variety of patterns, yet the ones commonly used among typical children, older than 6.6 years, are the dynamic tripod (Fig. 20.6J) and lateral tripod (Fig. 20.6I). Bergmann (1990) found that 88% of adults used the dynamic tripod, while 9% used a lateral tripod grip. Adults and children with neurologic conditions often display awkward pencil grips. Once a consistent pattern has been identified, writing efficiency can be tested via timed copying tests at near and far points.

Manipulation and Release. Once an object is secured, it can be stabilized or manipulated. Stabilization requires sustained fingertip forces to prevent slips. Manipulation is object motion in space, or with reference to another object (Corbetta & Mounoud, 1990). It includes several types of tasks, such as tool use (e.g., scissors), dressing (buttoning), eating (use of a knife), or money handling. Skill with manipulation often requires hand motion in reference to an object, such as pushing, pulling, shaking, throwing, transferring, or releasing.

Regulation of fingertip forces during object manipulation has been shown to be impaired in individuals with neurologic conditions (Duff & Gordon, 2003; Muratori et al., 2006, 2008; Nowak et al., 2002; Quinn et al., 2001; Raghavan et al., 2006). Fingertip force regulation of stable objects can be measured with small force transducers. Yet, this lab-based assessment is costly and not feasible for clinic use. To clinically assess fingertip force regulation without force transducers requires keen observation of performance during grasp, lift, and release of objects of different sizes, shape, weight, and texture (Fig. 20.7). For example, clients may be asked to grasp and lift, grasp and throw, or grasp and place (into or on top of) various objects. Observation of the client's performance can determine whether the grip pattern is sufficiently modified to accommodate object properties. Explicitly, is there evidence of errors such as excess squeeze (grip) forces for objects of varying texture, slips when lifting heavy/large objects, or overshoots during lifts with lightweight objects? Also, how much voluntary ROM does the individual display through the wrist, finger, and thumb extensors for object release? What is the release pattern used (e.g., tenodesis)? Can the individual grade release to place one object on top of another? Observations can be made during functional tasks, dexterity testing, or tests of in-hand manipulation (TIHM), since require variable hand movement.

Jean, our chronic stroke client, makes frequent errors grading fingertip forces, and has difficulty

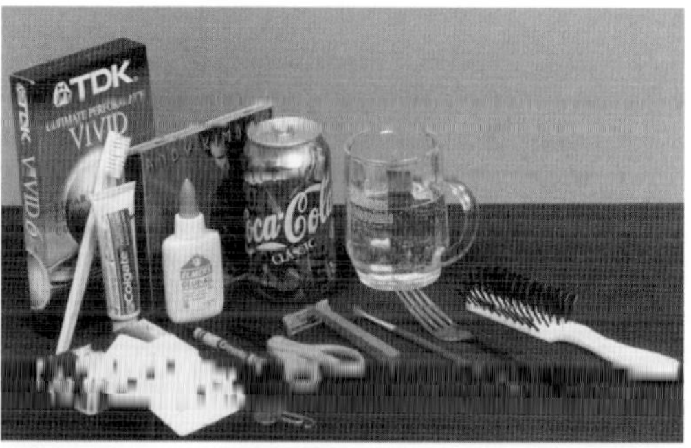

Figure 20.7 Objects of varied size, shape, weight, and texture can be used to roughly estimate available prehension patterns, the ability an individual has to form an anticipatory grip pattern and scale the fingertip forces during object manipulation.

releasing objects. For instance, she typically uses too much force when grasping and lifting a paper cup, causing compression of the sides of the cup and spilling of the liquid inside. This suggests significant errors in anticipatory scaling of the grip and load force.

The Strength–Dexterity Test or SD Test (Valero-Cuevas et al., 2003) was developed to examine manipulation of unstable objects. This task requires control of fingertip force direction and magnitude to compress a slender and compliant spring without buckling it. Dynamic compression force can be captured by fitting the spring with miniature load cells (ELB4-10, Measurement Specialties, Hampton, VA). A dexterity index (tendency of spring to buckle) in grams of force (gmf) is calculated from the mean sustained grip force (~ 5 seconds) for three maximal trials (Dayanidhi et al., 2013). The SD Test has been used to assess dexterity in children with CP (Vollmer et al., 2010) and persons with Parkinson's disease (PD; Lawrence et al., 2014; Peppoloni et al., 2017). Further work is needed to bring this tool into clinical practice.

In-Hand Manipulation. In-hand manipulation is the process of adjusting an object in one hand after grasping it (Exner, 1989; Pehoski, 1995). Figure 20.8 shows elements of in-hand manipulation including: (a) *translation*, moving an object from the fingers to the palm and back, as when picking up a coin and moving it to the palm; (b) *shift*, adjusting the position of an object held in the finger/thumb pads with thumb opposition (e.g., moving a pen closer to the point to write); and (c) *rotation* (simple or complex), rotating then stabilizing an object (e.g., turning a spoon for use after picking it up). Finger individuation and activation of hand muscles (Kwon et al., 2018) are essential for successful in-hand manipulation.

Assessment of in-hand manipulation provides insight into dexterity and handwriting problems and allows documentation of gains (Case-Smith, 1996; Cornhill & Case-Smith, 1996). Methods to examine translation, shift, and rotation include: (a) placing a pencil in a subject's palm and asking them to adjust it for use; and (b) placing a quarter in a subject's palm and asking them to use the fingers to place it into the coin slot of a machine. The TIHM (Case-Smith, 2000; Pont et al., 2008) uses the Nine-Hole Peg Test (NHPT) to assess translation with stabilization and rotation in children from 3 to 6 years of age. The TIHM was recently shown reliable and valid (Pont et al., 2008). Since the TIHM has not been adapted for adults, an observation of performance is recommended as outlined above.

Dexterity and Fine Motor Tests

The assessment of dexterity differs by age and condition. For those with unilateral dysfunction, skill for the affected and less-affected sides should be assessed. Common tests with normative data for diverse ages and populations are the NHPT (Mathiowetz et al., 1985a; Oxford et al., 2003; Poole et al., 2005), the Purdue Pegboard test (Mathiowetz et al., 1986; Tiffin, 1968), the Minnesota Rate of Dexterity test (Desrosiers et al., 1997; Surrey et al., 2003), and the Box and Block test (Desrosiers et al., 1994; Jongbloed-Pereboom et al., 2013; Mathiowetz et al., 1985b). Dexterity tests recommended by the APTA StrokEDGE II Taskforce are the NHPT and

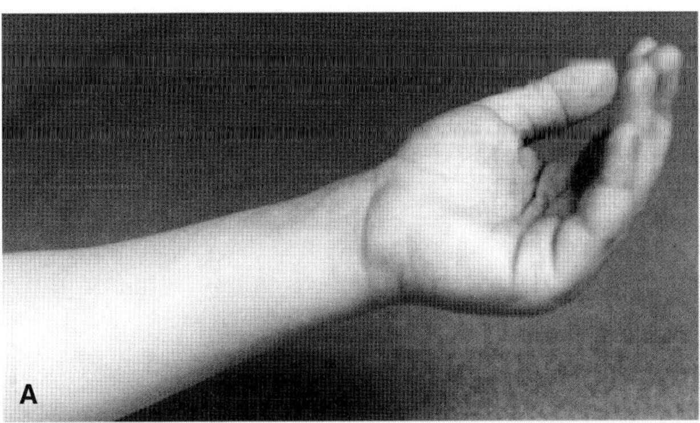

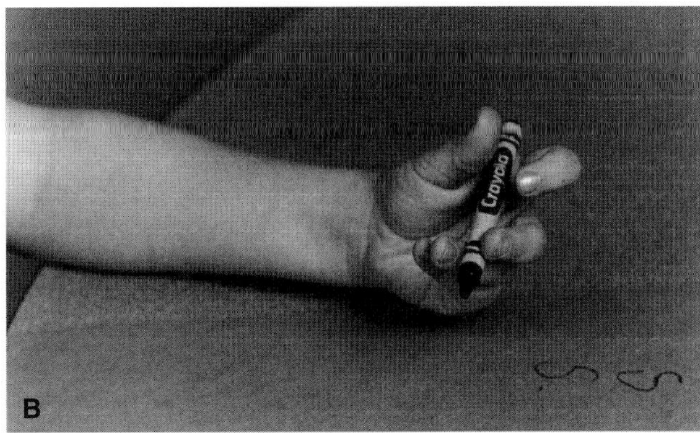

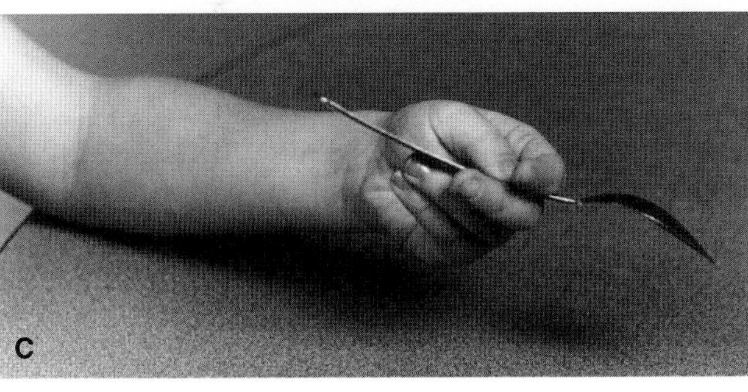

Figure 20.8 Elements of in-hand manipulation include: translation **(A)**, shift **(B)**, and rotation (simple or complex) **(C)**.

the Box and Block test. In the UE section of the video case study of Sue, our client with multiple sclerosis (MS), you can see her performance on the NHPT.

The Functional Dexterity Test (FDT; Aaron et al., 2003) is a timed pegboard test requiring two features of in-hand manipulation, shift, and rotation. The FDT is validated with excellent test–retest (ICC = 0.95) and intrarater (ICC = 0.91) reliability in adults. For children interrater (ICC = 0.99) and test–retest reliability (ICC = 0.90) have been established and it has discriminant validity between typically developing and children with congenital differences (Tissue et al., 2017). Updated adult (Satorio et al., 2013) and pediatric (Gogola et al., 2013) norms are available. The FDT would be useful to assess performance in all of our cases since the pegs are larger, allowing greater ease of manipulation for persons at various skill levels.

Developmental Fine Motor Tests. The fine motor section of developmental tests is often used to assess prehensile skill in typical and atypical children. Common tests normalized for infants and young children include the Peabody Fine Motor Scale—2nd edition (birth to 5 years) (Folio & Fewell, 2000; van Hartingsveldt et al., 2005; Wang et al., 2006), the Gesell Developmental Schedules (birth to 2.5 years) (Gesell et al., 1940), the Bayley Scale of Infant and Toddler Development® III (Bayley, 2006), Bayley™-4 (Bayley & Aylward, 2019) for birth to 42 months, and the Erhardt Developmental Prehension Assessment (up to 6 years) (Erhardt, 1984). The Bruininks-Oseretsky Test of Motor Proficiency-Fine Motor section, 2nd edition (BOT-2; Bruininks & Bruininks, 2005), has unimanual and bimanual items and is normed for children 4.5 to 14.5 years of age. Finally, the Movement Assessment Battery for Children, 2nd edition (Movement ABC-2), has sections on manual dexterity and ball skills (Henderson & Sugden, 2007), normed for those 3 to 16 years of age. Clinicians should examine the validity of a tool for a specific condition (Gill et al., 2019). Most tools would be appropriate for use with Tim.

Bilateral Coordination

Bilateral or bimanual tasks can be symmetrical, with both limbs performing the same action, or asymmetrical, with one limb stabilizing an object while the other limb performs an action on it. Common symmetrical tasks are ball throwing and towel folding. Many self-care tasks are asymmetrical such as holding a toothbrush with one hand and squeezing toothpaste onto the brush with the other. Some tools, such as the BOT-2, have items designed to test bilateral coordination in children (Bruininks & Bruininks, 2005). Versions of the AHA assess performance of the more affected hand during bimanual tasks.

Efficiency in bilateral task performance can be examined with a stopwatch. Yet, to quantify bilateral coordination, videotaping, kinematics or capturing motion with inertial sensors may be best (Miller et al., 2018, 2020). Wiesendanger and colleagues (Kazennikov et al., 2002) designed a clever test of asymmetrical skill entitled the "drawer-pulling" task often used in conjunction with videotape, kinematics and force transducers to assess performance at different ages and conditions (Hung et al., 2004, 2010; Kantak et al., 2016; Serrien & Wiesendanger, 2001). Performance of bimanual tasks would be important to assess with Jean and Genise, our two individuals with stroke, and in both Tim and Malachi.

Examination of Underlying Impairments

The third level of examination identifies factors that limit or enhance performance and planning of task-specific movements. In the ICF framework, these factors reflect examination of *Body Structure and Function*. Chapter 5 provides an overview of the examination of impairments. This section reviews features specific to reach, grasp, and manipulation.

Perception and Cognition

Impairments in this category relevant to UE dyscontrol include selective attention, visual neglect, planning, sequencing, apraxia/dyspraxia, and visual perception. Deficits in any of these areas can significantly influence hand and arm function. Research has shown that apraxia and deficits in sequencing can significantly affect hand and UE function in adults after left hemispheric stroke (Jax et al., 2013) and in children with developmental coordination disorder (Chang & Yu, 2016; Goyen et al., 2011). See Chapter 5 for a full review.

Musculoskeletal and Neuromuscular Factors

One's ability to move may be restricted by available joint motion, weakness, difficulty making isolated movements, or spasticity. The American Society of Hand Therapists (ASHT) publication *Clinical Assessment Recommendations* (MacDermid et al., 2015) provides a guide to tests of grip and pinch strength, ROM, sensibility, pain, edema, and sympathetic function, which could be useful to assess select items for any of our cases.

Range of Motion. The ASHT guidelines enhance reliability of UE ROM measures (MacDermid et al., 2015). Variations in wrist and forearm measures are reliable (Flowers et al., 2001; LaStayo & Wheeler, 1994). Smartphone applications using accelerometers and/or magnetometers are also valid and reliable to assess shoulder (Johnson et al., 2015) and wrist ROM (Pourahmadi et al., 2017). Finger ROM taken with smartphone photography are consistent with manual goniometry (ICC = 0.92, margin of error 3.2–5°) and, thus, may be useful for telerehabilitation (Zhao et al., 2020). Composite finger and hook fist flexion are best measured with the

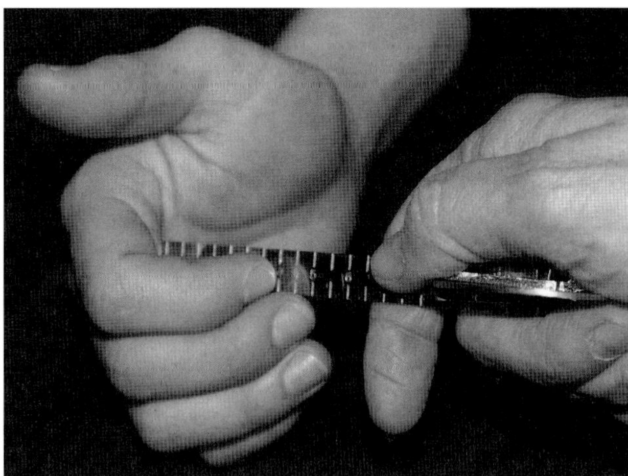

Figure 20.9 Measuring composite flexion with the ruler of a finger goniometer.

ruler of a finger goniometer (Fig. 20.9), as the distance between the finger pulp and distal palmar crease (De Tullio et al., 2021). Thumb opposition can be measured with the ruler from the volar thumb IP joint to the third metacarpal. Variability can exist depending on age or condition. It would be important to assess ROM in all of our cases.

Strength. The generation of sufficient force (strength) and power (rate of force generation) is essential to active UE function in persons with neurological conditions (Moreau, 2020; Starosta et al., 2017). Manual muscle testing or dynamometry can assess large muscles and grip and pinch strength (Wadsworth & Krishman, 1987). Grip dynamometers (Fig. 20.10) (Jamar Dynamometer, Asimow Engineering, Los Angeles, CA) adjust for hand width and should be calibrated. To measure grip strength, recording the mean of three trials in 90° elbow flexion in forearm and wrist neutral is recommended (Shechtman & Sindhu, 2015). In cases of weak grip or difficulty gripping the handle, a bulb dynamometer or a blood pressure cuff rolled to 5 cm and inflated to 5 mm Hg can measure grip strength. Change in the millimeters of mercury is recorded as the power of grip.

Pinch strength can be evaluated using electronic pinch meters (Pinch Gauge, B & L Engineering, Santa Ana, CA). Three types of pinch can be assessed (Fig. 20.11): (a) *tip-to-tip* (thumb tip to index finger tip), (b) *three-jaw chuck* (thumb pulp to index and long finger pulp), and (c) key or lateral pinch (thumb pulp to lateral index). Two measurements are taken and compared to baseline or norms (De Tullio et al., 2021).

Variability in muscle strength and grip/pinch strength exists across different conditions and ages (i.e., Jansen et al., 2008; Lee-Valkov et al., 2003; McQuiddy et al., 2015). In neurologic conditions, pinch strength may be more closely associated with manual skills than grip strength (Chen et al., 2007). In addition to Jean and

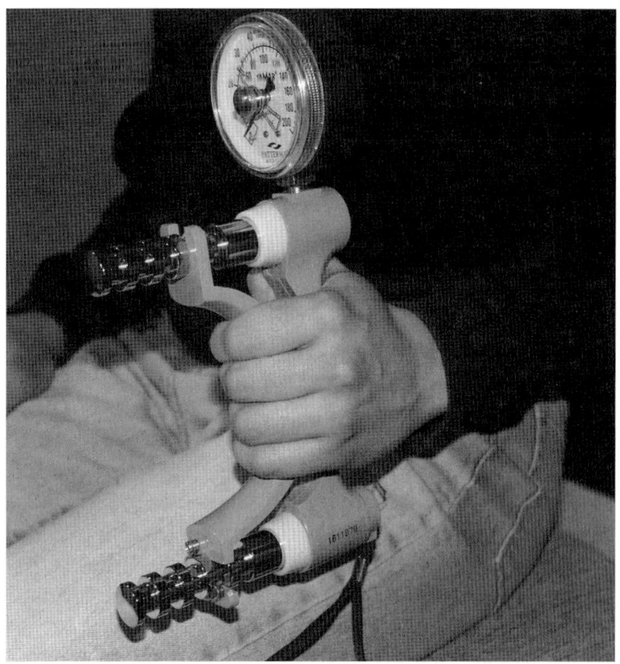

Figure 20.10 A Jamar dynamometer in the recommended position for testing yields an objective measure of grip strength.

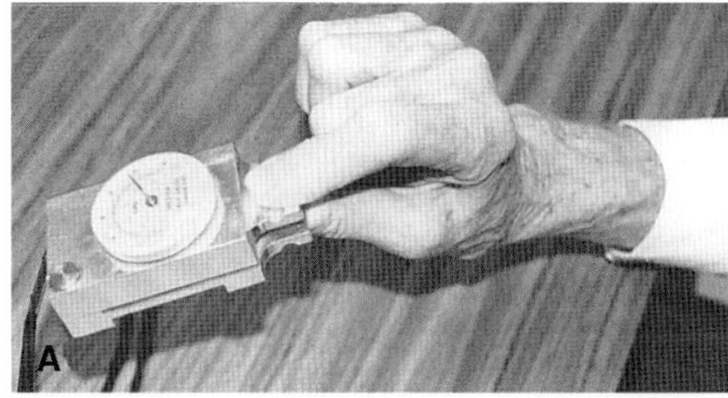

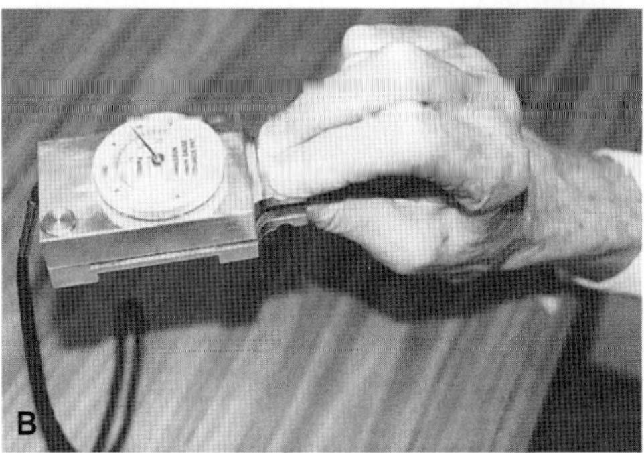

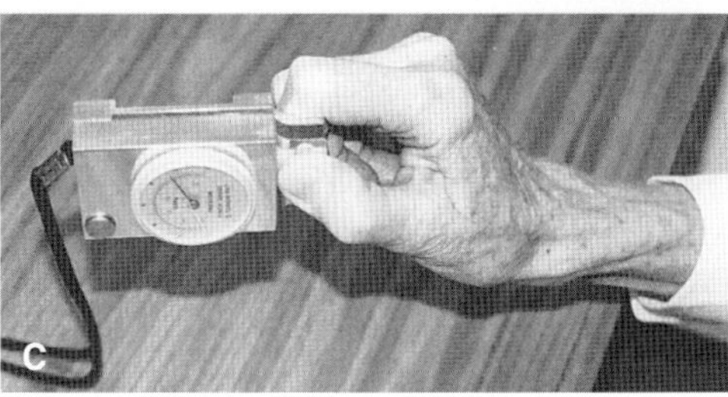

Figure 20.11 Use of a pinch meter to measure precision grip strength. Three types of pinch are examined: tip to tip **(A)**, three-jaw chuck **(B)**, key or lateral pinch **(C)**.

Genise, it would be important to assess Tim's grip and pinch strength as needed for school-based tasks and ADLs.

Motor Status. The Fugl–Meyer Motor Assessment-Upper Extremity (FMA-UE) section is designed to assess motor recovery poststroke (Fugl-Meyer et al., 1975). Chapter 5 reviews test details. A standardized scoring and training approach, used in a phase II trial, increased accuracy and reduced variability (See et al., 2013). Portions of the FMA-UE may be viewed in the video case study of Genise, our client with acute stroke.

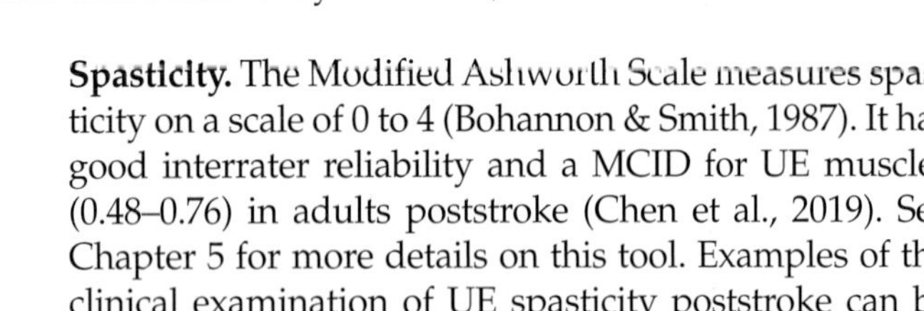
Spasticity. The Modified Ashworth Scale measures spasticity on a scale of 0 to 4 (Bohannon & Smith, 1987). It has good interrater reliability and a MCID for UE muscles (0.48–0.76) in adults poststroke (Chen et al., 2019). See Chapter 5 for more details on this tool. Examples of the clinical examination of UE spasticity poststroke can be seen in the impairment section of the video case study on Genise, our client with acute stroke.

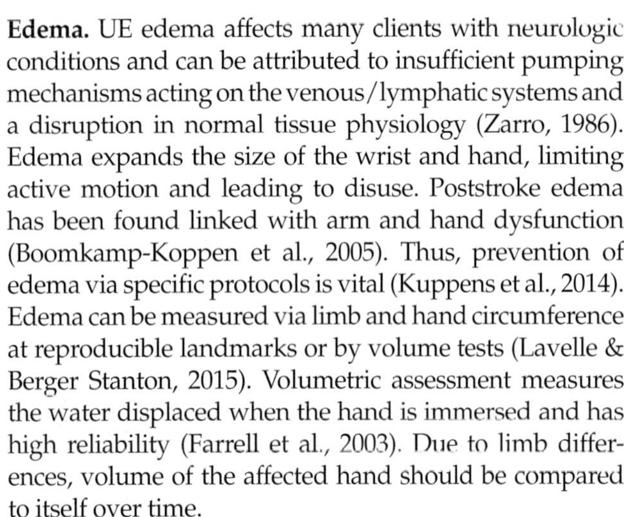
Edema. UE edema affects many clients with neurologic conditions and can be attributed to insufficient pumping mechanisms acting on the venous/lymphatic systems and a disruption in normal tissue physiology (Zarro, 1986). Edema expands the size of the wrist and hand, limiting active motion and leading to disuse. Poststroke edema has been found linked with arm and hand dysfunction (Boomkamp-Koppen et al., 2005). Thus, prevention of edema via specific protocols is vital (Kuppens et al., 2014). Edema can be measured via limb and hand circumference at reproducible landmarks or by volume tests (Lavelle & Berger Stanton, 2015). Volumetric assessment measures the water displaced when the hand is immersed and has high reliability (Farrell et al., 2003). Due to limb differences, volume of the affected hand should be compared to itself over time.

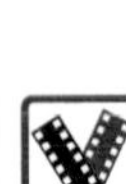
Sensibility. UE sensibility tests often focus on the fingertips and are key to understanding impairments affecting UE control (see Fig. 20.12 A,B and impairment section of video case studies). See Chapter 5 for a full review. Detailed descriptions are available in the ASHT Clinical Assessment Recommendations (MacDermid et al., 2015) and in a chapter by Jerosch-Herold (2011).

Pain. Pain can reduce recovery of UE function and participation regardless of origin (Vasudevan & Browne, 2014). Subjective pain can be gathered via self report, body diagrams, or pain rating scales (MacDermid et al., 2015). The McGill Pain Questionnaire (Melzack, 1975) examines pain quality and intensity. Body diagrams allow visualization of pain location and type. The Visual Analog Scale and Faces Pain Rating Scale (Wong & Baker, 1988) have good predictive and high concurrent validity in adults (Price et al., 1983) and children (Jedlinsky et al., 1999). The Face, Legs, Activity, Cry, Consolability (FLACC) scale is validated for use with infants and children from 2 months to 7 years of age (Merkel et al., 2002) and children with cognitive deficits (Malviya et al., 2006).

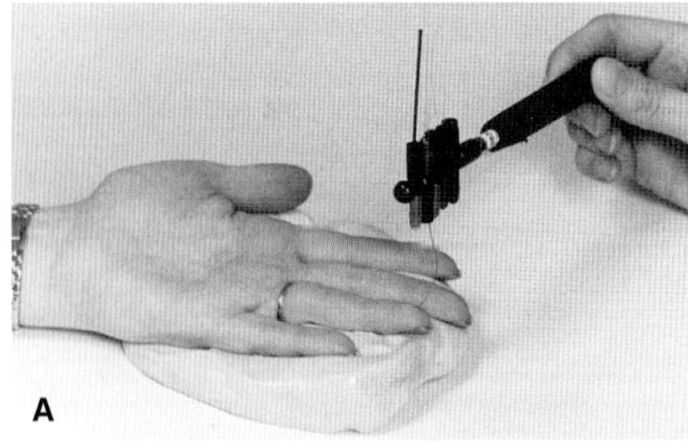

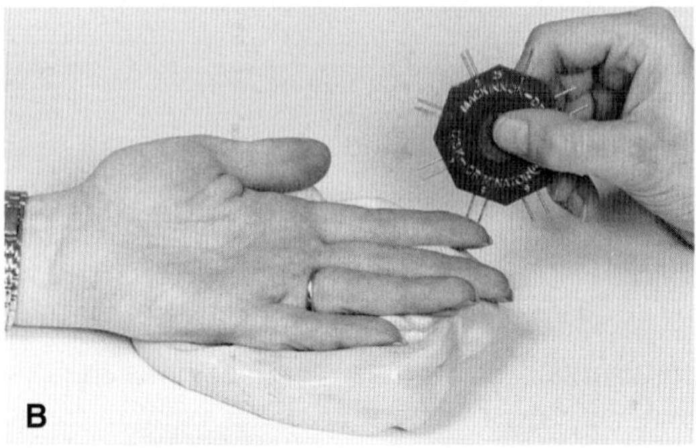

Figure 20.12 Tests of sensibility. **(A)** Weinstein Enhanced Sensory Test to examine touch pressure sensibility. **(B)** 2-point discrimination using the Disk-Criminator, a commercially available testing instrument.

In summary, when examining UE control, it is essential to assess areas across the ICF including: (a) *Activities and Participation*, to determine functional capability in a standard environment like the clinic (*capacity* in the ICF) and in one's actual environment (*performance* in the ICF); (b) strategies used to accomplish key components of UE function; and (c) underlying impairments (*Body Structure and Function* in the ICF). Since the list of measures is extensive, it is important to focus on areas that restrict UE function as relevant to life roles and participation. Tables 20.1 and 20.2 summarize evaluation profiles for Jean and Tim. The list highlights key areas of function, with participation, underlying components, and impairments, and specific tests that could be used for assessment.

EVALUATION: INTERPRETING THE RESULTS OF THE EXAMINATION

A task-oriented approach to retraining UE control in clients with neurologic dysfunction begins with harnessing strengths to modify (prevent) impairments,

TABLE 20.1 Summary of Evaluation Profile for Jean

<table>
<tr><th>Function (capacity and performance)</th><th>Strategy</th><th>Impairments of body structure</th></tr>
<tr><td>1. Documentation of frequency of social participation</td><td rowspan="4">Qualitative Movement:
• Eye–head coordination
• Anticipatory reach to grasp
• Prehension patterns available
• Grading of fingertip forces
• In-hand manipulation skill</td><td rowspan="4">• Cognition: Mini-Mental Status Examination
• Visual perception (MVPT-4) (Colarusso et al., 2015)
• Musculoskeletal: ROM, strength, power
• Isolated finger motion
• Spasticity in RUE
• Sensibility in RUE
• Edema in RUE
• Pain at rest and with active motion/sustained grip</td></tr>
<tr><td>2. Level of self-care independence: dressing, grooming, bathing, toileting</td></tr>
<tr><td>3. Level of independence in cooking and self-feeding</td></tr>
<tr><td>4. Level of mobility with an assistive device</td></tr>
<tr><td>5. Level of independence in handwriting</td><td>• Pencil grip or writing tool
• Efficiency of near and far copying with or without a writing tool</td><td></td></tr>
</table>

MVPT-4, Motor-Free Visual Test, 4th edition; ROM, range of motion; RUE, right upper extremity.

increase strategies to achieve function, and fostering functional capability (task frequency and independence in context [participation]). Understanding contextual factors, both environmental and personal, that impact treatment decisions is important. Personal factors (age, desires educational level, ethnicity, gender, personal interests, self-efficacy, and outcomes expectations) can all impact goals, choice of therapeutic strategies, and response to intervention. Environmental factors (social support, available technology, and other factors) also influence treatment.

Long-Term Goals

As proposed in Chapter 6, long-term goals should be objective and measurable, and expressed in terms of participation in self-care, work, or leisure activities executed to fulfill life roles. For example, a long-term goal for Jean could be "Jean will prepare a morning meal independently (to fulfill her homemaker role)." A long-term goal for Tim could be "Tim will be able to independently and efficiently don clothing for recess (to fulfill his student role)."

Short-Term Goals

Short-term goals should be objective and measurable. They may be described to resolve impairments and recover key motor strategies. They may include motor planning, sequencing, and adaptive strategies so functional tasks can be performed in changing environments. They also may be described as interim steps to achieving independence in a functional task. Tables 20.3 and 20.4 illustrate how identification of problems progress to the formation of goals and treatment planning in our two case studies. Examples are not all-inclusive, yet allow the close examination of the concepts.

Client-Identified Goals

In this era of client-centered practice, the COPM (Song et al., 2019) or the GAS (Debreceni-Nagy et al., 2019) can be used for clients or caregivers to set goals.

Cognition and Perception

Cognitive and perceptual deficits can restrict movement and are a major factor in lack of progress in those with neurologic insults (Cumming et al., 2013; Titus et al., 1991). Yet, research has shown that UE functional recovery poststroke can occur despite diminished cognition (Skidmore et al., 2012). See Table 5.3 for a review. Programs that include cognitive interventions within a task-oriented approach such as the Cognitive Orientation to daily Occupational Performance (CO-OP) program (McEwen et al., 2014; Wolf et al., 2016) may be beneficial. Music-based programs can also be effective to improve cognition and UE function in neurological conditions (Moumdjian et al., 2017; Pohl et al., 2018).

TABLE 20.2 Summary of Evaluation Profile for Tim

Function (capacity and performance)	Strategy	Impairments (body structure and function)
1. Documentation of frequency of play and social interaction during UE classroom and recess activities	Manipulation skills: • Prehension patterns available and frequency used • Pencil grip • In-hand manipulation skill • Efficiency of prehension (task duration)	• Cognition: Visual/auditory memory ABCs and numbers • Perception: VMI (Beery et al., 2004), TVPS-4 (Martin, 2017) • Musculoskeletal: Strength, isolated movement of fingers and thumb, power • Sensibility in both hands • Pain after prolonged hand use (endurance) (MacDermid et al., 2015)
2. Level of self-care independence: don/doff coat with, shoe tying/untying, handwashing, toileting		
3. Level of independence in manipulation of materials: pencils, scissors, glue, tape		
4. Level of independence in handwriting	• Efficiency of near and far copying skill with and without pencil grip (task duration) • Method used to hold paper steady	

UE, upper extremity; VMI, Visual–motor integration; TVPS-4, Test of Visual Perceptual Skills, 4th edition.

Attention and Unilateral Neglect. To promote the identification of an object's characteristics, clients can be encouraged to explore them visually and haptically, attending to relevant features used to shape their hand and scale fingertip forces. Before clients grasp objects, they can be asked about the relevant features such as, "Do you think that object is heavy or light?" "Is it slippery or not?" "Can you open your hand wide enough to secure the object?" In persons with hemiparesis and unilateral neglect, a clinician can promote motion into that workspace by placing visual and auditory objects in the area then asking them to locate those objects. Affected arm movement could be fostered by having the client perform tasks with the less-affected arm in a mirror or by observing another person. Visual mirror

feedback training is shown in the treatment video of Genise, our client with acute stroke.

Research evidence. A systematic review of RCTs examining the effect of cognitive training on spatial neglect (Bowen et al., 2013) had inconclusive results. Yet, retraining perceptual aspects of prehension is important to motor control (Desanghere & Marotta, 2008) and may be feasible with activation of the mirror neuron system. Mirror neurons found in the premotor, parietal, and primary motor cortex (M1) are active during action and observation of action (Bonaiuto & Arbib, 2010; Dushanova & Donoghue, 2010). Thus, viewing action causes enough activity to predict the direction and trajectory of observed motion online. Mirror-based action observation training in persons with conditions such as stroke can increase the neuronal response (Brunner et al., 2014; Garrison et al., 2010), improve UE function (Mao et al., 2020), and improve reaching time (Harmsen et al., 2015).

Tapping into the auditory system through music-based training or auditory cueing is currently being explored as a method to increase attention in the neglected visual field (Kang & Thaut, 2019; Schenke et al., 2020; Van Vleet & DeGutis, 2013). Research for

TABLE 20.3 Problems, Goals, and Methods Suitable for a 1-Hour Session—Jean

Level	Problems	Long-term goals	Short-term goals	Methods
1: Function (Capacity and Performance)	1. Jean is unable to prepare meals for herself and her husband. 2. Jean is unable to hold kitchen utensils. 3. Jean is unable to perform self-grooming.	1. Jean will prepare three 2-person meals independently, using utensils. 2. Jean will be able to groom herself in preparation for guests or outings.	1. Jean will prepare a simple one-person 3-step meal by herself. 2. Jean will manage utensils, hairbrush, toothbrush, and tooth-paste tube independently or with adaptive devices.	1. Provide written step-by-step directions 2. Modeling, task- practice, intrinsic/extrinsic feedback 3. Adapt tools such as adding foam to handles of utensils hairbrush, toothbrush to allow her to use a gross grasp or a lateral pinch.
2: Strategy	1. Jean can achieve a gross grasp only in her affected hand 2. Jean seems to wait until she contacts objects before closing her fingers (poor anticipatory control).		1. Jean will grasp objects of various sizes and shapes using a gross grasp and other pinch patterns. 2. Jean will prepare for object contact during reaches by opening and partly closing her hand	1. Practice reaching for stable objects requiring a gross grasp and progress to use of a lateral pinch. 2. During reaches, provide verbal cues to open then close fingers to prepare for object contact. 3. Video review of taped sessions talking through action in advance.
3: Impairments (Body structure and function)	1. Jean has visual and auditory memory deficits. 2. Jean is unable to sequence tasks greater than 2 steps in length. 3. Jean has partial isolated movement of the thumb and fingers. 4. Jean has weak finger and wrist extensors. 5. Sensibility is impaired in volar fingers and thumb pads		1. Jean will be verbally state the 3-step sequence of one meal preparation. 2. Jean will read sequence of one meal preparation independently. 3. Jean will isolate her thumb to achieve a lateral pinch. 4. Jean will extend her MPs actively to neutral and her wrist to 25 degrees. 5. Jean will use tactile and proprioceptive cues to identify objects.	1. Verbal rehearsal of meal preparation sequence prior to task practice. 2. Video review of taped sessions, discussing steps taken during performance. 3. Place and hold small objects and utensils in a lateral pinch. 4. Biofeedback, NMES and resistive equipment (1- to 3-lb weights). Cotton balls and Velcro boards Theraputty to foster active finger extension. 5. Place familiar objects on the table and have her practice identifying them via touch with and without vision.

FES, functional electrical stimulation; MP, metacarpophalangeal, NMES, neuromuscular electrical stimulation.

TABLE 20.4 Problems, Goals, and Methods Appropriate for Tim

Level	Problems	Long-term goals	Short-term goals	Methods
1: Function	1. Tim takes too long donning his coat and boots, limiting his play time at recess. 2. Tim requires moderate assistance to complete art projects that require use of scissors.	1. Tim will don his outdoor gear independently and efficiently allowing him to attend full recess. 2. Tim will complete art projects requiring use of scissors independently.	1. Tim will increase his efficiency for donning his coat / boots by reducing the task duration 25% per week. 2. Tim will trace a circle, cut it out, and paste it on paper as described in the directions.	1a. Therapist/peer modeling 1b. Timed task practice donning coat/ boots, and securing buttons. 1c. Variable intrinsic/extrinsic feedback. 1d. Large boots. 2. Use scissors with smaller finger openings to enhance stability. 3. Peer modeling with varied verbal feedback.
2: Strategy	1. Tim has trouble solving motor problems such as learning to secure fasteners on a new jacket. 2. Tim has limited in-hand manipulation skills.		1. Tim will secure and open a range of coat fasteners in 2 months. 2. Tim will shift a pencil along his fingerpads to write and rotate the pencil to erase in 1 month.	1a. Teacher/peer modeling 1b. Task practice with different fasteners on various jackets. 1c. Variable intrinsic/extrinsic feedback on solutions used. 2. Task practice moving varied writing tools in one hand.
3: Impairments	1. Tim has weak intrinsic hand muscles, reducing his pinch/grip strength.		1. Tim will increase pinch strength by 1/2 lb in 2 months (lateral pinch, 3-jaw chuck).	1. Therapeutic putty exercises at school and home. 2. 3-D object construction such as Legos.

this type of training is promising, yet, further work is warranted. Based on the evidence, using visual mirror feedback training or auditory cueing may be effective in both Jean and Genise.

Problem Solving and Apraxia. Learning to solve movement problems is a major step toward the development or recovery of motor skills (Adolph, 1994). To promote this, the clinician can ask the client to offer a verbal or motor solution to a select problem such as "how to hold the fork to get the potatoes on it." In clients without perceptual deficits, modeling an alternate strategy may be best. If they have perceptual issues, one could model the task then provide verbal or manual cues to guide them through suitable movement(s). Whenever manual assistance is given, the therapist (or helper) becomes part of the solution. Thus, any assistance should be followed by independent task practice to give clients the opportunity to plan and perform the movement themselves.

Research evidence. Requiring clients of any age to solve movement problems can foster motor learning (Harbourne & Berger 2019). Two examples are robotic training in adults poststroke and use of contingent reinforcement (CR) in infants at risk for UE dysfunction. Fasoli and Adans-Dester (2019) compared those who underwent UE robotic training (RT) only against those who received upper limb RT plus task-oriented training (RT-TOT). Both programs used the protocol, Active Learning Program for Stroke, which integrates cognitive strategies. All showed significant change in the FMA-UE,

MAL, WMFT, and the SIS-hand section supporting the inclusion of cognitive strategies within robotic training.

The paradigm of CR (Rovee & Rovee, 1969; Rovee Collier & Sullivan, 1980) initially engaged young infants by linking motion of a mobile with kicking or arm movement, via tethering of the mobile to the leg or arm of the infant. The CR paradigm has been used to assess learning and coordination in different infant groups (Heathcock et al., 2004; Sargent et al., 2014). Technological advances now allow expansion of the CR paradigm to reinforce self-generated muscle activation (Duff et al., 2017) or arm motion (Duff et al., 2020) detected with surface electromyography (EMG) or inertial sensors to drive motion of overhead mobiles or toys.

Training to Improve Musculoskeletal and Neuromuscular System Characteristics

Numerous methods are available to enhance ROM and strength, reduce the effects of spasticity, and increase isolated movement. Passive and active exercises, myofascial release (Manheim & Lavett, 1989), the Feldenkrais method (Apel, 1992), Tai Chi (Hogan, 2005; Venglar, 2005) yoga (Schmid et al., 2014), and other approaches (Wanning, 1993) can help mobilize structures essential to UE control. Participation in enjoyable recreational activities have been found to increase physical function and cognition (Han et al., 2017; Hogan, 2005).

Manual Techniques. Many sources describe in detail approaches to mobilize the trunk and UE structures to enhance movement in clients with neurologic dysfunction (Boehme, 1988; Carr & Shepard, 1992, 1998; Landel, 2018; Voss et al., 1985). Active movement should always follow passive strategies to promote carryover. For example, UE flexor tightness often develops in clients with hemiplegia who habitually hold the affected arm in a mass flexion pattern, limiting return of active movement. Thus, after passively stretching the flexors, a clinician could set-up a task to have the client touch or grasp stable objects placed below shoulder height yet within reach (Fig. 20.13). This could foster wrist and elbow extension while minimizing activation of a flexor synergy pattern. Target height could gradually be raised toward shoulder level as movement strategy improves.

Orthotics. Remediation of musculoskeletal tightness and shortening of arm and hand structures often includes casts and orthoses (Fess et al., 2005; Malick, 1980; Neuhaus et al., 1981). Sustained low-load stretch to joints and muscle, via orthotics, can change noncontractile tissue length (e.g., ligaments) and increase the number of sarcomeres (Blanchard et al., 1985; Tardieu et al., 1988). Orthotics that restrict joint motion can reduce the degrees of freedom that one has to control thus adding to functional ability.

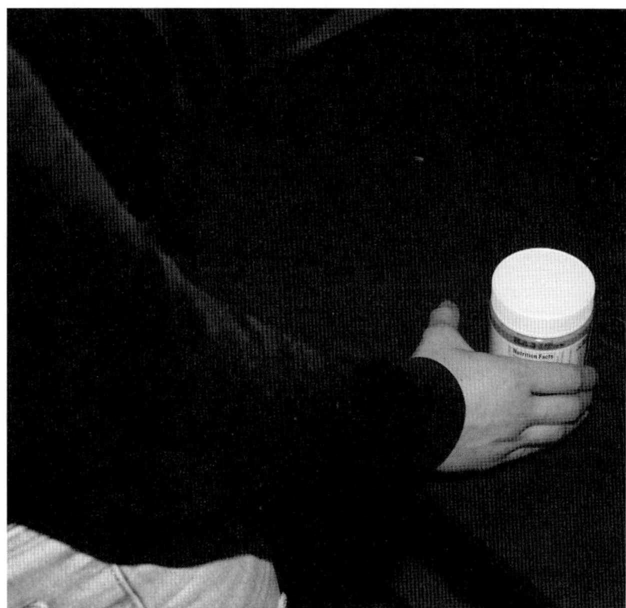

Figure 20.13 To prevent activation of an undesirable flexor synergy pattern, set up tasks to allow reach-to-grasp into gravity in sitting or standing as shown.

Orthoses or straps that minimize joint restriction or allow more functional hand use are optimal. Positions that reduce development of undesirable contractures linked with flaccidity or inactive hand movement, are preferred. For example, an intrinsic plus position of the hand (Fig. 20.14A) places the finger metacarpophalangeal joints in flexion and interphalangeal joints in extension ensuring that ligaments are taut, preventing shortening while the thumb remains in neutral. For persons with excessive wrist flexion that interferes with active grasp, a semiflexible orthotic (Fig. 20.14B) may be useful. This allows for partial wrist motion and weight bearing in the case of infants, while preventing extreme wrist flexion. Thumbs straps or adjustable splints placing the thumb in opposition (Fig. 20.14C) facilitate successful pinch patterns. Doucet and Mettler (2013) found that custom-fit dynamic progressive orthotics increase wrist PROM and reduce resistance to passive movement in adults with chronic stroke and hypertonicity. As feasible, nonaffected structures should move freely, preventing secondary deficits due to immobility. At 1 month poststroke, Genise is developing finger and wrist flexor tightness. It may be important to consider the use of a hand orthotic to prevent further loss of motion.

Augmented Motion and Feedback

Various methods are available to augment motion and provide feedback to reduce impairments and expand resources. These include robotic training, biofeedback, electrical stimulation, transcranial magnetic stimulation (TMS), transcranial direct current stimulation (tDCS), transcutaneous spinal stimulation, and sensory

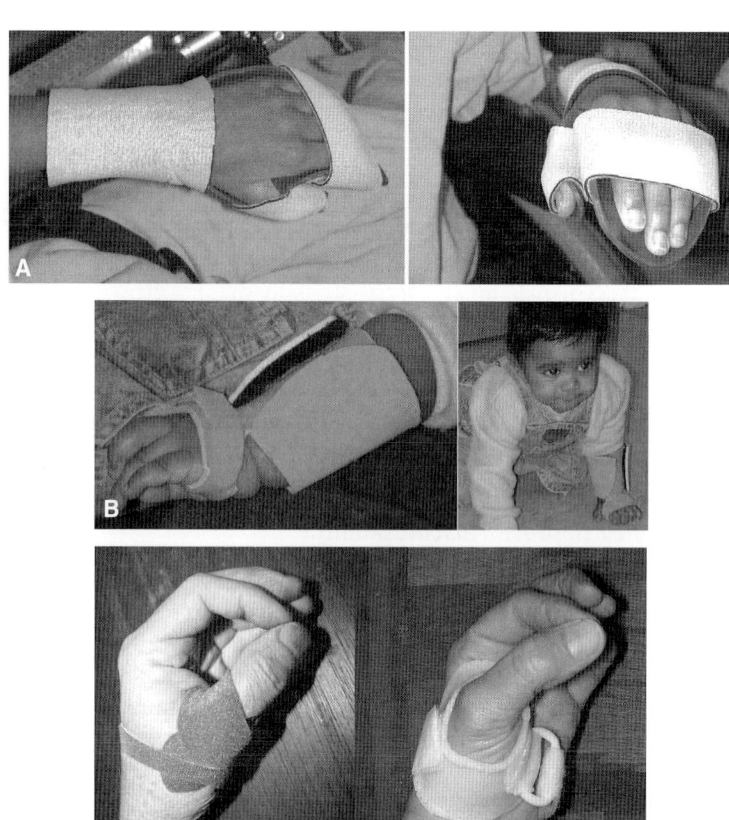

Figure 20.14 Orthotics and straps used to alter hand or wrist position, including an intrinsic plus position with the thumb in neutral **(A)**, a semiflexible wrist orthotic **(B)** can be used for weight bearing, and a thumb opposition strap and splint **(C)**.

reeducation. These methods can be used to prime the neural system in preparation for movement or be used to augment the effect of other training programs (Cassidy et al., 2014; Pomeroy et al., 2011; Stoykov & Madhavan, 2015). All of our cases may benefit from one or more of the methods reviewed subsequently.

Robotic Training. To augment passive/active training provided by therapists, and to increase movement repetitions and intensity during therapy, studies have explored robotic training (Bertani et al., 2017; Chen & Howard, 2016; Raghavan et al., 2020; Veerbeek et al., 2017). In a systematic review Zhang et al. (2017) found that RT and RT combined with conventional therapy led to better outcomes particularly in those with chronic stroke. Since robotic devices provides support for heavy limbs, training could begin earlier in the rehabilitation process (Raghavan et al., 2020).

Despite potential benefits, many studies have found that the effects of robotic therapy are comparable to those achieved with conventional therapy. Stein et al. (2004) compared a 6-week program (3 times per week) of robotic training in the form of progressive resistive exercise (PRE) to active assistive training on functional and motor recovery. Results ($n = 46$) revealed improvements in FMA UE and maximal force. While there were no group differences, those with better motor control before training made the most gains with PRE robotic training based on the FMA-UE. Reinkensmeyer et al. (2009) found that 4 to 5 weeks of robotic or nonrobotic training improved strength, speed, and coordination. A single-blind RCT (McCabe et al., 2015) compared the effect of three training programs run for 12 weeks, 5 hours per day, 5 days per week in persons with severe impairment poststroke: (a) robotic training with motor learning, (b) functional electrical stimulation plus motor learning, and (c) motor learning alone. While the authors did not find group differences all participants improved on the FMA-UE and the Arm Motor Ability Test. Wolf et al. (2015) conducted a single-blinded, multisite RCT comparing a home-based robotic system (Hand Mentor Pro) within a home exercise program (HEP) to HEP alone in 99 adults with hemiplegia. Both groups improved on the ARAT, WMFT, and FMA-UE. Rodgers et al. (2019) ran a multisite RCT in persons 1 to 5 years poststroke with moderate-to-severe UE dysfunction. They compared RT to enhanced upper limb therapy (EULT) and usual care and compared performance on the ARAT at 3 months post-training. Compared to usual care, RT and EULT did not improve UE function. Thus, robotic therapy alone may not significantly improve UE function beyond usual care.

To enhance outcomes from robotic therapy the parameters may need to be modified. In adults poststroke, Reinkensmeyer et al. (2012) compared conventional therapy to RT (using less motion assistance than needed for optimal performance) over 24 sessions in 2 months. Both groups improved FMA-UE score, at the 3-month follow-up, yet the robot-trained group improved grip strength and on the Box and Block test, whereas the control group did not. A unique study examined robotic assistance for finger movements during a 3-hour per week, 3-week training program using a musical game (Reinkensmeyer et al., 2017). The findings showed significant improvement in scores on the Box and Blocks and measures of depression and self-efficacy. Participants receiving high assistance during training showed significant change on the FMA-UE and lateral pinch strength. Hsieh et al. (2012) examined the effect of 4 weeks of high- versus low-intensity robotic training compared to control treatment. The high-intensity training had a greater number of repetitions. The results show that high-intensity RT led to significant improvement on the FMA-UE versus other forms of treatment. Thus, robotic therapy may be most beneficial if motion assistance ensures effort or guidance is sufficient (Reinkensmeyer et al., 2012; Rowe et al., 2017), and if it is employed at a significant intensity (Hsieh et al., 2012). Further work on ways to best augment robotic therapy with TMS, tDCS to further enhance UE function is needed. Genise, our client with acute stroke with profound paresis and little voluntary motion in her paretic limb, may benefit from RT to foster arm motion.

Robotic training studies done with children are favorable, yet clear benefits are not yet known. Gilliaux et al. (2015) compared two different 8-week programs provided 5 days per week in children with CP. One program used conventional therapy, and the other provided a program of conventional and robot-assisted sessions. The results revealed significant improvement in smoothness of movement based on kinematic analysis and improved dexterity based on the Box and Block test for the group engaged in conventional and robot-assisted training.

Biofeedback and Neuromuscular Electrical Stimulation. Biofeedback and neuromuscular electrical stimulation (NMES) augments motion in those with reduced UE function. NMES can be provided via surface, percutaneous, or implanted electrodes. Since treatment timelines vary based on the dysfunction, clinical judgment must guide scheduling. Research supports the integration of biofeedback and NMES into clinical practice to develop and recover active UE movement in adults and children (Alon et al., 2003, 2008; Garzon et al., 2016; Yang et al., 2019). Surface NMES is often used to successfully facilitate wrist extension (Fig. 20.15) yet ideally is followed up with active motion. Protocols studying the benefit of stimulation continue to evolve.

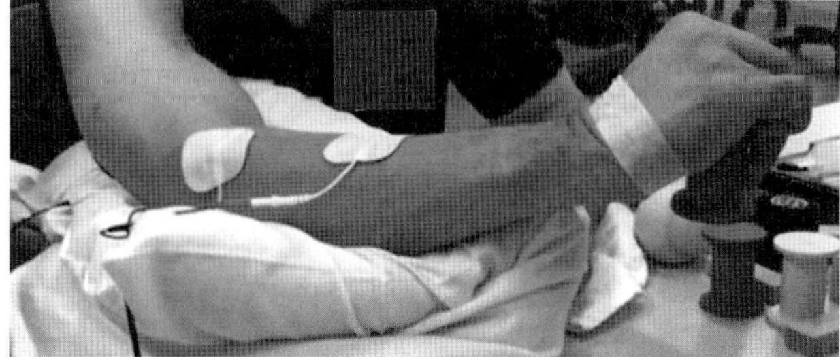

Figure 20.15 Augmenting wrist extension during grasp and lift of objects with neuromuscular electrical stimulation.

Doucet and Griffin (2013) examined the effect of high- (40 Hz) versus low-frequency (20 Hz) NMES in high functioning (HF) and low functioning (LF) adults with chronic stroke. The program ran 4 times per week for 1 month. Only the HF subjects showed significant improvement in outcome. HF subjects who received high-frequency NMES improved in strength, whereas those who received low-frequency NMES improved in dexterity and endurance. Knutson et al. (2012) compared a 6-week program of contralaterally controlled FES (CCFES) to cyclic NMES on UE impairment and performance in 17 adults poststroke. Participants wore a glove on the less-affected hand that controlled hand opening in the affected hand. The results revealed that CCFES led to improvements on the FMA-UE, Box and Block test, and Arm Motor Ability Test. There was also a significant increase in finger extension in the CCFES group. The CCFES protocol has now been shown to reduce impairment in persons with chronic stroke (Knutson et al., 2014) and increase the rate of recovery of wrist and finger extension in the acute phase poststroke (Zheng et al., 2019).

Studies examining NMES are limited in children. Wright and Granat (2000) applied 30 minutes of NMES for 6 weeks to the wrist extensors of children with unilateral CP (mean 10 years) and found active wrist extension and hand function improved and was maintained at the 6-week follow-up. Another study (Garzon et al., 2016) trained grasp and manipulation via NMES in three children with unilateral CP for 48 sessions in 16 weeks. All improved grip strength and two improved the QUEST grasp score with mixed results for the other measures.

Combining NMES with orthotics has been shown effective. Ozer et al. (2006) found the use of NMES and elbow/wrist/hand dynamic bracing (Ultraflex, Pottstown, PA) in children with unilateral CP led to improvement in scores on the Melbourne Assessment of Unilateral Limb Function, greater grip strength, and improved hand/wrist posture evaluation based on Zancolli's classification. The effects of the combined program lasted for 2 months posttreatment. A 3-week training program that included NMES in combination with a wrist orthotic (Hybrid Assistive Neuromuscular Dynamic Stimulation [HANDS]) was found to improve UE motor function and reduce spasticity in 20 adults with chronic stroke immediately and after a 3-month follow-up (Fujiwara et al., 2009).

The combination of NMES with other methods has also been shown effective. A pilot study examined the benefit of an integrated system of NMES and robotics on hand function and tracking in adults with chronic stroke (Rong et al., 2015). After 20 sessions, scores on the FMA-UE, ARAT, and WMFT improved and spasticity reduced, based on the Modified Ashworth Scale. An RCT in children with unilateral CP (Xu et al., 2015) compared outcomes from a 2-week, five times per week training program among three groups: Constraint Induced Movement Therapy (CIMT) alone, CIMT with NMES to the wrist and finger extensors, or traditional unimanual and bimanual training in Occupational Therapy (OT). Results showed that the group that underwent CIMT plus NMES had the highest rate of improvement in integrated EMG of the wrist extensors. Thus, the combined use of NMES with orthotics, RT, or CIMT may be most effective to improve UE function.

Technology in Brain-Computer Interface (BCI) or EEG-triggered NMES offers a way to synchronize cortical signals with movement initiated with electrical stimulation (Milosevic et al., 2020). Research has begun to explore the benefits of BCI to restore voluntary arm function in persons poststroke. Marquez-Chin et al. (2016a, 2016b) employed BCI in a 64-year-old male with chronic stroke and severe left hemiplegia. The BCI was used to trigger a neuroprosthesis to initiate reaching forward/laterally and reaching to the mouth for 40 sessions (60-minute active sessions, 3 times per week). The results revealed a clinically significant increase in the FMA-UE of 6 points (13–18) and a 7-point increase in the FIM self-care subscore (104–118). The TRI Hand Function Test Object Manipulation subscore and the ARAT score remained at zero since these tests require hand function, which were not programed within the neuroprosthesis. Further work in this exciting area is ongoing.

Cortical Stimulation. Stimulation of the cortex can be used to prime the nervous system and used in conjunction with practice-based methods. Recovery of arm and hand motion have been examined via implanted electrode methodology, external TMS, and tDCS. Levy et al. (2016) examined the use of cortical implanted stimulation to foster recovery of arm function poststroke. This multicenter RCT (Everest Phase III trial) included a 6-week task-oriented UE training program with the experimental group also receiving electrical epidural motor cortex stimulation (EECS). Select participants in the experimental group had serious adverse events related to EECS. The findings at 4 weeks post-training did not reveal efficacy for the EECS procedure. Yet, select group differences were found at 24 weeks. Further study of the procedures related to and the benefits of invasive cortical stimulation are recommended.

A pilot study with 10 clients examined the benefits of tDCS in combination with robotic therapy and found significant improvement in a small number of clients and little change in the majority of clients (Hesse et al., 2007). The authors concluded that the techniques were safe but required further examination. Giacobbe et al. (2013) examined the benefits of tDCS provided before, during, or after a 20-minute session of robotic training in persons with chronic stroke. Kinematic performance (speed and smoothness) improved most when tDCS was delivered before the robotic practice.

Low-frequency rTMS (≤1 Hz) provided to the nonlesioned hemisphere is theorized to provide an inhibitory effect in an attempt to reduce the interhemispheric suppression of activity in the lesioned hemisphere. Gillick et al. (2014) examined the benefits of low-frequency, repetitive TMS combined with CIMT (reviewed below) to improve hand function in children with unilateral CP. The results showed a significant improvement in the AHA score after low-frequency rTMS/CIMT training. Tretriluxana et al. (2013) examined the use of repetitive TMS (rTMS) given at a low frequency for the inhibitory effect on the nonlesioned hemisphere with regard to reach-to-grasp recovery in the affected arm of adults poststroke. This 2-day treatment demonstrated the feasibility of rTMS to improve reach-to-grasp function in those with hemiparesis.

The benefits of TMS, tDCS, and programs combining TMS or tDCS with other modes of therapy continue to expand. Gillick et al. (2018) conducted a small RCT during a 10 consecutive weekday session of CIMT. Children in group one received tDCS to the nonlesioned hemisphere for 20 minutes concurrently with 120 minutes of CIMT, whereas group two underwent CIMT only for 120 minutes. This study found the procedures feasible and safe with a subset of children with an intact corticospinal tract (CST) showing an improvement in hand function. Noninvasive brain stimulation is being explored with infants at risk, yet there are challenges (Behan et al., 2020; Kowalski et al., 2019). The benefits of noninvasive cortical stimulation after stroke are enhanced if combined with TOT or specific prehensile training (Bravi & Stoykov, 2007). Further work in this area is recommended.

Spinal Stimulation. Transcutaneous spinal cord (SC) stimulation introduced to enhance trunk stability and locomotion in persons with spinal cord injury (SCI; Gad et al. 2017; Gerasimenko et al., 2015) has now expanded to children with CP (Solopova et al. 2017). Cervical SC stimulation combined with training over 4 weeks in eight participants with complete and incomplete SCI increased grip strength and selective distal UE motor control (Gad et al., 2018). Research examining the effectiveness of cervical neuromodulation with training on UE skill and function in children and adults with hemiparesis is forthcoming.

Sensory Reeducation

Sensory reeducation makes use of neuroplasticity and higher cortical functions, including attention, learning, and memory, to facilitate sensory detection, recognition, and localization (Dellon et al., 1974; Zink & Philip, 2020). It is unclear whether sensory reeducation teaches clients how to use remaining sensibility to their advantage, or if it alters the physiologic basis for sensation. Investigators involved in training sensory function report that improvement is highly dependent on one's motivation and the training methods. Clients who are willing to use the affected limb are often better able to recover function.

A safe guideline for sensory training is related to one's performance on the Semmes–Weinstein Monofilaments test (see Chapter 5). If an individual cannot detect a 4.83 pressure rating, he or she is considered to have diminished protective sensation and treatment should focus on strategies to protect the limb from harmful stimuli (Brand, 1980) (Table 20.5). Vision can compensate for tactile deficits; as when viewing the hand when reaching for objects (Bell-Krotoski et al., 1993). Returning or developing sensibility is noted once touch pressure is above a pressure rating of 4.83. Then, treatment can focus on detection and localization of moving and stationary stimuli. As clients learn to perceive moving then constant touch, sensory reeducation can shift to stereognosis (e.g., object recognition).

TABLE 20.5 Summary of Guidelines Aimed at Protecting the Hand and Arm from Injury

1. Avoid exposure to thermal extremes and sharp objects.
2. Do not use excessive force when gripping a tool or object.
3. Build up small handles to distribute force and avoid localized increase in pressure.
4. Avoid tasks that require the use of a uniform grip over long periods.
5. Change tools frequently to alter grip pattern and to rest tissues.
6. Observe skin for signs of excess pressure.
7. Treat blisters and lacerations quickly and with care to avoid infection.
8. Maintain daily skin care, including soaking and oil massage to maintain optimal skin condition.

Source: Adapted from Brand PW. Management of sensory loss in the extremities. In: Omer E, Spinner M, eds. *Management of peripheral nerve problems.* Philadelphia, PA: Saunders, 1980:862–872.

Initiating training early in rehabilitation or using sensory substitution may improve motor function. In a multicenter RCT, Rosén et al. (2015) compared the timing of sensory reeducation after median and ulnar nerve repair. The experimental group began with mirror visual feedback and observation of touch the first week post-repair, whereas the control group began when reinnervation was detected. Greater improvement was noted in the experimental group. Rosén and Lundborg (2003) examined the use of artificial sensibility in the form of vibrotactile cues to replace absent sensibility after median and ulnar nerve repair in a single case study. They placed microphones on the tips of a sensor glove to pick up friction cues during object manipulation. Functional outcomes at 6 and 12 months showed higher performance levels than usual for nerve repair. Using neural imaging, Lundborg et al. (2005) verified that typical adults trained with vibrotactile input had greater activation of the somatosensory cortex than untrained adults. Further study of the timing of sensory reeducation and vibrotactile feedback training with other neural conditions is warranted.

The benefit of sensory and motor training was found effective in a study by Byl and Mckenzie (2000) in a clinic- and home-based program for persons with focal hand dystonia. Clinic treatment included (a) sensory training with and without biofeedback; and (b) stress-free hand use, mirror imagery, and mental practice designed to halt the atypical movements and facilitate typical hand motor control. The home program aimed to reduce neural tension, improve posture, facilitate relaxation, and promote aerobic capacity. Motor control, motor accuracy, sensory discrimination, and physical ability were improved post-training. Functional improvement was noted 3 to 6 months later with 11/12 subjects back to work.

Edema and Pain

Methods to reduce hand edema include compression (i.e., stretchy gloves), ice, elevation above heart level, or active muscle pumping. Reduction in edema with an increase in active movement may assist pain reduction. Methods to reduce pain are heat, cold, or transcutaneous electrical nerve stimulation (TENS; Mannheimer & Lampe, 1984).

Intervention for Sensorimotor Strategies

A task-oriented approach to retraining may begin by easing impairments that constrain task performance and participation. Reducing impairments may allow use of prior UE control strategies. Key components of UE motion such as a smooth hand path and hand pre-shaping may be best elicited if real tasks versus simulated ones are used (Wu et al., 1998). Since context drives retraining these components they must be done with purposeful tasks and real-life situations. The amount of time spent training different components will vary depending on the skill level present. Sensorimotor strategies would be useful for all of our cases.

Eye–Head Coordination

An important part of UE control is training or retraining eye–head coordination, essential to locate and stabilize gaze on a targets. Problems associated with object localization and gaze stabilization may influence reaching accuracy. Since different control mechanisms underlie motion of eyes, head, and trunk, these systems may be trained separately and in combination.

A progression of exercises for retraining eye–head coordination and gaze stabilization in clients with vestibular dysfunction were proposed by Susan Herdman, a PT, and David Zee, MD (Herdman et al., 2001; Zee, 1985). These exercises can retrain eye–head coordination in clients with central neurologic disorders. A literature review (Herdman, 2013) and clinical practice guidelines (Hall et al., 2016) summarize exercises vestibular training exercises (Table 20.6). The program begins with retraining saccadic and smooth-pursuit eye movements while the head is still. The exercises progress to training coordinated eye and head movements to peripheral targets and maintaining a stable gaze on objects moving in phase with the head. Finally, actions involving eye, head, and trunk motion are practiced as clients learn to locate targets in the far periphery while sitting, standing, and walking (Herdman et al., 2001; Zee, 1985).

Research in visual–perceptual training in persons with neurological lesions are expanding. In an RCT, Van Wyk et al. (2014) examined the effect of task-specific training on saccadic eye movement and

TABLE 20.6 Exercises to Retrain Saccadic and Smooth-Pursuit Eye Movements While the Head Is Still

Stage I. Eye Exercises
A. Exercises to improve visual following (smooth pursuit)
1. Sit in a comfortable position; do not move your head.
2. Hold a small target (2 × 2 inches) with written material at arm's length in front of you.
3. Keep your head still.
4. Move your arm slowly from side to side about 45 degrees. Focus on the words as you move.
5. Move your arm to the left, then right, then center. Rest for 3 seconds. Repeat 5 times.
6. Move your arm up and down about 30 degrees. Move your arm up, down, then center. Rest for 3 seconds. Repeat 5 times.
B. Exercises to improve gaze redirection (saccade)
1. Sit in a comfortable position; do not move your head.
2. Hold two small targets (2 × 2 inches), one in each hand, about 12 inches apart in front of you.
3. Move your eyes only from one target to the other.
4. Move right, move left. Stop and rest.
5. Repeat 5 times.
6. Hold two targets in front of you vertically, above and below the midline. Keep your head still; move your eyes only from one target to the other.
7. Move eyes up, eyes down. Stop and rest.
8. Repeat 5 times.

TABLE 20.6 Exercises to Retrain Saccadic and Smooth-Pursuit Eye Movements While the Head Is Still (*continued*)

Stage II. Head Exercises
A. Move head, object still
1. Side-to-side movements: Hold a small target at arm's length. Focus clearly on the words;; move your head slowly side to side. Move head to the right, left, then center. Rest. Repeat 5 times.
2. Up-and-down movements: Move your head up and down while keeping your eyes on the target held in front of you. Move head up; down; then center. Stop and rest. Repeat 5 times.
3. To progress, move your head faster and faster until you can no longer read the words. Repeat using a target that is attached to the wall 6 feet away.
4. Practice steps 1 and 2 with your eyes closed. Visualize the target as if your eyes were open.
Stage III. Eye–Head Exercises
A. Move eyes and head to stationary objects
1. Side-to-side movements: Hold two small targets (2 × 2 inches), one in each hand, 3-feet apart in front of you. Move your head and eyes toward one target, then the other. Clearly focus on the words on each target when you move your head and eyes. Look left; right; then rest. Repeat 5 times.
2. Up-and-down movements: Hold the two targets in front of you vertically, above and below the midline, 3-feet apart. Move your head and eyes toward one target, then the other. Clearly on the words on each target when you move your head and eyes. Look left; right; then rest. Repeat 5 times.
3. To progress, repeat steps 1 and 2, moving your head at faster and faster speeds until you can no longer read the words. Repeat using a target that is attached to the wall 6 feet away.
B. Move eyes, head, and object in phase together
1. Side-to-side movements: Hold a small target (2 × 2 inches) containing written material at arm's length in front of you. Move your arm and head together from side to side. Clearly focus on the words while you move your arm and head together slowly from side to side (about 15 degrees). Move left, right, center, then rest. Repeat 5 times.
2. Up-and-down movements: Hold a small target (2 × 2 inches) containing written material at arm's length in front of you. Move your arm and head together up and down. Clearly focus on the words while you move your arm and head together slowly up and down about 30 degrees. Move up; down; center; then rest. Repeat 5 times.
3. To progress, repeat steps 1 and 2, moving your head at faster and faster speeds until you can no longer read the words. Repeat using a target which is attached to the wall 6 feet away.

Modified with permission from Zee DS. Vertigo. In: Johnson RT, ed. *Current therapy in neurological diseases.* St. Louis, MO: C.V. Mosby, 1985:8–13.

scanning in adults poststroke with unilateral spatial neglect. The findings revealed that the King-Devick Test, Star Cancellation Test, and the Barthel Index had significant group differences favoring the group who underwent training. Another RCT (Wang et al., 2015) examined the effect of visual–spatial training on motor control in adults poststroke and found the training group significantly improved on an inattention test and the FMA-UE. Tsai et al. (2016) used a computer-based visual stimulation (VERSUS) program in young children with visual impairment to see if it could improve visual acuity (VA). The children made significant gains in VA suggesting that the VERSUS program is a viable option to improve VA in children with impairments.

Treatment strategies for visual neglect were reviewed earlier, yet the study of visual neglect/perception and the relationship they have to motor control requires further study. Training studies done in healthy populations may be relevant for persons with neurological conditions (Chen et al., 2016; Nyquist et al., 2016; Schuster et al., 2013). If training methods are beyond the scope of practice for clinicians at select clinical sites, it may be best to refer clients to a developmental optometrist or a clinician specializing in vision therapy.

Reach and Grasp

Reach-to-grasp movements require the ability to move the arm in all directions. They involve transporting the hand to an object to be grasped, forming the grip appropriately, stabilizing or manipulating the object, and possibly moving the object to a new location.

Facilitation of Active Motion. Training or retraining control of UE movement in cases of congenital or acquired paresis varies depending on the starting point. Several authors have laid out a progression of activities for retraining arm function (Boehme, 1988; Carr & Shepard, 1992; Voss et al., 1985). It may be easiest to begin by activating muscles through isolated joint movements via "place-and-hold" techniques in supine, sitting, and standing. Once muscle activation is achieved retraining active arm or hand control in a concentric or eccentric manner can begin in various positions. With partial UE control part to whole task practice may be feasible. Based on the difficulty transferring tasks learned in isolation to task performance in context, the demands may need to be modified.

The inclusion of targets or target objects in UE movement activities often engage clients more successfully than movement alone, because it makes the task more goal directed. Targets and target objects should vary depending on capabilities and program goals. For example, practice of select movements can be focused yet targeted as shown for reaching in Figure 20.13 and for supination in Figure 20.16. In persons with weakness or without grasping abilities, simply pointing to pictures with the whole hand, knocking down blocks or pushing balls will suffice. Thus, shoulder horizontal abduction and elbow extension could be practiced in sitting by asking a client to knock over a series of cardboard blocks with the dorsum of the hand, with arm support then progressing to the same action without support. As grasp improves, the type of objects used can be expanded. Examples of treatments which minimize the effects of gravity when practicing reaching with a paretic limb can be seen in the treatment video of Genise.

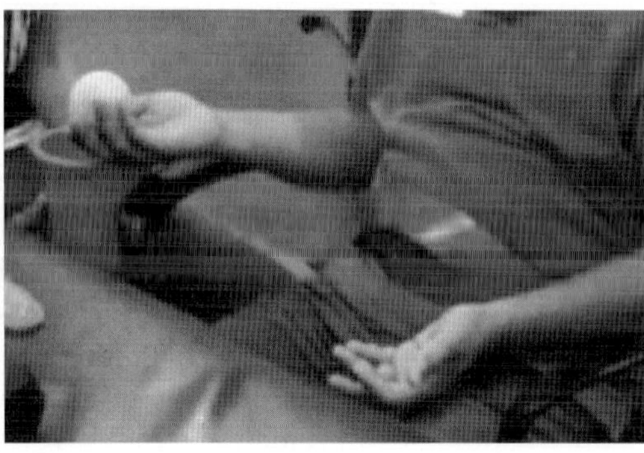

Figure 20.16 Targeted supination task.

Retraining Task-Dependent Characteristics of Reach. Features of arm transport vary with tasks, so intervention should be structured so clients can adapt reach used in a task-dependent way. The following are optional ways to train reaching based on research.

1. The transport phase of pointing, reaching and grasping, and grasping-manipulating objects all have very different features, thus training should be task specific.
2. Visual and auditory input can aid scanning for relevant cues of object location and features before movement onset. Initially, practice can be slower, drawing attention to visual cues for hand shaping, chiefly thumb position in relation to target location.
3. Reaching to new positions in space without visual input relies is guided by proprioception. To enhance performance, one might have a client initially locate a target visually then remove vision. Reaching accuracy would then provide evidence regarding the client's ability to control arm trajectory via proprioceptive cues only.
4. To facilitate force modulation during reaching, the clinician could ask the client to reach slowly, then quickly, to targets at various distances and locations. Reaching could then be practiced with cuff weights. In this way, the client can learn to program forces for slow and fast motion and movements requiring greater force and accuracy.
5. To reduce trunk compensation and foster reach extent and speed in the affected arm of persons poststroke, trunk motion could be dampened during reach training.
6. Visual modeling can take advantage of the Mirror Neuron System to enhance movement strategies. These strategies conducted prior to active movement may require longer processing and preparation time.

Verbal and Auditory Cues. Fasoli et al. (2002) studied the impact of verbal instructions on functional reach in individuals with stroke. They found reaches of those given externally focused or task-related instructions were shorter, with a higher peak velocity for all three tasks than the group who received internally focused or movement-related instructions. The effect of visual cueing to enhance movement in those with PD has been well documented yet less is known about the impact of auditory cueing. Nowak et al. (2006) trained individuals with PD on a grasp modulation task using auditory cues or stimulation of the subthalamic nucleus (SN). They found auditory cues were more effective than SN stimulation at improving akinesia. SN stimulation caused subjects to use excessive grip force during self-paced and externally paced conditions. More research is needed on the impact of scheduling verbal and auditory cueing during treatment in neurologic populations.

Postural Training. Many persons poststroke engage the trunk during reaching to compensate for insufficient UE motor control. Prevention of excess trunk activation may aid reach raining during recovery of the paretic arm. Yet, how is it best to set-up training of reach-and-grasp behaviors to reduce compensatory trunk motion?

Michaelsen et al. (2004b, 2006), examined the effectiveness of trunk restraint (TR) during reach-to-grasp training. Initially, Michaelsen and Levin (2004) had participants perform a reach-to-grasp task for 60 trials over a 1-day session. In the RCT, the experimental group wore a TR during reaches and the control group was asked not to move the trunk during reaches. The results indicated that the TR group used less trunk motion after training than controls. Elbow extension increased in both groups, yet was greater in the TR group at retention. A Temporal Coordination Index (TCI) was used to calculate the difference between elbow- and shoulder-phase angles (velocity against angle) at each moment in time (phase angle against time) throughout the reach. Multiple small peaks in the TCI provide evidence for a disruption in temporal coordination. TCI amplitude (TCI plotted against time) was found to correlate with the FMA-UE. In a follow-up RCT (Michaelsen et al., 2006), TR was compared against a control group. Thirty participants engaged in the supervised home program 3 times per week for 5 weeks. Results indicated that the TR group showed greater improvement than controls, on the FMA-UE and the Upper-Extremity Performance Assessment, particularly those with moderate hemiparesis. Kinematics revealed a decrease in trunk motion and increased elbow extension in the experimental group and the opposite finding in controls.

Thielman et al. (2004, 2008, 2010, 2012, 2013) examined various methods to retrain reach-to-grasp behaviors while restricting trunk motion. Thielman et al. (2008) compared task-related training (TRT) and resistive exercise (RE) in 11 adults after stroke for twelve 4-week sessions. For both groups, the trunk was restrained during training. After training, the hand path was straighter for the TRT group but not for the RE group. Also, trunk flexion decreased after both TRT and RE, yet arm flexion increased in the TRT group while reaching toward midline and contralateral targets. After training, FMA-UE scores improved in both groups, yet there was no change on the WMFT. In a 1-year follow-up study, the group that underwent TRT maintained straighter hand paths and spent less time in deceleration during reach (Thielman et al., 2013). Thielman and Bonsall (2012) used a crossover design in a case series to examine the benefit of REO Therapy (robot-assisted virtual training device) versus TRT in persons with moderate-to-severe hemiparesis poststroke. During REO training and TRT, a TR or auditory feedback was provided if the participant's shoulder was lifted off the anterior surface of the chairback. Auditory feedback was found feasible for both REO training and TRT yet needs further study to determine efficacy. These studies suggest that treatment aimed at reducing trunk compensation may lead to more efficient reach strategies and subsequent function.

Adaptive Positioning. Adaptive positioning is a frequently used to improve UE function. Seating programs are based on three assumptions: (a) adaptive seats will reduce abnormal muscle tone, (b) improved muscle tone will improve postural stability, and (c) increased postural stability will enhance UE control (McPherson et al., 1991; Waksvik & Levy, 1979). Several studies have examined the effect of altered seat angles on arm motion in children with and without CP. One study showed that arm motion was faster in children with CP with a backrest set at 90 degrees (Nwaobi et al., 1983). Another study (Angsupaisal et al., 2019) showed that foot supports with an anterior or neutral seat incline enhanced modulation of trunk extensor activity and improved reaching quality in children with spastic CP. Thus, children with CP may benefit from pelvic and trunk support with slight anterior neck flexion to foster visual–motor control. Furthermore, experience and body position are constraints that should be considered when examining the development of reaching behaviors (Carvalho et al., 2007, 2008).

Retraining Anticipatory Aspects of Reach and Grasp. Despite the importance of planning reaching trajectory and forces in advance, it can be challenging to train anticipatory control. Therapists can encourage its development by enhancing resources and providing opportunities to practice, reach to grasp of items varying in size, weight, and texture with placement in various locations with/without preparatory cues and feedback.

What can be done to assist clients who under- or overestimate the location and properties of target objects? First, related components such as vision and hand sensibility should be examined. We rely on sensory feedback to develop and strengthen our internal representations of object properties, used for anticipatory control of grip formation and force scaling. The potential to resolve visual or sensibility deficits should be determined first. Then visual and/or sensory reeducation techniques can be implemented (see above). Until hand sensibility improves, or if it remains poor, clients should be allowed extended practice or be taught compensatory techniques. Clients with underdeveloped or impaired anticipatory control demonstrate significant improvement with extended practice (Crajé et al., 2010; Dawson et al., 2010; Duff & Gordon, 2003). Interlimb transfer can also improve anticipatory force scaling in persons with hemiparesis (Gordon et al., 1999; Raghavan et al., 2006).

Grasp and Manipulation

Training grasp function in clients with paresis and dyscontrol often begins with the establishment of simple patterns such as the power grip (i.e., cylindrical), or lateral pinch depending on muscle activation and finger/thumb individuation (Duff, 2012; Erhardt, 1982). Power grip use simultaneous finger flexion with or without finger abduction to hold objects with wrist stabilization. Power grips also play an important role in holding and manipulating assistive mobility devices. It is probably best to retrain a power grip or a lateral pinch first, since finger fractionation (used with other precision grip patterns) may be limited.

Grip and pinch retraining can begin by placing objects in the hand to encourage an isometric contraction (Fig. 20.17A). This action alone often activates the wrist extensors to stabilize via the tenodesis effect. Training can move to active assistive motion by molding the hand around objects engaging finger flexion and thumb opposition while attempting active wrist extension. Grasp retraining could then progress to practice of active power and precision grip patterns as feasible (Fig 20.17A–C). Power grips include a cylindrical, spherical, or hook grasp. Precision grip patterns include a lateral pinch (thumb to lateral index), three-jaw chuck (thumb to radial two fingers), and a pincer grasp (index to thumb opposition, tip to tip, or pad to pad) (Duff, 2012). Practice of any pattern could be done in the vertical and horizontal planes to vary forearm and wrist orientation.

Many elements of grasp are planned in advance of object contact. Hand orientation, shape, and force characteristics are planned based on previous grasping experience, in conjunction with our ability to perceive relevant object cues (Fisk, 1990; Forssberg et al., 1991; Jeannerod, 1986; Westling & Johansson, 1984). Retraining grip formation is difficult if thumb and finger isolation and strength are limited as shown in Figure 20.18 which depicts a child with unilateral CP attempting a pincer grasp with limited thumb opposition. Errors in grasp control, such as gripping too loosely allowing slip or gripping too tightly thus crushing objects, result from deficits in grading forces. Yet, it may be tough to determine if inaccurate force scaling results from poor muscle control or diminished perception of object properties.

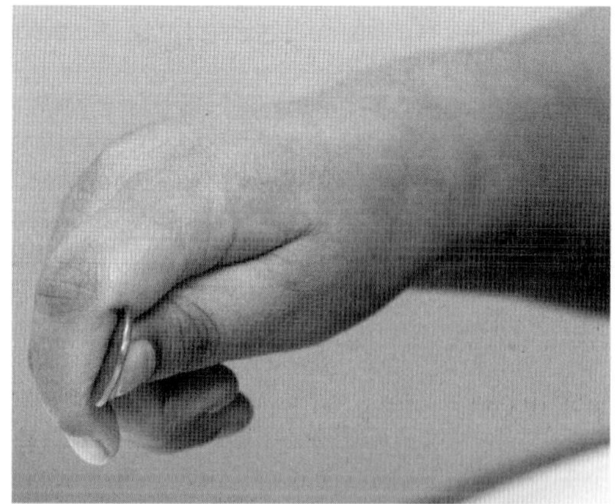

Figure 20.18 A child with unilateral cerebral palsy attempting a pincer grasp.

Elements of skilled grasp and manipulation include (a) active control over extrinsic and intrinsic hand muscles, (b) keen perceptual cues critical to anticipatory hand shaping and force scaling, and (c) accurate gradation of grip and fingertip forces. Thus, retraining of grasp control should address strength, coordination, and perceptual aspects of the task. Once isolated finger and thumb motion is available light strengthening can begin as shown in Figure 20.19A–C. Once basic strength is achieved, further training and strengthening intrinsic hand muscles can be accomplished with resistive therapy. Other tasks, such as lacing cardboard or leather with pipe cleaners or plastic laces, may be useful strengthening tasks. One could train fingertip force control by having the client drop a number of water drops from an eyedropper or pick up and replace objects such as paper cups without denting them. Skill requires learning to modify grasp to changing task demands via practice.

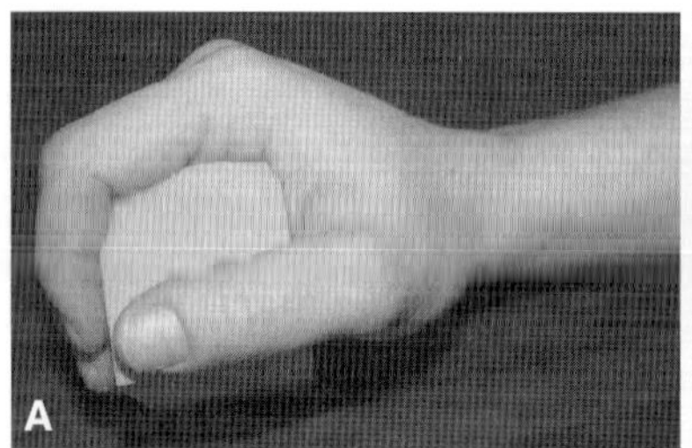

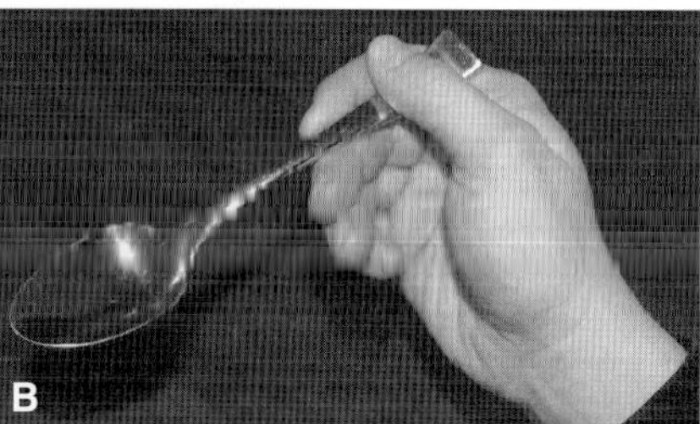

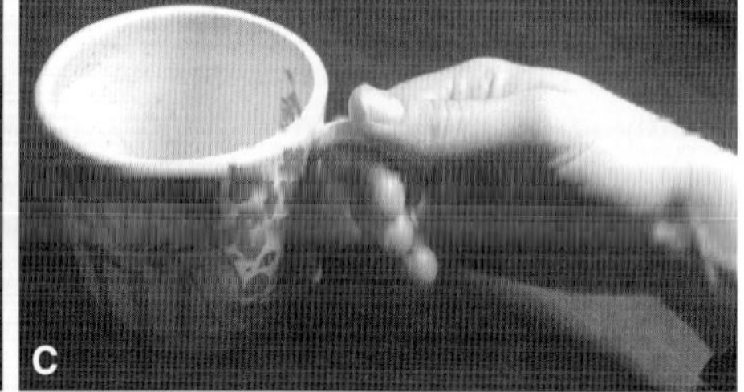

Figure 20.17 Retraining grasp and pinch progressing from place and holds to self-initiated grasps: power grasp **(A)**, lateral pinch on utensils **(B)**, and hook grip with a lateral pinch to secure a mug handle **(C)**.

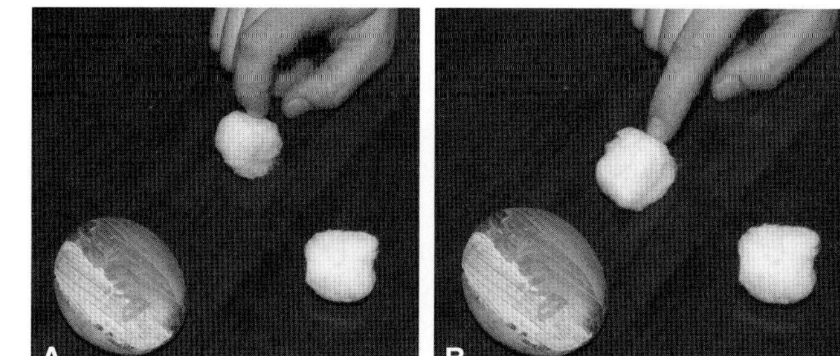
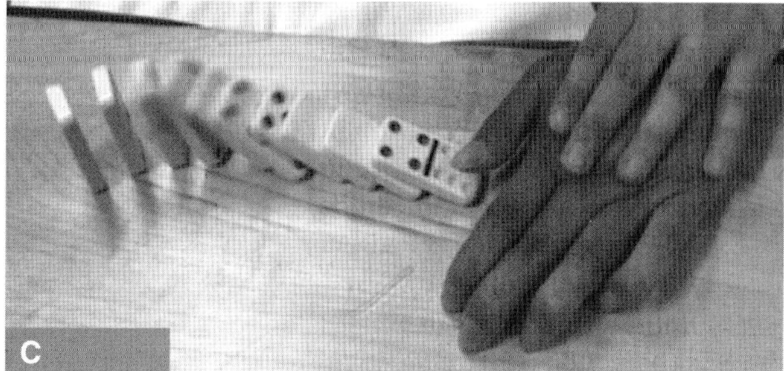

Figure 20.19 (A–C) Targeted practice of finger and thumb extension with low resistance.

Contextual Interference. To examine the impact of practice on learning, researchers have separated practice into blocked, random (contextual interference), and mixed schedules. Hanlon (1996) measured retention of a five-step functionally oriented movement sequence in the affected limb of 24 clients poststroke. The clients practiced a task in a blocked or random manner or were placed in a control group. The results showed greater improvement in the random-practice group on the first and second retention tests, supporting the positive effects of contextual interference on learning in this population. Pohl et al. (2006) examined whether adults with moderate stroke in the subacute phase could learn a motor sequence task implicitly in a single session. The task was to close an illuminated switch by reaching to touch it as quickly as possible in a random and repeated sequence organized separately in six blocks of 80 trials. Task practice for those poststroke was done with the less-affected arm and for controls with the right dominant or left nondominant arm. While the results show that response time for those with moderate stroke was greater than those with mild stroke and controls; the findings showed that implicit motor learning is maintained in those with moderate stroke and, thus, may be a useful training option.

Various studies have examined which practice schedule is best to improve UE function. Duff and Gordon (2003) studied the effect of blocked versus random practice on refining anticipatory force scaling during a grip–lift task in the affected hand of children with unilateral CP. While the blocked group performed better during acquisition, immediate and delayed retention was similar for the two forms of practice, yet the children may have needed more practice time to determine which schedule would ultimately lead to better retention. A study by Cauraugh and Kim (2003) found that blocked and random practice during an NMES program were effective at improving hand function. The effect of contextual interference on learning of a computer maze task in a single session was studied in children with CP (Prado et al., 2017) and adults poststroke (Moliterno et al., 2020). All participants performed the task with the most capable hand. In both studies random practice led to better performance in the transfer phase. Further work must determine the best UE practice schedule.

Finger Fractionation and In-Hand Manipulation. Limitations in finger fractionation (finger and thumb isolated movement) often stem from diminished corticomotoneuronal mechanisms as found in persons with neural deficits (Rothwell, 1994). Without finger fractionation it is difficult to manipulate objects in one hand entitled in-hand manipulation. If one shows some finger movement and has basic grasp-and-release patterns they are candidates for in-hand manipulation training (Exner & Henderson, 1995).

Treatment over multiple sessions could focus on all three forms of in-hand manipulation (translation, rotation, and shift) using small manipulatives (Exner, 1990). For example, one could have a client pick up pennies one at a time, move them to the palm, and hold them in the ulnar side of the hand. Or, pennies could be placed one at a time into an individual's palm with the instruction that each penny be translated to the fingertips then shifted to the thumb and index pads; then each coin could be placed in a slot or open container. Rotation and shift could be practiced by placing a pencil into the palm of a client's hand instructing them to rotate and adjust it to rest between the pads of the thumb, index, and long fingers. The two sides of the hand can learn separate roles by practicing tasks that require the power (ulnar) side to stabilize and the skill (radial) side to manipulate. One such task requires one to roll putty between the thumb and index finger while the ring and small fingers hold a small item. Another task is to squeeze the trigger of a spray bottle with the index and long fingers while the ring and small hold the bottle neck. As skill improves, task complexity can increase.

In-hand manipulation training should be graded. It can begin with easy tasks such as using objects of high friction and multiple points of contact, then progress to more challenging tasks such as using slippery objects with minimal points of contact. As tolerated, the size and shape of objects and the cues and the intensity of practice should be varied. While one person may be able to begin training at the level of object rotation, another may need to begin with finger-to-palm translation. Sensory reeducation and intrinsic muscle strengthening are coincident tasks.

Individuals with focal hand dystonia often lose motor control of one or more fingers stemming from highly repetitive, intensive hand use and atypical learning (Byl, 2003). The usual discrete finger representation found in the somatosensory cortex changes. For musicians with dystonia, the distance between finger representation is reduced and often begins to blend, resulting in a lack of finger fractionation and difficulty localizing light pressure. Sensory and motor training programs have been effective to foster change. One study had 10 clients with focal hand dystonia undergo a 4-week motor training program to increase finger fractionation emphasizing a decrease in undesirable movement overflow to fingers not involved in selected tasks (Zeuner et al., 2005). After training, there was a trend toward better handwriting and improvement on the Fahn dystonia scale. Yet, no changes were found in cortical excitability based on electroencephalography and TMS.

A 6-week training program using an activated virtual keypad (AVK) was examined for its benefit on finger individuation in adults with chronic stroke (Thielbar et al., 2014). Despite improvements in the AVK group and controls, only the AVK group improved finger individuation. A unique set-up for training finger individuation has been developed by McCall et al. (2019) for children with CP. Technology-driven programs to foster finger individuation and hand function continue to emerge, yet further research is warranted.

Release

While many clients with neurologic lesions can grasp objects, they may be unable to actively extend the fingers to release them without assistance of the other hand. To release effectively, they may need to use wrist flexion to passively extend the fingers or a tenodesis (Boehme, 1988; Erhardt, 1982). Even if a client can release objects actively, it may be inefficient. While children with unilateral CP can actively release objects, they often do so abruptly, with minimal grading of the action (Gordon et al., 2003; Lewis et al., 2002). Addressing release in treatment via NMES, practice or both may enhance effectiveness.

Rhoda Erhardt, an OT published an extensive developmental sequence for object release (Erhardt, 1982), designed to train and retrain release in persons with a neurologic dysfunction (Boehme, 1988). Her sequence begins with object release given external stabilization and progresses to release without it. This approach is based on how children learn to release objects when stabilized on a supporting surface before releasing objects in space (Boehme, 1988). Clients also practice releasing objects using a pattern of finger extension with the wrist in neutral (active or supported). As wrist stabilization increases and release improves, practice can progress to the release of objects into a container and stacking objects.

Training Proximal and Distal Function: Should One Precede the Other?

Should proximal function such as reaching be trained prior to distal function such as grasp? Development of the trunk and proximal UE neuromuscular system precedes the distal component (Kuypers, 1981). This developmental feature may contribute to the predominance of the trunk and proximal muscle activation in infant reaching (Berthier et al., 1999). Yet, because proximal control is not a necessary precursor to distal hand function, the two can be addressed concurrently in therapy, versus sequentially (Harbourne & Kamm, 2015). Thus, one should not wait for shoulder control to emerge before working on hand function.

Select CNS areas can substitute for injured regions (see Chapter 4; Merzenich & Jenkins, 1993). Proximal functions involving transport or shoulder stability may be substituted via alternative neural pathways. In contrast, damage to the CST often results in profound loss of precise hand movement because alternative pathways are not as readily available (Rothwell, 1994). Thus, limits in isolated thumb and finger movement and precision grip are common after CST lesions (Lang & Schieber, 2004; Raghavan et al., 2005).

Interventions at the Functional Level

A task-oriented approach to intervention requires that gains made in resolving impairments and refining key components of UE skill extend into improving the function. A key part of a task-oriented approach to treatment is task-specific practice of functional activities under changing environmental and task demands. Dunn et al. (1994) designed a therapeutic framework for practice—*The Ecology of Human Performance* (EHP)—that considers the effect of context. This model stems from the theory that ecology, or the interaction between person(s) and the environment, affects human behavior and performance. See the application of EHP to our case study, Jean, in Assessment Tool 20.8.

Integrating familiar or enjoyable tasks into therapeutic practice aids recovery of many aspects of function. Ma and Trombly (2002) reported that there was greater improvement in cognitive function following intervention that incorporated functional tasks and activities familiar and enjoyable to the individual. For example, many homemaking tasks, such as doing laundry, incorporate the UEs and simple cognitive/perceptual skills. Sorting clothes prior to washing requires classification and identification of fabric color and texture. Loading clothes into the washer/dryer and folding them afterward incorporates bimanual coordination, trunk stabilization, and large proximal and distal movements activating related muscle groups. While adults may be quite motivated to work on ADLs, children often require the added element of integrating practice into games to make ADLs more enjoyable.

Assessment Tool 20.8

Framework of Ecology of Human Performance

This framework considers the interaction between the person, the environment, and human task performance. This framework can be applied to retraining UE control in Jean in her role as a homemaker. The activities used during treatment depend on the individualized goals for the intervention and the status of the person's recovery. Note the subsequent examples used.

Goal	Interpretation	Activity Example
Establish/ restore	Improve person's skills and experiences	Introduce tasks/exercises to strengthen finger flexors and wrist extensors. With more strength, Jean could better engage in bimanual tasks (e.g., hold a bowl with her affected hand while stirring contents with the less-affected hand).
Alter	Select context that enables performance. Place person in different setting	Have Jean assist in meal preparation by setting the table in her home, using her affected hand and arm to hold items before placing them on the table with her less-affected hand.
Adapt	Change aspects of context and/or tasks to allow person to perform task	Introduce tools with large handles that allow Jean to hold them with her affected hand (e.g., stir bowl contents using her affected hand while the less-affected hand holds the bowl).
Prevent	Change course of events based on predictions of barriers to performance	Since Jean's affected arm tends to fatigue and her balance is only fair, have her prepare meals while sitting at a table with her elbows supported.
Create	Provide enriched contextual and task experiences to enhance performance	Have Jean prepare lunch for her family that requires use of her affected hand to manipulate pots, pans, dishes, and utensils unimanually and bimanually. The items could be retrieved from their original locations in cupboards, etc., to expand reach-and-grasp demands as well as trunk and balance requirements.

Reprinted with permission from Dunn W, Brown C, McGuigan A. The ecology of human performance: a framework for considering the effect of context. *Am J Occup Ther.* 1994;48:595–607.

Task-Oriented Training

TOT has been studied in various neurological conditions. Thielman et al. (2004) compared the effect of two 4-week training programs on reaching in clients > 6 months poststroke. Participants were placed in a low- or high-level group based on the Motor Assessment Scale and randomly assigned to a TRT group or a PRE group (resistive tubing used in planes/distances similar to TRT tasks). Kinematic findings for the low-level group had an increase in trunk use during ipsilateral targeted reaching after TRT and for midline and contralateral targeted reaching after PRE. With TRT, hand paths straightened in the low-level group, suggesting better interjoint coordination. Subjects in the high-level group showed the most change after PRE training, revealing less-compensatory trunk use, thus gains in the extent of reach. As stated under *postural training*, a 1-year follow-up was run (Thielman et al., 2013) from the two studies that incorporated TRT (Thielman et al., 2004, 2008). The TRT group maintained straighter hand paths and spent less time in deceleration during reaching. Further study of TRT and methods to restrict compensatory trunk motion continues including study of the efficacy of auditory feedback versus a trunk constraint (Thielman, 2010; Thielman & Bonsall, 2012).

Winstein et al. (2004) compared immediate and long-term benefits of two UE protocols for stroke, functional task practice (FT) and strength training (ST) with standard care (SC). The authors classified 64 clients by severity using the Orpington Prognostic Scale then randomly assigned them to one of three treatment groups. All subjects participated in the 4- to 6-week inpatient and outpatient program, while the FT and ST groups received 20 hours of treatment beyond SC. Outcome measures included the FMA-UE, isometric torque strength, and Functional Test of the Hemiparetic Upper Extremity (FTHUE). Those in the less severe category of the FT and ST groups, showed the most improvement in FMA-UE, isometric torque strength, and FTHUE immediately after treatment. Yet, at 6 months, isometric muscle torque in the FT group progressed significantly beyond that of the ST group. As reported by Duncan et al. (2003) the authors found that both task specificity and severity of stroke are important factors to consider during UE rehabilitation in the acute phase poststroke.

Recently, a phase III multisite study in adults poststroke was run to determine if there is greater improvement in arm and hand recovery after participation in an Accelerated Skill Acquisition Program (ASAP) versus those who receive dose equivalent usual care or standard usual care (Winstein et al., 2016). The primary measure, WMFT-time, did not differ between groups at long-term follow-up, thus the ASAP was not deemed superior. Yet, interestingly the findings suggest that the rate of improvement during training based on secondary measures was greater for the participants in the ASAP group.

Combined Training. Weakness can limit the gains made with task-specific practice in any population. Patten et al. (2013) conducted a crossover study comparing functional task-specific practice (FTP) to a hybrid program of strengthening and FTP in adults poststroke. Along with gains in muscle power, the authors found significantly greater WMFT-FAS scores and minimally important differences on the FMA-UE and FIM after the hybrid program. Conroy et al. (2019) ran an RCT with 12 weeks of training comparing one group who received 60 minutes of RT to one who received 45 minutes of RT with 15 minutes of transition to task practice (TTT). After training, no significant group differences were found on the FMA-UE. Yet, the RT plus TTT group had greater improvement on the log WMFT and the SIS-hand. A hybrid program with the inclusion of principles from the ASAP program would be beneficial for Jean and Genise.

Learning to Sequence Complex Functional Tasks. Modeling and verbal/mental rehearsal may be effective methods to improve sequencing of complex functional tasks (McCullagh et al., 1989). For example, Jean has difficulty sequencing the steps associated with meal preparation. During therapy sessions in a given week, the therapist could model the multistep process, such as making a sandwich and preparing a cup of tea, while giving simple verbal cues along the way. Before Jean attempts to repeat the same task, she could be asked to verbalize the sequence (explicit learning) then imagine herself performing the sequence (mental rehearsal). During practice, the therapist could initially coach a client through the task (verbally and/or manually), progress to practice from a written list (given intact vision) then to practice without verbal or written cues.

Tim's sequencing problems may include classroom art projects. In those situations, peer modeling would be effective only if a child can filter out irrelevant cues allowing focus on cues essential to sequence the task (Exner & Henderson, 1995; Vygotsky, 1978). It is possible that Tim has difficulty for many reasons (e.g., distractibility when given verbal instructions/visual demonstrations, constructional apraxia, or diminished visual perception).

If peer modeling of task sequences is ineffective for Jean or Tim, they may need alternate strategies such as verbal rehearsal prior to task performance (Vygotsky, 1978). For example, during the construction of an art project, one could begin by showing Tim the end product and have him verbally state how to complete it step by step. If he fails to give a correct response, the therapist could verbally interject, reviewing a missed step(s). Once the project is complete, the therapist may need to model the task sequence. It may be reinforcing for him to teach a fellow student how to complete the same task by demonstration and verbal cueing.

Practicing Functional Activities in Virtual Environments. Virtual reality (VR) alone or combined with other therapies has been found effective in fostering UE recovery in adults with neurologic disorders (Karamians et al., 2019) and in children (Eng et al., 2007; Levin et al., 2015; Rathinam et al., 2019; Ravi et al., 2017).

Research evidence. Holden et al. (2001) trained four persons 3 to 18 years of age after an acquired brain injury in real-world tasks using virtual-world pouring tasks. Subjects imitated the "teacher" on a screen while holding a "real" cup during training sessions (1 hour, 3 times/week = 16 sessions). Post-training, three of four subjects, had smoother, straighter, and more accurate trajectories of the pouring motion. Two showed transfer of the pouring trajectory into a novel workspace area. Tsoupikova et al. (2015) used VR to offer repetitive task practice in six adults with chronic hemiparesis. All improved performance on VR tasks with training, but only lateral pinch strength improved after 18 sessions.

A pilot study (Golomb et al., 2010) was run in three children with unilateral CP to examine the benefit of a remotely monitored, home-based video game. All children participated 5 days per week for 3 months. To monitor use, all subjects wore a sensor glove on the affected hand. All children improved ROM, hand and arm function, and bone density of the radius. In another pilot study (Qiu et al., 2009) VR was combined with robotic training in two children with CP within a clinic-based program 3 times per week for 3 weeks. Both children improved on the Melbourne Assessment of Unilateral Upper Limb, active ROM, grip and pinch strength, and kinematics of a VR reaching task (smoothness, hand path length, and duration). A study in adults with chronic stroke (Housman et al., 2009) compared the benefit of a computer-based VR system combined with a robotic device to a tabletop exercise program. Findings showed that all made improvements on the FMA-UE, active range-of-reaching motion, and the MAL, which remained 6 months after training. Yet, improvements on the FMA-UE at 6 months were greater for the experimental group. The benefits of affordable VR programs continue to be developed and marketed (King et al., 2010; Sucar et al., 2014) and some are being used within telerehabilitation programs (Cramer et al., 2019).

Rehabilitation using VR and gaming often increases engagement in treatment. A recent systematic review of 37 trials provided evidence that VR and gaming improve UE and ADL function in adults poststroke (Laver et al., 2015). Research is needed to further examine the efficacy of VR intervention (Brunner et al., 2014; Proffitt & Lange, 2015).

Dominance Training or Retraining. Bilateral UE tasks are symmetrical or asymmetrical. For symmetrical tasks, both arms and hands attempt to perform the same function as when throwing a large ball or folding a large towel. During asymmetrical tasks, one hand stabilizes an object while the other performs some form of manipulation or action on the object. For example, when chopping an onion, the nondominant hand may stabilize the onion while the other uses a knife to slice it. The nondominant or stabilizing limb often acts to control impedance, while the dominant controls the limb trajectory during a reach or the manipulative component of an action (Sainburg, 2005). A child who fails to develop a strong dominance or a person who suffers a stroke and loses substantial control of the dominant limb may benefit from dominance training or retraining (Sainburg & Duff, 2006).

Rehabilitation strategies should focus on training both limbs. Thus, if a right-handed individual suffers a left hemisphere stroke, the dominant right limb will be affected and often must take on the role of the nondominant limb while the less-affected nondominant left limb must take on the role of the dominant limb. In essence, years of practice performing bimanual tasks one way must now be relearned. To promote retraining, therapists could design activities to allow the right limb to practice impedance control by stabilizing objects while the left limb practices trajectory control or manipulative acts (Sainburg & Duff, 2006). Sample tasks could be: (a) holding a glass with the right hand while pouring water from a pitcher with the left, (b) stabilizing a piece of paper with the right while drawing using the left, and (c) holding a bagel with the right while cutting it in half with the left.

Research continues to focus on the less-affected arm and hand in persons poststroke. Jang and Jang (2016) used diffusion tensor imaging (DTI) to examine changes in the CST of the unaffected hemisphere in persons poststroke. Clinical UE tests were also taken at two time points; Day 1 (mean 23 ± 15.4 days poststroke) and Day 2 (mean 472 ± 449.17 days poststroke). Three groups were compared: (a) right hand dominance maintained, (b) dominance changed right to left, and (c) right hand dominance maintained since left hand was more affected. For those who changed dominance from right to left there was a significant increase in voxel number (fiber) found in the CST. Moderate correlations were also found in this group for clinical tests: grip strength ($r = 0.499$, $P < 0.05$), Purdue Peg Board Test ($r = 0.531$, $P < 0.05$), and MBI ($r = 0.551$, $P < 0.05$). Maenza et al. (2020) found that persons poststroke with the most severe paretic arm impairment based on clinical measures also have the greatest motor deficit in the less-affected arm. Since they must rely on the less-affected arm for daily activities the authors recommend that greater attention be given to that limb in therapy. Based on the work on Jang and Jang (2016) methods to improve function in the less-affected arm and hand may also increase fiber number in the CST. Future research should be directed at uncovering the best methods to enhance dominant and nondominant limb performance during development and after neurologic injury.

Ipsilesional Limb Training. Researchers are now closely examining control of the less-affected or ipsilesional limb. Pohl and Winstein (1999) studied the effects of reaching practice with the ipsilesional limb in 10 right-handed subjects who had had a stroke and 10 age-matched controls. The protocol varied the target width and the distance between targets, resulting in an easy and complex aiming task. After practice, movement times were faster for all in both reach conditions, yet, persons poststroke were slower than controls. Peak velocity only increased in the easy condition. Sainburg et al. (2016) ran a 3-week pilot training study in three adults poststroke focusing on speed and coordination in the nonparetic arm. All participated in nine 1-½ hour sessions of intense practice in real-life and VR tasks. After training, a straighter hand path in the nonparetic arm was noted by a reduction in direction error and aspect ratio. There also was a 25.8% mean reduction in time to perform the JHFT and a 9.5% mean reduction in score on the FMA-UE. The self care portion of the FIM improved by a mean of 22.6%. Further research is needed to examine the full benefits of training the nonparetic limb including the potential contribution from the paretic upper limb post-training with regard to ADL independence.

Training Handwriting. Training in handwriting is essential for persons with unrefined or lost skill. Writing implements such as pencil grips or orthotics may help a client sustain a hold on a writing implement to maximize function (Fig. 20.20A,B). While manipulating writing implements can initially be awkward, performance often improves with practice.

For children with unrefined handwriting skills, there are well-designed manuscript and cursive programs useful in school-based therapy programs or classrooms. Three such programs are Benbow's "Loops and Other Groups" (1991, 1992), Olsen and Knapton's "Handwriting without Tears" (2008), and the "Size Matters Handwriting Program" (SMHP; Moskowitz et al., 2017). Benbow's

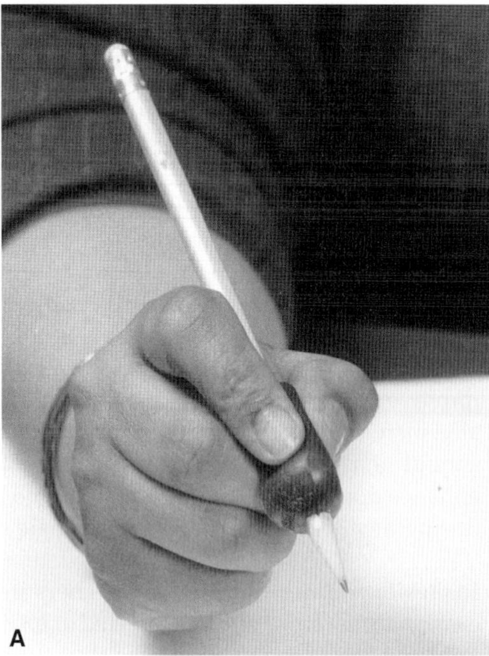

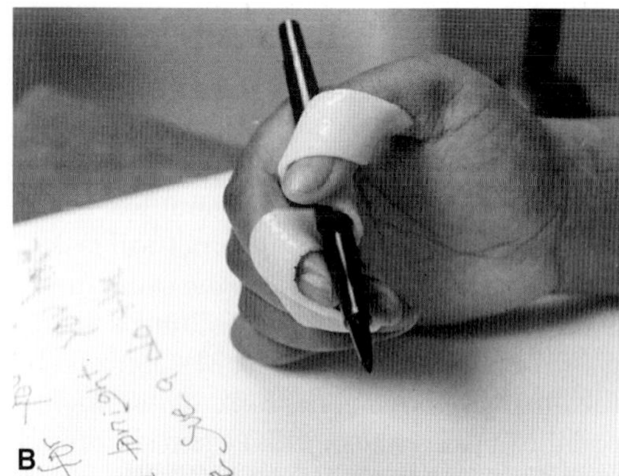

Figure 20.20 Assistive devices such as a pencil grip **(A)** and a custom-made writing utensil (design by Bobbie Ciocco, OTR/L) **(B)** used for handwriting.

program teaches cursive from a kinesiologic perspective via creative clustering of letters into "kites" and other subgroups; with ease of instruction and ample practice time for each grouping. Olsen's program emphasizes multisensory experiences and features gray blocks and simple line structure to visually guide printing and cursive. The SMHP is a curricular model that emphasizes size and progresses from blocked to random practice. These programs are effective in typical and atypically developing children in curricular and consultative models (Donica, 2015; Engel et al., 2018; Hape et al., 2014; Shimel et al., 2009; Zylstra & Pfeiffer, 2016).

Bryant et al. (2018) examined the feasibility of a home-based hand/arm resistance program to modify the size and quality of handwriting in persons with PD and essential tremor (ET). While grip strength improved in PD, it did not in those with ET. The size of handwriting did not change after participation. In addition to focusing on components related to handwriting, the opportunity for handwriting practice is essential.

Interventions to Increase Frequency of Arm and Hand Use

There are several therapeutic methods designed to enhance the frequency of arm and hand use, with a positive effect on the frequency of participation and independence in ADL tasks. These methods include CIMT, bimanual training, interlimb transfer, and combined programs.

Constraint-Induced Movement Therapy. CIMT is a form of massed practice designed to improve function in individuals with hemiplegia by constraining the less-affected limb and eliciting shaping behaviors in the affected limb. The efficacy of CIMT has been well studied in adults poststroke (see Dromerick et al., 2009; Pierce et al., 2003; Takebayashi et al., 2015; Taub et al., 1993; Wolf et al., 1989, 2006b), persons with TBI (see Karman et al., 2003), and in children with unilateral CP (Eliasson et al., 2005; Gordon et al., 2005; Pierce et al., 2002; Taub et al., 2004). CIMT fosters arm function in infants at risk for unilateral CP (Eliasson et al., 2018) and is currently being studied in toddlers (Chorna et al., 2015).

Neural changes are evident after CIMT (Matusz et al., 2018; Sawaki et al., 2008) yet adult kinematic studies suggest that improvements are primarily due to compensatory strategies versus an improvement in motor control (Kitago et al., 2013). Since the causal link between motor gains and changes in brain function and structure after CIMT are not fully understood (Wittenberg & Schaechter, 2009), further research in this area is warranted.

Research evidence. Early work provided significant evidence that CIMT may be effective (Taub et al., 1993; Wolf et al., 1989). More recently the findings are substantial. Wolf et al. (2006b) conducted a multisite study of CIMT, entitled the EXCITE trial, to compare the effect of a 2 week program of CIMT versus usual and customary care on UE function 3 to 9 months after stroke. Findings taken immediately, 1, and 2 years after training showed greater improvements in the CIMT group than controls on the WMFT-time and the amount of use on the MAL. Also, after training self-perceived hand function based on the SIS was lower in the CIMT group than controls. Gains were maintained over the next 12 months in the strength component of the WMFT and SIS (Wolf et al., 2008). In an analysis of a subset of data from the EXCITE trial (Alberts et al., 2004) the CIMT group were shown to have improved hand function more than controls, as revealed by greater pinch strength and regulation of fingertip forces, with less force rate variability during precision grip tasks.

The benefit of very early constraint-induced movement in stroke rehabilitation (VECTORS) was compared with traditional therapy in 52 adults poststroke (Dromerick et al., 2009). CIMT and traditional therapy were found equally beneficial during in-clinic treatment. Yet, at 3 months the CIMT group had less motor gains, suggesting that higher doses of therapy early may not be beneficial. Another RCT examined the benefits of CIMT in 47 adults within 4 weeks poststroke compared to usual care (Thrane et al., 2015). While WMFT-time and NHPT scores were significantly better immediately after CIMT, at the 6-month follow-up, there were no significant group differences on any measure.

CIMT has been found effective for infants and children with unilateral CP (Charles & Gordon, 2007; Eliasson et al., 2005, 2018; Gordon et al., 2005, 2006; Taub et al., 2004). Gordon et al. (2005) adapted the CIMT program for children aged 4 to 14 years of age with unilateral CP by restraining the less-affected limb in a sling 6 hours a day for 10 days. Shaping activities and repetitive practice were run in groups of two to three children to allow socialization and encouragement, yet the ratio of interventionist to child was 1:1. Motion(s) stressed were individualized based on deficits and potential for improvement. Modifications made to the adult program were well tolerated by the children. Findings revealed gains in dexterity and coordination and the amount and quality of use of the affected limb. At 1 year follow up further improvement was found in this same group of children (Charles & Gordon, 2007). The initial program by Gordon and colleagues was modified to a 15-day camp model (Hung et al., 2020). Goodwin et al. (2020) examined the use ratio (paretic/nonparetic arm) calculated from accelerometry in seven children with CP gathered during a 30-hour CIMT program. The authors found the use ratio increased during training, yet gains were not sustained after program completion. Crajé et al. (2010) showed that after participation in an 8-week CIMT or bimanual training program, children with unilateral CP improved their action planning for a sequential UE movement task based on grip choice at object contact. While promising methods to sustain the benefits gained from CIMT need further exploration.

Research evidence. Page and Levine (2003) used CIMT to study improvements in three individuals with TBI with documented learned nonuse. Their protocol included restraint of the affected limb five times per week, 5 hours per day for 10 weeks during periods of frequent use, with the addition of shaping activities during PT and OT. After treatment, subjects showed improvement on the MAL (amount and quality of use), improvement on the ARAT, and decreased time and better performance on the WMFT. This study provides preliminary support for using CIMT to foster use and function in the affected limb after TBI.

Modified CIMT has been shown to be effective. Pierce et al. (2003) had 17 clients with chronic stroke and one with subacute stroke engage home-based forced use in addition to seven 1-hour outpatient OT and PT sessions over a 2- to 3-week period. At follow-up, completion time for 12/17 subtests on the WMFT was reduced suggesting that this program was easy to implement and had a positive effect on function. Page et al. (2005, 2008, 2011) conducted studies with follow-up for a modified form of CIMT with shaping activities for the affected arm; in-clinic sessions of 30 minutes, 3 days per week combined with home-based constraint of the less-affected arm 5 to 6 hours per day, 5 days per week for 10 weeks. Immediate differences post-training revealed significant improvements on the ARAT and MAL (amount and quality of use) for those engaged in modified CIMT. Changes found on the ARAT and FMA-UE immediately after training were maintained 3 months post-training. Byl et al. (2003) studied the treatment effect of an UE crossover training program in 21 stable clients poststroke. The 8-week program (4 weeks sensory and 4 weeks motor training) required placing a glove on the less-affected limb and graded, repetitive sensory and motor activities for the affected limb. The results revealed a 20% improvement in functional independence, fine motor function, sensory discrimination, and musculoskeletal performance. Thus, a modified CIMT program may be suitable for clinic and home-use with good potential outcomes.

Bimanual Training. Bilateral training engages both limbs simultaneously to encourage interlimb coordination and motion in a limb with hemiparesis (see Abdollahi et al., 2018; Cauraugh et al., 2005; Charles & Gordon, 2006; Hung et al., 2017, 2018a; McCombe-Waller & Whitall, 2014; Mudie & Matyas, 2000, 2001; van Delden et al., 2015). Bimanual training can include symmetrical (e.g., both limbs performing the same action) and asymmetrical (e.g., one limb stabilizes an object or item while the other limb performs an action on it) tasks. Both functional and recreational bimanual tasks should be practiced (see Fig. 20.21A,B). Charles and Gordon (2006) developed The Hand–Arm Bilateral Training (HABIT) program for systematically training bimanual activities in children with unilateral CP. HABIT provides structured practice of progressively more challenging functional tasks that require bimanual hand use (see Table 20.7 for sample tasks). Task difficulty is graded as performance improves, by requiring greater speed or accuracy, or

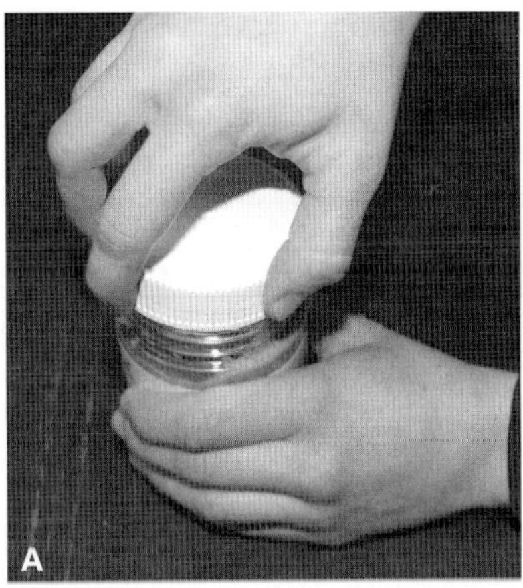

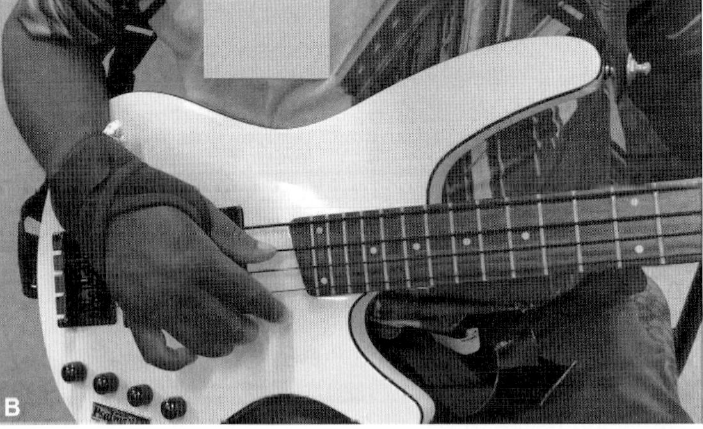

Figure 20.21 Asymmetrical bimanual practice for functional and recreational tasks. **(A)** Opening jars. **(B)** Playing guitar with a wrist strap for support.

TABLE 20.7 Bimanual Activities

Activity category	Repetitive task practice	Whole-task practice	Type of involved hand use	Graded constraints
Manipulative games and tasks	Precision grasp in symmetrical bimanual tasks	Precision grasp, wrist extension, and supination	Stabilizer, manipulator, active/passive assist, symmetrical and asymmetrical movements	Changing spatial and temporal constraints of task, for symmetrical tasks increasing frequency task is completed within a fixed time period
Card games	Active wrist supination in symmetrical bimanual tasks	Grasp, wrist stabilization, and supination	Stabilizer, manipulator, active/passive assist, symmetrical and asymmetrical movements	Changing spatial and temporal constraints of task, for symmetrical tasks increasing frequency task is completed within a fixed time period
Video games	Finger individuation	Finger individuation	Manipulator, active assist, symmetrical movements	Changing temporal constraints of task
Functional tasks	All movements	Precision grasp, wrist extension, and supination	Stabilizer, manipulator, active/passive assist, symmetrical and asymmetrical movements	Stabilizer, manipulator, active/passive assist, symmetrical and asymmetrical movements
Gross motor	Shoulder, upper-extremity movement, shoulder flexion abduction, and elbow–wrist extension	Shoulder, upper-extremity movement, shoulder flexion abduction, and elbow–wrist extension	Stabilizer, manipulator, active/passive assist, symmetrical and asymmetrical movements	Stabilizer, manipulator, active/passive assist, symmetrical and asymmetrical movements
Arts and crafts	Wrist and finger extension in symmetrical bimanual tasks	Precision grasp, wrist extension and supination	Stabilizer, manipulator, active/passive assist, symmetrical and asymmetrical movements	Stabilizer, manipulator, active/passive assist, symmetrical and asymmetrical movements

Reprinted with permission from Charles J, Gordon AM. Development of hand-arm bimanual intensive training (HABIT) for improving bimanual coordination in children with hemiplegic cerebral palsy. *Dev Med Child Neurol.* 2006;48:933, Table 1.

by providing tasks that require more skilled use of the affected hand and arm. Children practice tasks for 6 hours per day for 10 to 15 days, similar to the CIMT model. During bimanual task practice, children are asked to use the affected arm in the same manner as the nondominant limb of a typically developing child. HABIT uses part- and whole-practice and is designed of sufficient intensity to induce neuroplastic changes in the motor cortex. Outcomes from HABIT programs support the benefit of bimanual training to improve dexterity, hand and arm function and the amount of use in the affected arm and hand (Charles & Gordon, 2006).

In a clinic-based study, Hung et al. (2017) compared performance pre- and post-training in children with unilateral CP for two versions of HABIT for 15 days, 6 hours per day; group one engaged in structured practice with skill progression and the other in unstructured practice without skill progression. Kinematics during an asymmetrical drawer opening task were assessed. While both groups improved the timing of bimanual performance, only the group engaged in structured practice had less trunk involvement, greater elbow joint excursion, and less variability during the task after training. Hung et al. (2018) also studied the effectiveness of a home-based version of HABIT that ran 5 days per week for 9 weeks in seven children with unilateral CP. Kinematics assessed performance during the drawer opening task. Timing and movement quality improved in all children post training for this task, providing further support for bimanual training as an intervention for children with hemiparesis. Friel et al. (2016) studied neural changes via TMS in 20 children with unilateral CP before and after camp held for 6 hours per day, 5 days per week, for 3 weeks. Ten children received structured HABIT and 10 unstructured bimanual training. After training there was only a significant increase in the map size of the affected hand in the structured group.

Abdollahi et al. (2018) ran an RCT to study bimanual training in adults with chronic stroke. Two groups underwent three 45 minutes sessions per week for 2 weeks. Both groups underwent bimanual reach training, but one group received error augmentation enhanced with a robot. The results showed an advantage in the FMA-UE, the WMFT-FAS, and the MAL for the group receiving error augmentation. A unique bilateral arm training system has been designed by Xu et al. (2017) with a haptic interface and motion sensor to train manipulation. While this system has been tested with healthy persons, further research is needed to examine the efficacy for improve UE function in persons with UE dysfunction.

Research evidence. Is bimanual training is superior to unimanual arm training in adults or children with hemiparesis? Mudie and Matyas (2000) reported on data from 12 single-case studies in persons with hemiparesis poststroke; using a multiple-baseline design across three reach-to-grasp tasks. All 12 clients showed significant improvements in the affected arm after bilateral versus unilateral training; specific to the task trained and maintained for 6 months. The authors suggest that after stroke, the undamaged hemisphere might provide a template of appropriate neural responses for a restored neural network; available via transcortical communications that are uninhibited during bilateral symmetrical performance.

Cauraugh et al. (2005) compared unilateral and bilateral training for three groups: (a) a coupled bilateral group (concurrent wrist and finger movements with less-affected limb coupled with electrical stimulation to wrist and finger extensors on affected arm), (b) unilateral group with triggered stimulation to affected wrist and finger extensors, and (c) a control group. The program ran for 90 minutes, 4 days per week for 2 weeks. Post-training kinematics revealed an increase in peak velocity and shorter deceleration in bimanual reaching only for the bilateral group. Whereas the unilateral group increased peak velocity for the unilateral reach and had longer deceleration for the bimanual reach. The results showed that coupled bilateral training led to intralimb transfer from distal to proximal joints better than unilateral training.

McCombe-Waller et al. (2014) compared two training programs in persons with moderately severe hemiparesis poststroke. Group one engaged in 6 weeks of bilateral proximal training (BATRAC Tailwind device, Encore Path Inc.) then 6 weeks of unilateral TOT (Combo) whereas group two engaged in unilateral training for 12 weeks (SAEBO). Post-training the COMBO group had greater gains on the WMFT-time, and increased motor cortex activation during hand movement. Both groups improved on the FMA-UE and Maryland Arm Questionnaire for Stroke. Despite positive effects including the neural changes, from bilateral training, some studies reveal few differences in functional outcomes between usual treatment and bilateral practice (Desrosiers et al., 2005) or bimanual versus unimanual training (Gordon et al., 2008; van Delden et al., 2015; Stoykov et al., 2009). Further examination of the underlying mechanisms is needed to determine whether bimanual training is superior to unimanual.

Constraint Induced Movement Therapy—Bimanual Training. Studies comparing CIMT to bimanual training are being conducted in children and adults. In one study, 64 children with unilateral CP (mean age 10 years), were randomized to a 3-week CIMT or bimanual training program (Sakzewski et al., 2011). Both groups improved on self-selected goals gathered with the COPM, increased function based on the SFA and increased participation based on the Assessment of Life Habits and CAPE. In another study (Facchin et al., 2011), 105 children with unilateral CP were randomized into a 10-week program of modified CIMT or bimanual training (3 hours daily, 7 days per week) versus standard treatment (ST; 1-hour, twice a week). Findings showed that both experimental groups significantly improved affected hand function based on the QUEST and Besta Scale whereas the ST group did not. The younger bimanual group had greater change in ADL function and bimanual play whereas the modified CIMT group had greater change in grasp function. Another RCT compared kid-CIMT to bimanual training in 47 children with hemiplegia provided for 80 hours in 4 weeks (Deppe et al., 2013). The kid-CIMT led to greater affected arm use based on the Melbourne Assessment of Unilateral Upper Limb Function (Randall et al., 2001) yet, both led to increased use based on the AHA. Hung et al. (2020) ran an RCT comparing outcomes from CIMT or HABIT run for 15 days, 6 hours per day in children with unilateral CP. Kinematics revealed both groups had shorter movement times, less trunk rotation, and greater elbow and wrist motion in the affected arm during a reach–grasp–eat cookie task after training. Yet, only the CIMT group had a straighter hand path and lower hand position during the grasp portion of the task after training. Group differences may stem from the intensity obtained from CIMT versus HABIT.

It is possible that after stroke, bilateral training is fitting during early recovery, when rapid cortical reorganization is occurring and new networks to control movement are being formed. CIMT may then be appropriate in ensuring that new networks are used, avoiding the development of learned disuse. Further research is needed to determine the timing and efficacy of combining bimanual training and CIMT in sequence.

Interlimb Transfer. Intuitively, therapists have clients perform tasks with the less-affected limb first to promote more frequent use of the affected limb. The efficacy of this approach for the improvement of movement and function in the affected limb of those with hemiparesis will likely depend on the side of the lesion and the task under consideration.

Interlimb transfer can improve anticipatory force scaling during grasp and manipulation in adults and children with hemiplegia (Dawson et al., 2010; Gordon et al., 1999a, Raghavan et al., 2006; Steenbergen et al., 2008). Gordon et al. (1999) showed that if children with unilateral CP lift objects with the less-affected hand first, they show evidence of anticipatory force scaling on the first lift of a grip device with the affected hand. Steenbergen et al. (2008) studied performance of unimanual and bimanual performance during a grip–lift, transport, and release task. The authors found that temporal phase durations with the less-affected hand were longer during bimanual versus unimanual performance yet were closely aligned with affected hand. The force related variables exhibited by the affected hand were slightly better during the bimanual versus unimanual task suggesting some evidence of interlimb transfer. Camus et al. (2009) used TMS to examine the neural mechanisms of interlimb transfer in typical young adults during a sequential pinch force task. All right-handed subjects practiced the task with the right hand. After practice, performance in the left hand was measured. The authors found task speed and accuracy improved in both hands. These changes coincided with an increase in recruitment curves in the left M1 and decreased short intracortical inhibition in the left and right M1.

Interlimb transfer of visuomotor learning and novel force conditions after training in a reaching task have been found for typical young adults (Criscimagna-Hemminger et al., 2003; Malfait & Ostry, 2004; Sainburg & Wang, 2002; Wang & Sainburg, 2004a, b, 2006a, b). Specifics of the transfer depend on workspace location and handedness. Neva et al. (2019) studied the effect of acute aerobic exercise on learning and interlimb transfer after training over 4 days in a 2-week timespan. Based on kinematics and time-based reaching movements, the acute bout of aerobic exercise did enhance visuomotor adaptation and learning, and shortened reaction time during interlimb transfer. Support for the efficacy of interlimb transfer to improve prehension in those with dysfunction and the benefit of aerobic exercise on interlimb transfer and motor learning needs further study.

Lab Activity 20.1 will help you practice applying a task-oriented approach to treating a client with UE problems. In this lab, you will develop a treatment plan for Jean, our chronic stroke client, and identify the research evidence to support your treatment choices.

Improving Participation

The ability to adapt functional skills to the environment is essential to the recovery of participation, thus the context in which functional tasks are practiced should be considered. As function improves, the opportunity to resume life roles (e.g., homemaker, student) increases, and recovery of participation begins. Research examining factors inherent in fostering participation is ongoing (Reedman et al., 2017).

LAB ACTIVITY 20.1

Objective: Apply a task-oriented approach to retrain reach, grasp, and manipulation in a client with post-stroke hemiparesis. To identify the research evidence to support clinical decisions regarding specific treatment interventions.

Procedure: Reread the case study presented in Table 20.1. Review the list of functional problems, strategies, and impairments outlined.

Assignment: Create a table identifying the various treatments you will use to improve hand function in Jean. List the component to be targeted (column 1), the task or activity to be practiced (column 2), the environmental conditions under which practice will occur (column 3), and the research evidence supporting this aspect of treatment (column 4). For example, you may select to do CIMT since she tends to disuse her affected UE during functional tasks. The individual component listed in the table is Motor: Frequency of hand use, the task is massed practice, the specific environmental conditions you choose may be CIMT. Several research studies supports your decision to use CIMT with Jean, including the EXCITE trials by Wolf and colleagues and the modified program by Page and colleagues. Is increasing frequency alone enough to ensure recovery of hand function? What other aspects of hand function will you train? What research supports your decision?

Individual component of upper-extremity function	Task or activity	Environmental conditions	Research evidence
Motor: Frequency of affected hand use	Massed practice—shaping tasks	CIMT—three times a week in an outpatient program	Page et al. (2005, 2008), Pierce et al. (2003), Taub et al. (1993), Wolf et al. (2006b, 2008)

SUMMARY

1. Retraining UE control is important to most areas of rehabilitation. While both PT and OT retrain UE control, PTs tend to focus on postural and mobility aspects of UE function, while OTs tend to focus on age appropriate occupations or everyday activities considering the cognitive, visual–perceptual and psychosocial components inherent in prehensile skill and task performance.
2. A task-oriented approach to assessment of UE function requires a battery of tests that measure: (a) function, including capacity (behavior in a standardized environment) and performance (participation in real-world contexts); (b) strategies or the qualitative components of function, including eye–head coordination, transport, grasp and release, and manipulation; and (c) underlying sensory, motor, musculoskeletal, cognitive, visual–perceptual and psychosocial impairments.
3. Clinical research continues to support the use of a task-oriented approach alone and in combination with other therapies to treat neurologic disorders. Yet, the implementation of research findings into current clinical practice lags behind.
4. Preparing treatment plans to retrain UE control requires identification of a targeted list of client problems, including limitations in function, strategy, and impairments that constrain function. From this list, short- and long-term treatment goals are established, and therapeutic strategies are developed to meet those goals.
5. A task-oriented approach to retraining UE control seeks to minimize impairments, while maximizing the client's capacity for function and participation. Retraining involves the development of therapeutic strategies to: (a) remediate as many sensory, motor, cognitive, visual–perceptual and psychosocial impairments as possible; (b) generate strategies to improve qualitative and quantitative performance in the components of UE function; and (c) develop the capacity to perform functional tasks in a variety of environmental contexts to enhance participation.
6. Research suggests that the development of control over proximal body segments is not a necessary precursor to the emergence of distal hand function. Thus, proximal and distal UE segments can be retrained simultaneously, rather than sequentially.
7. Hand function requires the ability to grasp, release, and manipulate objects, as well as the capacity to

adapt grasp in response to object characteristics. Elements of grasp, include hand pre-shaping and force and use of internal representations we hold of an object's physical properties. Thus, retraining hand function requires attention to both perceptual and motor aspects of the task.

8. Sensory reeducation programs focus on protective and discriminative sensibility. Programs can teach a client how to harness remaining sensibility or to alter the physiological basis for sensation. The capacity to adapt to diminished sensibility depends on the client's motivation as well as training. Studies have shown that clients willing to use an affected limb were better able to recover function.
9. A major constraint to recovery of arm function may be the unwillingness of clients to use the affected UE when the less-affected extremity is available. Bilateral, unilateral, and interlimb transfer training may be effective methods to promote use separately or in combination. Further research is needed to determine the best sequence and timing of training for different ages and conditions. Cooperative bilateral training in which the limbs take on different roles during task performance may be a useful approach to increasing function but also requires more research.
10. Hand dominance plays a key role in the rehabilitation of unimanual and bimanual skill. Research suggests that the dominant limb has an advantage for control of reaching and the nondominant limb for stabilization. Due to the influence these advantages have on skill, they should be addressed during intervention. Research is needed to examine methods of enhancing skill considering limb asymmetry.

ANSWERS TO LAB ACTIVITY ASSIGNMENTS

Lab Activity 20.1

There is no single correct way to train UE function in Jean. It is essential that all aspects of arm and hand motor control be included in her rehabilitation program and that a range of tasks and conditions be used to help her develop a variety of strategies to grasp and manipulate different objects for a wide array of tasks and conditions. The specific order, duration, and timing of each activity is bound to vary.

We begin by determining Jean's main concern and aiding her identification of therapy goals related to hand function. She expresses concern that she can perform ADLs using her hands without dropping items and without the assistance of her spouse. She is confident that she can use her less-affected hand, but some bimanual tasks as used in cooking, may be tough.

So, our approach to training hand function will focus on reducing her impairments (weakness, diminished sensibility) and on practicing everyday tasks in context. We will try to incorporate principles of participation and motor learning into her program. Initially, we will have her participate in a CIMT program that is offered 3 times per week to increase use of her affected hand. As the frequency of use of her affected hand improves, we will shift to interlimb transfer tasks having her grasp and lift objects with the less-affected hand first followed by the affected hand. The physical properties of the objects will vary. At the same time, we will attempt to strengthen her hand through finger exercises using lightweight items then progress to Theraputty. We will employ sensory reeducation strategies for her hand via tactile discrimination and stereognosis tasks. Finally, to improve her participation in everyday tasks and sequencing, she will practice simple three-step tasks in the simulated kitchen.

Research to support our clinical decision making regarding this approach to treatment is steadily increasing. The following table presents some examples. What other research can you find to support your evidence-based rehabilitation program to improve hand function?

Individual component of upper-extremity function	Task or activity	Environmental conditions	Research evidence
Cognition: Goal setting	Interview	Context dependent	Combs et al. (2010), Dunn et al. (1994), Graham et al. (2010), Law et al. (2015), Quinn et al. (2014)
Motor: Activation of distal musculature	Place and hold, active distal movement	Action observation on less-affected hand with mirror training—followed by imitation or place and hold with the affected hand	Brunner et al. (2014), Harmsen et al. (2015)
Motor: Frequency of affected hand use	Massed practice—shaping tasks	CIMT—three times a week in an outpatient program or ASAP training	Page et al. (2005, 2008), Pierce et al. (2003), Taub et al. (1993), Wolf et al. (2006b, 2008), Winstein et al. (2016)
Motor: Anticipatory force scaling	Grasp and lift of stationary objects	Interlimb transfer—lift objects with less-affected hand first then by affected hand or ASAP training	Camus et al. (2009), Dawson et al. (2010), Raghavan et al. (2006), Winstein et al. (2016)
Motor: Wrist and finger extension activation and strength	Wrist and finger/thumb extension used to pre-shape hand before grasping	NMES to wrist and finger/thumb extensors in conjunction with grasp-and-release activities with objects of various sizes	Doucet and Griffin (2013), Fujiwara et al. (2009), Hara et al. (2008), Knutson et al. (2014), Zheng et al. (2019)
Motor: Sustained grip	Grasp and hold utensils	Blocked and random practice using grooming utensils in context with and without NMES	Cauraugh and Kim (2003), Dunn et al. (1994), Trombly and Ma (2002)
Cognitive and Sensory: Memory and tactile discrimination	Tactile discrimination tasks and object identification tasks	Identify textures and objects first with eyes open then with eyes closed or after placed in a box	Byl et al. (2003), Decker (2010)
Cognitive: Memory and sequencing	Simple three-step meal preparation	Making a cup of tea given verbal or written directions at first progressing to independence	Dunn et al. (1994), McEwen et al. (2014), Skidmore et al. (2018), Trombly and Ma (2002)

REFERENCES

A

Aaron DH, Stegink Jansen CW. Development of the Functional Dexterity Test (FDT): construction, validity, reliability, and normative data. J Hand Ther 2003;16:12–21.

Aartolahti E, Häkkinen A, Lönnroos E, et al. Relationship between functional vision and balance and mobility performance in community-dwelling older adults. Aging Clin Exp Res 2013;25(5):545–552.

Abbruzzese G, Berardelli A. Sensorimotor integration in movement disorders. Mov Disord 2003;18:231–240.

Abd El-Nabie WAE, Saleh MSM. Trunk and pelvic alignment in relation to postural control in children with cerebral palsy. J Back Musculoskelet Rehabil 2019;32(1):125–130. doi: 10.3233/BMR-181212.

Abdollahi F, Corrigan M, Lazzaro EDC, Kenyon RV, Patton JL. Error-augmented bimanual therapy for stroke survivors. NeuroRehabilitation 2018;43(1):51–61. doi: 10.3233/NRE-182413.

Abrams TW, Kandel ER. Is contiguity detection in classical conditioning a system or a cellular property? Learning in aplysia suggests a possible molecular site. Trends Neurosci 1988;11:128–135.

Ada L, Dean CM, Hall JM, et al. A treadmill and overground walking program improves walking in persons residing the community after stroke: a placebo controlled randomized trial. Arch Phys Med Rehabil 2003;84:1486–1491.

Ada L, Dorsch S, Canning CG. Strengthening interventions increase strength and improve activity after stroke: a systematic review. Aust J Physiother 2006;52:241–248.

Adkin AL, Bloem BR, Allum JH. Trunk sway measurements during stance and gait tasks in Parkinson's disease. Gait Posture 2005;22:240–249.

Adolph KE. Learning to solve the problem of moving: exploration, experience, and control. Paper presented at the Annual Conference in the Movement Sciences: Development of Skill in Infancy and Early Childhood, Teacher's College, Columbia University, New York, 1994.

Adolph KE, Berger SE. Motor development. In: Damon W, Lerner R, series eds.; Kuhn D, Siegler RS, vol. eds. Handbook of child psychology, vol. 2. Cognition, perception, and language, 6th ed. New York: Wiley, 2006:161–213.

Adolph KE, Berger SE, Leo AJ. Developmental continuity? Crawling, cruising, and walking Dev Sci 2011;14(2):306–318.

Adolph KE, Cole WG, Komati M, et al. How do you learn to walk? Thousands of steps and dozens of falls per day. Psychol Sci 2012;23(11):1387–1394.

Adolph KE, Hoch JE. Motor development: embodied, embedded, enculturated, and enabling. Annu Rev Psychol 2019;70:141–164.

Adolph KE, Vereijken B, Denny MA. Learning to crawl. Child Dev 1998;69:1299–1312.

Afschrift M, van Deursen R, De Groote F, Jonkers I. Increased use of stepping strategy in response to medio-lateral perturbations in the elderly relates to altered reactive tibialis anterior activity. Gait Posture 2019;68:575–582.

Agnew PJ, Dip OT, Maas F. Hand function related to age and sex. Arch Phys Med Rehabil 1982;63:269–271.

Ahmed S, Mayo NE, Higgins J, et al. The Stroke Rehabilitation Assessment of Movement (STREAM): a comparison with other measures used to evaluate the effects of stroke and rehabilitation. Phys Ther 2003;83:617–660.

Ailshire JA, Crimmins EM. Psychosocial factors associated with longevity in the United States: age differences between the old and oldest-old in the health and retirement study. J Aging Res 2011;2011:530534.

Albanese A, Bhatia K, Bressman S, Delong M, Fahn S, et al. Phenomenology and classification of dystonia: a consensus update. Mov Disord 2013;28:863–873.

Alberts JL, Butler AJ, Wolf SL. The effects of constraint-induced therapy on precision grip: a preliminary study. Neurorehabil Neural Repair 2004;18:250–258.

Alberts JL, Saling M, Adler CH, et al. Disruptions in the reach-to-grasp actions of Parkinson's patients. Exp Brain Res 2000;134:353–362.

Alexander GE, Crutcher MD. Functional architecture of basal ganglia circuits: neural substrates of parallel processing. Trends Neurosci 1990;13:266–271.

Alexander NB, Mollo JM, Giordani B, et al. Maintenance of balance, gait patterns and obstacle clearance in Alzheimer's disease. Neurology 1995;45:908–914.

Alexander NB, Schultz AB, Warwick DN. Rising from a chair: effect of age and functional ability on performance biomechanics. J Gerontol 1991;46:M91–M98.

Allet L, Leemann B, Guyen E, et al. Effect of different walking aids on walking capacity of patients with poststroke hemiparesis. Arch Phys Med Rehabil 2009;90:1408–1413.

Allin LJ, Brolinson PG, Beach BM, Kim S, Nussbaum MA, Roberto KA, Madigan ML. Perturbation-based balance training targeting both slip- and trip-induced falls among older adults: a randomized controlled trial. BMC Geriatrics 2020;20:1–13.

Allison L. Balance disorders. In: Umphred DA, ed. Neurological rehabilitation. St. Louis, MO: Mosby Year Book, 1995:802–837.

Allum JHJ, Honegger F, Schicks H. The influence of a bilateral vestibular deficit on postural synergies. J Vestib Res 1994;4:49–70.

Allum JHJ, Pfaltz CR. Visual and vestibular contributions to pitch sway stabilization in the ankle muscles of normals and patients with bilateral peripheral vestibular deficits. Exp Brain Res 1985;58:82–94.

Almli RB, Finger S. Toward a definition of recovery of function. In: Le Vere TE, Almli RB, Stein DG, eds. Brain injury and recovery: theoretical and controversial issues. New York: Plenum, 1988:1–4.

Alon G, Levitt AF, McCarthy PA. Functional electrical stimulation (FES) may modify the poor prognosis of stroke survivors with severe motor loss of the upper extremity: a preliminary study. Am J Phys Med Rehabil 2008;87(8):627–636. doi: 10.1097/PHM.0b013e31817fabc1.

Alon G, Sunnerhagen KS, Geurts AC, et al. A home-based self-administered stimulation program to improve selected hand functions in chronic stroke. NeuroRehabilitation 2003;18:215–225.

Alstermark B, Isa T, Ohki Y, Saito Y. Disynaptic pyramidal excitation in forelimb motoneurons mediated via C3-C4 propriospinal neurons in the Macaca fuscata. J Neurophysiol 1999;82:3580–3585.

Altman DG, Bland JM. Diagnostic tests. 1: Sensitivity and specificity. BMJ 1994;308:1552.

Alt Murphy M, Willen C, Sunnerhagen KS. Kinematic variables quantifying upper extremity performance after stroke during reaching and drinking from a glass. Neurorehabil Neural Repair 2011;25:71–80.

Alzghoul MB, Gerrard D, Watkins BA, et al. Ectopic expression of IGF-I and Shh by skeletal muscle inhibits disuse-mediated skeletal muscle atrophy and bone osteopenia in vivo. FASEB J 2004;18:221–223.

Amaral D. The anatomical organization of the central nervous system. In: Kandel ER, Schwartz JH, Jessell TM, eds. Principles of neural science, 4th ed. New York: McGraw-Hill, 2000:317–336.

American Physical Therapy Association. Guide to physical therapy practice, 3.0. Alexandria, VA: APTA, 2014. Retrieved from http://guidetoptpractice.apta.org/

Amiel-Tison C, Grenier A. Evaluation neurologique du nouveau-né et du nourrisson. [Neurological evaluation of the human infant.] New York: Masson, 1980:81–102.

Ammann-Reiffer C, Bastianen CH, van Hedel HJ. Measuring change in gait performance of children with motor disorders: assessing the functional mobility scale and the gillette functional assessment questionnaire walking scale. Dev Med Child Neurol 2019;61:717–724.

Amundson S. Evaluation Tool of Children's Handwriting (ETCH). Morganville, NJ: ETCH Administration, 1995.

An M, Dusing SC, Harbourne RT, Sheridan SM, START-Play Consortium. What really works in intervention? Using fidelity measures to support optimal outcomes. Phys Ther 2020;100:757–765.

Anaby DR, Law M, Feldman D, Majnemer A, Avery L. The effectiveness of the Pathways and Resources for Engagement and Participation (PREP) intervention: improving participation of adolescents with physical disabilities. Dev Med Child Neurol 2018;60(5):513–519. doi: 10.1111/dmcn.13682.

Anacker SL, DiFabio RP. Influence of sensory inputs on standing balance in community dwelling elders with a recent history of falling. Phys Ther 1992;72:575–584.

Anastasi D, Carpinella I, Gervasoni E, Matsuda PN, Bovi G, Ferrarin M, Cattaneo D. Instrumented version of the modified dynamic gait index in patients with neurologic disorders. PMR 2019;11:1312–1319.

van Andel S, Cole MH, Pepping GJ. Regulation of locomotor pointing across the lifespan: investigating age-related influences on perceptual-motor coupling. PLoS One 2018;13(7):e0200244.

Andel SV, Cole MH, Pepping GJ. Regulation of locomotor pointing across the lifespan: Investigating age-related influences on perceptual-motor coupling. PloS One 2018;13:1–16.

Andersen RA. The role of the inferior parietal lobule in spatial perception and visual-motor integration. In: Mountcastle VB, Plum F, Geiger SR, eds. Higher functions of the brain, part 2: the nervous system, vol. 5, Handbook of physiology, section 1. Bethesda, MD: American Physiological Association, 1987:483–518.

Andersen RA, Andersen KN, Hwang EJ, Hauschild M. Optic ataxia: from Bálint's syndrome to the parietal reach region. Neuron 2014;81:967–983.

Andersen RA, Buneo CA. Intentional maps in posterior parietal cortex. Annu Rev Neurosci 2002;25:189–220.

Andersen RA, Cui H. Intention, action planning, and decision making in parietal-frontal circuits. Neuron 2009;63:568–583.

Andersson G, Hagman J, Talianzadeh R, et al. Effect of cognitive load on postural control. Brain Res Bull 2002;58:135–139.

Anderson JB, Sinkjaer T. Stretch reflex variations during gait. In: Pedotti A, Ferrarin M, Quintern J, Riener R, eds. Neuroprosthetics. Berlin, Germany: Springer, 1996:45–50.

Anderson JL, Terzis G, Kryger A. Increase in the degree of coexpression of myosin heavy chain isoforms in skeletal muscle fibers of the very old. Muscle Nerve 1999;22:449–454.

Andersson G, Magnusson M. Neck vibration causes short-latency electromyographic activation of lower leg muscles in postural reactions of the standing human. Acta Otolaryngol 2002;122:284–288.

Andrews AW. Hand-held dynamometry for measuring muscle strength. J Hum Muscle Perform 1991;1:35–50.

Andrews AW. Self-report measures of mobility. Top Geriatr Rehabil 2012;28:2–10.

Andrews AW, Bohannon RW. Distribution of muscle strength impairments following stroke. Clin Rehabil 2000;14:79–87.

Andrews CJ, Burke D, Lance JW. The response to muscle stretch and shortening in Parkinsonian rigidity. Brain 1972;95:795–812.

Angsupaisal M, Dijkstra LJ, la Bastide-van Gemert S, et al. Effects of forward tilted seating and foot-support on postural adjustments in children with spastic cerebral palsy: an EMG-study. Eur J Paediatr Neurol 2019;23(5):723–732. doi: 10.1016/j.ejpn.2019.07.001.

Aniansson A, Grimby F, Gedberg A. Muscle function in old age. Scand J Rehabil Med 1978;6(Suppl):43–49.

Aniansson A, Hedberg M, Henning G, et al. Muscle morphology, enzymatic activity and muscle strength in elderly men: a follow up study. Muscle Nerve 1986;9:585–591.

Anson E, Pineault K, Bair W, Studenski S, Agrawal Y. Reduced vestibular function is associated with longer, slower steps in healthy adults during normal speed walking. Gait Posture 2019;68:340–345.

Antal A, Nitsche MA, Kincses TZ, et al. Facilitation of visuo-motor learning by transcranial direct current stimulation of the motor and extrastriate visual areas in humans. Eur J Neurosci 2004;19(10):2888–2892.

Aoki O, Otani Y, Morishita S, Domen K. The effects of various visual conditions on trunk control during ambulation in chronic post stroke patients. Gait Posture 2017;52:301–307.

Apel U. The Feldenkrais method: awareness through movement. WHO Reg Publ Eur Ser 1992;44:324–327.

Appasamy M, De Witt ME, Patel N, Yeh N, Bloom O, Oreste A. Treatment strategies for genu recurvatum in adult patients with hemiparesis: a case series. PMR 2015;7(2):105–112.

Araneda R, Ebner-Karestinos D, Paradis J, et al. Reliability and responsiveness of the Jebsen-Taylor test of hand function and the box and block test for children with cerebral palsy. Dev Med Child Neurol 2019;61(10):1182–1188. doi: 10.1111/dmcn.14184.

Aras MD, Gokkaya NK, Comert D, et al. Shoulder pain in hemiplegia: results from a national rehabilitation hospital in Turkey. Am J Phys Med Rehabil 2004;83:713–719.

Arce FI, Katz N, Sugarman H. The scaling of postural adjustments during bimanual load-lifting in traumatic brain-injured adults. Hum Mov Sci 2004;22:749–768.

Argetsinger LC, Trimble SA, Roberts MT, Thompson JE, Ugiliweneza B, Behrman AL. Sensitivity to change and responsiveness of the Segmental Assessment of Trunk Control (SATCo) in children with spinal cord injury. Dev Neurorehabil 2019;22:260–271.

Armand S, Decoulon G, Bonnefoy-Mazure A. Gait analysis in children with cerebral palsy. EFORT Open Rev 2016;1(12):448–460.

Arnold AJ, Liddy JJ, Harris RC, Claxton LJ. Task-specific adaptations of postural sway in sitting infants. Dev Psychobiol 2020;62(1):99–106.

Arshavsky Yu I, Berkinblit MB, Fukson OI, et al. Recordings of neurones of the dorsal spinocerebellar tract during evoked locomotion. Brain Res 1972a;43:272–275.

Arshavsky Yu I, Berkinblit MB, Gelfand IM, et al. Activity of the neurones of the ventral spino-cerebellar tract during locomotion. Biophysics 1972b;17:926–935.

Aruin AS, Almeida LH. Organization of a simple two joint synergy in individuals with Down syndrome. Am J Ment Retard 1996;101:256–268.

Aruin AS, Rao N. Ankle-Foot orthoses: proprioceptive inputs and balance implications. J Prosthet Ortho 2010;22(4 Suppl):34–37.

Arutyunyan GH, Gurfnkel VS, Mirskii ML. Organization of movements on execution by man of an exact postural task. Biophysics 1969;14:1162–1167.

Asai H, Fujiwara K, Tachino K. Limiting factor for moveable range of the center of foot pressure in backward direction. In: Taguchi K, Igarashi M, Mori S, eds. Vestibular and neural front. Amsterdam, The Netherlands: Elsevier Science BV, 1994:525–528.

Asanuma H, Keller A. Neuronal mechanisms of motor learning in mammals. Neuroreport 1991;2:217–224.

Asboth L, Friedli L, Beauparlant J, Martinez-Gonzalez C, Anil S, Rey E, Baud L, Pidpruzhnykova G, Anderson MA, Shkorbatova P, Batti L, Stephane P, Kreider J, Schneider BL, Barraud Q, Courtine G. Cortico–reticulo–spinal circuit reorganization enables functional recovery after severe spinal cord contusion. Nat Neurosci 2018;21:576–588.

Ashburn A, Hyndman D, Pickering R, et al. Predicting people with stroke at risk of falls. Age Ageing 2008;37:270–276.

Ashburn A, Stack E, Pickering RM, et al. A community dwelling sample of people with Parkinson's disease: characteristics of fallers and non-fallers. Age Ageing 2001;30:47–52.

Ashe MC, Miller WC, Eng JJ, et al. Older adults, chronic disease and leisure-time physical activity. Gerontology 2009;55:64–72.

Ashmead DH, Hill EW, Talor CR. Obstacle perception by congenitally blind children. Percept Psychophys 1989;46:425–433.

Aslin RN. Development of smooth pursuit in human infants. In: Fisher DF, Monty RA, Senders JW, eds. Eye movements: cognition and visual perception. Hillsdale, NJ: Erlbaum, 1981.

Assaiante C, Amblard B. An ontogenetic model for the sensorimotor organization of balance control in humans. Hum Mov Sci 1995;14:13–43.

Assaiante C, Mallau S, Viel S, et al. Development of postural control in healthy children: a functional approach. Neural Plast 2005;12:109–118.

Assaiante C, Woollacott M, Amblard B. Development of postural adjustment during gait initiation: kinematic and EMG analysis. J Motor Behav 2000;32:211–226.

Astill S, Utley A. Coupling of the reach and grasp phase during catching in children with developmental coordination disorder. J Motor Behav 2008;40:315–323.

Atkeson CG, Hollerbach JM. Kinematic features of unrestrained vertical arm movements. J Neurosci 1985;5:2318–2330.

Atun-Einy O, Berger SE, Scher A. Pulling to stand: common trajectories and individual differences in development. Dev Psychobiol 2012;54(2):187–198.

Atun-Einy O, Berger SE, Scher A. Assessing motivation to move and its relationship to motor development in infancy. Infant Behav Dev 2013;36(3):457–469.

Augurelle AS, Smith AM, Lejeune T, Thonnard JL. Importance of cutaneous feedback in maintaining a secure grip during manipulation of hand-held objects. J Neurophysiol 2003;89:665–671.

Au-Yeung SS, Hui-Chan CW. Predicting recovery of dextrous hand function in acute stroke. Disabil Rehabil 2009;31:394–401.

Avers D, Brown M. Daniels and Worthingham's muscle testing: techniques of manual examination and performance testing, 10th ed. St. Louis, MO: Elsevier, 2019.

Awad LN, Binder-Macleod SA, Pohlig RT, et al. Paretic propulsion and trailing limb angle are key determinants of long-distance walking function after stroke. Neurorehabil Neural Repair 2015;29:499–508. pii: 1545968314554625. [Epub ahead of print].

Awad LN, Kesar TM, Reisman D, et al. Effects of repeated treadmill testing and electrical stimulation on post-stroke gait kinematics. Gait Posture 2013;37:67–71.

Awad LN, Reisman DS, Kesar TM, et al. Targeting paretic propulsion to improve poststroke walking function: a preliminary study. Arch Phys Med Rehabil 2014;95:840–848.

Ayres AJ. Sensory integration and learning disorders. Los Angeles, CA: Western Psychological Services, 1972.

B

Baars BJ. How does a stream of consciousness that is relatively simple, serial, and limited in capacity emerge from a brain that is largely unconscious, complex, and massively parallel? In: Marsh E, ed. Ciba Symposium on Experimental and Theoretical Foundations of Consciousness (#174). London, UK: Wiley Interscience, 1993.

Babin-Ratte S, Sirigu A, Gilles M, et al. Impaired anticipatory finger grip-force adjustments in a case of cerebellar degeneration. Exp Brain Res 1999;128:81–85.

Bach-y-Rita P, Balliet R. Recovery from stroke. In: Duncan P, Badke MB, eds. Stroke rehabilitation: the recovery of motor control. Chicago, IL: Year Book, 1987:79–107.

Badell-Ribera A. Cerebral palsy: postural-locomotor prognosis in spastic diplegia. Arch Phys Med Rehabil 1985;66:614–619.

Badke MB, DiFabio RP. Balance deficits in patients with hemiplegia: considerations for assessment and treatment. In: Duncan P, ed. Balance: proceedings of the APTA Forum. Alexandria, VA: American Physical Therapy Association, 1990:73–78.

Baert I, Freeman J, Smedal T, et al. Responsiveness and clinically meaningful improvement, according to disability level, of five walking measures after rehabilitation in multiple sclerosis: a European multicenter study. Neurorehabil Neural Repair 2014;28(7):621–631.

Baert I, Vanlandewijck Y, Feys H, Vanhees L, Beyens H, Daly D. Determinants of cardiorespiratory fitness at 3, 6 and 12 months poststroke. Disabil Rehabil 2012;34(21):1835–1842.

Bailey CH, Chen M. Morphological basis of long-term habituation and sensitization in Aplysia. Science 1983;220(4592):91–93.

Bailey CH, Kandel ER. Synaptic growth and the persistence of long-term memory: a molecular perspective. In: Gazzaniga, MS, ed. The cognitive neurosciences, 3rd ed. Cambridge, MA: MIT Press, 2004.

Bair WN, Kiemel T, Jeka JJ, et al. Development of multisensory reweighting for posture control in children. Exp Brain Res 2007;183:435–446.

Baker PS, Bodner EV, Allman RM. Measuring life space mobility in community-dwelling older adults. J Am Geriatr Soc 2003;51:1610–1614.

Baker MP, Hudson JE, Wolf SL. A "feedback" cane to improve the hemiplegic patient's gait. Phys Ther 1979;59:170–171.

Bakker M, Verstappen CCP, Bloem BB, et al. Recent advances in functional neuroimaging of gait. J Neural Transm 2007;114:1323–1331.

Baldan AMS, Alouche SR, Araujo IMG, Freitas SMSF. Effect of light touch on postural sway in individuals with balance problems: a systematic review. Gait Posture 2014;40:1–10.

Balint R. Seelenhamung des "Schauens," optische Ataxie, raumliche Storung des Aufmersamkeit. Monatshr Psychiatr Neurol 1909;25:51–81.

Ballard CG, Shaw F, Lowery K, et al. The prevalence, assessment and associations of falls in dementia with Lewy bodies and Alzheimer's disease. Dement Geriatr Cogn Disord 1999;10(2):97–103.

Baloh RW. Dizziness, hearing loss and tinnitus: the essentials of neurotology. Philadelphia, PA: FA Davis, 1984.

Balzini L, Vannucchi L, Benvenuti F, et al. Clinical characteristics of flexed posture in elderly women. J Am Geriatr Soc 2003;51:1419–1426.

Ban´kosz Z, Winiarski S. Using wearable inertial sensors to estimate kinematic parameters and variability in the table tennis topspin forehand stroke. Appl Bionics Biomech 2020;2020:8413948. doi: 10.1155/2020/8413948.

Barbu-Roth M, Anderson DI, Streeter RJ, et al. Why does infant stepping disappear and can it be stimulated by optic flow? Child Dev 2015;86(2):441–455.

Barclay R, Jacquie Ripat J, Mayo N. Factors describing community ambulation after stroke: a mixed methods study. Clin Rehabil 2015;29:509–521. pii: 0269215514546769.

Barclay-Goddard RE, Stevenson TJ, Poluha W, et al. Force platform feedback for standing balance training after stroke. Cochrane Database Syst Rev 2004;(4):CD004129.

Barela AMF, Caporicci S, de Freitas PB, Jeka JJ, Barela JA. Light touch compensates peripheral somatosensory degradation in postural control of older adults. Hum Mov Sci 2018;60:122–130.

Barnes MR, Crutchfield CA, Heriza CB. The neurophysiological basis of patient treatment, vol. II: Reflexes in motor development. Morgantown, WV: Stokesville, 1978.

Barra J, Marquer A, Joassin R, et al. Humans use internal models to construct and update a sense of verticality. Brain 2010;133:3552–3563.

Barra J, Oujamaa L, Chauvineau V, et al. Asymmetric standing posture after stroke is related to a biased egocentric coordinate system. Neurology 2009;72;1582–1587.

Barreca S, Gowland CK, Stratford P, et al. Development of the Chedoke Arm and Hand Activity Inventory: theoretical constructs, item generation, and selection. Top Stroke Rehabil 2004;11(4):31–42.

Barreca SR, Stratford PW, Masters LM, et al. Comparing 2 versions of the Chedoke Arm and Hand Activity Inventory with the Action Research Arm Test. Phys Ther 2006;86:245–253.

Barrett RS, Cronin NJ, Lichtwark GA, et al. Adaptive recovery responses to repeated forward loss of balance in older adults. J Biomech. 2012;45(1):183–187.

Barthelemy D, Nielsen JB. Corticospinal contribution to arm muscle activity during human walking. J Physiol 2010;588:967–979.

Bartlett D, Birmingham T. Validity and reliability of a pediatric reach test. Pediatr Phys Ther 2003;15:84–92.

Bartlett D, Purdie B. Testing of the spinal alignment and range of motion measure: a discriminative measure of posture and flexibility for children with cerebral palsy. Dev Med Child Neurol 2005;47:739–743.

Bartolic A, Pirtosek Z, Rozman J, et al. Postural stability of Parkinson's disease patients is improved by decreasing rigidity. Eur J Neurol 2005;12:156–159.

Basford JR, Chou LS, Kaufman KR, et al. An assessment of gait and balance deficits after traumatic brain injury. Arch Phys Med Rehabil 2003;84:343–349.

Basler H, Luckmann J, Wolf U, et al. Fear-avoidance beliefs, physical activity, and disability in elderly individuals with chronic low back pain and healthy controls. Clin J Pain 2008;24:604–610.

Basmajian JV, De Luca CJ. Muscles alive: their functions revealed by electromyography, 5th ed. Baltimore, MD: Lippincott Williams & Wilkins, 1985.

Basmajian JV, Kukulka CG, Narayan MD, et al. Biofeedback treatment of foot-drop after stroke compared with standard rehabilitation technique: effects on voluntary control and strength. Arch Phys Med Rehabil 1975;56:231–236.

Bassile CC, Dean C, Boden-Albala B, et al. Obstacle training programme for individuals post stroke: feasibility study. Clin Rehabil 2003;17:130–136.

Bastian AJ. Cerebellar limb ataxia: abnormal control of self generated and external forces. Ann N Y Acad Sci 2002;978:16–27.

Bastian AJ, Martin TA, Keating JG, et al. Cerebellar ataxia: abnormal control of interaction torques across multiple joints. J Neurophysiol 1996;76:492–509.

Bastian AJ, Zackowski KM, Thach WT. Cerebellar ataxia: torque deficiency or torque mismatch between joints? J Neurophysiol 2000;83:3019–3030.

Bateni H, Heung E, Zettel J, et al. Can use of walkers or canes impede lateral compensatory stepping movements? Gait Posture 2004a;20:74–83.

Bateni H, Maki BE. Assistive devices for balance and mobility: benefits, demands, and adverse consequences. Arch Phys Med Rehabil 2005;86:134–145.

Bateni H, Zecevic A, McIlroy WE, et al. Resolving conflicts in task demands during balance recovery: does holding an object inhibit compensatory grasping? Eve Brain Res 2004b;157:49–58.

Bates D, Pruess K, Souney P, et al. Serious falls in hospitalized patients: correlates and resource utilization. Am J Med 1995;99:137–143.

Battaglia-Mayer A. A brief history of the encoding of hand position by the cerebral cortex: implications for motor control and cognition. Cereb Cortex 2019;29:716–731.

Battaglia-Mayer A, Babicola L, Satta E. Parieto-frontal gradients and domains underlying eye and hand operations in the action space. Neurosci 2016;334:76–92.

Bayley, N. Bayley scales of infant and toddler development, 3rd ed. San Antonio, TX: Harcourt Assessment, 2006.

Bayley N, Aylward GP. Bayley scales of infant and toddler development, 4th ed. technical manual. Bloomington, MN: NCS Pearson, 2019.

Bayouk JF, Boucher JP, Leroux A. Balance training following stroke: effects of task-oriented exercises with and without altered sensory input. Int J Rehabil Res 2006;29:51–59.

Bean JF, Kiely DK, Herman S, et al. The relationship between leg power and physical performance in mobility-limited older people. J Am Geriatr Soc 2002;50: 461–467.

Bean JF, Leveille SG, Kiely DK, et al. A comparison of leg power and leg strength within the InCHIANTI study: which influences mobility more? J Gerontol Med Sci 2003;58A:728–733.

Beauchet O, Dubost V, Herrmann FR, et al. Stride-to-stride variability while backward counting among healthy young adults. J Neuroeng Rehabil 2005;2:26.

Beauchet O, Dubost V, Herrman F, Rabilloud M, Gonthier R, Kressig RW. Relationship between dual-task related gait changes and intrinsic risk factors for falls among transitional frail older adults. Aging Clin Exp Res 2005;17:270–275.

Bechly KE, Carender WJ, Myles JD, et al. Determining the preferred modality for real-time biofeedback during balance training. Gait Posture 2013;37:391–396.

Beckung E, Hagberg G. Neuroimpairments, activity limitations, and participation restrictions in children with cerebral palsy. Dev Med Child Neurol 2002;44:309–316.

Beckung E, Hagberg G. Neuroimpairments, activity limitations, and participation restrictions in children with cerebral palsy. Dev Med Child Neurol 2002;44(5):309–316. doi: 10.1017/s0012162201002134.

Beebe JA, Lang CE. Relationships and responsiveness of six upper extremity function tests during the first six months of recovery after stroke. J Neurol Phys Ther 2009;33(2):96–103. doi: 10.1097/NPT.0b013e3181a33638.

Beer RF, Dewald JP, Rymer WZ. Deficits in the coordination of multijoint arm movements in patients with hemiparesis: evidence for disturbed control of limb dynamics. Exp Brain Res 2000;131:305–319.

Behan M, Nawshin T, Nemanich S, et al. A crossed-disciplinary evaluation of parental perceptions surrounding pediatric non-invasive brain stimulation research. Int J Pharm Healthcare Market 2020;14(4):623–640. doi-org.libproxy.chapman.edu/10.1108/IJPHM-01-2020-0005

Behrman AL, Teitelbaum P, Cauraugh JH. Verbal instructional sets to normalise the temporal and spatial gait variables in Parkinson's disease. J Neurol Neurosurg Psychiatry 1998;65:580–582.

Beilock SL, Carr TH, MacMahon C, et al. When paying attention becomes counterproductive: impact of divided versus skill-focused attention on novice and experienced performance of sensorimotor skills. J Exp Psychol Appl 2002;8:6–16.

Bekkers EMJ, Dockx K, Devan S, et al. The impact of dual-tasking on postural stability in people with parkinson's disease with and without freezing of gait. Neurorehabil Neural Repair 2018;32(2):166–174.

Beldarrain MG, Gafman J, deVelasco IR, et al. Prefrontal lesions impair the implicit and explicit learning of sequences on visualmotor tasks. Exp Brain Res 2002;142:529–538.

Belen'kii VY, Gurfinkel VS, Paltsev YI. Elements of control of voluntary movements. Biofizika 1967;12:135–141.

Bell-Krotoski J, Weinstein S, Weinstein C. Testing sensibility, including touch-pressure, two-point discrimination, point localization, and vibration. J Hand Ther 1993;2:114–123.

Benaim C, Pérennou DA, Villy J, et al. Validation of a standardized assessment of postural control in stroke patients: the Postural Assessment Scale for Stroke Patients (PASS). Stroke 1999;30:1862–1868.

Benbow M. Loops and other groups: a kinesthetic writing system, instructor's manual. Randolph, NJ: OT Ideas, 1991.

Benda BJ, Riley PO, Krebs DE. Biomechanical relationship between center of gravity and center of pressure during standing. IEEE Trans Rehabil Eng 1994;2:3–10.

Beninato M, Gill-Body KM, et al. Determination of the minimal clinically important difference in the FIM instrument in patients with stroke. Arch Phys Med Rehabil 2006;87(1):32–39.

Bennett KM, Castiello U. Reorganization of prehension components following perturbation of object size. Psychol Aging 1995;10:204–214.

Bensoussan L, Viton JM, Schieppati M, et al. Changes in postural control in hemiplegic patients after stroke performing a dual task. Arch Phys Med Rehabil 2007;88:1009–1015.

Bentzel K. Evaluation of sensation. In: Trombly CA, ed. Occupational therapy for physical dysfunction, 4th ed. Baltimore, MD: Lippincott Williams & Wilkins, 1995.

Berardelli A, Rothwell JC, Thompson PD, Hallett M. Pathophysiology of bradykinesia in parkinson's disease. Brain 2001;124:2131–2146.

Berardelli A, Sabra AF, Hallett M. Physiological mechanisms of rigidity in Parkinson's disease. J Neurol Neurosurg Psychiatry 1983;46:45–53.

Berg K. Measuring balance in the elderly: validation of an instrument. Dissertation. Montreal: McGill University, 1993.

Berg K, Wood-Dauphinee S, Williams JT, et al. Measuring balance in the elderly: preliminary development of an instrument. Physiother Can 1989;41:304–308.

Berg K, Wood-Dauphinee SL, Williams JT. Measuring balance in the elderly: validation of an instrument. Can J Public Health 1992;83:S9–S11.

Berger SE, Adolph KE. Learning and development in infant locomotion. Prog Brain Res 2007;164:237–255.

Berger W, Altenmueller E, Dietz V. Normal and impaired development of children's gait. Hum Neurobiol 1984a;3:163–170.

Berger SE, Harbourne RT, Guallpa Lliguichuzhca CL. Sit still and pay attention! Trunk movement and attentional resources in infants with typical and delayed development. Phys Occup Ther Pediatr 2019;39(1):48–59.

Berger W, Horstmann GA, Dietz VL. Tension development and muscle activation in the leg during gait in spastic hemiparesis: the independence of muscle hypertonia and exaggerated stretch reflexes. J Neurol Neurosurg Psychiatry 1984b;47:1029–1033.

Berger W, Quintern J, Dietz V. Stance and gait perturbations in children: developmental aspects of compensatory mechanisms. Electroencephalogr Clin Neurophysiol 1985;61:385–395.

Bergen G, Stevens MR, Burns ER. Falls and fall injuries among adults aged ≥65 years—United States, 2014. MMWR Morb Mortal Wkly Rep 2016;65:993–998.

Bergmann K. Incidence of atypical pencil grasps among nondysfunctional adults. Am J Occup Ther 1990;44:736–740.

Bernard-Demanze L, Vuillerme N, Ferry M, et al. Can tactile plantar stimulation improve postural control of persons with superficial plantar sensory deficit? Aging Clin Exp Res 2009;21:62–68.

Bernier PM, Grafton ST. Human posterior parietal cortex flexibly determines reference frames for reaching based on sensory context. Neuron 2010;68:776–788.

Bernstein N. The coordination and regulation of movement. London, UK: Pergamon, 1967.

Bertani R, Melegari C, De Cola MC, Bramanti A, Bramanti P, Calabrò RS. Effects of robot-assisted upper limb rehabilitation in stroke patients: a systematic review with meta-analysis. Neurol Sci 2017;38(9):1561–1569. doi: 10.1007/s10072-017-2995-5.

Bertenthal B, von Hofsten C. Eye, head and trunk control: the foundation of manual development. Neurosci Biobehav Rev 1998;22:515–520.

Bertenthal BI, Rose JL, Bai DL. Perception-action coupling in the development of visual control of posture. J Exp Psychol 1997;23:1631–1643.

Bertera EM, Bertera RL. Fear of falling and activity avoidance in a national sample of older adults in the United States. Health Soc Work 2008;33:54–62.

Berthier NE, Clifton RK, McCall DD, et al. Proximodistal structure of early reaching in human infants. Exp Brain Res 1999;127:259–269.

Berthier NE, Keen R. Development of reaching in infancy. Exp Brain Res 2006;169:507–518.

Berthoz A, Pozzo T. Head and body coordination during locomotion and complex movements. In: Swinnen SP, Heuer H, Massion J, et al., eds. Interlimb coordination: neural, dynamical and cognitive constraints. San Diego, CA. Academic, 1994:147–165.

Bertram CP, Lemay M, Stelmach GE. The effect of Parkinson's disease on the control of multi-segmental coordination. Brain Cogn 2005;57:16–20.

Beuter A, Hernández R, Rigal R, et al. Postural sway and effect of levodopa in early Parkinson's disease. Can J Neurol Sci 2008;35:65–68.

Bhat AN, Galloway JC. Toy-oriented changes during early arm movements: hand kinematics. Infant Behav Dev 2006;29:358–372.

Bhatt T, Pai YC. Generalization of gait adaptation for fall prevention: from moveable platform to slippery floor. J Neurophysiol 2009;101:948–957.

Bhatt H, Pieruccini-Faria F, Almeida QJ. Dynamics of turning sharpness influences freezing of gait in Parkinson's disease. Parkinsonism Relat Disord 2013;19:181–185.

Bhatt T, Wening JD, Pai YC. Adaptive control of gait stability in reducing slip-related backward loss of balance. Exp Brain Res 2006;170:61–73.

Bhatt T, Yang F, Pai Y-C. Learning to resist gait-slip falls: long-term retention in community-dwelling older adults. Arch Phys Med Rehabil 2012;93:557–564.

Biernaskie J, Chernenko G, Corbett D. Efficacy of rehabilitative experience declines with time after focal ischemic brain injury. J Neurosci 2004;24(5):1245–1254.

Biguer B, Prablanc C, Jeannerod M. The contribution of coordinated eye and head movements in hand pointing accuracy. Exp Brain Res 1984;55:462–469.

Bijoch L, Borczyk M, Czajkowski R. Bases of Jerzy Konorski's theory of synaptic plasticity. Eur J Neurosci 2019;51:1857–1866.

Bilney BE, Morris ME, Denisenko S. Physiotherapy for people with movement disorders arising from basal ganglia dysfunction. N Z J Physiotherapy 2003;31:94–100.

Bilodeau EA, Bilodeau IM, Schumsky DA. Some effects of introducing and withdrawing knowledge of results early and late in practice. J Exp Psychol 1959;58:142–144.

Binkofski F, Dohle C, Posse S, et al. Human anterior intraparietal area subserves prehension. Neurology 1998;50:1253–1259.

Birren JE, Cunningham W. Research on the psychology of aging: principles, concepts and theory. In: Birren JE, Schaie KW, eds. Handbook of the psychology of aging, 2nd ed. New York: Van Nostrand Reinhold, 1985:3–34.

Birren JE, Riegel KF, Morrison DF. Age differences in response speed as a function of controlled variations of stimulus conditions: evidence of a general speed factor. Gerontologia 1962;6:1–18.

Bisdorff AR, Wolsley CJ, Anastasopoulos D, et al. The perception of body vertically (subjective postural vertical) in peripheral and central vestibular disorders. Brain 1996;119:1523–1534.

Bishop B. Neurophysiology of motor responses evoked by vibratory stimulation. Phys Ther 1974;54:1273–1282.

Bishop M, Brunt D, Pathare N, et al. Changes in distal muscle timing may contribute to slowness during sit to stand in Parkinsons disease. Clin Biomech (Bristol, Avon) 2005;20(1):112–117.

Bisi MC, Stagni R. Evaluation of toddler different strategies during the first six-months of independent walking: a longitudinal study. Gait Posture 2015;41(2):574–579.

Bisson E, Contant B, Sveistrup H, et al. Functional balance and dual-task reaction times in older adults are improved by virtual reality and biofeedback training. Cyberpsychol Behav 2007;10:16–23.

Bjorklund A. Long distance axonal growth in the adult central nervous system. J Neurol 1994;241:S33–S35.

Black P, Markowitz RS, Cianci SN. Recovery of motor function after lesions in motor cortex of monkeys. Ciba Found Symp 1975;34:65–83.

Black FO, Nashner LM. Postural control in four classes of vestibular abnormalities. In: Igarashi M, Black FO, eds. Vestibular and visual control of posture and locomotor equilibrium. Basel, Switzerland: Karger, 1985:271–281.

Black FO, Nashner LM. Postural disturbance in patients with benign paroxysmal positional nystagmus. Ann Otol Rhinol Laryngol 1984a;93(6 Pt 1):595–599.

Black FO, Nashner LM. Vestibulospinal control differs in patients with reduced versus distorted vestibular function. Acta Otolaryngol (Stockh) Suppl 1984b;406:110–114.

Black FO, Shupert C, Horak FB, et al. Abnormal postural control associated with peripheral vestibular disorders. In: Pompeiano O, Allum J, eds. Vestibulospinal control of posture and movement. Progress in brain research, vol. 76. Amsterdam, The Netherlands: Elsevier Science, 1988:263–275.

Black K, Zafonte R, Millis S, et al. Sitting balance following brain injury: does it predict outcome? Brain Inj 2000;14:141–152.

Blanchard O, Cohen-Solal L, Tardieu C, et al. Tendon adaptation to different long term stresses and collagen reticulation in soleus muscle. Connect Tissue Res 1985;13(3):261–267.

Blank R, Heizer W, von Voss H. Development of externally guided grip force modulation in man. Neurosci Lett 2000;286:187–190.

Blanton S, Wolf AL. An application of upper-extremity constraint-induced movement therapy in a patient with subacute stroke. Phys Ther 1999;79:847–853.

Bleck EE. Locomotor prognosis in cerebral palsy. Dev Med Child Neurol 1975;17:18–25.

Blenkinsop GM, Pain MTG, Hiley MJ. Balance control strategies during perturbed and unperturbed balance in standing and handstand. R Soc Open Sci 2017;4:1–12.

Blennerhassett JM, Matyas TA, Carey LM. Impaired discrimination of surface friction contributes to pinch grip deficit after stroke. Neurorehabil Neural Repair 2007;21:263–272.

Bleyenheuft C, Bleyenheuft Y, Hanson P, et al. Treatment of genu recurvatum in hemiparetic adult patients: a systematic literature review. Ann Phys Rehabil Med 2010;53:189–199.

Bleyenheuft Y, Arnould C, Brandao MB, Bleyenheuft C, Gordon AM. Hand and arm bimanual intensive therapy including lower extremity (HABIT-ILE) in children with unilateral spastic cerebral palsy. Neurorehabil Neural Repair 2015;29:645–657.

Bleyenheuft Y, Dricot L, Ebner-Karestinos D, et al. Motor skill training may restore impaired corticospinal tract fibers in children with cerebral palsy. Neurorehabil Neural Repair 2020;34:533–546.

Bliem BR, Grimbergen YA, Cramer M, et al. Prospective assessment of falls in Parkinson's disease. J Neurol 2001;248: 950–958.

Blin O, Ferrandez AM, Pailhous J, et al. Dopa-sensitive and dopa-resistant gait parameters in Parkinson's disease. J Neurol Sci 1991;103:51–54.

Blin O, Ferrandez AM, Serratrice G. Quantitative analysis of gait in Parkinson patients: increased variability of stride length. J Neurosci 1990;98:91–97.

Blinch J, Doan JB, Gonzalez CLR. Complexity of movement preparation and the spatiotemporal coupling of bimanual reach-to-grasp movements. Exp Brain Res 2018;236:1801–1813.

Bliss TVP, Lomo T. Long-lasting potentiation of synaptic transmission in the dentate area of the anaesthetized rabbit following stimulation of the perforant path. J Physiol (Lond) 1973;232:331–356.

Bloem BR, Beckley DJ, van Dijk JG. Are automatic postural responses in patients with Parkinson's disease abnormal due to their stooped posture? Exp Brain Res 1999;124:481–488.

Bloem BR, Grimbergen YA, Cramer M, et al. "Stops Walking When Talking" does not predict falls in Parkinson's disease. Ann Neurol 2000;48:268.

Bloem BR, Grimbergen YA, van Dijk JG, et al. The "posture second" strategy: a review of wrong priorities in Parkinson's disase. J Neurol Sci 2006;248:196–204.

Bloom R, Przekop A, Sanger TD. Prolonged electromyogram biofeedback improves upper extremity function in children with cerebral palsy. J Child Neurol 2010;25(12); 1480–1484.

Blumenfeld H. Neuroanatomy through clinical cases, 3rd ed. Oxford: University Press Incorporated, 2010.

Bobath B. Abnormal postural reflex activity caused by brain lesions. London, UK: Heinemann, 1965.

Bobath B, Bobath K. Motor development in different types of cerebral palsy. London, UK: Heinemann, 1975.

Bobath K, Bobath B. The neuro-developmental treatment. In: Scrutton D, ed. Management of the motor disorders of children with cerebral palsy. Oxford: Blackwell Scientific Publications Ltd., 1984:6–18.

Bodranghien F, Bastian A, Casali C, et al. Consensus paper: revisiting the symptoms and signs of cerebellar syndrome. Cerebellum 2016;15:369–391.

Boehme R. Improving upper body control. Tucson, AZ: Therapy Skill Builders, 1988.

Boenig DD. Evaluation of a clinical method of gait analysis. Phys Ther 1977;7:795–798.

Bogen B, Aaslund MK, Ranhoff AH, Moe-Nilssen R. Two-year changes in gait variability in community-living older adults. Gait Posture 2019;72:142–147.

Bohannon RW. Hand-held compared with isokinetic dynamometry for measurement of static knee extension torque (parallel reliability of dynamometers). Clin Phys Physiol Meas 1990;11:217–222.

Bohannon RW. Comfortable and maximum walking speed of adults aged 20–79 years: reference values and determinants. Age Ageing 1997;26:15–19.

Bohannon RW, Andrews AW. Correlation of knee extensor muscle torque and spasticity with gait speed in patients with stroke. Arch Phys Med Rehabil 1990;71:330–333.

Bohannon RW, Crouch R. Minimal clinically important difference for change in 6-minute walk test distance of adults with pathology: a systematic review. J Eval Clin Pract 2017;23:377–381.

Bohannon RW, Glenney SS. Minimal clinically important difference for change in comfortable gait speed of adults with pathology: a systematic review. J Eval Clin Pract 2014;20:295–300.

Bohannon RW, Smith MB. Interrater reliability of a modified Ashworth scale of muscle spasticity. Phys Ther 1987;67(2):206–207.

Bohannon RW, Walsh S. Nature, reliability, and predictive value of muscle performance measures in patients with hemiparesis following stroke. Arch Phys Med Rehabil 1992;73:721–725.

Bohm H, Hosl M, Schwameder H, Doderlein L. Stiff-knee gait in cerebral palsy: how do patients adapt to uneven ground? Gait Posture 2014;39(4).1028–1033.

Bonaiuto J, Arbib MA. Extending the mirror neuron system model, II: what did I just do? A new role for mirror neurons. Biol Cybern 2010;102(4):341–359.

Bonan IV, Colle FM, Guichard JP, et al. Reliance on visual information after stroke. Part I. Balance on dynamic posturography. Arch Phys Med Rehabil 2004;85:268–273.

Bonan IV, Guettard E, Leman MC, et al. Subjective visual vertical perception relates to balance in acute stroke. Arch Phys Med Rehabil 2006;87: 642–646.

Boomkamp-Koppen HG, Visser-Meily JM, Post MW, et al. Poststroke hand swelling and oedema: prevalence and relationship with impairment and disability. Clin Rehabil 2005;19:552–559.

Boonyong S, Siu KC, van Donkelaar P, et al. Development of postural control during gait in typically developing children: the effects of dual-task conditions. Gait Posture 2012;35(3):428–434.

Booth ATC, Buizer AI, Meyns P, Oude Lansink ILB, Steenbrink F, van der Krogt MM. The efficacy of functional gait training in children and young adults with cerebral palsy: a systematic review and meta-analysis. Dev Med Child Neurol 2018;60:866–883.

Borrelli J, Creath RA, Pizac D, Hsiao H, Sanders OP, Rogers MW. Perturbation-evoked lateral steps in older adults: why take two steps when one will do? Clin Biomech (Bristol, Avon) 2019;63:41–47.

Borrelli JR, Zabukovec J, Jones S, Junod CA, Maki BE. Age-related changes in the capacity to select early-onset upper-limb reactions to either recover balance or protect against impact. Exp Gerontol 2019;125:110676.

Bortz WM IV, Bortz WM II. How fast do we age? Exercise performance over time as a biomarker. J Gerontol A Biol Sci Med Sci 1996;51:M223–M225.

Bosch-Bouju C, Hyland BI, Parr-Brownlie LC. Motor thalamus integration of cortical, cerebellar and basal ganglia information: implications for normal and parkinsonian conditions. Front Comput Neurosci 2013;7:1–21.

Boudreau MJ, Smith AM. Activity in rostral motor cortex in response to predictable force-pulse perturbations in a precision grip task. J Neurophysiol 2001;86:1079–1085.

Bovend'Eerdt TJ, Newman M, Barker K, et al. The effects of stretching in spasticity: a systematic review. Arch Phys Med Rehabil 2008;89:1395–13406.

Bowden MG, Balasubramanian CK, Neptune RR, et al. Anterior- posterior ground reaction forces as a measure of paretic leg contribution in hemiparetic walking. Stroke 2006;37:872–876

Bowen A, Wenman R, Mickelborough J, et al. Dual-task effects of talking while walking on velocity and balance following a stroke. Age Ageing 2001;30:319–323.

Bower TGR, Broughton JM, Moore MK. The coordination of visual and tactual input in infants. Percept Psychophys 1970a;8:51–53.

Bower TGR, Broughton JM, Moore MK. Demonstration of intention in the reaching behavior of neonate humans. Nature 1970b;228:679–681.

Bowler JV, Wade JP, Jones BE, et al. Contribution of diaschisis to the clinical deficit in human cerebral infarction. Stroke 1995;26:1000–1006.

Boxum AG, La Bastide-Van Gemert S, Dijkstra LJ, Furda A, Reinders-Messelink HA, Hadders-Algra

M. Postural control during reaching while sitting and general motor behaviour when learning to walk. Dev Med Child Neurol 2019;61(5):555–562.

Boyd LA, Winstein CJ. Implicit motor sequence learning in humans following unilateral stroke: the impact of practice and explicit knowledge. Neurosci Lett 2001;298:65–69.

Boyd LA, Winstein CJ. Impact of explicit information on implicit motor sequence learning following middle cerebral artery stroke. Phys Ther 2003;83:976–989.

Boyne P, Maloney T, DiFrancesco M, et al. Resting-state functional connectivity of subcortical locomotor centers explains variance in walking capacity. Hum Brain Mapp 2018;39(12):4831–4843.

Brach JS, Berlin JE, Van Swearingen JM, et al. Too much or too little step width variability is associated with a fall history in older persons who walk at or near normal gait speed. J Neuroeng Rehabil 2005;2:21.

Bradley NS, Bekoff A. Development of locomotion: animal models. In: Woollacott MH, Shumway-Cook A, eds. Development of posture and gait across the lifespan. Columbia: University of South Carolina, 1989:48–73.

Bradley NS, Smith JL. Neuromuscular patterns of stereotypic hindlimb behaviors in the first two postnatal months. I. Stepping in normal kittens. Dev Brain Res 1988;38:37–52.

Brady RA, Pavol MJ, Owings TM, et al. Foot displacement but not velocity predicts the outcome of a slip induced in young subjects while walking. J Biomech 2000;33:803–808.

Brændvik SM, Elvrum AK, Vereijken B, et al. Relationship between neuromuscular body functions and upper extremity activity in children with cerebral palsy. Dev Med Child Neurol 2010;52:29–34.

Brand PW. Management of sensory loss in the extremities. In: Omer E, Spinner M, eds. Management of peripheral nerve problems. Philadelphia, PA: Saunders, 1980:862–872.

Brandão MB, Ferre C, Kuo H-C, et al. Comparison of structured skill and unstructured practice during intensive bimanual training in children with unilateral spastic cerebral palsy. Neurorehabil Neural Repair 2014;28:452–461.

Brandão MB, Oliveira RH, Mancini MC. Functional priorities reported by parents of children with cerebral palsy: contribution to the pediatric rehabilitation process. Braz J Phys Ther 2014;18(6):563–571.

Brandstater M, deBruin H, Gowland C, et al. Hemiplegic gait: analysis of temporal variables. Arch Phys Med Rehabil 1983;64:583–587.

Brandt T, Daroff RB. The multisensory physiological and pathological vertigo syndromes. Ann Neurol 1979;7:195–197.

Brandt T, Wenzel D, Dichgans J. Die Entwicklung der visuellen Stabilisation des aufrechten Standes bein Kind: Ein Refezeichen in der Kinderneurologie (Visual stabilization of free stance in infants: a sign of maturity). Arch Psychiatr Nervenkr 1976;223:1–13.

Brashear A, Zafonte R, Corcoran M, et al. Inter- and intrarater reliability of the Ashworth scale and the disability assessment scale in patients with upper limb post stroke spasticity. Arch Phys Med Rehabil 2002;83:1349–1354.

Brauer S, Morris ME. Effects of dual task interference on postural control, movement and physical activity in healthy older people and those with movement disorders. In: Morris ME, Schoo A, eds. Optimizing exercise and physical activity in older people. London, UK: Butterworth Heinemann, 2004:2672–2687.

Brauer SG, Broome A, Stone C, et al. Simplest tasks have greatest dual task interference with balance in brain injured adults. Hum Mov Sci 2004;23:489–502.

Brauer SG, Woollacott M, Shumway-Cook A. The influence of a concurrent cognitive task on the compensatory stepping response to a perturbations in balance-impaired and healthy elders. Gait Posture 2002;15:83–93.

Brauer SG, Woollacott M, Shumway-Cook A. The interacting effects of cognitive demand and recovery of postural stability in balance-impaired elderly. J Gerontol Med Sci 2001;56:489–496.

Braun JJ, Meyer PM, Meyer DR. Sparing of a brightness habit in rats following visual decortication. J Comp Physiol Psychol 1986;61:79–82.

Braun S, Granger CV. A practical approach to functional assessment in pediatrics. Occup Ther Pract 1991;2:46–51.

Bravi L, Stoykov ME. New directions in occupational therapy: implementation of the task-oriented approach in conjunction with cortical stimulation after stroke. Top Stroke Rehabil 2007;14(6):68–73.

Breniere Y, Bril B. Development of postural control of gravity forces in children during the first 5 years of walking. Exp Brain Res 1998;121:255–262.

Breniere Y, Do MC, Sanchez J. A biomechanical study of the gait initiation process. J Biophys Med Nucl 1981;5:197–205.

Breniere Y, Do MC. When and how does steady state gait movement induced from upright posture begin? J Biomech 1986;19:1035–1040.

Brien M, Sveistrup H. An intensive virtual reality program improves functional balance and mobility of adolescents with cerebral palsy. Pediatr Phys Ther 2011;23:258–266.

Bril B, Breniere Y. Posture and independent locomotion in childhood: learning to walk or learning dynamic postural control? In: Savelsbergh GJP, ed. The development of coordination in infancy. Amsterdam, The Netherlands: North-Holland, 1993:337–358.

Brochier T, Boudreau MJ, Parc M, et al. The effects of muscimol inactivation of small regions of motor and somatosensory cortex on independent finger movements and force control in the precision grip. Exp Brain Res 1999;128:31–40.

Brod M, Mendelsohn GA, Roberts B. Patients' experiences of Parkinson's disease. J Gerontol B Psychol Sci Soc Sci 1998;53:213–222.

Broderick MP, Newell KM. Coordination patterns in ball bouncing as a function of skill. J Motor Behav 1999;31:165–189.

Broeder S, Nackaerts E, Nieuwboer A, et al. The effects of dual tasking on handwriting in patients with Parkinson's disease. Neuroscience 2014;263:193–202.

Broekmans T, Gijbels D, Eijnde BO, et al. The relationship between upper leg muscle strength and walking capacity in persons with multiple sclerosis. Mult Scler 2013;19:112–119.

Brogren E, Forssberg H, Hadders-Algra M. Influence of two different sitting positions on postural adjustments in children with spastic diplegia. Dev Med Child Neurol 2001;43:534–546.

Brogren E, Hadders-Algra M, Forssberg H. Postural control in children with spastic diplegia: muscle activity during perturbations to sitting. Dev Med Child Neurol 1996;38:379–388.

Brogren E, Hadders-Algra M, Forssberg H. Postural control in sitting children with cerebral palsy. Neurosci Biobehav Rev 1998;22:591–596.

Bronstein AM, Guerraz M. Visual-vestibular control of posture and gait: physiological mechanisms and disorders. Curr Opin Neurol 1999;12:5–11.

Brooks DC. The pixelated brain. 2011. Retrieved from www.pixelatedbrain.com

Brooks VB. The neural basis of motor control. New York: Oxford University Press, 1986.

Brown JK. Science and spasticity. Dev Med Child Neurol 1993;35:471–472.

Brown TG. The intrinsic factors in the act of progression in the mammal. Proc R Soc Lond B 1911;84:308–319.

Brown T, Thyer L. The convergent validity of the Children's Leisure Assessment Scale (CLASS) and Children's Assessment of Participation and Enjoyment and Preferences for Activities of Children (CAPE/PAC). Scand J Occup Ther 2020;27(5):349–363. doi: 10.1080/11038128.2019.1672784.

Brownstone RM, Chopek JW. Reticulospinal systems for tuning motor commands. Front Neural Circuits 2018;12:1–10.

Brown DM, Cullers CM, McMonigal LL, et al. The use of neuromuscular electrical stimulation for facilitation of task-oriented exercise in the upper extremity to achieve functional improvement in an individual with chronic post-stroke hemiparesis: a case study. Neurol Rep 2000;24:198–199.

Brown M, Dijkers M, Gordon WA, et al. Participation objective, participation subjective: a measure of participation combining outsider and insider perspectives. J Head Trauma Rehabil 2004;19:459–481.

Brown LA, McKenzie NC, Doan JB. Age-dependent differences in the attentional demands of obstacle negotiation. J Gerontol 2005;60A:924–927.

Brown JV, Sepehr MM, Ettlinger G, et al. The accuracy of aimed movements to visual targets during development: the role of visual information. J Exp Child Psychol 1986;41:443–460.

Brown LA, Shumway-Cook A, Woollacott MH. Attentional demands and postural recovery: the effects of aging. J Gerontol 1999;54A:M165–M171.

Brown LA, Sleik RJ, Winder TR. Attentional demands for static postural control after stroke. Arch Phys Med Rehabil 2002;83:1732–1735.

Bruce MF. The relation of tactile thresholds to histology in the fingers of the elderly. J Neurol Neurosurg Psychiatry 1980; 43:730.

Bruijn SM, Meijer OG, van Dieën JH, et al. Coordination of leg swing thorax rotations, and pelvis rotations during gait: the organisation of total body angular momentum. Gait Posture 2008;27: 455–462.

Bruininks RH, Bruininks BD. Bruininks-Oseretsky test of motor proficiency, 2nd ed. Circle Pines, MN: American Guidance Service, 2005.

Bruininks RH. Bruininks-Oseretsky Test of motor proficiency. Circle Pines, MN: American Guidance Service, 1978.

Bruner JS, Koslowski B. Visually pre-adapted constituents of manipulatory action. Perception 1972;1:3–14.

Brunner IC, Skouen JS, Ersland L, et al. Plasticity and response to action observation: a longitudinal FMRI study of potential mirror neurons in patients with subacute stroke. Neurorehabil Neural Repair 2014;28(9):874–884.

Brunner I, Skouen JS, Hofstad H, et al. Virtual reality training for upper extremity in subacute stroke (VIRTUES): study protocol for a randomized controlled multicenter trial. BMC Neurol 2014;14(1):186.

Brunnstrom S. Motor testing procedures in hemiplegia: based on sequential recovery stages. Phys Ther 1966;46:357–375.

Brunnstrom S. Movement therapy in hemiplegia: a neurophysiological approach. New York: Harper & Row, 1970.

Brunt D, VanderLinden DW, Behrman AL. The relation between limb loading and control parameters of gait initiation in persons with stroke. Arch Phys Med Rehabil 1995;76:627–634.

Bryant MS, Workman CD, Jamal F, Meng H, Jackson GR. Feasibility study: effect of hand resistance exercise on handwriting in Parkinson's disease and essential tremor. J Hand Ther 2018;31(1):29–34. doi: 10.1016/j.jht.2017.01.002.

Buchner DM, DeLateur BJ. The importance of skeletal muscle strength to physical function in older adults. Ann Behav Med 1991;13:1–12.

Buchner DM, Larson EB. Falls and fractures in patients with Alzheimer-type dementia. JAMA 1987;257:1492–1495.

Buchner DM, Larson EB, Wagner EH, et al. Evidence for a non-linear relationship between leg strength and gait speed. Age Ageing 1996;25:386–391.

Buckingham G, Bien´kiewicz M, Rohrbach N, et al. The impact of unilateral brain damage on weight perception, sensorimotor anticipation, and fingertip force adaptation. Vision Res 2015;115(Pt B):231–237. pii: S0042-6989(15)00046-2. doi: 10.1016/j.visres.2015.02.005.

Budisavljevic S, Castiello U. Reaching and grasping. In: Encyclopedia of Neuroscience. Elsevier, 2017.

Bullinger A. Cognitive elaboration of sensorimotor behaviour. In: Butterworth G, ed. Infancy and epistemology: an evaluation of Piaget's theory. London, UK: Harvester, 1981:173–199.

Bullinger A, Jouen F. Sensibilite du champ de detection peripherique aux variations posturales chez le bebe. Arch Psychol 1983;51:41–48.

Bultmann U, Pierscianek D, Gizewski ER, et al. Functional recovery and rehabilitation of postural impairment and gait ataxia in patients with acute cerebellar stroke. Gait Posture 2014;39:563–569.

Bumin G, Kavak ST. An investigation of the factors affecting handwriting skill in children with hemiplegic cerebral palsy. Disabil Rehabil 2010;32:692–703.

Bunday KL, Bronstein AM. Locomotor adaptation and aftereffects in patients with reduced somatosensory input due to peripheral neuropathy. J Neurophysiol 2009;102:3119–3128.

Bunco CA, Andersen RA. The posterior parietal cortex: sensorimotor interface for the planning and online control of visually guided movements. Neuropsychologia 2006;44:2594–2606.

Burgess PR, Clark FJ. Characteristics of knee-joint receptors in the cat. J Physiol Lond 1969;203:317–325.

Burke D, Wissel J, Donnan GA. Pathophysiology of spasticity in stroke. Neurology. 2013;80:S20–S26.

Bürkle A, Brabeck C, Diefenbach J, et al. The emerging role of poly(ADP-ribose) polymerase-1 in longevity. Int J Biochem Cell Biol 2005;37(5):1043–1053.

Burridge JH, Wood DE, Hermens HJ, et al. Theoretical and methodological considerations in the measurement of spasticity. Disabil Rehabil 2005;27:69–80.

Burns SP, Spanier DE. Break-technique handheld dynamometry: relation between angular velocity and strength measurements. Arch Phys Med Rehabil 2005;86(7):1420–1426.

Burtner PA, Woollacott MH, Craft GL, et al. The capacity to adapt to changing balance threats: a comparison of children with cerebral palsy and typically developing children. Dev Neurorehabil 2007;10:249–260.

Burtner PA, Woollacott MH, Qualls C. Stance balance control with orthoses in a select group of children with and without spasticity. Dev Med Child 1999;41:748–757.

Bushnell C, Bettger JP, Cockroft KM, et al. Chronic stroke outcome measures for motor function intervention trials: expert panel recommendations. Circ Cardiovasc Qual Outcomes 2015;8(6 Suppl 3):S163–S169. doi: 10.1161/CIRCOUTCOMES.115.002098.

Bütefisch C, Khurana V, Kopylev L, et al. Enhancing encoding of a motor memory in the primary motor cortex by cortical stimulation. J Neurophysiol 2004;91:2110–2116.

Butland RJA, Pang J, Gross ER, et al. Two-, six-, and 12-minute walking tests in respiratory disease. BMJ 1982;284:1607–1608.

Butler PB. A preliminary report on the effectiveness of trunk targeting in achieving independent sitting balance in children with cerebral palsy. Clin Rehabil 1998;12:281–293.

Butler PB, Saavedra S, Sofranac M, et al. Refinement, reliability, and validity of the segmental assessment of trunk control. Pediatr Phys Ther 2010;22:246–257.

Butterworth G, Cicchetti D. Visual calibration of posture in normal and motor retarded Down's syndrome infants. Perception 1978;7:513–525.

Butterworth G, Hicks L. Visual proprioception and postural stability in infancy: a developmental study. Perception 1977;6:255–262.

Butterworth G, Pope M. Origine et fonction de la proprioception visuelle chez l'enfant. In: de Schonen S, ed. Le developpement dans la premiere année. Paris, UK: Presses Universitaires de France, 1983:107–128.

Byl N, Roderick J, Mohamed O, et al. Effectiveness of sensory and motor rehabilitation of the upper limb following the principles of the upper limb following the principles of neuroplasticity: patients stable poststroke. Neurorehabil Neural Repair 2003;17(3):176–191.

Byl NN, McKenzie A. Treatment effectiveness for patients with a history of repetitive hand use and focal hand dystonia: a planned, prospective follow-up study. J Hand Ther 2000;13:289–301.

C

Cahill BM, Carr JH, Adams R. Intersegmental co-ordination in sit-to-stand: an age cross-sectional study. Physiother Res Int 1999;4:12–27.

Cailliet R. The shoulder in hemiplegia. Philadelphia, PA: FA Davis, 1980.

Cakit BD, Saracoglu M, Genc H, et al. The effects of incremental speed-dependent treadmill training on postural instability and fear of falling in Parkinson's disease. Clin Rehabil 2007;21:698–705.

Cakrt O, Chovanec M, Funda T, et al. Exercise with visual feedback improves postural stability after vestibular schwannoma surgery. Eur Arch Otorhinolaryngol 2010;267(9):1355–1360.

Cakrt O, Vyhnálek M, Slabý K, et al. Balance rehabilitation therapy by tongue electrotactile biofeedback in patients with degenerative cerebellar disease. NeuroRehabilitation. 2012;31(4):429–434. doi: 10.3233/NRE-2012-00813.

Cameron DM, Bohannon RW, Garrett GE, et al. Physical impairments related to kinetic energy during sit-to-stand and curb-climbing following stroke. Clin Biomech (Bristol, Avon) 2003;18(4):332–340.

Cameron M, Horak FB, Herndon RR, et al. Imbalance in multiple sclerosis: a result of slowed spinal somatosensory conduction. Somatosens Motor Res 2008;25:113–122.

Camicioli R, Howieson D, Lehman S. Talking while walking: the effects of a dual task on aging and Alzheimer's disease. Neurology 1997;48:955–958.

Camicioli R, Licis L. Motor impairment predicts falls in specialized Alzheimer care units. Alzheimer Dis Assoc Disord 2004;18:214–218.

Campanini I, Merlo A, Damiano B. A method to differentiate the causes of stiff-knee gait in stroke patients. Gait Posture 2013;38:165–169.

Campbell SK. Measurement of motor performance in cerebral palsy. In: Forssberg H, Hirschfeld H, eds. Movement disorders in children. Basel, Switzerland: Karger, 1991:264–271.

Campbell SK. Are models of disability useful in real cases? Pediatric case examples realized in research, clinical practice, and education. Phys Ther 2006;86:881–887.

Campbell AJ, Borrie MJ, Spears GF. Risk factors for falls in a community-based prospective study of people 70 years and older. J Gerontol 1989;44:M112–M117.

Campbell SK, Kolobe THA, Osten ET, et al. Construct validity of the Test of Infant Motor Performance. Phys Ther 1995;75:585–596.

Campbell AJ, Reinken J, Allen BC, et al. Falls in old age: a study of frequency and related clinical factors. Age Ageing 1981;10:264–279.

Campbell AJ, Robertson MC. Rethinking individual and community fall prevention strategies: a meta-regression comparing single and multifactorial interventions. Age Ageing 2007;36(6):656–662.

Campbell C, Rowse J, Ciol MA, et al. The effect of attentional demands on the Timed Up and Go Test in older adults with and without Parkinson's disease. Neurol Rep 2003;3:2–7.

Camus M, Ragert P, Vandermeeren Y, et al. Mechanisms controlling motor output to a transfer hand after learning a sequential pinch force skill with the opposite hand. Clin Neurophysiol 2009;120:1859–1865.

Cantin JF, McFadyen BJ, Doyon J, et al. Can measures of cognitive function predict locomotor behavior in complex environments following a traumatic brain injury? Brain Inj 2007;21:327–334.

Cappellini G, Sylos-Labini F, MacLellan MJ, et al. Locomotor patterns during obstacle avoidance in children with cerebral palsy. J Neurophysiol 2020;124(2):574–590.

Carey L, Matyas T, Oke L. Sensory loss in stroke patients: effective training of tactile and proprioceptive discrimination. Arch Phys Med Rehabil 1993;74:602–611.

Carlberg EB, Hadders-Algra M. Postural dysfunction in children with cerebral palsy: some implications for therapeutic guidance. Neural Plast 2005;12:221–228.

Carlsoo A. The initiation of walking. Acta Anat 1966;65:1–9.

Carlton LG. Processing visual feedback information for movement control. J Exp Psychol Hum Percept 1981;7:1019–1030.

Carpenter MG, Allum JHJ, Adkin AL, et al. Postural abnormalities to multidirectional stance perturbations in Parkinson's disease. J Neurol Neurosurg Psychiatry 2004;75:1245–1254.

Carpenter MG, Murnaghan CD, Inglis JT. Shifting the balance: evidence of an exploratory role for postural sway. Neuroscience 2010;171:196–204.

Carpinella I, Cattaneo D, Ferrarin M. Quantitative assessment of upper limb motor function in Multiple Sclerosis using an instrumented Action Research Arm Test. J Neuroeng Rehabil 2014;11:67.

Carpinella I, Gervasoni E, Anastasi D, Lencioni T, Cattaneo D, Ferrarin M. Instrumental assessment of stair ascent in people with multiple sclerosis, stroke, and parkinson's disease: a wearable-sensor-based approach. IEEE Trans Neural Syst Rehabil Eng 2018;26:2324–2332.

Carr JH, Shepherd RB. Motor relearning programme for stroke, 2nd ed. Rockville, MD. Aspen, 1992.

Carr JH, Shepherd RB. Neurologic rehabilitation: optimizing motor performance. Oxford, UK: Butterworth and Heinemann, 1998.

Carr JH, Shepherd RB, Nordholm L, et al. Investigation of a new motor assessment scale for stroke patients. Phys Ther 1985;65:175–180.

Carrera E, Tononi G. Diaschisis: past, present, future. Brain 2014;137:2408–2422.

Carswell A, McColl MA, Baptiste S, et al. The Canadian occupational performance measure: a research and clinical literature review. Can J Occup Ther 2004;71(4):210–222.

Carvalho I, Pinto SM, Chagas DV, Praxedes dos Santos JL, de Sousa Oliveira T, Batista LA. Robotic gait training for individuals with cerebral palsy: a systematic review and meta-analysis. Arch Phys Med Rehabil 2017;98:2332–2341.

Carvalho RP, Tudella E, Caljouw SR, Savelsbergh GJ. Early control of reaching: effects of experience and body orientation. Infant Behav Dev 2008;31(1):23–33. doi: 10.1016/j.infbeh.2007.06.001.

Carvalho RP, Tudella E, Savelsbergh GJ. Spatio-temporal parameters in infant's reaching movements are influenced by body orientation. Infant Behav Dev 2007;30(1):26–35. doi: 10.1016/j.infbeh.2006.07.006.

Cascarano GD, Loconsole C, Brunetti A, et al. Biometric handwriting analysis to support Parkinson's Disease assessment and grading. BMC Med Inform Decis Mak 2019;19(Suppl 9):252. doi: 10.1186/s12911-019-0989-3.

Case-Smith J. Fine motor outcomes in preschool children who receive occupational therapy services. Am J Occup Ther 1996;50(1):52–61.

Case-Smith J. Effects of occupational therapy services on fine motor and functional performance in preschool children. Am J Occup Ther 2000;54:372–380.

Cass SP, Borello-France D, Furman JM. Functional outcome of vestibular rehabilitation in patients with abnormal sensory organization testing. Am J Otol 1996;17:581–594.

Cassidy JM, Gillick BT, Carey JR. Priming the brain to capitalize on metaplasticity in stroke rehabilitation. Phys Ther 2014;94(1):139–150. doi: 10.2522/ptj.20130027.

Castiello U. The neuroscience of grasping. Nat Rev Neurosci 2005;6:726–736.

Catalano JF, Kleiner BM. Distant transfer and practice variability. Percept Mot Skills 1984;58:851–856.

Catena RD, van Donkelaar P, Chou LS. Altered balance control following concussion is better detected with an attention test during gait. Gait Posture 2007;25:406–411.

Catena RD, van Donkelaar P, Chou LS. Different gait tasks distinguish immediate vs. long-term effects of concussion on balance control. J Neuroeng Rehabil 2009;7:25–30.

Cattaneo D, DeNuzzo C, Fascia T, et al. Risks of falls in subjects with multiple sclerosis. Arch Phys Med Rehabil 2002;83:864–867.

Cattaneo D, Jonsdottir J. Sensory impairments in quiet standing in subjects with multiple sclerosis. Mult Scler 2009;15:59–67.

Cattaneo D, Jonsdottir J, Zocchi M, et al. Effects of balance exercises on people with multiple sclerosis: a pilot study. Clin Rehabil 2007;21:771–781.

Cauraugh JH, Kim SB. Stroke motor recovery: active neuromuscular stimulation and repetitive practice schedules. J Neurol Neurosurg Psychiatry 2003;74:1562–1566.

Cauraugh JH, Summers JJ. Neural plasticity and bilateral movements: a rehabilitation approach for chronic stroke. Prog Neurobiol 2005;75:309–320.

Cauraugh JH, Kim SB, Duley A. Coupled bilateral movements and active neuromuscular stimulation: intralimb transfer evidence during bimanual aiming. Neurosci Lett 2005;382(1–2):39–44.

Cavanagh PR, Gregor RJ. Knee joint torques during the swing phase of normal treadmill walking. J Biomech 1975;8:337–344.

Cernak K, Stevens V, Price R, et al. Locomotor training using body-weight support on a treadmill in conjunction with ongoing physical therapy in a child with severe cerebellar ataxia. Phys Ther 2008;88:88–97.

Centers for Disease Control and Prevention National Center for Injury Prevention and Control. Algorithm for Fall Risk Screening, Assessment, and Intervention 2009. www.cdc.gov/steadi.Cha J, et al. Locomotor ability in spinal rats is dependent on the amount of activity imposed on the hindlimbs during treadmill training. J Neurotrauma 2007;24:1000–1012.

Chakraborty S, Nandy A, Kesar TM. Gait deficits and dynamic stability in children and adolescents with cerebral palsy: a systematic review and meta analysis. Clin Biomech (Bristol, Avon) 2020;71:11–23.

Chalard A, Amarantini D, Tisseyre J, Marque P, Tallet J, Gasq D. Spastic co-contraction, rather than spasticity, is associated with impaired active function in adults with acquired brain injury: a pilot study. J Rehabil Med 2019;51:307–311.

Cham R, Redfern MS. Changes in gait when anticipating slippery floors. Gait Posture 2002;15:159–171.

Chambers AJ, Cham R. Slip-related muscle activation patterns in the stance leg during walking. Gait Posture 2007;25:565–572.

Chan PP, Si Tou JI, Tse MM, Ng SS. Reliability and validity of the timed up and go test with a motor task in people with chronic stroke. Arch Phys Med Rehabil 2017;98:2213–2220.

Chandler JM, Duncan PW, Studenski SA. Balance performance on the postural stress test: comparison of young adults, healthy elderly, and fallers. Phys Ther 1990;70:410–415.

Chandler JM, Hadley EC. Exercise to improve physiologic and functional performance in old age. In: Studenski S. Clinics in geriatric medicine: gait and balance disorders, vol. 12. Philadelphia, PA: Saunders, 1996:761–784.

Chang HA, Krebs DE. Dynamic balance control in elders: gait initiation assessment as a screening tool. Arch Phys Med Rehabil 1999;80:490–494.

Chang JJ, Wu TI, Wu WL, et al. Kinematical measure for spastic reaching in children with cerebral palsy. Clin Biomech (Bristol, Avon) 2005;20:381–388.

Chang SH, Yu NY. Comparison of motor praxis and performance in children with varying levels of developmental coordination disorder. Hum Mov Sci 2016;48:7–14. doi: 10.1016/j.humov.2016.04.001.

Chapman SB, McKinnon L. Discussion of developmental plasticity: factors affecting cognitive outcome after pediatric traumatic brain injury. J Commun Disord 2000;33:333–344.

Charles J, Gordon AM. Development of hand-arm bimanual intensive training (HABIT) for improving bimanual coordination in children with hemiplegic cerebral palsy. Dev Med Child Neurol 2006;48:931–936.

Charles JR, Gordon AM. A repeated course of constraint-induced movement therapy results in further improvement. Dev Med Child Neurol 2007;49:770–773.

Charles J, Lavinder G, Gordon A. Effects of constraint-induced therapy on hand function in children with hemiplegic cerebral palsy. Pediatr Phys Ther 2001;13:68–76.

Charness AL. Management of the upper extremity in the patient with hemiplegia. Course syllabus for the Annual Meeting of the Washington Physical Therapy Association, 1994.

Chemerinski E, Robinson RG, Kosier JT. Improved recovery in activities of daily living associated with remission of poststroke depression. Stroke 2001;32:113–117.

Chen HC. Factors underlying balance restoration after tripping: biomechanical model analyses. Doctoral dissertation, University of Michigan, 1993.

Chen X. Human Motion Analysis with Wearable Inertial Sensors. PhD diss., University of Tennessee, 2013. https://trace.tennessee.edu/utk_graddiss/2407

Chen H, Ashton-Miller JA, Alexander NB, et al. Stepping over obstacles: gait patterns of healthy young and old adults. J Gerontol 1991;46:M196–M203.

Chen CC, Bode RK, Granger CV, Heinemann AW. Psychometric properties and developmental differences in children's ADL item hierarchy: a study of the WeeFIM instrument. Am J Phys Med Rehabil 2005;84(9):671–679.

Chen N, Cai P, Zhou T, Thompson B, Fang F. Perceptual learning modifies the functional specializations of visual cortical areas. Proc Natl Acad Sci USA 2016;113(20):5724–5729. doi: 10.1073/pnas.1524160113.

Chen CL, Chen CY, Chen HC, et al. Responsiveness and minimal clinically important difference of Modified Ashworth Scale in patients with stroke. Eur J Phys Rehabil Med 2019;55(6):754–760. doi: 10.23736/S1973-9087.19.05545-X.

Chen CL, Chen HC, Tang SF, et al. Gait performance with compensatory adaptations in stroke patients with different degrees of motor recovery. Am J Phys Med Rehabil 2003a;82:925–935.

Chen KL, Chou YT, Yu WH, et al. A prospective study of the responsiveness of the original and the short form Berg Balance Scale in people with stroke. Clin Rehabil 2015;29:468–476. pii: 0269215514549032.

Chen R, Cohen LG, Hallett M. Nervous system reorganization following injury. Neuroscience 2002;4:761–773.

Chen CC, Granger CV, Peimer CA, et al. Manual Ability Measure (MAM-16): a preliminary report on a new patient-centered and task-oriented outcome measure of hand function. J Hand Surg Br 2005;30:207–216.

Chen YP, Howard AM. Effects of robotic therapy on upper-extremity function in children with cerebral palsy: a systematic review. Dev Neurorehabil 2016;19(1):64–71. doi: 10.3109/17518423.2014.899648.

Chen CC, Kasven N, Karpatkin HI, et al. Hand strength and perceived manual ability among patients with multiple sclerosis. Arch Phys Med Rehabil 2007;88:794–797.

Chen CH, Lin KH, Lu TW, et al. Immediate effect of lateral-wedged insole on stance and ambulation after stroke. Am J Phys Med Rehabil 2010;89:48–55.

Chen G, Patten C. Joint moment work during the stance to swing transition in hemiparetic subjects. J Biomech 2008;41:877–883.

Chen HC, Schultz AB, Ashton-Miller JA, et al. Stepping over obstacles: dividing attention impairs performance of old more than young adults. J Gerontol 1996;51(3):M116–M122.

Chen J, Woollacott MH. Lower extremity kinetics for balance control in children with cerebral palsy. J Mot Behav 2007;39(4):306–316.

Chen C-L, Yeung K-T, Bih L-I, Wang C-H, Chen M-I, Chien J-C. The relationship between sitting stability and functional performance in patients with paraplegia. Arch Phys Med Rehabil 2003b;84(9):1276–1281.

Chen H, Zhang SM, Schwarzschild MA, et al. Physical activity and the risk of Parkinson disease. Neurology 2005;64:664–669.

Cheng PT, Chen CL, Wang CM, et al. Leg muscle activation patterns of sit-to-stand movement in stroke patients. Am J Phys Med Rehabil 2004;83:10–16.

Cheng PT, Liaw MY, Wong MK, et al. The sit-to-stand movement in stroke patients and its correlation with falling. Arch Phys Med Rehabil 1998;79:1043–1046.

Cherng RJ, Su FC, Chen JJ, et al. Performance of static standing balance in children with spastic diplegic cerebral palsy under altered sensory environments. Am J Phys Med Rehabil 1999;78:336–343.

Chiarello LA, Palisano RJ, Wescott McCoy S, et al. Child engagement in daily life: a measure of participation for young children with cerebral palsy. Disabil Rehabil 2014;36(21):1804–1816.

Chiba R, Takakusaki K, Ota J, Yozu A, Haga N. Human upright posture control models based on multisensory inputs; in fast and slow dynamics. Neurosci Res 2016;104:96–104.

Chisari C, Venturi M, Bertolucci F, et al. Benefits of an intensive task-oriented circuit training in Multiple Sclerosis patients with mild disability. NeuroRehabilitation 2014;35(3):509–518.

Chiu H, Ada L, Bania T. Mechanically assisted walking training for walking, participation, and quality of life in children with cerebral palsy (Review). Cochrane Database Syst Rev 2020;11:1–86.

Cho KH, Lee WH. Effect of treadmill training based real-world video recording on balance and gait in chronic stroke patients: a randomized controlled trial. Gait Posture 2014;39:523–528.

Cho B, Scarpace D, Alexander NB. Tests of stepping as indicators of mobility, balance and fall risk in balance-impaired older adults. J Am Geriatr Soc 2004;52:1168–1173.

Choi Y, Kim Y, Kim M, Yoon B. Muscle synergies for turning during human walking. J Mot Behav 2019;51(1):1–9.

Choi NG, Bruce ML, DiNitto DM, Marti CN, Kunik ME. Fall worry restricts social engagement in older adults. J Aging Health 2020;32:422–431.

Chong RKY, Horak FB, Frank J, et al. Sensory organization for balance: specific deficits in Alzheimer's but not in Parkinson's disease. J Gerontol A Biol Sci Med Sci 1999;54:M122–M128.

Chong R, Horak F, Woollacott M. Parkinson's disease impairs the ability to change set quickly. J Neurol Sci 2000;175:57–70.

Chorna O, Heathcock J, Key A, et al. Early childhood constraint therapy for sensory/motor impairment in cerebral palsy: a randomised clinical trial protocol. BMJ Open 2015;5(12):e010212. doi: 10.1136/bmjopen-2015-010212.

Chou C, Chien C, Hsueh I, et al. Developing a short form of the Berg Balance Scale for people with stroke. Phys Ther 2006;86:195–204.

Chou L-S, Kaufman KR, Brey RH, et al. Motion of the whole body's center of mass when stepping over obstacles of different heights. Gait Posture 2001;13:17–26.

Chou L-S, Kaufman KR, Hahn ME, et al. Medio-lateral motion of the center of mass during obstacle crossing distinguishes elderly patients with imbalance. Gait Posture 2003;18:125–133.

Chou LS, Kaufman KR, Walker-Rabatin AE, et al. Dynamic instability during obstacle crossing following traumatic brain injury. Gait Posture 2004;20:245–254.

Chou P, Lee S. Turning deficits in people with Parkinson's disease. Tzu Chi Medical J 2013;25:200–202.

Chow JW, Stokic DS. Gait impairments in patients without lower limb hypertonia early poststroke are related to weakness of paretic knee flexors. Arch Phys Med Rehabil 2019;100(6):1091–1101.

Ciesla N, Dinglas V, Fan E, Kho M, Kuramoto J, Needham D. Manual muscle testing: a method of measuring extremity muscle strength applied to critically Ill patients. J Vis Exp 2011;50:2–6.

Cirstea MC, Mitnitski AB, Feldman AG, et al. Interjoint coordination dynamics during reaching in stroke. Exp Brain Res 2003;151:289–300.

Clark J, Lanphear A, Riddick C. The effects of videogame playing on the response selection processing of elderly adults. J Gerontol 1987;42:82–85.

Clark JE, Whitall J. Changing patterns of locomotion: from walking to skipping. In: Woollacott MH, Shumway-Cook A, eds. Development of posture and gait across the lifespan. Columbia: University of South Carolina, 1989:128–151.

Claverie P, Alexandre F, Nichol J, et al. L'activité tonique reflexe du nourisson. Pediatrie 1973;28:661–679.

Clifton RK, Muir DW, Ashmead DH, Clarkson MG. Is visually guided reaching in early infancy a myth? Child Dev 1993;64:1099–1110.

Cockburn J, Haggard P, Cock J, et al. Changing patterns of cognitive-motor interference (CMI) over time during recovery from stroke. Clin Rehabil 2003;17:167–173.

Cohen LG, Bandinelli S, Findlay TW, et al. Motor reorganization after upper limb amputation in man: a study with focal magnetic stimulation. Brain 1991;114:615–627.

Cohen H, Blatchly CA, Gombash LL. A study of the clinical test of sensory interaction and balance. Phys Ther 1993;73:346–351.

Cohen R, Gurfinkel V, Kwak E, Warden A, Horak F. Lighten up: specific postural instructions affect axial rigidity and step initiation in patients with Parkinson's disease. Neurorehabil Neural Repair 2015;29(9):878–888.

Colarusso RP, Hammill DD. Motor-Free Visual Perceptual Test-4th edition (MVPT-4). Novata, CA: Academic Therapy Publications, 2015.

Cole KJ. Grasp force control in older adults. J Mot Behav 1991;23:251–258.

Cole KJ. Age-related directional bias of fingertip force. Exp Brain Res 2006;175:285–291.

Cole KJ, Rotella DL. Old age affects fingertip forces when restraining an unpredictably loaded object. Exp Brain Res 2001;136:535–542.

Cole KJ, Rotella DL. Old age impairs the use of arbitrary visual cues for predictive control of fingertip forces during grasp. Exp Brain Res 2002;143:35–41.

Cole KJ, Rotella DL, Harper JG. Mechanisms for age-related changes of fingertip forces during precision gripping and lifting in adults. J Neurosci 1999;19:3228–3247.

Cole KJ, Rotella DL, Harper JG. Tactile impairments cannot explain the effect of age on a grasp and lift task. Exp Brain Res 1998;121:263–269.

Cole WG, Robinson SR, Adolph KE. Bouts of steps: the organization of infant exploration. Dev Psychobiol 2016;58(3):341–354.

Colebatch JG, Gandevia SC. The distribution of muscular weakness in upper motor neuron lesions affecting the arm. Brain 1989;112:749–763.

Colebatch JG, Govender S. Responses to anterior and posterior perturbations in Parkinson's disease with early postural instability: role of axial and limb rigidity. Exp Brain Res 2019;237(7):1853–1867.

Collen FM, Wade DT, Bradshaw CM. Mobility after stroke: reliability of measures of impairment and disability. Int Disabil Stud 1990;12:6–9.

Collignon O, Davare M, De Volder AG, et al. Time-course of posterior parietal and occipital cortex contribution to sound localization. J Cogn Neurosci 2008;20:1454–1463.

Collignon O, Voss P, Lassonde M, et al. Cross-modal plasticity for the spatial processing of sounds in visually deprived subjects. Exp Brain Res 2009;192:343–358.

Colman RJ, Anderson RM, Johnson SC, et al. Caloric restriction delays disease onset and mortality in rhesus monkeys. Science 2009;325(5937):201–204.

Colon-Emeric CS, Sloane R, Hawkes WG, et al. The risk of subsequent hip fracture in community-dwelling men and male veterans with hip fracture. Am J Med 2000;109:324–326.

Combs SA, Kelly SP, Barton R, et al. Effects of an intensive, task-specific rehabilitation program for individuals with chronic stroke: a case series. Disabil Rehabil 2010;32:669–678.

Connolly KJ. The development of competence in motor skills. In: Nadeau CH, Halliwell WR, Newell KM, et al., eds. Psychology of motor behavior and sport. Champaign, IL: Human Kinetics, 1979:229–250.

Conroy SS, Wittenberg GF, Krebs HI, Zhan M, Bever CT, Whitall J. Robot-assisted arm training in chronic stroke: addition of transition-to-task practice. Neurorehabil Neural Repair 2019;33(9):751–761. doi: 10.1177/1545968319862558.

Cook T, Cozzens B. Human solutions for locomotion: 3. The initiation of gait. In: Herman RM, Grillner S, Stein PSG, et al., eds. Neural control of locomotion. New York: Plenum, 1976:65–76.

Coote S, Finlayson M, Sosnoff JJ. Level of mobility limitations and falls status in persons with multiple sclerosis. Arch Phys Med Rehabil 2014;95:862–866.

Coppin AK, Shumway-Cook A, Saczynski JS, et al. Association of executive function and performance of dual-task physical tests among older adults: analyses from the InChianti study. Age Ageing 2006;35:619–624.

Corbetta D, Mounoud P. Early development of grasping and manipulation. In: Bard C, Fleury M, Hay L, eds. Development of eye-hand coordination across the lifespan. Columbia: University of South Carolina Press, 1990:188–213.

Corbetta M, Shulman GL. Spatial neglect and attention networks. Annu Rev Neurosci 2011;34:569–599.

Cordo P, Nashner L. Properties of postural adjustments associated with rapid arm movements. J Neurophysiol 1982;47:287–302.

Cornhill H, Case-Smith J. Factors that relate to good and poor handwriting. Am J Occup Ther 1996;50:732–729.

Costner W, Deeney T, Haltiwanger J, et al. School Function Assessment (SFA). San Antonio, TX: The Psychological Corporation of Harcourt Brace & Co., 1998.

Cote L, Crutcher MD. The basal ganglia. In: Kandel E, Schwartz JH, Jessell TM, eds. Principles of neuroscience, 3rd ed. New York: Elsevier, 1991.

Courtine G, Schieppati M. Human walking along a curved path. II. Gait features and EMG patterns. Eur J Neurosci 2003;18(1):191–205.

Courtine G, Schieppati M. Tunin of a basic coordination pattern constructs straight-ahead and curved walking in humans. J Neurophysiol 2004;91:1524–1525.

Craig CE, Doumas M. Slowed sensory reweighting and postural illusions in older adults: the moving platform illusion. J Neurophysiol 2019;121(2):690–700.

Craik R. Changes in locomotion in the aging adult. In: Woollacott MH, Shumway-Cook A, eds. Development of posture and gait across the lifespan. Columbia: University of South Carolina, 1989:176–201.

Craik RL. Recovery processes: maximizing function. In: Contemporary management of motor control problems. Proceedings of the II Step Conference. Alexandria, VA: American Physical Therapy Association, 1992:165–173.

Craik RL, Cozzens BA, Freedman W. The role of sensory conflict on stair descent performance in humans. Exp Brain Res 1982;45:399–409.

Crajé C, Aarts P, Nijhuis-van der Sanden M, Steenbergen B. Action planning in typically and atypically developing children (unilateral cerebral palsy). Res Dev Disabil 2010;31(5):1039–1046. doi: 10.1016/j.ridd.2010.04.007.

Crawford JD, Medendorp WP, Marotta JJ. Spatial transformations for eye-hand coordination. J Neurophysiol 2004;92:10–19.

Creath R, Kiemel T, Horak F, et al. A unified view of quiet and perturbed stance: simultaneous co-existing excitable modes. Neurosci Lett 2005;377:75–80.

Crenna P. Spasticity and "spastic" gait in children with cerebral palsy. Neurosci Biobehav Rev 1998;22:571–578.

Crenna P, Inverno M. Objective detection of pathophysiological factors contributing to gait disturbance in supraspinal lesions. In: Fedrizzi E, Avanzini G, Crenna P, eds. Motor development in children. New York: Libbey, 1994:103–118.

Criscimagna-Hemminger SE, Donchin O, Gazzaniga MS, et al. Learned dynamics of reaching movements generalize from dominant to non-dominant arm. J Neurophysiol 2003;89:168–176.

Crisostomo EA, Duncan PW, Propst MA, et al. Evidence that amphetamine with physical therapy promotes recovery of motor function in stroke patients. Ann Neurol 1988;23:94–97.

Crossman ERFW, Goodeve PJ. Feedback control of hand-movement and Fitts' law. Q J Exp Psychol 1983;35A:251–278.

Crow JL, Harmeling-van der Wel BC. Hierarchical properties of the motor function sections of the Fugl-Meyer Assessment Scale for people after stroke: a retrospective study. Phys Ther 2008;88:1554–1567.

Crowe TK, Dietz JC, Richardson PK, et al. Interrater reliability of the pediatric clinical test of sensory interaction for balance. Phys Occup Ther Pediatr 1990;10:1–27.

Cruz TH, Dhaher YY. Impaired lower limb muscle synergies post-stroke. Conf Proc IEEE Eng Med Biol Soc 2009;2009:3956–3959.

Cumming TB, Marshall RS, Lazar RM. Stroke, cognitive deficits, and rehabilitation: still an incomplete picture. Int J Stroke 2013;8(1):38–45.

Cuoco A, Callahan DM, Sayers S, et al. Impact of muscle power and force on gait speed in disabled older men and women. J Gerontol A Biol Sci Med Sci 2004;59:1200–1206.

Cupps C, Plescia MG, Houser C. The Landau reaction: a clinical and electromyographic analysis. Dev Med Child Neurol 1976;18:41–53.

Cunha BP, Freitas S, Gomes G, de Freitas PB. Hand grip and load force coordination of the ipsilesional hand of chronic stroke individuals. J Mot Behav 2019;51:610–621.

Curuk E, Lee Y, Aruin AS. Individuals with stroke improve anticipatory postural adjustments after a single session of targeted exercises. Hum Mov Sci 2020;69:102559.

Curtis DJ. PhD thesis: head and trunk postural control in moderate to severe cerebral palsy: a segmental approach to analysis and treatment. Faculty of Health and Medical Sciences, University of Copenhagen, Copenhagen, Denmark, Submitted February 2014.

Curtis DJ, Hansen L, Luun M, et al. Measuring postural sway in sitting: a new segmental approach. J Mot Behav 2015;47:427–435.

Curtis DJ, Woollacott M, Bencke J, et al. The functional effect of segmental trunk and head control training in moderate-to-severe cerebral palsy: a randomized controlled trial. Dev Neurorehabil 2018;21(2):91–100.

Cusick A, Lannin NA, Lowe K. Adapting the Canadian Occupational Performance Measure for use in a paediatric clinical trial. Disabil Rehabil 2007;30(29):761–766.

Cusick A, McIntyre S, Novak I, Lannin N, Lowe K. A comparison of goal attainment scaling and the Canadian occupational performance measure for paediatric rehabilitation research. Pediatr Rehabil 2006;9(2):149–157.

Cusick B, Sussman MD. Short leg casts: their role in the management of cerebral palsy. Phys Occup Ther Pediatr 1982;2:93–110.

Cyarto EV, Myers AM, Tudor-Locke C. Pedometer accuracy in nursing home and community-dwelling older adults. Med Sci Sports Exerc 2004;36:205–209.

D

D'Avella A, Lacquaniti F. Control of reaching movements by muscle synergy combinations. Front Comput Neurosci 2013;7:1–7.

da Costa CSN, Pavao SL, Visicato LP, de Campos AC, Rocha N. Effects of sensory manipulations on the dynamical structure of center-ofpressure trajectories of children with cerebral palsy during sitting. Hum Mov Sci 2019;63:1–9.

Da Costa CS, Rocha NA. Sit-to-stand movement in children: a longitudinal study based on kinematics data. Hum Mov Sci 2013;32(4):836–846.

Daley K, Mayo N, Wood-Dauphinee S. Reliability of scores on the Stroke Rehabilitation Assessment of Movement (STREAM). Phys Ther 1999;79(1):8–19.

Dall PM, Kerr A. Frequency of the sit to stand task: an observational study of free-living adults. Appl Ergon 2010;41(1):58–61.

Damiano DL, Abel MF. Functional outcomes of strength training in spastic cerebral palsy. Arch Phys Med Rehabil 1998;79:119–125.

Damiano DL, Arnold AS, Steele KM, et al. Can strength training predictably improve gait kinematics? a pilot study on the effects of hip and knee extensor strengthening on lower-extremity alignment in cerebral palsy. Phys Ther 2010;90:269–279.

Damiano DL, Prosser LA, Curatalo LA, et al. Muscle plasticity and ankle control after repetitive use of a functional electrical stimulation device for foot drop in cerebral palsy. Neurorehabil Neural Repair 2013;27:200–207.

Damiano DL, Quinlivan JM, Owen BF, et al. What does the Ashworth scale really measure and are instrumented measures more valid and precise? Dev Med Child Neurol 2002;44:112–118.

Danilov YP, Tyler ME, Skinner KL, et al. Efficacy of electrotactile vestibular substitution in patients with bilateral vestibular and central balance loss. Conf Proc IEEE Eng Med Biol Soc 2006;(Suppl):6605–6609.

Dannenbaum R, Dykes R. Sensory loss in the hand after sensory stroke: therapeutic rationale. Arch Phys Med Rehabil 1988;69:833–839.

Dargent-Molina P, Favier F, Grandjean H. Fall-related factors and risk of hip fracture: the EPIDOS prospective study. Lancet 1996;348:145–149.

Darrah J, Loomis J, Manns P, et al. Role of conceptual models in a physical therapy curriculum: application of an integrated model of theory, research, and clinical practice. Physiother Theory Pract 2006;22:239–250.

Darsaklis V, Snider LM, Majnemer A, Mazer B. Predictive validity of Prechtl's method on the qualitative assessment of general movements: a systematic review of the evidence. Dev Med Child Neurol 2011;53(10):896–906.

Das P, McCollum G. Invariant structure in locomotion. Neuroscience 1988;25:1023–1034.

Davies P. Aging and Alzheimer's disease: new light on old problems. Presented at the Annual Meeting of the Neuroscience Society, New Orleans, 1987.Davies PL, Soon PL, Young M, et al. Validity and reliability of the school function assessment in elementary school students with disabilities. Phys Occup Ther Pediatr 2004;24(3):23–43.

Dawson AM, Buxbaum LJ, Duff SV. The impact of left hemisphere stroke on force control with familiar and novel objects: neuroanatomic substrates and relationship to apraxia. Brain Res 2010;1317:124–136.

Day BL, Steiger MJ, Thompson PD, et al. Effect of vision and stance width on human body motion when standing: implications for afferent control of lateral sway. J Physiol 1993;469:479–499.

Dayanidhi S, Hedberg Å, Valero-Cuevas FJ, et al. Developmental improvements in dynamic control of fingertip forces last throughout childhood and into adolescence. J Neurophysiol 2013;110:1583–1592.

de Freitas PB, Freitas SMSF, Reschechtko S, Corson T, Lewis MM, Huang X, Latash ML. Synergic control of action in levodopanaive Parkinson's disease patients: I. Multi-finger interaction and coordination. Exp Brain Res 2020;238:229–245.

De Haan B, Karnath H-O, Driver J. Mechanisms and anatomy of unilateral extinction after brain injury. Neuropsychologia 2012;50:1045–1053.

de Haart M, Geurts AC, Huidekoper SC, et al. Recovery of standing balance in postacute stroke patients: a rehabilitation cohort study. Arch Phys Med Rehabil 2004;85:886–895.

de Kam D, Roelofs JMB, Geurts ACH, Weerdesteyn V. Body configuration at first stepping-foot contact predicts backward balance recovery capacity in people with chronic stroke. PLoS One 2018;13(2):e0192961.

De Leon RD, Hodgson JA, Roy RR, et al. Locomotor capacity attributable to step training versus spontaneous recovery after spinalization in adult cats. J Neurophysiol 1998;79:1329–1340.

De Souza LH, Hewer RL, Miller S. Assessment of recovery of arm control in hemiplegic stroke patients. 1. Arm function tests. Int Rehabil Med 1980;2:3–9.

De Quervain IA, Simon SR, Leurgans S, et al. Gait pattern in the early recovery period after stroke. J Bone Joint Surg Am 1996;78:1506–1514.

De Tullio LM, Wolfe DM, Strohl AB. Clinical examination of the hand. In: Skirven TM, Osterman AL, Fedorczyk JM, Amadio PC, Feldscher SB, Shin EK, eds. Rehabilitation of the hand. St. Louis: Mosby, 2021:46–61.

De Vries JIP, Visser GHA, Prechtl HFR. The emergence of fetal behavior: 1. Qualitative aspects. Early Hum Dev 1982;7:301–322.

De Weerdt W, Harrison MA. Measuring recovery of arm-hand function in stroke patients: a comparison of the Brunnstrom-Fugl-Meyer test and the Action Research Arm test. Physiother Canada 1985;37:65–70.

Dean CM, Richards CL, Malouin F. Task-related circuit training improves performance of locomotor tasks in chronic stroke: a randomized, controlled pilot trial. Arch Phys Med Rehabil 2000;81:409–417.

Dean CM, Richards CL, Malouin F. Walking speed over 10 meters overestimates locomotor capacity after stroke. Clin Rehabil 2001;15:415–421.

Debaere F, Swinnen SP, Beatse E, et al. Brain areas involved in interlimb coordination: a distributed network. Neuroimage 2001;14:947–958.

DeBolt LS, McCubbin JA. The effects of home-based resistance exercise on balance, power and mobility in adult with multiple sclerosis. Arch Phys Med Rehabil 2004;85:290–297.

Debreceni-Nagy A, Horváth J, Nagy S, Bajusz-Leny Á, Jenei Z. Feasibility of six-point goal attainment scale among subacute and chronic stroke patients. Int J Rehabil Res 2019 ;42(4):365–370. doi: 10.1097/MRR.0000000000000372.

Decety J, Sjoholm H, Ryding E, et al. The cerebellum participates in mental activity: tomographic measurements of regional cerebral blood flow. Brain Res 1990;535:313–317.

Decker SL. Tactile measures in the structure of intelligence. Can J Exp Psychol 2010;64(1):53–59.

DeFabio R, Badke MB. Relationship of sensory organization to balance function in patients with hemiplegia. Phys Ther 1990;70:542–560.

Dehaene S, Changeux J-P. Neural mechanisms for access to consciousness. In: Gazzaniga MS, ed. The cognitive neurosciences III. Cambridge, MA: MIT Press, 2004:1145–1157.

DeJersey MC. Report on a sensory programme for patients with sensory deficits. Aust J Physiother 1979;25:165–170.

DeKleijn A. Experimental physiology of the labyrinth. J Laryngol Otol 1923;38:646–663.

Del Rey P, Whitehurst M, Wood J. Effects of experience and contextual interference on learning and transfer. Percept Mot Skills 1983;56:581–582.

Delabastita T, Bogaerts S, Vanwanseele B. Age-related changes in achilles tendon stiffness and impact on functional activities: a systematic review and meta-analysis. J Aging Phys Act 2018:1–12.

Delacour J. Neurobiology of consciousness: an overview. Behav Brain Res 1997;85:127–141.

Deliagina TG, Zelenin PV, Orlovsky GN. Physiological and circuit mechanisms of postural control. Curr Opin Neurobiol 2012;22:646–652.

Dellen TV, Kalverboer AF. Single movement control and information processing, a developmental study. Behav Brain Res 1984;12:237–238.

Dellon AL, Curtis RM, Edgerton MT. Reeducation of sensation in the hand following nerve injury. Plast Reconstr Surg 1974;53:297–305.

Dellon A, Kallman C. Evaluation of functional sensation in the hand. J Hand Surg 1983;8:865–870.

DeLong M. The basal ganglia. In: Kandel ER, Schwartz JH, Jessell TM, eds. Principles of neural science, 4th ed. New York: Elsevier, 2000: 853–867.

Delval A, Tard C, Defebvre L. Why we should study gait initiation in Parkinson's disease. Neurophysiol Clin 2014;44:69–76.

Demartino AM, Rodrigues LC, Gomes RP, Michaelsen SM. Hand function and type of grasp used by chronic stroke individuals in actual environment. Top Stroke Rehabil 2019;26:247–254.

DeMatteo C, Law M, Russell D, et al. Quality of upper extremity skill test. Ontario, Canada: Neurodevelopmental Clinical Research Unit, 1992.

Demers L, Ska B, Desrosiers J, Alix C, Wolfson A. Development of a conceptual framework for the assessment of geriatric rehabilitation outcomes. Arch Gerontol Geriatr 2004;38:221–237.

Den Otter AR, Geurts ACH, Mulder T, et al. Gait recovery is not associated with changes in the temporal patterning of muscle activity during treadmill walking in patients with post stroke hemiparesis. Clin Neurophysiol 2006;117:4–15.

Dennis A, Dawes H, Elsworth C. Fast walking under cognitive-motor interference conditions in chronic stroke. Brain Res 2009;1287:104–110.

Denommé LT, Mandalfino P, Cinelli ME. Strategies used by individuals with multiple sclerosis and with mild disability to maintain dynamic stability during a steering task. Exp Brain Res 2014;232:1811–1822.

Deppe W, Thuemmler K, Fleischer J, et al. Modified constraint-induced movement therapy versus intensive bimanual training for children with hemiplegia—a randomized controlled trial. Clin Rehabil 2013;27(10):909–920.

Desanghere L, Marotta JJ. The specificity of learned associations in visuomotor and perceptual processing. Exp Brain Res 2008;187:595–601.

Deshpande N, Metter E, Lauretani F, et al. Activity restriction induced by fear of falling and objective and subjective measures of physical function: a prospective cohort study. J Am Geriatr Soc 2008;56:615–620.

Desrosiers J, Bourbonnais D, Corriveau H, et al. Effectiveness of unilateral and symmetrical bilateral task training for arm during the subacute phase after stroke: a randomized controlled trial. Clin Rehabil 2005;19:581–593.

Desrosiers J, Bravo G, Gerbert R, et al. Validation of the box and block test as a measure of dexterity of elderly: reliability, validity and norms study. Arch Phys Med Rehabil 1994;75:751–755.

Desrosiers J, Noreau L, Rochette A, et al. Predictors of handicap situations following post-stroke rehabilitation. Disabil Rehabil 2002,24.774–785.

Desrosiers J, Rochette A, Hebert R, et al. The Minnesota Manual Dexterity Test: reliability, validity and reference values studies with healthy elderly people. Can J Occup Ther 1997;64:270–276.

Deuschl G, Bain P, Brin M. Consensus statement of the Movement Disorder Society on tremor. Mov Disord 1998;13:2–23.

DeVellis RF. Scale development: theory and applications, 4th ed. Los Angeles, US: SAGE, 2017.

Devita P, Hortobagyi T. Age causes a redistribution of joint torques and powers during gait. J Appl Physiol 2000;88:1804–1811.

Dewald JP, Beer RF. Abnormal joint torque patterns in the paretic upper limb of subjects with hemiparesis. Muscle Nerve 2001;24:273–283.

Dewald JP, Beer RF, Given JD, et al. Reorganization of flexion reflexes in the upper extremity of hemiparetic subjects. Muscle Nerve 1999;22:1209–1221.

Dibble LE, Foreman KB, Addison O, et al. Exercise and medication effects on persons with Parkinson disease across the domains of disability: a randomized clinical trial. J Neuro Phys Ther 2015;39:85–92.

Dibble LE, Hale TF, Marcus RL, et al. High intensity resistance training amplifies muscle hypertrophy and functional gains I npersonw with Parkinsons disease. Mov Disord 2006;21:1444–1452.

Dibble LE, Lange M. Predicting falls in individuals with Parkinson disease: a reconsideration of clinical balance measures. J Neurol Phys Ther 2006;30:60–67.

Dichgans J, Fetter M. Compartmentalized cerebellar functions upon the stabilization of body posture. Rev Neurol (Paris) 1993;149:654–664.

Dicken DC, Rose DJ. Sensory organization abilities during upright stance in late onset Alzheimer's-type dementia. Exp Aging Res 2004;30:373–390.

Dickstein R, Peterka RJ, Horak FB. Effects of light fingertip touch on postural responses in subjects with diabetic neuropathy. J Neurol Neurosurg Psychiatry 2003;74:620–626.

Dickstein R, Shefi S, Marcovitz E, et al. Anticipatory postural adjustments in selected trunk muscles in post stroke hemiparetic patients. Arch Phys Med Rehabil 2004;85:261–267.

Dickstein R, Shupert CL, Horak FB. Fingertip touch improves postural stability in patients with peripheral neuropathy. Gait Posture 2001;14:238–247.

Diedrichsen J, Verstynen T, Lehman S, et al. Cerebellar involvement in anticipating the consequences of self-produced actions during bimanual movements. J Neurophysiol 2005;93:801–812.

Diener HC, Dichgans J, Bacher M, et al. Quantification of postural sway in normals and patients with cerebellar diseases. Electroencephalogr Clin Neurophysiol 1984a;57:134–142.

Diener HC, Dichgans J, Bruzek W, et al. Stabilization of human posture during induced oscillations of the body. Exp Brain Res 1982;45:126–132.

Diener HC, Dichgans J, Guschlbauer B, et al. The significance of proprioception on postural stabilization as assessed by ischemia. Brain Res 1984b;296:103–109.

Dierick F, Lefebvre C, van den Hecke A, et al. Development of displacement of centre of mass during independent walking in children. Dev Med Child Neurol 2004;46:533–539.

Dietz V. Locomotor recovery after spinal cord injury. Trends Neurosci 1997;20:346–347.

Dietz V. Quadrupedal coordination of bipedal gait: implications for movement disorders. J Neurol 2011;258:1406–1412.

Dietz V, Fouad K, Bastiaanse CM. Neuronal coordination of arm and leg movements during human locomotion. Eur J Neurosci 2001;14(11):1906–1914.

Dietz V, Gollhofer A, Kleiber M, et al. Regulation of bipedal stance: dependency on "load" receptors. Exp Brain Res 1992;89(1):229–231.

Dietz V, Ketelsen UP, Berger W, et al. Motor unit involvement in spastic paresis: relationship between leg muscle activation and histochemistry. J Neurol Sci 1986;75:89–103.

Dietz V, Schmidtbleicher D, Noth J. Neuronal mechanisms of human locomotion. J Neurophysiol 1979;42:1212–1222.

Dietz V, Schubert M, Discher M, et al. Influence of visuoproprioceptive mismatch on postural adjustments. Gait Posture 1994;2:147–155.

Dietz V, Trippel M, Horstmann GA. Significance of proprioceptive and vestibulo-spinal reflexes in the control of stance and gait. In: Patla AE, ed. Adaptability of human gait. Amsterdam, The Netherlands: Elsevier, 1991:37–52.

DiFabio R, Badke MB. Relationship of sensory organization to balance function in patients with hemiplegia. Phys Ther 1990;70:543–552.

DiFabio RP, Badke MB. Stance duration under sensory conflict conditions in patients with hemiplegia. Arch Phys Med Rehabil 1991;72:292–295.

DiFabio FP, Badke MB, Duncan PW. Adapting human postural reflexes following a localized cerebrovascular lesion: analysis of bilateral long latency responses. Brain Res 1986;363:257–264.

Dimitrova D, Horak FB, Nutt JG. Postural muscle responses to multidirectional translations in patients with Parkinson's disease. J Neurophysiol 2004a;91:489–501.

Dimitrova D, Nutt J, Horak FB. Abnormal force patterns for multidirectional postural responses in patients with Parkinson's disease. Exp Brain Res 2004b;156:183–195.

Ding L, Yang F. Muscle weakness is related to slip-initiated falls among community-dwelling older adults. J Biomech 2016;49(2):238–243.

Dion L, Malouin F, McFadyen B, et al. Assessing mobility and locomotor coordination after stroke with the rise-to-walk task. Neurorehabil Neural Repair 2003;17:83–92.

Dispa D, Thonnard JL, Bleyenheuft Y. Impaired predictive and reactive control of precision grip in chronic stroke patients. Int J Rehabil Res 2014;37:130–137.

Divani AA, Vazquez G, Barrett AM, et al. Risk factors associated with injury attributable to falling among elderly population with history of stroke. Stroke 2009;40:3286–3292.

Dixon PC, Smith T, Taylor MJD, Jacobs JV, Dennerlein JT, Schiffman JM. Effect of walking surface, late-cueing, physiological characteristics of aging, and gait parameters on turn style preference in healthy, older adults. Hum Mov Sci 2019;66:504–510.

Dobkin BH. Neurologic rehabilitation. Philadelphia, PA: FA Davis, 1996.

Dobkin BH, Duncan PW. Should body weight-supported treadmill training and robotic-assistive steppers for locomotor training trot back to the starting gate? Neurorehabil Neural Repair 2012;26:308–317.

Dobrossy MD, Dunnett SB. The influence of environment and experience on neural grafts. Nat Rev Neuroscience 2001;2:871–879.

Dobson F, Morris ME, Baker R, et al. Gait classification in children with cerebral palsy: a systematic review. Gait Posture 2007;25:140–152.

Dodd KJ, Taylor NF, Damiano DL. A systematic review of the effectiveness of strength-training programs for people with cerebral palsy. Arch Phys Med Rehabil 2002;83:1157–1164.

Dodwell PC, Muir D, Difranco D. Responses of infants to visual presented objects. Science 1976;194:209–211.

Domagalska-Szopa M, Szopa A. Postural orientation and standing postural alignment in ambulant children with bilateral cerebral palsy. Clin Biomech (Bristol, Avon) 2017;49:22–27.

Dombovy ML, Duncan P, Badke MB. Stroke rehabilitation: the recovery of motor control. Chicago, IL: Year Book, 1987.

Domellof E, Backstrom A, Johansson AM, Ronnqvist L, von Hofsten C, Rosander K. Kinematic characteristics of second-order motor planning and performance in 6- and 10-year-old children and adults: effects of age and task constraints. Dev Psychobiol 2020;62(2):250–265.

Dominguez-Zamora FJ, Lajoie K, Miller AB, Marigold DS. Age-related changes in gaze sampling strategies during obstacle navigation. Gait Posture 2020;76:252–258.

Dominici N, Ivanenko YP, Cappellini G, Zampagni ML, Lacquaniti F. Kinematic strategies in newly walking toddlers stepping over different support surfaces. J Neurophysiol 2010;103:1673–1684.

Donica DK. Handwriting Without Tears®: general education effectiveness through a consultative approach. Am J Occup Ther 2015;69(6):6906180050p1-8. doi: 10.5014/ajot.2015.018366.

Donker SF, Roerdink M, Greven AJ, et al. Regularity of center-of-pressure trajectories depends on the amount of attention invested in postural control. Exp Brain Res 2007;181:1–11.

Donoghue JP. Plasticity of adult sensorimotor representations. Curr Opin Neurobiol 1995;5:749–754.

Donoghue D, Stokes EK. How much change is true change? The minimum detectable change of the Berg Balance Scale in elderly people. J Rehabil Med 2009;41:343–346.

dos Santos Soares LM, Rozane JMSG, Carvalho RP. Motor performance of children with cerebral palsy in anterior reach. Clin Biomech (Bristol, Avon) 2019;68:158–162.

Doucet BM, Griffin L. High-versus low-frequency stimulation effects on fine motor control in chronic hemiplegia: a pilot study. Top Stroke Rehabil 2013;20:299–307.

Doucet BM, Mettler JA. Effects of a dynamic progressive orthotic intervention for chronic hemiplegia: a case series. J Hand Ther 2013;26(2):139–146.

Doumas M, Smolders C, Krampe RT. Task prioritization in aging: effects of sensory information on concurrent posture and memory performance. Exp Brain Res 2008;187:275–281.

Dowling JE. The retina: an approachable part of the brain. Cambridge, MA: Belknap, 1987.

Doya K. What are the computations of the cerebellum, the basal ganglia and the cerebral cortex? Neural Netw 1999;12:961–974.

Doya K. Complementary roles of basal ganglia and cerebellum in learning and motor control. Curr Opin Neurobiol 2000;10:732–739.

Dozza M, Chiari L, Horak FB. Audio-biofeedback improves balance in patients with bilateral vestibular loss. Arch Phys Med Rehabil 2005;86(7):1401–1403.

Dragert K, Zehr EP. High-intensity unilateral dorsiflexor resistance training results in bilateral neuromuscular plasticity after stroke. Exp Brain Res 2013;225:93–104.

Drillis R. The influence of aging on the kinematics of gait: the geriatric amputee. Washington, DC: National Academy of Science, National Research Council, 1961. Publication 919.

Dromerick AW, Lang CE, Birkenmeier RL, et al. Very early constraint-induced movement during stroke rehabilitation. Neurology 2009;73:195–201.

Druz˙bicki M, Rusek W, Snela S, et al. Functional effects of robotic-assisted locomotor treadmill therapy in children with cerebral palsy. J Rehabil Med 2013;45(4):358–363.

Dubost V, Beauchet O, Manckoundia P, et al. Decreased trunk angular displacement during sitting down: an early feature of aging. Phys Ther 2005;85:404–412.

Duff S, Goyen TA. Reliability and validity of the Evaluation Tool of Children's Handwriting-Cursive (ETCH-C) using the general scoring criteria. Am J Occup Ther 2010;64(1):37–46.

Duff SV. Prehension. In: Cech D, Martin S, eds. Functional movement development across the life span, 3rd ed. Philadelphia, PA: WB Saunders, 2012.

Duff SV, Gordon AM. Learning of grasp control in children with hemiparetic cerebral palsy. Dev Med Child Neurol 2003;45:746–757.

Duff SV, He J, Nelsen MA, et al. Interrater reliability of the Wolf Motor Function Test-Functional Ability Scale: why it matters. Neurorehabil Neural Repair 2015;29:436–443. pii: 1545968314553030.

Duff SV, Heathcock J, Prosser L. Efficacy of activity-based interventions to expand motor function & mobility in infants & toddlers. 74th Annual Meeting of the AACPDM. Sept. 2020.Duff SV, Sargent B, Kutch JJ, Berggren J, Leiby BE, Fetters L. Using contingent reinforcement to augment muscle activation after perinatal brachial plexus injury: a pilot study. Phys Occup Ther Pediatr 2017;37(5):555–565. doi: 10.1080/01942638.2017.1290733.

Duffy CJ, Wurtz RH. Medial superior temporal area neurons respond to speed patterns in optic flow. J Neurosci 1997;17:2839–2851.

Duhamel JR, Colby CL, Goldberg ME. The updating of the representation of visual space in parietal cortex by intended eye movements. Science 1992a;255:90–92.

Duhamel JR, Goldberg ME, Fitzgibbon EJ, et al. Saccadic dysmetria in a patient with a right frontoparietal lesion. Brain 1992b;115:1387–1402.

Dumas HM, Fragala Pinkham MA, Haley SM, et al. Computer adaptive test performance in children with and without disabilities: prospective field study of the PEDI-CAT. Disabil Rehabil 2012;34(5):393–401.

Duncan J, Bundesen C, Olson A, et al. Systematic analysis of deficits in visual attention. J Exp Psychol Gen 1999;128:450–478.

Duncan PW, Chandler J, Studenski S, et al. How do physiological components of balance affect mobility in elderly men? Arch Phys Med Rehabil 1993;74:1343–1349.

Duncan PW, Lai SM, Tyler D, et al. Evaluation of proxy responses to the stroke impact study. Stroke 2002;33:2593–2599.

Duncan PW, Propst M, Nelson SG. Reliability of the Fugl-Meyer assessment of sensorimotor recovery following cerebrovascular accident. Phys Ther 1983;63:1606–1610.

Duncan P, Richards L, Wallace D, et al. A randomized, controlled pilot study of a home-based exercise program for individuals with mild and moderate stroke. Stroke 1998;29:2055–2060.

Duncan P, Studenski S, Chandler J, et al. Functional reach: a new clinical measure of balance. J Gerontol 1990;45:M192–M197.

Duncan P, Studenski S, Richards L, et al. Randomized clinical trial of therapeutic exercise in subacute stroke. Stroke 2003;34:2173–2180.

Duncan PW, Sullivan KJ, Behrman AL, et al.; LEAPS Investigative Team. Body-weight-supported treadmill rehabilitation after stroke. N Engl J Med 2011;364(21):2026–2036.

Dunn W, Brown C, McGuigan A. The ecology of human performance: a framework for considering the effect of contex. Am J Occup Ther 1994;48:595–607.

Duong TT, Englander J, Wright J, et al. Relationship between strength, balance and swallowing deficits and outcome after traumatic brain injury: a multicenter analysis. Arch Phys Med Rehabil 2004;85:1291–1297.

Dushanova J, Donoghue J. Neurons in primary motor cortex engaged during action observation. Eur J Neurosci 2010;31: 386–398.

Dyer JO, Maupas E, de Andrade Melo S, et al. Changes in activation timing of knee and ankle extensors during gait are related to changes in heteronymous spinal pathways after stroke. J Neuroeng Rehabil 2014;11:148–165.

E

Earhart GM, Bastian AJ. Selection and coordination of human locomotor forms following cerebellar damage. J Neurophysiol 2001;85:759–769.

Ebersbach G, Dimitrijevic MR, Poewe W. Influence of concurrent tasks on gait: a dual-task approach. Percept Mot Skills 1995;81:107–113.

Edwards AS. Body sway and vision. J Exp Psychol 1946;36:526–535.

Edwards JM, Elliott D, Lee TD. Contextual interference effects during skill acquisition and transfer in Down's syndrome adolescents. Adapt Phys Activ Q 1986;3:250–258.

Eichhorn J, Orner J, Rickard K, et al. Aging effects on dual-task methodology using walking and verbal reaction time. Issues Aging 1998;21:8–12.

Eidenmüller S, Randerath J, Goldenberg G, et al. The impact of unilateral brain damage on anticipatory grip force scaling when lifting everyday objects. Neuropsychologia 2014;61:222–234.

Einkauf DK, Gohdes ML, Jensen GM, et al. Changes in spinal mobility with increasing age in women. Phys Ther 1987;67:370–375.

Einspieler C, Prechtl HFR. Prechtl's assessment of general movements: a diagnostic tool of the functional assessment of the young nervous system. Ment Retard Dev Disabil Res Rev 2005;11:61–67.

Elbert T, Pantev C, Wienbruch C, Rockstroh B, Taub E. Increased cortical representation of the fingers of the left hand in string players. Science 1995;270:305–307.

Elble RJ, Cousins R, Leffler K, et al. Gait initiation by patients with lower-half parkinsonism. Brain 1996;119:1705–1706.

Elble RJ, Leffler K. Pushing and pulling with the upper extremities while standing: the effects of mild Alzheimer's dementia and Parkinson's disease. Mov Disord 2000;15:255–268.

El-Gohary M, McNames J. Human joint angle estimation with inertial sensors and validation with A Robot Arm. IEEE Trans Biomed Eng vol 62(7):1759–1767. doi: 10.1109/TBME.2015.2403368.

Eliasson A-C, Krumlinde-Sundholm L, Rösblad B, et al. The Manual Ability Classification System (MACS) for children with cerebral palsy: scale development and evidence of validity and reliability. Dev Med Child Neurol 2006;48:549–554.

Eliasson A-C, Nordstrand L, Ek L, Wang C. The effectiveness of Baby-CIMT in infants younger than 12 months with clinical signs of unilateral-cerebral palsy; an explorative study with randomized design. Res Dev Disabil 2018;72:191–201. doi: 10.1016/j.ridd.2017.11.006.

Eliasson A-C, Ullenhag A, Wahlström U, Krumlinde-Sundholm L.

Mini-MACS: development of the Manual Ability Classification System for children younger than 4 years of age with signs of cerebral palsy. Dev Med Child Neurol 2017;59(1):72–78. doi: 10.1111/dmcn.13162.

Elvrum A-G, Andersen GL, Himmelmann K, et al. Bimanual Fine Motor Function (BFMF) classification in children with cerebral palsy: aspects of construct and content validity. Phys Occup Ther Pediatr 2016;36(1):1–16. doi: 10.3109/01942638.2014.975314.

Elvrum A-G, Zethraeus BM, Vik T, Krumlinde-Sundholm L. Development and validation of the Both Hands Assessment for children with bilateral cerebral palsy. Phys Occup Ther Pediatr 2018;38(2):113–126. doi: 10.1080/01942638.2017.1318431

Elsworth-Edelsten C, Bonnefoy-Mazure A, Laidet M, et al. Upper limb movement analysis during gait in multiple sclerosis patients. Hum Mov Sci 2017;54:248–252.

Emos MC, Rosner J. Neuroanatomy, upper motor nerve signs. Florida: Treasure Island; 2020.

Eng JJ, Winter DA. Kinetic analysis of the lower limbs during walking: what information can be gained from a three-dimensional model? J Biomech 1995;28:753–758.

Eng JJ, Winter DA, Patla AE. Intralimb dynamics simplify reactive control strategies during locomotion. J Biomech 1997;30:581–588.

Eng JJ, Winter DA, Patla AE. Strategies for recovery from a trip in early and late swing during human walking. Exp Brain Res 1994;102:339–349.

Eng K, Siekierka E, Pyk P, et al. Interactive visuo-motor therapy system for stroke rehabilitation. Med Biol Eng Comput 2007;45:901–907.

Engel C, Lillie K, Zurawski S, Travers BG. Curriculum-based handwriting programs: a systematic review with effect sizes. Am J Occup Ther 2018,72(3).7203205010p1-7203205010p8. doi: 10.5014/ajot.2018.027110.

Enoka R. Neuromechanics of human movement, 3rd ed. Champaign, IL: Human Kinetics, 2002.

Era P, Schroll M, Ytting H, et al. Postural balance and its sensory-motor correlates in 75-year-old men and women: a cross-national comparative study. J Gerontol Med Sci 1996;51A:53–63.

Erhardt RP. Developmental hand dysfunction: theory, assessment and treatment. Tucson, AZ: Therapy Skill Builders, 1982.

Evarts EV. Relation of pyramidal tract activity to force exerted during voluntary movement. J Neurophysiol 1968;31:14–27.

Exner CE, Henderson A. Cognition and motor skill. In: Henderson A, Pehoski C, eds. Hand function in the child: foundations for remediation. Philadelphia, PA: Mosby, 1995.

Eyring EJ, Murray WR. The effect of joint position on the pressure of intra-articular effusion. J Bone Joint Surg Am 1964;46:1235–1241.

F

Facchin P, Rosa-Rizzotto M, Visonà Dalla Pozza L, et al.; GIPCI Study Group. Multisite trial comparing the efficacy of constraint-induced movement therapy with that of bimanual intensive training in children with hemiplegic cerebral palsy: postintervention results. Am J Phys Med Rehabil 2011;90:539–553.

Faddy K, McCluskey A, Lannin NA. Interrater reliability of a new handwriting assessment battery for adults. Am J Occup Ther 2008;62(5):595–599.

Fahn S. An open trial of high-dosage antioxidants in early Parkinson's disease. Am J Clin Nutr 1991;53(1 Suppl):380S–382S.

Fahn S. The freezing phenomenon in parkinsonism. Adv Neurol 1995;67:53–63.

Fahn S, Jankovic J, Hallett M. Principles and practice of movement disorders, 2nd ed. Philadelphia: Elsevier; 2011.

Fahn S, Marsden CD, Caine DB. Classification and investigation of dystonia. In: Marsden CD, Fahn S, eds. Movement disorders 2. London, UK: Butterworth, 1987.

Fait P, McFadyen BJ, Swaine B, Cantin JF. Alterations to locomotor navigation in complex environment at 7 and 30 days following a concussion in an elite athlete. Brain Inj 2009;23:362–369.

Falduto L, Baron A. Age-related effects of practice and task complexity on card sorting. J Gerontol 1986;41:659–661.

Fan J, McCandliss BD, Sommer T, et al. Testing the efficiency and independence of attentional networks. J Cogn Neurosci 2002;14;340–347.

Farag I, Sherrington C, Kamper SJ, Ferreira M, Moseley AM. Lord SR, Cameron ID. Measures of physical functioning after hip fracture: construct validity and responsiveness of performance-based and self-reported measures. Age Ageing 2012;41:659–661.

Faria CD, Teixeira-Salmela LF, Nadeau S. Effects of the direction of turning on the timed up & go test with stroke subjects. Top Stroke Rehabil 2009;16:196–206.

Farin E, Fleitz A, Frey C. Psychometric properties of an International Classification of Functioning, Disability and Health (ICF)-oriented, adaptive questionnaire for the assessment of mobility, self-care and domestic life. J Rehabil Med 2007;39:537–546.

Farley CT, Ferris DP. Biomechanics of walking and running: center of mass movements to muscle action. Exerc Sport Sci Rev 1998;26:253–285.

Farley BG, Koshland GF. Training BIG to move faster: the application of the speed-amplitude relation as a rehabilitation strategy for people with Parkinson's disease. Exp Brain Res 2005;167:462–467.

Farrell K, Johnson A, Duncan H, et al. The intertester and intratester reliability of hand volumetrics. J Hand Ther 2003;16(4):292–299.

Fasoli SE, Adans-Dester CP. A paradigm shift: rehabilitation robotics, cognitive skills training, and function after stroke. Front Neurol 2019;10:1088. doi: 10.3389/fneur.2019.01088.

Fasoli SE, Trombly CA, Tickle-Degnen L, et al. Effect of instructions on functional reach in persons with and without cerebrovascular accident. Am J Occup Ther 2002;56:380–390.

Faulkner KA, Redfern MS, Cauley JA, et al. Multitasking: association between poorer performance and a history of recurrent falls. J Am Geriatr Soc 2007;55:570–576.

Favilla M. Reaching movements in children: accuracy and reaction time development. Exp Brain Res 2005;21:1–4.

Feder KP, Majnemer A. Children's handwriting evaluation tools and their psychometric properties. Phys Occup Ther Pediatr. 2003;23:65–84.

Feeney DM. Pharmacological modulation of recovery after brain injury: a reconsideration of diaschisis. J Neurol Rehabil 1991;5:113–128.

Feeney DM, Baron JC. Diaschisis. Stroke 1986;17:817–830.

Feeney DM, Gonzalez A, Law WA. Amphetamine restores locomotor function after motor cortex injury in the rat. Proc West Pharmacol Soc 1981;24:15–17.

Feeney DM, Gonzalez A, Law WA. Amphetamine haloperidol and experience interact to affect the rate of recovery after motor cortex injury. Science 1982;217:855–857.

Feeney DM, Sutton RL. Pharmacology for recovery of function after brain injury. Crit Rev Neurobiol 1987;3:135–185.

Feigin L, Sharon B, Czaczkes B, et al. Sitting equilibrium 2 weeks after stroke can predict walking ability after 6 months. Gerontology 1996;42:348–353.

Feldman AG. Change in the length of the muscle as a consequence of a shift in equilibrium in the muscle-load system. Biofizika 1974;19:534–538.

Feldman AB, Haley SM, Coryell J. Concurrent and construct validity of the Pediatric Evaluation of Disability Inventory. Phys Ther 1990;70:602–610.

Fellows SJ, Noth J, Schwarz M. Precision grip and Parkinson's disease. Brain 1998;121:1171–1184.

Fentress JC. Development of grooming in mice with amputated forelimbs. Science 1973;179:704.

Ferber S, Karnath HO. How to assess spatial neglect—line bisection or cancellation tasks? J Clin Exp Neuropsychol 2001;23:599–607.

Ferber-Viart C, Ionescu E, Morlet T, et al. Balance in healthy individuals assessed with Equitest: maturation and normative data for children and young adults. Int J Pediatr Otorhinolaryngol 2007;71:1041–1046.

Ferguson OW, Polskaia N, Tokuno CD. The effects of foot cooling on postural muscle responses to an unexpected loss of balance. Hum Mov Sci 2017;54:240–247.

Fernie GR, Gryfe CI, Holliday PJ, et al. The relationship of postural sway in standing: the incidence of falls in geriatric subjects. Age Ageing 1982;11:11–16.

Ferre CL, Brandão MB, Hung YC, et al. Feasibility of caregiver-directed home-based hand-arm bimanual intensive training: a brief report. Dev Neurorehabil. 2015;18(1):69–74.

Ferris DP, Louie M, Farley CT. Running in the real world: adjusting leg stiffness for different surfaces. Proc Biol Sci 1998;265:989–994.

Fess EE. Assessment of the upper extremity: instrumentation criteria. Occup Ther Pract 1990;1:1–11.

Fess EE, Gettle K, Phillips C, et al. Hand and upper extremity splinting principles and methods, 3rd ed. St. Louis, MO: Elsevier/Mosby, 2005.

Fetter M. Vestibular system disorders. In: Herdman S, ed. Vestibular rehabilitation, 2nd ed. Philadelphia, PA: FA Davis, 2000:91–102.

Fiatarone MA, Marks EC, Ryan ND, et al. High-intensity strength training in nonagenarians: effects on skeletal muscle. JAMA 1990;263:3029–3034.

Fiatarone MA, O'Neill EF, Ryan ND, et al. Exercise training and nutritional supplementation for physical frailty in very elderly people. N Engl J Med 1994;330:1769–1775.

Fickey SN, Browne MG, Franz JR. Biomechanical effects of augmented ankle power output during human walking. J Exp Biol 2018;221(Pt 22).

Fiez, JA, Petersen SE, Cheney, MK, et al. Impaired non-motor learning and error detection associated with cerebellar damage. Brain 1992;115:155–178.

Finlayson ML, Peterson EW, Cho CC. Risk factors for falling among people aged 45 to 90 years with multiple sclerosis. Arch Phys Med Rehabil 2006;87:1274–1279.

Finley FR, Cody KA. Locomotive characteristics of urban pedestrians. Arch Phys Med Rehabil 1970;51:423–426.

Finley FR, Cody KA, Finizie RV. Locomotion patterns in elderly women. Arch Phys Med Rehabil 1969;50:140–146.

Finley JM, Perreault EJ, Dhaher YY. Stretch reflex coupling between the hip and knee: implications for impaired gait following stroke. Exp Brain Res 2008;188(4):529–540.

Fishkind M, Haley SM. Independent sitting development and the emergence of associated motor components. Phys Ther 1986;66:1509–1514.

Fishbein P, Hutzler Y, Ratmansky M, Treger I, Dunsky A. A preliminary study of dual-task training using virtual reality: influence on walking and balance in chronic poststroke survivors. J Stroke Cerebrovasc Dis 2019;28:1–8.

Fisk JD, Goodale MA. The organization of eye and limb movements during unrestricted reaching to targets in contralateral and ipsilateral visual space. Exp Brain Res 1985;60:159–178.

Fitts PM. The information capacity of the human motor system in controlling the amplitude of movement. J Exp Psychol 1954;47:381–391.

Fitts PM. Perceptual-motor skill learning. In: Melton AW, ed. Categories of human learning, New York: Academic Press, 1964:243–285.

Fitts PM, Posner MI. Human performance. Belmont, CA: Brooks/Cole, 1967.

Flansbjer U, Miller M, Downham D, et al. Progressive resistance training after stroke: effects on muscle strength, muscle tone, gait performance and perceived participation. J Rehabil Med 2008;40:42–48.

Floel A, Cohen LG. Translational studies in neurorehabilitation: from bench to bedside. Cogn Behav Neurol 2006;19(1):1–10.

Florence SL, Kaas JH. Large–scale reorganization at multiple levels of the somatosensory pathway follows therapeutic amputation of the hand in monkeys. J Neurosci 1995;15:8083–8095.

Flowers KR, Stephens-Chisar J, LaStayo P, Galante BL. Intrarater reliability of a new method and instrumentation for measuring passive supination and pronation: a preliminary study. J Hand Ther 2001;14(1):30–35.

Floyer-Lea A, Matthews PM. Changing brain networks for visuomotor control with increased movement automaticity. J Neurophysiol 2004;92:2405–2412.

Foerster O. The motor cortex in man in the light of Hughlings Jackson's

Doctrines. In: Payton OD, Hirt S, Newman, R, eds. Scientific bases for neurophysiologic approaches to therapeutic exercise. Philadelphia, PA: FA Davis, 1977:13–18.

Foki T, Vanbellingen T, Lungu C, et al. Limb-kinetic apraxia affects activities of daily living in Parkinson's disease: a multi-center study. Eur J Neurol 2016;23:1301–1307.

Folio MR, Fewell RR. Peabody developmental motor scales examiner's manual, 2nd ed. Austin, TX: Pro-Ed, 2000.

Fong SS, Guo X, Liu KP, et al. Task-specific balance training improves the sensory organisation of balance control in children with developmental coordination disorder: a randomised controlled trial. Sci Rep 2016;6:20945.

Ford MP, Wagenaar RC, Newell KM. Phase manipulation and walking in stroke. J Neurol Phys Ther 2007a;31:85–91.

Ford MP, Wagenaar RC, Newell KM. The effects of auditory rhythms and instruction on walking patterns in individuals post stroke. Gait Posture 2007b;26:150–155.

Ford-Smith CD, VanSant AF. Age differences in movement patterns used to rise from a bed in subjects in the third through fifth decades of age. Phys Ther 1993;73:300–309.

Forma V, Anderson DI, Provasi J, et al. What does prone skateboarding in the newborn tell us about the ontogeny of human locomotion? Child Dev 2019;90(4):1286–1302.

Forssberg H. Ontogeny of human locomotor control: I. Infant stepping, supported locomotion, and transition to independent locomotion. Exp Brain Res 1985;57:480–493.

Forssberg H, Eliasson AC, Kinoshita H, et al. Development of human precision grip. I. Basic coordination of forces. Exp Brain Res 1991;85:451–457.

Forssberg H, Eliasson AC, Kinoshita H, et al. Development of human precision grip. IV. Tactile adaptation of isometric finger forces to the frictional condition. Exp Brain Res 1995;104:323–330.

Forssberg H, Grillner S, Rossignol S. Phase dependent reflex reversal during walking in chronic spinal cats. Brain Res 1975;85:103–107.

Forssberg H, Grillner S, Rossignol S. Phasic gain control of reflexes from the dorsum of the paw during spinal locomotion. Brain Res 1977;132:121–139.

Forssberg H, Hirschfeld H. Postural adjustments in sitting humans following external perturbations: muscle activity and kinematics. Exp Brain Res 1994;97(3):515–527.

Forssberg H, Kinoshita H, Eliasson AC, et al. Development of human precision grip. II. Anticipatory control of isometric forces targeted for object's weight. Exp Brain Res 1992;90:393–398.

Forssberg H, Nashner L. Ontogenetic development of postural control in man: adaptation to altered support and visual conditions during stance. J Neurosci 1982;2:545–552.

Forsstrom A, von Hofsten C. Visually directed reaching in children with motor impairments. Dev Med Child Neurol 1982;24:653–661.

Forster A, Young J. Incidence and consequences of falls due to stroke: a systematic inquiry. BMJ 1995;311:83–86.

Foster E, Sveistrup H, Woollacott MH. Transitions in visual proprioception: a cross-sectional developmental study of the effect of visual flow on postural control. J Motor Behav 1996;28:101–112.

Foster RJ, Maganaris CN, Reeves ND, Buckley JG. Centre of mass control is reduced in older people when descending stairs at an increased riser height. Gait Posture 2019;73:305–314.

Foudriat BA, Di Fabio RP, Anderson JH. Sensory organization of balance responses in children 3–6 years of age: a normative study with diagnostic implications. Int J Pediatr Otorhinolaryngol 1993;27:255–271.

Fox MD, Delp SL. Contributions of muscles and passive dynamics to swing initiation over a range of walking speeds. J Biomech 2010;43:1450–1455.

Fradet L, Lee G, Dounskaia N. Origins of submovements in movements of elderly adults. J Neuroeng Rehabil 2008;5:28.

Franchignoni F, Horak F, Godi M, et al. Using psychometric techniques to improve the Balance Evaluation System's Test: the mini-BESTest. J Rehabil Med 2010;42:323–331.

Franjoine MR, Gunther JS, Taylor MJ. Pediatric balance scale: a modified version of the Berg balance scale for the school-age child with mild to moderate motor impairment. Pediatr Phys Ther 2003;15:114–128.

Frank JS, Patla AE. Balance and mobility challenges in older adults: implications for preserving community mobility. Am J Prev Med 2003 Oct;25(3 Suppl 2):157–163.

Frank JS, Patla AE, Brown JE. Characteristics of postural control accompanying voluntary arm movement in the elderly. Soc Neurosci Abstr 1987;13:335.

Frascarelli M, Mastrogregori L, Conforti L. Initial motor unit recruitment in patients with spastic hemiplegia. Electromyogr Clin Neurophysiol 1998;38:267–271.

Fraser C, Wing A. A case study of reaching by a user of a manually-operated artificial hand. Prosthet Orthot Int 1981;5:151–156.

Frazzitta G, Maestri R, Uccellini D, Bertotti G, Abelli P. Rehabilitation treatment of gait in patients with Parkinson's disease with freezing: a comparison between two physical therapy protocols using visual and auditory cues with or without treadmill training. Mov Disord 2009;24(8):1139–1143.

Fredericks CM, Saladin LK. Clinical presentations in disorders of motor function. In: Fredericks CM, Saladin LK, eds. Pathophysiology of the motor systems: principles and clinical presentations. Philadelphia, PA: FA Davis, 1996.

Friel KM, Kuo HC, Fuller J, et al. Skilled bimanual training drives motor cortex plasticity in children with unilateral cerebral palsy. Neurorehabil Neural Repair 2016;30(9):834–844. doi: 10.1177/1545968315625838.

Friel KM, Nudo RJ. Recovery of motor function after focal cortical injury in primates: compensatory movement patterns used during rehabilitative training. Somatosens Motor Res 1998;15:173–189.

Fries JF. Successful aging: an emerging paradigm of gerontology. Clin Geriatr Med 2002;18:371–382.

Fries W, Danek A, Scheidtmann K, et al. Motor recovery following capsular stroke: role of descending pathways from multiple motor areas. Brain 1993;116:369–382.

Fritz NE, Cheek F, Nichols-Larsen DS. Motor-cognitive dual-task trianing in neurologic disorders: a systematic review. J Neurol Phys Ther 2015;39:142–153.

Frontera WR, Hughes VA, Fielding RA, et al. Aging of skeletal muscle: a 12 yr longitudinal study. J Appl Physiol 2000;88:1321–1326.

Fugl-Meyer AR, Jääskö L, Leyman I, et al. The post-stroke hemiplegic patient 1. A method for evaluation of physical performance. Scand J Rehabil Med 1975;7:13–31.

Fujiwara T, Kasashima Y, Honaga K, et al. Motor improvement and corticospinal modulation induced by hybrid assistive neuromuscular dynamic stimulation (HANDS) therapy in patients with chronic stroke. Neurorehabil Neuroal Repair 2009;23(2):125–132.

Fukuyama H, Ouchi Y, Matsuzaki S, et al. Brain functional activity during gait in normal subjects: a SPECT study. Neurosci Lett 1997;228:183–186.

Fulk GD, He Y, Boyne P, Dunning K. Predicting home and community walking activity poststroke. Stroke 2017;48:406–411.

Fuster JM. The prefrontal cortex: anatomy, physiology and neuropsychology of the frontal lobe, 2nd ed. New York: Raven, 1989.

G

Gabell A, Nayak USL. The effect of age on variability in gait. J Gerontol 1984;39:662–666.

Gabell A, Simons MA, Nayak USL. Falls in the healthy elderly: predisposing causes. Ergonomics 1985;28:965–975.

Gad P, Gerasimenko Y, Zdunowski S, et al. Weight bearing over-ground stepping in an exoskeleton with non-invasive spinal cord neuromodulation after motor complete paraplegia. Front Neurosci 2017;11L133. doi: 10.3389/fnins.2017.00333

Gad P, Lee S, Terrafranca N, Zhong H, et al. Non-invasive activation of cervical spinal networks after severe paralysis. J Neurotrauma 2018;35:2145–2158. doi: 10.1089/neu.2017.5461

Gadotti IC, Elbaum L, Jung Y, et al. Evaluation of eye, head and trunk coordination during target tracking tasks. Ergonomics 2016;59(11):1420–1427. doi: 10.1080/00140139.2016.1146345.

Gadotti I, Hernandez L, Manguson J, Sanchez L, Cevallos F. A pilot study on the evaluation of eye, head, and trunk coordination in subjects with chronic whiplash during a target-tracking task: a driving context approach. Musculoskelet Sci Pract 2020;46:102124. doi: 10.1016/j.msksp.2020.102124.

Gage JR. Gait analysis. An essential tool in the treatment of cerebral palsy. Clin Orthop Relat Res 1993;288:126–134.

Gage, WH, Zabjek KF, Hill SW, et al. Parallels in control of voluntary and perturbation-evoked reach-to-grasp movements: EMG and kinematics. Exp Brain Res 2007;181:627–637.

Gagnon I, Swaine B, Forget R. Exploring the comparability of the Sensory Organization Test and the Pediatric Clinical Test of Sensory Interaction for Balance in children. Phys Occup Ther Pediatr 2006;26:23–41.

Gagnon I, Swaine B, Friedman D, et al. Children show decreased dynamic balance after mild traumatic brain injury. Arch Phys Med Rehabil 2004;85:444–452.

Gahery Y, Massion J. Coordination between posture and movement. Trends Neurosci 1981;4:199–202.

Gallahue DL. Understanding motor development: infants, children, adolescents. Indianapolis, IN: Benchmark, 1989.

Galletly R, Brauer SG. Does the type of concurrent task affect preferred and cued gait in people with Parkinson's disease? Aust J Physiother 2005;51:175–180.

Galli M, Cimolin V, Crivellini M, et al. Quantification of upper limb motion during gait in children with hemiplegic cerebral palsy. J Dev Phys Disabil 2011;24:1–8.

Galloway JC, Thelen E. Feet first: object exploration in young infants. Infant Behav Dev 2004;27:107–112.

Galna B, Peters A, Murphy AT, et al. Obstacle crossing deficits in older adults: a systematic review. Gait Posture 2009;30:270–275.

Gan SM, Tung LC, Tang YH, et al. Psychometric properties of functional balance assessment in children with cerebral palsy. Neurorehabil Neural Repair 2008;22:745–753.

Gantschnig BE, Page J, Nilsson I, et al. Detecting differences in activities of daily living between children with and without mild disabilities. Am J Occup Ther 2013;67(3):319–327.

Gardner EP, Johnson KO. Touch. In: Kandel ER, Schwartz JH, Jessell TM, et al., eds. Principles of neural science. vol. E. New York: McGraw-Hill, 2013a:498–529.

Gardner EP, Johnson KO. The somatosensory system: receptors and central pathways. In: Kandel ER, Schwartz JH, Jessell TM, et al., eds. Principles of neural science. vol. E. New York: McGraw-Hill, 2013b:473–497.

Gardner EP, Kandel ER. Touch. In: Kandel ER, Schwartz JH, Jessell TM, eds. Principles of neural science, 4th ed. New York: McGraw-Hill, 2000:451–471.

Gardner EP, Martin JH, Jessell TM. The bodily senses. In: Kandel ER, Schwartz JH, Jessell TM, eds. Principles of neural science, 4th ed. New York: McGraw-Hill, 2000:430–450.

Garland SJ, Willems DA, Ivanova TD, et al. Recovery of standing balance and functional mobility after stroke. Arch Phys Med Rehabil 2003;84:1753–1759.

Garraghty PE, Hanes DP, Florence SL, et al. Pattern of peripheral deafferentation predicts reorganizational limits in adult primate somatosensory cortex. Somatosens Motor Res 1994;11:109–117.

Garrison KA, Winstein CJ, Aziz-Zadeh L. The mirror neuron system: a neural substrate for methods in stroke rehabilitation. Neurorehabil Neural Repair 2010;24:404–412.

Gates PE, Banks D, Johnston TE, et al. Randomized controlled trial assessing participation and quality of life in a supported speed treadmill training exercise program vs. a strengthening program for children with cerebral palsy. J Pediatr Rehabil Med 2012;5(2):75–88.

Gatev P, Thomas S, Lou JS, et al. Effects of diminished and conflicting sensory information on balance in patients with cerebellar deficits. Mov Disord 1996;11:654–664.

Gatts SK, Woollacott MH. How Tai Chi improves balance: biomechanics of recovery to a walking slip in impaired seniors. Gait Posture 2007;25:205–214.

Gatts SK, Woollacott MH. Neural mechanisms underlying balance improvement with short term Tai Chi training. Aging Clin Exp Res 2006;18:7–19.

Gauthier GM, Vercher JL, Ivaldi FM, et al. Oculo-manual tracking of visual targets: control learning, coordination control and coordination model. Exp Brain Res 1988;73:127–137.

Gebruers N, Truijen S, Engelborghs S, et al. Prediction of upper limb recovery, general disability, and rehabilitation status by activity measurements assessed by accelerometers or the Fugl-Meyer score in acute stroke. Am J Phys Med Rehabil 2014;93:245–252.

Gehlsen GM, Whaley MH. Falls in the elderly: part I, gait. Arch Phys Med Rehabil 1990;71:735–738.

Geldhof E, Cardon G, Bourdeaudhuij ID, et al. Static and dynamic standing balance: test-retest reliability and reference values in 9 to 10 year old children. Eur J Pediatr 2006;165:779–786.

Genthon N, Rougier P, Gissot AS, et al. Contribution of each lower limb to upright standing in stroke patients. Stroke 2008;39:1793–1799.

Gentile AM. Skill acquisition. In: Carr JH, Shepherd RB, Gordon J, Gentile AM, Held JM, eds. Foundations for physical therapy: Movement science. London: Heineman Physiotherapy, 1987:93–154.

Gentile AM. Skill acquisition: action movement, and neuromotor processes. In: Carr JA, Shepherd RB, eds. Movement science: foundations for physical therapy in rehabilitation. Rockville, MD: Aspen Publishers, 2000:111–187.

Gentile AM. Skill acquisition: action movement, and neuromotor processes. In: Carr J, Shepherd R, Gentile AM. Movement organization and delayed alternation behavior of monkeys following selective ablation of frontal cortex. Acta Neurobiol Exp (Wars) 1972;32(2):277–304.

Georgiou N, Iansek R, Bradshaw JL, et al. An evaluation of the role of internal cues in the pathogenesis of Parkinsonian hypokinesia. Brain 1993;116:1575–1587.

Georgopoulos AP, Kalaska JF, Caminiti R, et al. On the relations between the direction of two-dimensional arm movements and cell discharge in primate motor cortex. J Neurosci 1982;2:1527–1537.

Gerasimenko Y, Gorodnichev R, Moshonkina T, Sayenko D, Gad P, Edgerton VR. Transcutaneous electrical spinal-cord stimulation in humans. Annals Phys Rehabil Med 2015;58:225–231.

Gesell A. The ontogenesis of infant behavior. In: Carmichael L, ed. Manual of child psychology. New York: Wiley, 1946:335–373.

Gesell, A. The ontogenesis of infant behavior. In: Carmichael L, ed. Manual of child psychology. New York, NY: John Wiley, 1946:295–331.

Gesell A. Behavior patterns of fetal-infant and child. In: Hooker D, Kare C, eds. Genetics and inheritance of neuropsychiatric patterns. Res Publ Assoc Res Nerv Ment Dis 1954;33:114–126.

Gesell A, Amatruda CS. Developmental diagnosis, 2nd ed. New York: Paul B. Hoeber, 1947.

Gesell A, Halverson HM, Thompson H, et al. The first five years of life. New York: Harper & Row, 1940.

Geurts AC, de Haart M, van Nes IJ, et al. A review of standing balance recovery from stroke. Gait Posture 2005;22:267–281.

Ghai S, Ghai I, Effenberg A. Effects of dual tasks and dual-task training on postural stability: a systematic review and meta-analysis. Clin Interv Aging 2017;12:557–577.

Ghamkhar L, Kahlaee AH. The effect of trunk muscle fatigue on postural control of upright stance: a systematic review. Gait Posture 2019;72:167–174.

Ghez C. Contributions of central programs to rapid limb movement in the cat. In: Asanuma H, Wilson VJ, eds. Integration in the nervous system. Tokyo, Japan: Igaku-Shoin, 1979:305–320.

Ghez C. The cerebellum. In: Kandel E, Schwartz JH, Jessell TM, eds. Principles of neuroscience, 3rd ed. New York: Elsevier, 1991:633.

Ghez C, Krakauer J. The organization of movement. In: Kandel E, Schwartz J, Jessel T, eds. Principles of neuroscience, 4th ed. New York: McGraw-Hill, 2000:653–673.

Ghez C, Thatch WT. The cerebellum. In: Kandel E, Schwartz J, Jessel T, eds. Principles of neuroscience, 4th ed. New York: McGraw-Hill, 2000:832–852.

Giacobbe V, Krebs HI, Volpe BT, et al. Transcranial direct current stimulation (tDCS) and robotic practice in chronic stroke: the dimension of timing. NeuroRehabilitation 2013;33(1):49–56.

Giacomo R, Kalaska JF. Voluntary movement: the parietal and premotor cortex. In: Kandel ER, Schwartz JH, Jessell TM, Siegelbaum SA, Hudspeth AJ, eds. Principles of neural science, 5th ed. New York, NY: McGraw-Hill, 2013:2109–2178.

Gibson JJ. The senses considered as perceptual systems. Boston, MA: Houghton Mifflin, 1966.

Gibson AR, Horn KM, Van Kan PLE. Grasping cerebellar function. In: Bennett KMB, Castiello U, eds. Insights into the reach to grasp movement. Amsterdam, The Netherlands: Elsevier, 1994:129–150.

Gibson E, Walker AS. Development of knowledge of visual-tactual affordance of substance. Child Dev 1984;55:453–460.

Giladi N, Kao R, Fahn S. Freezing phenomenon in patients with parkinsonian syndromes. Mov Disord 1997;12:302–305.

Gilbert PFC, Thatch WT. Purkinje cell activity during motor learning. Brain Res 1977;128:309–328.

Gilchrist AL, Cowan N, Naveh-Benjamin M. Working memory capacity for spoken sentences decreases with adult aging: recall of fewer, but not smaller chunks in older adults. Memory 2008;16:773–787.

Gill K, Oslovich A, Synnes A, et al. Concurrent validity of the Bayley-III and the peabody developmental motor scales-2 at 18 Months. Phys Occup Ther Pediatr 2019;39(5):514–524. doi: 10.1080/01942638.2018.1546255.

Gill SV, Yang Z, Hung YC. Effects of singular and dual task constraints on motor skill variability in childhood. Gait Posture 2017;53:121–126.

Gill-Body KM, Popat RA, Parker SW, et al. Rehabilitation of balance in two patients with cerebellar dysfunction. Phys Ther 1997;77:534–552.

Gillespie LD, Robertson MC, Gillespie WJ, et al. Interventions for preventing falls in older people living in the community Cochrane Database Syst Rev 2009;(2):CD007146.

Gilliaux M, Renders A, Dispa D, et al. Upper limb robot-assisted therapy in cerebral palsy: a single-blind randomized controlled trial. Neurorehabil Neural Repair 2015;29(2):183–192.

Gillick B, Krach LE, Feyma T, et al. Primed low-frequency repetitive transcranial magnetic stimulation and constraint-induced movement therapy in pediatric hemiparesis: a randomized trial. Dev Med Child Neurol 2014;56(1):44–52.

Gillick B, Rich T, Nemanich S, et al. Transcranial direct current stimulation and constraint-induced therapy in cerebral palsy: a randomized, blinded, sham-controlled clinical trial. Eur J Paediatr Neurol 2018;22(3):358–368. doi: 10.1016/j.ejpn.2018.02.001.

Gilman S. Fusimotor fiber responses in the decerebellate cat. Brain Res 1969;14:218–221.

Gilman S. The spinocerebellar ataxias. Clin Neuropharmacol 2000;23:296–303.

Gilman S, Ebel HC. Fusimotor neuron responses to natural stimuli as a function of prestimulus fusimotor activity in decerebellate cats. Brain Res 1970;21:367–384.

Giuliani CA. Dorsal rhizotomy for children with cerebral palsy: support for concepts of motor control. Phys Ther 1991;71:248–259.

Gladstone DJ, Danells CJ, Black SE. The Fugl-Meyer assessment of motor recovery after stroke: a critical review of its measurement properties. Neurorehabil Neural Repair 2002;16:232–240.

Glaister BC, Bernatz GC, Klute GK, et al. Video task analysis of turning during activities of daily living. Gait Posture 2007;25:289–294.

Godges JJ, MacRae PG, Engelke KA. Effects of exercise on hip range of motion, trunk muscle performance and gait economy. Phys Ther 1993;73:468–477.

Gordon AM, Hung Y-C, Brandao M, et al. Bimanual training and constraint-induced movement therapy in children with hemiplegic cerebral palsy. Neurorehabil Neural Repair 2011;25:692–702.

Gordon J, ed. Movement science: foundations for physical therapy in rehabilitation. Rockville, MD: Aspen, 1987.

Gogola GR, Velleman PF, Zu S, et al. Hand dexterity in children: administration and normative values of the functional dexterity test. J Hand Surg Am 2013;38(12):2426–2431.

Goldberg ME, Hudspeth AJ. The vestibular system. In: Kandel ER, Schwartz JH, Jessell TM, eds. Principles of neural science, 4th ed. New York: McGraw-Hill, 2000:801–815.

Goldberg SR, Anderson FC, Pandy MG, Delp SL. Muscles that influence knee flexion velocity in double support: implications for stiff-knee gait. J Biomech 2004;37(8):1189–1196.

Goldstein LB. Basic and clinical studies of pharmacologic effects on recovery from brain injury. J Neural Transplant Plast 1993;4:175–192.

Goldstein LB. Neuropharmacology of TBI-induced plasticity. Brain Injury 2003;17:685–694.

Goldstein LB. Pharmacology of recovery after stroke. Stroke 1990;21(Suppl III):139–142.

Goldstein LB, Davis JN. Physician prescribing patterns after ischemic stroke. Neurology 1988;38:1806–1809.

Gollhofer A, Schmidtbleicher D, Quintem J, et al. Compensatory movements following gait perturbations: changes in cinematic and muscular activation patterns. Int J Sports Med 1986;7:325–329.

Golomb MR, McDonald BC, Warden SJ, et al. In-home virtual reality videogame telerehabilitation in adolescents with hemiplegic cerebral palsy. 2010;9:1e1–8e1.

Gomes MM, Barela JA. Postural control in Down syndrome: the use of somatosensory and visual information to attenuate body sway. Motor Control 2007;11:224–234.

Gong H, Sun L, Yang R, et al. Changes of upright body posture in the sagittal plane of men and women occurring with aging: a cross sectional study. BMC Geriatr 2019;19(1):71.

Gonshor A, Melville-Jones G. Short-term adaptive changes in the human vestibulo-ocular reflex arc. J Physiol (Lond) 1976;256:361–379.

González-Alvarez C, Subramanian A, Pardhans S. Reaching and grasping with restricted peripheral vision. Ophthalmic Physiol Opt 2007;27:265–274.

Goodale MA, Króliczak G, Westwood DA. Dual routes to action: contributions of the dorsal and ventral streams to adaptive behavior. Prog Brain Res 2005;149:269–283.

Goodale MA, Milner AD. Separate visual pathways for perception and action. Trends Neurosci 1992;15:20–25.

Goodale MA, Milner AD, Jakobson LS, et al. A neurological dissociation between perceiving objects and grasping them. Nature 1991;349:154–156.

Goode SL. The contextual interference effect in learning an open motor skill. Unpublished doctoral dissertation. Baton Rouge, LA: Louisiana State University, 1986.

Goodwin RD, Devanand DP. Stroke, depression, and functional health outcomes among adults in the community. J Geriatric Psychiatry Neurol 2008;21:41–46.

Goodwin BM, Sabelhaus EK, Pan YC, et al. Accelerometer measurements indicate that arm movements of children with cerebral palsy do not increase after Constraint-Induced Movement Therapy (CIMT). Am J Occup Ther 2020:7405205100p1-7405205100p9. doi: 10.5014/ajot.2020.040246.

Goodwin GM, McCloskey DI, Matthews PBC. The contribution of muscle afferents to kinaesthesia shown by vibration induced illusions of movement and by the effects of paralysing joint afferents. Brain 1972;95:705–748.

Goodworth AD, Mellodge P, Peterka RJ. Stance width changes how sensory feedback is used for multisegmental balance control. J Neurophysiol 2014;112:525–542.

Goodworth AD, Peterka RJ. Sensorimotor integration for multisegmental frontal plane balance control in humans. J Neurophysiol 2012;107:12–28.

Gordon J. Assumptions underlying physical therapy intervention: theoretical and historical perspectives. In: Carr JH, Shepherd RB, Gordon J, et al., eds. Movement sciences: foundations for physical therapy in rehabilitation. Rockville, MD: Aspen, 1987:1–30.

Gordon J. Motor control workshop for physical therapists, Umea, Sweden, June 1997.

Gordon AM. Development of hand motor control: handbook of brain and behavior in human development. Boston, MA: Kluwer, 2001:513–537.

Gordon AM, Charles J, Duff SV. Fingertip forces during object manipulation in children with hemiplegic cerebral palsy. II. Bilateral coordination. Dev Med Child Neurol 1999;41:176–185.

Gordon AM, Charles J, Steenbergen B. Fingertip force planning during grasp is disrupted by impaired sensorimotor integration in children with hemiplegic cerebral palsy. Pediatr Res 2006;60:587–591.

Gordon AM, Charles J, Wolf SL. Methods of constraint-induced movement therapy for children with hemiplegic cerebral palsy: development of a child-friendly intervention for improving upper-extremity function. Arch Phys Med Rehabil 2005;86(4):837–844.

Gordon AM, Chinnan A, Gill S, et al. Both constraint-induced movement therapy and bimanual training lead to improved performance of upper extremity function in children with hemiplegia. Dev Med Child Neurol 2008;50:957–958.

Gordon AM, Duff SV. Fingertip forces during object manipulation in children with hemiplegic cerebral palsy. I. Anticipatory scaling. Dev Med Child Neurol 1999a;41:166–175.

Gordon AM, Duff SV. Relationships between clinical measures and fine manipulative control in children with hemiplegic cerebral palsy. Dev Med Child Neurol 1999b;41:586–591.

Gordon J, Ghez C. Muscle receptors and spinal reflexes: the stretch reflex. In: Kandel E, Schwartz JH, Jessell TM, eds. Principles of neuroscience, 3rd ed. New York: Elsevier, 1991:564–580.

Gordon AM, Forssberg H, Johansson RS, et al. Development of human precision grip. III. Integration of visual size cues during the programming of isometric forces. Exp Brain Res 1992;90:399–403.

Gordon AM, Ingvarsson PE, Forssberg H. Anticipatory control of manipulative forces in Parkinson's disease. Exp Neurol 1997;145:477–488.

Gordon AM, Lewis S, Eliasson AC, et al. Object release under varying task constraints in children with hemiplegic cerebral palsy. Dev Med Child Neurol 2003;45:240–248.

Gorkovenko AV, Sawczyn S, Bulgakova NV, Jasczur-Nowicki J, Mishchenko VS, Kostyukov AI. Muscle agonist-antagonist interactions in an experimental joint model. Exp Brain Res. 2012;222:399–414.

Gormley ME, O'Brien CF, Yablon SA. A clinical overview of treatment decisions in the management of spasticity. Muscle Nerve Suppl 1997;6:S14–S20.

Gorniak SL, Plow M, McDaniel C, et al. Impaired object handling during bimanual task performance in multiple sclerosis. Mult Scler Int 2014;2014:450420.

Gosser SM, Rice MS. Efficiency of unimanual and bimanual reach in persons with and without stroke. Top Stroke Rehabil 2015;22:56–62.

Gottschall J, Kram R. Energy cost and muscular activity required for propulsion during walking. J Appl Physiol 2003;94: 1766–1772.

Gövert F, Deuschl G. Tremor entities and their classification: an update. Curr Opin Neurol 2015;28:393–399.

Gowland C, deBruin H, Basmajian JV, et al. Agonist and antagonist activity during voluntary upper-limb movement in patients with stroke. Phys Ther 1992;72:624–633.

Gowland C, Stratford P, Ward M, et al. Measuring physical impairment and disability wit the Chedoke-McMaster Stroke Assessment. Stroke 1993;24:58–63.

Goyen TA, Lui K, Hummell J. Sensorimotor skills associated with motor dysfunction in children born extremely preterm. Early Hum Dev 2011;87(7):489–493.

Grabiner MD, Bareither ML, Gatts S, et al. Task-specific training reduces trip-related fall risk in women. Med Sci Sports Exerc 2012;44:2410–2414.

Graci V, Elliott DB, Buckley JG. Peripheral visual cues affect minimum-foot-clearance during overground locomotion. Gait Posture 2009;30:370–374.

Graci V, Elliott DB, Buckley JG. Utility of peripheral visual cues in planning and controlling adaptive gait. Optom Vis Sci 2010;87:21–27.

Gracies JM. Pathophysiology of spastic paresis. I: paresis and soft tissue changes. Muscle Nerve 2005a;31:535–551.

Gracies JM. Pathophysiology of spastic paresis. II: emergence of muscle overactivity. Muscle Nerve 2005b;31:552–571.

Graham F, Rodger S, Ziviani J. Enabling occupational performance of children through coaching parents: three case reports. Phys Occup Ther Pediatr 2010;30(1):4–15.

Grasso R, Assaiante C, Prevost P, et al. Development of anticipatory orienting strategies during locomotor task in children. Neurosci Biobehav Rev 1998;22:533–539.

Gravem D, Singh M, Chen C, et al. Assessment of infant movement with a compact wireless accelerometer system. J Med Devices 2012;6:021013.

Gray DB, Hollingsworth HH, Stark SL, et al. Participation Survey/mobility: psychometric properties of a measure of participation for people with mobility impairments and limitations. Arch Phys Med Rehabil 2006;87:189–197.

Gray P, Hildebrand K. Fall risk factors in Parkinson's disease. J Neurosci Nurs 2000;32:222–228.

Greaves S, Imms C, Dodd K, et al. Development of the Mini-Assisting Hand Assessment: evidence for content and internal scale validity. Dev Med Child Neurol 2013;55:1030–1037.

Green LN, Williams K. Differences in developmental movement patterns used by active vs sedentary middle-aged adults coming from a supine position to erect stance. Phys Ther 1992;72:560–568.

Grefkes C, Fink GR. The functional organization of the intraparietal sulcus in humans and monkeys. J Anat 2005;207(1):3–17.

Gregson JM, Leathley M, Moor AP, et al. Reliability of the Tone Assessment Scale and the Modified Ashworth Scale as clinical tools for assessing poststroke spasticity. Arch Phys Med Rehabil 1999;80:1013–1016.

Gresty MA. Coordination of head and eye movements to fixate continuous and intermittent targets. Vision Res 1974;14: 395–403.

Griffin JM, Bradke F. Therapeutic repair for spinal cord injury: combinatory approaches to address a multifacted problem. EMBO Mol Med 2020;12:e11505.

Grillner S. Locomotion in the spinal cat. In: Stein RB, Pearson KG, Smith RS, et al., eds. Control of posture and locomotion. New York: Plenum, 1973:515–535.

Grillner S. Control of locomotion in bipeds, tetrapods, and fish. In: Brooks VB, ed. Handbook of physiology: the nervous system, vol. 2. Motor control. Baltimore, MD: Lippincott Williams & Wilkins, 1981:1179–1236.

Grillner S, Deliagnina T, Ekebuerg O, et al. Neural networks that coordinate locomotion and body orientation in lamprey. Trends Neurosci 1995;18:270–280.

Grillner S, Rossignol S. On the initiation of the swing phase of locomotion in chronic spinal cats. Brain Res 1978;146:269–277.

Grillner S, Zangger P. On the central generation of locomotion in the low spinal cat. Exp Brain Res 1979;34:241–261.

Gronley JK, Perry J. Gait analysis techniques: Rancho Los Amigos Hospital gait laboratory. Phys Ther 1984;64:1831–1837.

Grossman GE, Leigh RJ. Instability of gaze during locomotion in patients with deficient vestibular function. Ann Neurol 1990;27:528–532.

Guadagnin EC, Priario LAA, Carpes FP, Vaz MA. Correlation between lower limb isometric strength and muscle structure with normal and challenged gait performance in older adults. Gait Posture 2019;73:101–107.

Guadagnoli MA, Lee TD. Challenge point: a framework for conceptualizing the effects of various practice conditions in motor learning. J Motor Behav 2004;36:212–224.

Guarrera-Bowlby PL, Gentile AM. Form and variability during sit-to-stand transitions: children versus adults. J Motor Behav 2004;36:104–114.

Guccione AA. Physical therapy diagnosis and the relationship between impairments and function. Phys Ther 1991;71:499–504.

Guilbert J, Alamargot D, Morin MF. Handwriting on a tablet screen: role of visual and proprioceptive feedback in the control of movement by children and adults. Hum Mov Sci 2019;65:S0167-9457(18)30093-9. doi: 10.1016/j.humov.2018.09.001.

Guimarães AN, Ugrinowitsch H, Dascal JB, Porto AB, Okazaki VHA. Freezing degrees of freedom during motor learning: A systematic review. Motor Control 2020;24(3):457–471.

Guralnik JM, Simonsick EM, Ferrucci L, et al. A short physical performance battery assessing lower extremity function: association with self-reported disability and prediction of mortality and nursing home admission. J Gerontol A Biol Sci Med Sci 1994;49:M85–M94.

Gurfinkel V, Cacciatore TW, Cordo P, Horak F, Nutt J, Skoss R. Humans postural muscle tone in the body axis of healthy the influence of education and exercise on neck pain transition from sitting to standing. J Neurophysiol 2006;96:2678–2687.

Gurfinkel VS, Levik YS. Sensory complexes and sensorimotor integration. Fiziolog Cheloveka 1978;5:399–414.

Gurfinkel VS, Levick YS. Perceptual and automatic aspects of the postural body scheme. In: Paillard J, ed. Brain and space. New York: Oxford Science, 1991.

Gurfinkel VS, Lipshits MI, Popov KE. Is the stretch reflex the main mechanism in the system of regulation of the vertical posture of man? Biophysics 1974;19:761–766.

H

Haaland KY, Prestopnik JL, Knight RT, et al. Hemispheric asymmetries for kinematic and positional aspects of reaching. Brain 2004; 127(Pt 5):1145–1158.

Hackett ML, Köhler S, O'Brien JT, Mead GE. Neuropsychiatric outcomes of stroke. Lancet Neurol 2014;13:525–534.

Hadders-Algra M. Early human brain development: starring the subplate. Neurosci Biobehav Rev 2018;92:276–290.

Hadders-Algra M. Early human motor development: from variation to the ability to vary and adapt. Neurosci Biobehav Rev 2018;90:411–427.

Hadders-Algra, M, Brogren E, Forssberg H. Training affects the development of postural adjustments in sitting infants. J Physiology 1996;493:289–298.

Hadders-Algra M, Gramsberg A. Discussion on the clinical relevance of activity-dependent plasticity after an insult to the developing brain. Neurosci Biobehav Rev 2007;31:1213–1219.

Haffenden AM, Goodale MA. The effect of pictorial illusion on prehension and perception. J Cogn Neurosci 1998;10:122–136.

Hafström A. Perceived and functional balance control is negatively affected by diminished touch and vibration sensitivity in relatively healthy older adults and elderly. Gerontol Geriatr Med 2018;4:1–10.

Häger-Ross C, Schieber MH. Quantifying the independence of human finger movements: comparisons of digits, hands, and movement frequencies. J Neurosci 2000;20:8542–8550.

Haggerty S, Jiang LT, Galecki A, et al. Effects of biofeedback on secondary task response time and postural stability in older adults. Gait Posture 2012;35(4):523–528.

Hahn ME, Chou L-S. Can motion of individual body segments identify dynamic instability in the elderly? Clin Biomech (Bristol, Avon) 2003;18:737–744.

Hahn ME, Chou L-S. Age-related reduction in sagittal plane center of mass motion during obstacle crossing. J Biomech 2004;37:837–844.

Haley SM, Coster WJ, Ludlow LH, et al. Pediatric evaluation of disability inventory (PEDI). Boston, MA: New England Medical Center Hospitals, 1992.

Haley SM, Jette AM, Coster WJ, et al. Late life function and disability instrument. II. Development and evaluation of the disability component. J Gerontol A Biol Sci Med Sci 2002;57A:M217–M222.

Hall CD, Herdman SJ. Reliability of clinical measures used to assess patients with peripheral vestibular disorders J Neurol Phys Ther 2006;30:74–81.

Hall CD, Herdman SJ, Whitney SL, et al. Vestibular rehabilitation for peripheral vestibular hypofunction:

an evidence-based clinical practice guideline: from the American Physical Therapy Association Neurology Section. J Neurol Phys Ther 2016;40(2):124–155. doi: 10.1097/NPT.0000000000000120.

Hall LM, Brauer S, Horak F, Hodges PW. Adaptive changes in anticipatory postural adjustments with novel and familiar postural supports. J Neurophysiol 2010;103(2):968–976.

Hall LM, Brauer S, Horak F, Hodges PW. With novel and familiar postural supports adaptive changes in anticipatory postural adjustments adaptive changes in anticipatory postural adjustments with novel and familiar postural supports. J Neurophysiol 2010;103:968–976.

Hall KM, Bushnik T, Lakisic-Kazazic B, et al. Assessing traumatic brain injury outcome measures for long-term follow-up of community-based individuals. Arch Phys Med Rehabil 2001;82:367–374.

Hallemans A, Beccu S, Van Loock K, et al. Visual deprivation leads to gait adaptations that are age- and context-specific: I. Step-time parameters. Gait Posture 2009a;30(1):55–59.

Hallemans A, Beccu S, Van Loock K, et al. Visual deprivation leads to gait adaptations that are age- and context-specific: II. Kinematic parameters. Gait Posture 2009b;30(3):307–311.

Hallemans A, De Clercq D, Aerts P. Changes in 3D joint dynamics during the first 5 months after the onset of independent walking: a longitudinal follow-up study. Gait Posture 2006;24(3):270–279.

Hallemans A, Dhanis L, De Clercq D, et al. Changes in mechanical control of movement during the first 5 months of independent walking: a longitudinal study. J Motor Behav 2007;39:227–233.

Hallemans A, Verbecque E, Dumas R, Cheze L, Van Hamme A, Robert T. Developmental changes in spatial margin of stability in typically developing children relate to the mechanics of gait. Gait Posture 2018;63:33–38.

Hallett M. Physiology of basal ganglia disorders: an overview. Can J Neurol Sci 1993;20:177–183.

Hallett M. Overview of human tremor physiology. Mov Disord 1998;13:43–48.

Hallett M. Transcranial magnetic stimulation and the human brain. Nature 2000;406:147–150.

Hallett M, Shahani BT, Young RR. EMG analysis of stereotyped voluntary movements in man. J Neurol Neurosurg Psychiatry 1975;38:1154–1162.

Hamani C, Richter E, Schwalb JM, Lozano AM. Bilateral subthalamic nucleus stimulation for Parkinson's disease: a systematic review of the clinical literature. Neurosurgery 2005;56:1313–1324.

Hamburger V, Levi-Montalcini R. Proliferation, differentiation and degeneration in the spinal ganglia of the chick embryo under normal and experimental conditions. J Exp Zool 1949;111:457–501.

Hammer A, Nilsagard Y, Wallquist M. Balance training in stroke patients—a systematic review of randomized, controlled trials. Adv Physiother 2008;10:163–172.

Han, D, Adolph, KE. The impact of errors in infant development: falling like a baby. Dev Sci 2020:e13069. doi: 10.1111/desc.13069. Online ahead of print.

Han P, Zhang W, Kang L, et al. Clinical evidence of exercise benefits for stroke. Adv Exp Med Biol 2017;1000:131–151. doi: 10.1007/978-981-10-4304-8_9.

Hanakawa T, Katsumi Y, Fukuyama H, et al. Mechanisms underlying gait disturbance in Parkinson's disease: a single photon emission computed tomography study. Brain 1999;122:1271–1282.

Hanisch C, Konczak J, Dohle C. The effect of the Ebbinghaus illusion on grasping behaviour of children. Exp Brain Res 2001;137:237–245.

Hanlon RE. Motor learning following unilateral stroke. Arch Phys Med Rehabil 1996;77:811–815.

Hanna SE, Law MC, Rosenbaum PL, et al. Development of hand function among children with cerebral palsy: growth curve analysis for ages 16 to 70 months. Dev Med Child Neurol 2003;45:448–455.

Hara Y, Ogawa S, Tsujiuchi K, et al. A home-based rehabilitation program for the hemiplegic upper extremity by power-assisted functional electrical stimulation. Disabil Rehabil 2008;30(4):296–304.

Harada T, Goto F, Kanzaki S, et al. Vibrotactile neurofeedback for vestibular rehabilitation in patients with presbyvertigo. J Vestibul Res 2010;20(3–4):242–243.

Harbourne RT, Berger SE. Embodied cognition in practice: exploring effects of a motor-based problem-solving intervention. Phys Ther 2019;99(6):786–796. doi: 10.1093/ptj/pzz031.

Harbourne RT, Deffeyes JE, DeJong SL. Nonlinear variables can assist in identifying postural control deficits in infants. J Sport Exerc Psychol 2007;29(Suppl):S9.

Harbourne RT, Giuliani C, MacNeela, J. A kinematic and electromyographic analysis of the development of sitting posture in infants. Dev Psychobiol 1993;26:51–64.

Harbourne R, Kamm K. Upper extremity function: what's posture got to do with it? J Hand Ther 2015;28:106–112.

Harbourne RT, Stergiou N. Nonlinear analysis of the development of sitting postural control. Dev Psychobiol 2003;42:368–377.

Harbourne R, Stergiou N. Movement variability and the use of nonlinear tools: principles to guide physical therapist practice. Phys Ther 2009;89:267–282.

Hardy SE, Perera S, Roumani YF, et al. Improvement in usual gait speed predicts better survival in older adults. J Am Geriatr Soc 2007;55:1727–1734.

Haridas C, Zehr EP. Coordinated interlimb compensatory responses to electrical stimulation of cutaneous nerves in the hand and foot during walking. J Neurophysiol 2003;90(5):2850–2861.

Haridas C, Zehr EP, Misiaszek JE. Postural uncertainty leads to dynamic control of cutaneous reflexes from the foot during human walking. Brain Res 2005;1062:48–62.

Harley C, Boyd JE, Cockburn J, et al. Disruption of sitting balance after stroke: influence of spoken output. J Neurol Neurosurg Psychiatry 2006;77:674–676.

Harmsen WJ, Bussmann JB, Selles RW, et al. A mirror therapy-based action observation protocol to improve motor learning after stroke. Neurorehabil Neural Repair 2015;29:509–516. pii: 1545968314558598.

Harris JE, Eng JJ, Marigold DS, et al. Relationship of balance and mobility to fall incidence in people with chronic stroke. Phys Ther 2005;85:150–158.

Hase K, Stein RB. Turning strategies during human walking. J Neurophysiol 1999;81:2914–2922.

Hass G, Diener HC, Bacher M, et al. Development of postural control in children: short-, medium-, and long-latency EMG responses of leg muscles after perturbation of stance. Exp Brain Res 1986;64:127–132.

Hass G, Diener HC. Development of stance control in children. In: Amblard B, Berthoz A, Clarac F, eds. Development, adaptation and modulation of posture and gait. Amsterdam, The Netherlands: Elsevier, 1988:49–58.

Hauer K, Lamb SE, Jorstad EC, et al. Systematic review of definitions and methods of measuring falls in randomised controlled fall prevention trials. Age Ageing 2006;35:5–10.

Hauer K, Pfisterer M, Weber C, et al. Cognitive impairment decreased postural control during dual tasks in geriatric patients with a history of severe falls. J Am Geriatr Soc 2003;51:1638–1644.

Haugh AB, Pandyan AD, Johnson GR. A systematic review of the Tardieu Scale for the measurement of spasticity. Dis Rehabil 2006;28:899–907.

Hausdorff JM. Gait dynamics, fractals and falls: finding meaning in the stride-to-stride fluctuations of human walking. Hum Mov Sci 2007;26:555–589.

Hausdorff JM, Cudkowicz ME, Firtion R, et al. Gait variability and basal ganglia disorders: stride-to-stride variations of gait cycle timing in Parkinson's disease and Huntington's disease. Mov Disord 1998;13:428–437.

Hausdorff JM, Edelberg HK, Mitchell SL, et al. Increased gait unsteadiness in community-dwelling elderly fallers. Arch Phys Med Rehabil 1997;78:278–283.

Hausdorff JM, Rios DA, Edelberg HK. Gait variability and fall risk in community-living older adults: a 1-year prospective study. Arch Phys Med Rehabil 2001;82:1050–1056.

Hay L. Accuracy of children on an open-loop pointing task. Percept Motor Skills 1978;47:1079–1082.

Hay L. Spatial-temporal analysis of movements in children: motor programs versus feedback in the development of reaching. J Motor Behav 1979;11:189–200.

Hay L. Developmental changes in eye-hand coordination behaviors: Preprogramming versus feedback control. In: Bard C, Fleury M, Hay L, eds. Development of eye-hand coordination across the lifespan. Columbia: University of South Carolina Press, 1990:217–244.

Hay L, Bard C, Fleury M. Visuo-manual coordination from 6 to 10: specification, control and evaluation of direction and amplitude parameters of movement. In: Wade MG, Whiting HTA, eds. Motor development in children: aspects of coordination and control. Dordrecht, The Netherlands: Martinus Nijhoff, 1986.

Hayes KC, Riach CL. Preparatory postural adjustments and postural sway in young children. In: Woollacott MH, Shumway-Cook A, eds. Development of posture and gait across the life span. Columbia: University of South Carolina, 1989:97–127.

Hedberg A, Carlberg EB, Forssberg H, et al. Development of postural adjustments in sitting position during the first half year of life. Dev Med Child Neurol 2005;47:312–320.

Hedberg A, Forssberg H, Hadders-Algra M. Postural adjustments due to external perturbations during sitting in 1-month-old infants: evidence for the innate origin of direction specificity. Exp Brain Res 2004;157:10–17.

Hein A, Held R. Dissociation of the visual placing response into elicited and guided components. Science 1967;158:390–392.

Heinz F, Hesels K, Breitbach-Faller B, et al. Movement analysis by accelerometery of newborns and infants for the early detection of movement disorders due to infantile cerebral palsy. Med Biol Eng Comput 2010;48:765–772.

Heiman CM, Cole WG, Lee DK, Adolph KE. Object interaction and walking: integration of old and new skills in infant development. Infancy 2019;24(4):547–569.

Heitmann DK, Gossman MR, Shaddeau SA, et al. Balance performance and step width in non-institutionalized elderly female fallers and nonfallers. Phys Ther 1989;69:923–931.

Helbostad JL. Treadmill training and/or body weight support may not improve walking ability following stroke: commentary. Aust J Physiol 2003;49:278.

Held JM. Recovery of function after brain damage: theoretical implications for therapeutic intervention. In: Carr JH, Shepherd RB, Gordon J, et al., eds. Movement sciences: foundations for physical therapy in rehabilitation. Rockville, MD: Aspen, 1987: 155–177.

Held JM. Environmental enrichment enhances sparing and recovery of function following brain damage. Neurol Rep 1998;22:74–78.

Held JM, Gordon F, Gentile AM. Environmental influences on locomotor recovery following cortical lesions in rats. Behav Neurosci 1985;99:678–690.

Held JPO, Klaassen B, Eenhoorn A, van Beijnum BF, Buurke JH, Veltink PH, Luft AR. Inertial sensor measurements of upper-limb kinematics in stroke patients in clinic and home environment. Front Bioeng Biotechnol 2018;6:27. doi: 10.3389/fbioe.2018.00027.

Held R, Hein A. Movement-produced stimulation in the development of visually guided behavior. J Comp Physiol Psychol 1963;56:872–876.

Hellstrom K, Lindmark B, Wahlberg B, et al. Self-efficacy in relation to impairments and activities of daily living disability in elderly patients with stroke: a prospective investigation. J Rehabil Med 2003;35:202–207.

Henderson SE, Sugden DA. Movement Assessment Battery for Children (Movement ABC), 2nd ed. Upper Saddle River, NJ: Pearson, 2007.

Henry SM, Fung J, Horak FB. EMG responses to maintain stance during multidirectional surface translations. J Neurophysiol 1998;80:1939–1950.

Herbison GJ, Jaweed MM, Ditunno JF. Contractile properties of reinnervating skeletal muscle in the rat. Arch Phys Med Rehabil 1981;62:35–39.

Herdman SJ, ed. Vestibular rehabilitation, 3rd ed. Philadelphia, PA: FA Davis, 2007.

Herdman SJ. Vestibular rehabilitation. Curr Opin Neurol 2013;26(1):96–101. doi: 10.1097/WCO.0b013e32835c5ec4.

Herdman SJ, Schubert MC, Tusa RJ. Role of central preprogramming in dynamic visual acuity with vestibular loss. Arch Otolaryngol Head Neck Surg 2001;127:1205–1210.

Herman R. Augmented sensory feedback in control of limb movement. In: Fields WS, ed. Neural organization and its relevance to prosthetics. New York: Intercontinental Medical Book, 1973.

Herman R, Cook T, Cozzens B, et al. Control of postural reactions in man: the initiation of gait. In: Stein RB, Pearson KG, Smith RS, et al., eds. Control of posture and locomotion. New York: Plenum, 1973:363–388.

Herman S, Grillner R, Ralston HJ, et al., eds. Neural control of locomotion. New York: Plenum, 1976:675–705.

Herman T, Inbar-Borovsky N, Brozgol M, et al. The Dynamic Gait Index in healthy older adults: the role of stair climbing, fear of falling and gender. Gait Posture 2009;29:237–241.

Hermsdörfer J, Blankenfeld H, Goldenberg G. The dependence of ipsilesional aiming deficits on task demands, lesioned hemisphere, and apraxia. Neuropsychologia 2003;41:1628–1643.

Hermsdorfer J, Laimgruber K, Kerkhoff G, et al. Effects of unilateral brain damage on grip selection, coordination, and kinematics of ipsilesional prehension. Exp Brain Res 1999;128(1–2):41–51.

Hess JA, Woollacott M. Effect of high-intensity strength-training on functional measures of balance ability in balance-impaired older adults. J Manipulative Physiol Ther 2005;28:582–590.

Hess JA, Woollacott M, Shivitz N. Ankle force and rate of force production increase following high intensity strength training in frail older adults. Aging Clin Exp Res 2006;18:107–115.

Hesse S, Bertelt C, Jahnke MT, et al. Treadmill training with partial body weight support compared with physiotherapy in non ambulatory hemiparetic patients. Stroke 1995;26:976–981.

Hesse S, Bertelt C, Schaffrin A, et al. Restoration of gait in non ambulatory hemiparetic patients by treadmill training with partial weight support. Arch Phys Med Rehabil 1994;75:1087–1093.

Hesse S, Konrad M, Uhlenbroch D. Treadmill walking with partial body weight support versus floor walking in hemiparetic subjects. Arch Phys Med Rehabil 1999;80:421–427.

Hesse S, Reiter F, Jahnke M, et al. Asymmetry of gait initiation in hemiparetic stroke subjects. Arch Phys Med Rehabil 1997;78:719–724.

Hesse S, Werner C, Schonhardt EM, et al. Combined transcranial direct current stimulation and robot-assisted arm training in subacute stroke patients: a pilot study. Restor Neurol Neurosci 2007;25(1):9–15.

Hidler J, Nichols D, Pelliccio M, et al. Multicenter randomized clinical trial evaluating the effectiveness of the Lokomat in subacute stroke. Neurorehabil Neural Repair 2009;23:5–13.

Higgens JR, Spaeth RA. Relationship between consistency of movement and environmental conditions. Quest 1979;17:65.

Higginson JS, Zajac FE, Neptune RR, et al. Effect of equinus foot placement and intrinsic muscle response on knee extension during stance. Gait Posture 2006;23:32–36.

Hijmans JM, Geertzen JH, Dijkstra PU, et al. A systematic review of the effects of shoes and other ankle or foot appliances on balance in older people and people with peripheral nervous system disorders. Gait Posture 2007;25:316–323.

Hill K, Ellis P, Bernhardt J, et al. Balance and mobility outcomes for stroke patients: a comprehensive audit. Aust J Physiother 1997;43:173–180.

Hillel I, Gazit E, Nieuwboer A, et al. Is every-day walking in older adults more analogous to dual-task walking or to usual walking? Elucidating the gaps between gait performance in the lab and during 24/7 monitoring. Eur Rev Aging Phys Act 2019;16:6.

Hird JS, Landers DM, Thomas JR, et al. Physical practice is superior to mental practice in enhancing cognitive and motor task performance. J Sport Exerc Psychol 1991;13:281–293.

Hirschfeld H. On the integration of posture, locomotion and voluntary movement in humans: normal and impaired development. Dissertation. Karolinska Institute, Stockholm, 1992.

Hirschfeld H, Forssberg, H. Epigenetic development of postural responses for sitting during infancy. Exp Brain Res 1994;97:528–540.

Hirvensalo M, Rantanen T, Heikkinen E. Mobility difficulties and physical activity as predictors of mortality and loss of independence in the community-living older population. J Am Geriatr Soc 2000;48:493–498.

Himuro N, Abe H, Nishibu H, Seino T, Mori M. Easy-to-use clinical measures of walking ability in children and adolescents with cerebral palsy: a systematic review. Disabil Rehabil 2017;39:957–968.

Hoch JE, Rachwani J, Adolph KE. Where infants go: real-time dynamics of locomotor exploration in crawling and walking infants. Child Dev 2020;91(3):1001–1020.

Hodges PW, Gurfinkel VS, Brumagne S, et al. Coexistence of stability and mobility in postural control: evidence from postural compensation for respiration. Exp Brain Res 2002;144:293–302.

Hoehn MM, Yahr MD. Parkinsonism: onset, progression and mortality. Neurology 1967;17:433–450.

Hoffer MM, Feiwell E, Perry R, et al. Functional ambulation in patients with myelomeningocele. J Bone Joint Surg Am 1973;55:137–148.

Hoffmann T, Glasziou P, Boutron I, et al. Better reporting of interventions: template for intervention description and replication (TIDieR) checklist and guide. BMJ 2014;348:g1687.

Hofmeijer J, Algra A, Kappelle LJ, Van Der Worp HB. Predictors of life-threatening brain edema in middle cerebral artery infarction. Cerebrovasc Dis 2008;25:176–184.

Hogan M. Physical and cognitive activity and exercise for older adults: a review. Int J Aging Hum Dev 2005;60:95–126.

Hogan N, Bizzi E, Mussa-Ivaldi FA, et al. Controlling multijoint motor behavior. Exerc Sport Sci Rev 1987;15:15–90.

Hohtari-Kivimaki U, Salminen M, Vahlberg T, et al. Short Berg Balance

Scale: correlation to static and dynamic balance and applicability among the aged. Aging Clin Exp Res 2012;24:42–46.

Holbein MA, Redfern MS. Functional stability limits while holding loads in various positions. Int J Ind Ergon 1997;19:387–395.

Holbein-Jenny MA, McDermott K, Shaw C, Demchak J. Validity of functional stability limits as a measure of balance in adults aged 23-73 years. Ergonomics 2007;50(5):631–646.

Holden MK, Dettwiler A, Dyar T, et al. Retraining movement in patients with acquired brain injury using a virtual environment. Stud Health Technol Inform 2001;81:192–198.

Holsbeeke L, Ketelaar M, Schoemaker MM, Gorter JW. Capacity, capability, and performance: different constructs or three of a kind? Arch Phys Med Rehabil 2009;90(5):849–855.

Hollands KL, Agnihotri D, Tyson SF. Effects of dual task on turning ability in stroke survivors and older adults. Gait Posture 2014;40:564–569.

Hollands KL, Hollands MA, Zietz D, et al. Kinematics of turning 180 degrees during the timed up and go in stroke survivors with and without falls history. Neurorehabil Neural Repair 2010;24:358–367.

Hollerbach JM. Planning of arm movements. In: Osherson DN, Kosslyn SM, Hollerbach JM, eds. Visual cognition and action: an invitation to cognitive science, vol. 2. Cambridge, MA: MIT Press, 1990:183–211.

Hollman JH, McDade EM, Petersen RC. Normative spatiotemporal gait parameters in older adults. Gait Posture 2011;34(1):111–118.

Holmefur M, Aarts P, Hoare B, et al. Test-retest and alternate forms reliability of the assisting hand assessment. J Rehabil Med 2009;41(11):886–891.

Holmefur MM, Krumlinde-Sundholm L. Psychometric properties of a revised version of the Assisting Hand Assessment (Kids-AHA 5.0). Dev Med Child Neurol 2016;58(6):618–624. doi: 10.1111/dmcn.12939.

Hong SH, Jung SY, Oh HK, Lee SH, Woo YK. Effects of the immobilization of the upper extremities on spatiotemporal gait parameters during walking in stroke patients: a preliminary study. Biomed Res Int 2020;2:6157231. doi: 10.1155/2020/6157231.

Honeycutt CF, Nardelli P, Cope TC, et al. Muscle spindle responses to horizontal support surface perturbation in the anesthetized cat: insights into the role of autogenic feedback in whole body postural control. J Neurophysiol 2012;108(5):1253–1261.

Honeycutt CF, Nichols TR. Disruption of cutaneous feedback alters magnitude but not direction of muscle responses to postural perturbations in the decerebrate cat. Exp Brain Res 2010;203:765–771.

Hong M, Earhart GM. Effects of medication on turning deficits in individuals with Parkinson's disease. J Neurol Phys Ther 2010;34:11–16.

Horak F. Assumptions underlying motor control for neurologic rehabilitation. In: Contemporary management of motor control problems. Proceedings of the II Step Conference. Alexandria, VA: American Physical Therapy Association, 1991:11–27.

Horak F. Clinical measurement of postural control in adults. Phys Ther 1987;67:1881–1885.

Horak FB. Comparison of cerebellar and vestibular loss on scaling of postural responses. In: Brandt T, Paulus IO, Bles W, et al., eds. Disorders of posture and gait. Stuttgart, Germany: George Thieme Verlag, 1990:370–373.

Horak FB. Adaptation of automatic postural responses. In: Bloedel JR, Ebner TJ, Wise SP, eds. The acquisition of motor behavior in vertebrates. Cambridge, MA: MIT Press, 1996:57–85.

Horak FB, Anderson M, Esselman P, et al. The effects of movement velocity, mass displaced and task certainty on associated postural adjustments made by normal and hemiplegic individuals. J Neurol Neurosurg Psychiatry 1984;47:1020–1028.

Horak F, Diener HC. Cerebellar control of postural scaling and central set in stance. J Neurophysiol 1994;72:479–493.

Horak F, Diener HC, Nashner LM. Influence of central set on human postural responses. J Neurophysiol 1989a;62:841–853.

Horak FB, Dimitrova D, Nutt JG. Directional-specific postural instability in subjects with Parkinson's disease. Exp Neurol 2005;193:504–521.

Horak FB, Hlavacka F. Somatosensory loss increases vestibulospinal sensitivity. J Neurophsyiol 2001;86:575–585.

Horak F, Jones-Rycewicz C, Black FO, et al. Effects of vestibular rehabilitation on dizziness and imbalance. Otolaryngol Head Neck Surg 1992a;106:175–180.

Horak FB, Kluzik J, Hlavacka F. Velocity dependence of vestibular information for postural control on tilting surfaces. J Neurophysiol 2016;116:1468–1479.

Horak FB, Macpherson JM. Postural orientation and equilibrium. In: Shepard J, Rowell L, eds. Handbook of physiology, section 12. Exercise: regulation and integration of multiple systems. New York, Oxford University, 1996:255–292.

Horak F, Nashner L. Central programming of postural movements: adaptation to altered support surface configurations. J Neurophysiol 1986;55:1369–1381.

Horak FB, Nashner LM, Diener HC. Postural strategies associated with somatosensory and vestibular loss. Exp Brain Res 1990;82:167–177.

Horak FB, Nutt JG, Nashner LM. Postural inflexibility in parkinsonian subjects. J Neurol Sci 1992b;111:46–58.

Horak F, Shumway-Cook A. Clinical implications of postural control research. In: Duncan P, ed. Balance: proceedings of the APTA Forum. Alexandria, VA: American Physical Therapy Association, 1990:105–111.

Horak F, Shumway-Cook A, Black FO. Are vestibular deficits responsible for developmental disorders in children? Insights Otolaryngol 1988;3:2.

Horak F, Shupert C. The role of the vestibular system in postural control. In: Herdman S, ed. Vestibular rehabilitation. New York: Davis, 1994:22–46.

Horak FB, Shupert CL, Dietz V, et al. Vestibular and somatosensory contributions to responses to head and body displacements in stance. Exp Brain Res 1994;100:93–106.

Horak F, Shupert C, Mirka A. Components of postural dyscontrol in the elderly: a review. Neurobiol Aging 1989;10:727–745.

Horak FB, Wrisley DM, Frank J. The Balance Evaluation Systems test (BESTest) to differentiate balance deficits. Phys Ther 2009;89:484–498.

Hore J, Wild B, Diener HC. Cerebellar dysmetria at the elbow, wrist, and fingers. J Neurophysiol 1991;65:563–571.

Hornby TG, Campbell DD, Kahn JH, et al. Enhanced gait-related improvements after therapist- versus robotic-assisted locomotor training in subjects with chronic stroke: a randomized controlled study. Stroke 2008;39:1786–1792.

Hornby TG, Straube DS, Kinnaird CR, et al. Importance of specificity, amount, and intensity of locomotor training to improve ambulatory function in patients poststroke. Top Stroke Rehabil 2011;18(4):293–307.

Horowitz L, Sharby N. Development of prone extension postures in healthy infants. Phys Ther 1988;68:32–39.

Horslen BC, Murnaghan CD, Inglis JT, Chua R, Carpenter MG. Effects of postural threat on spinal stretch reflexes: evidence for increased muscle spindle sensitivity? J Neurophysiol 2013;110(4):899–906.

Horslen BC, Zaback M, Inglis JT, Blouin JS, Carpenter MG. Increased human stretch reflex dynamic sensitivity with height-induced postural threat. J Physiol 2018;596(21):5251–5265.

Housman SJ, Scott KM, Reinkensmeyer DJ. A randomized controlled trial of gravity-supported, computer-enhanced arm exercise for individuals with severe hemiparesis. Neurorehabil Neural Repair 2009;23(6):505–514.

Houwink A, Steenbergen B, Prange GB, et al. Upper-limb motor control in patients after stroke: attentional demands and the potential beneficial effects of arm support. Hum Mov Sci 2013;32:377–387.

Hovda DA, Feeney DM. Haloperidol blocks amphetamine induced recovery of binocular depth perception after bilateral visual cortex ablation in the cat. Proc West Pharmacol Soc 1985;28:209–211.

Howcroft J, Fehlings D, Zabjek K, et al. Wearable wrist activity monitor as an indicator of functional hand use in children with cerebral palsy. Dev Med Child Neurol 2011;53:1024–1029.

Howe TE, Rochester L, Jackson A, et al. Exercise for improving balance in older people. Cochrane Database Syst Rev 2007;(4):CD004963.

Howes D, Boller F. Simple reaction time: evidence for focal impairment from lesions of the right hemisphere. Brain 1975;98:317–332.

Hoy MG, Zernicke RF. Modulation of limb dynamics in the swing phase of locomotion. J Biomech 1985;18:49–60.

Hoy MG, Zernicke RF. The role of intersegmental dynamics during rapid limb oscillations. J Biomech 1986;19:867–877.

Hoy MG, Zernicke RF, Smith JL. Contrasting roles of inertial and muscle moments at knee and ankle during paw-shake response. J Neurophysiol 1985;54:1282–1294.

Hoyle G. Muscles and their neural control. New York: Wiley, 1983.

Hsieh Y, Hsueh I, Chou Y, et al. Development and validation of a short form of the Fugl-Meyer Motor Scale in patients with stroke. Stroke 2007;38:3052–3054.

Hsieh YW, Wu CY, Lin KC, et al. Dose–response relationship of robot-assisted stroke motor rehabilitation: the impact of initial motor status. Stroke 2012;43:2729–2734.

Hsu WL, Scholz JP, Schöner G, Jeka JJ, Kiemel T. Control and estimation of posture during quiet stance depends on multijoint coordination. J Neurophysiol 2007;97:3024–3035.

Hu M, Woollacott M. Multisensory training of standing balance in older adults. 1. Postural stability and one-leg stance balance. J Gerontol 1994a;49:M52–M61.

Hu M, Woollacott M. Multisensory training of standing balance in older adults. 2. Kinetic and electromyographic postural responses. J Gerontol 1994b;49:M62–M71.

Huang X, Mahoney JM, Lewis MM, et al. Both coordination and symmetry of arm swing are reduced in Parkinson's disease. Gait Posture 2012;35:373–377.

Hubel DH. Eye, brain and vision. New York: Scientific American, 1988.

Hubel DH, Wiesel TN. Receptive fields of single neurones in the cat's striate cortex. J. Physiol Lond 1959;148:574–591.

Hudson CC, Krebs DE. Frontal plane dynamic stability and coordination in subjects with cerebellar degeneration. Exp Brain Res 2000;132:103–113.

Hughes VA, Frontera WR, Wood M, et al. Longitudinal muscle strength changes in older adults: influence of muscle mass, physical activity and health. J Gerontol Biol Sci 2001;56A:B209–B217.

Huijbregts MPJ, Myers AM, Kay TM, et al. Systematic outcome measurement in clinical practice: challenges experienced by physiotherapists. Physiother Can 2002;54:25–36.

Huisinga JM, Filipi ML, Schmid KK, et al. Is there a relationship between fatigue questionnaires and gait mechanics in persons with multiple sclerosis? Arch Phys Med Rehabil 2011;92:1594–1601.

Huisinga JM, Schmid KK, Filipi ML, Stergiou N. Gait mechanics are different between healthy controls and patients with multiple sclerosis. J Appl Biomech 2013;29(3):303–311.

Hulliger M, Nordh E, Thelin AE, et al. The responses of afferent fibers from the glabrous skin of the hand during voluntary finger movements in man. J Physiol 1979;291:233–249.

Hung YC, Spingarn A. Whole body organization during a symmetric bimanual pick up task for children with unilateral cerebral palsy. Gait Posture 2018;64:38–42.

Hunnicutt JL, Gregory CM, Sciences H. Skeletal muscle changes following stroke: a systematic review and comparison to healthy individuals. Top Stroke Rehabil 2017;24:463–471.

Humm JL, Kozlowski DA, Bland ST, et al. Progressive expansion of brain injury by extreme behavior pressure: is glutamate involved? Exp Neurol 1999;157:349–358.

Hummel F, Celnik P, Giraux P, et al. Effects of non-invasive cortical stimulation on skilled motor function in chronic stroke. Brain 2005;128:490–499.

Humphrey NK, Weiskrantz L. Vision in monkeys after removal of the striate cortex. Nature 1969;215:595–597.

Hung YC, Brandão MB, Gordon AM. Structured skill practice during intensive bimanual training leads to better trunk and arm control than unstructured practice in children with unilateral spastic cerebral palsy.

Res Dev Disabil 2017;60:65–76. doi: 10.1016/j.ridd.2016.11.012.

Hung Y-C, Ferre CL, Gordon AM. Improvements in kinematic performance after home-based bimanual intensive training for children with unilateral cerebral palsy. Phys Occup Ther Pediatr 2018;38(4):370–381. doi: 10.1080/01942638.2017.1337663.

Hung Y-C, Meredith GS, Gill SV. Influence of dual task constraints during walking for children. Gait Posture 2013 Jul;38(3):450–454.

Hung Y-C, Spingarn A, Friel KM, Gordon AM. Intensive unimanual training leads to better reaching and head control than bimanual training in children with unilateral cerebral palsy. Phys Occup Ther Pediatr 2020;40(5):491–505. doi: 10.1080/01942638.2020.1712513.

Hutchinson KJ, Gómez-Pinilla F, Crowe MJ, Ying Z, Basso DM. Three exercise paradigms differentially improve sensory recovery after spinal cord contusion in rats. Brain 2004:127;1403–1414.

Huxham F, Baker R, Morris ME, et al. Head and trunk rotation during walking turns in Parkinson's disease. Mov Disord 2008;23:1391–1397.

Huxhold O, Li S-C, Schmiedek F, et al. Dual-tasking postural control: aging and the effects of cognitive demand in conjunction with focus of attention. Brain Res Bull 2006;69:294–305.

Hwang I, Tung L, Yang J, et al. Electromyographic analyses of global synkinsesis in the paretic upper limb after stroke. Phys Ther 2005;85:755–765.

Hyndman D, Ashburn A. People with stroke living in the community: attention deficits, balance, ADL ability, and falls. Disabil Rehabil 2003;25:817–822.

Hyndman D, Ashburn A. "Stops Walking When Talking" as a predictor of falls in people with stroke living in the community. J Neurol Neurosurg Psychiatry 2004;75:994–997.

Hyndman D, Ashburn A, Yardley L, et al. Interference between balance, gait and cognitive task performance among people with stroke living in the community. Dis Rehabil 2006;28:849–856.

Hyndman D, Pickering RM, Ashburn A. Reduced sway during dual task balance performance among people with stroke at 6 and 12 months after discharge from hospital. Neurorehabil Neural Repair 2009;23:847–854.

I

Ikai T, Kamikubo T, Takehara I, et al. Dynamic postural control in patients with hemiparesis. Am J Phys Med Rehabil 2003;82:463–469.

Imms FJ, Edholm OG. Studies of gait and mobility in the elderly. Age Ageing 1981;10:147–156.

Inacio M, Creath R, Rogers MW. Effects of aging on hip abductor-adductor neuromuscular and mechanical performance during the weight transfer phase of lateral protective stepping. J Biomech 2019;82:244–250.

Inglin B, Woollacott MH. Age-related changes in anticipatory postural adjustments associated with arm movements. J Gerontol 1988;43:M105–M113.

Inglis JT, Horak FB, Shupert CL, et al. The importance of somatosensory information in triggering and scaling automatic postural responses in humans. Exp Brain Res 1994;101:159–164.

Ingvarsson PE, Gordon AM, Forssberg H. Coordination of manipulative forces in Parkinson's disease. Exp Neurol 1997;145:489–501.

Inkster LM, Eng JJ. Postural control during a sit-to-stand task in individuals with mild Parkinson's disease. Exp Brain Res 2004;154:33–38.

Inkster LM, Eng JJ, MacIntyre DL, et al. Leg muscle strength is reduced in Parkinson's disease and relates to the ability to rise from a chair. Mov Disord 2003;18:157–162.

Inman VT, Ralston H, Todd F. Human walking. Baltimore, MD: Lippincott Williams & Wilkins, 1981.

Inness EL, Mansfield A, Lakhani B, et al. Impaired reactive stepping among patients ready for discharge from inpatient stroke rehabilitation. Phys Ther 2014;94:1755–1764.

Inoue A, Iwasaki S, Ushio M, et al. Effect of vestibular dysfunction on the development of gross motor function in children with profound hearing loss. Audiol Neurootol 2013;18(3):143–151.

Isa T, Ohki Y, Alstermark B, Pettersson LG, Sasaki S. Direct and indirect cortico- motoneuronal pathways and control of hand/arm movements. Physiology 2007;22:145–152.

Isa T, Ohki Y, Seki K, Alstermark B. Properties of propriospinal neurons in the C3-C4 segments mediating disynaptic pyramidal excitation to forelimb motoneurons in the macaque monkey. J Neurophysiol 2006;95:3674–3685.

Isles RC, Choy NL, Steer M, et al. Normal values of balance tests in women aged 20–80. J Am Geriatr Soc 2004;52:1367–1372.

Israely S, Carmeli E. Handwriting performance versus arm forward reach and grasp abilities among post-stroke patients, a case-control study. Top Stroke Rehabil 2017;24(1):5–11. doi: 10.1080/10749357.2016.1183383.

Ito M. The cerebellum and neural control. New York: Raven, 1984.

Ito M, Araki A, Tanaka H, et al. Muscle histopathology in spastic cerebral palsy. Brain Dev 1996;18:299–303.

Ivanenko YP, Dominici N, Cappellini C, et al. Development of pendulum mechanism and kinematic coordination from the first unsupported steps in toddlers. J Exp Biol 2004;207:3797–3810.

Ivanenko YP, Dominici N, Cappellini G, et al. Kinematics in newly walking toddlers does not depend upon postural stability. J Neurophysiol 2005;94:754–763.

Ivanenko Y, Gurfinkel VS. Human postural control. Front Neurosci 2018;12(171):1–9.

Ivry RB, Keele SW. Timing functions of the cerebellum. J Cogn Neurosci 1989;1:136–152.

Iyengar V, Santos MJ, Ko M, et al. Grip force control in individuals with multiple sclerosis. Neurorehabil Neural Repair 2009;23:855–861.

J

Jackson RT, Epstein CM, De L'Amme WR. Abnormalities in posturography and estimations of visual vertical and horizontal in multiple sclerosis. Am J Otol 1995;16:88–93.

Jacobs JV. A review of stairway falls and stair negotiation: lessons learned and future needs to reduce injury. Gait Posture 2016;49:159–167.

Jacobs JV, Horak FB, Van Tran K, et al. An alternative clinical postural stability test for patients with Parkinson's disease. J Neurol 2006;253:1404–1413.

Jacobs JV, Nutt JG, Carlson-Kuhta P, et al. Knee trembling during freezing of gait represents multiple anticipatory postural adjustments. Exp Neurol 2009;215:334–341.

Jamon M. The development of vestibular system and related functions in mammals: impact of gravity. Front Integr Neurosci 2014;8:11.

Jang SH, Jang WH. Change of the corticospinal tract in the unaffected hemisphere by change of the dominant hand following stroke: a cohort study. Medicine (Baltimore) 2016;95(6):e2620. doi: 10.1097/MD.0000000000002620.

Jansen CW, Niebuhr BR, Coussirat DJ, et al. Hand force of men and women over 65 years of age as measured by maximum pinch and grip force. J Aging Phys Act 2008;16(1):24–41.

Jayakaran P, Mitchell L, Johnson GM. Peripheral sensory information and postural control in children with strabismus. Gait Posture 2018;65:197–202.

Jeannerod M. The timing of natural prehension movements. J Motor Behav 1984;16:235–254.

Jeannerod M. The formation of finger grip during prehension: a cortically mediated visuomotor pattern. Behav Brain Res 1986;19:99–116.

Jeannerod M. Reaching and grasping: parallel specification of visuomotor channels. In: Handbook of perception and action, vol. 2. London, UK: Academic Press, 1996:405–460.

Jeannerod M. The neural and behavioral organization of goal-directed movements. Oxford, UK: Clarendon Press, 1990.

Jeannerod M, Arbib MA, Rizzolatti G, et al. Grasping objects: the cortical mechanisms of visuomotor transformation. Trends Neurosci 1995;18:314–320.

Jebsen RH, Taylor N, Trieschmann RB, et al. An objective and standard test of hand function. Arch Phys Med Rehabil 1969;50:311–319.

Jedlinsky BP, McCarthy CF, Michel TH. Validating pediatric pain measurement: sensory and affective components. Ped Phys Ther 1999;11:83–88.

Jeka JJ. Light touch contact as a balance aid. Phys Ther 1997;77:477–487.

Jeka JJ, Easton RD, Bentzen BL, et al. Haptic cues for orientation and postural control in sighted and blind individuals. Percept Psychophys 1996;58:409–423.

Jeka JJ, Lackner JR. Fingertip contact influences human postural control. Exp Brain Res 1994;100:495–502.

Jeka JJ, Lackner JR. The role of haptic cues from rough and slippery surfaces in human postural control. Exp Brain Res 1995;103:267–276.

Jeka J, Oie KS, Kiemel T. Multisensory information for human postural control: integrating touch and vision. Exp Brain Res 2000;134:107–125.

Jellinger KA. Neuropathology and pathogenesis of extrapyramidal movement disorders: a critical update. II. Hyperkinetic Disorders. J Neural Transm 2019;126: 997–1027.

Jellinger KA. Neuropathology of sporadic Parkinsons disease: evaluation and changes of concepts. Mov Disord 2012;27:8–30.

Jenkins WM, Merzenich MM. Reorganization of neocortical representations after brain injury: a neurophysiological model of the bases of recovery from stroke. Progr Brain Res 1987;71:249–266.

Jenkins, WM, Merzenich MM, Och MT, et al. Functional reorganization of primary somatosensory cortex in adult owl monkeys after behaviorally controlled tactile stimulation. J Neurophysiol 1990;63:82–104.

Jensen JL, Bothner KE, Woollacott MH. Balance control: the scaling of the kinetic response to accommodate increasing perturbation magnitudes. J Sport Exerc Psychol 1996;18:S45.

Jensen P, Jensen NJ, Terkildsen CU, Choi JT, Nielsen JB, Geertsen SS. Increased central common drive to ankle plantar flexor and dorsiflexor muscles during visually guided gait. Physiol Rep 2018;6(3):e13598.

Jensen JL, Thelen E, Ulrich BD, et al. Adaptive dynamics of the leg movement patterns in human infants: age-related differences in limb control. J Motor Behav 1995;27:366–374.

Jessell TM, Sanes JR. Differentiation and survival of nerve cells. In: Kandel ER, Schwartz JH, Jessell TM, Siegelbaum SA, Hudspeth AJ, eds. Principles of neural science, 5th ed. New York, NY: McGraw-Hill, 2013:2859–2906.

Jesus ST, Hoenig H. Postacute rehabilitation quality of care: toward a shared conceptual framework. Arch Phys Med Rehabil 2015;96:960–969.

Jethwa A, Mink J, Macarthur C, Knights S, Fehlings T, Fehlings D. Development of the Hypertonia Assessment Tool (HAT): a discriminative tool for hypertonia in children. Dev Med Child Neurol 2010;52:83–87.

Jette AM. Physical disablement concepts for physical therapy research and practice. Phys Ther 1994;74:380–386.

Jette AM. Assessing disability in studies on physical activity. Am J Prev Med 2003;25(3 Suppl 2):122–128.

Jette AM, Assmann SF, Rooks D, et al. Inter-relationships among disablement concepts. J Geron Med Sci 1998;20:M395–M404.

Jette DU, Bacon K, Batty C, et al. Evidence-based practice: beliefs, attitudes, knowledge, and behaviors of physical therapists. Phys Ther 2003;83:786–805.

Jette AM, Haley SM, Coster WJ, et al. Late life function and disability instrument: II. Development and evaluation of the function component. J Gerontol A Biol Sci Med Sci 2002;57A:M209–M216.

Jette AM, Haley SM, Coster WJ, et al. Late life function and disability instrument: I. development and evaluation of the disability component. J Gerontol A Biol Sci Med Sci 2002;57:209–216.

Jette DU, Stilphen M, Ranganathan VK, et al. Validity of the AM-PAC "6-Clicks" inpatient daily activity and basic mobility short forms. Phys Ther 2014;94:379–391.

Ji SG, Kim MK. The effects of mirror therapy on the gait of subacute stroke patients: a randomized controlled trial. Clin Rehabil 2015;29:348–354.

Jinnah HA, Factor SA. Diagnosis and treatment of dystonia. Neurol Clin 2015;33:77–100.

Jims C. Foot placement pattern, an aid in gait training: suggestions from the field. Phys Ther 1977;57:286.

Jo HJ, Maenza C, Good DC, Huang X, Park J, Sainburg RL, Latash ML.

Effects of unilateral stroke on multi-finger synergies and their feed-forward adjustments. Neuroscience 2016;319:194–205.

Johansson BB. Brain plasticity in health and disease. Keio J Med 2004;53:231–246.

Johansson RS. Sensory control of dexterous manipulation in humans. In: Wing AM, Haggard P, Flanagan J, eds. Hand and brain: the neurophysiology and psychology of hand movements. New York: Academic Press, 1996:381–414.

Johansson RS, Edin BB. Neural control of manipulation and grasp. In: Forssberg H, Hirschfeld H, eds. Movement disorders in children. Basel, Switzerland: Karger, 1992:107–112.

Johansson S, Ytterberg C, Claesson IM, et al. High concurrent presence of disability in multiple sclerosis. Associations with perceived health. J Neurol 2007;254:767–773.

Johnson J, Rodriguez MA, Snih SA. Life space mobility in the elderly: current perspectives. Clin Interv Aging 2020;15:1665–1674.

Johnson GR. Outcome measures in spasticity. Eur J Neurol 2002;9:10–16.

Johnson JK, Fritz JM, Brooke BS, et al. Physical function in the hospital is associated with patient-centered outcomes in an inpatient rehabilitation facility. Phys Ther 2020;100:1237–1248.

Johnson LB, Sumner S, Duong T, et al. Validity and reliability of smartphone magnetometer-based goniometer evaluation of shoulder abduction: a pilot study. Man Ther 2015. pii: S1356-689X(15)00052-1 [Epub ahead of print].

Johnston MV, Goverover Y, Dijkers M. Community activities and individual's satisfaction with them: quality of life in the first year after traumatic brain injury. Arch PMR 2005;86:735–745.

Johnston M, Nissim EN, Wood K, et al. Objective and subjective handicap following spinal cord injury: interrelationships and predictors. J Spinal Cord Med 2002;25:11–22.

Johnston TE, Watson KE, Ross SA, et al. Effects of a supported speed treadmill training exercise program on impairment and function for children with cerebral palsy. Dev Med Child Neurol 2011;53:742–750.

Jongbloed-Pereboom M, Nijhuis-van der Sanden MW, Steenbergen B. Norm scores of the box and block test for children ages 3–10 years. Am J Occup Ther 2013;67(3):312–318. doi: 10.5014/ajot.2013.006643.

Jonkers I, Delp S, Patten C. Capacity to increase walking speed is limited by impaired hip and ankle power generation in lower functioning persons post stroke. Gait Posture 2009;29:129–137.

Jonsdottir J, Cattaneo D. Reliability and validity of the Dynamic Gait Index in persons with chronic stroke. Arch Phys Med Rehabil 2007;88:1410–1415.

Jordan T, Rabbitt P. Response times to stimuli of increasing complexity as a function of ageing. Br J Psychol 1977;68:189–201.

Jørgensen L, Crabtree NJ, Reeve J, et al. Ambulatory level and asymmetrical weight bearing after stroke affects bone loss in the upper and lower part of the femoral neck differently: bone adaptation after decreased mechanical loading. Bone 2000;27:701–707.

Jouen F. Titres et travaux en vue de l'habilitation a diriger des recherches. State doctoral thesis, Universite Paris IV Paris, 1993:104.Jouen F, Lepecq J-C, Gapenne O, et al. Optic flow sensitivity in neonates. Infant Behav Dev 2000;23:271–284.

Judge JO, Underwood M, Gennosa T. Exercise to improve gait velocity. Arch Phys Med Rehabil 1993;74:400–406.

Judge J, Whipple R, Wolfson L. Effects of resistive and balance exercises on isokinetic strength in older persons. J Am Geriatr Soc 1994;42:937–946.

Juravle G, Colino FL, Meleqi X, Binsted G, Farnè A. Vision facilitates tactile perception when grasping an object. Sci Rep 2018;8:1–10.

Juvin L, Simmers J, Morin D. Propriospinal circuitry underlying interlimb coordination in mammalian quadrupedal locomotion. J Neurosci 2005;25(25):6025–6035.

K

Kaas JH, Florence SL, Jain N. Reorganization of sensory systems of primates after injury. Neuroscientist 1997;3:123–130.

Kabat H, Knott M. Proprioceptive facilitation therapy for paralysis. Physiotherapy 1954;40:171–176.

Kafri M, Laufer Y. Therapeutic effects of functional electrical stimulation on gait in individuals post-stroke. Ann Biomed Eng 2015;43:451–466.

Kajrolkar R, Yang F, Pai YC, et al. Dynamic stability and compensatory stepping responses during anterior gait slip perturbations in people with chronic hemiparetic stroke. J Biomech 2014;47:2751–2758.

Kalisch T, Ragert P, Schwenkreis P, et al. Impaired tactile acuity in old age is accompanied by enlarged hand representations in somatosensory cortex. Cereb Cortex 2009;19:1530–1538.

Kallin K, Gustafson Y, Sandman PO, et al. Factors associated with falls among older, cognitively impaired people in geriatric care settings: a population based study. Am J Geriatr Psychiatry 2005;13:501–509.

Kalron A, Nitzani D, Magalashvili D, et al. A personalized, intense physical rehabilitation program improves walking in people with multiple sclerosis presenting with different levels of disability: a retrospective cohort. BMC Neurol 2015;15:21.

Kamble N, Pal PK. Tremor syndromes: a review. Neurol India 2018;66:S36–S47.

Kaminski T, Bock C, Gentile AM. The coordination between trunk and arm motion during pointing movements. Exp Brain Res 1995;106:457–466.

Kamm K, Thelen E, Jensen J. A dynamical systems approach to motor development: In: Rothstein JM, ed. Movement science. Alexandria, VA: American Physical Therapy Association, 1991:11–23.

Kamble N, Pal PK. Tremor syndromes: a review. Neurology India 2018;66:36–47.

Kang TW, Oh DW, Lee JH, Cynn HS. Effects of integrating rhythmic arm swing into robot-assisted walking in patients with subacute stroke: a randomized controlled pilot study. Int J Rehabil Res 2018;41:57–62.

Kang K, Thaut MH. Musical neglect training for chronic persistent unilateral visual neglect post-stroke. Front Neurol 2019;10:474. doi: 10.3389/fneur.2019.00474.

Kandel ER. Cellular basis of behavior: an introduction to behavioral neurobiology. San Francisco, CA: Freeman, 1976.

Kandel ER. Genes, nerve cells, and the remembrance of things past. J Neuropsychiatry 1989;1:103–125.

Kandel ER. Cellular mechanisms of learning and the biological basis of individuality. In: Kandel ER, Schwartz JH, Jessell TM, eds. Principles of neural science, 4th ed. New York: McGraw-Hill, 2000a:1247–1279.

Kandel ER. The brain and behavior. In: Kandel ER, Schwartz JH, Jessell TM, eds. Principles of neural science, 4th ed. New York: McGraw-Hill, 2000b:5–17.

Kandel ER, Kupfermann I, Iversen S. Learning and memory. In: Kandel ER, Schwartz JH, Jessell TM, eds. Principles of neural science, 4th ed. New York: McGraw-Hill, 2000a:1231.

Kandel ER, Schwartz JH. Molecular biology of learning: modulation of transmitter release. Science 1982;218:433–443.

Kandel ER, Schwartz JH, Jessell TM, eds. Principles of neuroscience, 3rd ed. New York: Elsevier, 1991.

Kandel ER, Schwartz JH, Jessell TM, eds. Principles of neuroscience, 4th ed. New York: Elsevier, 2000b.

Kandel ER, Schwartz JH, Jessell TM, et al. Principles of neural science, 5th ed. New York: McGraw-Hill, 2013.

Kandel ER, Siegelbaum SA. Cellular mechanisms of implicit memory storage and the biological basis of individuality. In: Kandel ER, Schwartz JH, Jessel TM, et al., eds. Principles of neuroscience, 5th ed. New York: McGraw-Hill, 2013.

Kandel ER, Siegelbaum SA. Synaptic integration. In: Kandel ER, Schwartz JH, Jessell TM, eds. Principles of neural science, 4th ed. New York: McGraw-Hill, 2000:207–228.

Kang J, Martelli D, Vashista V, Martinez-Hernandez I, Kim H, Agrawal SK. Robot-driven downward pelvic pull to improve crouch gait in children with cerebral palsy. Sci Robot 2017,2.1–11.

Kantak SS, Zahedi N, McGrath RL. Task-dependent bimanual coordination after stroke: relationship with sensorimotor impairments. Arch Phys Med Rehabil 2016;97(5):798–806. doi: 10.1016/j.apmr.2016.01.020.

Kaplan CP. The community integration questionnaire with new scoring guidelines: concurrent validity and need for appropriate norms. Brain Inj 2001;15(8):725–731.

Kapteyn TS. Afterthought about the physics and mechanics of postural sway. Agressologie 1973;14:27–35.

Karasik LB, Adolph KE, Tamis-LeMonda CS, et al. Carry on: spontaneous object carrying in 13-month-old crawling and walking infants. Dev Psychol 2012;48(2):389–397.

Karasik D, Demissie S, Cupples A, et al. Disentangling the genetic determinants of human aging: biological age as an alternative to the use of survival measures. J Gerontol Biol Sci 2005;60A:574–587.

Karatas M, Çetin N, Bayramoglu M, Dilek A. Trunk muscle strength in relation to balance and functional disability in unihemispheric stroke patients. Am J Phys Med Rehabil 2004;83:81–87.

Karhula ME, Kanelisto KJ, Ruutiainen J, et al. The activities and participation categories of the ICF Core Sets for multiple sclerosis from the patient perspective. Disabil Rehabil 2013;35(6):492–497.

Karman N, Maryles J, Baker RW, et al. Constraint-induced movement therapy for hemiplegic children with acquired brain injuries. J Head Trauma Rehabil 2003;18(3):259–267.

Karnath HO, Broetz D. Understanding and treating "pusher syndrome." Phys Ther 2003;83:1119–1125.

Karnath HO, Ferber S, Dichgans J. The origin of contraversive pushing: evidence for a second graviceptive system in humans. Neurology 2000;55:1298–304.

Karst GM, Venema DM, Roehrs TG, et al. Center of pressure measures during standing tasks in minimally impaired persons with multiple sclerosis. J Neurol Phys Ther 2005;29:170–180.

Kasahara S, Saito H. The effect of aging on termination of voluntary movement while standing: a study on community-dwelling older adults. Hum Mov Sci 2019;64:347–354.

Katz S, Downs TD, Cash JR, et al. Progress in development of the index of ADL. Gerontologist 1970:20–30.

Katz R, Rondot P. Muscle reaction to passive shortening in normal man. Electroencephalogr Clin Neurophysiol 1978;45:90–99.

Katz RT, Rovai GP, Brait C, et al. Objective quantification of spastic hypertonia: correlation with clinical findings. Arch Phys Med Rehabil 1992;73:339–347.

Katz R, Rymer Z. Spastic hypertonia: mechanisms and measurement. Arch Phys Med Rehabil 1989;70:144–155.

Katz-Leurer M, Fisher I, Neeb M, et al. Reliability and validity of the modified functional reach test at the sub-acute stage post-stroke. Disabil Rehabil 2009;31:243–248.

Katzman WB, Sellmeyer DE, Stewart AL, et al. Changes in flexed posture, musculoskeletal impairments, and physical performance after group exercise in community-dwelling older women. Arch Phys Med Rehabil 2007;88:192–199.

Kautz SA, Patten C. Interlimb influences on paretic leg function in poststroke hemiparesis. J Neurophysiol 2005;93(5):2460–2473.

Kavounoudias A, Gilhodes JC, Roll R, et al. From balance regulation to body orientation: two goals for muscle proprioceptive information processing? Exp Brain Res 1999;124:80–88.

Kavounoudias A, Roll R, Roll JP. Foot sole and ankle muscle inputs contribute jointly to human erect posture regulation. J Physiol 2001;532:869–878.

Kawamura K, Tokuhiro A, Takechi H. Gait analysis of slope walking: a study on step length, stride width, time factors and deviation in the center of pressure. Acta Med Okayama 1991;45:179–184.

Kawato M. Internal models for motor control and trajectory planning. Curr Opin Neurobiol 1999;9:718–727.

Kay H. Some experiments on adult learning. In Old Age in the Modern World: Report of the third Congress of the International Association of Gerontology, London, UK 1954:259–267. Edinburgh: Livingstone, 1955.

Kay H. The effects of position in a display upon problem solving. Quart J Exper Psychol 1954;6:155–169.

Kazennikov O, Perrig S, Wiesendanger M. Kinematics of a coordinated goal-directed bimanual task. Behav Brain Res 2002;134(1–2):83–91.

Kearney K, Gentile AM. Prehension in young children with Down syndrome. Acta Psychol (Amst) 2003;112(1):3–16.

Keefe BD, Suray PA, Watt SJ. A margin for error in grasping: hand pre-shaping takes into account task-dependent changes in the probability of errors. Exp Brain Res 2019;237:1063–1075.

Keele S. Movement control in skilled motor performance. Psychol Bull 1968;70:387–403.

Keele SW. Behavioral analysis of movement. In: Brooks VB, ed. Handbook of physiology: I. The nervous system, vol. 2. Motor control, part 2. Baltimore, MD: Lippincott Williams & Wilkins, 1981:1391–1414.

Keele SW. Motor control. In: Kaufman L, Thomas J, Boff K, eds. Handbook of perception and performance. New York: Wiley, 1986:1–30.

Keele S, Ivry R. Does the cerebellum provide a common computation for diverse tasks? A timing hypothesis. In: Diamond A, ed. Developmental and neural bases of higher cognitive function. New York: New York Academy of Sciences, 1990:179–207.

Keele SW, Posner MI. Processing visual feedback in rapid movement. J Exp Psychol 1968;77:155–158.

Keenan MA, Perry J, Jordan C. Factors affecting balance and ambulation following stroke. Clin Orth Rel Res 1984;182:165–171.

Keith RA, Granger CV, Hamilton BB, et al. The functional independence measure: a new tool for rehabilitation. In: Eisenberg MG, Grzesiak RC, eds. Advances in clinical rehabilitation, vol. 1. New York: Springer Verlag, 1987:6–18.

Kelly VE, Bastian AJ. Antiparkinson medications improve agonist activation but not antagonist inhibition during sequential reaching movements. Mov Disord 2005;20:694–704.

Kelly VE, Hyngstrom AS, Rundle MM, et al. Interaction of levodopa and cues on voluntary reaching in Parkinson's disease. Mov Disord 2002;17(1):28–44.

Kelso JAS, Holt KG. Exploring a vibratory systems analysis of human movement production. J Neurophysiol 1980;43:1183–1196.

Kelso JA, Holt KG, Rubin P, et al. Patterns of human interlimb coordination emerge from the properties of non-linear, limit cycle oscillatory processes: theory and data. J Motor Behav 1981;13:226–261.

Kelso JAS, Southard DL, Goodman D. On the coordination of two-handed movements. J Exp Psychol Hum Percept 1979;5:229–238.

Kelso JAS, Tuller B. A dynamical basis for action systems. In: Gazanniga MS, ed. Handbook of cognitive neuroscience. New York: Plenum, 1984:321–356.

Kembhavi G, Darrah J, Magill-Evans J. Using the Berg Balance Scale to distinguish balance abilities in children with cerebral palsy. Pediatr Phys Ther 2002;14:92–99.

Kendall FP. Muscles: Testing and function with posture and pain. Baltimore, MD: Lippincott Williams & Wilkins, 2005.

Kendall FP, Kendall EM, Provance PG, Rodgers M, Romani W. Muscles: testing and function, with posture and pain, 5th ed. Baltimore, MD: Wolters Kluwer, 2014.

Kendall FP, McCreary EK. Muscles: testing and function, 3rd ed. Baltimore, MD: Lippincott Williams & Wilkins, 1983.

Kennard MA. Cortical reorganization of motor function: studies on a series of monkeys of various ages from infancy to maturity. Arch Neurol Psychiatr 1942;48:227–240.

Kennard MA. Relation of age to motor impairment in man and in subhuman primates. Arch Neurol Psychiatry 1940;44:377–398.

Kenny RA, Rubenstein LZ, Tinetti ME, et al. Summary of the updated American Geriatrics Society/British Geriatrics Society clinical practice guideline for prevention of falls in older persons. J Am Geriatr Soc 2011;59(1):148–157.

Kenshalo DR. Aging effects on cutaneous and kinesthetic sensibilities. In: Han SS, Coons DH, eds. Special senses in aging. Ann Arbor, MI: University of Michigan, 1979.

Kent JA, Sommerfeld JH, Mukherjee M, Takahashi KZ, Stergiou N. Locomotor patterns change over time during walking on an uneven surface. J Exp Biol 2019;222(Pt 14).

Keogh J, Morrison S, Barrett R. Age-related differences in inter-digit coupling during finger pinching. Eur J Appl Physol 2006;97:76–88.

Keogh J, Morrison S, Barrett R. Strength training improves the tri-digit finger-pinch force control of older adults. Arch Phys Med Rehabil 2007;88:1055–1063.

Kepple T, Siegel KL, Stanhope SJ. Relative contributions of the lower extremity joint moments to forward progression and support during gait. Gait Posture 1997;6:1–8.

Kerkhoff G, Schenk T. Rehabilitation of neglect: an update. Neuropsychologia 2012;50:1072–1079.

Kerns K, Mateer CA. Walking and chewing gum: the impact of attentional capacity on everyday activities. In: Sbordone RJ, Long CJ, eds. Ecological validity of neuropsychological testing. Delray Beach, FL: GR Press, 1996.

Kerr R. Movement control and maturation in elementary-grade children. Percept Motor Skills 1975;41:151–154.

Kerr R, Booth B. Skill acquisition in elementary school children and schema theory. In: Landers DM, Christina RW, eds. Psychology of motor behavior and sport, vol. 2. Champaign, IL: Human Kinetics, 1977.

Kerr B, Condon SM, McDonald LA. Cognitive spatial processing and the regulation of posture. J Exp Psychol 1985;11:617–622.

Kerrigan DC, Frates EP, Rogan S, Riley PO. Hip hiking and circumduction: quantitative definitions. Am J Phys Med Rehabil 2000;79(3):247–252. doi: 10.1097/00002060-200005000-00006.

Kerschensteiner M, Bareyre FM, Buddeberg BS, et al. Remodeling of axonal connections contributes to recovery in an animal model of multiple sclerosis. J Exp Med 2004;200(8):1027–1038.

Kerse N, Parag V, Feigin VL, et al. Falls after stroke: results from the Auckland regional Community Stroke (ARCOS) study, 2002 to 2003. Stroke 2008;39:1890–1893.

Kesar TM, Perumal R, Reisman DS, et al. Functional electrical stimulation of ankle plantarflexor and dorsiflexor muscles: effects on poststroke gait. Stroke 2009;40:3821–3827.

Kessler RM, Hertling D. Management of common musculoskeletal disorders. Philadelphia, PA: Harper & Row, 1983.

Ketelaar M, Vermeet A, Helders P. Functional motor abilities of children with CP: a systematic literature review of assessment measures. Clin Rehabil 1998;12:369–380.

Kim J, Chung Y, Kim Y, et al. Functional electrical stimulation applied to gluteus medius and tibialis anterior corresponding gait cycle for stroke. Gait Posture 2012a;36:65–67.

Kim CM, Eng JJ. The relationship of lower extremity muscle torque to locomotor performance in people with stroke. Phys Ther 2003;83:49–57.

Kim GY, Han MR, Lee HG. Effect of dual-task rehabilitative training on cognitive and motor function of stroke patients. J Phys Ther Sci 2014;26:1–6.

Kim MY, Kim JH, Lee JU, et al. The effects of functional electrical stimulation on balance of stroke patients in the standing posture. J Phys Ther Sci 2012b;24:77–81.

Kim S, Nussbaum MA, Mokhlespour Esfahani MI, Alemi MM, Jia B, Rashedi E. Assessing the influence of a passive, upper extremity exoskeletal vest for tasks requiring arm elevation: Part II—"Unexpected" effects on shoulder motion, balance, and spine loading. Appl Ergon 2018;70:323–330.

King M, Hale L, Pekkari A, et al. An affordable, computerized, table-based exercise system for stroke survivors. Disabil Rehabil Assist Technol 2010;5:288–293.

King LA, Horak FB. Lateral stepping for postural correction in Parkinson's disease. Arch Phys Med Rehabil 2008;89:492–499.

King G, Imms C, Stewart D, Freeman M, Nguyen T. A transactional framework for pediatric rehabilitation: shifting the focus to situated contexts, transactional processes, and adaptive developmental outcomes. Disabil Rehabil 2018;40:1829–1841.

King G, Law M, King S, et al. Children's Assessment of Participation and Enjoyment (CAPE) and Preferences for Activities of Children (PAC). San Antonio, TX: Harcourt Assessment, 2004.

King GA, Law M, King S, et al. Measuring children's participation in recreation and leisure activities: construct validation of the CAPE and PAC. Child Care Health Dev 2006;33:28–39.

Kingwell K. Informing tactics to combat MS. Nat Rev Neurol 2012;8:589.

Kinoshita H, Francis PR. A comparison of prehension force control in young and elderly individuals. Eur J Appl Physiol Occup Physiol 1996;74:450–460.

Kinsella S, Moran K. Gait pattern categorization of stroke participants with equinus deformity of the foot. Gait Posture 2008;27:144–151.

Kiresuk TJ, Sherman RE. Goal attainment scaling: a general method for evaluating comprehensive community mental health programs. Community Ment Health J 1968;4(6):443–453.

Kirshenbaum N, Riach CL, Starkes JL. Non-linear development of postural control and strategy use in young children: a longitudinal study. Exp Brain Res 2001;140:420–431.

Kitago T, Liang J, Huang VS, et al. Improvement after constraint-induced movement therapy: recovery of normal motor control or task-specific compensation? Neurorehabil Neural Repair 2013;27(2):99–109.

Kitazawa S, Kimura T, Ping-Bo Y. Cerebellar complex spikes encode both destinations and errors in arm movements. Nature 1998;392:494–497.

Klatzky RL, McCloskey B, Doherty S, et al. Knowledge about hand shaping and knowledge about objects. J Motor Behav 1987;19:187–213.

Klassen TD, Semrau JA, Dukelow SP, Bayley MT, Hill MD, Eng JJ. Consumer-based physical activity monitor as a practical way to measure walking intensity during inpatient stroke rehabilitation. Stroke 2017;48:2614–2617.

Kleim JA, Cooper NR, VandenBerg PM. Exercise induces angiogenesis but does not alter movement representations within rat motor cortex. Brain Res 2002;934:1–6.

Kleim JA, Jones TA. Principles of experience-dependent neural plasticity: implications for rehabilitation after brain damage. J Speech Lang Hear Res 2008;51:S225–S239.

Kleim JA, Jones TA, Schallert T. Motor enrichment and the induction of plasticity before or after brain injury. Neurochem Res 2003;28:1757–1769.

Kleim JA, Swain RA, Armstrong K, et al. Selective synaptic plasticity within the cerebellar cortex following complex motor skill learning. Neurobiol Learn Mem 1998;69:274–289.

Kleim JA, Vij K, Ballard DH, et al. Learning dependent synaptic modifications in the cerebellar cortex of the adult rat persist for at least four weeks. J Neurosci 1997;17:717–771.

Kleiner-Fisman G, Herzog J, Fisman DN, et al. Subthalamic nucleus deep brain stimulation: summary and meta-analysis of outcomes. Mov Disord 2006;21:S290–S304.

Klevberg GL, Elvrum AKG, Zucknick M, et al. Development of bimanual performance in young children with cerebral palsy. Dev Med Child Neurol 2018;60:490–497.

Klotz MC, Wolf SI, Heitzmann D, Maier MW, Braatz F, Dreher T. The association of equinus and primary genu recurvatum gait in cerebral palsy. Res Dev Disabil 2014;35(6):1357–1363.

Kluzik J, Horak FB, Peterka RJ. Differences in preferred reference frames for postural orientation shown by after-effects of stance on an inclined surface. Exp Brain Res 2005;162:474–489.

Kluzik J, Peterka RJ, Horak FB. Adaptation of postural orientation to changes in surface inclination. Exp Brain Res 2007;178:1–17.

Knaepen K, Goekint M, Heyman EM, Meeusen R. Neuroplasticity-exercise-induced response of peripheral brain-derived neurotrophic factor: a systematic review of experimental studies in human subjects. Sports Med 2010:40;765–801.

Knarr BA, Reisman DS, Binder-Macleod SA, et al. Understanding compensatory strategies for muscle weakness during gait by simulating activation deficits seen post stroke. Gait Posture 2013;38:270–275.

Knutsson E. An analysis of Parkinsonian gait. Brain 1972:475–486.

Knutsson E. Gait control in hemiparesis. Scand J Rehabil Med 1981;13:101–108.

Knutsson E. Can gait analysis improve gait training in stroke patients? Scand J Rehabil Med Suppl 1994;30:73–80.

Knudsen EI. Fundamental components of attention. Annu Rev Neurosci 2007;30:57–78.

Knutson JS, Harley MY, Hisel TZ, et al. Contralaterally controlled functional electrical stimulation for upper extremity hemiplegia: an early-phase randomized clinical trial in subacute stroke patients. Neurorehabil Neural Repair 2012;26(3):239–246.

Knutson JS, Harley MY, Hisel TZ, Makowski NS, Chae J. Contralaterally controlled functional electrical stimulation for recovery of elbow extension and hand opening after stroke: a pilot case series study. Am J Phys Med Rehabil 2014;93(6):528–539. doi: 10.1097/PHM.0000000000000066.

Knutsson E, Richards C. Different types of disturbed motor control in gait of hemiparetic patients. Brain 1979;102:405–430.

Ko M, Bishop MD, Behrman AL. Effects of limb loading on gait initiation in persons with moderate hemiparesis. Top Stroke Rehabil 2011;18:258–268.

Ko MS, Sim YJ, Kim DH, Jeon HS. Effects of three weeks of whole-body vibration training on joint-position sense, balance, and gait in children with cerebral palsy: A randomized controlled study. Physiother Canada 2016;68:99–105.

Ko SU, Jerome GJ, Simonsick EM, Ferrucci L. Obstacle-crossing task-related usual gait patterns of older adults differentiating falls and gait ability. J Aging Phys Act 2020:1–5. doi: 10.1123/japa.2019-0227.

Kobayashi M, Hutchinson S, Theoret H, et al. Repetitive TMS of the motor cortex improves ipsilateral sequential simple finger movements. Neurology 2004;62:91–98.

Kobayashi Y, Kawano K, Takemura AYA, et al. Temporal firing patterns of Purkinje cells in the cerebellar ventral paraflocculus during ocular following responses in monkeys II. Complex spikes. J Neurophysiol 1998;80:832–848.

Koch MW, Murray TJ, Fisk J, et al. Hand dexterity and direct disease related cost in multiple sclerosis. J Neurol Sci 2014;341:51–54.

Kochaneck KD, Xu, JQ, Murphy SL, Arias E. Mortality in the United States, 2013. NCHS Data Brief, No. 178. Hyattsville, MD: National Center for Health Statistics, Centers of Disease Control and Prevention, Department of Health and Human Services; 2014.

Koester J, Siegelbaum SA. Membrane potential. In: Kandel ER, Schwartz JH, Jessell TM, eds. Principles of neural science, 4th ed. New York: McGraw-Hill, 2000:125–139.

Kokkoni E, Haworth JL, Harbourne RT, Stergiou N, Kyvelidou A. Infant sitting postural control appears robust across changes in surface context. Somatosens Mot Res 2017;34(4):265–272.

Kollen B, Kwakkel G, Lindeman E. Time dependency of walking classification in stroke. Phys Ther 2006;86:618–625.

Kollen B, Port I, Lindeman E, et al. Predicting improvement in gait after stroke. Stroke 2005;36:2576–2680.

Kolobe THA, Bulanda M, Susman L. Predicting motor outcome at preschool age for infants tested at 7, 30, 60, and 90 days after term age using the Test of Infant Motor Performance. Phys Ther 2004;84:1144–1156.

Konczak J, Borutta M, Dichgans J. The development of goal-directed reaching in infants: 2. Learning to produce task-adequate patterns of joint torque. Exp Brain Res 1997;113:465–474.

Konczak J, Borutta M, Topka H, et al. The development of goal-directed reaching in infants: hand trajectory formation and joint torque control. Exp Brain Res 1995;106:156–168.

Konczak J, Dichgans J. The development toward stereotypic arm kinematics during reaching in the first 3 years of life. Exp Brain Res 1997;117:346–354.

Konczak J, Jansen-Osmann P, Kalveram KT. Development of force adaptation during childhood. J Motor Behav 2003;35:41–52.

Kong J, Kim K, Joung HJ, Chung CY, Park J. Effects of spastic cerebral palsy on multi-finger coordination during isometric force production tasks. Exp Brain Res 2019;237:3281–3295.

Konig M, Epro G, Seeley J, Potthast W, Karamanidis K. Retention and generalizability of balance recovery response adaptations from trip perturbations across the adult life span. J Neurophysiol 2019;122(5):1884–1893.

Komisar V, Maki BE, Novak AC. Effect of handrail height and age on the timing and speed of reach-to grasp balance reactions during slope descent. Appl Ergon 2019;81:102873.

Kosnik W, Winslow L, Kline D, et al. Visual changes in daily life throughout adulthood. J Gerontol 1988;43:P63–P70.

Kots YM, Syrovegin AV. Fixed set of variants of interactions of the muscles to two joints in the execution of simple voluntary movements. Biophysics 1966;11:1212–1219.

Koushyar H, Bieryla KA, Nussbaum MA, Madigan ML. Age-related strength loss affects non-stepping balance recovery. PLoS One 2019;14(1):e0210049.

Kowalski JL, Nemanich ST, Rao R, et al. Recruitment challenges in infant stroke and non-invasive brain stimulation research: demographics and factors. Brain Stim 2019;12(2):E38-E39.

Kozlowski DA, James DC, Schallert T. Use-dependent exaggeration of neuronal injury after unilateral sensorimotor cortex lesions. J Neurosci 1996;16:4776–4786.

Krakauer JW. Motor learning: its relevance to stroke recovery and neurorehabilitation. Curr Opin Neurol 2006;19:84–90.

Krakauer J, Ghez C. Voluntary movement. In: Kandel ER, Schwartz JH, Jessell TM, eds. Principles of neural science, 4th ed. New York: McGraw-Hill, 2000:756–779.

Kramer AF, Erickson KI, Colcombe SJ. Exercise, cognition and the aging brain. J Appl Physiol 2006;101:1237–1242.

Krasny-Pacini A, Hiebel J, Pauly F, Godon S, Chevignard M. Goal attainment scaling in rehabilitation: a literature-based update. Ann Phys Rehabil Med 2013;56(3):212–230. doi: 10.1016/j.rehab.2013.02.002.

Krebs DE, Edelstein JE, Fishman S. Reliability of observational kinematic gait analysis. Phys Ther 1985;65:1027–1033.

Krebs DE, Jette AM, Assmann SF. Moderate exercise improves gait stability in disabled elders. Arch Phys Med Rehabil 1998;79:1489–1495.

Kretch KS, Adolph KE. The organization of exploratory behaviors in infant locomotor planning. Dev Sci 2017;20(4).

Kriellaars DJ, Brownstone RM, Noga BR, et al. Mechanical entrainment of fictive locomotion in the decerebrate cat. J Neurophysiol 1994;71:2074–2086. doi:10.1111/desc.12421.

Krishnan V, de Freitas PB, Jaric S. Impaired object manipulation in mildly involved individuals with multiple sclerosis. Motor Control 2008;12:3–20.

Krishnan V, Jaric S. Hand function in multiple sclerosis: force coordination in manipulation tasks. Clin Neurophysiol 2008;119:2274–2281.

Kristinsdottir EK, Fransson PA, Magnusson M. Changes in postural control in healthy elderly subjects are related to vibration sensation, vision and vestibular asymmetry. Act Otolaryngol 2001;121:700–706.

Krumlinde-Sundholm L, Eliasson AC. Development of the assisting hand assessment: a Rasch-built measure intended for children with unilateral upper limb impairments. Scand J Occup Ther 2003;10(1):16–26.

Krumlinde-Sundholm L, Ek L, Sicola E, et al. Development of the hand assessment for infants: evidence of internal scale validity. Dev Med Child Neurol 2017a;59(12):1276–1283.

Krumlinde-Sundholm L, Lindkvist B, Plantin J, Hoare B. Development of the assisting hand assessment for adults following stroke: a Rasch-built bimanual performance measure. Disab Rehabil 2017b:1–9. doi: 10.1080/09638288.2017.1396365

Kugler PN, Kelso JAS, Turvey MT. On the control and coordination of naturally developing systems. In: Kelso JAS, Clark JE, eds. The development of movement control and coordination. New York: Wiley, 1982:5–78.

Kugler PN, Turvey MT. Information, natural law and self assembly of rhythmic movement. Hillsdale, NJ: Erlbaum, 1987.

Kuhtz-Buschbeck JP, Stolze H, Johnk K, et al. Development of prehension movements in children: a kinematic study. Exp Brain Res 1998;122:424–432.

Kunesch E, Schnitzler A, Tyercha C, et al. Altered force release control in Parkinson's disease. Behav Brain Res 1995;67:43–49.

Kung UM, Horlings CG, Honegger H, et al. Postural instability in cerebellar apraxia: correlations of knee, arm and trunk movements to center of mass velocity. Neuroscience 2009;159:390–404.

Kunimune S, Okada S. Contribution of vision and its age-related changes to postural stability in obstacle crossing during locomotion. Gait Posture 2019;70:284–288.

Kuo AD, Speers RA, Peterka RJ, et al. Effect of altered sensory conditions on multivariate descriptors of human postural sway. Exp Brain Res 1998;122:185–195.

Kuo AD, Zajac FE. A biomechanical analysis of muscle strength as a limiting factor in standing posture. J Biomech 1993;26:137–150.

Kupfermann I. Localization of higher cognitive and affective functions: the association cortices. In: Kandel E, Schwartz JH, Jessell TM, eds. Principles of neuroscience, 3rd ed. New York: Elsevier, 1991:823–838.

Kuppens SP, Pijlman HC, Hitters MW, van Heugten CM. Prevention and treatment of hand oedema after stroke. Disabil Rehabil 2014;36(11):900–906. doi: 10.3109/09638288.2013.824031.

Kurtzke JF. Rating neurologic impairment in multiple sclerosis: an expanded disability status scale (EDSS). Neurology 1983;33:1444–1452.

Kusmierz L, Isomura T, Toyoizumi T. Learning with three factors: modulating Hebbian plasticity with errors. Curr Opin Neurobiol 2017;46:170–177.

Kuypers HGJM. Corticospinal connections: postnatal development in rhesus monkey. Science 1962;138:678–680.

Kuypers HGJM. The descending pathways to the spinal cord, their anatomy and function. In: Eccles JC, ed. Organization of the spinal cord. Amsterdam, The Netherlands: Elsevier, 1964.

Kwakkel G, Wagenaar RC, Kollen BJ, et al. Predicting disability in stroke: a critical review of the literature. Age Ageing 1996;25:479–489.

Kwakkel G, Kollen BJ, Krebs HI. Effects of robot-assisted therapy on upper limb recovery after stroke: a systematic review. Neurorehabil Neural Repair 2008;22(2):111–121.

Kwon Y, Dwivedi A, McDaid AJ, Liarokapis M. On muscle selection for EMG based decoding of dexterous, in-hand manipulation motions. Annu Int Conf IEEE Eng Med Biol Soc 2018.;2018:1672–1675. doi: 10.1109/EMBC.2018.8512624.

Kyvelidou A, Stergiou N. Visual and somatosensory contributions to infant sitting postural control. Somatosens Mot Res 2018;35(3–4):240–246.

L

Lackner JR, DiZio P. Visual stimulation affects the perception of voluntary leg movements during walking. Perception 1988;17:71–80.

Lackner JR, DiZio P. Sensory-motor calibration processes constraining the perception of force and motion during locomotion. In: Woollacott MH, Horak FB, eds. Posture and gait: control mechanisms. Eugene, OR: University of Oregon, 1992:92–96.

Lajoie K, Drew T. Lesions of area 5 of the posterior parietal cortex in the cat produce errors in the accuracy of paw placement during visually guided locomotion. J Neurophysiol 2007;97:2339–2354.

Lajoie Y, Teasdale N, Bard C, et al. Attentional demands for static and dynamic equilibrium. Exp Brain Res 1993;97:139–144.

Lajoie Y, Teasdale N, Bard C, et al. Upright standing and gait: are there changes in attentional requirements related to normal aging? Exp Aging Res 1996;22(2):185–198.

Lakhani B, Mansfield A, Inness EL, et al. Compensatory stepping responses in individuals with stroke: a pilot study. Physiother Theory Pract 2011;27:299–309.

Lakie M, Campbell KS. Muscle thixotropy: where are we now? J Appl Physiol 2019;126:1790–1799.

Laliberte AM, Goltash S, Lalonde NR, Bui TV. Propriospinal neurons: essential elements of locomotor control in the intact and possibly the injured spinal cord. Front Cell Neurosci 2019; 13:1–16.

Lamb SE, Ferrucci L, Volapto S, et al. Risk factors for falling in home-dwelling older women with stroke: the Women's Health and Aging Study. Stroke 2003;34:494–501.

Lamont EV, Zehr EP. Earth-referenced handrail contact facilitates interlimb cutaneous reflexes during locomotion. J Neurophysiol 2007;98(1):433–442.

Lamontagne A, Malouin F, Richards CL, et al. Mechanisms of disturbed motor control in ankle weakness during gait after stroke. Gait Posture 2002;15:244–255.

Lance JW. Symposium synopsis. In: Feldman RG, Young RR, Koella WP, eds. Spasticity: disordered motor control. Chicago, IL: Year Book, 1980.

Landers MR, Hatlevig RM, Davis AD, et al. Does attentional focus during balance training in people with Parkinson's disease affect outcome? A randomised controlled clinical trial. Clin Rehabil 2015. pii: 0269215515570377 [Epub ahead of print].

Landel R. Managing post-concussion syndrome: the diagnostic dilemma, and where does manual therapy fit in? 18th Annual Patricia Leahy Lecture, University of the Sciences, Philadelphia PA. Sept. 2018.

Lang CE, Bastian AJ. Cerebellar subjects show impaired adaptation of anticipatory EMG during catching. J Neurophysiol 1999;82:2108–2119.

Lang CE, Bastian AJ. Additional somatosensory information does not improve cerebellar adaptation during catching. Clin Neurophysiol 2001;112:895–907.

Lang CE, Bastian AJ. Cerebellar damage impairs automaticity of a recently practiced movement. J Neurophysiol 2002;87:1136–1147.

Lang CE, DeJong SL, Beebe JA. Recovery of thumb and finger extension and its relation to grasp performance after stroke. J Neurophysiol 2009;102(1):451–459.

Lang C, Macdonald J, Gnip C. Counting repetitions: an observational study of outpatient therapy for people with hemiparesis post-stroke. J Neurol Phys Ther 2007;31:3–11.

Lang CE, et al. Observation of amounts of movement practice provided during stroke rehabilitation. Arch Phys Med Rehabil 2009;90:1692–1698.

Lang CE, Schieber MH. Reduced muscle selectivity during individuated finger movements in humans after damage to the motor cortex or corticospinal tract. J Neurophysiol 2004;91:1722–1733.

Lang CE, Wagner JM, Bastian AJ, et al. Deficits in grasp versus reach during acute hemiparesis. Exp Brain Res 2005;166:126–136.

Lang CE, Wagner JM, Edwards DF, et al. Recovery of grasp versus reach in people with hemiparesis poststroke. Neurorehabil Neural Repair 2006;20:444–454.

Lang CE, Wagner JW, Edwards DF, et al. Upper extremity use in people with hemiparesis in the first few weeks after stroke. J Neurologic Phys Ther 2007;31:56–63.

Lang W, Obrig H, Lindinger G, et al. Supplementary motor area activation while tapping bimanually different rhythms in musicians. Exp Brain Res 1990;79:504–514.

LaRocca NG. Impact of walking impairment in multiple sclerosis: perspectives of patients and care partners. Patient 2011;4:189–201.

La Scaleia V, Ivanenko Y, Fabiano A, et al. Early manifestation of arm-leg coordination during stepping on a surface in human neonates. Exp Brain Res 2018;236(4):1105–1115.

Lashley KS. Brain mechanism and intelligence. Chicago, IL: University of Chicago, 1929.

LaStayo PC, Wheeler DL. Reliability of passive wrist flexion and extension goniometric measurements: a multicenter study. Phys Ther 1994;74(2):162–174.

Latash ML. Muscle coactivation: definitions, mechanisms, and functions. J Neurophysiol 2018;120:88–104.

Latash ML, Anson JG. Synergies in health and disease: relations to adaptive changes in motor coordination. Phys Ther 2006;86:1151–1160.

Latash ML, Aruin AS, Neyman I, et al. Anticipatory postural adjustments during self inflicted and predictable perturbations in Parkinson's disease. J Neurol Neurosurg Psychiatry 1995;58(3):326–334.

Latash ML, Gelfand IM, Li ZM, et al. Changes in the force-sharing pattern induced by modifications of visual feedback during force production by a set of fingers. Exp Brain Res 1998;123(3):255–262.

Latash ML, Kang N, Patterson D. Finger coordination in persons with Down syndrome: atypical patterns of coordination and the effects of practice. Exp Brain Res 2002;146:345–355.

Latash ML, Krishnamoorthy V, Scholz J, et al. Postural synergies in development. Neural Plast 2005;12:119–130.

Latash ML, Scholz JP, Schöner G. Motor control strategies revealed in the structure of motor variability. Exerc Sport Sci Rev 2002;30:26–31.

Latash ML, Scholz JP, Schöner G. Toward a new theory of motor synergies. Motor Control 2007;11:276–308.

Latash ML, Turvey M. On dexterity and its development. Mahwah, NJ: Lawrence Erlbaum, 1996.

Laterra JJ, Goldstein GW. The blood-brain barrier, choroid plexus, and cerebrospinal fluid. In: Kandel ER, Schwartz JH, Jessell TM, Siegelbaum SA, Hudspeth AJ, eds. Principles of neural science, 5th ed. New York, NY: McGraw-Hill, 2013:[illegible].

Laufer Y. Effect of age on characteristics of forward and backward gait at preferred and accelerated walking speed. J Gerontol 2005;60A:627–632.

Laufer Y, Ashkenazi T, Josman N. The effects of a concurrent cognitive task on the postural control of young children with and wiout developmental coordination disorder. Gait Posture 2008;27:347–351.

Laufer Y, Elboim-Gabyzon M. Does sensory transcutaneous electrical stimulation enhance motor recovery following a stroke? A systematic review. Neural Rehabil Neural Repair 2011;25:799–809.

Laufer Y, Schwarzmann R, Sivan D, et al. Postural control of patients with hemiparesis: force plates measurements based on the clinical sensory organization test. Physiother Theory Pract 2005;21:163–171.

Laver KE, George S, Thomas S, et al. Virtual reality for stroke rehabilitation. Cochrane Database Syst Rev 2015;(2):CD008349.

Lavery JJ. Retention of simple motor skills as a function of type of knowledge of results. Can J Psychol 1962;16:300–311.

Lavelle K, Breger Stanton D. Measurement of edema in the hand clinic. In: MacDermid J, Solomon G, Valdes K, American Society of Hand

Therapists, eds. ASHT Clinical Assessment Recommendations 3rd ed. Mt. Laurel, NJ: American Society of Hand Therapists. 2015.

Law LS, Webb CY. Gait adaptation of children with cerebral palsy compared with control children when stepping over an obstacle. Dev Med Child Neurol 2005;47:321–328.

Law M, Anaby D, Imms C, et al. Improving the participation of youth with physical disabilities in community activities: an interrupted time series design. Aust Occup Ther J 2015;62.105–115. doi: 10.1111/1440-1630.12177.

Law M, Baptiste S, Carswell A, et al. Canadian occupational performance measure, 4th ed. Ottawa, ON: Canadian Association of Occupational Therapists, 2005.

Law M, King G, King S, et al. Patterns of participation in recreational and leisure activities among children with complex physical disabilities. Dev Med Child Neuro 2006;48:337–342.

Lawrence DG, Hopkins DA. Developmental aspects of pyramidal motor control in the rhesus monkey. Brain Res 1972;40:117–118.

Lawrence EL, Fassola I, Werner I, et al. Quantification of dexterity as the dynamical regulation of instabilities: comparisons across gender, age, and disease. Front Neurol 2014;5(53):1–13.

Lawton MP. The functional assessment of elderly people. J Am Geriatr Soc 1971;19:465–481.

Lay AN, Hass CJ, Gregor RJ. The effects of sloped surfaces on locomotion: a kinematic and kinetic analysis. J Biomech 2006;39:1621–1628.

Lazzari RD, Politti F, Belina SF, et al. Effect of transcranial direct current stimulation combined with virtual reality training on balance in children with cerebral palsy: a randomized, controlled, double-blind, clinical trial. J Mot Behav 2017;49:329–336.

Lebiedowska MK, Syczewska M. Invariant sway properties in children. Gait Posture 2000;12:200–204.

Ledebt A, Becher J, Kapper J, et al. Balance training with visual feedback in children with hemiplegic cerebral palsy: effect on stance and gait. Motor Control 2005;9:459–468.

Ledebt A, Bril B, Breniere Y. The build-up of anticipatory behavior: an analysis of the development of gait initiation in children. Exp Brain Res 1998;120:9–17.

Ledebt A, Bril B, Wiener-Vacher S. Trunk and head stabilization during the first months of independent walking. Neuroreport 1995;6:1737–1740.

Lee DK, Cole WG, Golenia L, Adolph KE. The cost of simplifying complex developmental phenomena: a new perspective on learning to walk. Dev Sci 2018;21(4):e12615.

Lee DN, Aronson E. Visual proprioceptive control of standing in human infants. Percept Psychophys 1974;15:529–532.

Lee HJ, Chou LS. Balance control during stair negotiation in older adults. J Biomech 2007;40:2530–2536.

Lee H-M, Galloway JC. Early intensive postural and movement training advances head control in very young infants. Phys Ther 2012;92(7):935–947.

Lee JW, Chung E, Lee BH. A comparison of functioning, activity, and participation in school-aged children with cerebral palsy using the manual ability classification system. J Phys Ther Sci 2015;27(1):243–246.

Lee JW, Chung E, Lee BH. A comparison of functioning, activity, and participation in school-aged children with cerebral palsy using the manual ability classification system. J Phys Ther Sci 2015;27(1):243–246. doi: 10.1589/jpts.27.243.

Lee BC, Kim J, Chen S, et al. Cell phone based real-time vibrotactile feedback for balance rehabilitation training. J Neuroeng Rehabil 2012;9(1):10.

Lee DN, Lishman R. Visual proprioceptive control of stance. J Hum Mov Studies 1975;1:87–95.

Lee I, Manson J, Hennekens C, et al. Body weight and mortality: a 27 year follow up of middle aged men. JAMA 1993;270:2623–2628.

Lee DN, Young DS. Gearing action to the environment. Experiments in Brain Research, Series 15. Berlin, Germany: Springer Verlag, 1986:217–230.

Lee RG, van Donkelaar P. Mechanisms underlying functional recovery following stroke. Can J Neurol Sci 1995;22:257–263.

Lee TD. Transfer-appropriate processing: a framework for conceptualizing practice effects in motor learning. In: Meijer OG, Roth K, eds. Complex movement behavior: the motor-action controversy. Amsterdam, The Netherlands: North-Holland, 1988.

Lee YH, Yong SY, Kim SH, et al. Functional electrical stimulation to ankle dorsiflexor and plantarflexor using single foot switch in patients with hemiplegia from hemorrhagic stroke. Ann Rehabil Med 2014;38:310–316.

Lee-Valkov PM, Aaron DH, Eladoumikdachi F, et al. Measuring normal hand dexterity values in normal 3-,4-, and 5-year-old children and their relationship with grip and pinch strength. J Hand Ther 2003;16(1):22–28.

Lefumat HZ, Miall RC, Cole JD, Bringoux L, Bourdin C, Vercher J, Sarlegna FR. Generalization of force-field adaptation in proprioceptively-deafferented subjects. Neurosci Lett 2016;616:160–165.

Leone C, Feys P, Moumdjian L, D'Amico E, Zappia M, Patti F. Cognitive-motor dual-task interference: a systematic review of neural correlates. Neurosci Biobehav Rev 2017;75:348–360.

Lehman D, Toole T, Lofald D, et al. Training with verbal instructional cues results in near-term improvement of gait in people with Parkinson's disease. J Neurol Phys Ther 2005;29(1):2–8.

Leipert J, Bauder H, Miltner WHR, Taub E, Weiller C. Treatment-induced cortical reorganization after stroke in humans. Stroke, 2000;31:1210–1216.

Lemon RN. Descending pathways in motor control. Annu Rev Neurosci 2008;31:195–218.

Lemon RN, Mantel GWH, Muir RB. Corticospinal facilitation of hand muscles during voluntary movements in the conscious monkey. J Physiol 1986;381:497–527.

Lemsky C, Miller CJ, Nevitt M, et al. Reliability and validity of a physical performance and mobility examination for hospitalized elderly. Soc Gerontol 1991;31:221.

Leonard CT, Sandholdt DY, McMillan JA, et al. Short- and long-latency contributions to reciprocal inhibition during various levels of muscle contraction of individuals with cerebral palsy. J Child Neurol 2006;21:240–246.

Lerner-Frankiel MB, Vargas S, Brown MB, et al. Functional community ambulation: what are your criteria? Clin Manage 1990;6:12–15.

Levin MF. Interjoint coordination during pointing movements is disrupted in spastic hemiparesis. Brain 1996;119(Pt 1):281–293.

Levin MF, Horowitz M, Jurrius C, et al. Trajectory formation and interjoint coordination of drawing movements in normal and hemiparetic subjects. Neurosci Abstr 1993;19:990.

Levin MF, Kleim JA, Wolf SF. What do motor "Recovery" and "Compensation" mean in patients following stroke? Neurorehabil Neural Repair 2009;23:313–319.

Levin MF, Michaelsen SM, Cirstea CM, et al. Use of the trunk for reaching targets placed within and beyond the reach in adult hemiparesis. Exp Brain Res 2002;143(2):171–180.

Levin MF, Weiss PL, Keshner EA. Emergence of virtual reality as a tool for upper limb rehabilitation: incorporation of motor control and motor learning principles. Phys Ther 2015;95:415-425.

Levy RM, Harvey RL, Kissela BM, et al. Epidural electrical stimulation for stroke rehabilitation: results of the prospective, multicenter, randomized, single-blinded everest trial. Neurorehabil Neural Repair 2016;30(2):107–119. doi: 10.1177/1545968315575613.

Lewald J. More accurate sound localization induced by short-term light deprivation. Neuropsychologia 2007;45:1215–1222.

Lewek MD, Poole R, Johnson J, et al. Arm swing magnitude and asymmetry during gait in the early stages of Parkinson's disease. Gait Posture 2010;31:256–260.

Lewis C, Bottomly J. Musculoskeletal changes with age. In: Lewis C, ed. Aging: health care's challenge, 2nd ed. Philadelphia, PA: Davis, 1990:145–146.

Lewis GN, Byblow WD. Bimanual coordination dynamics in post stroke hemiparetics. J Motor Behav 2004;36:174–186.

Li C, Verghese J, Holtzer R. A comparison of two walking while talking paradigms. Gait Posture 2014;40:415–419.

Li KZ, Roudaia E, Lussier M, et al. Benefits of cognitive dual-task training on balance performance in healthy older adults. J Gerontol A Biol Sci Med Sci 2010;65:1344–1352.

Li S-C, Huxhold O, Schmiedek F. Aging and attenuated processing robustness. Gerontology 2004;50:28–34.

Li X, He J, Yun J, Qin H. Lower limb resistance training in individuals with parkinson's disease: an updated systematic review and meta-analysis of randomized controlled trials. Front Neurol 2020;11:1–16.

Liao HF, Hwang AW. Relations of balance function and gross motor ability for children with cerebral palsy. Percept Motor Skills 2003;96(3 Pt 2):1173–1184.

Libertus K, Needham A. Teach to reach: the effects of active vs. passive reaching experiences on action and perception. Vision Res 2010;50(24):2750–2757.

Lieber RL, Runesson E, Einarsson F, et al. Inferior mechanical properties of spastic muscle bundles due to hypertrophic but compromised extracellular matrix material. Muscle Nerve 2003;28:464–471.

Liebesman JL, Carafelli E. Physiology of range of motion in human joints: a critical review. Crit Rev Phys Med Rehabil 1994;6:131–160.

Liepert J, Miltner WH, Bauder H, et al. Motor cortex plasticity during constraint-induced movement therapy in stroke patients. Neurosci Lett 1998;250:5–8.

Lin KC, Fu T, Wu CY, et al. Psychometric comparisons of the Stroke Impact Scale 3.0 and Stroke-Specific Quality of Life Scale. Qual Life Res 2010;19(3):435–443.

Lin S-I, Woollacott MH. Postrual muscle responses following changing balance threats in young stable older, and unstable older adults. J Motor Behav 2002;34:42.

Lin S-I, Woollacott MH, Jensen J. Postural response in older adults with different levels of functional balance capacity. Aging Clin Exp Res. 2004;16:373.

Lin YC, Chao YL, Wu SK, et al. Comprehension of handwriting development: Pen-grip kinetics in handwriting tasks and its relation to fine motor skills among school-age children. Aust Occup Ther J 2017;64(5):369–380. doi: 10.1111/1440 1630.12393.

Lindenberger U, Marsiske M, Baltes PB. Memorizing while walking: increase in dual-task costs from young adulthood to old age. Psychol Aging 2000;15:417–436.

Lima DP, de Almeida SB, de Carvalho Bonfadini J, et al. Clinical correlates of sarcopenia and falls in Parkinson's disease. PLoS One 2020;15:1–12.

Liphart J, Gallichio J, Tilson JK, et al. Concordance and discordance between measured and perceived balance and the effect on gait speed and falls following stroke. Clin Rehabil 2015. pii: 0269215515578294 [Epub ahead of print].

Lipsitz LA, Jonsson PV, Kelley MM, et al. Causes and correlates of recurrent falls in ambulatory frail elderly. J Gerontol 1991;46:M114–M122.

Lipsitz LA, Manor B, Habtemariam D, Iloputaife I, Zhou J, Travison TG. The pace and prognosis of peripheral sensory loss in advanced age: association with gait speed and falls. BMC Geriatr 2018;18(1):274.

Liu W, Lipsitz LA, Montero-Odasso M, et al. Noise-enhanced vibrotactile sensitivity in older adults, patients with stroke, and patients with diabetic neuropathy. Arch Phys Med Rehabil 2002;83:171–176.

Liu-Ambrose T, Katarynych LA, Ashe MC, et al. Dual-task gait performance among community-dwelling senior women: the role of balance confidence and executive functions. J Gerontol A Biol Sci Med Sci 2009;64:975–982.

Livingstone M, Hubel D. Segregation of form, color, movement and depth: anatomy, physiology, perception. Science 1988;240:740–749.

Lloréns R, Gil-Gómez JA, Alcañiz M, et al. Improvement in balance using a virtual reality-based stepping exercise: a randomized controlled trial involving individuals with chronic stroke. Clin Rehabil 2015;29:261–268.

Lo AC, Triche EW. Improving gait in multiple sclerosis using robot-assisted, body weight supported treadmill training. Neurorehabil Neural Repair 2008;22:661–671. doi: 10.1177/1545968308318473.

Lockhart TE, Smith JL, Woldstad JC. Effects of aging on the biomechanics of slips and falls. Hum Factors 2005;47:708–729.

Lockhart TE, Woldstad JC, Smith JL. Effects of age-related gait changes on the biomehcanics of slips and falls. Ergonomics 2003;46:1136–1160.

Lockman JJ, Ashmead DH, Bushnell EW. The development of anticipatory hand orientation during infancy. J Exp Child Psychol 1984;37:176–186.

Loewen SC, Anderson BA. Predictors of stroke outcomes using objective measurement scales. Stroke 1990;21:78–81.

Lomaglio MJ, Eng JJ. Muscle strength and weight-bearing symmetry relate to sit-to-stand performance in individuals with stroke. Gait Posture 2005;22:126–131.

Long H, Ma-Wyatt A. The distribution of spatial attention changes with task demands during goal-directed reaching. Exp Brain Res 2014;232:1883–1893. DOI 10.1007/s00221-014-3880-6.

Lopez C, Blanke O. The thalamocortical vestibular system in animals and humans. Brain Res Rev 2011;67:119–146.

Lord SE, Halligan PW, Wade DT. Visual gait analysis: the development of a clinical assessment and scale. Clin Rehabil 1998;12:107–119.

Lord SE, McPherson K, McNaughton HK, et al. Community ambulation after stroke: how important and obtainable is it and what measures appear predictive? Arch Phys Med Rehabil 2004;86:234–239.

Lord SR, Lloyd DG, Li SK. Sensorimotor function, gait patterns and falls in community-dwelling women. Age Ageing 1996;25:292–299.

Lord S, Rochester L. Measurement of community ambulation after stroke: current status and future developments. Stroke 2005;36:1457–1461.

Lord SE, Rochester L, Weatherall M, et al. The effect of environment and task on gait parameters after stroke: a randomized comparison of measurement conditions. Arch Phys Med Rehabil 2006;87:967–973.

Lord S, Sherrington C, Menz HB. Falls in older people. Cambridge, UK: Cambridge University Press, 2001:68.

Lord S, Ward J, Williams P, et al. An epidemiological study of falls in older community dwelling women: the Randwick falls and fracture study. Aust J Public Health 1993;17:240–245.

Louwers A, Beelen A, Holmefur M, Krumlinde-Sundholm L. Development of the Assisting Hand Assessment for adolescents (Ad-AHA) and validation of the AHA from 18 months to 18 years. Dev Med Child Neurol 2016;58:1303–1309.

Louwers A, Krumlinde-Sundholm L, Boeschoten K, Beelin A. Reliability of the assisting hand assessment in adolescents. Dev Med Child Neurol 2017;59(9):926–932. doi: 10.1111/dmcn.13465.

Lu T, Pan Y, Kao SY, et al. Gene regulation and DNA damage in the ageing human brain. Nature 2004;429:883–891.

Lu TW, Yen HC, Chen HL, et al. Symmetrical kinematic changes in highly functioning older patients post-stroke during obstacle-crossing. Gait Posture 2010;31:511–516.

Lum PS, Burgar CG, Shor PC. Evidence for strength imbalances as a significant contributor to abnormal synergies in hemiparetic subjects. Muscle Nerve 2003;27:211–221.

Lundborg G, Bjorkman A, Hansson T, et al. Artificial sensibility of the hand based on cortical audiotactile interaction: a study using functional magnetic resonance imaging. Scand J Plast Reconstr Surg Hand Surg 2005;39(6):370–372.

Lundgren-Lindquist B, Aniansson A, Rundgren A. Functional studies in 79 year olds: 3. Walking performance and climbing ability. Scand J Rehabil Med 1983;12:107–112.

Lundin-Olsson L, Nyberg L, Gustafson Y. Stops walking when talking as a predictor of falls in elderly people. Lancet 1997;349:617.

Luo TZ, Maunsell JHR. Attention can be subdivided into neurobiological components corresponding to distinct behavioral effects. PNAS 2019;116:26187–26194

Luria AR. Higher cortical functions in man. New York: Basic, 1966.

Lusardi MM, Fritz S, Middleton A, et al. Determining risk of falls in community dwelling older adults: a systematic review and meta-analysis using posttest probability. J Geriatr Phys Ther 2017;40:1–36.

Ly DH, Lockhart DJ, Lerner RA, et al. Mitotic misregulation and human aging. Science 2000;287:2486–2492.

Lyle RC. A performance test for assessment of upper limb function in physical rehabilitation treatment and research. Int J Rehabil Res 1981;4:483–492.

M

Ma HI, Trombly CA. A synthesis of the effects of occupational therapy for persons with stroke, part II: remediation of impairments. Am J Occup Ther 2002;56(3):260–274.

Macefield VG, Knellwolf TP. Functional properties of human muscle spindles. J Neurophysiol 2018;120,452–467.

Mackay CP, Kuys SS, Brauer SG. The effect of aerobic exercise on brain-derived neurotrophic factor in people with neurological disorders: a systematic review and meta-analysis. Neural Plast 2017;2017:4716197.

MacDermid J, Solomon G, Valdes K. American society of hand therapists. ASHT clinical assessment recommendations, 3rd ed. Mt. Laurel, NJ: American Society of Hand Therapists, 2015.

MacKay DG. The problem of flexibility, fluency, and the speed- accuracy trade-off in skilled behavior. Psychol Rev 1982;89:48–506.

MacKay-Lyons M. Variability in spatiotemporal gait characteristics over the course of the L-dopa cycle in people with advanced Parkinson disease. Phys Ther 1998;78:1083–1094.

Mackey AH, Walt SE, Stott NS. Deficits in upper-limb task performance in children with hemiplegic cerebral palsy as defined by 3-dimensional kinematics. Arch Phys Med Rehabil 2006;87:207–215.

Maddox WT, Ashby FG. Dissociating explicit and procedural-learning based systems of perceptual category learning. Behav Proc 2004;66:309–332.

Maenza C, Good DC, Winstein CJ, Wagstaff DA, Sainburg RL. Functional deficits in the less-impaired arm of stroke survivors depend on hemisphere of damage and extent of paretic arm impairment. Neurorehabil Neural Repair 2020;34(1):39–50. doi: 10.1177/1545968319875951.

Magee DJ. Orthopedic physical assessment. Philadelphia, PA: Saunders, 1987.

Magill R, Anderson D. Motor learning and control: concepts and applications, 10th ed. New York, NY: McGraw Hill, 2014.

Magill RA, Hall KG. A review of the contextual interference effect in motor skill acquisition. Hum Mov Sci 1990;9:241–289.

Magnus R. Animal posture (Croonian lecture). Proc R Soc Lond 1925;98:339.

Magnus R. Some results of studies in the physiology of posture. Lancet 1926;2:531–585.

Magnusson M, Enbom H, Johansson R, et al. Significance of pressor input from the human feet in lateral postural control: the effect of hypothermia on galvanically induced body-sway. Acta Otolaryngol 1990;110:321–327.

Mahon CE, Farris DJ, Sawicki GS, et al. Individual limb mechanical analysis of gait following stroke. J Biomech 2015;48:984–989.

Mahoney JR, Cotton K, Verghese J. Multisensory integration predicts balance and falls in older adults. J Gerontol A Biol Sci Med Sci 2019;74(9):1429–1435.

Majsak MJ, Kaminski T, Gentile AM, et al. Effects of a moving target versus a temporal constraint on reach and grasp in patients with Parkinson's disease. Exp Neurol 2008;210:479–488.

Mak MK, Hui-Chan CW. Switching of movement direction is central to parkinsonian bradykinesia in sit-to-stand. Mov Disord 2002;17:1188–1195.

Mak MK, Levin O, Mizrahi J, et al. Joint torques during sit-to-stand in healthy subjects and people with Parkinson's disease. Clin Biomech (Bristol, Avon) 2003;18:197–206.

Mak MK, Patla A, Hui-Chan C. Sudden turn during walking is impaired in people with Parkinson's disease. Exp Brain Res 2008;190:43–51.

Maki B, Holliday PJ, Topper AK. Fear of falling and postural performance in the elderly. J Gerontol 1991;46:M123–M131.

Maki BE, Holliday PJ, Topper AK. A prospective study of postural balance and risk of falling in an ambulatory and independent elderly population. J Gerontol 1994;49:M72–M84.

Maki BE, McIlroy WE. Control of rapid limb movements for balance recovery: age-related changes and implications for fall prevention. Age Ageing 2006;35(Suppl 2):ii12–ii18.

Maki BE, McIlroy WE, Fernie GR. Change-in-support reactions for balance recovery. IEEE Eng Med Biol Mag 2003;22:20–26.

Maldonado M, Allred RP, Felthauser EL, et al. Motor skill training, but not voluntary exercise, improves skilled reaching after unilateral ischemic lesions of the sensorimotor cortex in rats. Neurorehabil Neural Repair 2008;22:250–261.

Malfait N, Ostry DJ. Is interlimb transfer of force-field adaptation a cognitive response to the sudden introduction of load? J Neurosci 2004;24:8084–8089.

Malick M. Manual on static hand splinting. Pittsburgh, PA: Harmarville Rehab Center, 1980.

Malouin F, McFadyen B, Dion L, et al. A fluidity scale for evaluating the motor strategy of the rise to walk task after stroke [appendix]. Clin Rehabil 2003;17:674–684.

Malouin F, Pichard L, Bonneau C, et al. Evaluating motor recovery early after stroke: comparison of the Fugl-Meyer Assessment and the Motor Assessment Scale. Arch Phys Med Rehabil 1994;75:1206–1212.

Malviya S, Voepel-Lewis T, Burke C, et al. The revised FLACC observational pain tool: improved reliability and validity assessment in children with cognitive impairment. Paediatr Anaesth 2006;16(3):258–265.

Man'kovskii NB, Mints AY, Lysenyuk VP. Regulation of the preparatory period for complex voluntary movement in old and extreme old age. Hum Physiol Moscow 1980;6:46–50.

Manchester D, Woollacott M, Zederbauer-Hylton N, et al. Visual, vestibular and somatosensory contributions to balance control in the older adult. J Gerontol 1989;44:M118–M127.

Mancini M, Rocchi L, Horak FB, Chiari L. Effects of Parkinson's disease and levodopa on functional limits of stability. Clin Biomech (Bristol, Avon) 2008;23:450–458.

Mancini M, Zampieri C, Carlson-Kuhta P, et al. Anticipatory postural adjustments prior to step initiation are hypometric in untreated Parkinson's disease: an accelerometer-based approach. Eur J Neurol 2009;16:1028–1034.

Manheim CJ, Lavett DK. The myofascial release manual. Thorofare, NJ: Slack, 1989.

Mann RA, Hagy JL, White V, Liddell D. The initiation of gait. J Bone Joint Surg Am 1979;61:232–239.

Mann RA, Hagy JL, White V, et al. The initiation of gait. J Bone Joint Surg Am 1979;61:232–239.

Mannheimer JS, Lampe GN. Clinical transcutaneous electrical nerve stimulation. Philadelphia, PA: Davis, 1984.

Mansfield A, Inness EL, Komar J, et al. Training rapid stepping responses in an individual with stroke. Phys Ther 2011;91:958–969.

Mansfield A, Inness EL, Wong JS, et al. Is impaired control of reactive stepping related to falls during inpatient stroke rehabilitation? Neurorehabil Neural Repair 2013;27:526–533.

Mansfield A, Peters AL, Liu BA, et al. A perturbation-based balance training program for older adults: study protocol for a randomised controlled trial. BMC Geriatr 2007;7:12.

Mansfield A, Peters AL, Liu BA, et al. Effect of a perturbation-based balance training program on compensatory stepping and grasping reactions in older adults: a randomized controlled trial. Phys Ther 2010;90(4):476–491.

Manto M. Cerebellar motor syndrome from children to the elderly. In: Aminoff M, Boller F, Swaab D, eds. Handbook of clinical neurology. Netherlands: Elsevier, 2018:151–166.

Marchese R, Bove M, Abbruzzese G. Effect of cognitive and motor tasks on postural stability in Parkinson's disease: a posturographic study. Mov Disord 2003;18:652–658.

Marchetti GF, Whitney SL, Blatt PJ, et al. Temporal and spatial characteristics of gait during performance of the Dynamic Gait Index in people with and people without balance or vestibular disorders. Phys Ther 2008;88:640–651.

Marencakova J, Price C, Maly T, Zahalka F, Nester C. How do novice and improver walkers move in their home environments? An open-sourced infant's gait video analysis. PLoS One 2019;14(6):e0218665.

Mao H, Li Y, Tang L, Chen Y, Ni J, Liu L, Shan C. Effects of mirror neuron system-based training on rehabilitation of stroke patients. Brain Behav 2020;10(8):e01729. doi: 10.1002/brb3.1729.

Marigold DS, Eng JJ. Altered timing of postural reflexes contributes to falling in persons with chronic stroke. Exp Brain Res 2006;171:459–468.

Marigold DS, Eng JJ, Dawson AS, et al. Exercise leads to faster postural reflexes, improved balance and mobility, and fewer falls in older persons with chronic stroke. J Am Geriatr Soc 2005;53:416–423.

Marigold DS, Eng JJ, Tokuno CD, et al. Contribution of muscle strength and integration of afferent input to postural instability in persons with stroke. Neurorehabil Neural Repair 2004;18(4):222–229.

Marigold DS, Patla AE. Strategies for dynamic stability during locomotion on a slippery surface: effects of prior experience and knowledge. J Neurophysiol 2002;88:339–353.

Marigold DS, Patla AE. Adapting locomotion to different surface compliances: neuromuscular responses and changes in movement dynamics. J Neurophysiol 2005;94(3):1733–1750.

Marneweck M, Grafton ST. Neural substrates of anticipatory motor adaptation for object lifting. Sci Rep 2020a;10:1–10.

Marneweck M, Grafton ST. Representational neural mapping of dexterous grasping before lifting in humans. J Neurosci 2020b;40:2708–2716.

Marsico P, Frontzek-Weps V, Balzer J, Van Hedel HJA. Hypertonia assessment tool: reliability and validity in children with neuromotor disorders. J Child Neurol 2017;32:132–138.

Marque P, Felez A, Puel M, et al. Impairment and recovery of left motor function in patients with right hemiplegia. J Neurol Neurosurg Psychiatry 1997;62:77–81.

Marquez-Chin C, Marquis A, Popovic MR. BCI-triggered functional electrical stimulation therapy for upper limb. Eur J Transl Myol 2016;26(3):6222. doi: 10.4081/ejtm.2016.6222.

Marquez-Chin C, Marquis A, Popovic MR. EEG-triggered functional electrical stimulation therapy for restoring upper limb function in chronic stroke with severe hemiplegia. Case Rep Neurol Med 2016;2016:9146213. doi: 10.1155/2016/9146213.

Marsden CD. Slowness of movement in Parkinson's disease. Mov Disord 1989;4:26–37.

Marsden CD, Quinn NP. The dystonias. BMJ 1990;300:139–144.

Marteniuk RG, Leavitt JL, Mackenzie CL, et al. Functional relationships between grasp and transport components in a prehension task. Hum Mov Sci 1990;9:149–176.

Marteniuk RG, Mackenzie CL, Jeannerod M, et al. Constraints on human arm movements trajectories. Can J Psychol 1987;41:365–368.

Martin JP. The basal ganglia and posture. London, UK: Pitman, 1967.

Martin JH, Donarummo L, Hacking A. Impairments in prehension produced by early postnatal sensory motor cortex activity blockage. J Neurophysiol 2000;83:895–906.

Martin JH, Kably B, Hacking A. Activity-dependent development of cortical axon terminations in the spinal cord and brain stem. Exp Brain Res 1999;125:184–199.

Martin TA, Keating JG, Goodkin HP, et al. Storage of multiple gaze-hand calibrations. Neurosci Abstr 1993;19:980.

Martinelli AR, Coelho DB, Teixeira LA. Light touch leads to increased stability in quiet and perturbed balance: Equivalent effects between post-stroke and healthy older individuals. Hum Mov Sci 2018;58:268–278.

Martelli D, Xia B, Prado A, Agrawal SK. Gait adaptations during overground walking and multidirectional oscillations of the visual field in a virtual reality headset. Gait Posture 2019;67:251–256.

Marwaha R, Hall SJ, Knight CA, et al. Load and grip force coordination in static bimanual manipulation tasks in multiple sclerosis. Motor Control 2006;10:160–177.

Masani K, Sin VW, Vette AH, et al. Postural reactions of the trunk muscles to multidirectional perturbations in sitting. Clin Biomech (Bristol, Avon) 2009;24:176–182.

Massion J. Movement, posture and equilibrium: interaction and coordination. Prog Neurobiol 1992;38(1):35–36.

Massion J. Role of motor cortex in postural adjustments associated with movement. In: Asanuma H, Wilson VJ, eds. Integration in the nervous system. Tokyo, Japan: Igaku-Shoin, 1979:239–260.

Massion J, Woollacott M. Normal balance and postural control. In: Bronstein AM, Brandt T, Woollacott M, et al., eds. Clinical disorders of balance posture and gait, 2nd ed. London, UK: Edward Arnold, 2004.

Mathias S, Nayak U, Issacs B. Balance in elderly patients: the "Get-up and Go" test. Arch Phys Med Rehabil 1986;67:387–389.

Mathiowetz V, Rogers SL, Dowe-Keval M, et al. The Purdue Pegboard: norms for 14- to 19-year olds. Am J Occup Ther 1986;40(3):174–179.

Mathiowetz V, Weber K, Kashman N, et al. Adult norms for the Nine Hole Peg Test of finger dexterity. Occup Ther J Res 1985;5:24–38.

Matsuda PN, Bamer A, Shumway-Cook A, et al. Falls in multiple sclerosis: incidence, risk factors and provider response (Abstract). 61st Annual Meeting of the American Academy of Neurology, Seattle, WA, 2009.Matsuda PN, Taylor CS, Shumway-Cook A. Evidence for the validity of the modified dynamic gait index across diagnostic groups. Phys Ther 2014;94(7):996–1004.

Matsuda PN, Taylor C, Shumway-Cook A. Examining the relationship between medical diagnoses and patterns of performance on the modified Dynamic Gait Index. Phys Ther 2015;95(6):854–863.

Matsuda P, Shumway-Cook A Kraft G. Falls in multiple sclerosis: incidence, causes, risk factors and health care provider response. Phys Med Rehabil 2011;3(7):624–632.

Matthews A, Garry MI, Martin F, Summers J. Neural correlates of performance trade-offs and dual-task interference in bimanual coordination: an ERP investigation. Neurosci Lett 2006;400:172–176.

Matusz PJ, Key AP, Gogliotti S, et al. Somatosensory plasticity in pediatric cerebral palsy following constraint-induced movement therapy. Neural Plast 2018;2018:1891978. doi: 10.1155/2018/1891978.

Mauritz KH, Dichgans J, Hufschmidt A. Quantitative analysis of stance in late cortical cerebellar atrophy of the anterior lobe and other forms of cerebellar ataxia. Brain 1979;102:461–482.

May D, Nayak US, Isaacs B. The life space diary: a measure of mobility in old people at home. Int Rehabil Med 1985;7:182–186.

Mayer NH. Clinicophysiologic concepts of spasticity and motor dysfunction in adults with upper motoneuron lesion. Muscle Nerve 1997;6(Suppl):S1–S13.

Mayo NE, Anderson S, Barclay R, et al. Getting on with the rest of your life following stroke: a randomized trial of a complex intervention aimed at enhancing life participation post stroke. Clin Rehabil. 2015 Jan 27. pii: 0269215514565396. [Epub ahead of print]

Mayo NE, Goldberg MS, Levy AR, et al. Changing rates of stroke in the province of Quebec Canada: 1981–1988. Stroke 1991;22:590–595.

Mayo NE, Wood-Dauphinee S, Côté R, et al. Activity, participation, and quality of life six months post-stroke. Arch Phys Med Rehabil 2002;83:1035–1042.

Mayston M. The Bobath concept: evolution and application. In: Forssberg H, Hirschfeld H, eds. Movement disorders in children. Medicine and sport science, vol. 36. Basel, Switzerland: S. Karger, 1992:1–6.

McCabe J, Monkiewicz M, Holcomb J, et al. Comparison of robotics, functional electrical stimulation, and motor learning methods for treatment of persistent upper extremity dysfunction after stroke: a randomized controlled trial. Arch Phys Med Rehabil. 2015;96:981–990. pii: S0003-9993(14)01228-3. doi: 10.1016/j.apmr.2014.10.022.

McCabe J, Monkiewicz M, Holcomb J, et al. Comparison of robotics, functional electrical stimulation, and motor learning methods for treatment of persistent upper extremity dysfunction after stroke: a randomized controlled trial. Arch Phys Med Rehabil 2015;96(6):981–990. doi: 10.1016/j.apmr.2014.10.022.

McCall JV, Ludovice MC, Blaylock JA, Kamper DG. A platform for rehabilitation of finger individuation in children with hemiplegic cerebral palsy. IEEE Int Conf Rehabil Robot 2019 Jun;2019:343–348. doi: 10.1109/ICORR.2019.8779537.

McCarty ME, Clifton RK, Collard RR. Problem solving in infancy: the emergence of an action plan. Dev Psychol 1999;35:1091–1101.

McChesney JW, Woollacott MH. The effect of age-related declines in proprioception and total knee replacement on postural control. J Gerontol 2000;55:658–666.

McCombe Waller S, Whitall J, et al. Sequencing bilateral and unilateral task-oriented training versus task-oriented training alone to improve arm function in individuals with chronic stroke. BMC Neurol 2014;14:236. doi: 10.1186/s12883-014-0236-6.

McConvey J, Bennett SE. Reliability of the Dynamic Gait Index in individuals with multiple sclerosis. Arch Phys Med Rehabil 2005;86:130–133.

McCoy AO, VanSant AF. Movement patterns of adolescents rising from a bed. Phys Ther 1993;73:182–193.

McCrea DA, Rybak IA. Organization of mammalian locomotor rhythm and pattern generation. Brain Res Rev 2008;57:134–146.

McCrea PH, Eng JJ, Hodgson AJ. Saturated muscle activation contributes to compensatory reaching strategies after stroke. J Neurophysiol 2005;94:2999–3008.

McCullagh P, Weiss MR, Ross D. Modeling considerations in motor skill acquisition and performance: an integrated approach. Exerc Sport Sci Rev 1989;17:475–513.

McCulloch K. Attention and dual-task conditions: physical therapy implications for individuals with acquired brain injury. J Neurol Phys Ther 2007;31:104–118.

McDonnell PM. Patterns of eye-hand coordination in the first year of life. Can J Psychol 1979;33:253–267.

McDonnell MN, Hillier SL. Vestibular rehabilitation for unilateral peripheral vestibular dysfunction. Cochrane Database Syst Rev 2015;1:CD005397. doi:10.1002/14651858.CD005397.pub4.

McEwen D, Taillon-Hobson A, Bilodeau M, et al. Virtual reality exercise improves mobility after stroke: an inpatient randomized controlled trial. Stroke 2014;45:1853–1855.

McFadyen BJ, Malouin F, Dumas F. Anticipatory locomotor control for obstacle avoidance in mid-childhood aged children. Gait Posture 2001;13:7–16.

McFadyen BJ, Winter DA. An integrated biomechanical analysis of normal stair ascent and descent. J Biomech 1988;21:733–744.

McGavin CR, Gupta SP, McHardy GJR. Twelve minute walking test for assessing disability in chronic bronchitis. BMJ 1976;1:822–823.

McGraw M. The neuromuscular maturation of the human infant. New York: Hafner Press, 1945.

McGraw MB. From reflex to muscular control in the assumption of an erect posture and ambulation in the human infant. Child Dev 1932;3:291.

McGuire BA, Gilbert CD, Rivlin PK, et al. Targets of horizontal connections in macaque primary visual cortex. J Comp Neurol 1991;305:370–392.

McIlroy W, Maki B. Do anticipatory adjustments precede compensatory stepping reactions evoked by perturbation? Neurosci Lett 1993;164:199–202.

McIlroy WE, Maki BE. The control of lateral stability during rapid stepping reactions evoked by antero-posterior perturbation: does anticipatory control play a role? Gait Posture 1999;9:190–198.

McIntosh AS, Beatty KT, Dwan LN, et al. Gait dynamics on an inclined walkway. J Biomech 2006;39:2491–2502.

McKee KJ, Orbell S, Austin CA, et al. Fear of falling, falls efficacy, and health outcomes in older people following hip fracture. Disabil Rehabil 2002;24(6):327–333.

McKinnon CD, Winter DA. Control of body balance in the frontal plane during human walking. J Biomech 1993;26:633–644.

McMahon TA. Muscles, reflexes and locomotion. Princeton, NJ: Princeton University, 1984.

McNevin NH, Shea CH, Wulf G. Increasing the distance of an external focus of attention enhances learning. Psychol Res 2003;67:22–29.

McNevin NH, Wulf G. Attentional focus on supra-postural tasks affects postural control. Hum Mov Sci 2002;21:187–202.

McPherson J, Schild R, Spaulding SJ, et al. Analysis of upper extremity movement in four sitting positions: a comparison of persons with and without cerebral palsy. Am J Occup Ther 1991;2:123–129.

McPherson JJ, Schild R, Spaulding SJ, Barsamian P, Transon C, White SC. Analysis of upper extremity movement in four sitting positions: a comparison of persons with and without cerebral palsy. Am J Occup Ther 1991;45(2):123–129. doi: 10.5014/ajot.45.2.123.

McQuiddy VA, Scheerer CR, Lavalley R, McGrath T, Lin L. Normative values for grip and pinch strength for 6- to 19-year-olds. Arch Phys Med Rehabil 2015;96(9):1627–1633. doi: 10.1016/j.apmr.2015.03.018.

McVea DA, Pearson KG. Object avoidance during locomotion. Adv Exp Med Biol 2009;629:293–315.

Medina JJ. The clock of ages. New York: Cambridge University Press, 1996.

Medley A, Thompson M. Development, reliability, and validity of the Sitting Balance Scale. Physiother Theory Pract 2011;27:471–481.

Melmoth DR, Finlay AL, Morgan MJ, et al. Grasping deficits and adaptations in adults with stereo vision losses. Invest Ophthalmol Vis Sci 2009;50:3711–3720.

Melville-Jones G, Mandl G. Neurobionomics of adaptive plasticity: integrating sensorimotor function with environmental demands. In: Desmedt JE, ed. Motor control mechanisms in health and disease. Adv Neurol 1983;39:1047–1071.

Melzack R. The McGill Pain Questionnaire: major properties and scoring methods. Pain 1975;1:277–299.

Mentiplay BF, Perraton LG, Bower KJ, et al. Assessment of lower limb muscle strength and power using hand-held and fixed dynamometry: a reliability and validity study. PLoS One 2015;10:1–18.

Merkel S, Voepel-Lewis T, Malviya S. Pain assessment in infants and young children: the FLACC scale. Am J Nurs 2002;102(10):55–58.

Merzenich MM, Jenkins WM. Reorganization of cortical representation of the hand following alterations of skin inputs induced by nerve injury, skin island transfers & experience. J Hand Ther 1993;6(2):89–104.

Metaxiotis D, Accles W, Siebel A, et al. Hip deformities in walking patients with cerebral palsy. Gait Posture 2000;11:86–91.

Metrot J, Mottet D, Hauret I, et al. Changes in bimanual coordination during the first 6 weeks after moderate hemiparetic stroke. Neurorehabil Neural Repair 2013;27:251–259.

Meyer DE, Abrams RA, Kornblum S, et al. Optimality in human motor performance: ideal control of rapid aimed movements. Psychol Rev 1988;95:340–370.

Meyer JS, Obara K, Muramatsu K, et al. Cognitive performance after small strokes correlates with ischemia, not atrophy of the brain. Dementia 1995;6:312–322.

Meyer-Heim A, Ammann-Reiffer C, Schmartz A, et al. Improvement of walking abilities after robotic-assisted locomotion training in children with cerebral palsy. Arch Dis Child 2009;94:615–620.

Meyns P, Bruijn SM, Duysens J. The how and why of arm swing during human walking. Gait Posture 2013;13:555–562.

Meyns P, Desloovere K, Van Gestel L, et al. Altered arm posture in children with cerebral palsy is related to instability during walking. Eur J Paediatr Neurol 2012;16:528–535.

Meyns P, Van Gestel L, Bruijn SM, et al. Is interlimb coordination during walking preserved in children with cerebral palsy? Res Dev Disabil 2012;33:1418–1428.

Meyns P, Van Gestel L, Massaad F, et al. Arm swing during walking at different speeds in children with Cerebral Palsy and typically developing children. Res Dev Disabil 2011;32:1957–1964.

Mezzarane RA, Klimstra M, Lewis A, et al. Interlimb coupling from the arms to legs is differentially specified for populations of motor units comprising the compound H reflex during "reduced" human locomotion. Exp Brain Res 2011;208(2):157–168.

Miall RC, Ingram HA, Cole JD, Gauthier GM. Weight estimation in a "deafferented" man and in control subjects: are judgements influenced by peripheral or central signals? Exp Brain Res 2000;133:491–500.

Miall RC, Rosenthal O, Ørstavik K, Cole JD, Sarlegna FR. Loss of haptic feedback impairs control of hand posture: a study in chronically deafferented individuals when grasping and lifting objects. Exp Brain Res 2019;237:2167–2184.

Micera S, Carpaneto J, Posteraro F, et al. Characterization of upper arm synergies during reaching tasks in able-bodied and hemiparetic subjects. Clin Biomech (Bristol, Avon) 2005;20:939–946.

Michael KM, Allen JK, Macko RF. Reduced activity after stroke: the role of balance, gait, and cardiovascular fitness. Arch Phys Med Rehabil 2005;86:1552–1556.

Michaelsen SM, Dannenbaum R, Levin MF. Task-specific training with trunk restraint on arm recovery in stroke: randomized control trial. Stroke 2006;37:186–192.

Michaelsen SM, Jacobs S, Roby-Braimi A, et al. Compensation for distal impairments of grasping in adults with hemiparesis. Exp Brain Res 2004a;157:162–173.

Michaelsen SM, Levin MF. Short-term effects of practice with trunk restraint on reaching movements in patients with chronic stroke: a controlled trial. Stroke 2004b;35:1914–1919.

Michaelsen SM, Luta A, Roby-Brami A, et al. Effect of trunk restraint on the recovery of reaching movements in hemiparetic patients. Stroke 2001;32:1875–1883.

Michaelsen SM, Magdalon EC, Levin MF. Grip aperture scaling to object size in chronic stroke. Motor Control 2009;13:197–217.

Middleton A, Merlo-Rains A, Peters DM, et al. Body weight-supported treadmill training is no better than overground training for individuals with chronic stroke: a randomized controlled trial. Top Stroke Rehabil 2014;21:462–476.

Middleton FA, Strick PL. Anatomical evidence for cerebellar and basal ganglia involvement in higher cognitive function. Science 1994;266:458–461

Middleton FA, Strick PL. Basal ganglia and cerebellar loops: motor and cognitive circuits. Brain Res Rev. 2000;31:236–250.

Milani-Comparetti A, Gidoni EA. Pattern analysis of motor development and its disorders. Dev Med Child Neurol 1967;9:625–630.

Milardi D, Quartarone A, Bramanti A, Anastasi G, Bertino S, Basile GA, Buonasera P, Pilone G, Celeste G, Rizzo G, Bruschetta D, Cacciola A. The Cortico-Basal Ganglia-Cerebellar Network: past, present and future perspectives. Front Syst Neurosci 2019;13:1–14.

Milczarek JJ, Kirby RL, Harrison ER, et al. Standard and four-footed canes: their effect on the standing balance of patients with hemiparesis. Arch Phys Med Rehabil 1993;74:281–285.

Mileti I, Taborri J, Rossi S, et al. Reactive postural responses to continuous yaw perturbations in healthy humans: the effect of aging. Sensors (Basel) 2020;20(1):63.

Mille ML, Johnson-Hilliard M, Martine KM, et al. One-step, two steps, three steps more… Directional vulnerability to falls in community dwelling older people. J Gerontol A Biol Sci Med Sci 2013;68:1540–1548.

Miller A, Duff SV, Quinn L, et al. Development of sensor-based measures of upper extremity interlimb coordination. Annu Int Conf IEEE Eng Med Biol Soc 2018;2018:3160–3164. doi: 10.1109/EMBC.2018.8512903.

Miller A, Quinn L, Duff SV, Wade E. Comparison of machine learning approaches for classifying upper extremity tasks in individuals post-stroke. Annu Int Conf IEEE Eng Med Biol Soc 2020;2020:4330–4336. doi: 10.1109/EMBC44109.2020.9176331.

Miller EK, Buschman TJ. Cortical circuits for the control of attention. Curr Opin Neurobiol. 2013;23:216–222.

Miller PH. Theories of developmental psychology, 4th ed. New York: Worth Publishers, 2002.

Millington PJ, Myklebust BM, Shambes GM. Biomechanical analysis of the sit-to-stand motion in elderly persons. Arch Phys Med Rehabil 1992;73:609–617.

Mills R, Levac D, Sveistrup H. Kinematics and postural muscular activity during continuous oscillating platform movement in children and adolescents with cerebral palsy. Gait Posture 2018;66:13–20.

Milner AD, Goodale MA. Visual pathways to perception and action. Prog Brain Res 1993;95:317–337.

Milner AD, Ockleford EM, Dewar W. Visuo-spatial performance following posterior parietal and lateral frontal lesions in stumptail macaques. Cortex 1977;13:350–360.

Milner B. Amnesia following operation on the temporal lobes. In: Whitty CWM, Zangwill OL, eds. Amnesia. London, UK: Butterworths, 1966:109–133.

Milot MH, Nadeau S, Gravel D, et al. Effect of increases in plantarflexor and hip flexor muscle strength on the levels of effort during gait in individuals with hemiparesis. Clin Biomech (Bristol, Avon) 2008;23:415–423.

Milosevic M, Marquez-Chin C, Masani K, et al. Why brain-controlled neuroprosthetics matter: mechanisms underlying electrical stimulation of muscles and nerves in rehabilitation. Biomed Eng Online 2020;19(1):81. doi: 10.1186/s12938-020-00824-w.

Miltner W, Bauder H, Sommer M, et al. Effects of constraint induced movement therapy on patients with chronic motor deficits after stroke. Stroke 1999;30:586–592.

Milton JG, Small SS, Solodkin A. On the road to automatic: dynamic aspects in the development of expertise. J Clin Neurophysiol 2004;21:134–143.

Mirelman A, Maidan I, Herman T, et al. Virtual reality for gait training: can it induce motor learning to enhance complex walking and reduce fall risk in patients with Parkinson's disease? J Gerontol A Biol Sci Med Sci 2011;66:234–240.

Mishkin M, Ungerleider LG. Contribution of striate inputs to the visuospatial functions of parieto-preoccipital cortex in monkeys. Behav Brain Res 1982;6:57–77.

Miszko TA, Cress ME, Slade JM, et al. Effect of strength and power training on physical function in community-dwelling older adults. J Gerontol A Biol Sci Med Sci 2003;58:171–175.

Miyai I, Fujimoto Y, Yamamoto H, et al. Long term effect of body weight supported treadmill training in Parkinson's disease: a randomized controlled trial. Arch Phys Med Rehabil 2002;83:1370–1373.

Miyasike-daSilva V, McIlroy WE. Gaze shifts during dual-tasking stair descent. Exp Brain Res 2016;234(11):3233–3243.

Moberg E. The unsolved problem: how to test the functional value of hand sensibility. J Hand Ther 1991;4:105–110.

Mochon S, McMahon TA. Ballistic walking. J Biomech 1980;13:49–57.

Mockford M, Caulton JM. Systematic review of progressive strength training in children and adolescents with cerebral palsy who are ambulatory. Pediatr Phys Ther 2008;20(4):318–333.

Mok NW, Brauer SG, Hodges PW. Hip strategy for balance control in quiet standing is reduced in people with low back pain. Spine 2004;29:E107–E112.

Molen HH. Problems on the evaluation of gait. Dissertation, Free University, Institute of Biomechanics and Experimental Rehabilitation, Amsterdam, 1973.

Molinari M, Leggio MG, Solida A. Cerebellum and procedural learning: evidence from focal cerebellar lesions. Brain 1997;120:1753–1762.

Moliterno AH, Bezerra FV, Pires LA, et al. Effect of contextual interference in the practicing of a computer task in individuals poststroke. Biomed Res Int 2020;2020:2937285. doi: 10.1155/2020/2937285.

Moll I, Vles JSH, Soudant DLHM, et al. Functional electrical stimulation of the ankle dorsiflexors during walking in spastic cerebral palsy: a systematic review. Dev Med Child Neurol 2017;59:1230–1236.

Monbaliu E, Himmelmann K, Lin JP, et al. Clinical presentation and management of dyskinetic cerebral palsy. Lancet Neurol 2017;16:741–749.

Monger C, Carr JH, Fowler V. Evaluation of a home-based exercise and training programme to improve sit-to-stand in patients with chronic stroke. Clin Rehabil 2002;16:361–367.

Montgomery J. Assessment and treatment of locomotor deficits in stroke. In: Duncan PW, Badke MB. Stroke rehabilitation: the recovery of motor control. Chicago, IL: Year Book, 1987:223–259.

Monzee J, Lamarre Y, Smith AM. The effects of digital anesthesia on force control using a precision grip. J Neurophysiol 2003;89:672–683.

Monzee J, Smith AM. Responses of cerebellar interpositus neurons to predictable perturbations applied to an object held in a precision grip. J Neurophysiol 2004;91:1230–1239.

Moore CG, Schenkman M, Kohrt WM, et al. Study in Parkinson disease of exercise (SPARX): translating high-intensity exercise from animals to humans. Contemp Clin Trials 2013;36:90–98.

Moore JL, Roth EJ, Killian C, et al. Locomotor training improves daily stepping activity and gait efficiency in individuals poststroke who have reached a "plateau" in recovery. Stroke 2010;41(1):129–135.

Moore S, Brunt D, Nesbitt ML, et al. Investigation of evidence for anticipatory postural adjustments in seated subjects who performed a reaching task. Phys Ther 1992;72:335–343.

Morasso P. Spatial control of arm movements. Exp Brain Res 1981;42:223–227.

Moreau NG. Muscle performance in children and youth with cerebral palsy: implications for resistance training. In: Miller F, Bachrach S, Lennon N, O'Neil M, eds. Cerebral palsy, 2nd ed. Springer Pub, 2020.

Moreau NG, Bodkin AW, Bjornson K, Hobbs A, Soileau M, Lahasky K. Effectiveness of rehabilitation interventions to improve gait speed in children with cerebral palsy: systematic review and Meta-Analysis. Phys Ther 2016;96:1938–1954.

Morgan M, Phillips JG, Bradshaw JL, et al. Age-related motor slowness: simply strategic? J Gerontol 1994;49:M133–M139.

Morgan P. The relationship between sitting balance and mobility outcomes in stroke. Aust J Physiother 1994;40:91–96.

Morgen K, Kadom N, Sawaki L, et al. Training-dependent plasticity in patients with multiple sclerosis. Brain 2004;127:2506–2517.

Morris ME. Locomotor training in people with Parkinson disease. Phys Ther 2006;86:1426–1435.

Morris DM, Uswatte G, Crago JE, et al. The reliability of the Wolf motor function test for assessing upper extremity function after stroke. Arch Phys Med Rehabil 2001;82:750–755.

Morris JC, Rubin EH, Morris EJ. Senile dementia of the Alzheimer's type: an important risk factor for serious falls. J Gerontol 1987;42:412–417.

Morris ME, Iansek R, Matyas TA, et al. Stride length regulation in Parkinson's disease: normalization strategies and underlying mechanisms. Brain 1996;119:551–569.

Morris RGM, Anderson E, Lynch GS, et al. Selective impairment of learning and blockage of long-term potentiation by an N-methyl-D-aspartate receptor antagonist, AP5. Nature 1986;319:774–776.

Morris SL, Dodd KJ, Morris ME. Outcomes of progressive resistance strength training following stroke: a systematic review. Clin Rehabil 2004;18(1):27–39.

Mortenson PA, Eng JJ. The use of casts in the management of joint mobility and hypertonia following brain injury in adults: a systematic review. Phys Ther 2003;83:648–658.

Morton SM, Bastian AJ. Cerebellar control of balance and locomotion. Neuroscientist 2004;10:247–259.

Morton SM, Bastian AJ. Mechanisms of cerebellar gait ataxia. Cerebellum 2007;6:79–86.

Morton SM, Bastian AJ. Relative contributions of balance and voluntary leg-coordination deficits to cerebellar gait ataxia. J Neurophysiol 2003;89:1844–1856.

Moskowitz B, Beth Carswell B, Kitzmiller J, et al. The effectiveness of the size matters handwriting program. Am J Occup Ther 2017;71(4_Supplement_1):7111520304. Doi: org/10.5014/ajot.2017.71S1-PO5147

Moseley AM, Lanzarone S, Bosman JM, et al. Ecological validity of walking speed assessment after traumatic brain injury: a pilot study. J Head Trauma Rehabil 2004;19:341–348.

Motl RW, Smith DC, Elliott J, et al. Combined training improves walking mobility in persons with significant disability from multiple sclerosis: a pilot study. J Neurol Phys Ther 2012;36(1):32–37.

Motl RW, Suh Y, Dlugonski D, et al. Oxygen cost of treadmill and overground walking in mildly disabled persons with multiple sclerosis. J Neurol Sci 2011;32:255–262.

Mott FW, Sherrington CS. Experiments upon the influence of sensory nerves upon movement and nutrition of the limbs: preliminary communication. Proc R Soc Lond Biol 1895;57:481–488.

Mourey F, Grishin A, d'Athis P, et al. Standing up from a chair as a dynamic equilibrium task: a comparison between young and elderly subjects. J Gerontol 2000;55:B425–B431.

Moumdjian L, Sarkamo T, Leone C, Leman M, Feys P. Effectiveness of music-based interventions on motricity or cognitive functioning in neurological populations: a systematic review. Eur J Phys Rehabil Med 2017;53(3):466–482. doi: 10.23736/S1973-9087.16.04429-4.

Mozzafarian D, Benjamin eJ, Go AS, et al. On behalf of the American Heart Association Statistics Committee and Stroke Statistics Subcommittee. Heart disease and stroke statistics—2016 update: a report from the American Heart Association. Circulation 2016;133(4):e38–360.

Msall ME, DiGaudio K, Rogers BT, et al. Functional Independence Measure for Children (Wee-FIM): conceptual basis and pilot use in children with developmental disabilities. Clin Pediatr 1994;33:421–430.

Mudge S, Barber PA, Stott NS. Circuit-based rehabilitation improves gait endurance but not usual walking activity in chronic stroke: a randomized controlled trial. Arch Phys Med Rehabil 2009;90:1989–1994.

Mudge S, Stott NS. Timed walking tests correlate with daily step activity in persons with stroke. Arch Phys Med Rehabil 2009;90:296–301.

Mudie MH, Matyas TA. Can simultaneous bilateral movement involve the undamaged hemisphere in reconstruction of neural networks damaged by stroke? Disabil Rehabil 2000;22(1–2):23–37.

Mudie MH, Matyas TA. Responses of the densely hemiplegic upper extremity to bilateral training. Neurorehabil Neural Repair 2001;15:129–140.

Muir BC, Bodratti LA, Morris CE, Haddad JM, van Emmerik REA, Rietdyk S. Gait characteristics during inadvertent obstacle contacts in young, middle-aged and older adults. Gait Posture 2020;77:100–104.

Muir RB, Lemon RN. Corticospinal neurons with a special role in precision grip. Brain Res 1983;261:312–316.

Muir SW, Berg K, Chesworth B, et al. Use of the Berg Balance Scale for predicting multiple falls in community dwelling elderly people: A prospective study. Phys Ther 2008;88:449–459.

Mukherjee A, Chakravarty A. Spasticity mechanisms—for the clinician. Front Neurol 2010;1:149.

Mulder T, Berndt H, Pauwels J, et al. Sensorimotor adaptability in the elderly and disabled. In: Stelmach G, Homberg V, eds. Sensori-motor impairment in the elderly. Dordrecht, The Netherlands: Kluwer, 1993.

Müller ML, Redfern MS, Jennings JR. Postural prioritization defines the interaction between a reaction time task and postural perturbations. Exp Brain Res 2007;183:447–456.

Mullie Y, Duclos C. Role of proprioceptive information to control balance during gait in healthy and hemiparetic individuals. Gait Posture 2014;40:610–615.

Mulroy S, Gronley J, Weiss W, et al. Use of cluster analysis for gait pattern classification of patients in early and late recovery phases following stroke. Gait Posture 2003;18:114–125.

Mulroy SJ, Klassen T, Gronley JK, et al. Gait parameters associated with responsiveness to treadmill training with body weight support after stroke: an exploratory study. Phys Ther 2010;90:209–223.

Munton JS, Ellis MI, Chamberlain MA, et al. An investigation into the problems of easy chairs used by the arthritic and the elderly. Rheumatol Rehabil 1981;20:164–173.

Muratori LM, Dapul G, Bartels MN, et al. Effect of object transport on grasp coordination in multiple system atrophy. Mov Disord 2006;21:555–563.

Muratori LM, McIsaac TL, Gordon AM, et al. Impaired anticipatory control of force sharing patterns during whole-hand grasping in Parkinson's disease. Exp Brain Res 2008;185(1):41–52.

Murray M, Kory R, Sepic S. Walking patterns of normal women. Arch Phys Med Rehabil 1970;51:637–650.

Murray MP, Drought AB, Kory RC. Walking patterns of normal men. J Bone Joint Surg Am 1964;46:335–360.

Murray MP, Kory RC, Clarkson BH, et al. Comparison of free and fast speed walking patterns of normal men. Am J Phys Med 1966;45:8–24.

Murray MP, Kory RC, Clarkson BH. Walking patterns in healthy older men. J Gerontol 1969;24:169–178.

Murray MP, Mollinger LA, Gardner GM, et al. Kinematic and EMG patterns during slow, free, and fast walking. J Orthop Res 1984;2:272–280.

Murray MP. Gait as a total pattern of movement. Am J Phys Med 1967;46:290–333.

Mushiake H, Inase M, Tanji J. Neuronal activity in the primate premotor, supplementary and precentral motor cortex during visually guided and internally determined sequential movements. J Neurophysiol 1991;66:705–718.

Mushiake H, Strick P. Preferential activity of dentate neurons during limb movements guided by vision. J Neurophysiol 1993;70:2660–2664.

Mutlu A, Livanelioglu A, Gunel K. Reliability of Ashworth and Modified Ashworth Scales in children with spastic cerebral palsy. BMC Musculoskel Disord 2008;9:44–51.

Mutsaarts M, Steenbergen B, Bekkering H. Anticipatory planning deficits and task context effects in hemiparetic cerebral palsy. Exp Brain Res 2006;172:151–162.

N

Nadeau S, Gravel D, Arsenault AB, et al. Dynamometric assessment of the plantarflexors in hemiparetic subjects: relations between muscular, gait and clinical parameters. Scand J Rehabil Med 1997;29:137–146.

Nakahara H, Doya K, Hikosaka O. Parallel cortico-basal ganglia mechanisms for acquisition and execution of visuomotor sequences: a computational approach. J Cogn Neurosci 2001;13:626–647.

Nambu A, Tokuno H, Takada M. Functional significance of the cortico-subthalamo-pallidal 'hyperdirect' pathway. Neurosci Res 2002;43:111–117.

Nanhoe-Mahabier W, Allum JH, Pasman EP, et al. The effects of vibrotactile biofeedback training on trunk sway in Parkinson's disease patients. Parkinsonism Relat Disord 2012;18:1017–1021.

Napier JR. The prehensile movement of the human hand. J Bone Joint Surg Br 1956;38:902–913.

Narici MV, Maffulli N, Maganaris CN. Ageing of human muscles and tendons. Disabil Rehabil 2008;30:1548–1554.

Nasar JL, Troyer D. Pedestrian injuries due to mobile phone use in public places. Accid Anal Prev 2013;57:91–95.

Nascimento LR, da Silva LA, Araújo Barcellos JVM, Teixeira-Salmela LF. Ankle-foot orthoses and continuous functional electrical stimulation improve walking speed after stroke: a systematic review and meta-analyses of randomized controlled trials. Physiotherapy 2020;109:43–53.

Nashner L, Woollacott M, Tuma G. Organization of rapid responses to postural and locomotor-like perturbations of standing man. Exp Brain Res 1979;36:463–476.

Nashner L, Woollacott M. The organization of rapid postural adjustments of standing humans: an experimental-conceptual model. In: Talbott RE, Humphrey DR, eds. Posture and movement. New York: Raven, 1979:243–257.

Nashner L. Adapting reflexes controlling the human posture. Exp Brain Res 1976;26:59–72.

Nashner LM. Adaptation of human movement to altered environments. Trends Neurosci 1982;5:358–361.

Nashner LM. Balance adjustment of humans perturbed while walking. J Neurophysiol 1980;44:650–664.

Nashner LM. Fixed patterns of rapid postural responses among leg muscles during stance. Exp Brain Res 1977;30:13–24.

Nashner LM. Sensory, neuromuscular, and biomechanical contributions to human balance. In: Duncan P, ed. Balance: Proceedings of the APTA Forum. Alexandria, VA: American Physical Therapy Association, 1989:5–12.

Nashner LM, Shumway-Cook A, Marin O. Stance posture control in select groups of children with cerebral palsy: deficits in sensory organization and muscular coordination. Exp Brain Res 1983;49:393–409.

Nathan PW, Smith M, Deacon P. Vestibulospinal, reticulospinal and descending propriospinal nerve fibres in man. Brain 1996,119:1809–1833.

National Center for Health Statistics. Health, United States, 2016: with chartbook on long-term trends in health. Hyattsville, MD: US Department of Health and Human Services, CDC, National Center for Health Statistics; 2017.

Navarro MD, Lloréns R, Noé E, et al. Validation of a low-cost virtual reality system for training street-crossing. A comparative study in healthy, neglected and non-neglected stroke individuals. Neuropsychol Rehabil 2013;23(4):597–618.

Negrotti A, Secchi C, Gentilucci M. Effects of disease progression and L-dopa therapy on the control of reaching-grasping in Parkinson's disease. Neuropsychologia 2005;43:450–459.

Nelson SR, DiFabio RP, Anderson JH. Vestibular and sensory interaction deficits assessed by dynamic platform posturography in patients with multiple sclerosis. Ann Otol Rhinol Laryngol 1995;104:62–68.

Neptune RR, Kautz SA, Zajac FE. Contributions of the individual ankle plantar flexors to support, forward progression and swing initiation during walking. J Biomech 2001;34:1387–1398.

Neuhaus BE, Ascher B, Coullon M, et al. A survey of rationales for and against hand splinting in hemiplegia. Am J Occup Ther 1981;35:83–95.

Neurology Section Outcome Measures Recommendations, American Physical Therapy Association. http://www.neuropt.org/professional-resources/neurology-section-outcome-measures-recommendations. Accessed February 14, 2015.Neva JL, Ma JA, Orsholits D, Boisgontier MP, Boyd LA. The effects of acute exercise on visuomotor adaptation, learning, and inter-limb transfer. Exp Brain Res 2019;237(4):1109–1127. doi: 10.1007/s00221-019-05491-5.

Nevitt MC, Cummings SR, Kidd S, et al. Risk factors for reMW recurrent nonsyncopal falls. JAMA 1989;261:2663–2668.

Newell A, Rosenbloom PS. Mechanisms of skill acquisition and the law of practice. In: Anderson JR, ed. Cognitive skills and their acquisition. Hillsdale, NJ: Erlbaum, 1981:1–55.

Newell K. Degrees of freedom and the development of center of pressure profiles. In: Newell KM, Molenaar PMC, eds. Applications of nonlinear dynamics to developmental process modeling. Hillsdale, NJ: Erlbaum, 1997:63–84.

Newell K, van Emmerik REA. The acquisition of coordination: preliminary analysis of learning to write. Hum Mov Sci 1989;8: 17–32.

Newell KM. Motor skill acquisition. Annu Rev Psychol 1991;42:213–237.

Newell KM, Carlton LG, Hancock PA. Kinetic analysis of response variability. Psychol Bull 1984;96:133–151.

Newell KM, Kennedy JA. Knowledge of results and children's motor learning. Dev Psychol 1978;14:531–536.

Newell KM, Vaillancourt DE. Dimensional change in motor learning. Hum Mov Sci 2001;20:695–715.

Newton R. Validity of the multi-directional reach test: a practical measure for limits of stability in older adults. J Gerontol Med Sci 2001;56A:M248–M252.

Ng SS, Hui-Chan CW. The timed up & go test: its reliability and association with lower-limb impairments and locomotor capacities in people with chronic stroke. Arch Phys Med Rehabil 2005;86:1641–1647.

Ng SSM. Balance ability, not muscle strength and exercise endurance, determines the performance of hemiparetic subjects on the timed-sit-to-stand test. Am J Phys Med Rehabil 2010;89:497–504.

Nichols D, Case-Smith J. Reliability and validity of the pediatric evaluation of disability inventory. Ped Phys Ther 1996;8(1): 15–24.

Nicolai S, Mirelman A, Herman T, et al. Improvement of balance after audio-biofeedback. A 6-week intervention study in patients with progressive supranuclear palsy. Gerontol Geriatr 2010;43:224–228.

Niewczyk PM, Granger CV. Measuring function in young children with impairments. Pediatr Phys Ther 2010;22(1):42–51.

Nilsagård Y, Denison E, Gunnarsson LG, et al. Factors perceived as being related to accidental falls by persons with multiple sclerosis. Disabil Rehabil 2009a;31(16):1301–1310.

Nilsagård Y, Lundholm C, Denison E, et al. Predicting accidental falls in people with multiple sclerosis—a longitudinal study. Clin Rehabil 2009b;23(3):259–269.

Nitsche MA, Fricke K, Henschke U, et al. Pharmacological modulation of cortical excitability shifts induced by transcranial direct current stimulation in humans. J Physiol 2003;553:293–301.

Nogueira LA, Teixeira L, Sabino P, et al. Gait characteristics of multiple sclerosis patients in the absence of clinical disability. Disabil Rehabil 2013;35:1472–1478.

Norton BJ, Bromze HE, Saurmann SA, et al. Correlation between gait speed and spasticity at the knee. Phys Ther 1975;55:355–359.

Noseworthy JH, Lucchinetti C, Rodriguez M, et al. Multiple sclerosis. N Engl J Med 2000;343:938–952.

Noth J. Trends in the pathophysiology and pharmacotherapy of spasticity. J Neurol 1991;238:131–139.

Novacheck TF, Stout JS, Tervo R. Reliability and validity of the Gillette Functional Assessment Questionnaire as an outcome measure in children with walking disabilities. J Pediatr Orthop 2000;20(1): 75–86.

Nowak DA, Glasauer S, Hermsdorfer J. Grip force efficiency in long-term deprivation of somatosensory feedback. Neuroreport 2003;14:1803–1807.

Nowak DA, Grefkes C, Dafotakis M, et al. Dexterity is impaired at both hands following unilateral subcortical middle cerebral artery stroke. Eur J Neurosci 2007;25:3173–3184.

Nowak DA, Hermsdörfer J, Marquardt C, et al. Grip and load force coupling during discrete vertical arm movements with a grasped object in cerebellar atrophy. Exp Brain Res 2002;145(1):28–39.

Nowak DA, Tisch S, Hariz M, Limousin P, Topka H, Rothwell JC. Sensory timing cues improve akinesia of grasping movements in Parkinson's disease: a comparison to the effects of subthalamic nucleus stimulation. Mov Disord 2006;21(2):166–172. doi: 10.1002/mds.20657.

Nudo RJ. Mechanisms for recovery of motor function following cortical damage. Curr Opin Neurobiol 2006;16:638–644.

Nudo RJ. Neural bases of recovery after brain injury. J Commun Disord 2011;44: 515–520.

Nudo RJ. Postinfarct cortical plasticity and behavioral recovery. Stroke 2007;38:840–845.

Nudo RJ, Milliken GW, Jenkins WM, et al. Use-dependent alterations of movement representations in primary motor cortex of adult squirrel monkeys. J Neurosci 1996;16:785–807.

Nutt JG, Carter JH, Lea ES, et al. Motor fluctuations during continuous levodopa infusions in patients with Parkinson's disease. Mov Disord 1997;12:285–292.

Nutt JG, Carter JH, Woodward W, et al. Does tolerance develop to levodopa? Comparison of 2- and 21-H levodopa infusions. Mov Disord 1993;8:139–143.

Nutt JG, Woodward WR, Hammerstad JP, et al. The "on-off" phenomenon in Parkinson's disease. Relation to levodopa absorption and transport. N Engl J Med 1984;310:483–488.

Nwaobi OM, Brubaker CE, Cusick B, et al. Electromyographic investigation of extensor activity in cerebral-palsied children in different seating positions. Dev Med child Neurol 1983;25:175–183.

Nyberg L, Gustafson Y. Fall prediction index for patients in stroke rehabilitation. Stroke 1997;28:716–721.

Nyquist JB, Lappin JS, Zhang R, Tadin D. Perceptual training yields rapid improvements in visually impaired youth. Sci Rep 2016;6:37431. doi: 10.1038/srep37431.

O

O'Keefe J, Dostsrovsky J. The hippocampus as a spatial map: preliminary evidence from unit activity in the freely-moving rat. Brain Res 1971;34:171–175.

O'Shea S, Morris ME, Iansek R. Dual task interference during gait in people with Parkinson's disease: effects of motor versus cognitive secondary tasks. Phys Ther 2002;82:888–897.

O'Sullivan SB, Schmitz TJ. Physical rehabilitation assessment and treatment, 4th ed. Philadelphia, PA: Davis, 2001.

Oates AR, Awdhan A, Arnold C, Fung J, Lanovaz JL. Adding light touch while walking in older adults: biomechanical and neuromotor effects. J Aging Phys Act 20201–20206. doi: 10.1123/japa.2019-0270.

Obeso JA, Marin C, Rodriguez-Oroz C, et al. The basal ganglia in Parkinson's disease: current concepts and unexplained observations. Ann Neurol 2008;64:30–46.

Ochi A, Yokoyama S, Abe T, et al. Differences in muscle activation patterns during step recovery in elderly women with and without a history of falls. Aging Clin Exp Res 2014;26(2):213–220.

Ochs AL, Newberry J, Lenhardt ML, et al. Neural and vestibular aging associated with falls. In: Birren JE, Schaie KW, eds. Handbook of psychology of aging. New York: Van Nostrand & Reinholdt, 1985:378–399.

Ogden R, Franz SI. On cerebral motor control: the recovery from experimentally produced hemiplegia. Psychobiology 1917;1:33–49.

Ohata K, Tsuboyama T, Haruta T, et al. Relation between muscle thickness, spasticity, and activity limitations in children and adolescents with cerebral palsy. Dev Med Child Neurol 2008;50:152–156.

Oie KS, Kiemel T, Jeka JJ. Multisensory fusion: simultaneous re-weighting of vision and touch for the control of human posture. Cogn Brain Res 2002;14:164–176.

Okamoto T, Kumamoto M. Electromyographic study of the learning process of walking in infants. Electromyography 1972;12:149–158.

Okamoto T, Okamoto K. Electromyographic characteristics at the onset of independent walking in infancy. Electromyogr Clin Neurophysiol 2001b;41:33–41.

Okamoto T, Okamoto K, Andrew PD. Electromyographic study of newborn stepping in neonates and young infants. Electromyogr Clin Neurophysiol 2001a;41:289–296.

Okubo Y, Schoene D, Lord SR. Step training improves reaction time, gait and balance and reduces falls in older people: a systematic review and meta-analysis. Br J Sports Med 2017;51:586–593.

Oliver D, Britton M, Seed P, et al. Development and evaluation of evidence based risk assessment tool (STRATIFY) to predict which elderly inpatients will fall: case-control and cohort studies. BMJ 1997;315:1049–1053.

Oliver D, Daly F, Martin FC, et al. Risk factors and risk assessment tools for falls in hospital in-patients: a systematic review. Age Ageing 2004;33(2):122–130.

Olivier I, Cuisinier R, Vaugoyeau M, et al. Dual-task study of cognitive and postural interference in 7-year-olds and adults. Neuroreport 2007;18:817–821.

Olney SJ, Griffin MP, McBride ID. Temporal, kinematic and kinetic variables related to gait speed in subjects with hemiplegia: a regression approach. Phys Ther 1994;74:872–885.

Olney SJ, Griffin MP, Monga TN, et al. Work and power in gait of stroke patients. Arch Phys Med Rehabil 1991;72:309–314.

Olney SJ, Monga TN, Costigan PA. Mechanical energy of walking of stroke patients. Arch Phys Med Rehabil 1986;67:92–98.

Olney SJ, Richards CL. Hemiparetic gait following stroke. Part 1: characteristics. Gait Posture 1996;4:136–148.

Olsen J, Knapton E. Handwriting without tears, 3rd ed. Cabin John, MD: Western Psychological Services, 2008.

Onla-or S, Winstein CJ. Determining the optimal challenge point for motor skill learning in adults with moderately severe Parkinsons disease. Neurorehabil Neural Repair 2008;22:385–395.

Orendurff MS, Schoen JA, Bernatz GC, et al. How humans walk: bout duration, steps per bout, and rest duration. J Rehabil Res Dev 2008;45:1077–1089.

Orendurff MS, Segal AD, Klute GK, et al. The effect of walking speed on center of mass displacement. J Rehabil Res Dev 2004;41:829–834.

Ornitz E. Normal and pathological maturation of vestibular function in the human child. In: Romand R, ed. Development of auditory and vestibular systems. New York: Academic Press, 1983:479–536.

Orr R, Raymond J, Fiatarone Singh M. Efficacy of progressive resistance training on balance performance in older adults: a systematic review of randomized controlled trials. Sports Med 2008;38:317–343.

Ortiz-Rosario A, Berrios-Torres I, Adeli H, et al. Combined corticospinal and reticulospinal effects on upper limb muscles. Neurosci Lett 2014;561:30–34.

Ottenbacher KJ, Msall ME, Lyon N, et al. The WeeFIM instrument: its utility in detecting change in children with developmental disabilities. Arch Phys Med Rehabil 2000;81:1317–1326.

Ottenbacker KJ, Hsu Y, Granger CV, et al. The reliability of the functional independence measure: a quantitative review. Arch Phys Med Rehabil 1996;77(12):1226–1232.

Ouellette M, LeBrasseur NK, Beam JF, et al. High intensity resistance training improves muscle strength, self-reported function and disability in long term stroke survivors. Stroke 2004;35: 1404–1409.

Overstall PW, Exton-Smith AN, Imms FJ, et al. Falls in the elderly related to postural imbalance. BMJ 1977;1:261–264.

Oxford GK, Vogel LV, Mitchell A, et al. Adult norms for a commercially available nine hold peg test for finger dexterity. Am J Occup Ther 2003;57:570–573.

Ozer K, Chesher SP, Scheker LR. Neuromuscular electrical stimulation and dynamic bracing for the management of upper-extremity spasticity in children with cerebral palsy. Dev Med Child Neurol 2006;48(7):559–563.

Ozkul C, Guclu-Gunduz A, Eldemir K, Apaydin Y, Gulsen C, Yazici G, Soke F, Irkec C. Effect of task-oriented circuit training on motor and cognitive performance in patients with multiple sclerosis: a single-blinded randomized controlled trial. NeuroRehabilitation 2020;46:343–353.

P

Paci M, Baccini M, Rinaldi LA. Pusher behaviour: a critical review of controversial issues. Disabil Rehabil 2009;31:249–258.

Page S, Levine P. Forced use after TBI: promoting plasticity and function through practice. Brain Inj 2003;17:675–681.

Page SJ, Levine P, Leonard AC. Modified constraint-induced therapy in acute stroke: a randomized controlled pilot study. Neurorehabil Neural Repair 2005;19(1):27–32. doi: 10.1177/1545968304272701.

Page SJ, Levine P, Leonard A, Szaflarski JP, Kissela BM. Modified constraint-induced therapy in chronic stroke: results of a single-blinded randomized controlled trial. Phys Ther 2008;88(3):333–340. doi: 10.2522/ptj.20060029.

Page SJ, Murray C, Hermann V. Affected upper-extremity movement ability is retained 3 months after modified constraint-induced therapy. Am J Occup Ther 2011;65(5):589–593. doi: 10.5014/ajot.2011.000513.

Pai YC, Bhatt T, Wang F, et al. Inoculation against falls: rapid adaptation by young and older adults to slips during daily activities. Arch Phys Med Rehabil 2010;91:452–459.

Pai YC, Bhatt T, Yang F, et al. Perturbation training can reduce community-dwelling older adults' annual fall risk: a randomized controlled trial. J Gerontol A Biol Sci Med Sci 2014;69(12):1586–1594.

Pai Y-C, Maki BE, Iqbal K, et al. Thresholds for step initiation induced by support-surface translation: a dynamic center-of-mass model provides much better prediction than a static model. J Biomech 2000;33:387–392.

Pai Y-C, Naughton BJ, Chang RW, et al. Control of body center of mass momentum during sit-to-stand among young and elderly adults. Gait Posture 1994;2:109–116.

Pai Y-C, Wening JD, Runtz EF, et al. Role of feedforward control of movement stability in reducing slip-related balance loss and falls among older adults. J Neurophysiol 2003;90:755–762.

Paillard J. Cognitive versus sensorimotor encoding of spatial information. In: Ellen P, Thinus-Blanc C, eds. Cognitive processes and spatial orientation in animal and man: neurophysiology and developmental aspects. NATO ASI Series 37. The Hague, The Netherlands: Martinus Nijhoff, 1987:43–77.

Palisano RJ. Neuromotor and developmental assessment. In: Wilhelm IJ, ed. Physical therapy assessment in early infancy. New York: Churchill Livingstone, 1993:173–224.

Palisano RJ, Kang LJ, Chiarello LA, Orlin MN, Oeffinger D, Maggs J. Social and community participation of children and youth with cerebral palsy is associated with age and gross motor function classification. Phys Ther 2009;89:1304–1314.

Palliyath S, Hallett M, Thomas SL, et al. Gait in patients with cerebellar ataxia. Mov Disord 1998;13:958–964.

Palluel E, Chauvel G, Bourg V, et al. Effects of dual tasking on postural and gait performances in children with cerebral palsy and healthy children. Int J Dev Neurosci 2019;79:54–64.

Palombaro KM, Craik RL, Mangione KK, et al. Determining meaningful changes in gait speed after hip fracture. Phys Ther 2006;86:809–816.

Pan B, Sun Y, Xie B, Huang Z, Wu J, Hou J, Liu Y, Huang Z, Zhang Z. Alterations of muscle synergies during voluntary arm reaching movement in subacute stroke survivors at different levels of impairment. Front Comput Neurosci 2018;12:1–11.

Pandyan AD, Price CIM, Rodgers H, et al. Biomechanical examination of a commonly used measure of spasticity. Clin Biomech (Bristol, Avon) 2001;16:859–865.

Pang MY, Eng JJ, Dawson AS, et al. A community-based fitness and mobility exercise program for older adults with chronic stroke: a randomized, controlled trial. J Am Geriatr Soc 2005;53:1667–1674.

Pang MY, Lam T, Yang JF. Infants adapt their stepping to repeated trip-inducing stimuli. J Neurophysiol 2003;90:2731–2740.

Pang MY, Yang JF. Interlimb coordination in human infant stepping. J Physiol 2001;533(Pt 2):617–625.

Pang MY, Yang JF. Sensory gating for the initiation of the swing phase in different directions of human infant stepping. J Neurosci 2002;22:5734–5740.

Pang MY, Yang JF. The initiation of the swing phase in human infant stepping: importance of hip position and leg loading. J Physiol (Lond) 2000;528(Pt 2):389–404.

Papa E, Cappozzo A. Sit-to-stand motor strategies investigated in able-bodied young and elderly subjects. J Biomech 2000;33:1113–1122.

Papegaaij S, deLima-Pardini AC, Smith BA, et al. Keeping your balance while balancing a cylinder: interaction between postural and voluntary goals. Exp Brain Res 2012;223:79–87.

Pardasaney PK, Latham NK, Jette AM, Wagenaar RC, Ni P, Slavin MD, Bean JF. Sensitivity to change and responsiveness of four balance measures for community-dwelling older adults. Phys Ther 2012;92:388–397.

Pare M, Dugas C. Developmental changes in prehension during childhood. Exp Brain Res 1999;125:239–247.

Pare N, Rabin L, Fogel J, et al. Mild traumatic brain injury and its sequelae: characterisation of divided attention deficits. Neuropsychol Rehabil 2009;19: 110–137.

Parijat P, Lockhart TE. Effects of moveable platform training in preventing slip-induced falls in older adults. Ann Biomed Eng 2012;40:1111–1121.

Park ES, Park CI, Lee HJ, et al. The characteristics of sit-to-stand transfer in young children with spastic cerebral palsy based on kinematic and kinetic data. Gait Posture 2003;17:43–49.

Park EY, Kim WH, Choi YI. Factor analysis of the WeeFIM in children with spastic cerebral palsy. Disabil Rehabil 2013;35(17):1466–1471.

Park J, Lewis MM, Huang X, Latash ML. Effects of olivo-ponto-cerebellar atrophy (OPCA) on finger interaction and coordination. Clin Neurophysiol 2013;124:991–998.

Park J, Wu YH, Lewis MM, Huang X, Latash ML. Changes in multifinger interaction and coordination in Parkinson's disease. J Neurophysiol 2012;108:915–924.

Park SW, Wolf SL, Blanton S, et al. The EXCITE trial: predicting a clinically meaningful motor activity log outcome. Neurorehabil Neural Repair 2008;22: 486–493.

Parker TM, Osternig LR, Lee HJ, et al. The effect of divided attention on gait stability following concussion. Clin Biomech (Bristol, Avon) 2005;20:389–395.

Parker VM, Wade DT, Langton Hewer R. Loss of arm function after stroke: measurement, frequency, and recovery. Int Rehabil Med 1986;8:69–73.

Parkinson J. An essay on the shaking palsy. London: Whittingham and Rowland for Sherwood, Needly and Jones, 1817.

Parreira RB, Grecco LAC, Oliveira CS. Postural control in blind individuals: a systematic review. Gait Posture 2017;57:161–167.

Partridge CJ, Edwards SM, Mee R, et al. Hemiplegic shoulder pain: a study of two methods of physiotherapy treatment. Clin Rehabil 1990;4:43–49.

Parvathaneni A, Das JM. Balint Syndrome. In: StatPearls[internet]. StatPearls Publishing LLC, 2020.

Pascual-Leone A, Amedi A, Fregni F, et al. The plastic human brain cortex. Annu Rev Neurosci 2005;28:377–401.

Pascual-Leone A, Cammarota A, Wassermann EM, et al. Modulation of motor cortical outputs to the reading hand of Braille readers. Ann Neurol 1993;34:33–37.

Pascual-Leone A, Grafman J, Hallett M. Modulation of cortical motor output maps during development of implicit and explicit knowledge. Science 1994;263:1287–1289.

Passingham RE. Premotor cortex: sensory cues and movement. Behav Brain Res 1985;16:175–185.

Passingham RE, Chen YC, Thaler D. Supplementary motor cortex and self-initiated movement. In: Ito M, ed. Neural programming. Tokyo, Japan: Japan Scientific Society, 1989:13–24.

Pastalan LA, Mantz RK, Merrill J. The simulation of age-related sensory losses: a new approach to the study of environmental barriers. In: Preiser WFE, ed. Environment design research, vol. 1. Stroudsberg, PA: Dowden, Hutchinson & Ross, 1973:383–390.

Patel M, Fransson PA, Lush D, Petersen H, Magnusson M, Johansson R, Gomez S. The effects of foam surface properties on standing body movement. Acta Otolaryngol 2008;128:952–960.

Patla A, Sepulveda F, Quevedo A, et al. Visual sampling characteristics during quiet standing and walking in an individual with peripheral neuropathy. Proceedings of the 5th Annual Conference of the International Functional Electrical Stimulation Society, 2000; http://ifess.org/proceedings/IFESS2000/IFESS2000_037_Patla.pdf

Patla A, Shumway-Cook A. Dimensions of mobility: defining the complexity and difficulty associated with community mobility. J Aging Phys Act 1999;7:7–19.

Patla AE. Age-related changes in visually guided locomotion over different terrains: major issues. In: Stelmach G, Homberg V, eds. Sensorimotor impairment in the elderly. Dordrecht, The Netherlands: Kluwer, 1993:231–252.

Patla AE. Strategies for dynamic stability during adaptive human locomotion. IEEE Eng Med Biol Mag 2003;22:48–52.

Patla AE. Understanding the control of human locomotion: a prologue. In: Patla AE, ed. Adaptability of human gait. Amsterdam, The Netherlands: North-Holland, 1991:3–17.

Patla AE. Understanding the roles of vision in the control of human locomotion. Gait Posture 1997;5:54–69.

Patla AE, Adkin A, Martin C, et al. Characteristics of voluntary visual sampling of the environment for safe locomotion over different terrains. Exp Brain Res 1996;112:513–522.

Patla AE, Frank JS, Winter DA. Balance control in the elderly: implications for clinical assessment and rehabilitation. Can J Public Health 1992a;83(Suppl 2):S29–S33.

Patla AE, Prentice SD, Martin C, et al. The bases of selection of alternate foot placement during locomotion in humans. In: Woollacott MH, Horak F, eds. Posture and gait: control mechanisms. Eugene, OR: University of Oregon, 1992b:226–229.

Patla AE, Winter DA, Frank JS, et al. Identification of age-related changes in the balance-control system. In: Duncan P, ed. Balance: Proceedings of the APTA Forum, Alexandria, VA: American Physical Therapy Association, 1990:43–55.

Patla PE, Ishac MG, Winter DA. Anticipatory control of center of mass and joint stability during voluntary arm movement from a standing posture: interplay between active and passive control. Exp Brain Res 2002;143:318–327.

Patrick E, Ada L. The Tardieu Scale differentiates contracture from spasticity whereas the Ashworth Scale is confounded by it. Clin Rehabil 2006;20:173–182.

Patrick SK, Noah JA, Yang JF. Developmental constraints of quadrupedal coordination across crawling styles in human infants. J Neurophysiol 2012;107(11):3050–3061.

Patten C, Condlilffe EG, Dairaghi CA, et al. Concurrent neuromechanical and functional gains following upper-extremity power training post-stroke. J Neuroeng Rehabil 2013;10:1.

Patterson SL, Forrester LW, Rodgers MM, et al. Determinants of walking function after stroke: differences by deficit severity. Arch Phys Med Rehabil 2007;88:115–119.

Patton HD, Fuchs A, Hille B, et al. Textbook of physiology, vol. 1, 21st ed. Philadelphia, PA: Saunders, 1989.

Paulignan Y, McKenzie C, Marteniuk R, et al. The coupling of arm and finger movements during prehension. Exp Brain Res 1990;79:431–436.

Paulus W, Straube A, Brandt T. Visual stabilisation of posture. Brain 1984;107:1143–1163.

Paus T. Structural maturation of neural pathways in children and adolescents: In vivo study. Science 1999;283:1908–1911.

Pause M, Kunesch E, Binkofski F, et al. Sensorimotor disturbances in patients with lesions of the parietal cortex. Brain 1989;112:1599–1625.

Pavao SL, dos Santos AN, Woollacott MH, Rocha NA. Assessment of postural control in children with cerebral palsy: a review. Res Dev Disabil 2013;34(5):1367–1375.

Pavol MJ, Owings TM, Foley KT, et al. The sex and age of older adults influence the outcome of induced trips. J Gerontol 1999;54A:M103–M108.

Payton O, Melson C, Ozer M. Patient participation in program planning: a manual for therapists. Philadelphia, PA: FA Davis, 1990.

Pearson KG. Proprioceptive regulation of locomotion. Curr Opin Neurobiol 1995;5:786–791.

Pearson KG. Generating the walking gait: role of sensory feedback. Prog Brain Res 2004;143:123–129.

Pearson KG, Gordon JE. Spinal reflexes. In: Kandel ER, Schwartz JH, Jessell TM, Siegelbaum SA, Hudspeth AJ, eds. Principles of neural science, 5th ed. New York, NY: McGraw-Hill, 2013:1936–1984.

Pearson K, Gordon J. Locomotion. In: Kandel E, Schwartz JH, Jessell TM, eds. Principles of neural science, 4th ed. New York: McGraw-Hill, 2000:737–755.

Pearson KG, Ramirez JM, Jiang W. Entrainment of the locomotor rhythm by group Ib afferents from ankle extensor muscles in spinal cats. Exp Brain Res 1992;90:557–566.

Pedersen SW, Eriksson T, Oberg B. Effects of withdrawal of antiparkinson medication on gait and clinical score in the Parkinson patient. Acta Neurol Scand 1991;84:7–13.

Peel C, Sawyer Baker P, Roth DL, et al. Assessing mobility in older adults: the UAB Study of Aging Life-Space Assessment. Phys Ther 2005;85:1008–1019.

Pehoski C. Object manipulation in infants and children. In: Henderson A, Pehoski C., eds. Hand function in the child: foundations for remediation. St. Louis, MO: Mosby, 1995:136–153.

Peiper A. Cerebral functions in infancy and childhood. New York: Consultants Bureau, 1963.

Penfield W. Functional localization in temporal and deep Sylvian areas. Res Publ Assoc Res Nerv Ment Dis 1958;36:210–226.

Penfield W, Rassmussen T. The cerebral cortex of man: a clinical study of localization of function. New York: Macmillan, 1950.

Perell KL, Nelson A, Goldman RL, et al. Fall risk assessment measures: an analytic review. J Gerontol A Biol Sci Med Sci 2001;56:M761–M766.

Perenin MT, Jeannerod M. Residual vision in cortically blind hemifields. Neuropsychologia 1975;13:1–7.

Pérennou D. Weight bearing asymmetry in standing hemiparetic patients. J Neurol Neurosurg Psychiatry 2005;76:62.

Pérennou D. Postural disorders and spatial neglect in stroke patients: a strong association. Restor Neurol Neurosci 2006;24(4–6):319–334.

Pérennou DA, Amblard B, Leblond C, et al. Biased postural vertical in humans with hemispheric cerebral lesions. Neurosci Lett 1998;252.75–78.

Perera S, Mody SH, Woodman RC, et al. Meaningful change and responsiveness in common physical performance measures in older adults. J Am Geriatr Soc 2006;54:743–752.

Perkins-Ceccato N, Passmore SR, Lee TD. Effects of focus of attention depend on golfers' skill. J Sports Sci 2003;21:593–600.

Peppoloni L, Lawrence EL, Ruffaldi E, Valero-Cuevas FJ. Characterization of the disruption of neural control strategies for dynamic fingertip forces from attractor reconstruction. PLoS One. 2017;12(2):e0172025.

Perry J, Burnfield JM. Gait analysis: normal and pathological function. Thorofare, NJ: Slack, 2010.

Perry J, Garrett M, Gronley JK, et al. Classification of walking handicap in the stroke population. Stroke 1995;26:982–989.

Perry J. Gait analysis: normal and pathological function. Thorofare, NJ: Slack, 1992.

Perry SB. Clinical implications of a dynamical systems theory. Neurol Rep 1998;22: 4–10.

Peterka RJ. Sensorimotor integration in human postural control. J Neurophysiol 2002;88:1097–1118.

Peterka RJ. Sensory Integration for Human Balance Control, 1st ed. Elsevier BV;2018.

Peterka RJ, Black FO. Age-related changes in human posture control: sensory organization tests. J Vestib Res 1990–1991;1:73–85.

Peterka RJ, Loughlin PJ. Dynamic regulation of sensorimotor integration in human postural control. J Neurophysiol 2004;91:410–423.

Petersen SE, Posner MI. The attention system of the human brain: 20 years after. Annu Rev Neurosci 2012;35: 73–89.

Petersen TH, Willerslev-Olsen M, Conway BA, Nielsen JB. The motor cortex drives the muscles during walking in human subjects. J Physiol 2012;590(10):2443–2452.

Peterson CL, Hall AL, Kautz SA, et al. Pre-swing deficits in forward propulsion, swing initiation and power generation by individual muscles during hemiparetic walking. J Biomech 2010;43:2348–2355.

Peterson CL, Kautz SA, Neptune RR. Muscle work is increased in preswing during hemiparetic walking. Clin Biomech (Bristol, Avon) 2011;26:859–866.

Peterson EW, Cho CC, Finlayson ML. Fear of falling and associated activity curtailment among middle aged and older adults with multiple sclerosis. Mult Scler 2007;13:1168–1175.

Peterson EW, Cho CC, von Koch L, et al. Injurious falls among middle aged and older adults with multiple sclerosis. Arch Phys Med Rehabil 2008;89:1031–1037.

Petrarca M, Zanelli G, Patanè F, et al. Reach-to-grasp interjoint coordination for moving object in children with hemiplegia. J Rehabil Med 2009;41:995–100.

Pettersson AF, Olsson E, Wahlund LO. Motor function in subjects with mild cognitive impairment and early Alzheimer's disease. Dement Geriatr Cogn Disord 2005;19(5–6):299–304.

Petzinger GM, Fisher BE, McEwen S, et al. Exercise-enhanced neuroplasticity targeting motor and cognitive circuitry in Parkinson's disease. Lancet Neurol 2013;12:716–726.

Petzinger GM, Walsh JP, Akopian G, et al. Effects of treadmill exercise on dopaminergic transmission in the 1-methyl-4-phenyl-1,2,3,6-tetrahydropyridine-lesioned mouse model of basal ganglia injury. J Neurosci 2007;27:5291–5300.

Pham TM, Winblad B, Granholm AC, et al. Environmental influences on brain neurotrophins in rats. Pharmacol Biochem Behav 2002;73:167–175.

Phan PL, Blennerhassett JM, Lythgo N, et al. Over-ground walking on level and sloped surfaces in people with stroke compared to healthy matched adults. Dis Rehabil 2013;35:1302–1307.

Piaget J. The origins of intelligence in children. New York: Norton, 1951.

Picelli A, Melotti C, Origano F, et al. Robot-assisted gait training in patients with Parkinson disease: a randomized controlled trial. Neurorehabil Neural Repair 2012a;26:353–361.

Picelli A, Melotti C, Origano F, et al. Does robotic gait training improve balance in Parkinson's disease? A randomized controlled trial. Parkinsonism Relat Disord 2012b;18(8):990–993.

Picelli A, Melotti C, Origano F, et al. Robot-assisted gait training versus equal intensity treadmill training in patients with mild to moderate Parkinson's disease: a randomized controlled trial. Parkinsonism Relat Disord 2013;19(6):605–610.

Picelli A, Melotti C, Origano F, et al. Robot-assisted gait training is not superior to balance training for improving postural instability in patients with mild to moderate Parkinson's disease: a single-blind randomized controlled trial. Clin Rehabil 2015;29:339–347.

Pierce SR, Daly K, Gallagher KG, et al. Constraint-induced therapy for a child with hemiplegic cerebral palsy: a case report. Arch Phys Med Rehabil 2002;83(10):1462–1463.

Pierce SR, Gallagher KG, Schaumburg SW, et al. Home forced use in an outpatient rehabilitation program for adults with hemiplegia: a pilot study. Neurorehabil Neural Repair 2003;17(4):214–219.

Pieh C, Proudlock F, Gottlob I. Smooth pursuit in infants: maturation and the influence of stimulation. Br J Ophthalmol 2012;96(1):73–77.

Pierrot-Deseilligny E, Burke D. The circuitry of the human spinal cord. spinal and corticospinal mechanisms of movement. Cambridge: Cambridge University Press, 2009.

Pijnappels M, Bobbert MF, van Dieen JH. Control of support limb muscles in recovery after tripping in young and older subjects. Exp Brain Res 2005;160:326–333.

Pijnappels M, Van Wezel BM, Colombo G, et al. Cortical facilitation of cutaneous reflexes in leg muscles during human gait, Brain Res 1998;787:149–153.

Pilkar R, Yarossi M, Nolan KJ. EMG of the tibialis anterior demonstrates a training effect after utilization of a foot drop stimulator. NeuroRehabilitation 2014;35(2):299–305.

Piper, MC, Darrah, J. Motor assessment of the developing infant. Philadelphia, PA: WB Saunders, 1994.

Pitts DG. The effects of aging on selected visual functions: dark adaptation, visual acuity, stereopsis, and brightness contrast. In: Sekular R, Kline D, Dismukes K, eds. Modern aging research: aging and human visual function. New York: Liss, 1982:131–160.

Pin TW, Butler PB, Cheung HM, Shum SLF. Segmental assessment of trunk control in infants from 4 to 9 months of age- a psychometric study. BMC Pediatr 2018;18:1–8.

Pizzamiglio G, Zhang Z, Duta M, Rounis E. Factors influencing manipulation of a familiar object in patients with limb apraxia after stroke. Front Human Neurosci 2020;13:1–13.

Platt JR. Strong inference. Science 1964;146:347–352.

Platz T, Eickhof C, Nuyens G, et al. Clinical scales for the assessment of spasticity, associated phenomena, and function: a systematic review of the literature. Disabil Rehabil 2005;27:7–18.

Plotnik M, Giladi N, Hausdorff JM. Bilateral coordination of gait and Parkinson's disease: the effects of dual tasking. J Neurol Neurosurg Psychiatry 2009;80:347–350.

Plummer P, Apple S, Dowd C, et al. Texting and walking: effect of environmental setting and task prioritization on dual-task interference in healthy young adults. Gait Posture 2015;41(1):46–51.

Plummer P, Eskes G, Wallace S, et al. Cognitive-motor interference during functional mobility after stroke: state of the science and implications for future research. Arch Phys Med Rehabil 2013;94:2565–2574.

Plummer P, Meg E, Morris ME, et al. Assessment of unilateral neglect. Phys Ther 2003;83:732–740.

Plummer P, Villalobos RM, Vayda MS, et al. Feasibility of dual-task gait training for community-dwelling adults after stroke: a case series. Stroke Res Treat 2014;2014:538602.

Plummer-D'Amato P, Altmann LJP. Relationships between motor function and gait-related dual task interference after stroke: a pilot study. Gait Posture 2012;35:170–172.

Plummer-D'Amato P, Altmann LJP, Behrman AL, et al. Interference between cognition, double-limb support, and swing during gait in community-dwelling individuals poststroke. Neurorehabil Neural Repair 2010;24:542–549.

Plummer-D'Amato P, Altmann LJP, Saracino D, et al. Interactions between cognitive tasks and gait after stroke: a dual task study. Gait Posture 2008;27:683–688.

Podsiadlo D, Richardson S. The timed "Up and Go" test: a test of basic functional mobility for frail elderly persons. J Am Geriatr Soc 1991;39:142–148.

Poewe WH. Clinical aspects of motor fluctuations in Parkinson's disease. Neurology 1994;44(7 Suppl 6):S6–S9.

Pogetti LS, de Souza RM, Tudella E, Teixeira LA. Early infant's use of visual feedback in voluntary reaching for a spatial target. Front Psychol 2013;4:520.

Pohl P, Carlsson G, Bunketorp Käll L, Nilsson M, Blomstrand C. Experiences from a multimodal rhythm and music-based rehabilitation program in late phase of stroke recovery—A qualitative study. PLoS One 2018;13(9):e0204215. doi: 10.1371/journal.pone.0204215.

Pohl PS, Kemper S, Siengsukon CF, et al. Dual-task demands of hand movements for adults with stroke: a pilot study. Top Stroke Rehabil 2011;18:238–247.

Pohl PS, McDowd JM, Filion D, et al. Implicit learning of a motor skill after mild and moderate stroke. Clin Rehabil 2006;20:246–253.

Pohl PS, McDowd JM, Filion D, Richards LG, Stiers W. Implicit learning of a motor skill after mild and moderate stroke. Clin Rehabil 2006;20(3):246–253. doi: 10.1191/0269215506cr916oa.

Pohl PS, McDowd JM, Filion DL, et al. Implicit learning of a perceptual motor skill after stroke. Phys Ther 2001;81:1780–1789.

Pohl PS, Winstein CJ. Practice effects on the less-affected upper extremity after stroke. Arch Phys Med Rehabil 1999;80:668–675.

Pohl PS, Winstein CJ, Fisher BE. The locus of age-related movement slowing: sensory processing in continuous goal-directed aiming. J Gerontol 1996;51:P94–P102.

Poincare, H. Science and hypothesis. In: Gould SJ, ed. The value of science: Essential writings of Henri Poincare. New York: The Modern Library, 2001:7–180. Original work published 1905.

Poizner H, Mack L, Verfaellie M, et al. Three-dimensional computergraphic analysis of apraxia. Brain 1990;113:85–101.

Poldrack RA, Sabb FW, Foerde K, et al. Neural correlates of motor skill automaticity. J Neurosci 2005;25:5356–5364.

Polit A, Bizzi E. Characteristics of motor programs underlying arm movements in monkeys. J Neurophysiol 1979;42: 183–194.

Pollock CL, Hunt MA, Vieira TM, Gallina A, Ivanova TD, Garland SJ. Challenging standing balance reduces the asymmetry of motor control of postural sway poststroke. Motor Control 2019;23(3):327–343.

Pomeroy V, Aglioti SM, Mark VW, et al. Neurological principles and rehabilitation of action disorders: rehabilitation interventions. Neurorehabil Neural Repair 2011;25(5):33S–43S.

Pons TP, Garraghty PE, Mishkin M. Lesion induced plasticity in the second somatosensory cortex of adult macaques. Proc Natl Acad Sci USA 1988;85:5279–5281.

Pont K, Wallen M, Bundy A, et al. Reliability and validity of the test of in-hand manipulation in children ages 5 to 6 years. Am J Occup Ther 2008;62:384–392.

Poole JL, Burtner PA, Torres TA, et al. Measuring dexterity in children using the nine-hole peg test. J Hand Ther 2005;18:348–351.

Poole JL, Sadek J, Haaland KY. Ipsilateral deficits in 1-handed shoe tying after left or right hemisphere stroke. Arch Phys Med Rehabil 2009;90(10):1800–1805.

Poole JL, Whitney SL. Motor assessment scale for stroke patients: concurrent validity and interrater reliability. Arch Phys Med Rehabil 1988;69(3 Pt 1):195–197.

Poole KE, Vedi S, Debiram I, et al. Bone structure and remodelling in stroke patients: early effects of zoledronate. Bone 2009;44:629–633.

Popa LS, Ebner TJ. Cerebellum, predictions and errors. Front Cell Neurosci 2019;12:1–13.

Porro G, van der Linden D, van Nieuwenhuizen O, et al. Role of visual dysfunction in postural control in children with cerebral palsy. Neural Plast 2005;12:205–210.

Porter R. The corticomotoneuronal component of the pyramidal tract: corticomotoneuronal connections and functions in primates. Brain Res Rev 1985;10:1–26.

Porto JM, Freire Junior RC, Bocarde L, et al. Contribution of hip abductor-adductor muscles on static and dynamic balance of community-dwelling older adults. Aging Clin Exp Res 2019;31(5):621–627.

Potter K, Fulk GD, Salem Y, et al. Outcome measures in neurological physical therapy practice: part I. Making sound decisions. J Neurol Phys Ther 2011;35:57–64.

Pound P, Gompertz P, Ebrahim S. A patient-centered study of the consequences of stroke. Clin Rehabil 1998;12:338–347.

Pourahmadi MR, Ebrahimi Takamjani I, et al. Reliability and concurrent validity of a new iPhone® goniometric application for measuring active wrist range of motion: a cross-sectional study in asymptomatic subjects. J Anat 2017;230(3):484–495. doi: 10.1111/joa.12568.

Powell D, Threlkeld AJ, Fang X, Muthumani A, Xia R. Amplitude- and velocity-dependency of rigidity measured at the wrist in Parkinson's disease. Clin Neurophysiol 2012;123:764–773.

Powell J, Pandyan AD, Granat M, et al. Electrical stimulation of wrist extensors in poststroke hemiplegia. Stroke 1999;30:1384–1389.

Powell LE, Myers AM. The Activities-specific Balance Confidence (ABC) Scale. J Gerontol Med Sci 1995;50A(1):M28–M34.

Powers RK, Campbell DL, Rymer WZ. Stretch reflex dynamics in spastic elbow flexor muscles. Ann Neurol 1989;25:32–42.

Pozzo T, Berthoz A, Lefort L. Head stabilization during various locomotor tasks in humans. 1. Normal subjects. Exp Brain Res 1990;82:97–106.

Pozzo T, Berthoz A, Lefort L, et al. Head stabilization during various locomotor tasks in humans. II. Patients with bilateral peripheral vestibular deficits. Exp Brain Res 1991;85:208–217.

Pozzo T, Levik Y, Berthoz A. Head stabilization in the frontal plane during complex equilibrium tasks in humans. In: Woollacott M, Horak F, eds. Posture and gait: control mechanisms. Eugene, OR: University of Oregon, 1992:97–100.

Pradhan SD, Brewer BR, Carvell GE, et al. Assessment of fine motor control in individuals with Parkinson's disease using force tracking with a secondary cognitive task. J Neurol Phys Ther 2010;34:32–40.

Pradhan SD, Scherer R, Matsuoka Y, et al. Use of sensitive devices to assess the effect of medication on attentional demands of precision and power grips in individuals with Parkinson disease. Med Biol Eng Comput 2011;49:1195–1199.

Prado MTA, Fernani DCGL, Silva TDD, Smorenburg ARP, Abreu LC, Monteiro CBM. Motor learning paradigm and contextual interference in manual computer tasks in individuals with cerebral palsy. Res Dev Disabil 2017;64:56–63. doi: 10.1016/j.ridd.2017.03.006.

Prayson RA, Hannahoe BM. Clinicopathological findings in patients wtih infantile hemiparesis and epilepsy. Hum Pathol 2004;35:734–738.

Prechtl HF, Cioni G, Einspieler C, et al. Role of vision on early motor development: lessons from the blind. Dev Med Child Neurol 2001;43:198–201.

Prechtl HFR. Continuity and change in early neural development. In: Prechtl HFR, ed. Continuity of neural functions from prenatal to postnatal life. Clinics in Developmental Medicine 94. Oxford, UK: Blackwell Scientific, 1984:1–15.

Prechtl HFR. Prenatal motor development. In: Wade MC, Whiting HTA, eds. Motor development in children: aspects of coordination and control. Dordrecht, The Netherlands: Martinus Nijhoff, 1986:53–64.

Price DD, McGrath PA, Rafii A, et al. The validation of visual analogue scales as ratio scale measure for chronic and experimental pain. Pain 1983;17:45–56.

Priplata A, Niemi J, Salen M, et al. Noise enhanced human balance control. Phys Rev Lett 2002;89(23):238101.

Priplata AA, Niemi JB, Harry JD, et al. Vibrating insoles and balance control in elderly people. Lancet 2003;362:1123–1124.

Priplata AA, Patritti BL, Niemi JB, et al. Noise-enhanced balance control in patients with diabetes and patients with stroke. Ann Neurol 2006;59:4–12.

Profeta VLS, Turvey MT. Bernstein's levels of movement construction: a contemporary perspective. Hum Mov Sci 2018;57:111–133.

Proffitt R, Lange B. Considerations in the efficacy and effectiveness of virtual reality interventions for stroke rehabilitation: moving the field forward. Phys Ther 2015;95(3):441–448.

Prokop T, Berger W. Influence of optic flow on locomotion in normal subjects and patients with Parkinson's disease. Electroencephalogr Clin Neurophysiol 1996;99:402.

Proske U, Gandevia SC. The proprioceptive senses: their roles in signaling body shape, body position and movement, and muscle force. Physiol Rev 2012;92,1651–1697.

Prosperini L, Leonardi L, De Carli P, et al. Visuo-proprioceptive training reduces risk of falls in patients with multiple sclerosis. Mult Scler 2010;16:491–499.

Proud EL, Morris ME. Skilled hand dexterity in Parkinson's disease: effects of adding a concurrent task. Arch Phys Med Rehabil 2010;91(5):794–799.

Pua YH, Ong PH, Clark RA, Matcher DB, Lim ECW. Falls efficacy, postural balance, and risk for falls in older adults with falls related emergency department visits: prospective cohort study. BMC Geriatr 2017;17:1–7.

Q

Qiu Q, Ramirez DA, Saleh S, et al. The New Jersey Institute of Technology Robot-Assisted Virtual Rehabilitation (NJIT-RAVR) system for children with cerebral palsy: a feasibility study. J Neuroeng Rehabil 2009;6:40.

Quaney BM, Perera S, Maletsky R, et al. Impaired grip force modulation in the ipsilesional hand after unilateral middle cerebral artery stroke. Neurorehabil Neural Repair 2005;19:338–349.

Quinn L, Debono K, Dawes H, et al.; Members of the TRAIN-HD Project Group. Task-specific training in Huntington disease: a randomized controlled feasibility trial. Phys Ther 2014;94(11):1555–1568.

Quinn L, Gordon J. Functional outcomes: documentation for rehabilitation. Philadelphia, PA: Saunders, 2003.

Quinn L, Reilmann R, Marder K, et al. Altered movement trajectories and force control during object transport in Huntington's disease. Mov Disord 2001;16(3):469–480.

Quintana LA. Evaluation of perception and cognition. In: Trombly CA, ed. Occupational therapy for physical dysfunction, 4th ed. Baltimore, MD: Lippincott Williams & Wilkins, 1995.

R

Rabadi MH, Rabadi FM. Comparison of the Action Research Arm Test and the Fugl-Meyer Assessment as measures of upper-extremity motor weakness after stroke. Arch Phys Med Rehabil 2006;87:962–966.

Rabaglietti E, De Lorenzo A, Brustio PR. The role of working memory on dual-task cost during walking performance in childhood. Front Psychol 2019;10:1–8.

Rabbitt P, Birren JE. Age and responses to sequences of repetitive and interruptive signals. J Gerontol 1967;22:143–150.

Rabbitt PM, Rogers M. Age and choice between responses in a self-paced repetitive task. Ergonomics 1965;8:435–444.

Rachwani J, Herzberg O, Golenia L, Adolph KE. Postural, visual, and manual coordination in the development of prehension. Child Dev 2019;90(5):1559–1568.

Rachwani J, Kaplan BE, Tamis-LeMonda CS, Adolph KE. Children's use of everyday artifacts: Learning the hidden affordance of zipping. Dev Psychobiol In press.

Rachwani J, Santamaria V, Saavedra SL, et al. The development of trunk control and its relation to reaching in infancy: a longitudinal study. Front Hum Neurosci 2015;9:94. doi: 10.3389/fnhum.2015.00094. eCollection 2015.

Rachwani J, Santamaria V, Saavedra SL, Woollacott MH. The development of trunk control and its relation to reaching in infancy: a longitudinal study. Front Hum Neurosci 2015;9:94.

Rachwani J, Soska KC, Adolph KE. Behavioral flexibility in learning to sit. Dev Psychobiol 2017;59:937–948.

Rademaker GGJ. De Beteekenis der Roode Kernen en van the overige Mesencephalon voor Spiertonus, Lichaam-shouding en Labyrinthaire Reflexen. Leiden, The Netherlands: Eduarol Ijdo, 1924.

Raffalt PC, Spedden ME, Geertsen SS. Dynamics of postural control during bilateral stance—Effect of support area, visual input and age. Hum Mov Sci 2019;67:102462.

Raffegeau TE, Haddad JM, Huber JE, Rietdyk S. Walking while talking: young adults flexibly allocate resources between speech and gait. Gait Posture 2018;64:59–62.

Raghavan P. The nature of hand motor impairment after stroke and its treatment. Curr Treat Options Cardiovasc Med 2007;9:221–228.

Raghavan P, Bilaloglu S, Ali SZ, et al. The role of robotic path assistance and weight support in facilitating 3D movements in individuals with poststroke hemiparesis. Neurorehabil Neural Repair 2020;34(2):134–147. doi: 10.1177/1545968319887685.

Raghavan P, Krakauer JW, Gordon AM. Impaired anticipatory control of fingertip forces in patients with a pure motor or sensorimotor lacunar syndrome. Brain 2006;129(Pt 6):1415–1425.

Raghavan P, Petra E, Krakaer JW, et al. Patterns of impairment in digit independence after subcortical stroke. J Neurophysiol 2005;95:369–378.

Rahman S, Griffin HJ, Quinn NP, et al. On the nature of fear of falling in Parkinson's disease. Behav Neurol 2011;24:219–228.

Raibert M. Symmetry in running. Science 1986;231:1292–1294.Rallon CR, Chen CC. Performance-based and self-reported assessment of hand function. Am J Occup Ther 2008;62:574–579.

Ralston HJ. Energetics of human walking. In: Herman RM, Grillner S, Stein PSG, et al., eds. Neural control of locomotion. New York: Plenum, 1976:77–98.

Ramachandran VS, Stewart M, Rogers-Ramachandran DC. Perceptual correlates of massive cortical reorganization. Neuroreport 1992;3:583–586.

Ramnemark A, Nyberg L, Lorentzon R, et al. Progressive hemiosteoporosis on the paretic side and increased bone mineral density in the nonparetic arm the first year after severe stroke. Osteoporos Int 1999;9:269–275.

Ramon y Cajal SR, DeFelipe J, Jones EG. Cajal's degeneration and regeneration of the nervous system. New York, NY: Oxford University Press, 1991.

Rand D, Eng JJ. Predicting daily use of the affected upper extremity 1 year after stroke. J Stroke Cerebrovasc Dis 2015;24(2):274–283.

Rand MK, Lemay M, Squire LM, et al. Control of aperture closure initiation during reach-to-grasp movements under manipulations of visual feedback and trunk involvement in Parkinson's disease. Exp Brain Res 2009;201:509–525.

Rand MK, Shimansky Y, Stelmach GE, et al. Effects of accuracy constraints on reach-to-grasp movements in cerebellar patients. Exp Brain Res 2000;135:179–188.

Rand MK, Smiley-Oyen AL, Shimansky YP, et al. Control of aperture closure during reach-to-grasp movements in Parkinson's disease. Exp Brain Res 2006;168:131–142.

Randall M, Carlin JB, Chondros P, et al. Reliability of the Melbourne assessment of unilateral Upper Limb Function. Develop Med Child Neurol 2001;43(11):761–767.

Rankin JK, Woollacott MH, Shumway-Cook A, et al. Cognitive influence on postural stability: a neuromuscular analysis in young and older adults. J Gerontol 2000;55A:M112–M119.

Rantanen T, Guralnik JM, Ferrucci L, et al. Coimpairments: strength and balance as predictors of severe walking disability. J Gerontol 1999;54A:M172–M176.

Rapcsak SZ, Watson RT, Heilman KM. Hemispace-visual field interactions in visual extinction. J Neurol Neurosurg Psychiatry 1987;50:1117–1124.

Rasmussen IA, Xu J, Antonsen IK, et al. Simple dual tasking recruits prefrontal cortices in chronic severe traumatic brain injury patients, but not in controls. J Neurotrauma 2008;25:1057–1070.

Rathinam C, Mohan V, Peirson J, Skinner J, Nethaji KS, Kuhn I. Effectiveness of virtual reality in the treatment of hand function in children with cerebral palsy: a systematic review. J Hand Ther 2019;32(4):426–434.e1. doi: 10.1016/j.jht.2018.01.006.

Ravi DK, Kumar N, Singhi P. Effectiveness of virtual reality rehabilitation for children and adolescents with cerebral palsy: an updated evidence-based systematic review. Physiotherapy 2017;103(3):245–258. doi: 10.1016/j.physio.2016.08.004.

Rea P. Brainstem tracts. In: Rea P, ed. Essential clinical anatomy of the nervous system. Elsevier, 2015:177–192.

Reber RJ, Squire LR. Encapsulation of implicit and explicit memory in sequence learning. J Cogn Neurosci 1998;10:248–263.

Redfern MS, Jennings JR, Martin C, et al. Attention influences sensory integration for postural control in older adults. Gait Posture 2001;14:211–216.

Redfern MS, Müller ML, Jennings JR, et al. Attentional dynamics in postural control during perturbations in young and older adults. J Gerontol Biol Sci 2002;57A:298–303.

Reed ES. An outline of a theory of action systems. J Motor Behav 1982;14:98–134.

Reedman SE, Boyd RN, Elliott C, Sakzewski L. ParticiPAte CP: a protocol of a randomised waitlist-controlled trial of a motivational and behaviour change therapy intervention to increase physical activity through meaningful participation in children with cerebral palsy. BMJ Open 2017;7(8):e015918. doi: 10.1136/bmjopen-2017-015918.

Regnaux JP, David D, Daniel O, et al. Evidence for cognitive processes involved in the control of steady state of walking in healthy subjects and after cerebral damage. Neurorehabil Neural Repair 2005;19(2):125–132.

Rehabilitation Measures Database [May 20, 2014]. Available at: www.rehabmeasures.org

Reid KF, Naumova EN, Carabello RJ, et al. Lower extremity muscle mass predicts functional performance in mobility-limited elders. J Nutr Health Aging 2008;12:493–498.

Reilly D, van Donkelaar P, Saavedra S, et al. The effects of dual task conditions: the interaction between the development of postural control and executive attention. J Motor Behav 2008a;40:90–102.

Reilly DS, Woollacott MH, van Donkelaar P, et al. The interaction between executive attention and postural control in dual-task conditions: children with cerebral palsy. Arch Phys Med Rehabil 2008b;89:834–842.

Reimers J. Clinically based decision making for surgery. In: Sussman M, ed. The diplegic child. Rosemont, IL:

American Academy of Orthopedic Surgeons, 1992:155, 156, 158.

Reinbolt JA, Fox MD, Arnold AS, et al. Importance of preswing rectus femoris activity in stiff-knee gait. J Biomech 2008;41:2362–2369.

Reinkensmeyer DJ, Maier MA, Guigon E, et al. Do robotic and non-robotic arm movement training drive motor recovery after stroke by a common neural mechanism? Experimental evidence and a computational model. Conf Proc IEEE Eng Med Biol Soc 2009;2009:2439–2441.

Reinkensmeyer DJ, Wolbrecht ET, Chan V, et al. Comparison of three-dimensional, assist-as-needed robotic arm/hand movement training provided with Pneu-WREX to conventional tabletop therapy after chronic stroke. Am J Phys Med Rehabil 2012;91:S232–S241.

Reisman DS, Scholz JP. Aspects of joint coordination are preserved during pointing in persons with post-stroke hemiparesis. Brain 2003;126(Pt 11):2510–2527.

Remelius JG, Jones SL, House JD, et al. Gait impairments in persons with multiple sclerosis across preferred and fixed walking speeds. Arch Phys Med Rehabil 2012;93:1637–1642.

Remple MS, Bruneau RM, Vandenberg PM, et al. Sensitivity of cortical movement representations to motor experience: evidence that skill learning but not strength training induces cortical reorganization. Behav Brain Res 2001;123:133–141.

Reoli R, Cherry-Allen K, Therrien A, et al. Can the ARAT be used to measure arm function in people with cerebellar ataxia? Phys Ther 2020:pzaa203. doi: 10.1093/ptj/pzaa203.

Resnick HE, Vinik AI, Schwartz AV, et al. Independent effects of peripheral nerve dysfunction on lower-extremity physical function in old age: the Women's Health and Aging Study. Diabetes Care 2000;23(11):1642–1647.

Rey A. Le freinage volontaire du mouvement graphique chez l'enfant. In: Epreuves d'intelligence pratique et de psychomotricite. Neuchatel, Switzerland: Delachaux & Niestle, 1968.

Riach CL, Starkes JL. Velocity of center of pressure excursions as an indicator of postural control systems in children. Gait Posture 1994;2:167–172.

Rice MS, Newell KM. Interlimb coupling and left hemiplegia because of right cerebral vascular accident. Occup Ther J Res 2001;21:12–28.

Rice MS, Newell KM. Upper extremity interlimb coupling in persons with left hemiplegia due to stroke. Arch Phys Med Rehabil 2004;85:629–634.

Richards CL, Malouin F, Bravo G, et al. The role of technology in task-oriented training in persons with subacute stroke: a randomized controlled trial. Neurorehabil Neural Repair 2004;18(4):199–211.

Richards CL, Malouin F, Dumas F, et al. Early and intensive treadmill locomotor training for young children with cerebral palsy: a feasibility study. Pediatr Phys Ther 1997;9:158–165.

Richards CL, Malouin F, Dumas F, et al. Gait velocity as an outcome measure of locomotor recovery after stroke. In: Craik RL, Oatis C, eds. Gait analysis: theory and applications. St. Louis, MO: Mosby, 1995:355–364.

Richards CL, Olney SJ. Hemiparetic gait following stroke. Part II: recovery and physical therapy. Gait Posture 1996;4:149–162.

Richardson D. Physical therapy in spasticity. Eur J Neurol 2002;9:17–26.

Richardson PK, Atwater SW, Crowe TK, Dietz JC. Performance of preschoolers on the Pediatric Clinical Test of Sensory Interaction for Balance. Am J Occup Ther 1992;46:793–800.

Richter RR, VanSant AF, Newton RA. Description of adult rolling movements and hypothesis of developmental sequences. Phys Ther 1989;69:63–71.

Ricken AX, Bennett SJ, Savelsbergh GJ. Coordination of reaching in children with spastic hemiparetic cerebral palsy under different task demands. Motor Control 2005;9:357–371.

Rikli R, Jones CJ. Senior fitness test manual. Champaign, IL: Human Kinetics, 2001.

Riley MA, Baker AA, Schmit JM, et al. Effects of visual and auditory short-term memory tasks on the spatiotemporal dynamics and variability of postural sway. J Motor Behav 2005;37:311–324.

Riley MA, Wong S, Mitra S, et al. Common effects of touch and vision on postural parameters. Exp Brain Res 1997;117:165–170.

Rine RM, Braswell J, Disher D, et al. Improvement of motor development and postural control following intervention in children with sensorineural hearing loss and vestibular impairment. Int J Pediatr Otorhinolaryngol 2004;68:1133–1232.

Rine RM, Cornwall G. Evidence of progressive delay of motor development in children with sensorineural hearing loss and concurrent vestibular dysfunction. Percept Mot Skills 2000;90:1101–1112.

Ring C, Nayak USL, Isaacs B. Balance function in elderly people who have and who have not fallen. Arch Phys Med Rehabil 1988;69:261–264.

Rinne P, Hassan M, Goniotakis D, et al. Triple dissociation of attention networks in stroke according to lesion location. Neurology 2013;81:812–820.

Riolo L, Fisher K. Is there evidence that strength training could help improve muscle function and other outcomes without reinforcing abnormal movement patterns or increasing reflex activity in a man who has had a stroke? Phys Ther 2003;83:844–851.

Risedal A, Zeng J, Johansson BB. Early training may exacerbate brain damage after focal brain ischemia in the rat. J Cereb Blood Flow Metab 1999;19:997–1003.

Rizzo JR, Beheshti M, Naeimi T, Feiz F, Fatterpekar G, Balcer LJ, Galetta SL, Shaikh AG, Rucker JC, Hudson TE. The complexity of eye-hand coordination: a perspective on cortico-cerebellar cooperation. Cerebellum Ataxias 2020;7:1–9.

Rizzolatti G, Camarda R, Fogassi L, et al. Functional organization of inferior area 6 in the macaque monkey. Exp Brain Res 1988;71:491–597.

Roberts TDM. Neurophysiology of postural mechanisms. London, UK: Butterworths, 1979.

Robertson SL, Jones LA. Tactile sensory impairments and prehensile function in subjects with left-hemisphere cerebral lesions. Arch Phys Med Rehabil 1994;75:1108–1117.

Robinson CA, Matsuda PN, Ciol MA, et al. Understanding physical factors associated with participation in community walking following stroke. Disabil Rehabil 2011;33:1033–1042.

Robinson CA, Matsuda PN, Ciol MA, et al. Understanding the factors impacting participation in community mobility following stroke: physical characteristics of the individual. Abstract Presented at the World Congress of Physical Therapy, Vancouver, BC, Canada, 2007.

Robinson CA, Shumway-Cook A, Ciol MA, et al. Participation in community walking following stroke: subjective versus objective measures and the impact of personal factors. Phys Ther 2011b;91:1865–1876.

Robinson JL, Schmidt GL. Quantitative gait evaluation in the clinic. Phys Ther 1981;61:351–353.

Robinson RG, Jorge RE. Post-Stroke Depression: a review. Am J Psychiatry. 2016 1;173:221–231.

Rocchi L, Chiari L, Cappello A, et al. Comparison between subthalamic nucleus and globus pallidus internus stimulation for postural performance in Parkinson's disease. Gait Posture 2004;19:172–183.

Rocchi L, Chiari L, Cappello A, et al. Identification of distinct characteristics of postural sway in Parkinson's disease: a feature selection procedure based on principal component analysis. Neurosci Lett 2006;394:140–145.

Rocchi L, Chiari L, Horak FB. Effects of deep brain stimulation and levodopa on postural sway in Parkinson's disease. J Neurol Neurosurg Psychiatry 2002;73:267–274.

Roche N, Bonnyaud C, Geiger M, et al. Relationship between hip flexion and ankle dorsiflexion during swing phase in chronic stroke patients. Clin Biomech (Bristol, Avon) 2015;30:219–225. doi: 10.1016/j.clinbiomech.2015.02.001.

Rochester L, Hetherington V, Jones B, et al. Attending to the task: interference effects of functional tasks on walking in Parkinson's disease and the roles of cognition, depression, fatigue and balance. Arch Phys Med Rehabil 2004;85:1578–1585.

Rodgers H, Bosomworth H, Krebs HI, et al. Robot assisted training for the upper limb after stroke (RATULS): a multicentre randomised controlled trial. Lancet 2019;394(10192):51–62. doi: 10.1016/S0140-6736(19)31055-4.

Rodriguez-Oroz MC, Jahanshahi M, Krack P, et al. Initial clinical manifestations of Parkinson's disease: features and pathophysiological mechanisms. Lancet Neurol 2009;8:1128–1139.

Roerdink M, de Haart M, Daffertshofer A, et al. Dynamical structure of center-of-pressure trajectories in patients recovering from stroke. Exp Brain Res 2006;174:256–269.

Roerdink M, Geurts A, de Haart M, et al. On the relative contribution of the paretic leg to the control of posture after stroke. Neurorehabil Neural Repair 2009;23:267–274.

Roeles S, Rowe PJ, Bruijn SM, et al. Gait stability in response to platform, belt, and sensory perturbations in young and older adults. Med Biol Eng Comput 2018;56(12):2325–2335.

Rogers MW. Control of posture and balance during voluntary movements in Parkinson's disease. In: Duncan P, ed. Balance: proceedings of the APTA Forum. Alexandria, VA: American Physical Therapy Association, 1990:79–86.

Rogers MW. Motor control problems in Parkinson's disease. In: Contemporary management of motor control problems. Proceedings of the II Step Conference. Alexandria, VA: American Physical Therapy Association, 1991:195–208.

Rogge AK, Röder B, Zech A, et al. Balance training improves memory and spatial cognition in healthy adults. Sci Rep 2017;7:5661.

Rojas VG, Rebolledo GM, Muñoz EG, Cortés NI, Gaete CB, Delgado CM. Differences in standing balance between patients with diplegic and hemiplegic cerebral palsy. Neural Regen Res 2013;8(26):2478–2483. doi:10.3969/j.issn.1673-5374.2013.26.009

Roland PE, Larsen B, Lassen NA, et al. Supplementary motor area and other cortical areas in organization of voluntary movements in man. J Neurophysiol 1980;43:118–136.

Roll JP, Bard C, Paillard J. Head orienting contributes to directional accuracy of aiming at distant targets. Hum Mov Sci 1986;5:359–371.

Roll JP, Roll R. From eye to foot: a proprioceptive chain involved in postural control. In: Amblard B, Berthoz A, Clarac F, eds. Posture and gait: development, adaptation and modulation. Amsterdam, The Netherlands: Elsevier, 1988:155–164.

Romberg MH. Manual of nervous diseases of man. London, UK: Sydenham Society, 1853:395–401.

Romkes J, Peeters W, Oosterom AM, et al. Evaluating upper body movements during gait in healthy children and children with diplegic cerebral palsy. J Ped Ortho Part B 2007;16:175–180.

Roncesvalles MN, Woollacott MW, Burtner PA. Neural factors underlying reduced postural adaptability in children with cerebral palsy. Neuroreport 2002;13:2407–2410.

Roncesvalles MNC, Jensen J. The expression of weight-bearing ability in infants between four and seven months of age. Sport Exerc Psychol 1993;15:568.

Roncesvalles MNC, Woollacott MH, Jensen JL. Development of lower extremity kinetics for balance control in infants and young children. J Motor Behav 2001;33:180–192.

Roncesvalles MNC, Woollacott MH, Jensen JL. The development of compensatory stepping skills in children. J Motor Behav 2000;32:100–111.

Roncesvalles N, Woollacott M, Brown N, et al. An emerging postural response: is control of the hip possible in the newly walking child? J Motor Behav 2003;36:147–159.

Rong W, Tong KY, Hu XL, et al. Effects of electromyography-driven robot aided hand training with neuromuscular electrical stimulation on hand control performance after chronic stroke. Disabil Rehabil Assist Technol 2015;10(2):149–159.

Ronnqvist L, Rosblad B. Kinematic analysis of unimanual reaching and grasping movements in children with hemiplegic cerebral palsy. Clin Biomech (Bristol, Avon) 2007;22:165–175.

Roostaei M, Raji P, Morone G, Razi B, Khademi-Kalantari K. The effect of dual task conditions on gait and balance performance in children with cerebral palsy: a systematic review and meta-analysis of observational studies. J Bodyw Mov Ther 2021;26:448–462.

Rorden C, Jelsone L, Simon-Dack S, Baylis LL, Baylis GC. Visual extinction: the effect of temporal and spatial bias. Neuropsychologia 2009;47:321–329.

Rosander K, von Hofsten C. Development of gaze tracking of small and large objects. Exp Brain Res 2002;146:257–264.

Rosander K, von Hofsten C. Visual-vestibular interaction in early infancy. Exp Brain Res 2000;133:321–333.

Rose D. Fall proof: a comprehensive balance and mobility program. Champaign, IL: Human Kinetics, 2003.

Rose DJ. A multilevel approach to the study of motor control and learning. Boston, MA: Allyn & Bacon, 1997.

Rose DK, Winstein CJ. Bimanual training after stroke: are two hands better than one? Top Stroke Rehabil 2004;11:20–31.

Rose J, Wolff DR, Jones VK, et al. Postural balance in children with cerebral palsy. Dev Med Child Neurol 2002;44:58–63.

Rose SJ. Physical therapy diagnosis: role and function. Phys Ther 1989;69:535–537.

Rosen B, Vikstrom P, Turner S, et al. Enhanced early sensory outcome after nerve repair as a result of immediate post-operative re-learning: a randomized controlled trial. J Hand Surg Eur 2015;40:598–606. doi.org/10.1177/1753193414553163

Rosenbaum D. Human motor control. New York: Academic Press, 1991.

Rosenblum S, Sachs D, Schreuer N. Reliability and validity of the Children's Leisure Assessment Scale. Am J Occup Ther 2010;64(4):633–641 doi: 10.5014/ajot.2010.08173.

Rosenhall U, Rubin W. Degenerative changes in the human vestibular sensory epithelia. Acta Otolaryngol 1975;79:67–81.

Rosenkranz K, Nitsche MA, Tergau F, et al. Diminution of training-induced transient motor cortex plasticity by weak transcranial direct current stimulation in the human. Neurosci Lett 2000;296(1):61–63.

Rosenrot P, Wall JC, Charteris J. The relationship between velocity, stride time, support time and swing time during normal walking. J Hum Mov Stud 1980;6:323–335.

Rosenthal RB, Deutsch SD, Miller W, et al. A fixed-ankle, below-the-knee orthosis for the management of genu recurvatum in spastic cerebral palsy. J Bone Joint Surg Am 1975;57:545–547.

Rosin R, Topka H, Dichgans J. Gait initiation in Parkinson's disease. Mov Disord 1997;12:682–690.

Roskies A. The binding problem. Neuron 1999;24:7–9.

Ross SM, MacDonald M, Bigouette JP. Effects of strength training on mobility in adults with cerebral palsy: a systematic review. Disabil Health J 2016;9:375–384.

Rossetti Y, Revol P, McIntosh R, et al. Visually guided reaching: bilateral posterior parietal lesions cause a switch from fast visuomotor to slow cognitive control. Neuropsychologia 2005;43:162–177.

Rosso AL, Taylor JA, Tabb LP, Michael YL. Mobility, disability, and social engagement in older adults. J Aging Health 2013;25:617–637.

Rothstein J. Disability and our identity. Phys Ther 1994;74:375–377.

Rothstein JM, Echternach JL, Riddle DL. The Hypothesis-Oriented Algorithm for Clinicians II (HOAC II): a guide for patient management. Phys Ther 2003;83:455–470.

Rothstein JM, Echternach JL. Hypothesis-oriented algorithm for clinicians: a method for evaluation and treatment planning. Phys Ther 1986;66:1388–1394.

Rothwell JC. Brainstem myoclonus. Clin Neurosci 1995–1996;3(4):214–218.

Rothwell JC, Traub MM, Day BL, et al. Manual motor performance in a deafferented man. Brain 1982;105:515–542.

Rovee-Collier CK, Sullivan MW. Organization of infant memory. J Exp Psychol [Hum Learn] 1980;6:798–807.

Rovee CK, Rovee DT. Conjugate reinforcement of infant exploratory behavior. J Exp Child Psychol 1969;8(1):33–39. doi: 10.1016/0022-0965(69)90025-3.

Rowe JB, Chan V, Ingemanson ML, Cramer SC, Wolbrecht ET, Reinkensmeyer DJ. Robotic assistance for training finger movement using a hebbian model: a randomized controlled trial. Neurorehabil Neural Repair 2017;31(8):769–780. doi: 10.1177/1545968317721975.

Roy CW. Shoulder pain in hemiplegia: a literature review. Clin Rehabil 1988;2:35–44.

Rozendal RH. Biomechanics of standing and walking. Amsterdam, The Netherlands: Elsevier, 1986.

Rozumalski A, Schwartz MH. Crouch gait patterns defined using k-means cluster analysis are related to underlying clinical pathology. Gait Posture 2009;30:155–160.

Rubenstein LZ. Falls in older people: epidemiology, risk factors and strategies for prevention. Age Ageing 2006;35(S2):ii37–ii41.

Rubenstein LZ, Josephson KR. Guidelines for prevention of falls in older persons. J Am Geriatr Soc 2001;49:664–672.

Rubenstein LZ, Robbins AS, Schulman BL, et al. Falls and instability in the elderly. J Am Geriatr Soc 1988;36:266–278.

Rubenstein LZ, Vivrette R, Harker JO, et al. Validating an evidence-based, self-rated fall risk questionnaire (FRQ) for older adults. J Safety Res 2011;42:493–499.

Ruff HA. Infants' manipulative exploration of objects: effects of age and object characteristics. Dev Psychol 1984;20:9–20.

Runge CF, Shupert CL, Horak FB, et al. Postural strategies defined by joint torques. Gait Posture 1999;10:161–170.

Russell DJ, Rosenbaum PL, Gowland C, et al. Manual for the gross motor function measure. Hamilton, ON: McMaster University, 1993.

Rymer W, Katz RT. Mechanisms of spastic hypertonia. In: Katz RT, ed. Spasticity: state of the art review, vol. 8. Philadelphia, PA: Hanley & Belfus, 1994:441–154.

S

Saavedra S, Joshi A, Woollacott M, et al. Eye hand coordination in children with cerebral palsy. Exp Brain Res 2009;192:155–165.

Saavedra S, Woollacott MH. Contributions of spinal segments to trunk postural control during typical development. Dev Med Child Neurol 2009;51(Suppl.5):82.

Saavedra SL, van Donkelaar P, Woollacott MH. Learning about gravity: segmental assessment of upright control as infants develop independent sitting. J Neurophysiol 2012;108:2215–2229.

Saavedra SL, Woollacott MH. Segmental contributions to trunk control in children with moderate-to-severe cerebral palsy. Arch Phys Med Rehabil 2015;96(6):1088–1097.

Sackett DL, Rosenberg WMC, Muir Gray JA, et al. Evidence-based medicine: what it is and what it isn't. BMJ 1996;312:71–72.

Sadeghi H, Allard P, Duhaime M. Contributions of lower limb muscle power in gait of people without impairments. Phys Ther 2000;80:1188–1196.

Saether R, Helbostad JL, Ripagen II, et al. Clinical tools to assess balance in children and adults with cerebral palsy: a systematic review. Dev Med Child Neurol 2013;55:988–999.

Sahrmann SA, Norton BJ. The relationship of voluntary movement to spasticity in the upper motor neuron syndrome. Arch Neurol 1977;2:460–465.

Sahrmann SA. Diagnosis by the physical therapist: a prerequisite for treatment. Phys Ther 1988;68:1703–1706.

Said CM, Galea M, Lythgo N. Obstacle crossing performance does not differ between the first and subsequent attempts in people with stroke. Gait Posture 2009;30:455–458.

Said CM, Galea MP, Lythgo N. People with stroke who fail an obstacle crossing task have a higher incidence of falls and utilize different gait patterns compared with people who pass the task. Phys Ther 2013;93:334–344.

Said CM, Goldie PA, Culham E, et al. Control of lead and trail limbs during obstacle crossing following stroke. Phys Ther 2005;85:413–427.

Said CM, Goldie PA, Patla AE, et al. Balance during obstacle crossing following stroke. Gait Posture 2008;27:23–30.

Sainburg RL, Duff SV. Does motor lateralization have implications for stroke rehabilitation? J Rehabil Res Dev 2006;4:311–322.

Sainburg RL, Ghilardi MF, Poizner H, et al. Control of limb dynamics in normal subjects and patients without proprioception. J Neurophysiol 1995;73:820–835.

Sainburg RL, Maenza C, Winstein C, Good D. Motor lateralization provides a foundation for predicting and treating non-paretic arm motor deficits in stroke. Adv Exp Med Biol 2016;957:257–272. doi: 10.1007/978-3-319-47313-0_14.

Sainburg RL, Poizner H, Ghez C. Loss of proprioception produces deficits in interjoint coordination. J Neurophysiol 1993;70:2136–2147.

Sainburg RL, Wang J. Interlimb transfer of visuomotor rotations: independence of direction and final position information. Exp Brain Res 2002;145:437–447.

Sakata H, Shibutani H, Kawano K, et al. Neural mechanisms of space vision in the parietal association cortex of the monkey. Vision Res 1985;25:453–463.

Sakurada T, Ito K, Gomi H. Bimanual motor coordination controlled by cooperative interactions in intrinsic and extrinsic coordinates. Eur J Neurosci 2016;43:120–130.

Sakurada T, Kansaku K. Attention-dependent switching between intrinsic-muscle and extrinsic-visual coordinates during bimanual movements. Eur J Neurosci 2020. doi: 10.1111/ejn.15097.

Sakzewski L, Boyd R, Ziviani J. Clinimetric properties of participation measures for 5-to 13-year old children with cerebral palsy: a systematic review. Dev Med Child Neurol 2007;49:232–240.

Sakzewski L, Gordon A, Eliasson AC. The state of the evidence for intensive upper limb therapy approaches for children with unilateral cerebral palsy. J Child Neurol 2014;29:1077–1090.

Sakzewski L, Miller L, Ziviani J, et al. Randomized comparison trial of density and context of upper limb intensive group versus individualized occupational therapy for children with unilateral cerebral palsy. Dev Med Child Neurol 2015;57:539–547.

Sakzewski L, Ziviani J, Abbott DF, et al. Participation outcomes in a randomized trial of 2 models of upper-limb rehabilitation for children with congenital hemiplegia. Arch Phys Med Rehabil 2011;92(4):531–539.

Salbach NM, Mayo NE, Higgins J, et al. Responsiveness and predictability of gait speed and other disability measures in acute stroke. Arch Phys Med Rehabil 2001;82:1204–1212.

Salbach NM, Mayo NE, Robichaud-Ekstrand S, et al. Balance self-efficacy and its relevance to physical function and perceived health status after stroke. Arch Phys Med Rehabil 2006;87:364–370.

Salbach NM, Mayo NE, Wood-Dauphinee S, et al. A task oriented intervention enhances walking distance and speed in the first year post stroke: a randomized controlled trial. Clin Rehabil 2004;18:509–519.

Salimi I, Brochier T, Smith AM. Neuronal activity in somatosensory cortex of monkeys using a precision grip. II. Responses To object texture and weights. J Neurophysiol 1999a;81:835–844.

Salimi I, Brochier T, Smith AM. Neuronal activity in somatosensory cortex of monkeys using a precision grip. III. Responses to altered friction perturbations. J Neurophysiol 1999b;81:845–857.

Salmoni AW, Schmidt RA, Walter CB. Knowledge of results and motor learning: a review and critical reappraisal. Psychol Bull 1984;95:355–386.

Sandin KJ, Smith BS. The measure of balance in sitting in stroke rehabilitation prognosis. Stroke 1990;21:82–86.

Sandhaug M, Andelic N, Langhammer B, Mygland A. Community integration 2 years after moderate and severe traumatic brain injury. Brain Inj 2015;29(7–8):915–920. doi: 10.3109/02699052.2015.1022880.

Sanes JN, LeWitt PA, Mauritz KH. Visual and mechanical control of postural and kinetic tremor in cerebellar system disorders. J Neurol Neurosurg Psychiatry 1988;51:934–943.

Sanes JN, Mauritz KH, Dalakas MC, et al. Motor control in humans with large-fiber sensory neuropathy. Hum Neurobiol 1985;4:101–114.

Sanes JR, Jessell TM. Repairing the damaged brain. In: Kandel ER, Schwartz JH, Jessel TM, et al., eds. Principles of neuroscience, 5th ed. New York: McGraw-Hill, 2013.

Sanes JR, Jessell TM. Experience and the refinement of synaptic connections. In: Kandel ER, Schwartz JH, Jessell TM, Siegelbaum SA, Hudspeth AJ, eds. Principles of neural science, 5th ed. New York, NY: McGraw-Hill, 2013:3015–3080.

Sanford J, Moreland J, Swanson LR, et al. Reliability of the Fugl-Meyer assessment for testing motor performance in patients following stroke. Phys Ther 1993;73: 447–454.

Sanger TD. Basic and translational neuroscience of childhood-onset dystonia: a control-theory perspective. Annu Rev Neurosci 2018;41:41–59.

Sanger TD, Delgado MR, Gaebler-Spira D, et al. Classification and definition of disorders causing hypertonia in childhood. Pediatrics 2003;111:e89–e97.

Santamaria V. The effect of different levels of external trunk support on postural and reaching control in children with cerebral palsy. Ph.D. Dissertation, University of Oregon, 2015, 242 pages; 3700446. ProQuest; http://gradworks.Santamaria V, Khan M, Luna T, et al. Promoting functional and independent sitting in children with cerebral palsy using the robotic trunk support trainer. IEEE Trans Neural Syst Rehabil Eng 2020;28:2995–3004.

Santamaria V, Rachwani J, Manselle W, Saavedra SL, Woollacott M. The impact of segmental trunk support on posture and reaching while sitting in healthy adults. J Mot Behav 2018;5:51–64.

Santamaria V, Rachwani J, Saavedra S, Woollacott M. Effect of segmental trunk support on posture and reaching in children with cerebral palsy. Pediatr Phys Ther 2016;28(3):285–293.

Santamaria V, Rachwani J, Saussez G, Bleyenheuft Y, Dutkowsky J, Gordon AM, Woollacott MH. The seated postural & reaching control test in cerebral palsy: a validation study. Phys Occup Ther Pediatr 2020;40(4):441–469.

Sargent B, Schweighofer N, Kubo M, et al. Infant exploratory learning: influence on leg joint coordination. PLoS One 2014;9(3):e91500.

Satorio F, Bravini E, Vercelli S, et al. The Functional Dexterity Test: test-retest reliability analysis and up-to date reference norms. J Hand Ther 2013;26(1):62–67.

Saunders D. Evaluation, treatment and prevention of musculoskeletal disorders. Minneapolis, MN: Viking Press, 1991.

Saunders JB, Inman VT, Eberhart HD. The major determinants in normal and pathological gait. J Bone Joint Surg Am 1953 Jul;35(3):543–558.

Sawaki L, Butler AJ, Leng X, et al. Constraint-induced movement therapy results in increased motor map area in subjects 3 to 9 months after stroke. Neurorehabil Neural Repair 2008;22:505–513.

Sawers A, Bhatt T. Neuromuscular determinants of slip-induced falls and recoveries in older adults. J Neurophysiol 2018;120(4):1534–1546.

Schaefer S, Jagenow D, Verrel J, et al. The influence of cognitive load and walking speed on gait regularity in children and young adults. Gait Posture 2015;41(1):258–262.

Schaefer SY, Haaland KY, Sainburg RL. Dissociation of initial trajectory and final position errors during visuomotor adaptation following unilateral stroke. Brain Res 2009;1298:78–91.

Schallert T, Fleming SM, Woodlee MT. Should the injured and intact hemispheres be treated differently during the early phases of physical restorative therapy in experimental stroke or parkinsonism? Phys Med Rehabil Clin 2003;14:1–20.

Schallert T, Leasure JL, Kolb B. Experience associated structural events, subependymal cellular proliferative activity and functional recovery after injury to the central nervous system. J Cereb Blood Flow Metab 2000;20:1513–1528.

Schultenbrund C. The development of human motility and motor disturbances. Arch Neurol Psychiatry 1928;20:720.

Scheidt RA, Conditt MA, Secco EL, Mussa-Ivaldi FA. Interaction of visual and proprioceptive feedback during adaptation of human reaching movements. J Neurophysiol 2005;93:3200–3213.

Schenke N, Franke R, Puschmann S, et al. Can auditory cues improve visuo-spatial neglect? Results of two pilot studies. Neuropsychol Rehabil 2020:1–21. doi: 10.1080/09602011.2020.1727931.

Schenkman M. Interrelationships of neurological and mechanical factors in balance control. In: Duncan P, ed. Balance: proceedings of the APTA Forum. Alexandria, VA: American Physical Therapy Association, 1990:29–41.

Schenkman M, Butler RB. "Automatic Postural Tone" in posture, movement, and function. Forum on physical therapy issues related to cerebrovascular accident. Alexandria, VA: American Physical Therapy Association, 1992:16–21.

Schenkman M, Butler RB. A model for multisystem evaluation, interpretation, and treatment of individuals with neurologic dysfunction. Phys Ther 1989;69:538–547.

Schenkman M, Cutson TM, Zhu CW, et al. A longitudinal evaluation of patients' perceptions of Parkinson's disease. Gerontologist 2002;42:790–798.

Schenkman M, Deutsch JE, Gill-Body KM. An integrated framework for decision making in neurologic physical therapist practice. Phys Ther 2006;86:1681–1702.

Schenkman MA, Berger RA, Riley PO, et al. Whole-body movements during rising to standing from sitting. Phys Ther 1990;10:638–651.

Schettino LF, Adamovich SV, Hening W, et al. Hand preshaping in Parkinson's disease: effects of visual feedback and medication state. Exp Brain Res 2006;168:186–202.

Schuster D, Rivera J, Sellers BC, Fiore SM, Jentsch F. Perceptual training for visual search. Ergonomics 2013;56(7):1101–1115. doi: 10.1080/00140139.2013.790481.

Schieber MH. Muscular production of individuated finger movements: the roles of extrinsic finger muscles. J Neurosci 1995;15(1 Pt 1):284–297.

Schieppati M, Hugon M, Grasso M, et al. The limits of equilibrium in young and elderly normal subjects and in Parkinsonians. Electroencephalogr Clin Neurophysiol 1994;93:286–298.

Schillings AM, van Wezel BM, Mulder T, et al. Muscular responses and movement strategies during stumbling over obstacles. J Neurophysiol 2000;83:2093–2102.

Schloon H, O'Brien MJ, Scholten CA, et al. Muscle activity and postural behavior in newborn infants: a polymyographic study. Neuropadiatrie 1976;7:384–415.

Schloemer SA, Thompson JA, Silder A, Thelen DG, Siston RA. Age-related differences in gait kinematics, kinetics, and muscle function: a principal component analysis. Ann Biomed Eng 2017;45(3):695–710.

Scholtes VA, Becher JG, Comuth A, Dekkers H, Van Dijk L, Dallmeijer AJ. Effectiveness of functional progressive resistance exercise strength training on muscle strength and mobility in children with cerebral palsy: a randomized controlled trial. Dev Med Child Neurol. 2010 Jun;52(6):e107–e113.

Schmahmann JD, Guell X, Stoodley CJ, Halko MA. The theory and neuroscience of cerebellar cognition. Annu Rev Neurosci 2019;42:337–364.

Schmid AA, Miller KK, Van Puymbroeck M, et al. Yoga leads to multiple physical improvements after stroke, a pilot study. Complement Ther Med 2014;22(6):994–100.

Schmid AA, Van Puymbroeck M, Altenburger PA, et al. Balance and balance self-efficacy are associated with activity and participation after stroke: a cross-sectional study in people with chronic stroke. Arch Phys Med Rehabil 2012;93:1101–1107.

Schmidt R. Motor and action perspectives on motor behaviour. In: Meijer OG, Roth K, eds. Complex movement behavior: the motor-action controversy. Amsterdam, The Netherlands: Elsevier, 1988a:3–44.

Schmidt RA. A schema theory of discrete motor skill learning. Psychol Rev 1975;82:225–260.

Schmidt RA. Motor control and learning, 2nd ed. Champaign, IL: Human Kinetics, 1988b.

Schmidt RA. Motor learning principles for physical therapy. In: Lister M, ed. Contemporary management of motor control problems. Proceedings of the II Step Conference. Alexandria, VA: American Physical Therapy Association, 1991:49–63.

Schmidt RA, Lee TD. Motor control and learning: a behavioral emphasis, 5th ed. Champaign, IL: Human Kinetics, 2011.

Schmidt RA, Young DE, Swinnen S, Shapiro DC. Summary knowledge of results for skill acquisition: support for the guidance hypothesis. J Exp Psychol Learn Mem Cogn 1989;15:352–359.

Schmitz TJ. Coordination assessment. In: O'Sullivan S, Schmitz TM, eds. Physical rehabilitation: assessment and treatment, 4th ed. Philadelphia, PA: FA Davis, 2001:212.

Schmitz TJ. Gait training with assistive devices. In: O'Sullivan S, Schmitz TM, eds. Physical rehabilitation: assessment and treatment, 2nd ed. Philadelphia, PA: FA Davis, 1998.

Schneck CM, Henderson A. Descriptive analysis of the developmental progression of grip position for pencil and crayon control in nondysfunctional children. Am J Occup Ther 1990;44:893–900.

Schneiberg S, Sveistrup H, McFadyen B, et al. The development of coordination for reach-to-grasp movements in children. Exp Brain Res 2002;146(2):142–154.

Schneider K, Zernicke RF. Jerk-cost modulations during the practice of rapid arm movements. Biol Cybern 1989;60:221–230.

Schneider TR, Buckingham G, Hermsdörfer J. Torque-planning errors affect the perception of object properties and sensorimotor memories during object manipulation in uncertain grasp situations. J Neurophysiol 2019 121;1289–1299.

Schnitzler A, Kessler KR, Benecke R. Transcallosally mediated inhibition of interneurons within human primary motor cortex. Exp Brain Res 1996;112:381–391.

Scholtes VAB, Becher JG, Beelen A, et al. Clinical assessment of spasticity in children with cerebral palsy: a critical review of available instruments. Dev Med Child Neurol 2006;48:64–73.

Scholtes VAB, Becher JG, Beelen A, Lankhorst GJ. Clinical assessment of spasticity in children with cerebral palsy: a critical review of available instruments. Dev Med Child Neurol 2006;48:64–73.

Scholz JP, Danion F, Latash ML, et al. Understanding finger coordination through analysis of the structure of force variability. Biol Cybern 2002,86.29–39.

Scholz JP, Schöner G, Hsu WL, et al. Motor equivalent control of the center of mass in response to support surface perturbations. Exp Brain Res 2007;180:163–179.

Schultz A, Alexander NB, Gu MJ, et al. Postural control in young and elderly adults when stance is challenged: clinical versus laboratory measurements. Ann Otol Rhinol Laryngol 1993;102:508–517.

Schultz AB. Muscle function and mobility biomechanics in the elderly: an overview of some recent research. J Gerontol 1995;50A(special issue):60–63.

Schwab RS. Progression and prognosis in Parkinson's disease. J Nerv Ment Dis 1960;130:556–572.

Schwartz I, Sajin A, Fisher I, et al. The effectiveness of locomotor therapy using robotic-assisted gait training in subacute stroke patients: a randomized controlled trial. Phys Med Rehabil 2009;1:516–523.

Schwartz I, Sajin A, Moreh E, et al. Robot-assisted gait training in multiple sclerosis patients: a randomized trial. Mult Scler 2012;18:881–890.

Schwartz MF, Reed ES, Montgomery M, et al. The quantitative description of action disorganization after brain damage: a case study. Cogn Neuropsychol 1991;8:381–414.

Scianni A, Butler JM, Ada L, et al. Muscle strengthening is not effective in children and adolescents with cerebral palsy: a systematic review. Aust J Physiother 2009;55(2):81–87.

Sea MJC, Henderson A, Cermak SA. Patterns of visual spatial inattention and their functional significance in stroke patients. Arch Phys Med Rehabil 1993;74:355–360.

Sebastian MV, Hernandez-Gil L. Do 5-year-old children perform dual task coordination better than AD patients? J Atten Disord 2013. [Epub ahead of print].

See J, Dodakian L, Chou C, et al. A standardized approach to the Fugl-Meyer Assessment and its implications for clinical trials. Neurorehabil Neural Repair 2013;27:732.

Seidel B, Krebs DE. Base of support is not wider in chronic ataxic and unsteady patients. J Rehabil Med 2002;34(6):288–292.

Seo NJ, Rymer WZ, Kamper DG. Altered digit force direction during pinch grip following stroke. Exp Brain Res 2010;202:891–901.

Serra-Ano P, Pellicer-Chenoll M, Garcia-Masso X, Brizuela G, Garcia-Lucerga C, Gonzalez LM. Sitting balance and limits of stability in persons with paraplegia. Spinal Cord 2013;51(4):267–272.

Sertel M, Sakızlı E, Bezgin S, Demirci CS, Şahan TY, Kurtoğlu F. The effect of single-tasks and dual-tasks on balance in older adults. Cogent Soc Sci 2017;3:1330913.

Shah VV, McNames J, Mancini M, Carlson-Kuhta P, Spain RI, Nutt JG, El-Gohary M, Curtze C, Horak FB. Quantity and quality of gait and turning in people with multiple sclerosis, Parkinson's disease and matched controls during daily living. J Neurol 2020;267(4):1188–1196.

Shaltenbrand G. The development of human motility and motor disturbances. Arch Neurol Pyschiatr 1928;20:720–730.

Shambes GM, Gibson JM, Welker W. Fractured somatotopy in granule cell tactile areas of rat cerebellar hemispheres revealed by micromapping. Brain Behav Evol 1978;15:94–140.

Shapiro DC, Schmidt RA. The schema theory: recent evidence and developmental implications. In: Kelso JAS, Clark JE, eds. The development of movement control and coordination. New York: Wiley, 1982:113–173.

Shaughnessy M, Michael KM, Sorkin JD, et al. Steps after stroke: capturing ambulatory recovery. Stroke 2005;23:1305–1307.

Shea CH, Shebilske W, Worchel S. Motor learning and control. Englewood Cliffs, NJ: Prentice Hall, 1993.

Shea SL, Aslin RN. Oculomotor responses to step-ramp targets by young infants. Vision Res 1990;30:1077–1092.

Shechtman O, Sindhu BS. Grip strength. In: MacDermid J, Solomon G, Valdes K, American Society of Hand Therapists, eds. ASHT clinical assessment recommendations, 3rd ed. Mt. Laurel, NJ: American Society of Hand Therapists, 2015.

Sheldon JH. On the natural history of falls in older age. BMJ 1960;4:1685–1690.

Sheldon JH. The effect of age on the control of sway. Gerontol Clin 1963;5:129–138.

Shema SR, Brozgol M, Dorfman M, et al. Clinical experience using a 5-week treadmill training program with virtual reality to enhance gait in an ambulatory physical therapy service. Phys Ther 2014;94:1319–1326.

Shepard K. Theory: criteria, importance and impact. In: Contemporary management of motor control problems: Proceedings of the II Step Conference. Alexandria, VA. American Physical Therapy Association, 1991:5–10.

Shepherd RB, Crosbie J, Squires T. The contribution of the ipsilateral leg to postural adjustments during fast voluntary reaching in sitting. Abstract of International Society for Biomechanics, 14th Congress, Paris, 1993.

Sherrard RM, Bower AJ. BDNF and NT3 extend the critical period for developmental climbing fiber plasticity. Neuroreport 2001;12:2871–2874.

Sherrington C. The integrative action of the nervous system, 2nd ed. New Haven, CT: Yale University, 1947.

Sherrington C. The integrative action of the nervous system. New Haven, CT: Yale University, 1906.

Sherrington C, Whitney J, Lord SR, et al. Effective exercise for the prevention of falls: a systematic review and meta-analysis. J Am Geriatr Soc 2008;56:2234–2243.

Sherrington CS. Decerebrate rigidity, and reflex coordination of movements. J Physiol Lond 1898;22:319–332.

Shik ML, Severin FV, Orlovsky GN. Control of walking and running by means of electrical stimulation of the mid-brain. Biophysics 1966;11:756–765.

Shim JK, Lay BS, Zatsiorsky VM, Latash ML. Age-related changes in finger coordination in static prehension tasks. J Appl Physiol 2004;97:213–224.

Shimel K, Candler C, Neville-Smith M. Comparison of cursive handwriting instruction programs among students without identified problems. Phys Occup Ther Pediatr 2009;29(2):170–181. doi: 10.1080/01942630902784738.

Shin JH, Park G, Cho DY. Cognitive-motor interference on upper extremity motor performance in a robot-assisted planar reaching task among patients with stroke. Arch Phys Med Rehabil 2017;98:730–737.

Shore BJ, Allar BG, Miller PE, Matheney TH, Snyder BD, Fragala-Pinkham M. Measuring the reliability and construct validity of the pediatric evaluation of disability Inventory-Computer Adaptive Test (PEDI-CAT) in Children With Cerebral Palsy. Arch Phys Med Rehabil. 2019;100(1):45–51. doi: 10.1016/j.apmr.2018.07.427.

Shukla AW, Ounpraseuth S, Okun MS, Gray V, Schwankhaus J, Metzer WS. Micrographia and related deficits in Parkinson's disease: a cross-sectional study. BMJ Open 2012;2:1–6.

Shulman D, Spencer A, Ann Vallis L. Older adults exhibit variable responses in stepping behaviour following unexpected forward perturbations during gait initiation. Hum Mov Sci 2019;63:120–128.

Shumway-Cook A, Anson D, Haller S. Postural sway biofeedback for pre-training postural control following hemiplegia. Arch Phys Med Rehabil 1988;69:395–400.

Shumway-Cook A, Baldwin M, Pollisar N, et al. Predicting the probability of falls in community dwelling older adults. Phys Ther 1997a;77:812–819.

Shumway-Cook A, Brauer S, Woollacott M. Predicting the probability for falls in community-dwelling older adults using the Timed Up and Go Test. Phys Ther 2000;80:896–903.

Shumway-Cook A, Ciol M, Gruber W, et al. Incidence and risk factors for falls following hip fracture in community dwelling older adults. Phys Ther 2005a;85:648–655.

Shumway-Cook A, Ciol MA, Hoffman J, et al. Falls in the Medicare population: incidence, associated factors, and impact on health care. Phys Ther 2009;89:324–332.

Shumway-Cook A, Gruber W, Baldwin M, et al. The effect of multidimensional exercises on balance, mobility and fall risk in community dwelling older adults. Phys Ther 1997b;77:46–57.

Shumway-Cook A, Guralnik JM, Phillips CL, et al. Age-associated declines in complex walking task performance: the Walking InCHIANTI Toolkit. J Am Geriatr Soc 2007;55:58–65.

Shumway-Cook A, Horak F. Assessing the influence of sensory interaction on balance. Phys Ther 1986;66:1548–1550.

Shumway-Cook A, Horak F. Balance rehabilitation in the neurologic patient: course syllabus. Seattle, WA: Neuroscience Education and Research Associates, 1992.

Shumway-Cook A, Horak FB. Rehabilitation strategies for patients with vestibular deficits. Neurol Clin 1990;8:441–457.

Shumway-Cook A, Horak FB. Vestibular rehabilitation: an exercise approach to managing symptoms of vestibular dysfunction. Semin Hearing 1989;10:196–205.

Shumway-Cook A, Hutchinson S, Kartin D, et al. Effect of balance training on recovery of stability in children with cerebral palsy. Dev Med Child Neurol 2003;45:591–602.

Shumway-Cook A, Matsuda PN, Taylor C. Investigating the validity of the environmental framework underlying the original and modified Dynamic Gait Index. Phys Ther 2015 Jun;95(6):864–870.

Shumway-Cook A, McCollum G. Assessment and treatment of balance disorders in the neurologic patient. In: Montgomery T, Connolly B, eds. Motor control and physical therapy: theoretical framework and practical applications. Chattanooga, TN: Chattanooga, 1990:123–138.

Shumway-Cook A, Olmscheid R. A systems analysis of postural dyscontrol in traumatically brain-injured patients. J Head Trauma Rehabil 1990;5:51–62.

Shumway-Cook A, Patla A, Stewart A, et al. Assessing environmentally determined mobility disability: self-report versus observed community mobility. J Am Geriatr Soc 2005b;53:700–704.

Shumway-Cook A, Patla A, Stewart A, et al. Environmental components of mobility disability in community-living older persons. J Am Geriatr Soc 2003;51:393–398.

Shumway-Cook A, Patla A, Stewart A, et al. Environmental demands associated with community mobility in older adults with and without mobility disability. Phys Ther 2002;82:670–681.

Shumway-Cook A, Taylor CS, Matsuda PN, et al. Expanding the scoring system for the Dynamic Gait Index. Phys Ther 2013;93:1493–1506.

Shumway-Cook A, Woollacott M. Attentional demands and postural control: the effect of sensory context. J Gerontology 2000;55A:M10–M16.

Shumway-Cook A, Woollacott M. Postural control in the Down's syndrome child. Phys Ther 1985b;9:211–235.

Shumway-Cook A, Woollacott M. The growth of stability: postural control from a developmental perspective. J Motor Behav 1985a;17:131–147.

Shumway-Cook A, Woollacott M, Baldwin M, et al. The effects of cognitive demands on postural control in elderly fallers and non-fallers. J Gerontol 1997c;52:M232–M240.

Sibley KM, Beauchamp MK, Van Ooteghem K, et al. Using the systems framework for postural control to analyze the components of balance evaluated in standardized balance measures: a scoping review. Arch Phys Med Rehabil 2015;96:122–132.

Sidaway B, Anderson J, Danielson G, et al. Effects of long-term gait training using visual cues in an individual with Parkinson disease. Phys Ther 2006;86:186–194.

Sidiropoulos AN, Santamaria V, Gordon AM. Continuous inter-limb coordination deficits in children with unilateral spastic cerebral palsy. Clin Biomech (Bristol, Avon) 2021;81:105250. doi: 10.1016/j.clinbiomech.2020.105250.

Sienko KH, Balkwill MD, Oddsson LI, et al. The effect of vibrotactile feedback on postural sway during locomotor activities. J Neuroeng Rehabil 2013;10:93.

Silsupadol P, Lugade V, Shumway-Cook A, et al. Training-related changes in dual-task walking performance of elderly persons with balance impairment: a double-blind, randomized controlled trial. Gait Posture 2009a;29:634–639.

Silsupadol P, Shumway-Cook A, Lugade V, et al. Effects of single-task versus dual-task training on balance performance in older adults: a double-blind, randomized controlled trial. Arch Phys Med Rehabil 2009b;90:381–387.

Silsupadol P, Shumway-Cook A, Woollacott M. Training of balance under single and dual task conditions in older adults with balance impairment: three case reports. Phys Ther 2006;86:269–281.

Simoneau GG, Cavanagh PR, Ulbrecht JS, et al. The influence of visual factors on fall-related kinematic variables during stair descent by older women. J Gerontol 1991;46:188–195.

Singer RN. Motor learning and human performance, 3rd ed. New York: Macmillan, 1980.

Singh S, Mandziak A, Barr K, et al. Human string-pulling with and without a string: movement, sensory control, and memory. Exp Brain Res 2019;237:3431–3447.

Sinkjaer T, Andersen JB, Larsen B. Soleus stretch reflex modulation during gait in humans. J Neurophysiol 1996;76:1112–1120.

Siu KC, Catena RD, Chou LS, et al. Effects of a secondary task on obstacle avoidance in healthy young adults. Exp Brain Res 2008;184(1):115–120.

Siu KC, Chou LS, Mayr U, et al. Does inability to allocate attention contribute to balance constraints during gait in older adults? J Gerontol A Biol Sci Med Sci 2008;63:1364–1369.

Skidmore ER, Becker JT, Whyte EM, et al. Cognitive impairments and depressive symptoms did not impede upper limb recovery in a clinical repetitive task practice program after stroke: a pilot study. Am J Phys Med Rehabil 2012;91(4):327–331.

Slavin MD, Held JM, Basso DM, et al. Fetal brain tissue transplants and recovery of locomotion following damage to sensorimotor cortex in rats. Prog Brain Res 1988;78:33–38.

Slijper H, Latash, ML, Rao N, et al. Task-specific modulation of anticipatory postural adjustments in individuals with hemiparesis. Clin Neurophysiol 2002;113:642–655.

Sloane P, Baloh RW, Honrubia V. The vestibular system in the elderly. Am J Otolaryngol 1989;1:422–429.

Slobounov SM, Moss SA, Slobounova ES, et al. Aging and time to instability of posture. J Geronotol Biol Sci 1998;53:71–78.

Small SL, Hlustik P, Noll DC, et al. Cerebellar hemispheric activation ipsilateral to the paretic hand correlates with functional recovery after stroke. Brain 2002;125:1544–1557.

Smania N, Martini MC, Gambina G, et al. The spatial distribution of visual attention in hemineglect and extinction patients. Brain 1998;121:1759–1770.

Smania N, Picelli A, Gandolfi M, et al. Rehabilitation of sensorimotor integration deficits in balance impairment of patients with stroke hemiparesis: a before/after pilot study. Neurol Sci 2008;29:313–319.

Smidt GL, Rogers MW. Factors contributing to the regulation and clinical assessment of muscular strength. Phys Ther 1982;62:1283–1290.

Smith AW, Wong DP. Sagittal and frontal plane gait initiation kinetics in healthy, young subjects. J Hum Kinet 2019;67:85–100.

Smith BT, Mulcahey MJ, Betz RR. An implantable upper extremity neuroprosthesis in a growing child with a C5 spinal cord injury. Spinal Cord 2001;39:118–123.

Smith GV, Silver KH, Goldberg AP, et al. "Task-oriented" exercise improves hamstring strength and spastic reflexes in chronic stroke patients. Stroke 1999;30(10):2112–2118.

Smith JL. Programming of stereotyped limb movements by spinal generators. In: Stelmach GE, Requin J, eds. Tutorials in motor behavior. Amsterdam, The Netherlands: North-Holland, 1980:95–115.

Smith JL, Smith LA, Dahms KL. Motor capacities of the chronic spinal cat: recruitment of slow and fast extensors of the ankle. Neurosci Abstr 1979;5:387.

Smith JL, Zernicke RF. Predictions for neural control based on limb dynamics. Trends Neurosci 1987;10:123–128.

Smith-Ray RL, Makowski-Woidan B, Hughes SL. A randomized trial to measure the impact of a community-based cognitive training intervention on balance and gait in cognitively intact Black older adults. Health Educ Behav 2014;41(1 Suppl):62S–69S.

Smits-Engelsman BC, Blank R, van der Kaay AC, et al. Efficacy of interventions to improve motor performance in children with developmental coordination disorder: a combined systematic review and meta-analysis. Dev Med Child Neurol 2013;55:229–237.

Snapp-Childs W, Corbetta D. Evidence of early strategies in learning to walk. Infancy. 2009;14(1):101–116.

Snijders AH, Weerdesteyn V, Hagen YJ, et al. Obstacle avoidance to elicit freezing of gait during treadmill walking. Mov Disord 2010;25:57–63.

Snow BJ, Tsui JK, Bhart MH, et al. Treatment of spasticity with botulinum toxin: a double blind study. Ann Neurol 1990;28:512–515.

Soangra R, Lockhart TE. Dual-task does not increase slip and fall risk in healthy young and older adults during walking. Appl Bionics Biomech 2017;2017:1014784.

Sober SJ, Sabes PN. Multisensory integration during motor planning. J Neurosci 2003;23:6982–6992.

Socie MJ, Boes MK, Motl RW, et al. Monitoring spatiotemporal gait parameters during the 6-minute walk in people with multiple sclerosis. Int J MS Care 2011;13(S3).

Socie MJ, Sosnoff JJ. Gait variability and multiple sclerosis. Mult Scler Int 2013;2013:645197.

Sofuwa O, Nieuwboer A, Desloovere K, et al. Quantitative gait analysis in Parkinson's disease: comparison with a healthy control group. Arch Phys Med Rehabil 2005;86:1007–1013.

Sohlberg MM, Mateer C. Cognitive rehabilitation: an integrated neuropsychological approach. New York: Guilford Publication, 2001.

Sollerman C. Assessment of grip function: evaluation of a new method. Sweden: MITAB, 1984.

Sommerfeld DK, von Arbin MH. The impact of somatosensory function on activity performance and length of hospital stay in geriatric patients with stroke. Clin Rehabil 2004;18:149–155.

Song J, Sigward S, Fisher B, et al. Altered dynamic postural control during step turning in persons with early-stage parkinson's disease. Parkinsons Dis 2012;2012:386962.

Song H, Dai X, Li J, Zhu S. Hamstring co-contraction in the early stage of rehabilitation after anterior cruciate ligament reconstruction: a longitudinal study. Am J Phys Med Rehabil 2018;97(9):666–672.

Song CS, Lee ON, Woo HS. Cognitive strategy on upper extremity function for stroke: a randomized controlled trials. Restor Neurol Neurosci 2019;37(1):61–70. doi: 10.3233/RNN-180853.

Song J-H. The role of attention in motor control and learning. Current opinion in Psychology 2019;29:261–265.

Soska KC, Galeon MA, Adolph KE. On the other hand: overflow movements of infants' hands and legs during unimanual object exploration. Dev Psychobiol 2012;54(4):372–382.

Sosnoff JJ, Gappmaier E, Frame A, et al. Influence of spasticity on mobility and balance in persons with multiple sclerosis. J Neurol Phys Ther 2011b;35:129–132.

Sosnoff JJ, Weikert M, Dlugonski D, et al. Quantifying gait impairment in multiple sclerosis using GAITRite technology. Gait Posture 2011a;34:145–147.

Sousa AS, Silva A, Santos R. Ankle anticipatory postural adjustments during gait initiation in healthy and post-stroke subjects. Clin Biomech (Bristol, Avon) 2015;30(9):960–965.

Southard D, Higgins T. Changing movement patterns: effects of demonstration and practice. Res Q Exer Sport 1987;58:77–80.

Speechley M, Tinetti M. Assessment of risk and prevention of falls among elderly persons: role of the physiotherapist. Physiother Can 1990;2:75–79.

Speechley M, Tinetti M. Falls and injuries in frail and vigorous community elderly persons. J Am Geriatr Soc 1991;39:46–52.

Speers RA, Kuo AD, Horak FB. Contributions of altered sensation and feedback responses to changes in coordination of postural control in aging. Gait Posture 2002;16:20–30.

Spirduso W. Physical dimensions of aging. Champaign, IL: Human Kinetics, 1995.

Spirduso W, Francis K, MacRae PG. Physical dimensions of aging. Champaign, IL: Human Kinetics, 2005.

Squire LR. Mechanisms of memory. Science 1986;232:1612–1619.

Srygley JM, Herman T, Giladi N, et al. Self-report of missteps in older adults: a valid proxy of fall risk? Arch Phys Med Rehabil 2009;90:786–792.

Stack E, Ashburn A. Dysfunctional turning in Parkinson's disease. Disabil Rehabil 2008;30:1222–1229.

Stackhouse C, Shewokis PA, Pierce SR, et al. Gait initiation in children with cerebral palsy. Gait Posture 2007;26:301–308.

Stahnisch FW, Nitsch R. Santiago Ramon y Cajal's concept of neuronal plasticity: the ambiguity lives on. Trends Neurosci 2002;25:589–591.

Stalvey B, Owsley C, Sloane ME, et al. The life space questionnaire: a measure of the extent of mobility of older adults. J Appl Gerontol 1999;18:479–498.

Stapley PJ, Drew T. The pontomedullary reticular formation contributes to the compensatory postural responses observed following removal of the support surface in the standing cat. J Neurophysiol 2009;101:1334–1350.

Stapley PJ, Ting LH, Hulliger M, et al. Automatic postural responses are delayed by pyridoxine-induced somatosensory loss. J Neurosci 2002;22:5803–5807.

Stark T, Walker B, Phillips JK, Fejer R, Beck R. Hand-held dynamometry correlation with the gold standard isokinetic dynamometry: a systematic review. PM R 2011;3:472–479.

Starosta M, Kostka J, Redlicka J, Miller E. Analysis of upper limb muscle strength in the early phase of brain stroke. Acta Bioeng Biomech 2017;19(3):85–91.

Startzell JK, Owens DA, Mulfinger LM, Cavanagh PR. Stair negotiation in older people: a review. J Am Geriatr Soc 2000;48:567–580.

Steenbergen B, Hulstijn W, Lemmens IHL, et al. The timing of prehensile movements in subjects with cerebral palsy. Dev Med Child Neurol 1998;40:108–114.

Stehouwer DJ, Farel PB. Development of hindlimb locomotor behavior in the frog. Dev Psychobiol 1984;17:217–232.

Stein DG, Brailowsky S, Will B. Brain repair. New York: Oxford, 1995.

Stein J. Cerebellar forward models to control movement. J Physiol 2009;587:299.

Stein J, Krebs HI, Frontera WR, et al. Comparison of two techniques of robot-aided upper limb exercise training after stroke. Am J Phys Med Rehabil 2004;83:720–728.

Stein RB. Reflex modulation during locomotion: functional significance. In: Patla A, ed. Adaptability of human gait. Amsterdam, The Netherlands: North Holland, 1991:21–36.

Stephens MJ, Yang JF. Loading during the stance phase of walking in humans increases the extensor EMG amplitude but does not change the duration of the step cycle. Exp Brain Res 1999;124:363–370.

Stephenson JL, De Serres SJ, Lamontagne A. The effect of arm movements on the lower limb during gait after a stroke. Gait Posture 2010;31:109–115.

Stephenson JL, Lamontagne A, De Serres SJ. The coordination of upper and lower limb movements during gait in healthy and stroke individuals. Gait Posture 2009;29:11–16.

Stergiou N, Harbourne R, Cavanaugh J. Optimal movement variability: a new theoretical perspective for neurologic physical therapy. J Neurol Phys Ther 2006;30:120–129.

Stern EB. Stability of the Jebsen-Taylor hand function test across three test sessions. Am J Occup Ther 1992;7:647–649.

Stern GM, Lander CM, Lees AJ. Akinetic freezing and trick movements in Parkinson's disease. J Neural Transm Suppl 1980;16:137–141.

Stern Y, Mayeux R, Rosen J, et al. Perceptual motor dysfunction in Parkinson's disease: a deficit in sequential and predictive voluntary movement. J Neurol Neurosurg Psychiatry 1983;46:145–151.

Steward O. Reorganization of neuronal connections following CNS trauma: principles and experimental paradigms. J Neurotrauma [illegible].

Stillman B, McMeeken J. A video-based version of the pendulum test: technique and normal response. Arch Phys Med Rehabil 1995;76(2):166–176.

Stockmeyer S. An interpretation of the approach of Rood to the treatment of neuromuscular dysfunction. Am J Phys Med 1967;46:950–955.

Stoffregen TA, Adolph K, Thelen E, et al. Toddlers' postural adaptations to different support surfaces. Mot Control 1997;1:119–137.

Stoffregen TA, Pagulayan RJ, Bardy BG, et al. Modulating postural control to facilitate visual performance. Hum Mov Sci 2000;19:203–220.

Stoffregen TA, Riccio GE. An ecological theory of orientation and the vestibular system. Psychol Rev 1988;95(1):3–14.

Stoquart-Elsankari S, Bottin C, Roussel-Pieronne M. Motor and cognitive slowing in multiple sclerosis: an attentional deficit? Clin Neurol Neurosurg 2010;112:226–232.

Stott NS, Reynolds N, McNair P. Level versus inclined walking: ambulatory compensations in children with cerebral palsy under outdoor conditions. Pediatr Phys Ther 2014;26(4):428–435.

Stoykov ME, Lewis GN, Corcos DM. Comparison of bilateral and unilateral training for upper extremity hemiparesis in stroke. Neurorehabil Neural Repair 2009;23(9):945–953. doi: 10.1177/1545968309338190.

Stoykov ME, Madhavan S. Motor priming in neurorehabilitation. J Neurol Phys Ther 2015;39(1):33–42.

Strick PL. Anatomical organization of multiple areas of frontal lobe: implications for recovery of function. Adv Neurol 1988;47:293–312.

Strub RL, Black FW. The mental status examination in neurology. Philadelphia, PA: FA Davis, 1977.

Strupp M, Arbusow V, Pereira DB, et al. Subjective straight ahead during neck muscle vibration: effect of aging. Neuroreport 1999;10:3191–3194.

Studenski S, Duncan PW, Chandler J. Postural responses and effector factors in persons with unexplained falls: results and methodologic issues. J Am Geriatr Soc 1991;39:229–234.

Sturnieks DL, St George R, Lord SR. Balance disorders in the elderly. Clin Neurophysiol 2008;38:467–478.

Sucar LE, Orihuela-Espina F, Velazquez RL, Reinkensmeyer DJ, Leder R, Hernández-Franco J. Gesture therapy: an upper limb virtual reality-based motor rehabilitation platform. IEEE Trans Neural Syst Rehabil Eng 2014;22(3):634–643. doi: 10.1109/TNSRE.2013.2293673.

Sudarsky L, Ronthal M. Gait disorders among elderly patients: a survey study of 50 patients. Arch Neurol 1983;40:740–743.

Sudarsky L, Ronthal M. Gait disorders in the elderly: assessing the risk for falls. In: Vellas B, Toupet M, Rubenstein L, et al., eds. Falls, balance and gait disorders in the elderly. Amsterdam, The Netherlands: Elsevier, 1992:117–127.

Sudsawad P, Trombly CA, Henderson A, et al. Testing the effect of kinesthetic training on handwriting performance in first-grade students. Am J Occup Ther 2002;56(1): 26–33.

Sudsawad P, Trombly CA, Henderson A, et al. The relationship between the Evaluation Tool of Children's Handwriting and teacher's perceptions of handwriting legibility. Am J Occup Ther 2001;55(5):518–523.

Sugden DA. Movement speed in children. J Motor Behav 1980;12:125–132.

Sukal-Moulton T, Clancy T, Zhang LQ, et al. Clinical application of a robotic ankle training program for cerebral palsy compared to the research laboratory application: does it translate to practice? Arch Phys Med Rehabil 2014;95:1433–1440.

Sullivan E, Rose E, Pfefferbaum A. Effect of vision, touch and stance on cerebellar vermian-related sway and tremor: a quantitative physiological and MRI study. Cerebral Cortex 2006;16:1077–1086.

Sullivan JE, Hedman LD. A home program of sensory and neuromuscular electrical stimulation with upper-limb task practice in a patient 5 years after a stroke. Phys Ther 2004;84:1045–1054.

Sullivan KJ, Knowlton BJ, Dobkin BH. Step training with body weight support: effect of treadmill speed and practice paradigms on poststroke locomotor recovery. Arch Phys Med Rehabil 2002;83:683–691.

Sun J, Walters M, Svensson N, et al. The influence of surface slope on human gait characteristics: a study of urban pedestrians walking on an inclined surface. Ergonomics 1996;39:677–692.

Sunderland A. Recovery of ipsilateral dexterity after stroke. Stroke 2000;31(2):430–433.

Sundermeier L, Woollacott M, Jensen J, et al. Postural sensitivity to visual flow in aging adults with and without balance problems. J Gerontol A Biol Sci Med Sci 1996;51:M45–M52.

Sundermier L, Woollacott M, Roncesvalles N, et al. The development of balance control in children: comparisons of EMG and kinetic variables and chronological and developmental groupings. Exp Brain Res 2001;136:340–350.

Sur M, Pallas SL, Roe AW. Cross-modal plasticity in cortical development: differentiation and specification of sensory neocortex. Trends Neurosci 1990;13:227–233.

Surberg PR. Aging and effect of physical-mental practice upon acquisition and retention of a motor skill. J Gerontol 1976;31:64–67.

Surgent OJ, Dadalko OI, Pickett KA, Travers BG. Balance and the brain: a review of structural brain correlates of postural balance and balance training in humans. Gait Posture 2019;71:245–252.

Surrey LR, Nelson K, Delelio C, et al. A comparison of performance outcomes between the Minnesota Rate of Manipulation Test and the Minnesota Manual Dexterity Test. Work 2003;20(2):97–102.

Surkar SM, Hoffman RM, Davies B, Harbourne R, Kurz MJ. Impaired anticipatory vision and visuomotor coordination affects action planning and execution in children with hemiplegic cerebral palsy. Res Dev Disabil 2018;80:64–73.

Sütbeyaz S, Yavuzer G, Sezer N, et al. Mirror therapy enhances lower-extremity motor recovery and motor functioning after stroke: a randomized controlled trial. Arch Phys Med Rehabil 2007;88:555–559.

Sutherland DH, Olshen R, Cooper L, et al. The development of mature gait. J Bone Joint Surg Am 1980;62:336–353.

Suzuki E, Chen W, Kondo T. Measuring unilateral spatial neglect during stepping. Arch Phys Med Rehabil 1997;78:173–178.

Suzuki M, Miyai I, Ono T, et al. Prefrontal and premotor cortices are involved in adapting walking and running speed on the treadmill: an optical imaging study. Neuroimage 2004;23:1020–1026.

Svehlík M, Zwick EB, Steinwender G, et al. Gait analysis in patients with Parkinson's disease off dopaminergic therapy. Arch Phys Med Rehabil 2009;90:1880–1886.

Sveistrup H, Woollacott M. Practice modifies the developing automatic postural response. Exp Brain Res 1997;114:33–43.

Sveistrup H, Woollacott MH. Longitudinal development of the automatic postural response in infants. J Motor Behav 1996;28:58–70.

Sweatt JD, Kandel ER. Persistent and transcriptionally-dependent increase in protein phosphorylation in long-term facilitation of Aplysia sensory neurons. Nature 1989;339:51–54.

Sylos-Labini F, La Scaleia V, Cappellini G, et al. Distinct locomotor precursors in newborn babies. Proc Natl Acad Sci USA 2020;117(17):9604–9612.

Sylos-Labini F, Magnani S, Cappellini G, et al. Foot placement characteristics and plantar pressure distribution patterns during stepping on ground in neonates. Front Physiol 2017;8:784.

T

Taguchi K, Tada C. Change of body sway with growth of children. In: Amblard B, Berthoz A, Clarac F, eds. Posture and gait: development, adaptation and modulation. Amsterdam, The Netherlands: Elsevier, 1988:59–65.

Taira M, Milne S, Georgopoulos AP, et al. Parietal cortex neurons of the monkey related to the visual guidance of hand movement. Exp Brain Res 1990;83:29–36.

Tajali S, Shaterzadeh-Yazdi MJ, Negahban H, van Dieën JH, Mehravar M, Majdinasab N, Saki-Malehi A, Mofateh R. Predicting falls among patients with multiple sclerosis: Comparison of patient-reported outcomes and performance-based measures of lower extremity functions. Mult Scler Relat Disord 2017;17:69–74.

Takakusaki K. Neurophysiology of gait: from the spinal cord to the frontal lobe. Mov Disord 2013;28(11):1483–1491.

Takakusaki K. Functional neuroanatomy for posture and gait control. J Mov Disord 2017;10(1):1–17.

Takahashi M, Tsujita N, Akiyama I. Evaluation of the vestibulo-ocular reflex by gaze function. Acta Otolaryngol 1988;105:7–12.

Takakusaki K, Saitaoh K, Harada H, et al. Role of the basal ganglia-brainstem pathways in the control of motor behaviors. Neurosci Res 2004;50:137–151.

Takakusaki K, Tomita N, Yano M. Substrates for normal gait and pathophysiology of gait disturbances with respect to the basal ganglia dysfunction. J Neurol 2008;255:19–29.

Takebayashi T, Amano S, Hanada K, et al. A one-year follow-up after modified constraint-induced movement therapyfor chronic stroke patients with paretic arm: a prospective case series study. Top Stroke Rehabil 2015;22(1):18–25.

Takebe D, Kukulka C, Narayan G, et al. Peroneal nerve stimulator in rehabilitation of hemiplegic patients. Arch Phys Med Rehabil 1975;56:237–239.

Tamaru Y, Naito Y, Nishikawa T. Earlier and greater hand pre-shaping in the elderly: a study based on kinematic analysis of reaching movements to grasp objects. Psychogeriatrics 2017;17:382–388.

Tan Z, Liu H, Yan T, et al. The effectiveness of functional electrical stimulation based on a normal gait pattern on subjects with early stroke: a randomized controlled trial. Biomed Res Int 2014;2014:545408.

Tang A, Rymer WZ. Abnormal force—EMG relations in paretic limbs of hemiparetic human subjects. J Neurol Neurosurg Psychiatry 1981;44:690–698.

Tang PF, Woollacott MH. Inefficient postural responses to unexpected slips during walking in older adults. J Gerontol 1998;53:M471–M480.

Tang PF, Woollacott MH, Chong RKY. Control of reactive balance adjustments in perturbed human walking: roles of proximal and distal postural muscle activity. Exp Brain Res 1998;119:141–152.

Tang PF, Woollacott MH. Phase-dependent modulation of proximal and distal postural responses to slips in young and older adults. J Gerontol 1999;54:M89–M102.

Tardieu C, Lespargot A, Tabary C, et al. For how long must the soleus muscle be stretched each day to prevent contracture? Dev Med Child Neurol 1988;30(1):3–10.

Tatton WG, Eastman MJ, Bedingham W, et al. Defective utilization of sensory input as the basis for bradykinesia, rigidity and decreased movement repertoire in Parkinson's disease: a hypothesis. Can J Neurol Sci 1984;11:136–143.

Taub E. Motor behavior following deafferentation in the developing and motorically mature monkey. In: Herman S, Grillner R, Ralston HJ, et al., eds. Neural control of locomotion. New York: Plenum, 1976:675–705.

Taub E. Some anatomical observations following chronic dorsal rhizotomy in monkeys. Neuroscience 1980;5:389–401.

Taub E. Technique to improve chronic motor deficit after stroke. Arch Phys Med Rehabil 1993;74:347–354.

Taub E, Berman AJ. Movement and learning in the absence of sensory feedback. In: Freedman SJ, ed. The neurophysiology of spatially oriented behavior. Homewood, NJ: Dorsey, 1968:173–192.

Taub E, Crago JE, Uswatte G. Constraint-induced movement therapy: a new approach to treatment in physical rehabilitation. Rehabil Psychol 1998;43(2):152–170.

Taub E, Landesman Ramey S, DeLuca S, et al. Efficacy of constraint-induced movement therapy for children with cerebral palsy with asymmetric motor impairment. Pediatrics 2004;113:305–312.

Taub E, Miller NE, Novack TA, et al. Technique to improve chronic motor deficit after stroke. Arch Phys Med Rehabil 1993;74:347–354.

Taub E, Wolf SL. Constraint-induction techniques to facilitate upper extremity use in stroke patients. Top Stroke Rehabil 1997;3:38–61.

Taylor N, Sand PL, Jebsen RH. Evaluation of hand function in children. Arch Phys Med Rehabil 1973;54(3):129–135.

Teasdale N, Bard C, LaRue J, et al. On the cognitive penetrability of postural control. Exp Aging Res 1993;19:1–13.

Teasdale N, Simoneau M. Attentional demands for postural control: the effects of aging and sensory reintegration. Gait Posture 2001;14: 203–210.

Teasdale N, Stelmach GE, Breunig A. Postural sway characteristics of the elderly under normal and altered visual and support surface conditions. J Gerontol 1991;46: B238–B244.

Teasell R, McRae M, Foley N, et al. The incidence and consequences of falls in stroke patients during inpatient rehabilitation: factors associated with high risk. Arch Phys Med Rehabil 2002;83:329–333.

Teixeira-Salmela LF, Olney SJ, Nadeau S, et al. Muscle strengthening and physical conditioning to reduce impairment and disability in chronic stroke survivors. Arch Phys Med Rehabil 1999;80:1211–1218.

Ternes AM, Fielding J, Addamo PK, et al. Concurrent motor and cognitive function in multiple sclerosis: a motor overflow and motor stability study. Cogn Behav Neurol 2014;27(2):68–76.

Tessier-Lavigne M. Visual processing by the retina. In: Kandel ER, Schwartz JH, Jessell TM, eds. Principles of neural science, 4th ed. New York: McGraw-Hill, 2000:507–522.

Teulings HL, Contreras-Vidal JL, Stelmach GE, Adler CH. Adaptation of handwriting size under distorted visual feedback in patients with Parkinson's disease and elderly and young controls. J Neurol Neurosurg Psychiatry. 2002;72:315–324.

Teulings HL, Contreras-Vidal JL, Stelmach GE, Adler CH. Parkinsonism reduces coordination of fingers, wrist, and arm in fine motor control. Exp Neurol 1997;146(1):159–170.

Thacker EL, Chen H, Patel AV, et al. Recreational physical activity and risk of Parkinson's disease. Mov Disord 2008;23:69–74.

Thelen DG, Schultz AB, Alexander NB, et al. Effects of age on rapid ankle torque development. J Gerontol Med Sci 1996;51:M226–M232.

Thelen E, Corbetta D, Kamm K, et al. The transition to reaching: mapping intention and intrinsic dynamics. Child Dev 1993;64:1058–1098.

Thelen E, Fisher DM, Ridley-Johnson R. The relationship between physical growth and a newborn reflex. Infant Behav Dev 1984;7:479–493.

Thelen E, Fisher DM. Newborn stepping: an explanation for a disappearing reflex. Dev Psychol 1982;18:760–775.

Thelen E, Kelso JAS, Fogel A. Self-organizing systems and infant motor development. Dev Rev 1987;7: 39–65.

Thelen E, Spencer JP. Postural control during reaching in young infants: a dynamic systems approach. Neurosci Biobehav Rev 1998;22:507–514.

Thelen E, Ulrich BD. Hidden skills: a dynamic systems analysis of treadmill stepping during the first year. Monogr Soc Res Child Dev 1991;56(1):1–104.

Thelen E, Ulrich, BD, Jensen JL. The developmental origins of locomotion. In: Woollacott MH, Shumway-Cook A, eds. Development of posture and gait across the life span. Columbia: University of South Carolina, 1989:25–47.

Therrien AS, Bastian AJ. The cerebellum as a movement sensor. Neurosci Lett 2019;688:37–40.

Thielbar KO, Lord TJ, Fischer HC, et al. Training finger individuation with a mechatronic-virtual reality system leads to improved fine motor control post-stroke. J Neuroeng Rehabil 2014;11(1):171.

Thielman G. Rehabilitation of reaching poststroke: a randomized pilot investigation of tactile versus auditory feedback for trunk control. J Neurol Phys Ther 2010;34(3):138–144. doi: 10.1097/NPT.0b013e3181efa1e8.

Thielman G, Kaminski T, Gentile AM. Rehabilitation of reaching after stroke: comparing 2 training protocols utilizing trunk restraint. Neurorehabil Neural Repair 2008;22:697–705.

Thielman GT, Dean CM, Gentile AM. Rehabilitation of reaching after stroke: task-related training versus progressive resistive exercise. Arch Phys Med Rehabil 2004;85:1613–1618.

Thieme H, Mehrholz J, Pohl M, et al. Mirror therapy for improving motor function after stroke. Cochrane Database Syst Rev 2012;(3):CD008449.

Thilmann AF, Fellows SJ, Garms E. The mechanism of spastic muscle hypertonus. Brain 1991;114:233–244.

Thomas NDA, Gardiner JD, Crompton RH, Lawson R. Keep your head down: Maintaining gait stability in challenging conditions. Hum Mov Sci 2020;73:102676.

Thomas RL, Williams AK, Lundy-Ekman L. Supine to stand in elderly persons: relationship to age, activity level, strength and range of motion. Issues Aging 1998;21: 9–18.

Thompson M, Medley A. Forward and lateral sitting functional reach in younger, middle aged, and older adults. J Ger Phys Ther 2007;30:43–48.

Thornton M, Marshall S, McComas J, et al. Benefits of activity and virtual reality based balance exercise programmes for adults with traumatic brain injury: perceptions of participants and their caregivers. Brain Inj 2005;19:989–1000.

Tiffin J. Purdue pegboard examiner manual. Chicago, IL: Science Research Associates, 1968.

Tillerson JL, Cohen AD, Philhower J, et al. Forced limb-use effects on the behavioral and neurochemical effects of 6-hydroxydopamine. J Neurosci 2001;21:4427–4435.

Tilson JK, Sullivan KJ, Cen SY, et al. Meaningful gait speed improvement during the first 60 days poststroke: minimal clinically important difference. Phys Ther 2010;90:196–208.

Timiras P. Aging of the skeleton, joints and muscles. In: Timiras PS, ed. Physiological basis of aging and geriatrics, 2nd ed. Ann Arbor, MI: CRC Press, 1994.

Tinetti ME. Performance-oriented assessment of mobility problems in elderly patients. J Am Geriatr Soc 1986;34:119–126.

Tinetti ME, Doucette JT, Claus EB. The contribution of predisposing and situational risk factors to serious fall injuries. J Am Geriatr Soc 1995;43:1207–1213.

Tinetti ME, Ginter SF. Identifying mobility dysfunctions in elderly patients: standard neuromuscular examination or direct assessment? JAMA 1988;259:1190–1193.

Tinetti ME, Richman D, Powell L. Falls efficacy as a measure of fear of falling. J Gerontol 1990;45:P239–P243.

Tinetti ME, Speechley M, Ginter SF. Risk factors for falls among elderly persons living in the community. N Engl J Med 1988;319:1701–1707.

Tinetti ME, Williams TF, Mayewski R. Fall risk index for elderly patients based on numbers of chronic disabilities. Am J Med 1986;80:429–434.

Ting LH, Macpherson JM. A limited set of muscle synergies for force control during a postural task. J Neurophysiol 2005;93:609–613.

Ting LH, McKay JL. Neuromechanics of muscle synergies for posture and movement. Curr Opin Neurobiol 2007;17:622–628.

Tissue CM, Velleman PF, Stegink-Jansen CW, et al. Validity and reliability of the functional dexterity test in children. J Hand Ther 2017;30(4):500–506. doi: 10.1016/j.jht.2016.08.002.

Titus MND, Gall NG, Yerxa EJ, et al. Correlation of perceptual performance and activities of daily living in stroke patients. Am J Occup Ther 1991;45:410–418.

Tobis JS, Lowenthal M. Evaluation and management of the brain damaged patient. Springfield, IL: Charles C. Thomas, 1960.

Tohyama T, Kinoshita M, Kobayashi K, Isa K, Watanabe D, Kobayashi K, Liu M, Isa T, Strick PL. Contribution of propriospinal neurons to recovery of hand dexterity after corticospinal tract lesions in monkeys. Proc Natl Acad Sci USA 2017;114,604–609.

Tomassini V, Johansen-Berg H, Jbabdi S, et al. Relating brain damage to brain plasticity in patients with multiple sclerosis. Neurorehabil Neural Repair 2012;26:581–593.

Tomassini V, Matthews PM, Thompson AJ, et al. Neuroplasticity and functional recovery in multiple sclerosis. Nat Rev Neurol 2012a;8:635–646.

Tomita H, Fukaya Y, Ueda T, et al. Deficits in task-specific modulation of anticipatory postural adjustments in individuals with spastic diplegic cerebral palsy. J Neurophysiol 2011;105(5):2157–2168.

Torres-Oviedo G, Macpherson JM, Ting LH. Muscle synergy organization is robust across a variety of postural perturbations. J Neurophysiol 2006;96:1530–1546.

Torres-Oviedo G, Ting LH. Muscle synergies characterizing human postural responses. J Neurophysiol 2007;98:2144–2156.

Toupet M, Gagey PM, Heuschen S. Vestibular patients and aging subjects lose use of visual input and expend more energy in static postural control. In: Vellas B, Toupet M, Rubenstein L, et al., eds. Falls, balance and gait disorders in the elderly. Paris, France: Elsevier, 1992:183–198.

Towen B. Neurological development in infancy. Clinics in developmental medicine 58. Philadelphia, PA: JF Lippincott, 1976.

Travis AM, Woolsey CN. Motor performance of monkeys after bilateral partial and total cerebral decortication. Am J Phys Med 1956;35:273–310.

Treisman A. Solutions to the binding problem: progress through controversy and convergence. Neuron 1999;24:105–110, 111–125.

Trejo-Gabriel-Galan JM, Rogel-Melgosa V, Gonzalez S, Sedano J, Villar JR, Arenaza-Basterrechea N. Rehabilitation of hemineglect of the left arm using movement detection bracelets activating a visual and acoustic alarm. J Neuroeng Rehabil 2016;13:79.

Tretriluxana J, Gordon J, Fisher BE, et al. Hemisphere specific impairments in reach-to-grasp control after stroke: effects of object size. Neurorehabil Neural Repair 2009;23:679–691.

Tretriluxana J, Gordon J, Winstein CJ. Manual asymmetries in grasp pre-shaping and transport-grasp coordination. Exp Brain Res 2008;188:305–315.

Tretriluxana J, Kantak S, Tretriluxana S, et al. Low frequency repetitive transcranial magnetic stimulation to the non-lesioned hemisphere improves paretic arm reach-to-grasp performance after chronic stroke. Disabil Rehabil Assist Technol 2013;8(2):121–124.

Trombly C. Anticipating the future: assessment of occupational function. Am J Occup Ther 1993;47:253–257.

Trombly CA. Theoretical foundations for practice. In: Trombly CA, ed. Occupational therapy for physical dysfunction, 4th ed. Baltimore, MD: Lippincott Williams & Wilkins, 1995:15–28.

Tsai LT, Hsu JL, Wu CT, Chen CC, Su YC. A new visual stimulation program for improving visual acuity in children with visual impairment: a pilot study. Front Hum Neurosci 2016;10:157. doi: 10.3389/fnhum.2016.00157.

Tsai WC, Lien HY, Liu WY, Guo SL, Lin YH, Yang TF. Early and anticipatory postural adjustments in healthy subjects under stable and unstable sitting conditions. J Electromyogr Kinesiol. 2018;43(259):21–27.

Tsang WW, Ng SS, Lee MW, et al. Does postural stability affect the performance of eye-hand coordination in stroke survivors? Am J Phys Med Rehabil 2013;92:781–788.

Tse T, Douglas J, Lentin P, Carey L. Measuring participation after stroke: a review of frequently used tools. Arch Phys Med Rehabil 2013;94:177–192.

Tseng SC, Morton SM. Impaired interlimb coordination of voluntary leg movements in poststroke hemiparesis. J Neurophysiol 2010;104(1):248–257.

Tsoupikova D, Stoykov NS, Corrigan M, et al. Virtual immersion for post-stroke hand rehabilitation therapy. Ann Biomed Eng 2015;43:467–477.

Tur BS, Küçükdeveci AA, Kutlay S, et al. Psychometric properties of the WeeFIM in children with cerebral palsy in Turkey. Dev Med Child Neurol 2009;51(9):732–738.

Turner-Stokes L, Williams H. Goal attainment scaling: a direct comparison of alternative rating methods. Clin Rehabil. 2010;24(1):66–73. doi: 10.1177/0269215509343846.

Turvey MT, Carello C. Dynamics of Bernstein's levels of synergies. In: Latash ML, Turvey MT, eds. Dexterity and its development. Mahwah, NJ: Erlbaum, 1996:339–377.

Tuthill JC, Azim E. Proprioception. Curr Biol 2018;28:R194–R203.

Twitchell T. Reflex mechanisms and the development of prehension. In: Connolly K, ed. Mechanisms of motor skill development. New York: Academic Press, 1970.

Twitchell TE. The restoration of motor function following hemiplegia in man. Brain 1951;74:443.

Tyson SF, Hanley M, Chillala J. Sensory loss in hospital-admitted people with stroke: characteristics, associated factors and relationship with function. Neurorehabil Neural Repair 2008;22:166–172.

U

Ugur C, Gucuyener D, Uzuner N, et al. Characteristics of falling in patients with stroke. J Neurol Neurosurg Psychiatry 2000;69:649–651.

Ullman MT. Contributions of memory circuits to language: the declarative/procedural model. Cognition 2004;92:231–270.

Ulrich DA, Ulrich BD, Angulo-Kinzler RM, et al. Treadmill training of infants with Down syndrome: evidence-based developmental outcomes. Pediatrics 2001;108(5):E84.

Ungerleider LG, Brody BA. Extrapersonal spatial orientation: the role of posterior parietal, anterior frontal, and inferotemporal cortex. Exp Neurol 1977;56:265–280.

Urbin MA, Bailey RR, Lang CE. Validity of body-worn sensor acceleration metrics to index upper extremity function in hemiparetic stroke. J Neurol Phys Ther 2015;39(2):111–118.

Uswatte G, Foo WL, Olmstead H, et al. Ambulatory monitoring of arm movement using accelerometry: An objective measure of upper-extremity rehabilitation in persons with chronic stroke. Arch Phys Med Rehabil 2005;86:1498–1501.

Uswatte G, Giuliani C, Winstein C, et al. Validity of accelerometry for monitoring real-world arm activity in patients with subacute stroke: Evidence from the extremity constraint-induced therapy evaluation trial. Arch Phys Med Rehabil 2006;87(10):1340–1345.

Uswatte G, Taub E, Griffin A, Vogtle L, Rowe J, Barman J. The pediatric motor activity log-revised: assessing real-world arm use in children with cerebral palsy. Rehabil Psychol 2012;57(2):149–158. doi: 10.1037/a0028516.

Uswatte G, Taub E, Morris D, et al. The Motor Activity Log-28: assessing daily use of the hemiparetic arm after stroke. Neurology 2006;67:1189–1194.

Utley A, Sugden D. Interlimb coupling in children with hemiplegic cerebral palsy during reaching and grasping at speed. Dev Med Child Neurol 1998;40:396–404.

V

Vagge A, Pellegrini M, Iester M, et al. Motor skills in children affected by strabismus. Eye 2021;35:544–547.

Valero-Cuevas FJ, Smaby N, Venkadesan M, et al. The strength-dexterity test as a measure of dynamic pinch performance. J Biomech 2003;36(2):265–270.

Vallis LA, McFadyen BJ. Children use different anticipatory control strategies than adults to circumvent an obstacle in the travel path. Exp Brain Res 2005;167:119–127.

van de Winckel A, Gauthier L. A revised motor activity log following rasch validation (Rasch-Based MAL-18) and consensus methods in chronic stroke and multiple sclerosis. Neurorehabil Neural Repair 2019;33(10):787–791. doi: 10.1177/1545968319868717.

van Delden AL, Beek PJ, Roerdink M, et al. Unilateral and bilateral upper-limb training interventions after stroke have similar effects on bimanual coupling strength. Neurorehabil Neural Repair 2015;29(3):255–267.

van der Fits IBM, Klip AWJ, vanEykern LA, et al. Postural adjustments accompanying fast pointing movements in standing, sitting and lying adults. Exp Brain Res 1998;120:202–216.

van der Heide JC, Begeer C, Fock JM, et al. Postural control during reaching in preterm children with cerebral palsy. Dev Med Child Neurol 2004;46:253–266.

van der Heide JC, Otten B, Stremmelaar E, et al. Kinematic characteristics of reaching movements in preterm children with cerebral palsy. Pediatr Res 2005;57:883–889.

Van der Krogt M, Doorenbosch, A, Becher JG, et al. Walking speed modifies spasticity effects in gastrocnemius and soleus in cerebral palsy gait. Clin Biomech (Bristol, Avon) 2009;24:422–428.

van der Krogt MM, Sloot LH, Harlaar J. Overground versus self-paced treadmill walking in a virtual environment in children with cerebral palsy. Gait Posture 2014;40:587–593.

van der Lee JH, Beckerman H, Lankhorst GJ, et al. The responsiveness of the Action Research Arm Test and the Fugl-Meyer Assessment Scale in chronic stroke patients. J Rehabil Med 2001;33:110–113.

van der Linden ML, Scott SM, Hooper JE, et al. Gait kinematics of people with multiple sclerosis and the acute application of functional electrical stimulation. Gait Posture 2014;39:1092–1096.

van der Meer AL, van der Weel FR, Lee DN. The functional significance of arm movements in neonates. Science 1995;267:693–695.

van Dieën JH, van Leeuwen M, Faber GS. Learning to balance on one leg: motor strategy and sensory weighting. J Neurophysiol 2015;114:2967–2982.

Van Donkelaar P, Lee RG. Interactions between the eye and hand motor systems: disruptions due to cerebellar dysfunction. J Neurophysiol 1994;72:1674–1684.

van Eijck MM, Schoonman GG, van der Naalt J, de Vries J, Roks G. Diffuse axonal injury after traumatic brain injury is a prognostic factor for functional outcome: a systematic review and meta-analysis. Brain Inj 2018;32:395–402.

van Hartingsveldt MJ, Cup EH, Oostendorp RA. Reliability and validity of the fine motor scale of the Peabody Developmental Motor Scales-2. Occup Ther Int 2005;12(1):1–13.

van Ooijen MW, Heeren A, Smulders K, et al. Improved gait adjustments after gait adaptability training are associated with reduced attentional demands in persons with stroke. Exp Brain Res 2015;233:1007–1018.

van Peppen RPS, Kortsmit M, Lindeman E, et al. Effects of visual feedback therapy on postural control in bilateral standing after stroke: a systematic review. J Rehabil Med 2006;38:3–9.

van Polanen V, Tibold R, Nuruki A, Davare M. Visual delay affects force scaling and weight perception during object lifting in virtual reality. J Neurophysiol 2019;121:1398–1409.

van Praag H. Exercise and the brain: something to chew on. Trends Neurosci 2009;32:283–290.

VanSwearingen JM, Paschal KA, Bonino P, Yang JF. The modified gait abnormality rating scale for recognizing the risk of recurrent falls in community-dwelling elderly adults. Phys Ther 1996;76:994–1002.

Van Thiel E, Meulenbroek RG, Hulstijn W, et al. Kinematics of fast hemiparetic aiming movements toward stationary and moving targets. Exp Brain Res 2000;132:230–242.

Van Thiel E, Steenbergen B. Shoulder and hand displacements during hitting, reaching, and grasping movements in hemiparetic cerebral palsy. Motor Control 2001;5:166–182.

Van Vleet TM, DeGutis JM. Cross-training in hemispatial neglect: auditory sustained attention training ameliorates visual attention deficits. Cortex 2013;49(3):679–690. doi: 10.1016/j.cortex.2012.03.020.

van Vliet PM, Sheridan MR. Ability to adjust reach extent in the hemiplegic arm. Physiotherapy 2009;95:176–184.

van Vliet PM, Sheridan MR. Coordination between reaching and grasping in patients with hemiparesis and healthy subjects. Arch Phys Med Rehabil 2007;88:1325–1331.

van Wegen EE, van Emmerik RE, Wagenaar RC, et al. Stability boundaries and lateral postural control in Parkinson's disease. Motor Control 2001;5:254–269.

Van Woerkom TC, Minderhoud JM, Gottschal T, et al. Neurotransmitters in the treatment of patients with severe head injuries. Eur Neurol 1982;21:227–234.

van Wyk A, Eksteen CA, Rheeder P. The effect of visual scanning exercises integrated into physiotherapy in patients with unilateral spatial neglect poststroke: a matched-pair randomized control trial. Neurorehabil Neural Repair 2014;28(9):856–873. doi: 10.1177/1545968314526306.

Vandervoort AA, Chesworth BM, Cunningham DA, et al. Age and sex effects on mobility of the human ankle. J Gerontol 1992;47:17–21.

Vaney C, Gattlen B, Lugon-Moulin V, et al. Robotic-assisted step training (lokomat) not superior to equal intensity of over-ground rehabilitation in patients with multiple sclerosis. Neurorehabil Neural Repair 2012;26:212–221.

VanSant AF. Age differences in movement patterns used by children to rise from a supine position to erect stance. Phys Ther 1988a;68:1130–1138.

VanSant AF. Concepts of neural organization and movement. In: Connolly BH, Montgomery PC, eds. Therapeutic exercise in developmental disabilities. Chattanooga, TN: Chattanooga, 1987:1–8.

VanSant AF. Life-span development in functional tasks. Phys Ther 1990;70:788–798.

VanSant AF. Rising from a supine position to erect stance: description of adult movement and a developmental hypothesis. Phys Ther 1988b;68:185–192.

Vasudevan JM, Browne BJ. Hemiplegic shoulder pain: an approach to diagnosis and management. Phys Med Rehabil Clin N Am 2014;25(2):411–437. doi: 10.1016/j.pmr.2014.01.010.

Vearrier LA, Langan J, Shumway-Cook A, et al. An intensive massed practice approach to retraining balance post-stroke. Gait Posture 2005;22:154–163.

Veerbeek JM, Langbroek-Amersfoort AC, van Wegen EE, Meskers CG,

Kwakkel G. Effects of robot assisted therapy for the upper limb after stroke. Neurorehabil Neural Repair 2017;31(2):107–121. doi: 10.1177/1545968316666957.

Venglar M. Case report: Tai Chi and Parkinsonism. Physiother Res Int 2005;10(2):116–121.

Ventre-dominey J. Vestibular function in the temporal and parietal cortex: distinct velocity and inertial processing pathways. Front Integr Neurosci 2014;8:1–13.

Verbrugge L, Jette A. The disablement process. Soc Sci Med 1994;38:1–14.

Vercher JL, Gauthier GM, Guedon O, et al. Self-moved target eye tracking in control and deafferented subjects: roles of arm motor command and proprioception in arm-eye coordination. J Neurophysiol 1996;76:1133–1144.

Vereijken B, van Emmerik REA, Whiting HTA, et al. Freezing degrees of freedom in skill acquisition. J Motor Behav 1992;24:133–142.

Verrel J, Bekkering H, Steenbergen B. Eye-hand coordination during manual object transport with the affected and less affected hand in adolescents with hemiparetic cerebral palsy. Exp Brain Res 2008;187:107–116.

Vidoni ED, Boyd LA. Preserved motor learning after stroke is related to the degree of proprioceptive deficit. Behav Brain Funct 2009;5:36.

Viitasalo MK, Kampman V, Sotaniemi KA, et al. Analysis of sway in Parkinson's disease using a new inclinometry-based method. Mov Disord 2002;17:663–669.

Vilenchik MM, Knudson AG. Inverse radiation dose-rate effects on somatic and germ-line mutations and DNA damage rates. Proc Natl Acad Sci U S A 2000;97:5381–5386.

Vilis T, Hore J. Central neural mechanisms contributing to cerebellar tremor produced by limb perturbations. J Neurophysiol 1980;43:279–291.

Vinter A. Manual imitations and reaching behaviors: an illustration of action control in infancy. In: Bard C, Fleury M, Hay L, eds. Development of eye-hand coordination across the lifespan. Columbia: University of South Carolina, 1990:157–187.

Viosca E, Martinez JL, Almagro PL, et al. Proposal and validation of a new functional ambulation classification scale for clinical use. Arch Phys Med Rehabil 2005;86:1234–1238.

Visser H. Gait and balance in senile dementia of Alzheimer's type. Age Ageing 1983;12:296–301.

Vitório R, Pieruccini-Faria F, Stella F, et al. Effects of obstacle height on obstacle crossing in mild Parkinson's disease. Gait Posture 2010;31:143–146.

Voelcker-Rehage C, Alberts JL. Age-related changes in grasping force modulation. Exp Brain Res 2005;166:61–70.

Voelcker-Rehage C, Alberts JL. Effect of motor practice on dual-task performance in older adults. J Gerontol B Psychol Sci Soc Sci 2007;62:P141–P148.

Voepel-Lewis T, Merkel S, Tait AR, et al. The reliability and validity of the Face, Legs, Activity, Cry, Consolability observational tool as a measure of pain in children with cognitive impairment. Anesth Analg 2002;95:1224–1229.

Vollmer B, Holmström L, Forsman L, et al. Evidence of validity in a new method to measure dexterity in children and adolescents. Dev Med Child Neurol 2010;52:948–954.

von Hofsten C. Eye-hand coordination in the newborn. Dev Psychol 1982;18:450–461.

von Hofsten C. Developmental changes in the organization of prereaching movements. Dev Psychol 1984;3:378–388.

von Hofsten C. Action in development. Dev Sci 2007;10:54–60.

von Hofsten C. On the development of perception and action. In: Valsiner J, Connolly K, eds. Handbook of developmental psychology. Thousand Oaks, CA: Sage, 2003.

von Hofsten C. Studying the development of goal-directed behavior. In: Kalverboer AF, Hopkins B, Geuze R, eds. Motor development in early and later childhood: longitudinal approaches. Cambridge, UK: Cambridge University, 1993:109–124.

von Hofsten C, Fazel-Zandy S. Development of visually guided hand orientation in reaching. J Exp Child Psychol 1984;38:208–219.

von Hofsten C, Lindhagen K. Observations on the development of reaching for moving objects. J Exp Child Psychol 1979;28:158–173.

von Hofsten C, Ronnqvist L. Preparation for grasping an object: a developmental study. J Exp Psychol 1988;14:610–621.

von Hofsten C, Rosander K. Development of smooth pursuit tracking in young infants. Vision Res 1997;37:1799–1810.

von Hofsten C, Rosander K. The development of gaze control and predictive tracking in young infants. Vision Res 1996;36:81–96.

von Monakow C. Die Localization im Grosshirn und der Abbau der Funktion durch korticale Herde. Wiesbaden, Germany: JF Bergmann, 1914.

Voss D, Ionata M, Myers B. Proprioceptive neuromuscular facilitation: patterns and techniques, 3rd ed. Philadelphia, PA: Harper & Row, 1985.

Vrtunski PB, Patterson MB. Psychomotor decline can be described by discontinuities in response trajectories. Int J Neurosci 1985;27:265–275.

Vuillerme N, Nafati G. How attentional focus on body sway affects postural control during quiet standing. Psychol Res 2007;71:192–200.

Vygotsky LS. Mind in society: the development of higher psychological processes. Cambridge, MA: Harvard University Press, 1978.

W

Wade MG, Lindquist R, Taylor JR, Treat-Jacobson D. Optical flow, spatial orientation, and the control of posture in the elderly. J Gerontol 1995;50B:P51–P58.

Wadsworth PT, Krishman R. Intrarater reliability of manual muscle testing and hand held dynamometric muscle testing. Physiol Rev 1987;67:1342–1347.

Wakeling J, Delaney R, Dudkiewicz I. A method for quantifying dynamic muscle dysfunction in children and young adults with cerebral palsy. Gait Posture 2007;25:580–589.

Waksvik K, Levy R. An approach to seating for the cerebral palsied. Can J Occup Ther 1979;46:147–152.

Walchli M, Keller M, Ruffieux J, Mouthon A, Taube W. Age-dependent adaptations to anticipated and non-anticipated perturbations after balance training in children. Hum Mov Sci 2018;59:170–177.

Walker C, Brouwer BJ, Culham EG. Use of visual feedback in retraining balance following acute stroke. Phys Ther 2000;80(9):886–895.

Walker N, Mellick D, Brooks CA, et al. Measuring participation across impairment groups using the Craig Handicap Assessment Reporting Technique. Am J Phys Med Rehabil 2003;82(12):936–941.

Walker-Batson D, Smith P, Unwin H, et al. Use of amphetamine in the treatment of aphasia. Restor Neurol Neurosci 1992;4:47–50.

Wall C III, Kentala E. Control of sway using vibrotactile feedback of body tilt in patients with moderate and severe postural control deficits. J Vestib Res 2005;15:313–325.

Wallace PS, Whishaw IQ. Independent digit movements and precision grip patterns in 1–5-month-old human infants: hand-babbling, including vacuous then self-directed hand and digit movements, precedes targeted reaching. Neuropsychologia 2003;41:1912–1918.

Wallace SA, Weeks DL, Kelso JAS. Temporal constraints in reaching and grasping behavior. Hum Mov Sci 1990;9:69–93.

Wallen M, Bundy A, Pont K, et al. Psychometric properties of the Pediatric Motor Activity Log for children with cerebral palsy. Dev Med Child Neurol. 2009;51:200–208.

Wallen P. Cellular bases of locomotor behaviour in lamprey: coordination and modulatory control of spinal circuitry. In: Ferrell WR, Proske U, eds. Neural control of movement. New York: Plenum, 1995:125–133.

Walston JD. Sarcopenia in older adults. Curr Opin Rheumatol 2012;24:623–627.

Wang CH, Hsieh CL, Dai MH, et al. Interrater reliability and validity of the Stroke Rehabilitation Assessment of Movement (STREAM) instrument. J Rehabil Med 2002;34(1):20–24.

Wang HH, Liao HF, Hsieh CL. Reliability, sensitivity to change, and responsiveness of the peabody developmental motor scales-second edition for children with cerebral palsy. Phys Ther 2006;86(10):1351–1359. doi: 10.2522/ptj.20050259.

Wang J, Bohan M, Leis BC, et al. Altered coordination patterns in parkinsonian patients during trunk-assisted prehension. Parkinsonism Relat Disord 2006;12: 211–222.

Wang J, Sainburg RL. Interlimb transfer of novel inertial dynamics is asymmetrical. J Neurophysiol 2004a;92:349–360.

Wang J, Sainburg RL. Interlimb transfer of visuomotor rotations depends on handedness. Exp Brain Res 2006a;175(2):223–230.

Wang J, Sainburg RL. Limitations in interlimb transfer of visuomotor rotations. Exp Brain Res 2004b;155:1–8.

Wang J, Sainburg RL. The symmetry of interlimb transfer depends on workspace locations. Exp Brain Res 2006b;170:464–471.

Wang TY, Bhatt T, Yang F, et al. Generalization of motor adaptation to repeated-slip perturbation across tasks. Neuroscience 2011;180:85–95.

Wang W, Ji X, Ni J, et al. Visual spatial attention training improve spatial attention and motor control for unilateral neglect patients. CNS Neurol Disord Drug Targets 2015;14(10):1277–1282. doi: 10.2174/1871527315666151111122926.

Wanning T. Healing and the mind/body arts: massage, acupuncture, yoga, t'ai chi, and Feldenkrais. AAOHN J 1993;41(7):349–351.

Ward AB. A summary of spasticity management—a treatment algorithm. Eur J Neurol 2002;9:48–55.

Ward NS, Brown MM, Thompson AJ, et al. Neural correlates of motor recovery after stroke: a longitudinal fMRI study. Brain 2003;126:2476–2496.

Ward NS, Cohen LG. Mechanisms underlying recovery of motor function after stroke. Arch Neurol 2004;61:1844–1848.

Warren WH. Action modes and laws of control for the visual guidance of action. In: Meijer OG, Roth K, eds. Complex movement behavior: the motor-action controversy. Amsterdam, The Netherlands: North-Holland, 1988:339–380.

Wartenberg R. Pendulousness of the legs as a diagnostic test. Neurology 1951;1:8–24.

Washington K, Shumway-Cook A, Price R, et al. Muscle responses to seated perturbations for typically developing infants and those at risk for motor delays. Dev Med Child Neurol 2004;46:681–688.

Waters R, McNeal DR, Tasto J. Peroneal nerve conduction velocity after chronic electrical stimulation. Arch Phys Med Rehabil 1975;56:240–243.

Waters RL, Barnes G, Husserl T, et al. Comparable energy expenditure after arthrodesis of the hip and ankle. J Bone Joint Surg Am 1988;70:1032–1037.

Waters RL, Mulroy S. The energy expenditure of normal and pathologic gait. Gait Posture 1999;9:207–231.

Weber PC, Cass SP. Clinical assessment of postural stability. Am J Otol 1993;14:566–569.

Weiller C, Chollet F, Friston KJ, et al. Functional reorganization of the brain in recovery from striatocapsular infarction in man. Ann Neurol 1992;31:463–472.

Weiller C, Ramsay SC, Wise RJS, et al. Individual patterns of functional reorganization in the human cerebral cortex after capsular infarction. Ann Neurol 1993;33:181–189.

Weiskrantz L, Warrington ER, Sanders MD, et al. Visual capacity in the hemianopic field following a restricted occipital ablation. Brain 1974;97:709–728.

Weiss PH, Dafotakis M, Metten L, Noth J. Distal and proximal prehension is differentially affected by Parkinson's disease. The effect of conscious and subconscious load cues. J Neurol 2009;256:450–456.

Weisz S. Studies in equilibrium reaction. J Nerv Ment Dis 1938;88:150–162.

Welford AT. Motor performance. In: Birren G, Schaie K, eds. Handbook of the psychology of aging. New York: Van Nostrand Reinhold, 1977:3–20.

Welford AT. Motor skills and aging. In: Mortimer J, Pirozzolo FJ, Maletta G, eds. The aging motor system. New York: Praeger, 1982:152–187.

Werner WG, Gentile AM. Improving gait and promoting retention in individuals with Parkinson's disease: a pilot study. J Neurol 2010;257(11):1841–1847.

Westlake KP, Patten C. Pilot study of Lokomat versus manual-assisted treadmill training for locomotor recovery post-stroke. J Neuroeng Rehabil 2009;6:18–29.

Westling G, Johansson RS. Factors influencing the force control during precision grip. Exp Brain Res 1984;53:277–284.

Wetter S, Poole JL, Haaland KY. Functional implications of ipsilesional motor deficits after unilateral stroke. Arch Phys Med Rehabil 2005;86:776–781.

Whanger A, Wang HS. Clinical correlates of the vibratory sense in elderly psychiatric patients. J Gerontol 1974;29:39–45.

Whipple RH, Wolfson LI, Amerman PM. The relationship of knee and ankle weakness to falls in nursing home residents: an isokinetic study. J Am Geriatr Soc 1987;35:13–20.

White BL, Castle P, Held R. Observations on the development of visually-directed reaching. Child Dev 1964;35:349–364.

Whiteneck GG, Charlifue SW, Gerhart KA, et al. Quantifying handicap: a new measure of long-term rehabilitation outcomes. Arch Phys Med Rehabil 1992;73:519–526.

Whitney S, Wrisley D, Furman J. Concurrent validity of the Berg Balance Scale and the Dynamic Gait Index in people with vestibular dysfunction. Physiotherapy Res Int 2003;8:178–186.

Whitney SL, Hudak MT, Marchetti GF. The Dynamic Gait Index relates to self reported fall history in individuals with vestibular dysfunction. J Vestib Res 2000;10:99–105.

Whitney SL, Wrisley DM. The influence of footwear on timed balance scores of the modified clinical test of sensory interaction and balance. Arch Phys Med Rehabil 2004;85:439–443.

Whyte J, Hart T. It's more than a black box; it's a Russian doll: defining rehabilitation treatments. Am J Phys Med Rehabil 2003;82:639–652.

Wichman T, DeLong MR. Basal Ganglia. In: Kandel ER, Schwartz JH, Jessell TM, Siegelbaum SA, Hudspeth AJ, eds. Principles of neural science, 5th ed. New York, NY: McGraw-Hill, 2013:2397–2435.

Wielinski CL, Erickson-Davis C, Wichmann R, et al. Falls and injuries resulting from falls among patients with Parkinson's disease and other Parkinsonian syndromes. Mov Disord 2005;20:410–415.

Wiener-Vacher SR, Hamilton DA, Wiener SI. Vestibular activity and cognitive development in children: perspectives. Front Integr Neurosci 2013;7:92.

Wiener-Vacher SR, Toupet F, Narcy P. Canal and otolith vestibulo-ocular reflexes to vertical and off vertical axis rotations in children learning to walk. Acta Otolaryngol 1996;116:657–656.

Wiesendanger M, Serrien DJ. Neurological problems affecting hand dexterity. Brain Res Rev 2001;36:161–168.

Wiley ME, Damiano DL. Lower-extremity strength profiles in spastic cerebral palsy. Dev Med Child Neurol 1998;40:100–107.

Wilkins AJ, Shallice T, McCarthy R. Frontal lesions and sustained attention. Neuropsychologia 1987;25:359–365.

Willer B, Rosenthal M, Kreutzer J S. et al. Assessment of community integration following rehabilitation for traumatic brain injury. J Head Trauma Rehabil 1993;8: 75–87.

Williams EN, Carrll SG, Reddihough DS, et al. Investigation of the timed "up and go" test in children. Dev Med Child Neurol 2005;47:518–524.

Williams H. Aging and eye-hand coordination. In: Bard C, Fleury M, Hay L, eds. Development of eye-hand coordination across the lifespan. Columbia: University of South Carolina, 1990: 327–357.

Williamson GL, Leiper CI, Mayer NH. Beaver College Assessment of speed and accuracy of movement in older adults using Fitts' tapping test. Neurosci Abstr 1993;19:556.

Wilmut K, Wann JP, Brown JH. Problems in the coupling of eye and hand in the sequential movements of children with Developmental Coordination Disorder. Child Care Health Dev 2006;32:665–678.

Wilson DM. The central nervous control of flight in a locust. J Exp Biol 1961;38:471–490.Wing AM, Frazer C. The contribution of the thumb to reaching movements. Q J Exp Psychol 1983;35A:297–309.

Windhorst U. Muscle proprioceptive feedback and spinal networks. Brain Res Bull 2007;73:155–202.

Winograd CH, Lemsky CM, Nevitt MC, et al. Development of a physical performance and mobility examination. J Am Geriatr Soc 1994;42:743–749.

Winogrodzka A, Wagenaar RC, Booij J, et al. Rigidity and bradykinesia reduce interlimb coordination in Parkinsonian gait. Arch Phys Med Rehabil 2005;86:183–189.

Winstein C, Gardner ER, McNeal DR, et al. Standing balance training: effect on balance and locomotion in hemiparetic adults. Arch Phys Med Rehabil 1989;70: 755–762.

Winstein C, Lewthwaite R, Blanton SR, et al. With case exemplar from the accelerated skill acquisition program. J Neuro Phys Ther 2014;38:190–200.

Winstein C, Wolf SL. Task-oriented training to promote upper extremity recovery. In: Stein J, ed. Stroke recovery and rehabilitation. New York: Demos, 2009.

Winstein CJ. Designing practice for motor learning: clinical implications: contemporary management of motor control problems. Proceedings of the II Step Conference. Alexandria, VA: American Physical Therapy Association, 1991.

Winstein CJ, Wolf SL, Dromerick AW, et al. Interdisciplinary Comprehensive Arm Rehabilitation Evaluation (ICARE) investigative team. Effect of a task oriented rehabilitation program on upper extremity recovery following motor stroke: the ICARE randomized clinical trial. JAMA 2016;315(6):571–581. doi: 10.1001/jama.2016.0276.

Winstein CJ, Merians AS, Sullivan KJ. Motor learning after unilateral brain damage. Neuropsychologia 1999;27:975–987.

Winstein CJ, Pohl PS. Effects of unilateral brain damage on the control of goal directed hand movements. Exp Brain Res 1995;105:163–174.

Winstein CJ, Schmidt RA. Reduced frequency of knowledge of results enhances motor skill learning. J Exp Psychol Learn Memory Cogn 1990;16:677–691.

Winter D. Energy generation and absorption at the ankle and knee during fast, natural and slow cadences. Clin Orthop Relat Res 1983a;175:147–154.

Winter DA. Biomechanical motor patterns in normal walking. J Motor Behav 1983b;15:302–330.

Winter DA. Biomechanics and motor control of human movement. New York: Wiley, 1990:80–84.

Winter DA. Kinematic and kinetic patterns of human gait: variability and compensating effects. Hum Mov Sci 1984;3:51–76.

Winter DA. Knowledge base for diagnostic gait assessments. Med Prog Technol 1993;19:61–81.

Winter DA. Overall principle of lower limb support during stance phase of gait. J Biomech 1980;13:923–927.

Winter DA, McFadyen BJ, Dickey JP. Adaptability of the CNS in human walking. In: Patla AE, ed. Adaptability of human gait. Amsterdam, The Netherlands: Elsevier, 1991:127–144.

Winter DA, Patla AE, Frank JS, et al. Biomechanical walking pattern changes in the fit and healthy elderly. Phys Ther 1990;70:340–347.

Winter DA, Prince F, Frank JS, et al. Unified theory regarding A/P and M/L balance in quiet stance. J Neurophysiol 1996;75:2334–2343.

Wise RA, Brown CD. Minimal clinically important differences in the six-minute walk test and the incremental shuttle walking test. COPD 2005;2:125–129.

Wisleder D, Zernicke RF, Smith JL. Speed-related changes in hindlimb intersegmental dynamics during the swing phase of cat locomotion. Exp Brain Res 1990;79:651–660.

Witchel HJ, Oberndorfer C, Needham R, et al. Thigh-Derived Inertial Sensor Metrics to Assess the Sit-to-Stand and Stand-to-Sit Transitions in the Timed Up and Go (TUG) Task for quantifying mobility impairment in multiple sclerosis. Front Neurol 2018;9:684.

Witherington DC, von Hofsten C, Rosander K, et al. The development of anticipatory postural adjustments in infancy. Infancy 2002;3:495–517.

Witney AG, Wing A, Thonnard JL, et al. The cutaneous contribution to adaptive precision grip. Trends Neurosci 2004;27:638–643.

Wittenberg GF, Schaechter JD. The neural basis of constraint-induced movement therapy. Curr Opin Neurol 2009;22(6):582–588. doi: 10.1097/WCO.0b013e3283320229.

Wolf SL, Catlin PA, Ellis M, et al. Assessing Wolf motor function test as outcome measure for research in patients after stroke. Stroke 2001;32:1635.

Wolf SL, Lecraw DE, Barton LA, et al. Forced use of hemiplegic upper extremities to reverse the effect of learned nonuse among chronic stroke and head injured patients. Exp Neurol 1989b;104(2):125–132.

Wolf SL, McJunkin JP, Swanson ML, et al. Pilot normative database for the Wolf motor function test. Arch Phys Med Rehabil 2006;87(2):443–445.

Wolf SL, Sahu K, Bay RC, et al. The HAAPI (Home Arm Assistance Progression Initiative) Trial: a Novel robotics delivery approach in stroke rehabilitation. Neurorehabil Neural Repair 2015;29(10):958–968. doi: 10.1177/1545968315575612.

Wolf SL, Winstein CJ, Miller JP, et al. Retention of upper limb function in stroke survivors who have received constraint-induced movement therapy: the EXCITE randomized trial. Lancet Neurol 2008;7(1):33–40.

Wolf TJ, Polatajko H, Baum C, et al. Combined cognitive-strategy and task-specific training affects cognition and upper-extremity function in subacute stroke: an exploratory randomized controlled trial. Am J Occup Ther 2016;70(2):7002290010p1-7002290010p10. doi: 10.5014/ajot.2016.017293.

Wolfson L, Judge J, Whipple R, et al. Strength is a major factor in balance, gait and the occurrence of falls. J Geronotol 1995;50A:64–67.

Wolfson L, Whipple R, Amerman P, et al. Gait and balance in the elderly. Clin Geriatr Med 1985;1:649–659.

Wolfson L, Whipple R, Amerman P, et al. Gait assessment in the elderly: a gait abnormality rating scale and its relation to falls. J Gerontol 1990;45:M12–M19.

Wolfson L, Whipple R, Derby C, et al. Balance strength training in older adults: Intervention gains and Tai Chi maintenance. J Am Geriatr Soc 1996;44:498–506.

Wolfson L, Whipple R, Derby CA, et al. A dynamic posturography study of balance in healthy elderly. Neurology 1992;42:2069–2075.

Wong DL, Baker CM. Pain in children: comparison of assessment scales. Pediatr Nurs 1988;14:9–17.

Wood BH, Bilclough JA, Bowron A, et al. Incidence and predition of falls in Parkinson's disease: a prospective multidisciplinary study. J Neurol Neurosurg Psychiatry 2002;72:721–725.

Wood DE, Burridge JH, VanWijck FM, et al. Biomechanical approaches applied to the lower and upper limb for the measurement of spasticity: a systematic review of the literature. Disabil Rehabil 2005;27:19–32.

Woodbury ML, Velozo CA, Richards LG, et al. Dimensionality and construct validity of the Fugl-Meyer assessment of the upper extremity. Arch Phys Med Rehabil 2007;88:715–723.

Wood-Dauphinee SL, Williams JI, Shapiro SH. Examining outcome measures in a clinical study of stroke. Stroke 1990;21(5):731–739.

Woodford H, Walker R. Emergency hospital admissions in idiopathic Parkinson's disease. Mov Disord 2005;20:1104–1108.

Woollacott M. Aging, posture control and movement preparation. In: Woollacott MH, Shumway-Cook A, eds. Development of posture and gait across the life span. Columbia: University of South Carolina, 1989:155–175.

Woollacott M. Gait and postural control in the aging adult. In: Bles W, Brandt T, eds. Disorders of posture and gait. Amsterdam, The Netherlands: Elsevier, 1986:325–336.

Woollacott M. Unbounded potentialities of resonance—the dynamic interface between mind and brain: perspectives from neuroscience and meditative traditions, and research at their common frontiers. Master's thesis, University of Oregon, 2005.

Woollacott M, Burtner P, Jensen J, et al. Development of postural responses during standing in healthy children and in children with spastic diplegia. Neurosci Biobehav Rev 1998;22:583–589.

Woollacott M, Debu B, Mowatt M. Neuromuscular control of posture in the infant and child: is vision dominant? J Motor Behav 1987;19:167–186.

Woollacott M, Roseblad B, von Hofsten C. Relation between muscle response onset and body segmental movements during postural perturbations in humans. Exp Brain Res 1988;72:593–604.

Woollacott M, Shumway-Cook A, Hutchinson S, et al. The effect of balance training on the organization of muscle activity used in the recovery of stability in children with cerebral palsy: a pilot study. Dev Med Child Neurol 2005;47:455–461.

Woollacott M, Shumway-Cook A. Attention and the control of posture and gait: a review of an emerging area of research. Gait Posture 2002;16:1–14.

Woollacott M, Shumway-Cook A. Changes in posture control across the life span: a systems approach. Phys Ther 1990;70:799–807.

Woollacott M, Shumway-Cook A. Clinical research methodology for the study of posture and balance. In: Masdeu JC, Sudarsky L, Wolfson L, eds. Gait disorders of aging: falls and therapeutic strategies. Philadelphia, PA: Lippincott-Raven, 1997: 107–121.

Woollacott M, Shumway-Cook A. The development of the postural and voluntary motor control system in Down's syndrome children. In: Wade M, ed. Motor skill acquisition of the mentally handicapped: issues in research and training. Amsterdam, The Netherlands: Elsevier, 1986:45–71.

Woollacott MH, Jensen J. Posture and locomotion. In: Heuer H, Keele S, eds. Handbook of perception and action, vol. 2. New York: Academic Press, 1996:333–403.

Woollacott MH, Shumway-Cook A, Nashner L. Aging and posture control: changes in sensory organization and muscular coordination. Int J Aging Hum Dev 1986;23:97–114.

Woollacott MH, Sveistrup H. Changes in the sequencing and timing of muscle response coordination associated with developmental transitions in balance abilities. Hum Mov Sci 1992;11:23–36.

World Health Organization. International classification of functioning, disability and health. Geneva, Switzerland: World Health Organization, 2001.

World Health Organization. International classification of impairment, activity and participation ICIDH-2. Geneva, Switzerland: World Health Organization, 1980.

World Health Organization (WHO). Clinician form for international classification of functioning, disability and health. ICF Checklist Version 2.1a, Clinician Form, (2003). Wright BD, Masters GN. Rating scale analysis. Chicago, IL: MESA, 1982.

Wright DL, Kemp TL. The dual-task methodology and assessing the attentional demands of ambulation with walking devices. Phys Ther 1992;72:306–315.

Wright JM von. A note on the role of 'guidance' in learning. Br J Psychol 1957;48:133–137.

Wright PA, Granat MH. Therapeutic effects of functional electrical stimulation of the upper limb of eight children with cerebral palsy. Dev Med Child Neurol 2000;42:724–727.

Wrisley DM, Kumar NA. Functional gait assessment: concurrent, discriminative, and predictive validity in community-dwelling older adults. Phys Ther 2010;90:761–773.

Wrisley DM, Marchetti GF, Kuharsky DK, et al. Reliability, internal consistency and validity of data obtained with the functional gait assessment. Phys Ther 2004;84:906–918.

Wrisley DM, Walker ML, Echternach JL, et al. Reliability of the Dynamic Gait Index in people with vestibular disorders. Arch Phys Med Rehabil 2003;84:1528–1533.

Wrisley DM, Whitney SL, Furman JM. Vestibular rehabilitation outcomes in patients with a history of migraine. Otol Neurotol 2002;23:483–487.

Wu AR, Kuo AD. Determinants of preferred ground clearance during swing phase of human walking. J Exp Biol 2016;219(Pt 19): 3106–3113.

Wu C, Trombly CA, Lin K, et al. Effects of object affordances on reaching in persons with and without cerebrovascular accident. Am J Occup Ther 1998;52:447–456.

Wu CY, Chou SH, Kuo MY, et al. Effects of object size on intralimb and interlimb coordination during a bimanual prehension task in patients with left cerebral vascular accidents. Motor Control 2008;12:296–310.

Wu CY, Trombly CA, Lin KC. The relationship between occupational form and occupational performance: a kinematic perspective. Am J Occup Ther 1994;48:679–687.

Wu M, Kim J, Arora P, et al. Locomotor training through a 3D cable-driven robotic system for walking function in children with cerebral palsy: a pilot study. Conf Proc IEEE Eng Med Biol Soc 2014;2014: 3529–3532.

Wu T, Hallett M. Neural correlates of dual task performance in patients with Parkinsons disease. J Neurol Neurosurg Psychiatry 2008;79:760–766.

Wu T, Hallett M. The influence of normal human aging on automatic movements. J Physiol 2005;562:605–615.

Wu T, Kansaku K, Hallett M. How self-initiated memorized movements become automatic: a functional MRI study. J Neurophysiol 2004a;91:1690–1698.

Wu YW, Day SM, Strauss DJ, et al. Prognosis for ambulation in cerebral palsy: a population-based study. Pediatrics 2004b;114:1264–1271.

Wulf G, Prinz W. Directing attention to movement effects enhances learning: a review. Psychon Bull Rev 2001;8:648–660.

Wulf G, Shea C, Park JH. Attention and motor performance: preferences for and advantages of an external focus. Res Q Exerc Sport 2001;72: 335–244.

Wulf G, Weigelt C. Instructions about physical principles in learning a complex motor skill: to tell or not to tell. Res Q Exerc Sport 1997;68:362–367.

Wurtz RH, Kandel ER. Central visual pathways. In: Kandel ER, Schwartz JH, Jessell TM, eds. Principles of neural science, 4th ed. New York: McGraw-Hill, 2000a:523–547.

Wurtz RH, Kandel ER. Perception of motion, depth and form. In: Kandel ER, Schwartz JH, Jessell TM, eds. Principles of neural science, 4th ed. New York: McGraw-Hill, 2000b: 548–571.

X

Xia R, Rymer WZ. The role of shortening reaction in mediating rigidity in Parkinson's disease. Exp Brain Res 2004;156:524–528.

Xia R, Sun J, Threlkeld AJ. Analysis of interactive effect of stretch reflex and shortening reaction on rigidity in Parkinson's disease. Clin Neurophysiol 2009;120:1400–1407.

Xu C, Li S, Wang K, Hou Z, Yu N. Quantitative assessment of paretic limb dexterity and interlimb coordination during bilateral arm rehabilitation training. IEEE Int Conf Rehabil Robot 2017;2017:634–639. doi: 10.1109/ICORR.2017.8009319.

Xu K, He L, Mai J, Yan X, Chen Y. Muscle recruitment and coordination following constraint-induced movement therapy with electrical stimulation on children with hemiplegic cerebral palsy: a randomized controlled trial. PLoS One 2015;10(10):e0138608. doi: 10.1371/journal.pone.0138608.

Y

Yan K, Fang J, Shahani BT. An assessment of motor unit discharge patterns in stroke patients using surface electromyographic technique. Muscle Nerve 1998a;21:946–947.

Yan K, Fang J, Shahani BT. Motor unit discharge behaviors in stroke patients. Muscle Nerve 1998b;21:1502–1506.

Yanagisawa N. Functions and dysfunctions of the basal ganglia in humans. Proc Jpn Acad Ser B Phys Biol Sci 2018;94:275–304.

Yancosek KE, Mullineaux DR. Stability of handwriting performance following injury-induced hand-dominance transfer in adults: a pilot study. J Rehabil Res Dev 2011;48(1):59–68.

Yang DJ, ParK SK, Kim JH, Heo JW, Lee YS, Uhm YH. Effect of changes in postural alignment on foot pressure and walking ability of stroke patients. J Phys Ther Sci 2015;27:2943–2945.

Yang F, Bhatt T, Pai YC. Generalization of treadmill-slip training to prevent a fall following a sudden (novel) slip in over-ground walking. J Biomech 2013;46:63–69.

Yang JD, Liao CD, Huang SW, et al. Effectiveness of electrical stimulation therapy in improving arm function after stroke: a systematic review and a meta-analysis of randomised controlled trials. Clin Rehabil 2019;33(8):1286–1297. doi: 10.1177/0269215519839165.

Yang JF, Stephens MJ, Vishram R. Transient disturbances to one limb produce coordinated, bilateral responses during infant stepping. J Neurophysiol 1998;79:2329–2337.

Yang YR, Chen YC, Lee CS, et al. Dual-task-related gait changes in individuals with stroke. Gait Posture 2007;25:185–190.

Yang YR, Wang RY, Chen YC, et al. Dual-task exercise improves walking ability in chronic stroke: a randomized controlled trial. Arch Phys Med Rehabil 2007b;88:1236–1240.

Yang YR, Mi PL, Huang SF, Chiu SL, Liu YC, Wang RY. Effects of neuromuscular electrical stimulation on gait performance in chronic stroke with inadequate ankle control. A randomized controlled trial. PLoS One 2018;13:1–13.

Yamaguchi T, Masani K. Effects of age-related changes in step length and step width on the required coefficient of friction during straight walking. Gait Posture 2019;69:195–201.

Yamazaki Y, Ohkuwa T, Itoh H, Suzuki M. Reciprocal activation and coactivation in antagonistic muscles during rapid goal-directed movements. Brain Res Bull 1994;34:587–593.

Yardley L, Smith H. A prospective study of the relationship between feared consequences of falling and avoidance of activity in community-living older people. Gerontologist 2002;42:17–23.

Yekutiel M. Sensory reeducation of the hand after stroke. London, UK: Whurr, 2000.

Yogev G, Giladi N, Peretz C, et al. Dual tasking, gait rhythmicity, and Parkinson's disease: which aspects of gait are attention demanding? Eur J Neurosci 2005;22:1248–1256.

Yogev G, Plotnik M, Peretz C. Gait asymmetry in patients with Parkinson's disease and elderly fallers: when does the bilateral coordination of gait require attention? Exp Brain Res 2007;177:336–346.

Yorkston KM, Kuehn CM, Johnson KL, et al. Measuring participation in multiple sclerosis: a comparison of the domains of frequency, importance, and self-efficacy. Disabil Rehabil 2008;30:88–97.

Young A. Exercise physiology in geriatric practice. Acta Scand 1986;711(Suppl): 227–232.

Z

Zaaimi B, Edgley SA, Soteropoulos DS, et al. Changes in descending motor pathway connectivity after corticospinal tract lesion in macaque monkey. Brain 2012;135 (Pt 7):2277–2289.

Zackowski KM, Dromerick AW, Sahrmann SA, et al. How do strength, sensation, spasticity and joint individuation relate to the reaching deficits of people with chronic hemiparesis? Brain 2004;127:1035–1046.

Zaino CA, McCoy SW. Reliability and comparison of electromyographic and kinetic measurements during a standing reach task in children with and without cerebral palsy. Gait Posture 2008;27:128–137.

Zang Y, Schutter ED. Climbing fibers provide graded error signals in cerebellar learning. Front Syst Neurosci 2019;13:1–11.

Zarkou A, Lee SCK, Prosser LA, Hwang S, Jeka J. Stochastic resonance stimulation improves balance in children with cerebral palsy: a case control study. J Neuroeng Rehabil 2018;15(1):115.

Zarro VJ. Mechanisms of inflammation and repair. In: Michlovitz SL, ed. Thermal agents in rehabilitation. Philadelphia, PA: Davis, 1986.

Zarrugh MY, Todd FN, Ralston HJ. Optimization of energy expenditure during level walking. Eur J Appl Physiol 1974;33:293–306.

Zee DS. Vertigo. In: Johnson RT, ed. Current therapy in neurologic disease. St. Louis, MO: CV Mosby, 1985:8–13.

Zehr EP, Balter JE, Ferris DP, et al. Neural regulation of rhythmic arm and leg movement is conserved across human locomotor tasks. J Physiol 2007b;582(Pt 1):209–227.

Zehr EP, Duysens J. Regulation of arm and leg movement during human locomotion. Neuroscientist 2004;10:347–361.

Zehr EP, Klimstra M, Dragert K, et al. Enhancement of arm and leg locomotor coupling with augmented cutaneous feedback from the hand. J Neurophysiol 2007a;98(3):1810–1814.

Zehr EP, Komiyama T, Stein RB. Cutaneous reflexes during human gait: electromyographic and kinematic responses to electrical stimulation. J Neurophysiol 1997;77:3311–3325.

Zehr EP, Loadman PM. Persistence of locomotor-related interlimb reflex networks during walking after stroke. Clin Neurophysiol 2012;123(4):796–807.

Zelazo PR, Zelazo NA, Kolb S. Newborn walking. Science. 1972;177:1058–1059.

Zeller W. Konstitution und Entwicklung. Göttingen, Germany: Verlag fur Psychologic, 1964.

Zettel JL, McIlroy WE, Maki BE. Gaze behavior of older adults during rapid balance-recovery reactions. J Gerontol 2008;63A:885–891.

Zeuner KE, Shill HA, Sohn YH, et al. Motor training as treatment in focal hand dystonia. Mov Disord 2005;20:335–341.

Zhang C, Li-Tsang CW, Au RK. Robotic approaches for the rehabilitation of upper limb recovery after stroke: a systematic review and meta-analysis. Int J Rehabil Res 2017;40(1):19–28. doi: 10.1097/MRR.0000000000000204.

Zhang Y, Brenner E, Duysens J, Verschueren S, Smeets JBJ. Effects of aging on postural responses to visual perturbations during fast pointing. Front Aging Neurosci 2018;10:401.

Zhao JZ, Blazar PE, Mora AN, Earp BE. Range of motion measurements of the fingers Via Smartphone photography. Hand (NY) 2020;15(5):679–685. doi: 10.1177/1558944718820955.

Zheng Y, Mao M, Cao Y, Lu X. Contralaterally controlled functional electrical stimulation improves wrist dorsiflexion and upper limb function in patients with early-phase stroke: a randomized controlled trial. J Rehabil Med 2019;51(2):103–108. doi: 10.2340/16501977-2510.

Zigmond MJ, Cameron JL, Leak RK, et al. Triggering endogenous neuroprotective processes through exercise in models of dopamine deficiency. Parkinsonism Relat Disord 2009;15:S42–S45.

Zigmond MJ, Smeyne RJ. Exercise: is it a neuroprotective and if so, how does it work? Parkinsonism Relat Disord 2014;20:S123–S127.

Zihl J, Werth R. Contributions to the study of "blindsight": 2. The role of specific practice for saccadic localization in patients with postgeniculate visual field defects. Neuropsychologia 1984;22:13–22.

Zijlmans JC, Poels PJ, Duysens J, et al. Quantitative gait analysis in patients with vascular parkinsonism. Mov Dis 1996;11:501–508.

Zijlstra A, Mancini M, Chiari L, et al. Biofeedback for training balance and mobility tasks in older populations: a systematic review. J Neuroeng Rehabil 2010;7:58.

Zimny ML. Mechanoreceptors in articular tissues. Am J Anat 1988;182:16–32.

Zink PJ, Philip BA. Cortical plasticity in rehabilitation for upper extremity peripheral nerve injury: a scoping review. Am J Occup Ther 2020;74(1):7401205030p1-7401205030p15. doi: 10.5014/ajot.2020.036665.

Zucker RS, Regehr WG. Short term synaptic plasticity. Annu Rev Physiol 2002;64:355–405.

Zylstra SE, Pfeiffer B. Effectiveness of a handwriting intervention with at-risk kindergarteners. Am J Occup Ther 2016;70(3):7003220020p1-8. doi: 10.5014/ajot.2016.018820.

INDEX

B

C

D

N

Q

R

S

T

U

V

W

Z